M000201236

# User's Guide to the Book

**Introductory pages:**

- The introductory pages provide all relevant anatomical informations concerning the subject of the chapter. Important details and connections are explained easily to understand.
- The Dissection Link for each chapter comprises brief and concise tips essential for the dissection of the respective body region.
- Exam Check Lists provide all keywords for possible exam questions.

**Atlas pages:**

- The menu bar on top indicates the topics of each chapter, the bold print shows the subject of the respective pages.
- Important anatomical structures in the figures are highlighted in bold print.
- Small supplement sketches located next to complex views show visual angles and intersecting planes and, thus, facilitate orientation.
- Detailed figure captions explain the relationships of anatomical structures.
- Bulleted lists in figure captions as well as in tables help structuring complex facts and provide a better overview.
- Figures, tables and text boxes are interconnected by cross-references.
- Cross-references link the figures to the separate Table Booklet with tables of muscles, joints, and nerves, thus providing a sufficient anatomical knowledge for the exam.
- Clinical Remarks boxes provide clinical background knowledge concerning the anatomical structures illustrated on the page.

**Appendix:**

- List of abbreviations as well as general terms of direction and position can be found at the end of the book.
- The color chart depicting the different colors of the cranial bones used in a number of illustrations can be found inside the back cover of this volume.

# Perfect Orientation – the New Navigation System

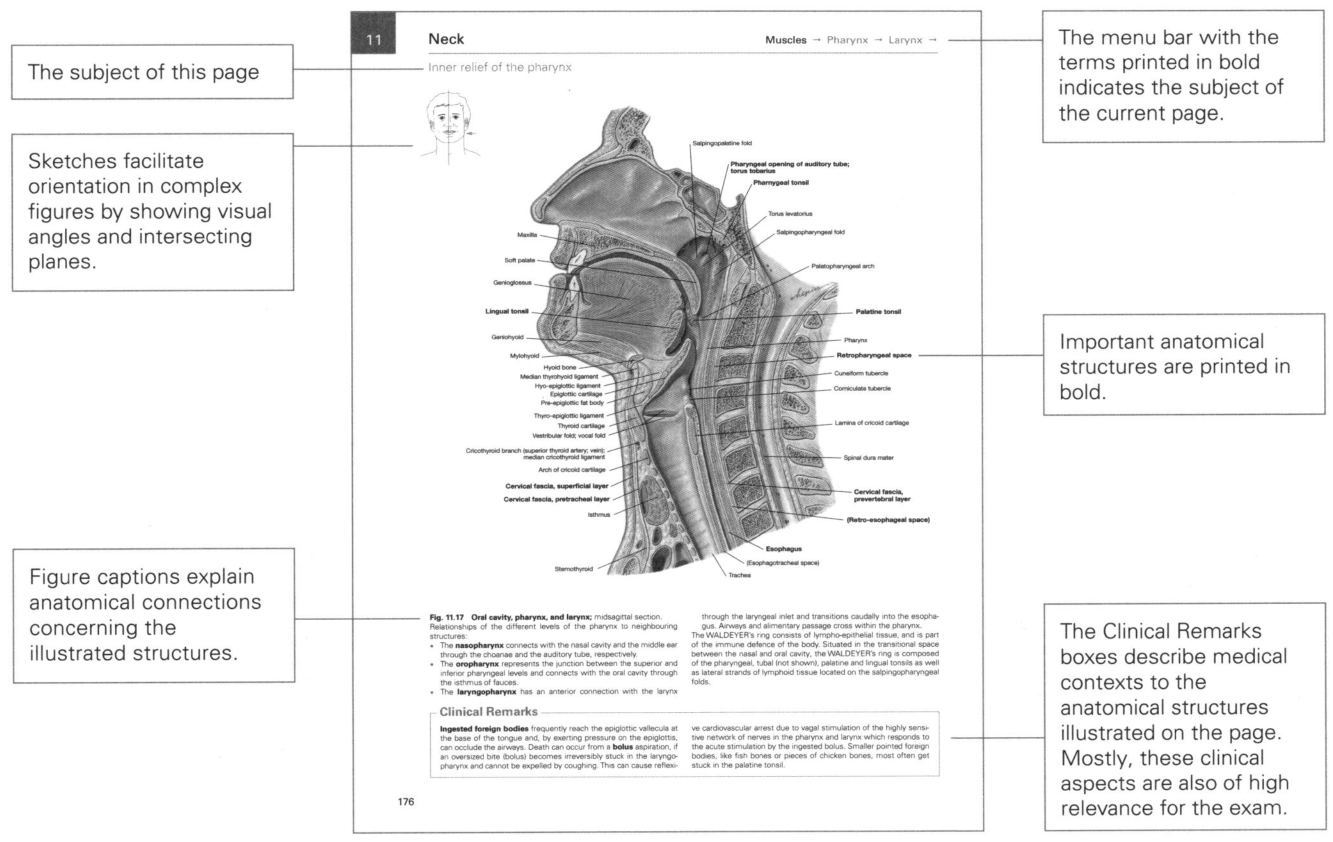
The subject of this page
Sketches facilitate orientation in complex figures by showing visual angles and intersecting planes.
Figure captions explain anatomical connections concerning the illustrated structures.
The menu bar with the terms printed in bold indicates the subject of the current page.
Important anatomical structures are printed in bold.
The Clinical Remarks boxes describe medical contexts to the anatomical structures illustrated on the page. Mostly, these clinical aspects are also of high relevance for the exam.
11
Neck
Muscles → Pharynx → Larynx →
Inner relief of the pharynx
Clinical Remarks
176

## The following contents can be found in the other two volumes:

Vol. 1 General Anatomy and Musculoskelal System

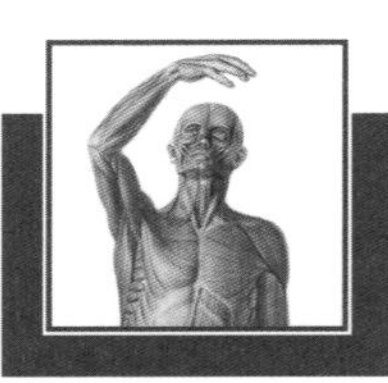

### 1 General Anatomy

Orientation on the Body → Surface Anatomy → Development → Muskuloskeletal System → Vessels and Nerves → Imaging Techniques → Integumentary System

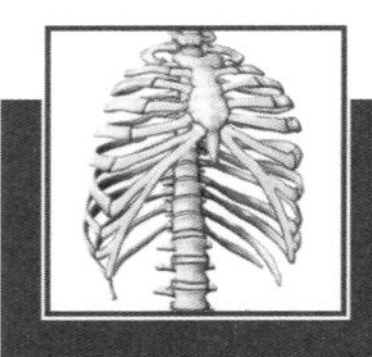

### 2 Trunk

Surface Anatomy → Development → Skeleton → Imaging → Muscles → Vessels and Nerves → Topography, Back → Female Breast → Topography, Abdomen and Abdominal Wall

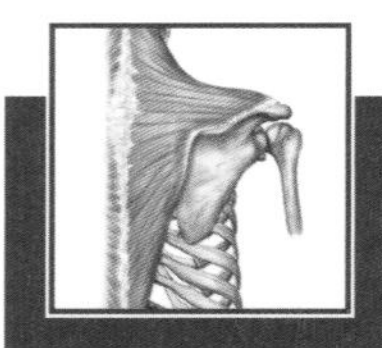

### 3 Upper Extremity

Surface Anatomy → Development → Skeleton → Imaging → Muscles → Topography → Sections

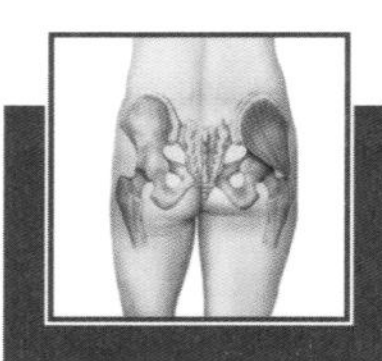

### 4 Lower Extremity

Surface Anatomy → Skeleton → Imaging → Muscles → Topography → Sections

Vol. 2 Internal Organs

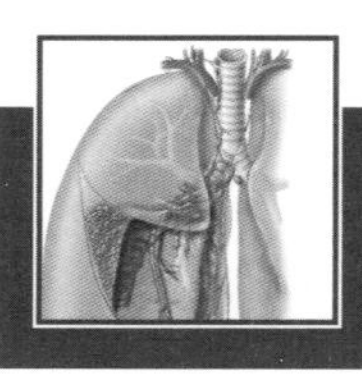

### 5 Viscera of the Thorax

Heart → Lungs → Esophagus → Thymus → Topography → Sections

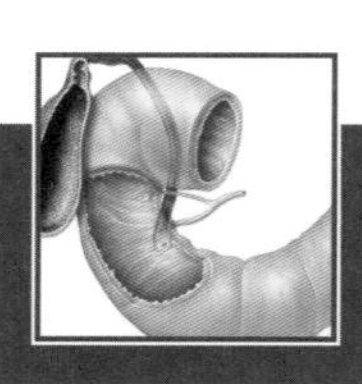

### 6 Viscera of the Abdomen

Development → Stomach → Intestines → Liver and Gallbladder → Pancreas → Spleen → Topography → Sections

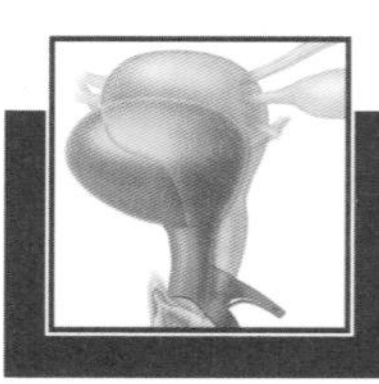

### 7 Pelvis and Retroperitoneal Space

Kidney and Adrenal Gland → Efferent Urinary System → Genitalia → Rectum and Anal Canal → Topography → Sections

Paulsen, Waschke

# Sobotta

Atlas of Human Anatomy
English Nomenclature

**Head, Neck, and Neuroanatomy**

Translated by
T. Klonisch and S. Hombach-Klonisch

# Editors

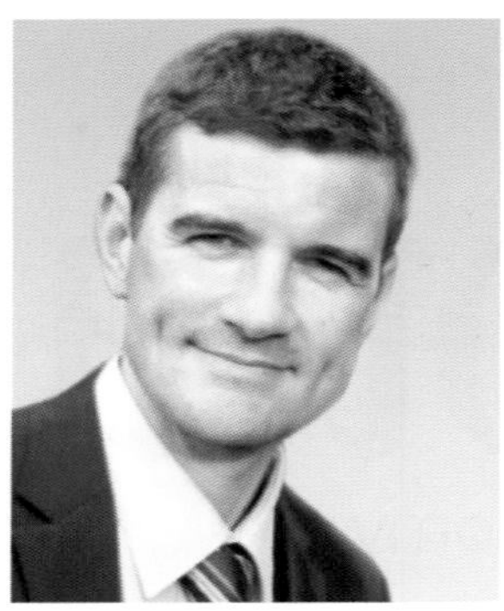

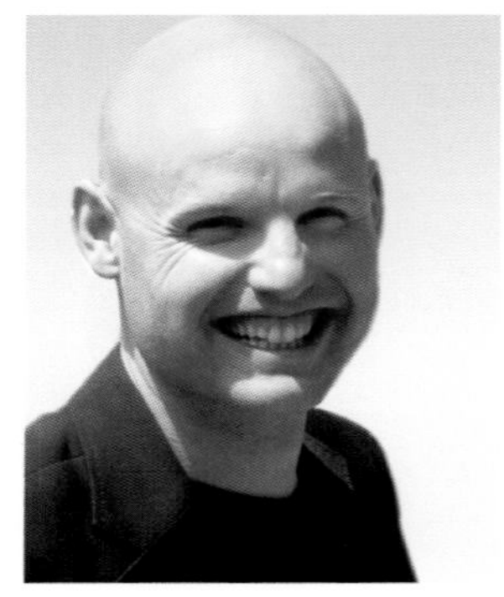

## Prof. Dr. Friedrich Paulsen

### Dissecting Courses for Students

*In his teaching, Friedrich Paulsen puts great emphasis on the fact that students can actually dissect on cadavers of body donors. "The hands-on experience in dissection is extremely important not only for the three-dimensional understanding of anatomy and as the basis for virtually every medical profession, but for many students also clearly addresses the issue of death and dying for the first time. The members of the dissection team not only study anatomy but also learn to deal with this special issue. At no other time medical students will have such a close contact to their classmates and teachers again."*

Professor Friedrich Paulsen (born 1965 in Kiel) passed the 'Abitur' in Brunswick and trained successfully as a nurse. After studying human medicine in Kiel, he became scientific associate at the Institute of Anatomy, Department of Oral and Maxillofacial Surgery and the Department of Otolaryngology, Head and Neck Surgery of the Christian-Albrechts-Universität Kiel. In 2002, together with his colleagues, he was awarded the Teaching Award for outstanding teaching in the field of anatomy at the Medical Faculty of the University of Kiel. On several occasions he gained work experience abroad in the academic section of the Department of Ophthalmology, University of Bristol, UK, where he did research for several months.

From 2004 to 2010 as a University Professor, he was head of the Macroscopic Anatomy and Prosector Section at the Department of Anatomy and Cell Biology of the Martin-Luther-Universität Halle-Wittenberg. Starting in April 2010, Professor Paulsen became the Chairman at the Institute of Anatomy II of the Friedrich-Alexander-Universität Erlangen. Since 2006, Professor Paulsen is a board member of the Anatomical Society and 2009 he was elected the general secretary of the International Federation of Associations of Anatomy (IFAA).

His main research area concerns the innate immune system. Topics of special interest are antimicrobial peptides, trefoil factor peptides, surfactant proteins, mucins, corneal wound healing, as well as stem cells of the lacrimal gland and diseases such as eye infections, dry eye, or osteoarthritis.

## Prof. Dr. Jens Waschke

### More Clinical Relevance in Teaching

*From March 2011 on, Professor Jens Waschke is Chairman of department I at the Institute of Anatomy and Cell Biology at the Ludwig-Maximilians-Universität(LMU) Munich. " For me, teaching at the department of vegetative anatomy, which is responsible for the dissection courses of both Munich's large universities LMU and TU, emphasizes the importance of teaching anatomy with clear clinical relevance," says Jens Waschke.*
*"The clinical aspects in the Atlas introduce students to anatomy in the first semesters. At the same time, it indicates the importance of this subject for future clinical practice, as understanding human anatomy means more than just memorization of structures."*

Professor Jens Waschke (born in 1974) habilitated in 2007 after graduation from Medical School and completing a doctoral thesis in Anatomy at the University of Wuerzburg. From 2003 to 2004 he joined Professor Fitz-Roy Curry at the University of California in Davis for a nine months research visit. In 2006, Jens Waschke was awarded the Investigator Prize of the "Anatomische Gesellschaft" (Anatomical Society).

Starting in June 2008, he became the Chairman of the newly established department III at the Institute of Anatomy and Cell Biology at the University of Wuerzburg. In March 2011, Professor Jens Waschke changed to the Ludwig-Maximilians-Universität (LMU) in Munich to become Chairman of department I of the "Anatomische Anstalt" as the successor of Professor Reinhard Putz, the former editor of Sobotta Atlas.

His main research area concerns cellular mechanisms that control the adhesion between cells and the cellular junctions establishing the outer and inner barriers of the human body. The attention is focused on the regulations of the endothelial barrier in inflammation and the mechanisms, which lead to the formation of fatal epidermal blisters in pemphigus, an autoimmune skin disease. The goal is to gain a better understanding of cell adhesion as a basis for the development of new therapeutic strategies.

# Sobotta

## Atlas of Human Anatomy

**Head, Neck, and Neuroanatomy**

15th edition
Edited by F. Paulsen and J. Waschke

Translated by T. Klonisch and
S. Hombach-Klonisch, Winnipeg, Canada

569 Colored Plates with 627 Figures

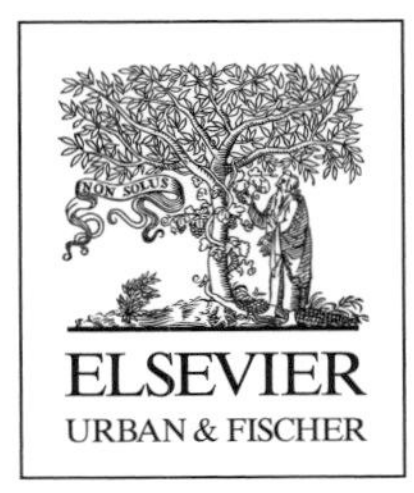
ELSEVIER
URBAN & FISCHER

URBAN & FISCHER
München

**All business correspondence should be made with:**
Elsevier GmbH, Urban & Fischer Verlag, Hackerbrücke 6, 80335 Munich, Germany, mail to: medizinstudium@elsevier.de

**Addresses of the editors:**
Professor Dr. med. Friedrich Paulsen
Institut für Anatomie II (Chairman)
Universität Erlangen-Nürnberg
Universitätsstraße 19
91054 Erlangen
Germany

Professor Dr. med. Jens Waschke
Institut für Anatomie I (Chairman)
Ludwig-Maximilians-Universität
Pettenkoferstraße 11
80333 München
Germany

**Addresses of the translators:**
Professor Dr. med. Sabine Hombach-Klonisch
Professor Dr. med. Thomas Klonisch
Faculty of Medicine
Department of Human Anatomy and Cell Science
University of Manitoba
745 Bannatyne Avenue
Winnipeg Manitoba R3E 0J9
Canada

**Bibliographic information published by the Deutsche Nationalbibliothek**
The Deutsche Nationalbibliothek lists this publication in the Deutsche Nationalbibliografie; detailed bibliographic data are available in the Internet at http://www.d-nb.de.

**All rights reserved**
15th Edition 2013
© Elsevier GmbH, Munich
Urban & Fischer Verlag is an imprint of Elsevier GmbH.

13 14 15 16 17 5 4 3 2 1

For copyright concerning the pictorial material see picture credits.

All rights, including translation, are reserved. No part of this publication may be reproduced, stored in a retrieval system, or transmitted in any other form or by any means, electronic, mechanical, photocopying, recording, or otherwise without the prior written permission of the publisher.

Acquisition editor: Alexandra Frntic, Munich; Dr. Katja Weimann, Munich
Development editor: Dr. Andrea Beilmann, Munich
Editing: Ulrike Kriegel, buchundmehr, Munich
Production manager: Sibylle Hartl, Munich; Renate Hausdorf, buchundmehr, Gräfelfing
Composed by: abavo GmbH, Buchloe
Printed and bound by: Firmengruppe appl, Wemding
Illustrators: Dr. Katja Dalkowski, Buckenhof; Sonja Klebe, Aying-Großhelfendorf; Jörg Mair, Munich; Stephan Winkler, Munich
Cover illustration: Nicola Neubauer, Puchheim
Cover design: SpieszDesign, Neu-Ulm
Printed on 115 g Quatro Silk

ISBN 978-0-7020-5253-8

This atlas was founded by Johannes Sobotta †, former Professor of Anatomy and Director of the Anatomical Institute of the University in Bonn, Germany.

*German editions:*
1st edition: 1904–1907 J. F. Lehmanns Verlag, Munich
2nd–11th edition: 1913–1944 J. F. Lehmanns Verlag, Munich
12th edition: 1948 and following editions Urban & Schwarzenberg, Munich
13th edition: 1953, editor H. Becher
14th edition: 1956, editor H. Becher
15th edition: 1957, editor H. Becher
16th edition: 1967, editor H. Becher
17th edition: 1972, editors H. Ferner and J. Staubesand
18th edition: 1982, editors H. Ferner and J. Staubesand
19th edition: 1988, editor J. Staubesand
20th edition: 1993, editors R. Putz and R. Pabst Urban & Schwarzenberg, Munich
21st edition: 2000, editors R. Putz and R. Pabst Urban & Fischer, Munich
22nd edition: 2006, editors R. Putz and R. Pabst Urban & Fischer, Munich
23rd edition: 2010, editors F. Paulsen and J. Waschke Elsevier, Munich

*Foreign editions:*
**Arabic edition**
Modern Technical Center, Damaskus
**Chinese edition (complex characters)**
Ho-Chi Book Publishing Co, Taiwan
**Chinese edition (simplified Chinese edition)**
Elsevier, Health Sciences Asia, Singapore
**Croatian edition**
Naklada Slap, Jastrebarsko
**Czech edition**
Grada Publishing, Prague
**Dutch edition**
Springer Media, Houten
**English edition (with nomenclature in English)**
Elsevier Inc., Philadelphia
**English edition (with nomenclature in Latin)**
Elsevier GmbH, Urban & Fischer
**French edition**
Tec & Doc Lavoisier, Paris
**Greek edition (with nomenclature in Greek)**
Parisianou, S.A., Athen
**Greek edition (with nomenclature in Latin)**
Parisianou, S.A., Athen
**Hungarian edition**
Medicina Publishing, Budapest
**Indonesian edition**
Penerbit Buku Kedokteran EGC, Jakarta
**Italian edition**
Elsevier Masson STL, Milan
**Japanese edition**
Igaku Shoin Ltd., Tokyo
**Korean edition**
Elsevier Korea LLC
**Polish edition**
Elsevier Urban & Partner, Wroclaw
**Portuguese edition (with nomenclature in English)**
Editora Guanabara Koogan, Rio de Janeiro
**Portuguese edition (with nomenclature in Latin)**
Editora Guanabara Koogan, Rio de Janeiro
**Russian edition**
Reed Elsevier LLC, Moscow
**Spanish edition**
Elsevier España S.L.
**Turkish edition**
Beta Basim Yayim Dagitim, Istanbul
**Ukrainian edition**
Elsevier Urban & Partner, Wroclaw

Current information by www.elsevier.de and www.elsevier.com

# Table of contents

# Translators

## Prof. Dr. Thomas Klonisch

Professor Thomas Klonisch (born 1960) studied human medicine at the Ruhr-Universität Bochum and the Justus-Liebig-Universität (JLU) Giessen. He successfully completed his doctoral thesis at the Institute of Biochemistry at the Faculty of Medicine of the JLU Giessen and became a scientific associate at the Institute of Medical Microbiology, University of Mainz (1989–1991). As an Alexander von Humboldt Fellow he joined the University of Guelph, Ontario, Canada, from 1991–1992 and, in 1993–1994, continued his research at the Ontario Veterinary College, Guelph, Ontario. From 1994–1996, he joined the immunoprotein engineering group at the Department of Immunology, University College London, UK, as a senior research fellow. From 1996–2004 he was a scientific associate at the Department of Anatomy and Cell Biology, Martin-Luther-Universität Halle-Wittenberg, where he received his accreditation as anatomist (1999), completed his habilitation (2000), and held continuous national research funding by the German Research Council (DFG) and German Cancer Research Foundation (Deutsche Krebshilfe). In 2004, he was appointed Full Professor and Head at the Department of Human Anatomy and Cell Science at the Faculty of Medicine, University of Manitoba, Winnipeg, Canada, where he is currently serving his second term as department chairman.

His research areas concern the mechanisms employed by cancer cells and their cancer stem/progenitor cells to enhance tissue invasiveness and survival strategies in response to anticancer treatments. One particular focus is on the role of endocrine factors, such as the relaxin-like ligand-receptor system, in promoting carcinogenesis.

## Prof. Dr. Sabine Hombach-Klonisch

Teaching clinically relevant anatomy and clinical case-based anatomy learning are the main teaching focus of Sabine Hombach-Klonisch at the Medical Faculty of the University of Manitoba. Since her appointment in 2004, Professor Hombach has been nominated annually for teaching awards by the Manitoba Medical Student Association.

Sabine Hombach (born 1963) graduated from Medical School at the Justus-Liebig-Universität Giessen in 1991 and successfully completed her doctoral thesis in 1994. Following a career break to attend to her two children she re-engaged as a sessional lecturer at the Department of Anatomy and Cell Biology of the Martin-Luther-Universität Halle-Wittenberg in 1997 and received a post-doctoral fellowship by the province of Saxony-Anhalt from 1998–2000. Thereafter, she joined the Department of Anatomy and Cell Biology as a scientific associate. Professor Hombach received her accreditation as anatomist in 2003 by the German Society of Anatomists and by the Medical Association of Saxony-Anhalt and completed her habilitation at the Medical Faculty of the Martin-Luther-Universität Halle-Wittenberg in 2004. In 2004, Professor Hombach was appointed Assistant Professor at the Department of Human Anatomy and Cell Science, Faculty of Medicine of the University of Manitoba. She has been the recipient of the Merck European Thyroid von Basedow Research Prize by the German Endocrine Society in 2002 and received the Murray L. Barr Young Investigator Award by the Canadian Association for Anatomy, Neurobiology and Cell Biology in 2009.

Her main research interests are in the field of cancer research and environmental toxicants. Her focus in cancer research is to identify the molecular mechanisms that regulate cancer cell migration and metastasis. She employs unique cell and animal models and human primary cells to study epigenetic and transgenerational effects facilitated by environmental chemicals.

# Preface

In the preface to the first edition of his Atlas, Johannes Sobotta wrote in May 1904: "Many years of experience in anatomical dissection led the author to proceed with the presentation of the peripheral nervous system and the blood vessels such that the illustrations of the book are presented to the student exactly in the same manner as body parts are presented to them in the dissection laboratories, i.e. simultaneous presentation of blood vessels and nerves of the same region. Alternating descriptive and image materials are distinctive features of this atlas. The images are the core piece of the atlas. Apart from table legends, auxiliary and schematic drawings, the descriptive material includes short and concise text parts suitable for use of this book in the gross anatomy laboratory."

As with fashions, reading and study habits of students change periodically. The multimedia presence and availability of information as well as stimuli are certainly the main reasons of ever changing study habits. These developments and changing demands of students to textbooks and atlases, which they utilise, as well as the availability of digital media of textbook contents, is accounted for by editors and publishers. Apart from interviews and systematic surveys of students, the textbook sector is occasionally an indicator enabling the evaluation of expectations of students. Detailed textbooks with the absolute claim of completeness are exchanged in favour of educational books that are tailored to the didactic needs of students and the contents of the study of human medicine, dentistry, and biomedical sciences, as well as the corresponding examinations. Similarly, illustrations in atlases such as the Sobotta, which contain exact naturalistic depiction of real anatomical specimens, fascinate doctors and associated medical professions for many generations throughout the world. However, students sometimes perceive them as too complicated and detailed. This awareness requires the consideration of how the strength of the atlas, which is known for its standards of accuracy and quality during its centennial existence featuring 14 editions, can be adapted to modern educational concepts without compromising the oeuvre's unique characteristics and authenticity. Elsevier and the editors Professor Reinhard Putz and Professor Reinhard Pabst, who were in charge of the atlas up to its 14th edition, have concluded after due consideration that a new editorial team resembling the great enthusiasm for anatomy and anatomy lessons of colleagues Putz and Pabst, will meet the new/increased requirements best. Together with the Elsevier publishing house, we are extremely pleased to be charged with the new composition of the 15th edition of Sobotta. In redesigning, a very clear outline of contents and a didactic introduction to the pictures was taken into account. Not every fashion is accompanied with something entirely new. Under didactical aspects we have revisited the old concept of a three-volume atlas, as used in Sobotta's first edition, with: General Anatomy and Musculoskeletal System (vol. 1), Internal Organs (vol. 2), and Head, Neck, and Neuroanatomy (vol. 3). Referring back to the approach mentioned in the preface of the first edition, which is devoted to an old trend of combining the image atlas with explanatory text, is currently en vogue, which we have adopted in a modified fashion. Each image is accompanied by a short explanatory text, which serves to introduce students to the image, explaining why the particular preparation and presentation of a region was selected. The individual chapters were systematically organised in terms of current subject matter and prevailing study habits; omitted and incomplete illustrations – particularly the systematics of the neurovascular pathways – were supplemented or replaced. The majority of these new figures are conceptualised to facilitate studying the relevant pathways of blood supply and innervation by didactical aspects. We have also reviewed many existing figures, reduced figure legends, and highlighted keywords by bold print to simplify access to the anatomical contents. Numerous clinical examples are used to enhance the "lifeless anatomy", present the relevance of anatomy for the future career to the student, and provide a taste of what's to come. Introductions to the individual chapters received a new conceptual design, covering in brief a summary of the content, the associated clinical aspects, and relevant dissection steps for the covered topic. It serves as a checklist for the requirements of the Institute of Medical and Pharmaceutical Examination Questions (IMPP) and is based on the German oral part of the preclinical medical examination (Physikum). Also new are brief introductions to each topic in embryology and the online connections of the atlas with the ability to download all images for reports, lectures, and presentations. We want to emphasize two points:

1. The "new" Sobotta in the 15th edition is not a study atlas, claiming completeness of a comprehensive knowledge and, thus, does not try to convey the intention to replace an accompanying textbook.
2. No matter how good the didactic approach, it cannot relieve the students of studying, but aid in visualization. Anatomy is not difficult to study, but very time-consuming. Sacrificing this time is worthwhile, since physicians and patients will benefit from it.

The goal of the 15th edition of Sobotta is not only to facilitate learning, but also to make learning exciting and attracting, so that the atlas is consulted during the study period as well as in the course of professional practice.

Erlangen and Wuerzburg, summer 2010, exactly 106 years after the first edition.

Friedrich Paulsen and Jens Waschke

# Acknowledgements

First, we would like to express that the work on the Sobotta was exciting and challenging. During stages, at which one could see the progress of development of individual chapters and newly developed pictures with a slight detachment, one obtained satisfaction, was elated with pride and identified oneself evermore with the Sobotta.

The redesign of Sobotta is obviously not the sole work of two inexperienced editors, but rather requires more than ever a well-attuned team under the coordination of the publisher. Without the long experience of Dr. Andrea Beilmann, who supervised several editions of the Sobotta and exerted the calming influence of the Sobotta team, many things would have been impossible. We thank her for all the help and support.

Ms. Alexandra Frntic, who is also part of the four-member Sobotta team, pursued the first major project of her career and tackled it with passion and enthusiasm. Her liveliness and management by motivation have enlivened and cheered the editors. We express our gratitude to Ms. Frntic. We like to reflect back on the Sobotta initialisation week in Parsberg and weekly conference calls, in which Dr. Beilmann and Ms. Frntic supported us in the composition of the Sobotta and presented an admirable way to merge the variety of two personalities to achieve a single layout. Without the assertiveness, the calls for perseverance and the protective hand of Dr. Dorothea Hennessen, who directed the project of the "15th edition of Sobotta" and always believed in her Sobotta team and the tight schedule, this edition would have not been published. Like a number of previous productions, the routinier Renate Hausdorf led the successful reproduction of the atlas. Other people involved in the editing process and the success of the 15th edition of the Sobotta and whom we sincerely thank are Ms. Susanne Szczepanek (manuscript editing), Ms. Julia Baier, Mr. Martin Kortenhaus and Ms. Ulrike Kriegel (editing), Ms. Amelie Gutsmiedl (formal text editing), Ms. Sibylle Hartl (internal production), Ms. Claudia Adam and Mr. Michael Wiedorn (formal figure editing and typesetting), Ms. Nicola Neubauer (layout development and refining the typesetting data) and the students Doris Bindl, Derkje Hockertz, Lisa Link, Sophia Poppe, Cornelia Rippl and Katherina and Florian Stumpfe. For the compilation of the index, we express our gratitude to Dr. Ursula Osterkamp-Baust. Special thanks are expressed to the illustrators Dr. Katja Dalkowski, Ms. Sonja Klebe, Mr. Jörg Mair and Mr. Stephan Winkler, who in addition to revising existing illustrations have developed a variety of excellent figures. Priv.-Doz. Dr. rer. nat. Helmut Wicht, Senkenberg Anatomy, Goethe-Universität Frankfurt/Main, has revived the lifelessness of the introductions to the chapters indited by the two editors through his unique style of writing. We express our gratitude to Priv.-Doz. Dr. rer. nat. Wicht.

A big help to us was the advisory council, which in addition to the former editors Prof. Dr. med. Dr. h. c. Reinhard Putz, Ludwig-Maximilians-Universität Munich, and Prof. Dr. med. Reinhard Pabst, Hannover Medical School, and colleagues Prof. Dr. med. Peter Kugler, Julius-Maximilians-Universität Wuerzburg, and Prof. Dr. rer. nat. Gottfried Bogusch, Charité Berlin, supported us strongly with advice and critical comments. We would like to specifically emphasise the effort of Ms. Renate Putz, who corrected the manuscript very carefully; her comments were of crucial importance for the consistency of the work in itself and with the earlier editions.

For support with corrections and revisions, we express our sincere thanks to Ms. Stephanie Beilicke, Dr. rer. nat. Lars Bräuer, Ms. Anett Diker, Mr. Fabian Garreis, Ms. Elisabeth George, Ms. Patricia Maake, Ms. Susann Möschter, Mr. Jörg Pekarsky and Mr. Martin Schicht.

For assistance in creating clinical fi gures, we express our gratitude to Priv.-Doz. Dr. med. Hannes Kutta, Clinic and Polyclinic for Oto-Rhino-Laryngology at the University Hospital Hamburg-Eppendorf, Prof. Dr. med. Norbert Kleinsasser, University Clinic for Oto-Rhino-Laryngo-Pathology, Julius-Maximilians-Universität Wuerzburg, Prof. Dr. med. Andreas Dietz, Head of Clinic and Polyclinic for Oto-Rhino-Laryngology at the University Leipzig, Dr. med. Dietrich Stoevesandt, Clinic for Diagnostic Radiology at the Martin-Luther-Universität Halle-Wittenberg, Prof. Dr. med. Stephan Zierz, Director of the University Hospital and Polyclinic for Neurology at the Martin-Luther-Universität Halle-Wittenberg, Dr. med. Berit Jordan, Hospital and Polyclinic for Neurology at the Martin-Luther-Universität Halle-Wittenberg, Dr. med. Saadettin Sel, University Hospital for Ophthalmology at the Martin-Luther-Universität Halle-Wittenberg, Mr. cand. med. Christian Schroeder, Eckernförde, and Mr. Denis Hiller, Bad Lauchstädt.

We also would like to express our thanks to our anatomical mentors Prof. Dr. med. Bernhard Tillmann, Christian-Albrechts-Universität Kiel, and Prof. Dr. med. Detlev Drenckhahn, Julius-Maximilians-Universität Wuerzburg, whom we not only owe our anatomical training, the motivation for subject matter, and the sense of mission, but also have been great role models in their design of textbooks and atlases, as well as in their teaching excellence.

Our deepest gratitude to our parents, Dr. med. Ursula Paulsen and Prof. Dr. med. Karsten Paulsen, and also Annelies Waschke and Dr. med. Dieter Waschke, who intensely supported and sustained the Sobotta project. Karsten Paulsen, who passed away in May 2010, studied anatomy as a medical student from the 4th edition of Sobotta. Dieter Waschke used the 16th edition of Sobotta and continues to attain knowledge with medical literature even during retirement. The 23rd edition is dedicated to our fathers.

Last but not least, we thank our wives Dr. med. Dana Paulsen and Susanne Waschke, who not only had to share us with the Sobotta in the last year, but also were on hand with help and advice on many issues and have been strongly supportive.

# Head



8

# The Head – Leading from the Top

The skeleton of the head (caput/cephalon), i.e. the skull (cranium), consists of two parts: the facial bones (viscerocranium) and the skull (neurocranium). The border between the two – the roof of one and the floor of the other – is the base of the skull, which lies roughly in an oblique plane defined by the eyebrows, the external opening of the outer ear canal and the base of the occiput.

## Skull Cap (Calvaria) and Scalp

The highly arched **calvaria** (skull cap, cranial cap) forms a longitudinal oval dome over the cranial base and protects the cranial cavity, in which the brain (cerebrum) surrounded by hard and soft meninges floats in the cerebrospinal fluid (CSF). The calvaria is divided in frontal, parietal, temporal, and occipital regions formed by identically named bones (frontal, parietal, temporal and occipital bone).

The skin of the calvaria is tough **("scalp")** and firmly adherent to a flat tendon, which spans from the forehead to the occiput. This tendon (epicranial aponeurosis) is part of the occipitofrontalis, a mimic muscle that raises eyebrows and wrinkles the skin of the forehead horizontally. Skin and tendon are movable on the skull cap and can be relatively easily lifted off and removed as the scalp. Vascular injuries of the scalp can lead to a severe but usually not-life threatening bleeding.

## Skull Base

The base of the skull forms the roof of the two orbits and the nasal cavity, but also the roof of the throat (pharynx, reaching up to the base of the skull) and the base of the occiput which articulates at the occipital foramen (foramen magnum) with the first cervical vertebra. Numerous foramina, canals, and fissures cover the cranial base and serve as passageways for many nerves and blood vessels. At the bottom side of the skull base, pointing towards the viscerocranium, numerous processes, spines, and notches are present, to which muscles and ligaments are attached. The upper side of the skull base, the floor of the neurocranium, is less irregular and resembles terraces on three floors: the top floor, the anterior cranial fossa, is positioned above the orbits. One step down, the middle cranial fossa is located at the level of the temporal bones. The last step leads down into the posterior cranial fossa with the foramen magnum.

## Facial Bones and Cavities

The largest **facial bone,** the maxillary bone (maxilla), is placed in the center of the viscerocranium. The maxilla forms the floor of the orbits most of the sidewalls of the nasal cavity, the anterior part of the palate, and carries the maxillary row of teeth. Like many other bones of the skull, the maxilla is "pneumatized", i.e. it is hollow and filled with air which is drawn from the nasal cavity (maxillary sinus, paranasal sinuses). Besides the maxilla, half a dozen other smaller bones are involved in the construction of the viscerocranium.

Breathing, smelling, tasting, chewing, swallowing, speaking, seeing, and being seen – these are the tasks of the **organs** that are supported and protected by the viscerocranium.

The eyes and their auxiliary apparatus (visual system, → p. 98) are responsible for vision. Being seen is the responsibility of the facial muscles. The permanent activity of these muscles, which do not control bones but the facial skin, is responsible for the formation of wrinkles.

The olfactory sense is up to the nose, even though it only performs it with its smallest part, the olfactory epithelium at the roof of the nasal cavity under the base of the skull. The outer cartilage-framed nasal vestibule and the far more spacious bony inner nasal cavity serve for breathing: Through the inner nostrils (choanae), the nasal cavity opens behind the throat (pharynx) which in turn communicates much more caudally with the larynx and the windpipe (trachea).

Biting, chewing, talking, tasting, and swallowing are the functions of the oral cavity and the accompanying organs. Similar to the nose, the oral cavity also has a vestibule, the space between lips and cheeks on one side and the teeth on the other side.

Behind the teeth lies the larger oral cavity proper which is almost completely filled by the tongue at a closed bite. At its posterior aspect, the oral cavity opens towards the pharynx and, at the price of choking, the respiratory tract and ingestive tract cross here. The roof of the mouth, the palate, also forms the floor of the nasal cavity. In the front, the palate is rigid and bony, while dorsally towards the pharynx it becomes soft, flexible, and muscular. The uvula dangles from the soft part of the palate. The floor of the mouth, which is surrounded by the movable mandible and which carries the tongue, is made of muscle plates. During speech almost all of these structures act together (along with many other structures), whereby the nose is used as an additional resonator.

Two **pits** of the facial skeleton are important: If one removes (first imaginary, later on in reality during the dissection sessions) the ascending bony branch of the mandible (ramus of mandible), which leads to the temporomandibular joint, one enters the soft tissues of the lateral aspect of the head from "behind the cheek" and enters a space that is referred to as the infratemporal fossa. Positioned in this region are masticatory muscles (medial and lateral pterygoid) and several branches of nerves. In addition, the terminal branches of the large external carotid artery lead towards the center of the viscerocranium.

In the direction of the orbit, the infratemporal fossa extends further inwards and cranially into a wider space, the pterygopalatine fossa. It is essential to locate this cavity during dissection and its contents and multiple pathways are important to remember. This cavity is a "key distributor" for vessels and nerves of the viscerocranium. Since it is hidden and its anatomy is extremely complex, all anatomists adore it and like to examine students on it.

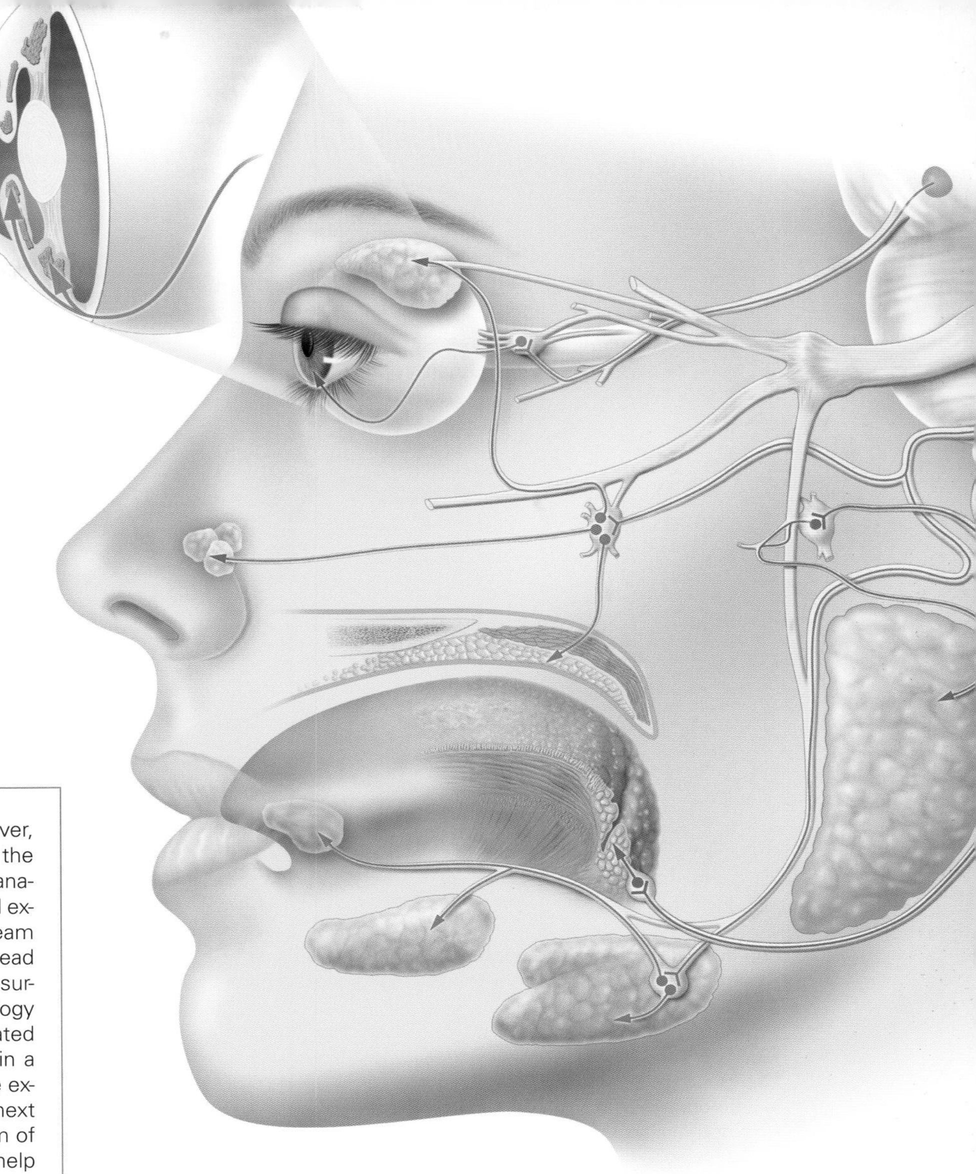

## Clinical Remarks

Ailments and injuries of the head are frequent events; however, diseases affecting the skull base are rare. Common to all is the fact that they are often life-threatening. Since the head is an anatomically complex system, consultation by a variety of medical experts is required to ensure optimal care of the patient. This team of experts includes medical disciplines like otolaryngology, head and neck surgery, neurosurgery, oral, dental, facial and plastic surgery, ophthalmology, radiation therapy, and diagnostic radiology and neuroradiology. Some patients with a severe head-related ailment (e.g. unclear headache or impaired blood perfusion in a region of the brain stem resulting in vertigo and nausea) have experienced an odyssey of referrals from one doctor to the next before encountering the one physician or, even better, a team of medical experts who identify the problem and are able to help this patient. As a response to this, some university medical centers now offer a co-ordinated, multidisciplinary team approach to provide quality treatment and follow-up for such patients. Thus, therapeutic strategies are discussed and co-ordinated among the members of the different medical disciplines involved in each particular case in order to provide the most optimal patient care and allow for a speedy recovery of the patient.

→ ***Dissection Link***

The dissection of the **superficial facial region** at the lateral sagittal plane of the head (head in a lateral position) is showing the facial arteries and veins, muscles of facial expression, all branches of the facial nerve, and the peripheral branches of the trigeminal nerve.

The dissection of the **deep facial region** includes the removal of the parotid gand, the presentation of the parotid plexus (facial nerve [VII]), the dissection of the retromandibular fossa, the representation of all four masticatory muscles, and the demonstration of the course of the maxillary artery up to its terminal branches, as well as the preparation of the temporomandibular joint with presentation of the articular disc and identification of the chorda tympani.

Dissection of the **midsagittal** planes of the head (head in medial position): The dissection of the nasal septum with its cartilaginous and bony parts as well as the olfactory nerves and the nasopalatine nerve is followed by the removal of the nasal septum and the presentation of the lateral nasal wall with openings of the paranasal sinuses and the nasolacrimal duct. The pterygopalatine fossa is opened and its contents are displayed. Finally, the sphenopalatine artery at the sphenopalatine foramen is located, followed by the full dissection of the oral cavity with representation of the submandibular and sublingual glands, lingual, hypoglossal, and glossopharyngeal nerves, as well as the dissection of the palatal muscles beneath the auditory tube cartilage, and of the tonsillar fossa.

## **EXAM** CHECK LIST

• Development: neurocranium, viscerocranium, cranial nerves, sensory organs, face, cranium with calvaria, base of the skull, exit points with penetrating structures, temporomandibular joint and infratemporal fossa • head and neck muscles, fascia and facial muscles, masticatory muscles, fascia of the head, hyoid bone and suprahyal muscles • components of the head: nasal cavity (with orifices), paranasal sinuses, topographic relationships, oral cavity, teeth, tongue, glands of the mouth, palate and function of the soft palate (cleft formation), isthmusof fauces, WALDEYER's tonsillar ring, tonsils, pharynx, pterygopalatine fossa, innervation and supply of all structures, facial paralysis and course of the cranial nerves [V, VII–XII]

## Regions of head and neck

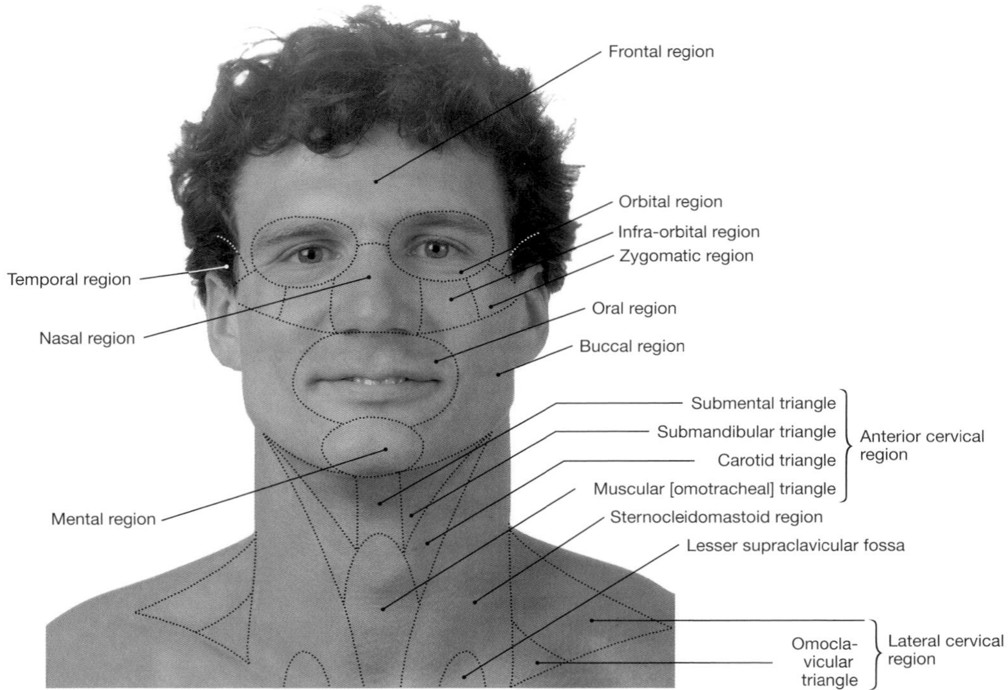
Frontal region
Orbital region
Infra-orbital region
Zygomatic region
Temporal region
Nasal region
Oral region
Buccal region
Submental triangle
Submandibular triangle
Carotid triangle
Muscular [omotracheal] triangle
Anterior cervical region
Mental region
Sternocleidomastoid region
Lesser supraclavicular fossa
Omocla-vicular triangle
Lateral cervical region

**Fig. 8.1 Regions of the head and neck;** frontal view.
The **head** is divided into the following topographic regions:

- frontal region
- temporal region
- orbital region
- nasal region
- infraorbital region
- zygomatic region
- oral region
- buccal region
- mental region
- parietal region
- occipital region
- parotideomasseteric region

The **neck** is divided into the following topographic regions:

- anterior cervical region, composed of submental, submandibular, carotid, and muscular (omotracheal) triangle
- sternocleidomastoid region with lesser supraclavicular fossa
- lateral cervical region with omoclavicular triangle
- posterior cervical region

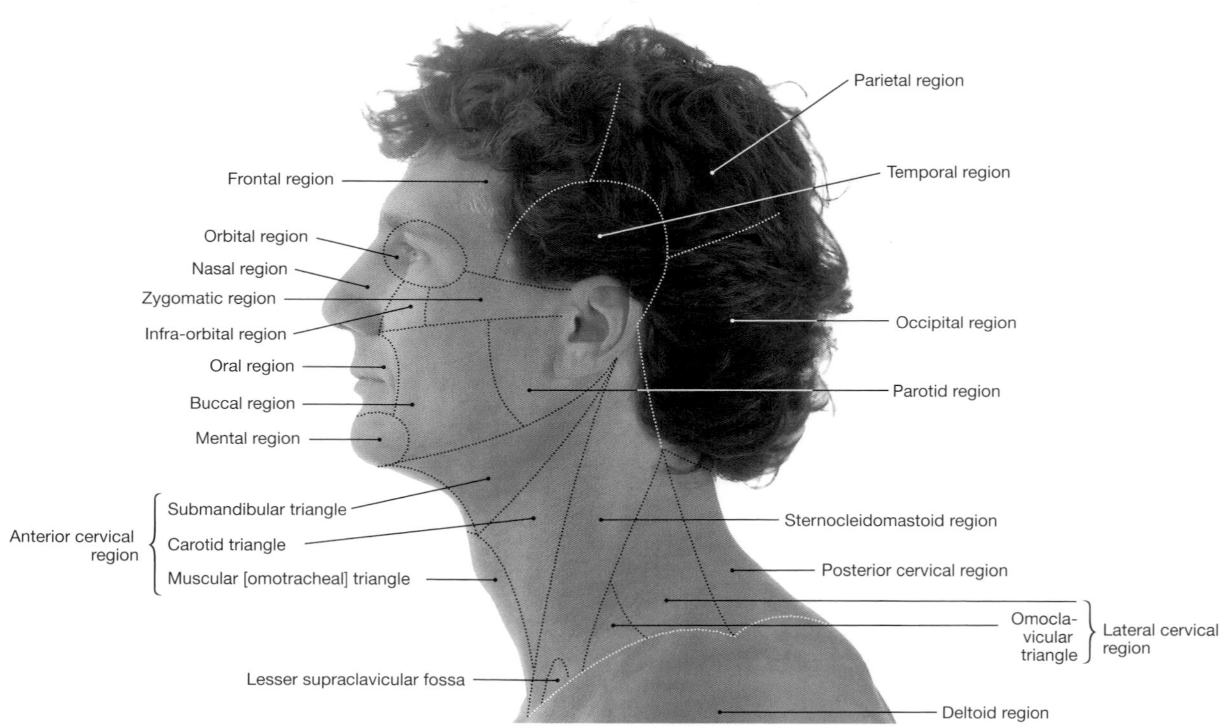
Parietal region
Frontal region
Temporal region
Orbital region
Nasal region
Zygomatic region
Infra-orbital region
Occipital region
Oral region
Parotid region
Buccal region
Mental region
Anterior cervical region
Submandibular triangle
Carotid triangle
Muscular [omotracheal] triangle
Sternocleidomastoid region
Posterior cervical region
Omocla-vicular triangle
Lateral cervical region
Lesser supraclavicular fossa
Deltoid region

**Fig. 8.2 Regions of the head and neck;** lateral view.

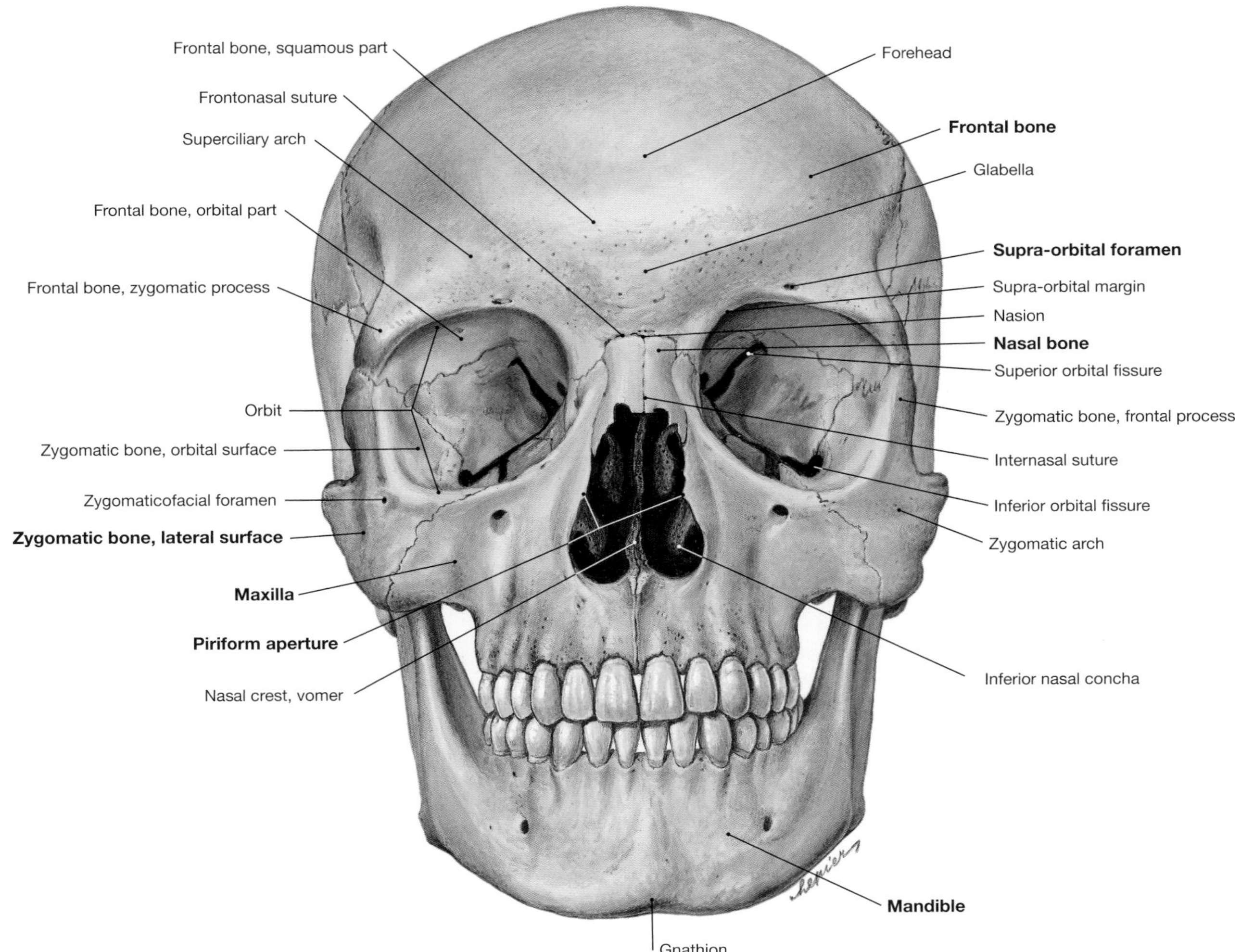
Frontal bone, squamous part
Frontonasal suture
Superciliary arch
Frontal bone, orbital part
Frontal bone, zygomatic process
Orbit
Zygomatic bone, orbital surface
Zygomaticofacial foramen
Zygomatic bone, lateral surface
Maxilla
Piriform aperture
Nasal crest, vomer
Forehead
Frontal bone
Glabella
Supra-orbital foramen
Supra-orbital margin
Nasion
Nasal bone
Superior orbital fissure
Zygomatic bone, frontal process
Internasal suture
Inferior orbital fissure
Zygomatic arch
Inferior nasal concha
Mandible
Gnathion

**Fig. 8.3 Skull, cranium;** frontal view.
From bottom to top one can see the lower jaw or mandible, the two upper jaws or maxillary bones, the nasal bones located between the maxillary bone and the orbit as well as the frontal bone above the orbit. The **frontal bone** consists of four parts (→ Fig. 8.23). Above the supra-orbital margin the bilateral superciliary arch bulges out. A part of the frontal bone protrudes medially downwards and forms a portion of the medial margin of the orbit. At the lateral aspect, the zygomatic process has contact with the frontal process of the zygomatic bone. Both form the lateral margin of the orbit.
The **zygomatic bone** constitutes the major part of the lateral and lower margins of the orbit.
The pair of **nasal bones** is connected to the frontal bone by the fronto-nasal suture and to each other by the internasal suture.

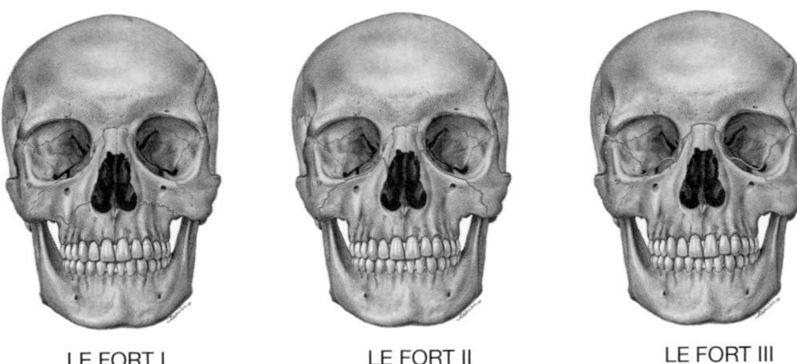
LE FORT I
LE FORT II
LE FORT III

**Fig. 8.4 LE FORT's fractures.**

## Clinical Remarks

Car accidents are among the most frequent causes of midfacial fractures, which are classified according to LE FORT (→ Fig. 8.4):
- LE FORT I: horizontal fracture line with isolated detachment of the maxillary alveolar rim ("floating palate")
- LE FORT II: pyramidal fracture line involving the maxillary bone in the region of the floor of the orbit; involvement of the ethmoidal bones, anterior skull base, and nasal bones is also possible
- LE FORT III: transverse fracture line with craniofacial dissociation

## Skull bones

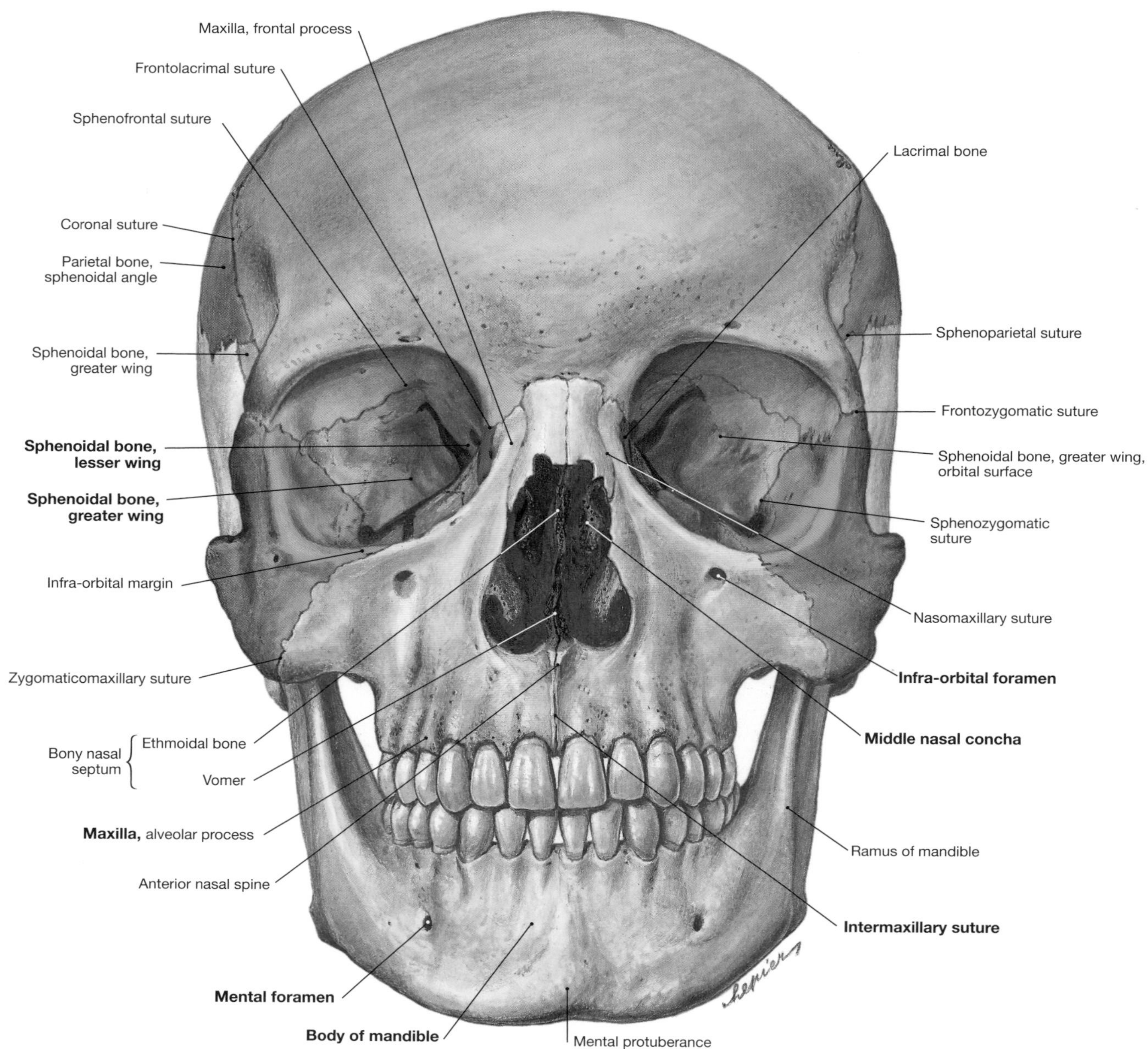
Maxilla, frontal process
Frontolacrimal suture
Sphenofrontal suture
Coronal suture
Parietal bone, sphenoidal angle
Sphenoidal bone, greater wing
Sphenoidal bone, lesser wing
Sphenoidal bone, greater wing
Infra-orbital margin
Zygomaticomaxillary suture
Bony nasal septum
Ethmoidal bone
Vomer
Maxilla, alveolar process
Anterior nasal spine
Mental foramen
Body of mandible
Mental protuberance
Lacrimal bone
Sphenoparietal suture
Frontozygomatic suture
Sphenoidal bone, greater wing, orbital surface
Sphenozygomatic suture
Nasomaxillary suture
Infra-orbital foramen
Middle nasal concha
Ramus of mandible
Intermaxillary suture

**Fig. 8.5 Skull bones;** frontal view; color chart see inside of the back cover of this volume.

The upper jaw or maxillary bone **(maxilla)** is located between the orbit and the oral cavity. The maxillary bone participates in the formation of the lower and medial margins of the orbit and has a lateral border with the zygomatic bone. The frontal process of the maxilla connects with the frontal bone. The infraorbital foramen is located below the lower margin of the orbit in the body of the maxillary bone. The anterior nasal spine protrudes in the midline. The alveolar process creates the lower margin of the maxilla and supports the teeth. In the orbit, the maxilla creates the lower margin of the inferior orbital fissure and, together with the zygomatic bone, forms the lateral margin of the orbit.

The lower jaw or **mandible** consists of a body and the rami of mandible, which merge in the mandibular angle. The body of mandible is composed of the alveolar parts with teeth and the base of mandible beneath. The latter protrudes in the midline as mental protuberance. In addition, the mental foramen is shown.

### Clinical Remarks

**Fractures of the nasal bone and the supporting cartilaginous nasal framework** are among the most frequent fractures of the facial region. One can distinguish closed and open nasal fractures. Open fractures involve bony parts piercing through the skin and soft tissue. The nasal septum and nasal conchae can also be affected. Fractures of the nasal framework are typically a result of violent physical disputes, car accidents, martial arts like karate, boxing, and of a variety of team sports.

## Skull bones

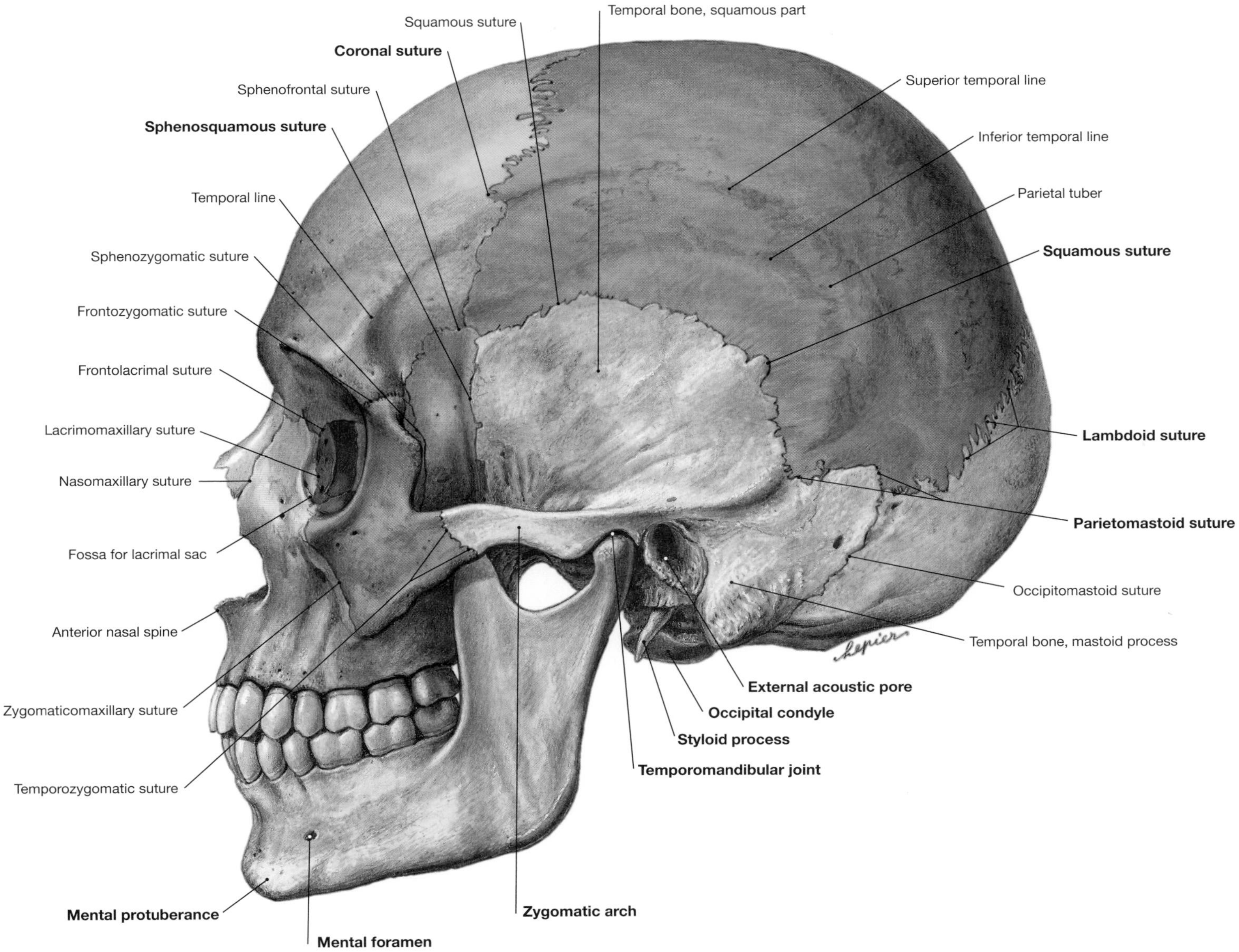

Squamous suture
Temporal bone, squamous part
**Coronal suture**
Sphenofrontal suture
Superior temporal line
**Sphenosquamous suture**
Inferior temporal line
Temporal line
Parietal tuber
Sphenozygomatic suture
**Squamous suture**
Frontozygomatic suture
Frontolacrimal suture
Lacrimomaxillary suture
**Lambdoid suture**
Nasomaxillary suture
**Parietomastoid suture**
Fossa for lacrimal sac
Occipitomastoid suture
Anterior nasal spine
Temporal bone, mastoid process
**External acoustic pore**
Zygomaticomaxillary suture
**Occipital condyle**
**Styloid process**
**Temporomandibular joint**
Temporozygomatic suture
**Mental protuberance**
**Zygomatic arch**
**Mental foramen**

**Fig. 8.6 Skull bones;** lateral view; color chart see inside of the back cover of this volume.
The lateral view displays parts of the frontal, parietal, occipital, sphenoidal, and temporal bones, parts of the viscerocranium (nasal, lacrimal, maxillary, and zygomatic bones) as well as the lateral side of the lower jaw (mandible).
In the viscerocranium, the **nasal bone** has its cranial and posterior borders with the frontal bone and the maxilla, respectively. The upper part of the **lacrimal bone** forms the fossa for lacrimal sac between **maxilla** and ethmoidal bone. The alveolar process of the maxilla contains the upper teeth. The medial aspect of the maxilla connects with the frontal bone, its lateral aspect contacts the zygomatic bone. The anterior nasal spine protrudes in the anterior midline. The **zygomatic bone** is responsible for the contour of the region of the cheek.
The head of mandible articulates with the temporal bone in the temporomandibular joint.
In its upper frontal aspect, the **frontal bone** is connected with the parietal bone and the sphenoidal bone via the coronal suture. The **parietal bone** connects with the occipital bone in the lambdoid suture and with the **sphenoidal bone** in the shenoparietal suture. The sphenoidal bone and the **temporal bone** form the sphenosquamous suture. The temporal and occipital bones connect in the posterior occipitomastoid suture. The major part of the lateral wall of the skull is formed by the squamous part of the temporal bone.

The temporal bone and the zygomatic bone form the zygomatic arch, which bridges the temporal fossa. The tympanic part of the temporal bone is located below the base of the zygomatic process and directly adjacent to the squamous part. At its surface lies the external acoustic opening.

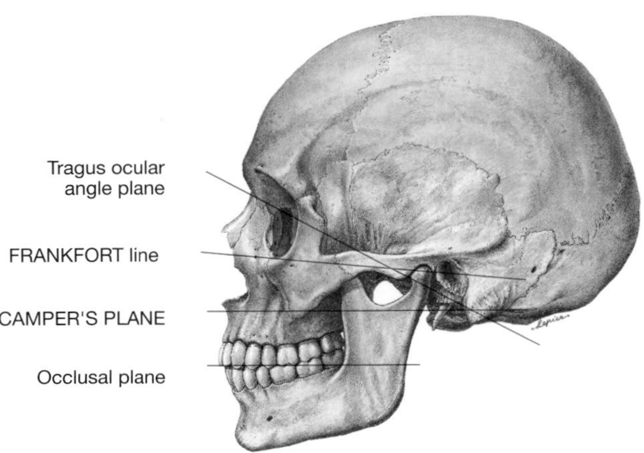
Tragus ocular angle plane
FRANKFORT line
CAMPER'S PLANE
Occlusal plane

**Fig. 8.7 Reference lines for the teeth.**

## Skull bones

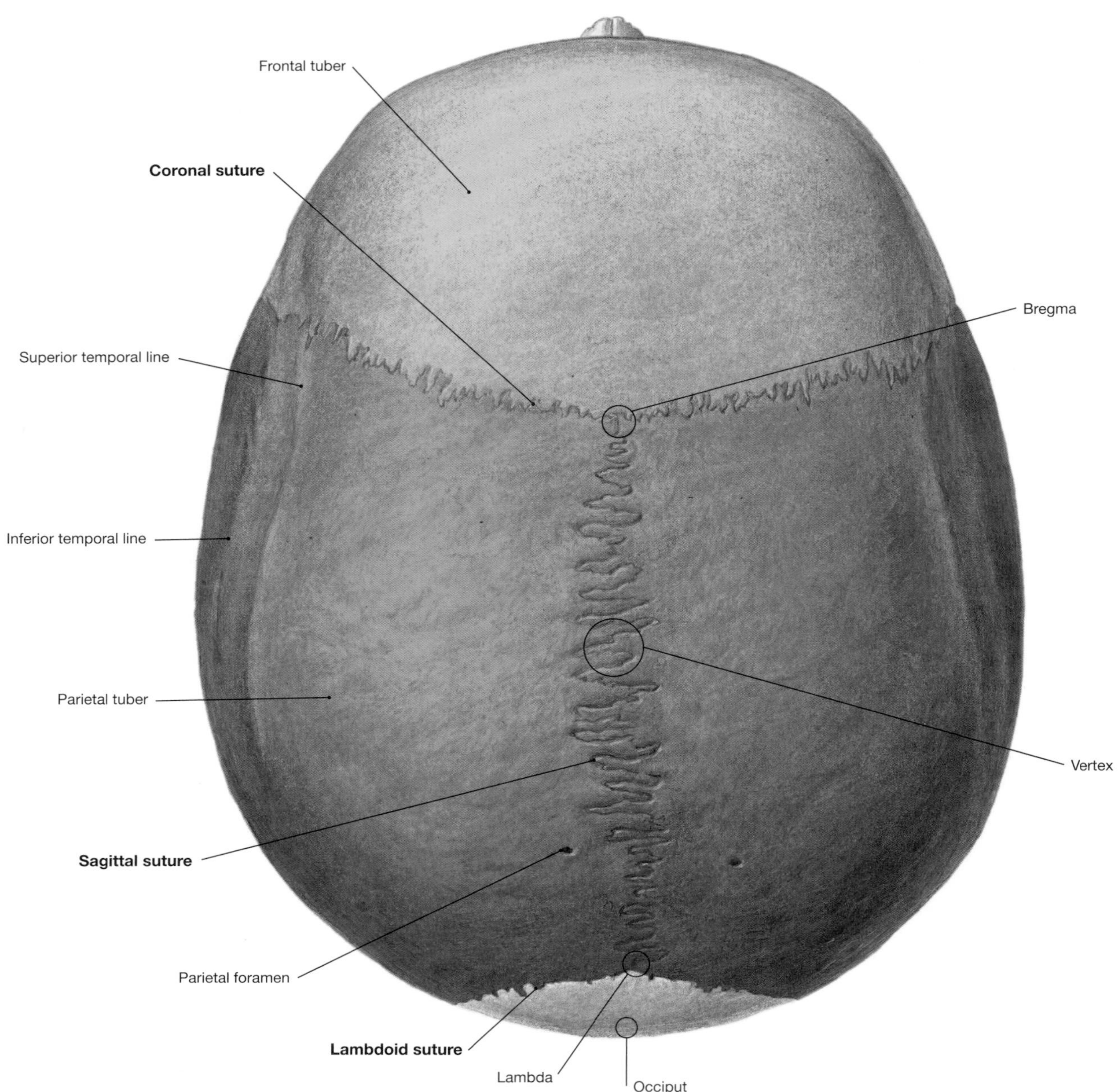
Frontal tuber
Coronal suture
Superior temporal line
Inferior temporal line
Parietal tuber
Sagittal suture
Parietal foramen
Lambdoid suture
Lambda
Occiput
Vertex
Bregma

**Fig. 8.8 Skull bones;** superior view; color chart see inside of the back cover of this volume.

A view on the upper part of the skull (skull cap, calvaria) reveals the frontal bone, the parietal bones, and the occipital bone. The frontal bone and the parietal bones are separated by the **coronal suture.** Both parietal bones meet at the **sagittal suture.** The occipital bone connects with the two parietal bones by the **lambdoid suture.** The contact point between the coronal and sagittal sutures is called **bregma,** the contact point of the sagittal and lambdoid sutures is named **lambda.** In the dorsal part of the parietal bones and bilaterally in close proximity to the sagittal suture are the paired parietal foramina for the passage of the emissary veins.

### Clinical Remarks

Extensive external physical force can lead to skull fractures. **Skull fractures** are further differentiated into:

- **linear** fractures presenting with clear fracture lines
- **split** skull fractures with multiple bony fragments (impression fracture with inward pointing bony parts which can cause a compression or tear of the Dura mater as well as an injury to brain tissue)
- **diastatic** fractures (with fracture lines including sutures and result in a widening of the suture)
- **basal skull fractures.**

All fractures associated with an open wound of the skin of the head and fractures involving the paranasal sinuses or the middle ear are considered to be open fractures with a risk of infection. They require a surgical intervention.

## Skull bones

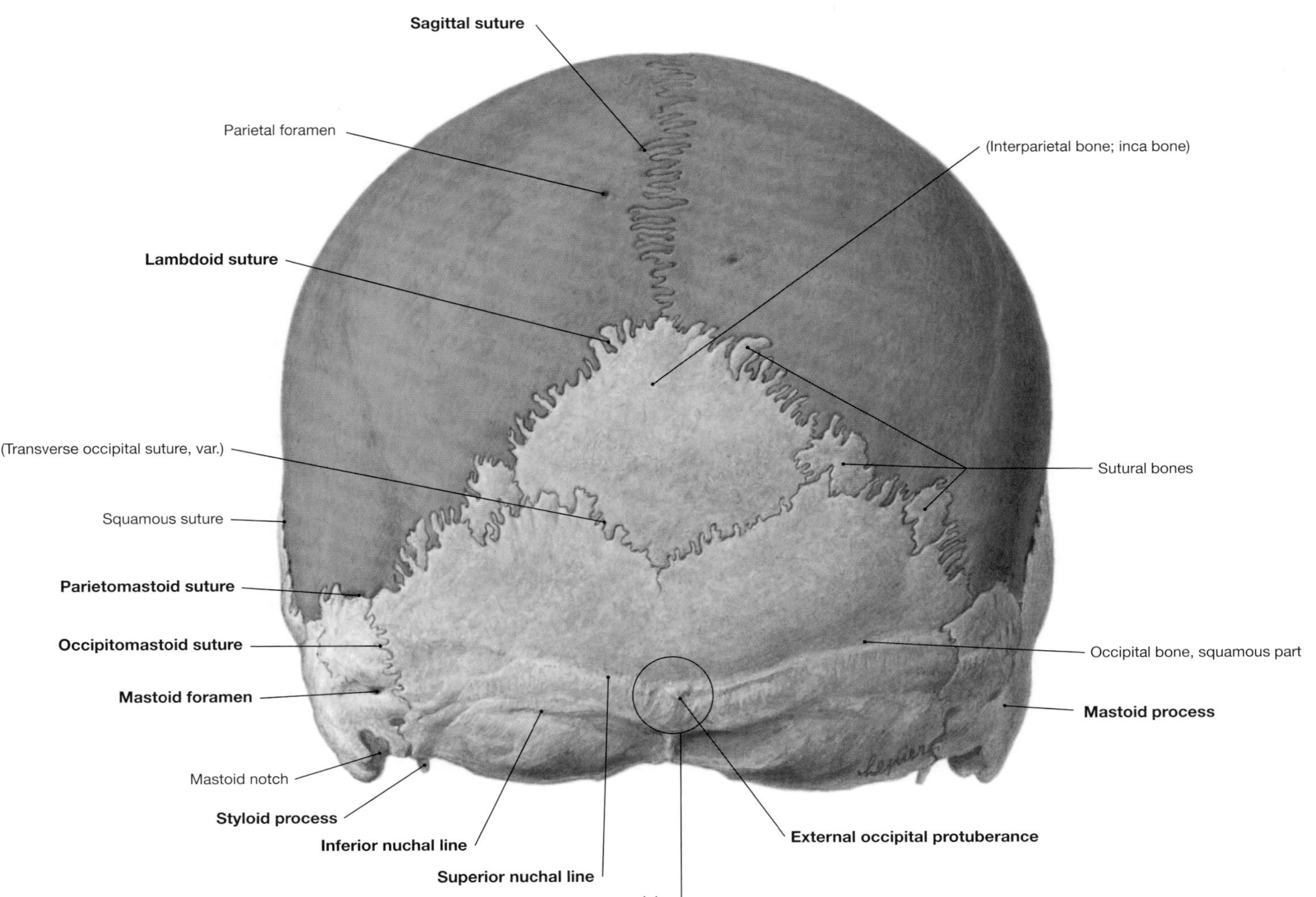
Sagittal suture
Parietal foramen
(Interparietal bone; inca bone)
Lambdoid suture
(Transverse occipital suture, var.)
Sutural bones
Squamous suture
Parietomastoid suture
Occipitomastoid suture
Occipital bone, squamous part
Mastoid foramen
Mastoid process
Mastoid notch
Styloid process
Inferior nuchal line
External occipital protuberance
Superior nuchal line
Inion

**Fig. 8.9 Skull bones;** posterior view; color chart see inside of the back cover of this volume.
This view from the posterior side shows the temporal, parietal, and the occipital bones. To both sides of the **temporal bone** the mastoid process is visible. At the lower medial margin of the mastoid process lies the mastoid notch; this notch serves as attachment point for the posterior belly of the digastric muscle.
Shown from posterior, both **parietal bones** meet in the midline in the sagittal suture, connect posteriorly with the occipital bone in the lambdoid suture, and are separated laterally from the temporal bones by the parietomastoid suture.

The **occipital bone** occupies most of the posterior part of the skull. The central structure is the squamous part of occipital bone. Frequently, sutural bones are found along the lambdoid suture. The external occipital protuberance is an easily palpable bony reference point on the occipital bone. Its most protruding point is the inion. The protuberance extends bilaterally in an arch-shaped line as superior nuchal line, a bony crest which serves for the attachment of the autochthonous (intrinsic) muscles of the back. At approximately 2–2.5 cm below the external occipital protuberance, the inferior nuchal line runs in a similar arch-shaped fashion, serving as additional attachment sites for muscles.

## Skull bones

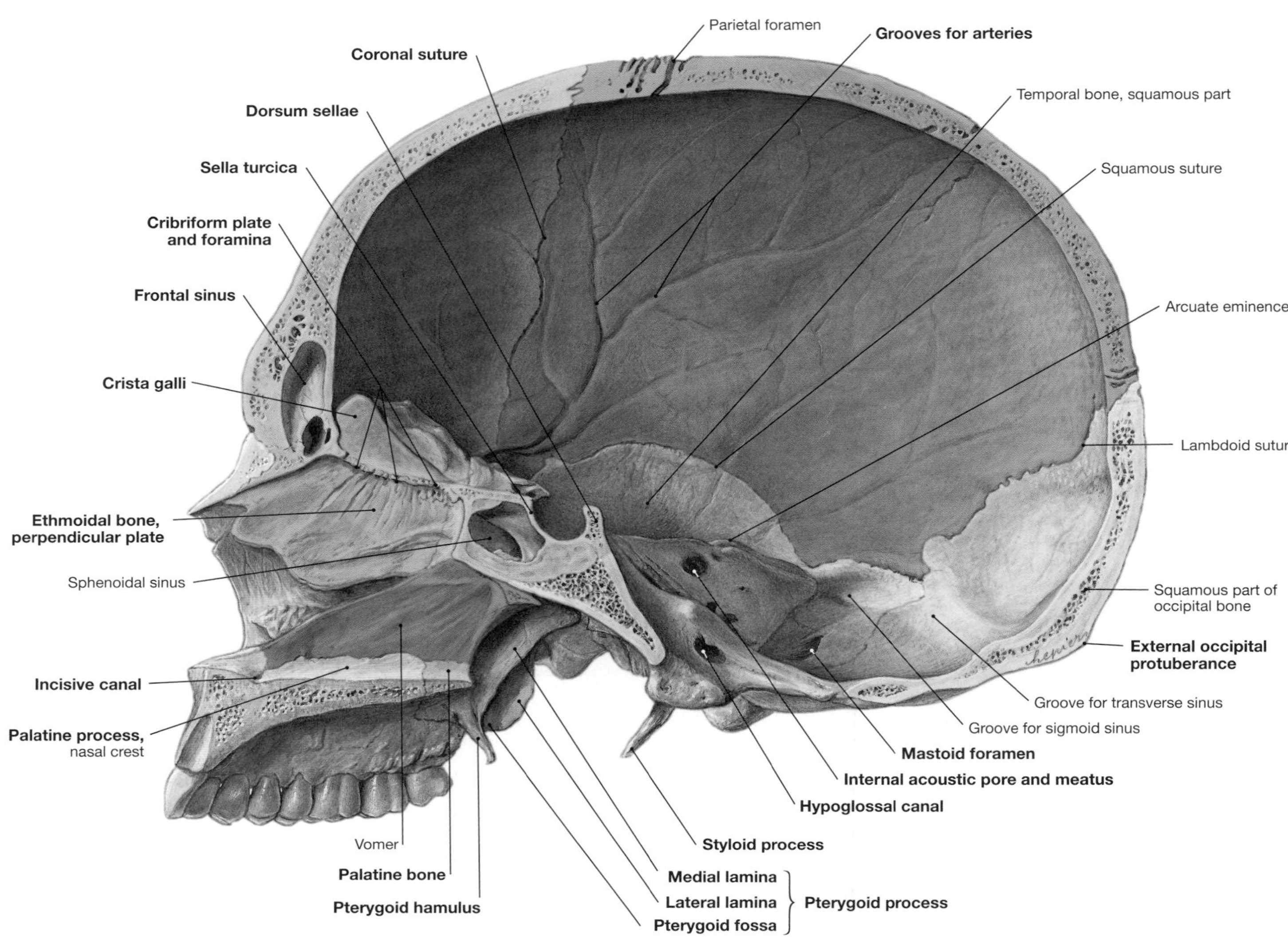
Parietal foramen
Grooves for arteries
Coronal suture
Temporal bone, squamous part
Dorsum sellae
Squamous suture
Sella turcica
Cribriform plate and foramina
Frontal sinus
Arcuate eminence
Crista galli
Lambdoid suture
Ethmoidal bone, perpendicular plate
Sphenoidal sinus
Squamous part of occipital bone
External occipital protuberance
Incisive canal
Groove for transverse sinus
Palatine process, nasal crest
Groove for sigmoid sinus
Mastoid foramen
Internal acoustic pore and meatus
Hypoglossal canal
Styloid process
Vomer
Palatine bone
Medial lamina
Lateral lamina
Pterygoid fossa
Pterygoid process
Pterygoid hamulus

**Fig. 8.10 Skull bones, right side;** medial view; color chart see inside of the back cover of this volume.
The cranial cavity includes the skull cap (calvaria) and the base of the skull which is composed of the anterior, middle, and posterior cranial fossae. The cranial cavity surrounds the brain with its meninges and encloses the proximal portion of the cranial nerves, including the blood vessels and the venous sinuses. On the inside of the cranial cavity, the pulsations of the medial meningeal artery have carved out grooves for arteries. The perpendicular plate of the ethmoidal bone and the vomer, the bony part of the nasal septum, are located at the transition region from neurocranium to viscerocranium. The palatine processes of the maxillary and palatine bone form the hard palate.

## Skull bones

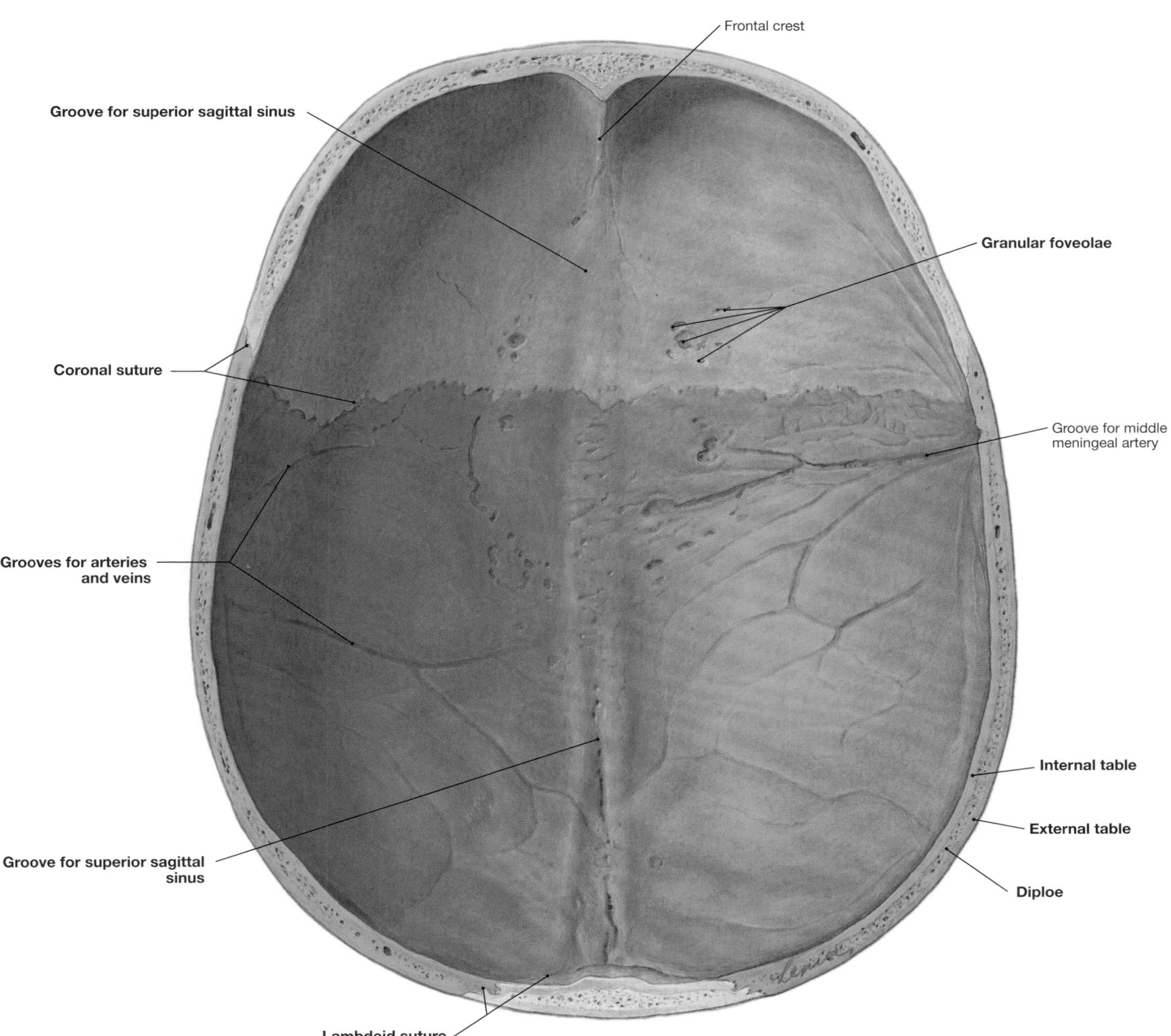
Frontal crest
Groove for superior sagittal sinus
Granular foveolae
Coronal suture
Groove for middle meningeal artery
Grooves for arteries and veins
Internal table
External table
Groove for superior sagittal sinus
Diploe
Lambdoid suture

**Fig. 8.11 Roof of the skull, calvaria;** inner aspect; color chart see inside of the back cover of this volume.

The inside of the skull cap reveals the coronal suture between frontal bone and parietal bones and the lambdoid suture between parietal bones and occipital bone. Also visible at the inside of the frontal bone is the frontal crest which serves as an attachment for the falx cerebri (duplication of the dura mater composed of tough fibrous tissue; separates both cerebral hemispheres). The frontal crest transitions into the groove of the superior sagittal sinus (location of the superior sagittal sinus) which becomes wider and deeper in its posterior part. It extends across the lambdoid suture onto the occipital bone.

Bilaterally and alongside the entire length of the groove of the superior sagittal sinus, irregularly grouped small depressions (granular foveolae, location of the cauliflower-like arachnoid granulations [PACCHIONIAN granulations]) are identified. The lateral part of the calvaria contains multiple arterial and venous grooves.

The **bones of the calvaria** possess a special **structure.** They consist of a thick outer and thin inner compact layer, named external and internal table, and a thin layer of spongiosa, known as diploë.

## Clinical Remarks

The internal table of the calvarian bones is thin and can be easily damaged by **external forces** that result in a bending fracture of the table. If thereby branches of the medial meningeal artery (which course in the groove for medial meningeal artery of the internal table) are injured, an **epidural hematoma** may occur (→ Fig. 12.11).

## Inner aspect of the base of the skull

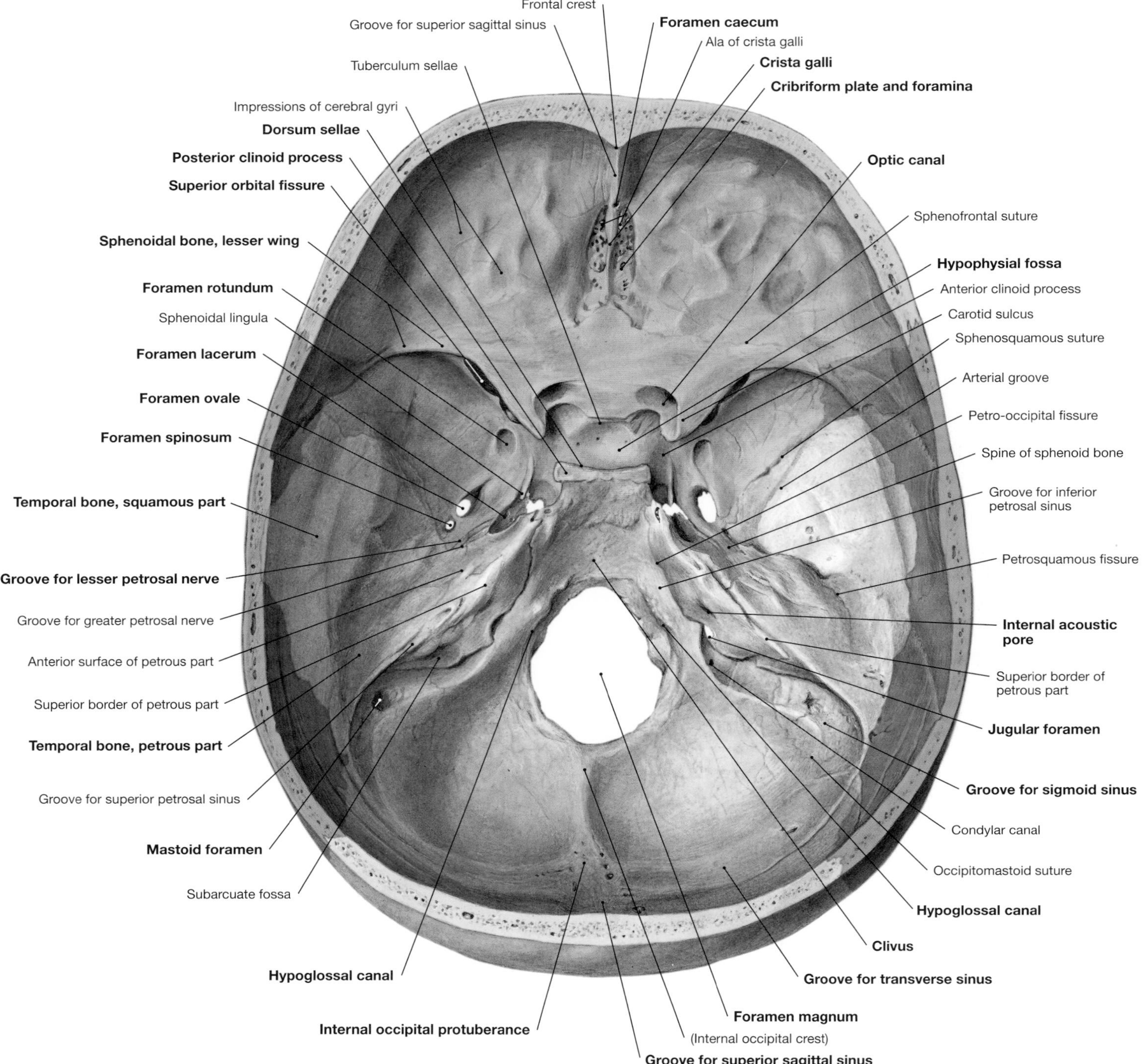
Frontal crest
Groove for superior sagittal sinus
Foramen caecum
Ala of crista galli
Tuberculum sellae
Crista galli
Cribriform plate and foramina
Impressions of cerebral gyri
Dorsum sellae
Posterior clinoid process
Optic canal
Superior orbital fissure
Sphenofrontal suture
Sphenoidal bone, lesser wing
Hypophysial fossa
Foramen rotundum
Anterior clinoid process
Sphenoidal lingula
Carotid sulcus
Sphenosquamous suture
Foramen lacerum
Arterial groove
Foramen ovale
Petro-occipital fissure
Foramen spinosum
Spine of sphenoid bone
Groove for inferior petrosal sinus
Temporal bone, squamous part
Petrosquamous fissure
Groove for lesser petrosal nerve
Internal acoustic pore
Groove for greater petrosal nerve
Anterior surface of petrous part
Superior border of petrous part
Superior border of petrous part
Jugular foramen
Temporal bone, petrous part
Groove for sigmoid sinus
Groove for superior petrosal sinus
Condylar canal
Mastoid foramen
Occipitomastoid suture
Subarcuate fossa
Hypoglossal canal
Clivus
Hypoglossal canal
Groove for transverse sinus
Foramen magnum
Internal occipital protuberance
(Internal occipital crest)
Groove for superior sagittal sinus

**Fig. 8.12 Inner aspect of the base of the skull;** superior view; color chart see inside of the back cover of this volume.

The anterior, middle, and posterior cranial fossae form the inner base of the skull. The frontal, ethmoidal, and sphenoidal bones participate in the structure of the **anterior cranial fossa.** The latter is located above the nasal cavity and orbit and contains the foramen cecum, the crista galli (attachment point for the falx cerebri), and the bilateral cribriform plate. Posterior to the frontal bone and ethmoidal bones, the body and the lesser wings of the sphenoidal bone form the base of the anterior cranial fossa. The body also forms the border to the middle cranial fossa.

The **middle cranial fossa** is composed of the sphenoidal and temporal bones. Its floor is elevated in the midline, and at this point it becomes part of the body of the sphenoidal bone. The pit-shaped lateral portions are parts of the greater wing of the sphenoidal bone and the squamous part of the temporal bone. Located in the middle cranial fossa are the saddle-shaped sella turcica with the hypophysial fossa and, on both sides the optic canal, the superior orbital fissure, and the foramina rotundum, ovale, spinosum, and lacerum. The anterior surface of petrous part demarcates the posterior aspect of the middle cranial fossa.

## Inner aspect of the base of the skull

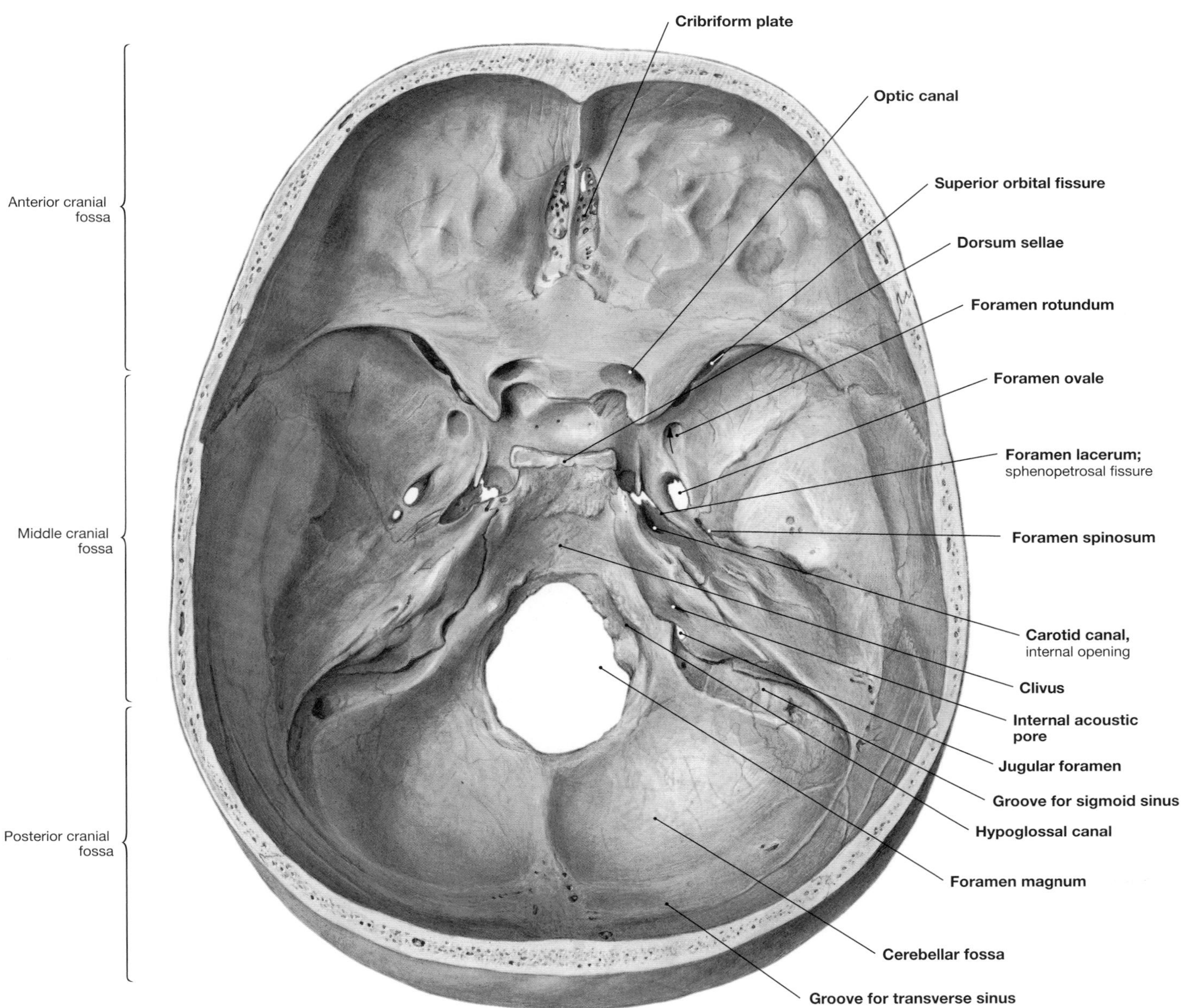
Cribriform plate
Optic canal
Superior orbital fissure
Dorsum sellae
Foramen rotundum
Foramen ovale
Foramen lacerum; sphenopetrosal fissure
Foramen spinosum
Carotid canal, internal opening
Clivus
Internal acoustic pore
Jugular foramen
Groove for sigmoid sinus
Hypoglossal canal
Foramen magnum
Cerebellar fossa
Groove for transverse sinus
Anterior cranial fossa
Middle cranial fossa
Posterior cranial fossa

**Fig. 8.13 Inner aspect of the base of the skull;** superior view.
Of the three cranial fossae, the **posterior cranial fossa** is the biggest. It is composed of the temporal bones, the occipital bone, and, to a smaller extent, of the sphenoidal bone and the parietal bones.
In the midline, its anterior margin is formed by the dorsum sellae and the clivus. The clivus is an oblique bony rim, which creates a slope from the dorsum sellae to the foramen magnum. The clivus is composed of parts of the body of the sphenoidal bone and the basilar part of the occipital bone. The posterior aspect of the posterior cranial fossa consists mainly of the groove for transverse sinus. The foramen magnum is the largest opening of the posterior cranial fossa.
Additional structures of the posterior cranial fossa include the hypoglossal canal, the internal acoustic pore, and the jugular foramen. The groove for sigmoid sinus approaches the jugular foramen from lateral. The central depression in the posterior cranial fossa is the cerebellar fossa.

## Outer aspect of the base of the skull

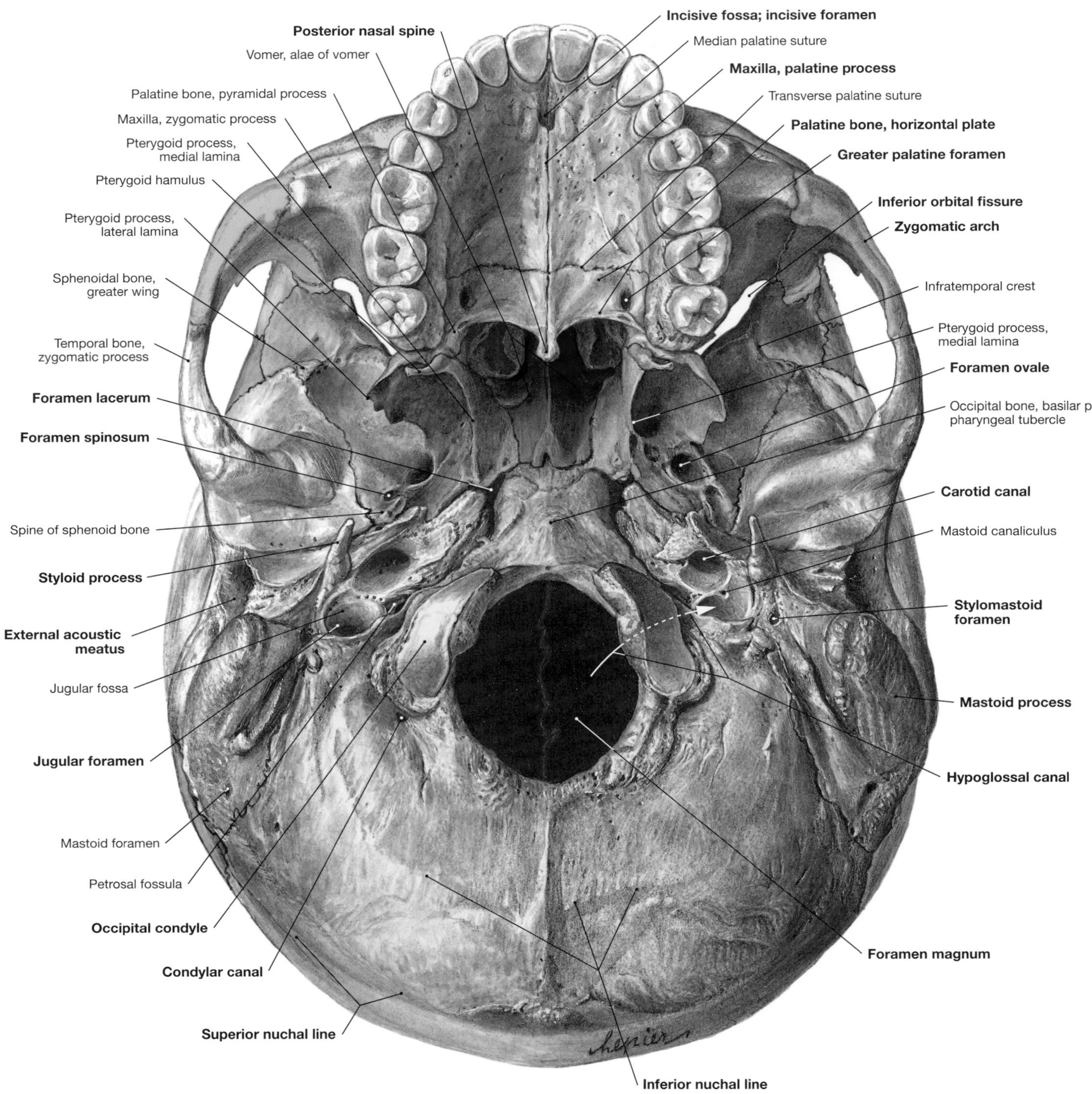
Posterior nasal spine
Vomer, alae of vomer
Palatine bone, pyramidal process
Maxilla, zygomatic process
Pterygoid process, medial lamina
Pterygoid hamulus
Pterygoid process, lateral lamina
Sphenoidal bone, greater wing
Temporal bone, zygomatic process
Foramen lacerum
Foramen spinosum
Spine of sphenoid bone
Styloid process
External acoustic meatus
Jugular fossa
Jugular foramen
Mastoid foramen
Petrosal fossula
Occipital condyle
Condylar canal
Superior nuchal line
Inferior nuchal line
Incisive fossa; incisive foramen
Median palatine suture
Maxilla, palatine process
Transverse palatine suture
Palatine bone, horizontal plate
Greater palatine foramen
Inferior orbital fissure
Zygomatic arch
Infratemporal crest
Pterygoid process, medial lamina
Foramen ovale
Occipital bone, basilar part, pharyngeal tubercle
Carotid canal
Mastoid canaliculus
Stylomastoid foramen
Mastoid process
Hypoglossal canal
Foramen magnum

**Fig. 8.14 Outer aspect of the base of the skull;** inferior view.
The cranial base extends to the middle incisors in the front, bilaterally to the mastoid process and the zygomatic arch, and to the superior nuchal lines in the back. The cranial base divides into three compartments:

- anterior compartment with upper teeth and hard palate
- middle compartment posterior to the palate up to the anterior margin of the foramen magnum
- posterior compartment from the anterior margin of the foramen magnum to the superior nuchal lines

**Anterior cranial base:** encompasses the palate (→ Fig. 8.26).
**Middle cranial base:** the anterior part of this middle compartment is composed of the vomer and the sphenoidal bone; the temporal bones and the occipital bone form the posterior part. The vomer is located in the frontal part of the midline, rides on the sphenoidal bone, and constitutes the posterior part of the nasal septum.
The sphenoidal bone is composed of a central body and the paired greater and lesser wings (not visible from below).
Following directly the body of the sphenoidal bone is the basilar part of the occipital bone, which represents the beginning of the posterior cranial base. The basilar part extends up to the foramen magnum. Here, the pharyngeal tubercle protrudes. It constitutes the bony attachment point for parts of the pharynx.
(continuation → Fig. 8.15)

## Outer aspect of the base of the skull

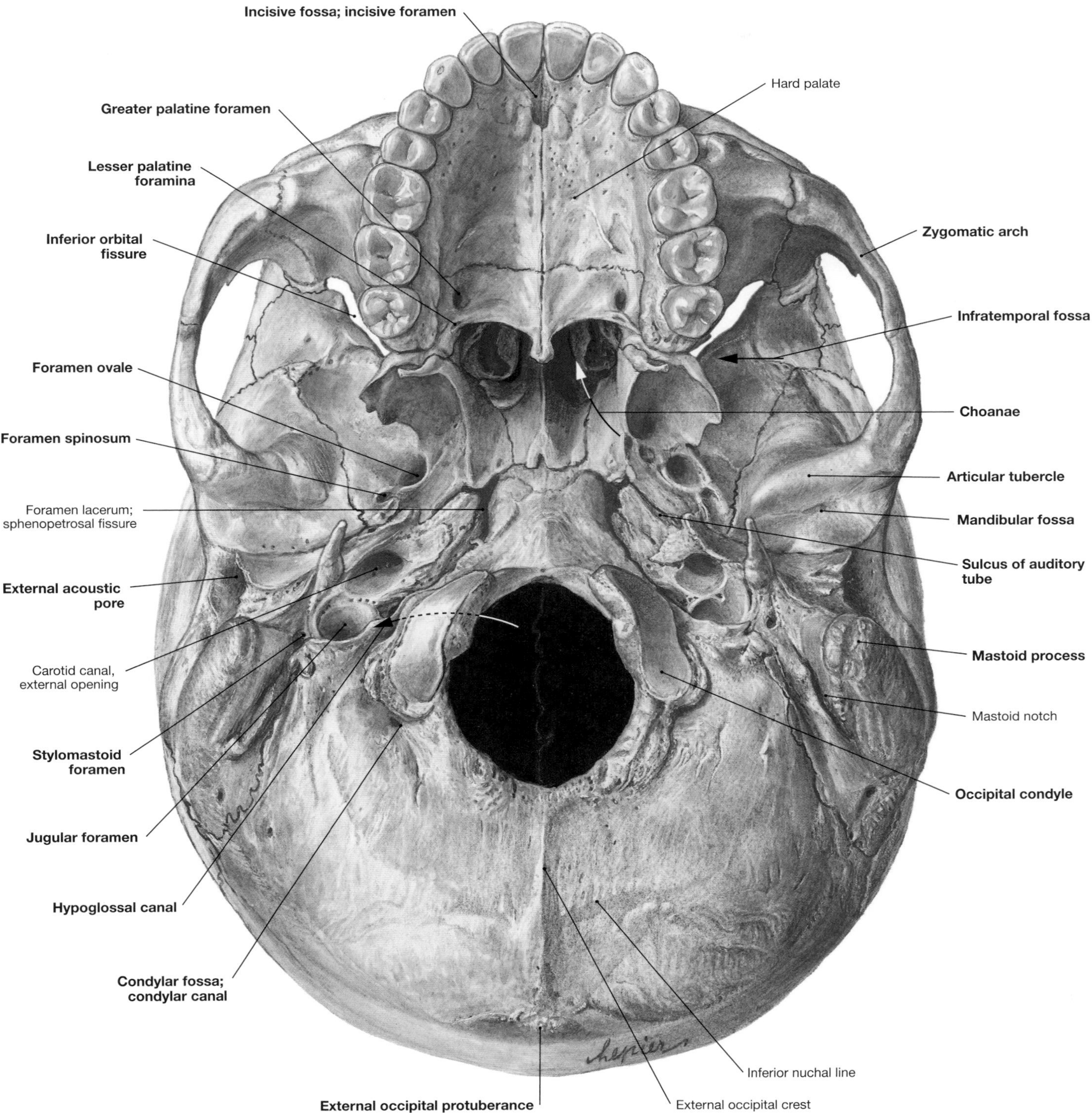
Incisive fossa; incisive foramen
Hard palate
Greater palatine foramen
Lesser palatine foramina
Inferior orbital fissure
Zygomatic arch
Infratemporal fossa
Foramen ovale
Choanae
Foramen spinosum
Articular tubercle
Foramen lacerum; sphenopetrosal fissure
Mandibular fossa
Sulcus of auditory tube
External acoustic pore
Mastoid process
Carotid canal, external opening
Mastoid notch
Stylomastoid foramen
Occipital condyle
Jugular foramen
Hypoglossal canal
Condylar fossa; condylar canal
Inferior nuchal line
External occipital protuberance
External occipital crest

**Fig. 8.15 Outer aspect of the base of the skull;** inferior view.
**Middle cranial base** (continuation of → Fig. 8.14): The sulcus of auditory tube is positioned at the border between the greater wing of the sphenoidal bone and the petrous part of the temporal bone and forms the entrance into the bony part of the auditory tube (→ p. 145). The bony canal continues through the petrous part of the temporal bone to the tympanic cavity. Located laterally is the squamous part of the temporal bone which is involved in the formation of the temporomandibular joint. The mandibular fossa is part of the articular surface of the temporomandibular joint (→ pp. 36–39). The articular tubercle is located at the anterior margin of the mandibular fossa.
**Posterior cranial base:** The posterior compartment extends from the anterior margin of the foramen magnum to the superior nuchal lines and consists of parts of the occipital and temporal bones. Each of the paired lateral parts possesses an occipital condyle for the articulation with the atlas. Located behind the condyle is the condylar fossa, which contains the condylar canal; anterior to the condyle the hypoglossal canal is situated. Immediately lateral thereof lies the jugular foramen.

## Foramina of the outer base of the skull

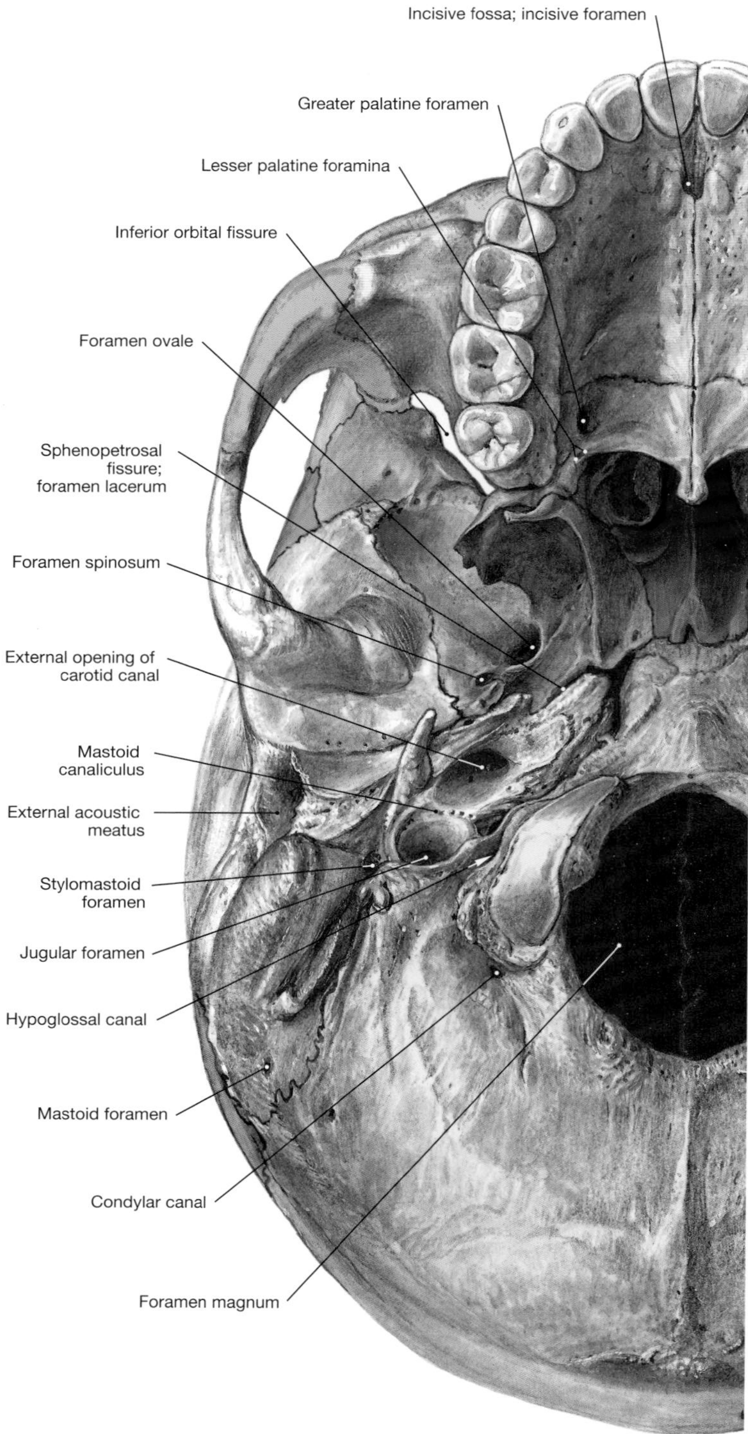
Incisive fossa; incisive foramen
Greater palatine foramen
Lesser palatine foramina
Inferior orbital fissure
Foramen ovale
Sphenopetrosal fissure; foramen lacerum
Foramen spinosum
External opening of carotid canal
Mastoid canaliculus
External acoustic meatus
Stylomastoid foramen
Jugular foramen
Hypoglossal canal
Mastoid foramen
Condylar canal
Foramen magnum

**Fig. 8.16 Outer aspect of the base of the skull with foramina;** inferior view; color chart see inside of the back cover of this volume.

**Foramina of the Outer Base of the Skull and their Content**

| Foramina | Content |
|---|---|
| **Incisive foramen** | • Nasopalatine nerve (maxillary nerve [V/2]) |
| **Greater palatine foramen** | • Greater palatine nerve (maxillary nerve [V/2])<br>• Greater palatine artery (descending palatine artery) |
| **Lesser palatine foramen** | • Lesser palatine nerves (maxillary nerve [V/2])<br>• Lesser palatine arteries (descending palatine artery) |
| **Inferior orbital fissure** | • Infraorbital artery (maxillary artery)<br>• Inferior ophthalmic vein<br>• Infraorbital nerve (maxillary nerve [V/2])<br>• Zygomatic nerve (maxillary nerve [V/2]) |
| **Foramen rotundum** (→ p. 12) | • Maxillary nerve [V/2] |
| **Foramen ovale** | • Mandibular nerve [V/3]<br>• Venous plexus of foramen ovale |
| **Foramen spinosum** | • Meningeal branch (mandibular nerve [V/3])<br>• Medial meningeal artery (maxillary artery) |
| **Sphenopetrosal fissure and foramen lacerum** | • Lesser petrosal nerve (glossopharyngeal nerve [IX]))<br>• Greater petrosal nerve (facial nerve [VII]<br>• Deep petrosal nerve (internal carotid plexus) |
| **External opening of carotid canal and carotid canal** | • Internal carotid artery, petrous part<br>• Internal carotid venous plexus<br>• Internal carotid plexus (sympathetic trunk, superior cervical ganglion) |
| **Stylomastoid foramen** | • Facial nerve [VII] |
| **Jugular foramen** | Anterior part:<br>• Inferior petrosal sinus<br>• Glossopharyngeal nerve [IX]<br>Posterior part:<br>• Posterior meningeal artery (ascending pharyngeal artery)<br>• Sigmoid sinus (superior bulb of jugular vein)<br>• Vagus nerve [X]<br>• Meningeal nerve (vagus nerve [X])<br>• Accessory nerve [XI] |
| **Mastoid canaliculus** | • Auricular branch of vagus nerve (vagus nerve [X]) |
| **Hypoglossal canal** | • Hypoglossal nerve [XII]<br>• Venous plexus of hypoglossal canal |
| **Condylar canal** | • Condylar emissary vein |
| **Foramen magnum** | • Meninges<br>• Internal vertebral venous plexus (marginal sinus)<br>• Vertebral arteries (subclavian arteries)<br>• Anterior spinal artery (vertebral arteries)<br>• Medulla oblongata/spinal cord<br>• Spinal roots (accessory nerve [XI]) |

### Clinical Remarks

In **basilar skull fractures** the fracture lines traverse the openings at the base of the skull. Thus, blood vessels and nerves passing through these openings can be injured with resulting nerve palsies and bleedings as frequent complications. In addition, basilar skull fractures can involve the frontal, sphenoidal, and ethmoidal sinuses (cerebrospinal fluid [CSF] and/or blood exiting through the nose). Lateral basilar skull fractures often involve the petrous bone (CSF exiting from the outer ear canal).

## Foramina of the inner base of the skull

| Foramina of the Inner Aspect of the Base of the Skull and their Content | |
|---|---|
| **Foramina** | **Content** |
| **Cribriform plate** | • Olfactory nerves [I]<br>• Anterior ethmoidal artery (ophthalmic artery) |
| **Optic canal** | • Optic nerve [II]<br>• Ophthalmic artery (internal carotid artery)<br>• Meninges; sheath of optic nerve |
| **Superior orbital fissure** | Middle part:<br>• Nasociliary nerve (ophthalmic nerve [V/1])<br>• Oculomotor nerve [III]<br>• Abducent nerve [VI]<br>Lateral part:<br>• Trochlear nerve [IV]<br>mutual origin of:<br>– frontal nerve (ophthalmic nerve [V/1])<br>– lacrimal nerve (ophthalmic nerve [V/1])<br>• Orbital branch (medial meningeal artery)<br>• Superior ophthalmic artery |
| **Foramen rotundum** | • Maxillary nerve [V/2] |
| **Foramen ovale** | • Mandibular nerve [V/3]<br>• Venous plexus of foramen ovale |
| **Foramen spinosum** | • Meningeal branch (mandibular nerve [V/3])<br>• Medial meningeal artery (maxillary artery) |
| **Sphenopetrosal fissure and foramen lacerum** | • Lesser petrosal nerve (glossopharyngeal nerve [IX])<br>• Greater petrosal nerve (facial nerve [VII])<br>• Deep petrosal nerve (internal carotid plexus) |
| **Internal opening of carotid canal and carotid canal** | • Internal carotid artery, petrous part<br>• Internal carotid venous plexus<br>• Internal carotid plexus (sympathetic trunk, superior cervical ganglion) |
| **Pore and internal acoustic meatus** | • Facial nerve [VII]<br>• Vestibulocochlear nerve [VIII]<br>• Labyrinthine artery (basilar artery)<br>• Labyrinthine veins |
| **Jugular foramen** | Anterior part:<br>• Inferior petrosal sinus<br>• Glossopharyngeal nerve [IX]<br>Posterior part:<br>• Posterior meningeal artery (ascending pharyngeal artery)<br>• Sigmoid sinus (superior bulb of jugular vein)<br>• Vagus nerve [X]<br>• Accessory nerve [XI]<br>• Meningeal branch (vagus nerve [X]) |
| **Hypoglossal canal** | • Hypoglossal nerve [XII]<br>• Venous plexus of hypoglossal canal |
| **Condylary canal** | • Condylar emissary vein |
| **Foramen magnum** | • Meninges<br>• Internal vertebral venous plexus (marginal sinus)<br>• Vertebral arteries (subclavian arteries)<br>• Anterior spinal artery (vertebral arteries)<br>• Medulla oblongata/spinal cord<br>• Spinal roots (accessory nerve [XI]) |

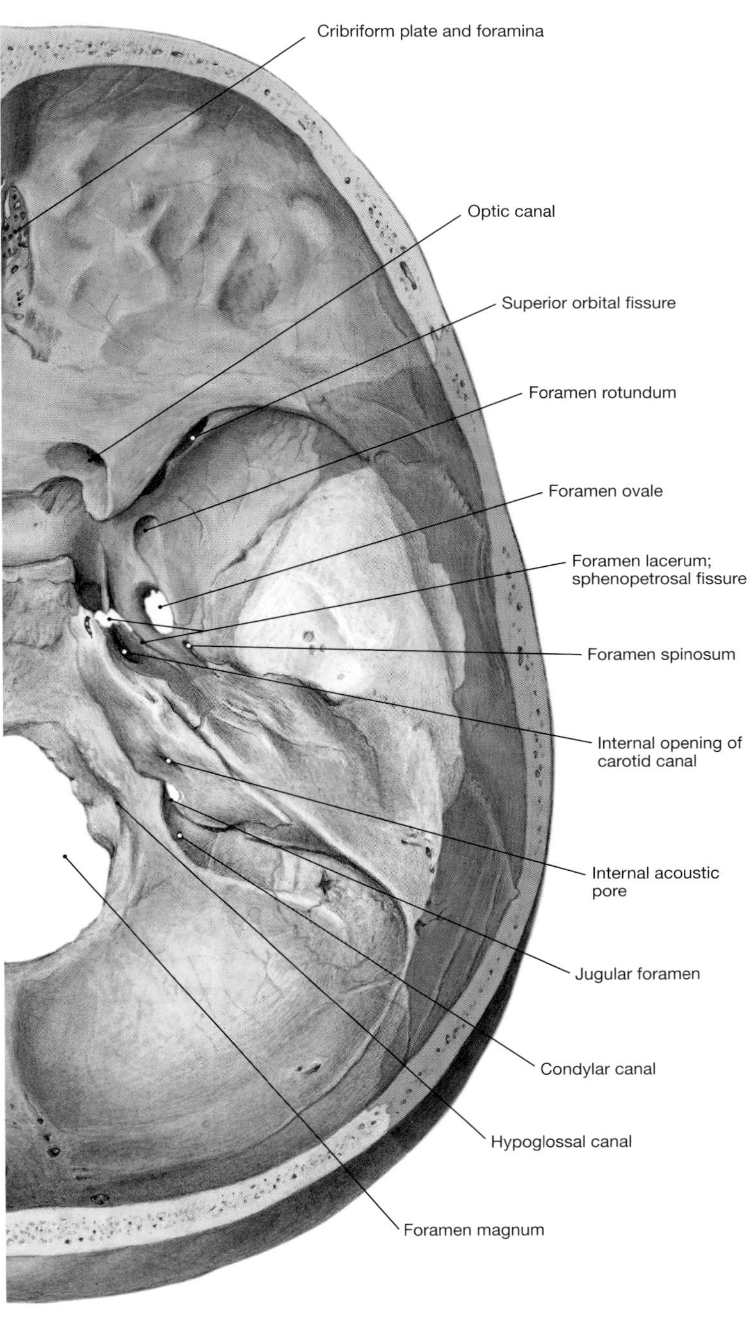
Cribriform plate and foramina
Optic canal
Superior orbital fissure
Foramen rotundum
Foramen ovale
Foramen lacerum; sphenopetrosal fissure
Foramen spinosum
Internal opening of carotid canal
Internal acoustic pore
Jugular foramen
Condylar canal
Hypoglossal canal
Foramen magnum

**Fig. 8.17 Inner aspect of the base of the skull with foramina;** superior view; color chart see inside of the back cover of this volume.

## Development of the skull

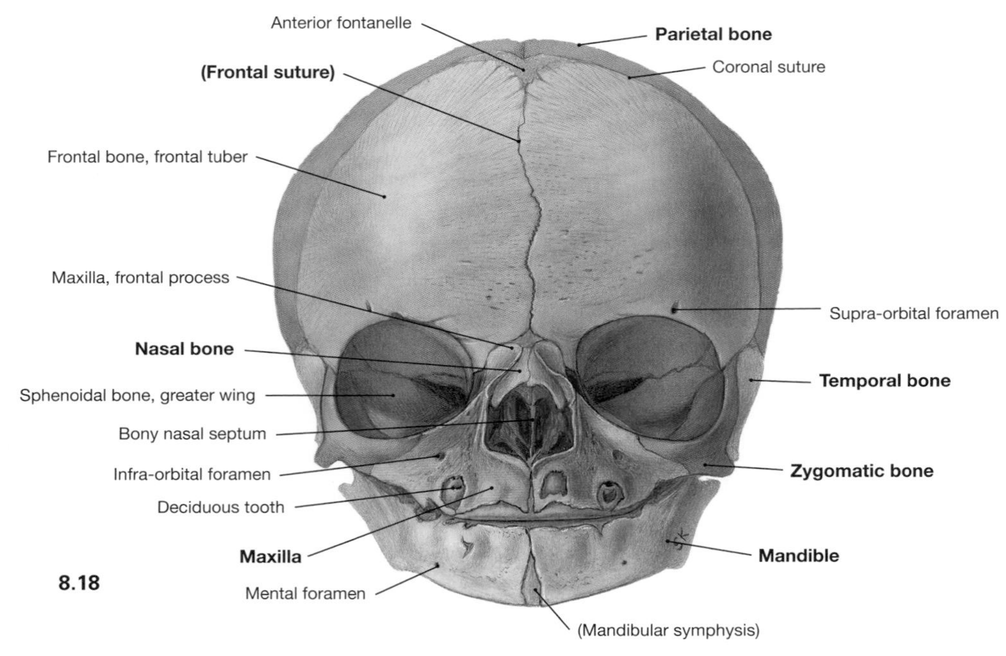
Anterior fontanelle
Parietal bone
(Frontal suture)
Coronal suture
Frontal bone, frontal tuber
Maxilla, frontal process
Supra-orbital foramen
Nasal bone
Temporal bone
Sphenoidal bone, greater wing
Bony nasal septum
Infra-orbital foramen
Zygomatic bone
Deciduous tooth
Maxilla
Mandible
Mental foramen
(Mandibular symphysis)

8.18

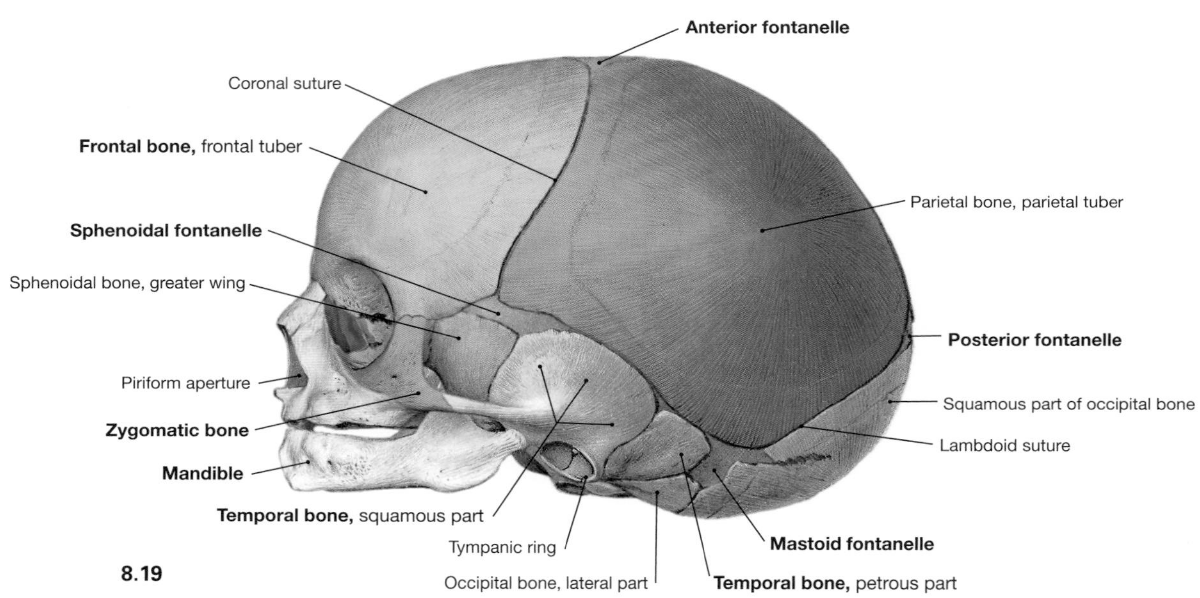
Anterior fontanelle
Coronal suture
Frontal bone, frontal tuber
Parietal bone, parietal tuber
Sphenoidal fontanelle
Sphenoidal bone, greater wing
Posterior fontanelle
Piriform aperture
Squamous part of occipital bone
Zygomatic bone
Lambdoid suture
Mandible
Temporal bone, squamous part
Tympanic ring
Mastoid fontanelle
Occipital bone, lateral part
Temporal bone, petrous part

8.19

**Fig. 8.18 and Fig. 8.19 Skull of a newborn;** frontal (→ Fig. 8.18) and lateral (→ Fig. 8.19) views; color chart see inside of the back cover of this volume.

At birth, the newborn has six fontanelles, two unpaired (anterior and posterior fontanelle) and two paired (sphenoidal and mastoid fontanelles). During **delivery,** sutures and fontanelles serve as reference structures to assess the location and position of the fetal head. Shortly before birth, the posterior fontanelle becomes the leading part of the head in the case of a normal cephalic presentation.

In concert with the sutures, the fontanelles allow a limited deformation of the fetal skull during delivery. The remarkable postnatal growth results in the fontanelles becoming rapidly smaller and complete closure will occur by the end of the third year of life.

## Development of the skull

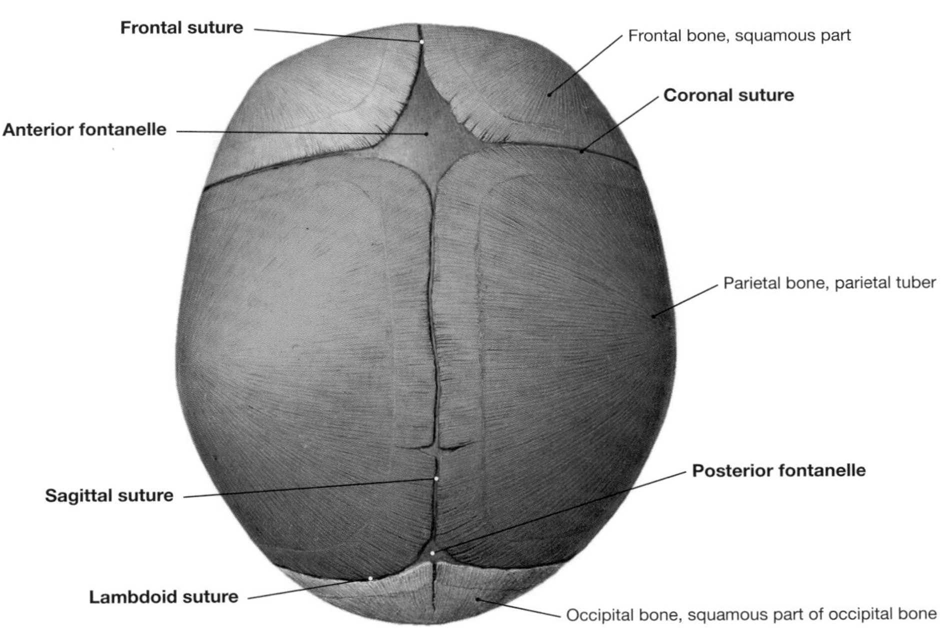
Frontal suture
Anterior fontanelle
Frontal bone, squamous part
Coronal suture
Parietal bone, parietal tuber
Posterior fontanelle
Sagittal suture
Lambdoid suture
Occipital bone, squamous part of occipital bone

**Fig. 8.20 Skull of a newborn;** superior view; color chart see inside of the back cover of this volume.

At birth, the bony plates of the skull cap (calvaria) are still separated by the interstitial tissue located in the cranial sutures. The sutures are widened to fontanelles in regions where more than two bones meet. During life, most sutures, fontanelles, and synchondroses ossify. Important sutures include the **lambdoid suture, frontal suture, sagittal suture,** and **coronal suture** which gradually fuse up to about 50 years of age (the frontal suture already between the first and second year of life).

| **Fontanelles** | | |
|---|---|---|
| **Fontanelle** | **Number** | **Closure [month of life]** |
| Anterior fontanelle (large fontanelle) | 1 | Approx. 36 |
| Posterior fontanelle (small fontanelle) | 1 | Approx. 3 |
| Sphenoidal fontanelle (anterior lateral fontanelle) | Paired | Approx. 6 |
| Mastoid fontanelle (posterior lateral fontanelle) | Paired | Approx. 18 |

## Development of the skull

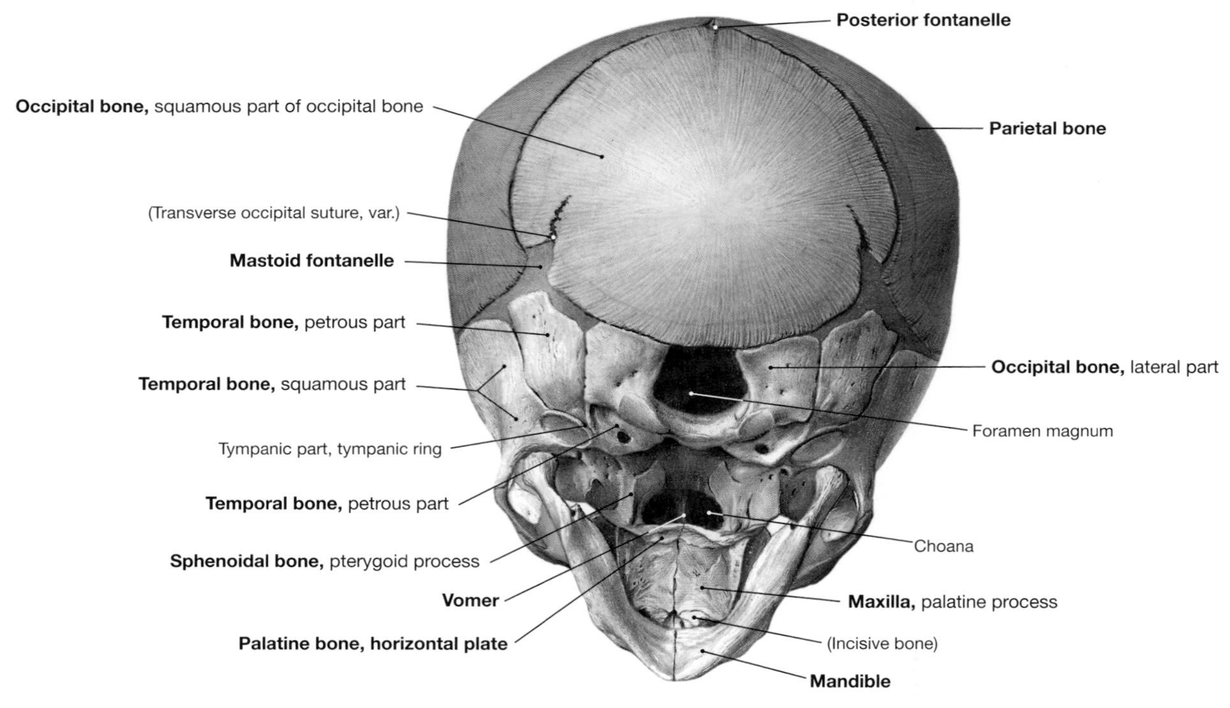
Posterior fontanelle
Occipital bone, squamous part of occipital bone
Parietal bone
(Transverse occipital suture, var.)
Mastoid fontanelle
Temporal bone, petrous part
Temporal bone, squamous part
Occipital bone, lateral part
Foramen magnum
Tympanic part, tympanic ring
Temporal bone, petrous part
Choana
Sphenoidal bone, pterygoid process
Vomer
Maxilla, palatine process
Palatine bone, horizontal plate
(Incisive bone)
Mandible

**Fig. 8.21 Skull, cranium, of a newborn;** posterior inferior view; color chart see inside of the back cover of this volume.
The development of the skull involves a desmal and an enchondral ossification mode (→ table). The mesenchyme of the head is the primordial building material that derives from the prechordal mesoderm, the occipital somites, and the neural crest. At the time of birth, some cranial bones are linked by cartilaginous joints (cranial synchondroses).

| Ossification Mode of the Skull Bones | | | |
|---|---|---|---|
| | **Viscerocranium** | **Neurocranium** | **Ossicles** |
| **Desmal** | Mandibular bone except for condylar process, maxilla, zygomatic bone, palatine bone, nasal bone, vomer, lacrimal bone | Medial plate of the pterygoid process of the sphenoidal bone, squamous part of the temporal bone, squamous part of occipital bone, frontal bone, parietal bone | |
| **Chondral** | Condylar process of the mandibular bone, ethmoidal bone, inferior nasal concha | Sphenoidal bone except for medial plate of the pterygoid process, petrous part and tympanic part of the temporal bone, lateral part and basilar part of the occipital bone | |
| **MECKEL's cartilage** | | | Malleus, incus |
| **REICHERT's cartilage** | | Styloid process of the temporal bone | Stapes |

## Craniostenoses

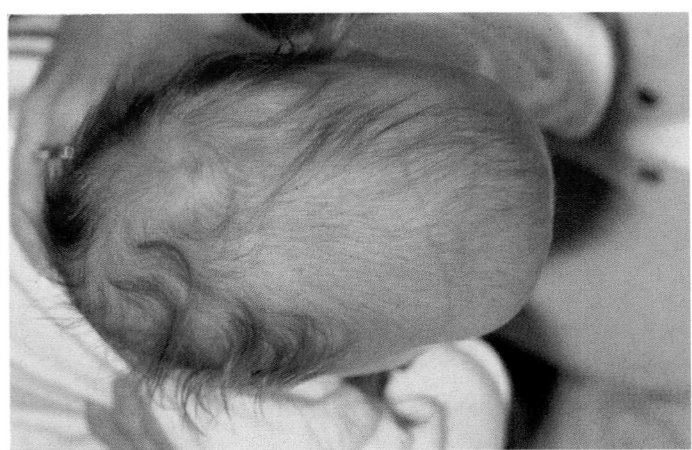

a

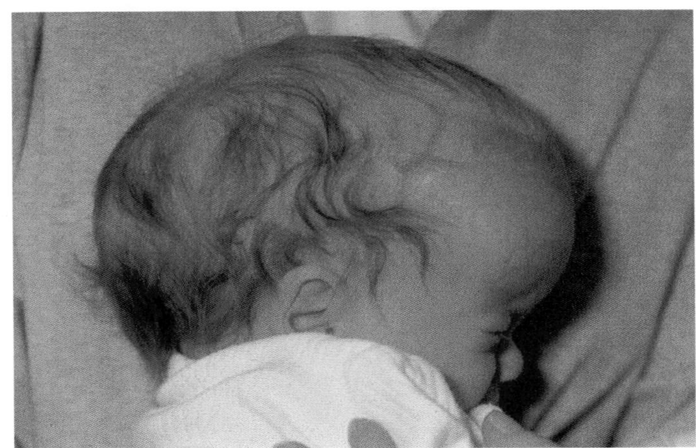

b

**Figs. 8.22a and b Craniostenoses;** child with scaphocephalus. [20]
This clinical picture is the result of a premature closure of the sagittal suture. The skull cap is disproportionally long.
**a** superior view
**b** view from the right side

### Clinical Remarks

A dysostosis is a deviation from normal bony growth. The premature closure of one or more sutures results in **craniosynostoses.** Premature closure of the sagittal suture results in the extension of the skull in the frontal and occipital region. The skull becomes longer and narrower **(scaphocephaly).** The premature closure of the coronal sutures results in **acrocephaly** (also named turricephaly). Asymmetric craniosynostosis **(plagiocephaly)** results from unilateral premature occlusion of the coronal and lambdoid sutures. **Microcephaly** results from impaired growth of the brain because the growth of the skull bones adjusts to the size of the brain. Thus, small brain size causes an underdeveloped neurocranium and mental retardation in children with microcephaly.

## Frontal and ethmoidal bones

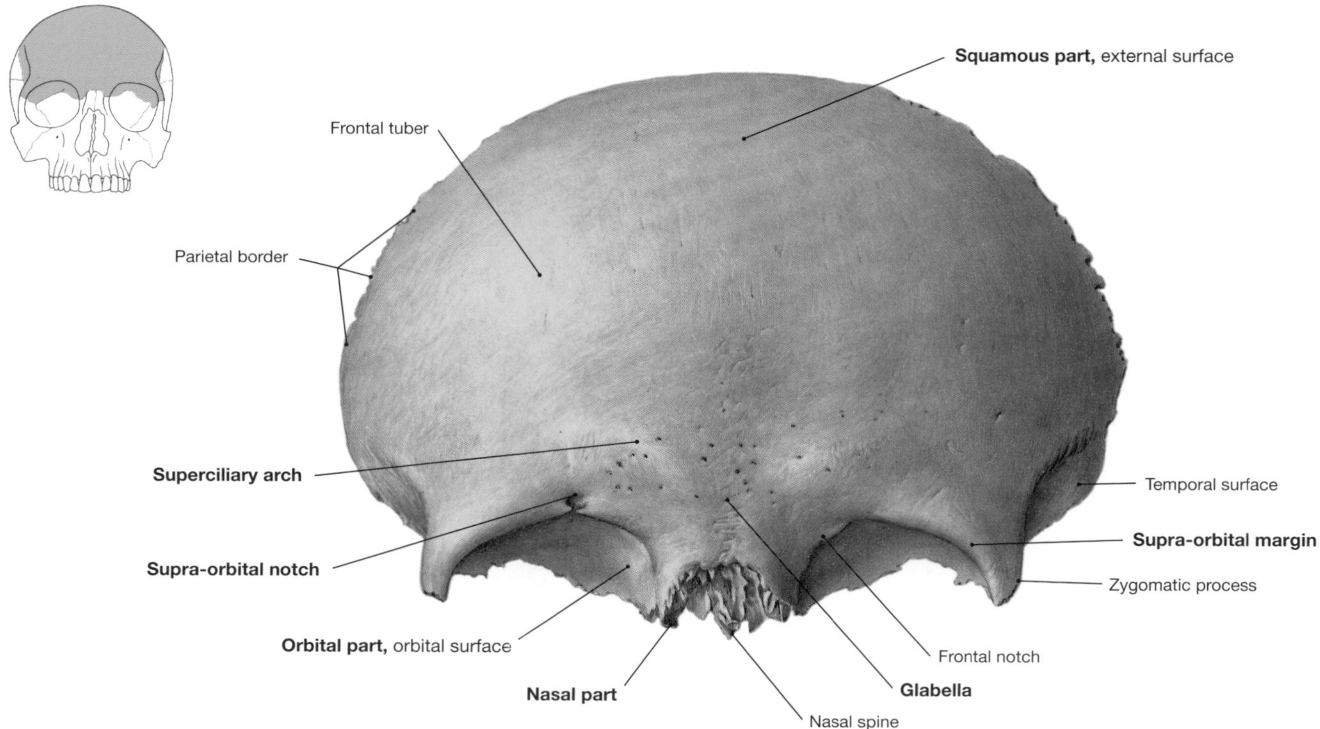
Squamous part, external surface
Frontal tuber
Parietal border
Superciliary arch
Temporal surface
Supra-orbital margin
Supra-orbital notch
Zygomatic process
Orbital part, orbital surface
Frontal notch
Nasal part
Glabella
Nasal spine

**Fig. 8.23 Frontal bone;** frontal view; color chart see inside of the back cover of this volume.
Located most anterior in the skull cap, the frontal bone participates in the formation of the walls of the orbital and nasal cavity. The unpaired frontal bone has **four parts:**

- the unpaired squamous part
- the paired orbital parts and
- the unpaired nasal part

Above the upper margin of the orbit (supra-orbital margin) the prominent superciliary arch protrudes, a phenotype commonly more developed in men than in women. In the midline between the two arches, the bone is flat and creates the glabella (area between the eyebrows). Frequently, a supraorbital foramen, more rarely a frontal notch, is present at the medial margin of the orbit.

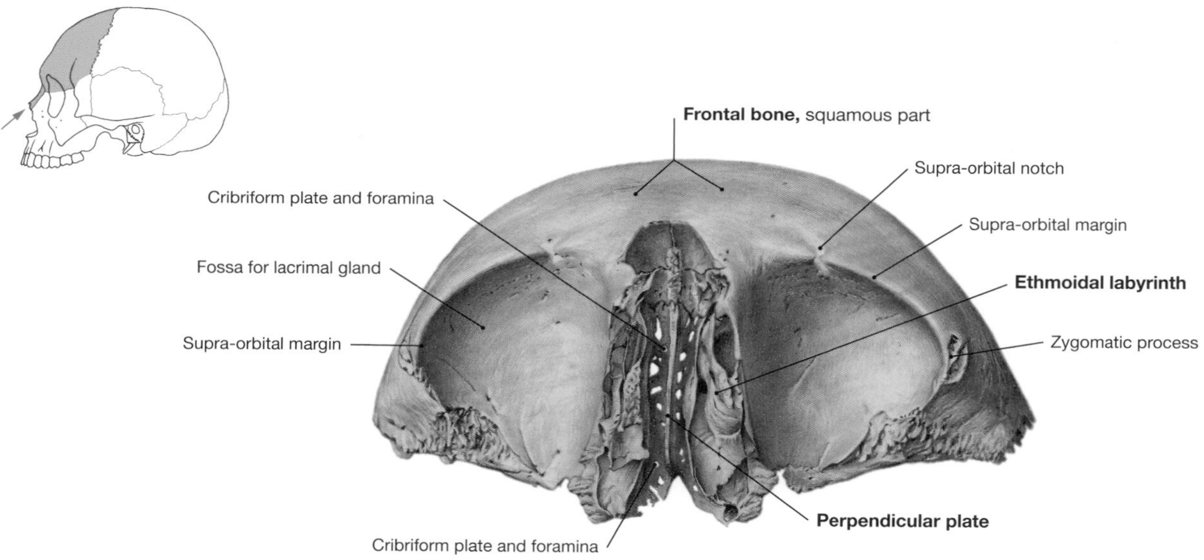
Frontal bone, squamous part
Supra-orbital notch
Cribriform plate and foramina
Supra-orbital margin
Fossa for lacrimal gland
Ethmoidal labyrinth
Supra-orbital margin
Zygomatic process
Perpendicular plate
Cribriform plate and foramina

**Fig. 8.24 Frontal bone, ethmoidal bone, and nasal bones;** inferior view; color chart see inside of the back cover of this volume.
The ethmoidal bone and nasal bones connect with the frontal bone in a medial anterior and caudal position and form part of the nasal skeleton. The frontal sinus is located within the frontal bone.

## Upper jaw and palatine bone

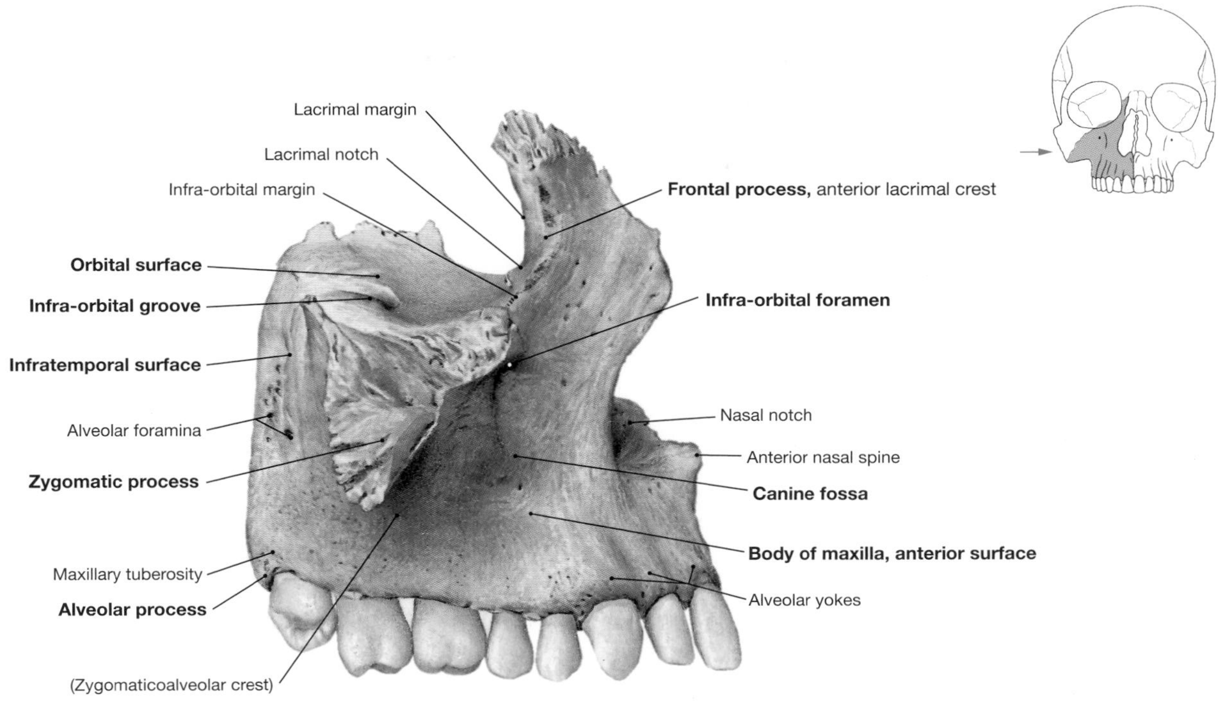
Lacrimal margin
Lacrimal notch
Infra-orbital margin
Frontal process, anterior lacrimal crest
Orbital surface
Infra-orbital groove
Infra-orbital foramen
Infratemporal surface
Alveolar foramina
Nasal notch
Anterior nasal spine
Zygomatic process
Canine fossa
Body of maxilla, anterior surface
Maxillary tuberosity
Alveolar process
Alveolar yokes
(Zygomaticoalveolar crest)

**Fig. 8.25 Upper jaw, maxilla, right side;** lateral view.
The upper jaw can be divided into the body of maxilla, frontal process (connects with the frontal bone), zygomatic process (connects with the zygomatic bone), palatine process (anterior part of the palate, → Fig. 8.26), and alveolar process. The latter creates the lower margin of the maxilla and is composed of the dental alveoli which contain the roots of the teeth. The protruding anterior rim of these dental sockets are named alveolar yokes. The infraorbital foramen is located in the body of maxilla, immediately below the lower orbital margin.

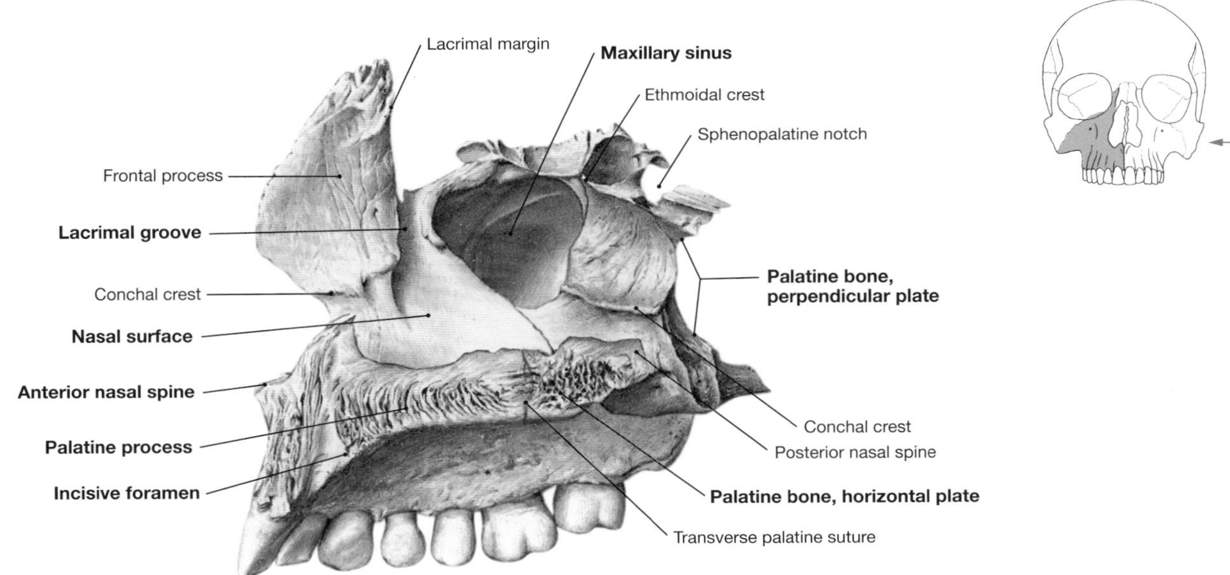
Lacrimal margin
Maxillary sinus
Ethmoidal crest
Sphenopalatine notch
Frontal process
Lacrimal groove
Palatine bone, perpendicular plate
Conchal crest
Nasal surface
Anterior nasal spine
Conchal crest
Posterior nasal spine
Palatine process
Incisive foramen
Palatine bone, horizontal plate
Transverse palatine suture

**Fig. 8.26 Upper jaw, maxilla, and palatine bone, right side;** medial view into the maxillary sinus; color chart see inside of the back cover of this volume.
Posterior to the maxilla lies the palatine bone which is composed of two plates: The **horizontal plate** creates the posterior part of the palate (bony palate), the **perpendicular plate** extends vertically upright (perpendicular to the horizontal plate) and is the posterior medial margin of the maxillary sinus.

## Nasal cavity

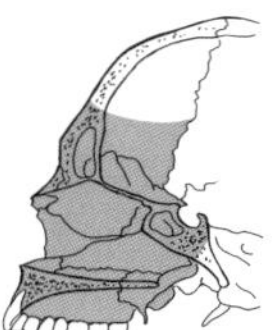

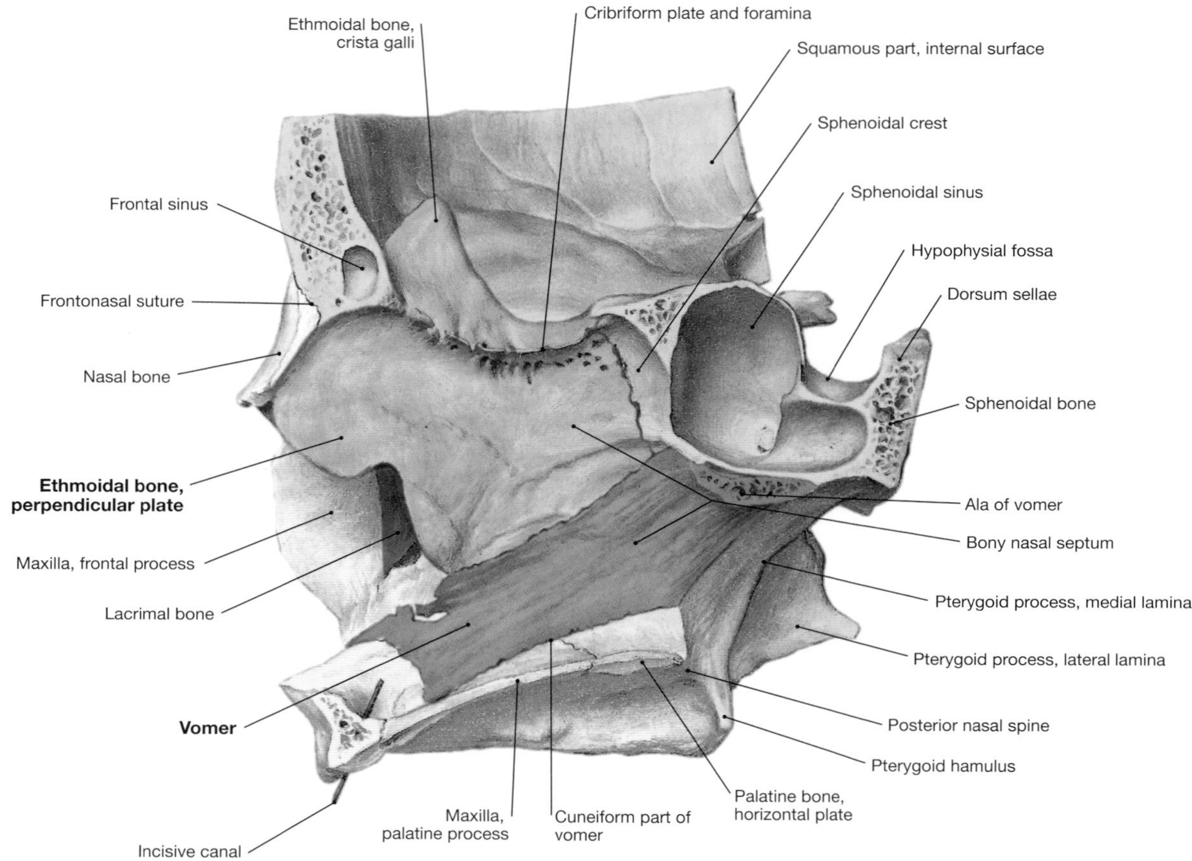
Ethmoidal bone, crista galli
Cribriform plate and foramina
Squamous part, internal surface
Sphenoidal crest
Sphenoidal sinus
Hypophysial fossa
Dorsum sellae
Sphenoidal bone
Ala of vomer
Bony nasal septum
Pterygoid process, medial lamina
Pterygoid process, lateral lamina
Posterior nasal spine
Pterygoid hamulus
Palatine bone, horizontal plate
Cuneiform part of vomer
Maxilla, palatine process
Incisive canal
Vomer
Lacrimal bone
Maxilla, frontal process
Ethmoidal bone, perpendicular plate
Nasal bone
Frontonasal suture
Frontal sinus

**Fig. 8.27 Bony septum of the nose;** lateral view; color chart see inside of the back cover of this volume.

The perpendicular plate of the ethmoidal bone and the vomer create the bony septum of the nose. The **ethmoidal bone** is located between the frontal bone and the maxilla and is also connected with the nasal, lacrimal, sphenoidal, and palatine bones. At its top, the ethmoidal bone forms the crista galli. Perforated with multiple holes, the cribriform plate is the roof of the nasal cavity and part of the floor of the anterior cranial fossa. The perpendicular plate of the ethmoidal bone is located below the crista galli, divides the bony labyrinth of the ethmoidal bone into a right and left part, and constitutes the upper part of the bony nasal septum.

The **vomer** forms the largest part of the bony nasal septal skeleton. This flat and trapezoid bone connects cranially with the perpendicular plate of the ethmoidal bone and at its posterior aspect via the ala of vomer with the sphenoidal bone. Caudally, the cuneiform part of vomer borders at the palatine process of the maxilla and at the horizontal plate of the palatine bone.

### Clinical Remarks

Traumatic events (punched nose or falls onto the nose) or abnormal growth of the maxilla can cause a **septum deviation.** More than 60% of the population has at least a mild septum deviation. Septum deviations mainly impair breathing through the nose. This can affect the ability of the nose to warm up, clean, and moisturize the air passing through the nose. In turn, patients with impaired nasal breathing are forced to breathe through their mouth, which results in snoring and an increased susceptibility for infections. Insufficient ventilation of the paranasal sinuses may cause sinusitis with post-nasal drip and potential inflammation of the larynx and the bronchial tree. At an advanced age, this can lead to hypoxia and subsequently results in cardiovascular diseases.

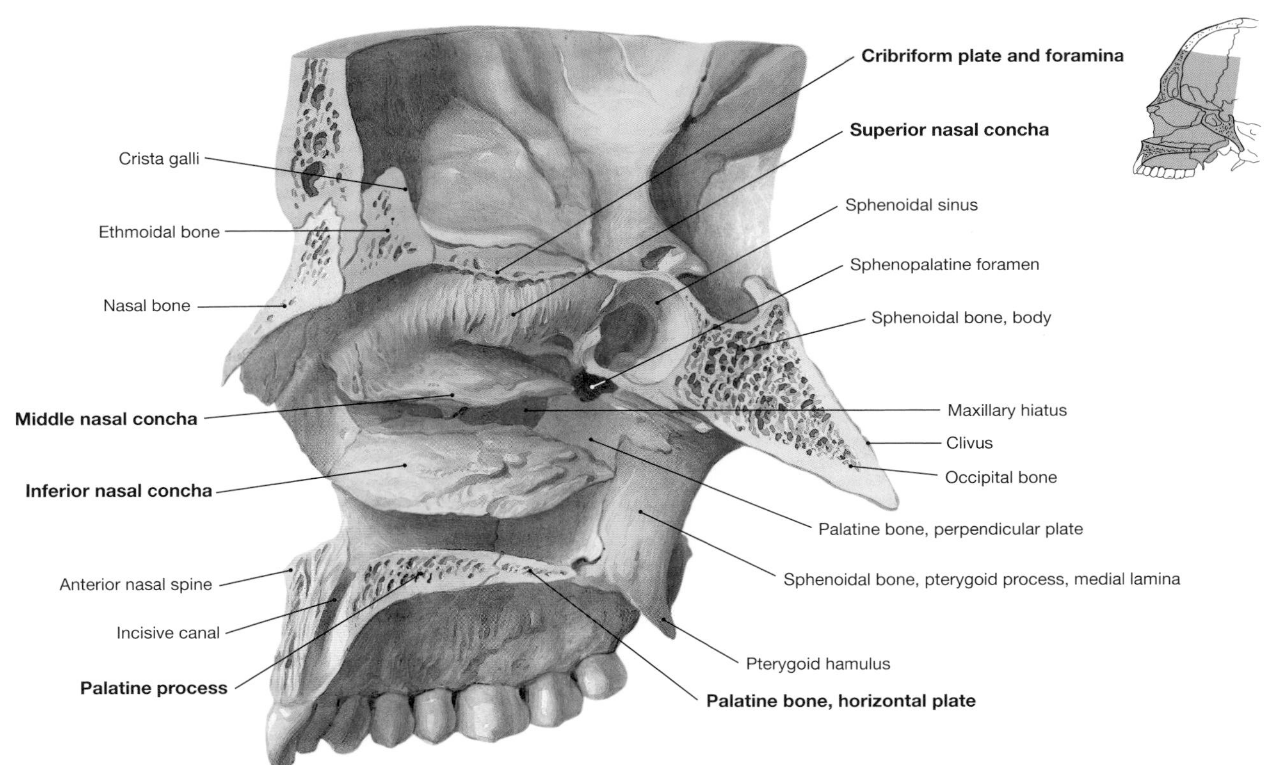
Cribriform plate and foramina
Superior nasal concha
Sphenoidal sinus
Sphenopalatine foramen
Sphenoidal bone, body
Maxillary hiatus
Clivus
Occipital bone
Palatine bone, perpendicular plate
Sphenoidal bone, pterygoid process, medial lamina
Pterygoid hamulus
Palatine bone, horizontal plate
Crista galli
Ethmoidal bone
Nasal bone
Middle nasal concha
Inferior nasal concha
Anterior nasal spine
Incisive canal
Palatine process

**Fig. 8.28 Lateral wall of the nasal cavity, right side;** view from the left side; color chart see inside of the back cover of this volume.
The view onto the lateral wall of the nasal cavity reveals the roof created by the cribriform plate of the ethmoidal bone which also forms the superior and middle nasal concha. The upper nasal passage (superior nasal meatus) is located between the two nasal conchae. Below sits the inferior nasal concha as a separate bone.

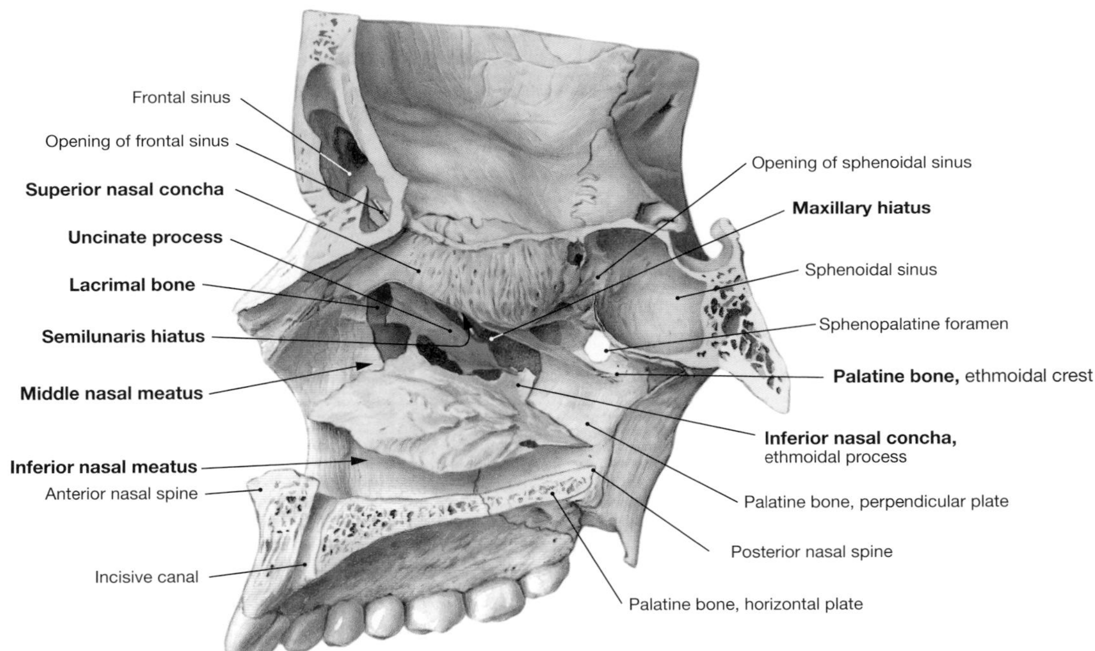
Frontal sinus
Opening of frontal sinus
Superior nasal concha
Uncinate process
Lacrimal bone
Semilunaris hiatus
Middle nasal meatus
Inferior nasal meatus
Anterior nasal spine
Incisive canal
Opening of sphenoidal sinus
Maxillary hiatus
Sphenoidal sinus
Sphenopalatine foramen
Palatine bone, ethmoidal crest
Inferior nasal concha, ethmoidal process
Palatine bone, perpendicular plate
Posterior nasal spine
Palatine bone, horizontal plate

**Fig. 8.29 Lateral wall of the nasal cavity, right side;** medial view after the middle nasal concha was removed; color chart see inside of the back cover of this volume.
Beneath the middle nasal concha, a thin bony lamella, the **uncinate process,** is part of the ethmoidal bone. It provides only an incomplete closure of the medial wall of the maxillary sinus. Many openings remain above and below the uncinate process and one of them is the maxillary hiatus.

The **maxilla** and the **palatine bone** create the floor and parts of the lateral wall (floor: horizontal plate; lateral wall: perpendicular plate). The **lacrimal bone** is also part of the lateral wall and contributes to the anterior margin of the maxillary sinus. The inferior nasal concha is anchored to all of these three bones and divides the nasal wall in a middle (medial nasal meatus) and an inferior nasal passage (inferior nasal meatus) which are located above and below this nasal concha, respectively.

## Hard palate

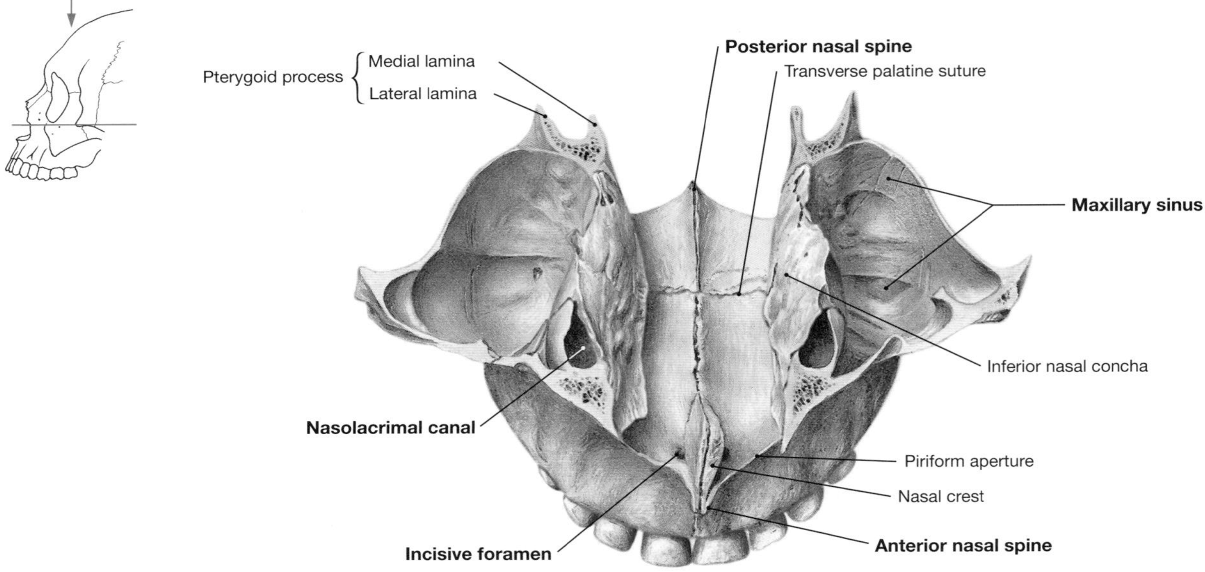
Pterygoid process
Medial lamina
Lateral lamina
Posterior nasal spine
Transverse palatine suture
Maxillary sinus
Inferior nasal concha
Nasolacrimal canal
Piriform aperture
Nasal crest
Anterior nasal spine
Incisive foramen

**Fig. 8.30 Hard palate; maxillary sinus, and inferior nasal concha;** superior view; color chart see inside of the back cover of this volume. The hard palate represents a horizontal bony plate created by the maxilla and the palatine bone. It separates the oral front from the nasal cavity. The incisive foramen creates a connection between both cavities. The present image shows the floor of the nasal cavity. Located laterally are the maxillary sinuses.

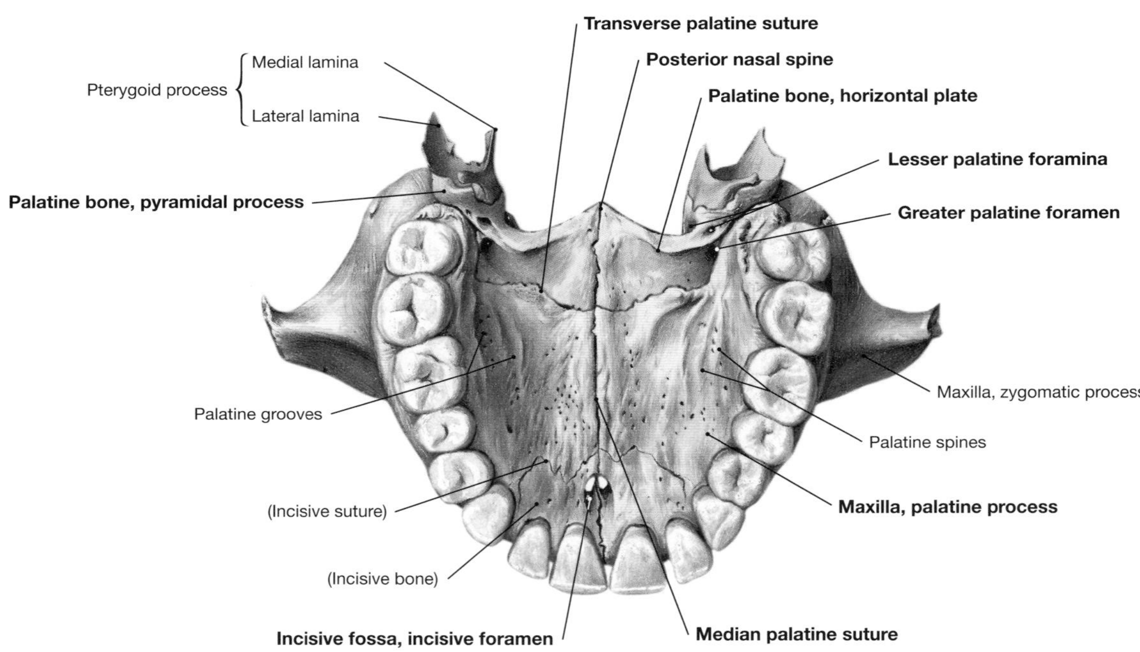
Transverse palatine suture
Posterior nasal spine
Palatine bone, horizontal plate
Pterygoid process
Medial lamina
Lateral lamina
Lesser palatine foramina
Greater palatine foramen
Palatine bone, pyramidal process
Maxilla, zygomatic process
Palatine grooves
Palatine spines
(Incisive suture)
Maxilla, palatine process
(Incisive bone)
Incisive fossa, incisive foramen
Median palatine suture

**Fig. 8.31 Hard palate;** inferior view; color chart see inside of the back cover of this volume.
The hard palate is part of the **anterior cranial fossa.** The teeth are attached to the two maxillary alveolar arches. These arches are the anterior and lateral margins of the hard palate. Its rostral part consists of the palatine processes of the two maxillae and the horizontal plates of the palatine bones in its posterior aspect. In the midline, the **palatine processes** are connected by the median palatine suture and dorsally they connect via the transverse palatine suture with the palatine bones. The **horizontal plates** of the palatine bones are connected in the midline by the interpalatine suture (a continuation of the median palatine suture). Located behind the incisures in the frontal part of the midline are the paired **incisive fossae** which become the incisive foramina and the incisive canals. Near the posterior margin to both sides of the hard palate are the **greater palatine foramina,** which become the greater palatine canals, and the **lesser palatine foramina.** The latter are located in the pyramidal process of the palatine bone and open into the lesser palatine canals. In the posterior aspect of the midline, the **posterior nasal spine** protrudes as a pointed process of the hard palate.

## Orbit and pterygopalatine fossa

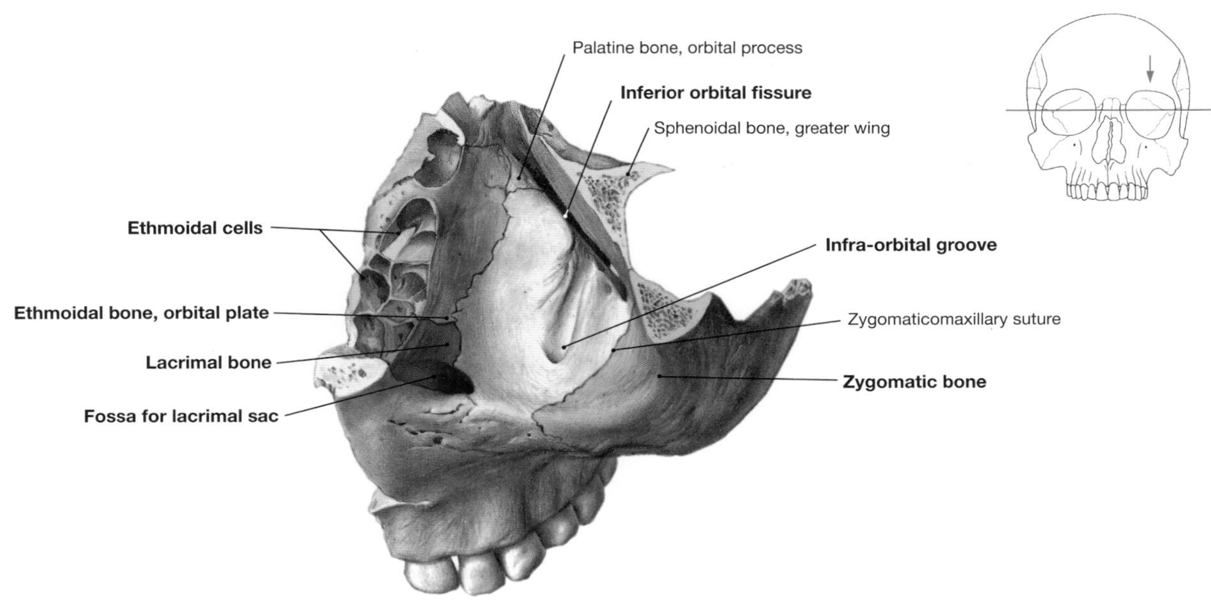

Palatine bone, orbital process
Inferior orbital fissure
Sphenoidal bone, greater wing
Ethmoidal cells
Infra-orbital groove
Ethmoidal bone, orbital plate
Zygomaticomaxillary suture
Lacrimal bone
Zygomatic bone
Fossa for lacrimal sac


**Fig. 8.32 Floor of the orbital cavity, left side;** superior view; color chart see inside of the back cover of this volume.

The floor of the orbit is the roof of the maxillary sinus. In it lies the infraorbital sulcus, which becomes a bony canal below the floor of the orbit and ends in the infraorbital foramen. It contains the infraorbital nerve and the corresponding blood vessels. The zygomatic bone forms the lateral part of the floor of the orbit and the medial part is composed of the orbital plate of the ethmoidal and lacrimal bone. Together with the maxilla, the latter creates the fossa of lacrimal gland containing the lacrimal gland. For the orbital cavity → Figs. 9.9 to 9.13.

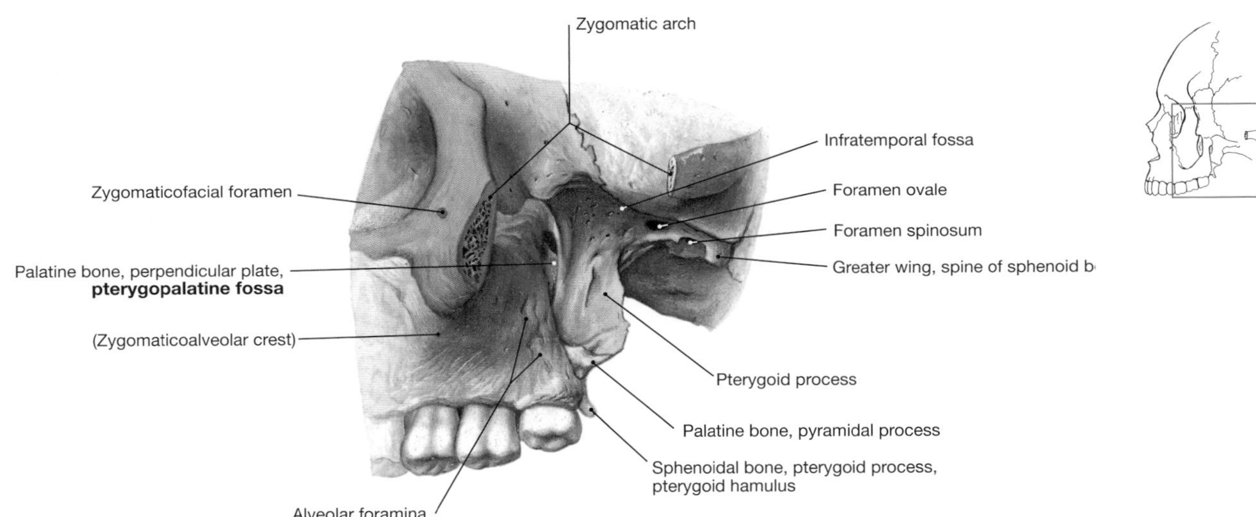

Zygomatic arch
Infratemporal fossa
Foramen ovale
Zygomaticofacial foramen
Foramen spinosum
Greater wing, spine of sphenoid b
Palatine bone, perpendicular plate,
pterygopalatine fossa
(Zygomaticoalveolar crest)
Pterygoid process
Palatine bone, pyramidal process
Sphenoidal bone, pterygoid process,
pterygoid hamulus
Alveolar foramina


**Fig. 8.33 Pterygopalatine fossa, left side;** lateral view; color chart see inside of the back cover of this volume.

The pterygopalatine fossa is the medial continuation of the infratemporal fossa. Its bony margins are the maxilla, the palatine bone, and the sphenoidal bone. This fossa is an important **relais station** connecting the middle cranial fossa, the orbit, and the nasal cavity. It serves as a conduit for many nerves and blood vessels located in these structures (→ pp. 78 and 79).

The **lateral access route to the pterygopalatine fossa** is a common surgical strategy for the resection of tumors in this region, such as nasopharyngeal fibroma.

## Orbit

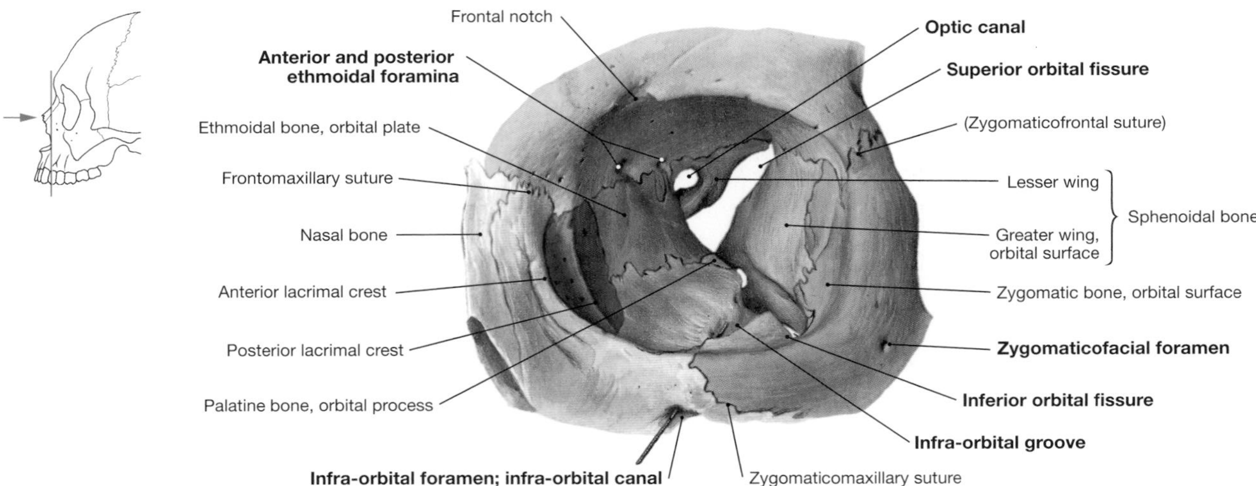

Frontal notch
Anterior and posterior ethmoidal foramina
Ethmoidal bone, orbital plate
Frontomaxillary suture
Nasal bone
Anterior lacrimal crest
Posterior lacrimal crest
Palatine bone, orbital process
Infra-orbital foramen; infra-orbital canal
Optic canal
Superior orbital fissure
(Zygomaticofrontal suture)
Lesser wing
Greater wing, orbital surface
Sphenoidal bone
Zygomatic bone, orbital surface
Zygomaticofacial foramen
Inferior orbital fissure
Infra-orbital groove
Zygomaticomaxillary suture


**Fig. 8.34 Orbit, left side;** frontal view; probe in the infraorbital canal; color chart see inside of the back cover of this volume.

The ethmoidal, lacrimal, palatine, sphenoidal, zygomatic, and maxillary bones create the margins of the orbital cavity. Passages to and from the orbit are the superior and inferior orbital fissures, the optic canal, and the anterior and posterior ethmoidal foramina. Located in the posterior part of the orbital floor, the infraorbital sulcus becomes the infraorbital canal which projects towards the front of the orbit and ends as infraorbital foramen located below the inferior margin of the orbit. Positioned laterally, the zygomatic bone regularly contains a zygomaticofacial foramen. For the orbital cavity → Figs. 9.9 to 9.13.

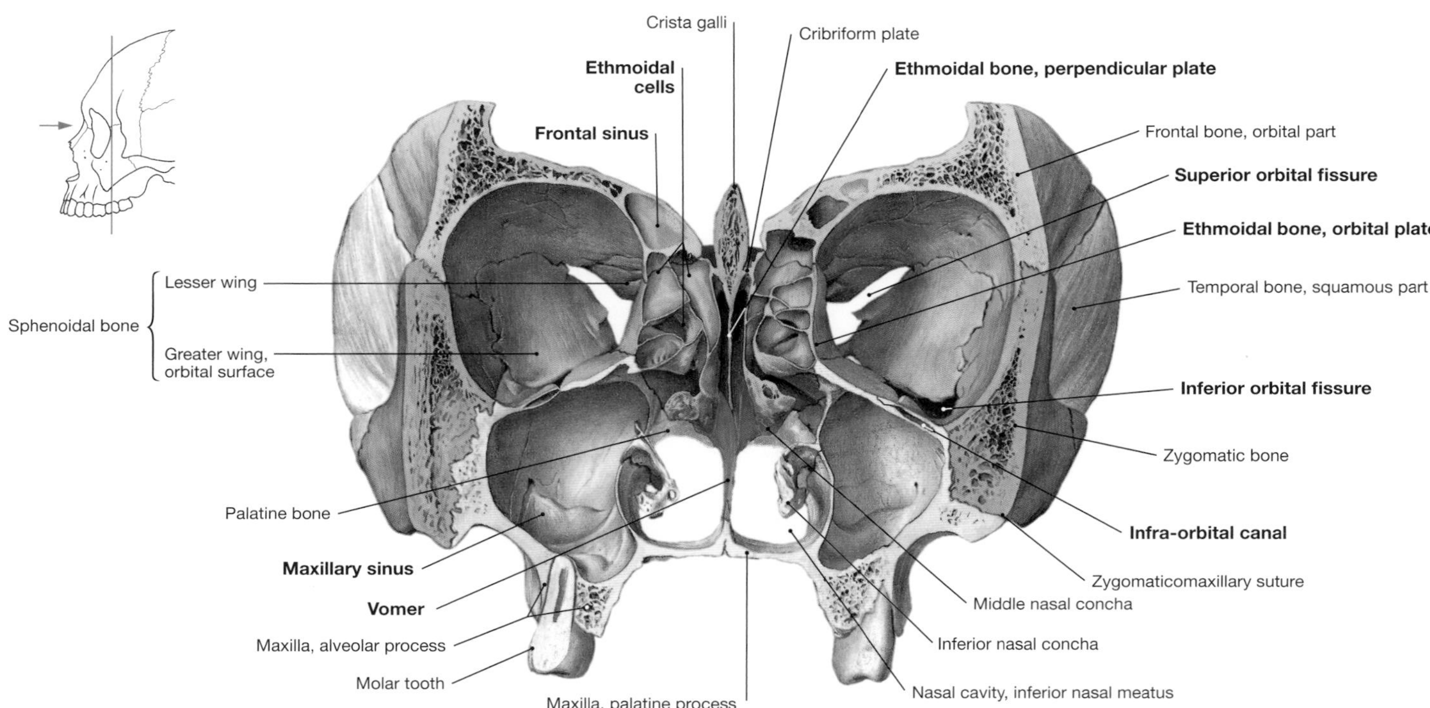

Crista galli
Cribriform plate
Ethmoidal cells
Ethmoidal bone, perpendicular plate
Frontal sinus
Frontal bone, orbital part
Superior orbital fissure
Ethmoidal bone, orbital plate
Temporal bone, squamous part
Lesser wing
Sphenoidal bone
Greater wing, orbital surface
Inferior orbital fissure
Zygomatic bone
Palatine bone
Infra-orbital canal
Maxillary sinus
Zygomaticomaxillary suture
Vomer
Middle nasal concha
Maxilla, alveolar process
Inferior nasal concha
Molar tooth
Nasal cavity, inferior nasal meatus
Maxilla, palatine process


**Fig. 8.35 Viscerocranium;** frontal section at the level of the two orbits; frontal view; color chart see inside of the back cover of this volume.

The unpaired ethmoidal bone contains the anterior and posterior **ethmoidal cells.** The perpendicular plate of the ethmoidal bone lies immediately beneath the crista galli, separates the bony labyrinth of the ethmoidal bone into a right and a left half, and participates in the upper part of the bony nasal septum. At its posterior aspect it is followed by the vomer. The lateral walls of the ethmoidal cells consist of a thin **orbital lamina,** known as **lamina papyracea,** constituting the major part of the medial wall of the orbit. The maxillary sinus is located directly below the orbit. The infraorbital canal is located in its roof, which also constitutes the floor of the orbit. The cribriform plate positions clearly below the roof of the orbit. For the orbital cavity → Figs. 9.9 to 9.13.

## Clinical Remarks

The paper-thin orbital lamina (lamina papyracea) of the ethmoidal bone between the orbit and the ethmoidal sinuses represents no barrier to the spreading of an **inflammation from the ethmoidal cells** into the orbit which can escalate into an orbital phlegmon. Figure 8.35 demonstrates the close proximity between a roots of a molar tooth and the maxillary sinus. Inflammations of the second premolars and/or the first molars can lead to an odontogenic inflammation of the maxillary sinus (maxillary sinusitis).

## Orbit

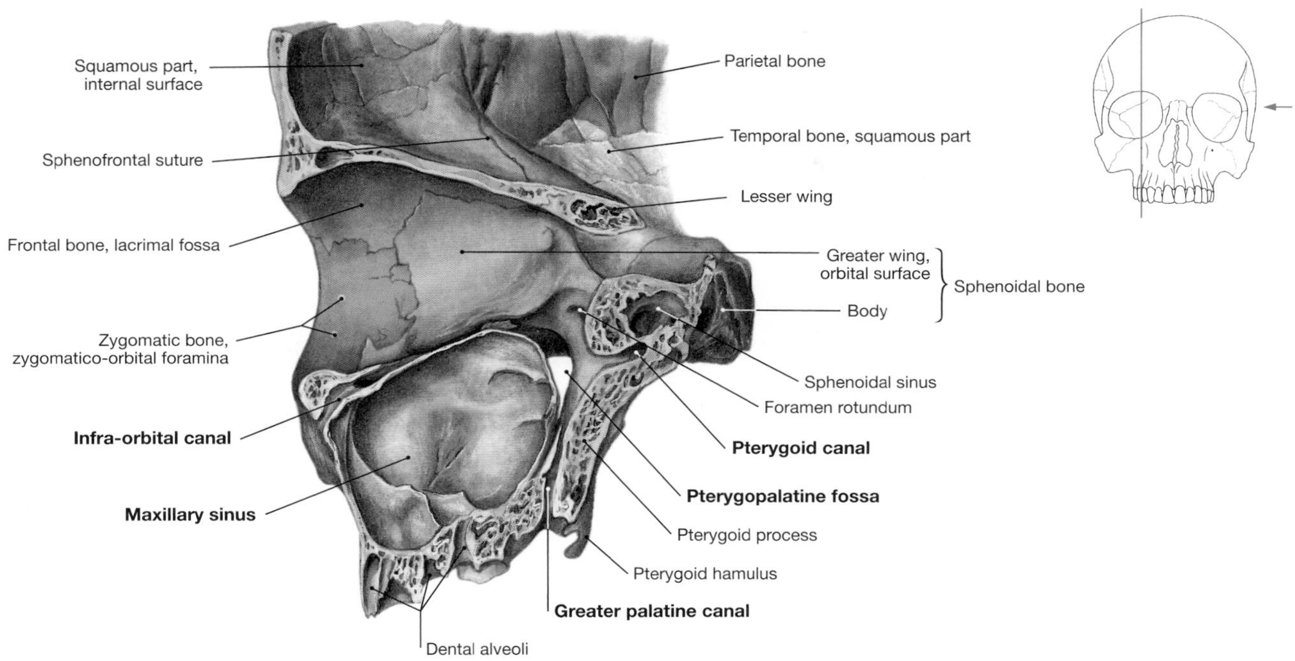
Squamous part, internal surface
Parietal bone
Temporal bone, squamous part
Sphenofrontal suture
Lesser wing
Frontal bone, lacrimal fossa
Greater wing, orbital surface
Body
Sphenoidal bone
Zygomatic bone, zygomatico-orbital foramina
Sphenoidal sinus
Foramen rotundum
Infra-orbital canal
Pterygoid canal
Pterygopalatine fossa
Maxillary sinus
Pterygoid process
Pterygoid hamulus
Greater palatine canal
Dental alveoli

**Fig. 8.36 Lateral wall of the orbit, right side;** medial view; color chart see inside of the back cover of this volume.
The zygomatic, frontal, sphenoidal, and maxillary bones form the lateral wall of the orbit. The infraorbital canal is depicted clearly in the anterior third of the orbital floor, as is the very thin bony layer separating the orbit from the maxillary sinus. The pterygopalatine fossa is located posteriorly to the maxillary sinus and connects laterally to the infratemporal fossa, cranially to the orbit, and in its inferior aspect connects to the oral cavity via the greater palatine canal. From a posterior cranial position, the pterygoid canal exits into the pterygopalatine fossa.

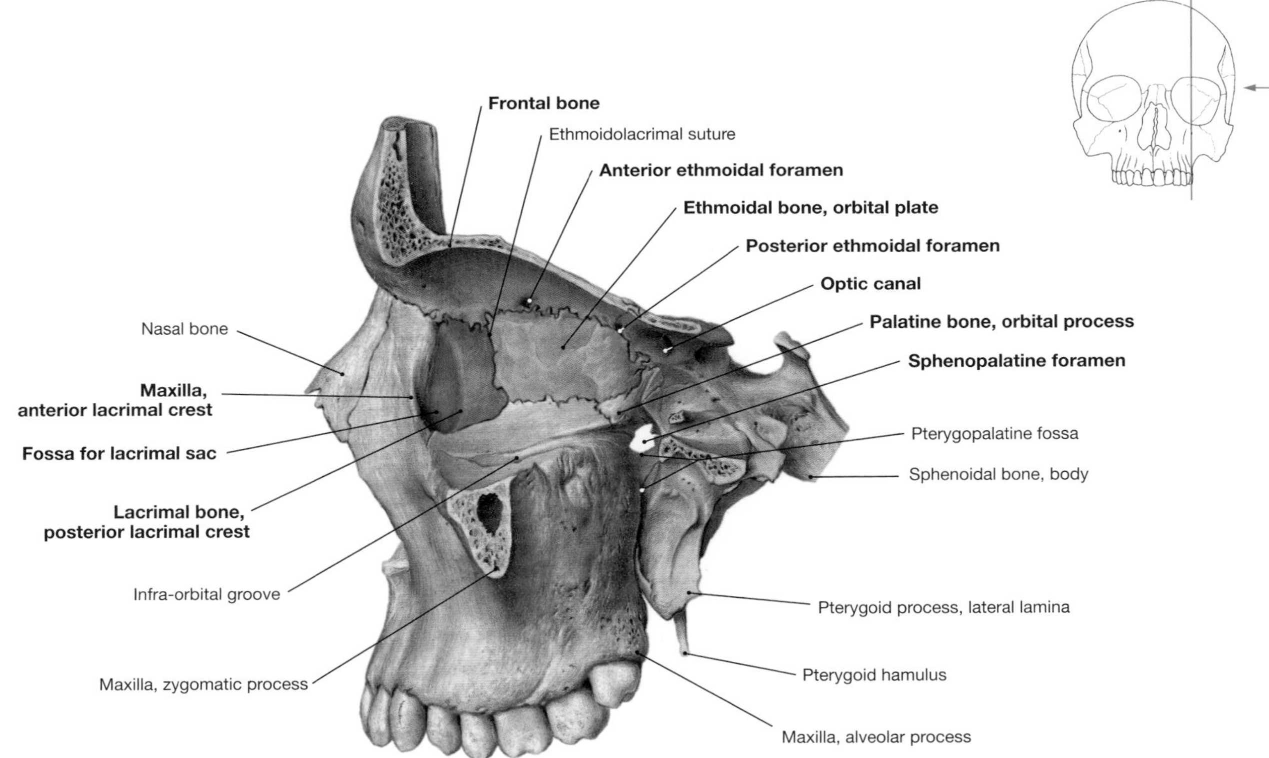
Frontal bone
Ethmoidolacrimal suture
Anterior ethmoidal foramen
Ethmoidal bone, orbital plate
Posterior ethmoidal foramen
Optic canal
Palatine bone, orbital process
Sphenopalatine foramen
Nasal bone
Maxilla, anterior lacrimal crest
Fossa for lacrimal sac
Pterygopalatine fossa
Sphenoidal bone, body
Lacrimal bone, posterior lacrimal crest
Infra-orbital groove
Pterygoid process, lateral lamina
Pterygoid hamulus
Maxilla, zygomatic process
Maxilla, alveolar process

**Fig. 8.37 Medial wall of the orbit, left side;** lateral view; color chart see inside of the back cover of this volume.
The lacrimal bone, the maxilla, and the frontal bone form the anterior part of the medial wall of the orbit, whereas in the posterior part the orbital lamina of the ethmoidal bone (lamina papyracea), the orbital process of the palatine bone, and the sphenoidal bone are placed between the frontal bone and the maxilla. Both, the anterior lacrimal crest of the maxilla and the posterior lacrimal crest of the lacrimal bone provide the margins for a depression (fossa for lacrimal gland) of the lacrimal sac. Located in the medial wall of the orbit are the anterior and posterior ethmoidal foramina and the optic canal. The sphenopalatine foramen is located at the top of the pterygopalatine fossa.

# Sphenoidal bone

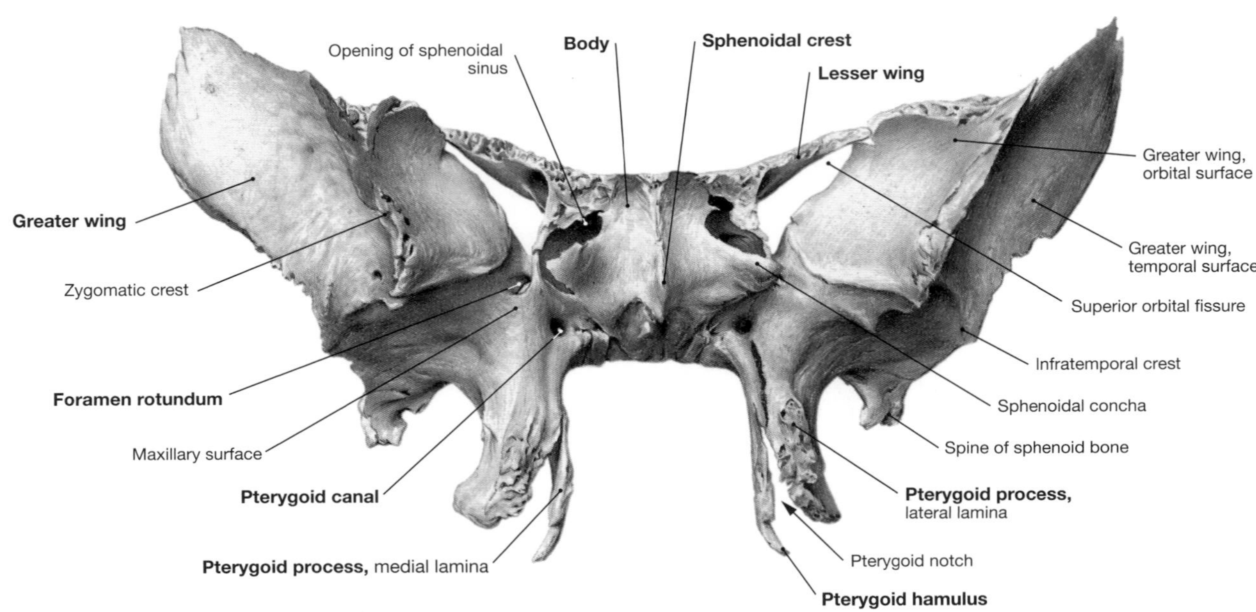
Opening of sphenoidal sinus
Body
Sphenoidal crest
Lesser wing
Greater wing, orbital surface
Greater wing, temporal surface
Superior orbital fissure
Infratemporal crest
Sphenoidal concha
Spine of sphenoid bone
Pterygoid process, lateral lamina
Pterygoid notch
Pterygoid hamulus
Greater wing
Zygomatic crest
Foramen rotundum
Maxillary surface
Pterygoid canal
Pterygoid process, medial lamina

**Fig. 8.38 Sphenoidal bone;** frontal view.
The unpaired sphenoidal bone connects the viscerocranium with the neurocranium. Two pairs of wing-shaped bones extend from the body of the sphenoidal bone. The **lesser wings** sit on the top, the **greater wings** at the bottom, and below the **pterygoid processes** project. The center of the sphenoidal bone contains the **sphenoidal sinuses.** The sphenoidal crest subdivides the anterior part of the body into two halves.

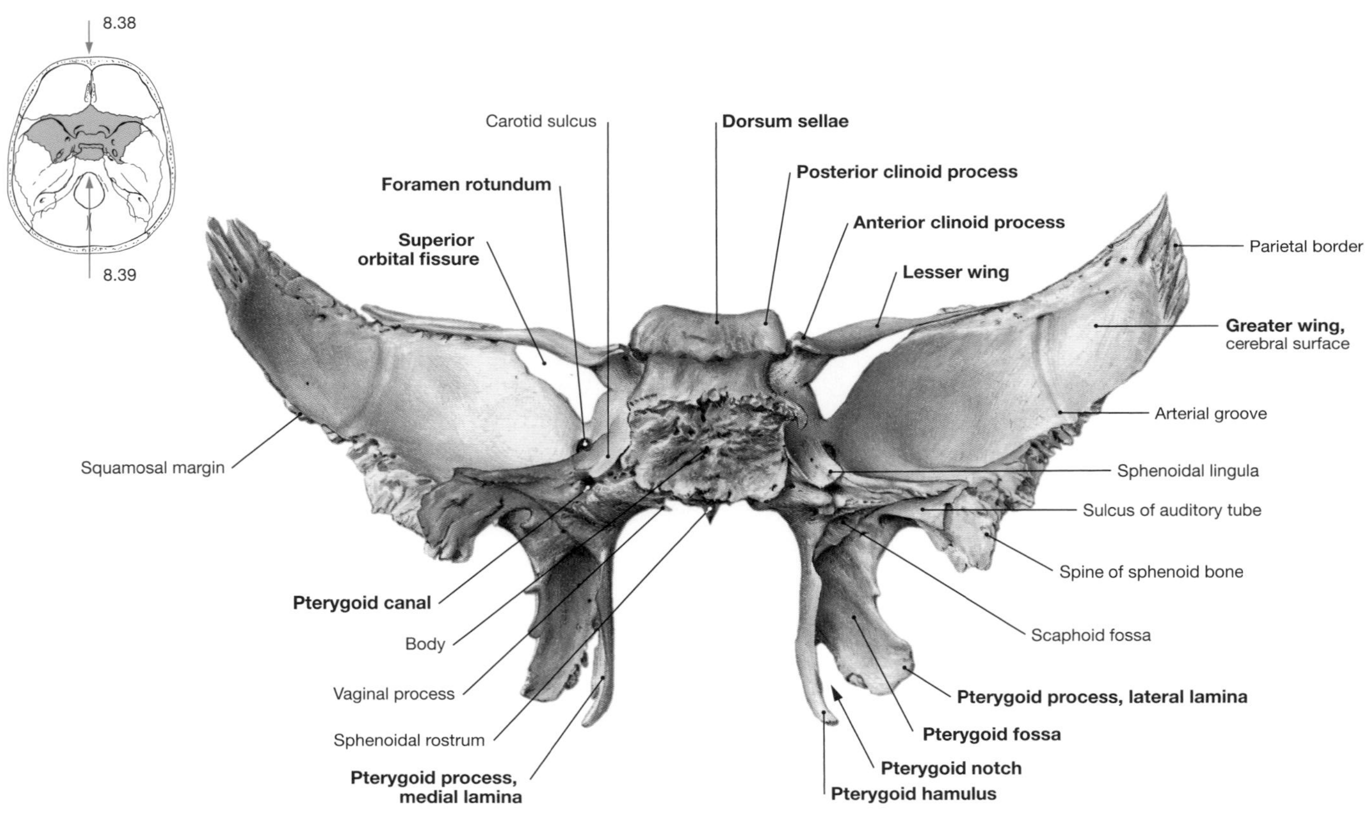
8.38
8.39
Carotid sulcus
Dorsum sellae
Foramen rotundum
Posterior clinoid process
Superior orbital fissure
Anterior clinoid process
Lesser wing
Parietal border
Greater wing, cerebral surface
Arterial groove
Squamosal margin
Sphenoidal lingula
Sulcus of auditory tube
Spine of sphenoid bone
Pterygoid canal
Scaphoid fossa
Body
Vaginal process
Pterygoid process, lateral lamina
Pterygoid fossa
Sphenoidal rostrum
Pterygoid notch
Pterygoid process, medial lamina
Pterygoid hamulus

**Fig. 8.39 Sphenoidal bone;** posterior view.
The lesser and greater wings of the sphenoidal bone participate in the formation of the **superior orbital fissure.** On both sides, the pterygoid process divides into a smaller medial lamina and a larger lateral lamina, which create the **pterygoid notch** and enclose the pterygoid fossa. The **pterygoid hamulus** is the caudal extension of the medial lamina. At its base, the pterygoid canal perforates the sphenoidal bone and enters into the pterygopalatine fossa.

## Sphenoidal bone and occipital bone

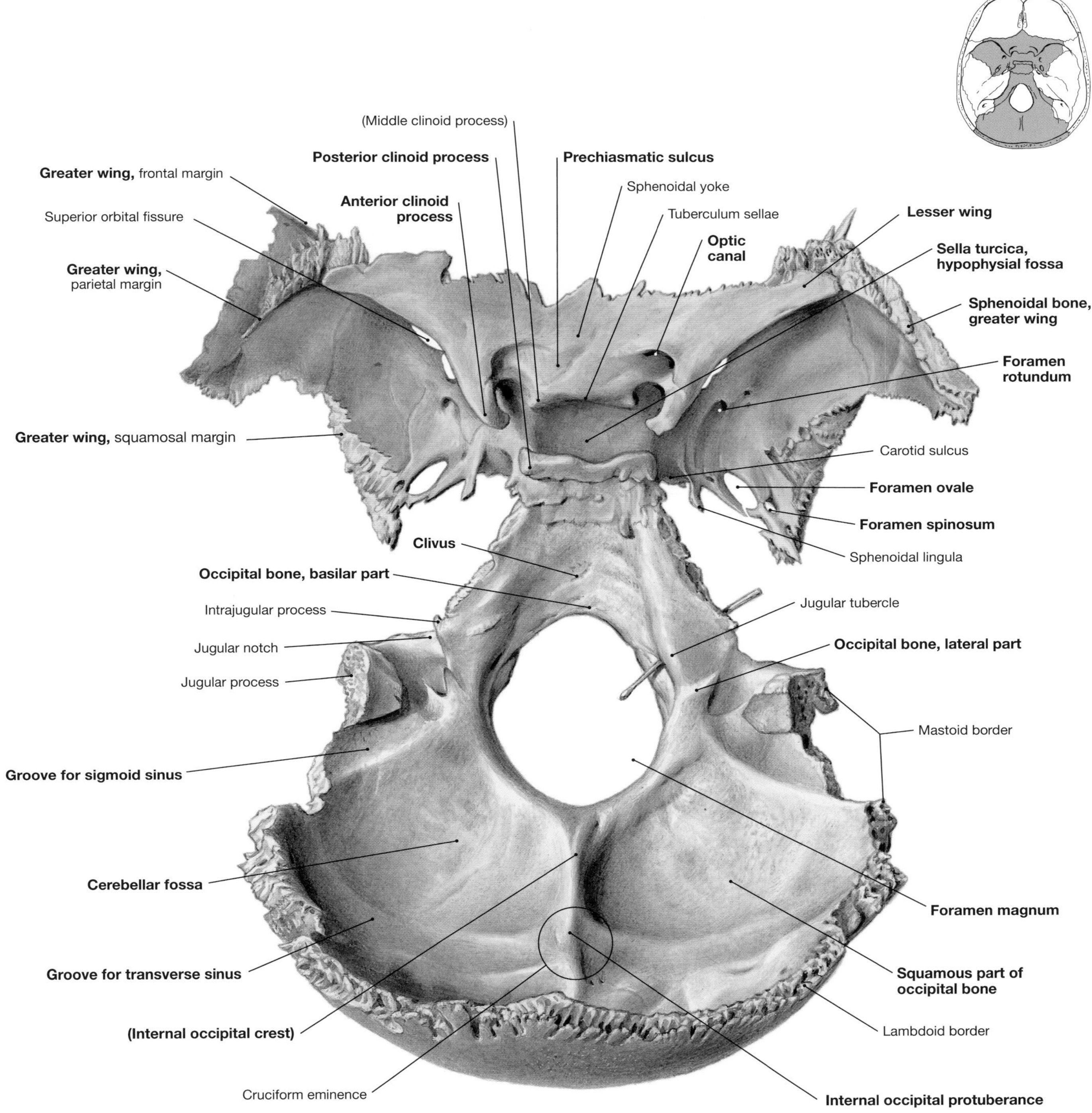
(Middle clinoid process)
Posterior clinoid process
Prechiasmatic sulcus
Greater wing, frontal margin
Sphenoidal yoke
Anterior clinoid process
Tuberculum sellae
Superior orbital fissure
Lesser wing
Optic canal
Sella turcica, hypophysial fossa
Greater wing, parietal margin
Sphenoidal bone, greater wing
Foramen rotundum
Greater wing, squamosal margin
Carotid sulcus
Foramen ovale
Foramen spinosum
Clivus
Sphenoidal lingula
Occipital bone, basilar part
Jugular tubercle
Intrajugular process
Occipital bone, lateral part
Jugular notch
Jugular process
Mastoid border
Groove for sigmoid sinus
Cerebellar fossa
Foramen magnum
Groove for transverse sinus
Squamous part of occipital bone
Lambdoid border
(Internal occipital crest)
Cruciform eminence
Internal occipital protuberance

**Fig. 8.40 Sphenoidal bone and occipital bone;** superior view; color chart see inside of the back cover of this volume.

The center of the **sphenoidal bone** is composed of the **sella turcica** with the hypophysial fossa. The Tuberculum sellae creates the anterior rim of the hypophysial fossa and extends laterally into the medial clinoid process. The prechiasmatic sulcus and the jugum sphenoidale (sphenoidal yoke) are located in front of the Tuberculum sellae. The clivus forms the posterior part of the saddle-shaped sella turcica and the posterior clinoid process represents the lateral elevated end of its upper rim. In the region of the sella turcica and at its anterior rim, the optic canal perforates the lesser wing. The foramina rotundum, ovale, and spinosum pierce the greater wing bilaterally in an anterior cranial to posterior caudal direction.

The unpaired **occipital bone** is composed of the squamous part, two lateral parts, and one basilar part. These four parts delimit the **foramen magnum.** At the inner surface of the squamous part of occipital bone, the groove of the superior sagittal sinus and the grooves for the transverse sinus meet at the internal occipital protuberance. Further, the grooves for the sigmoid sinus and the occipital sinus are visible at the inner surface. Above and below the occipital protuberance, the inner surface of the squamous part of the occipital bone forms the cerebral fossa and the cerebellar fossa, respectively. Together with the body of the sphenoidal bone, the basilar part of the occipital bone generates the clivus.

## Temporal bone

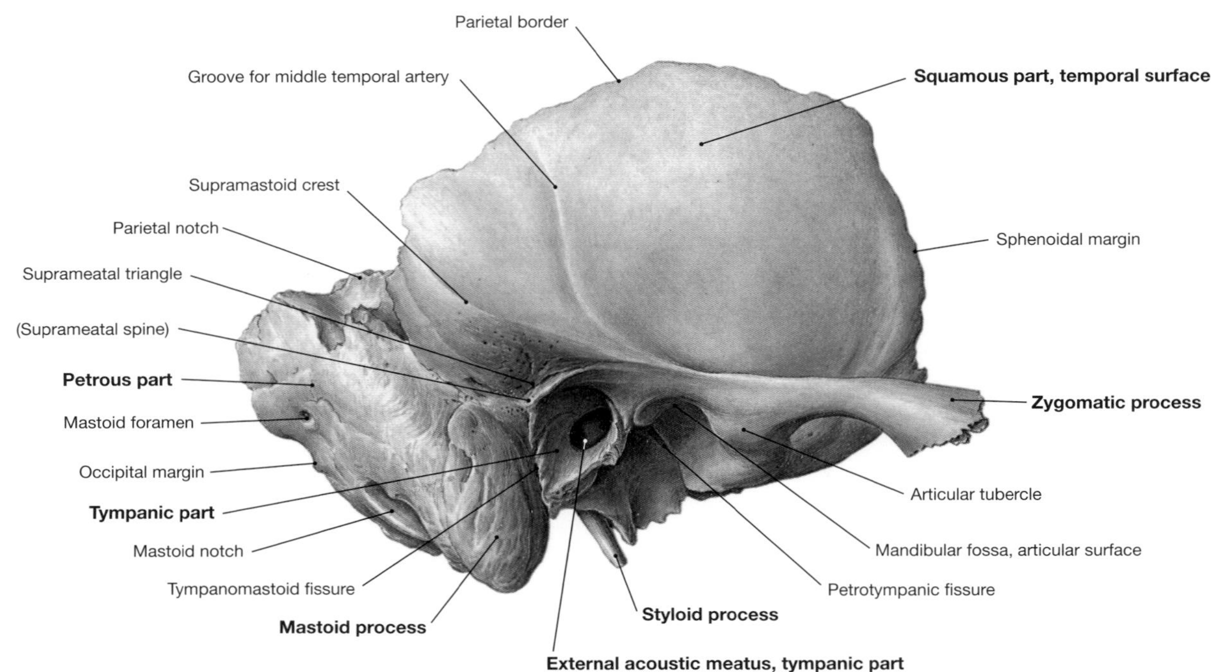
Parietal border
Groove for middle temporal artery
Squamous part, temporal surface
Supramastoid crest
Parietal notch
Sphenoidal margin
Suprameatal triangle
(Suprameatal spine)
Petrous part
Zygomatic process
Mastoid foramen
Occipital margin
Articular tubercle
Tympanic part
Mastoid notch
Mandibular fossa, articular surface
Tympanomastoid fissure
Petrotympanic fissure
Mastoid process
Styloid process
External acoustic meatus, tympanic part

**Fig. 8.41 Temporal bone, right side;** lateral view.
The paired temporal bone is part of the viscerocranium and neurocranium. It participates in the formation of the lateral side and the base of the cranium. The squamous part, the tympanic part, and the petrous part (petrous bone) can be distinguished.
Through its parietal border, the **squamous part** connects with the parietal bone. The zygomatic process protrudes anterior and superior of the meatus and extends in an anterior direction.
The **petrous part** borders at the parietal and occipital bones. The central outer opening is the external acoustic meatus. Located at its posterior caudal aspect is the mastoid process. Middle and inner ear are located within the petrous part (not visible). Access routes are the internal acoustic meatus, → p. 17), the stylomastoid foramen (→ p. 16) and the musculotubal canal (→ Figs. 10.30 and 10.37).
The **tympanic part** forms the bony wall of the external acoustic meatus. As a ring-shaped structure, it is associated with the squamous and petrous parts. The tympanic part delimits the external acoustic meatus at its frontal, caudal, and posterior side and extends to the tympanic membrane (→ Figs. 10.15 and 10.25).

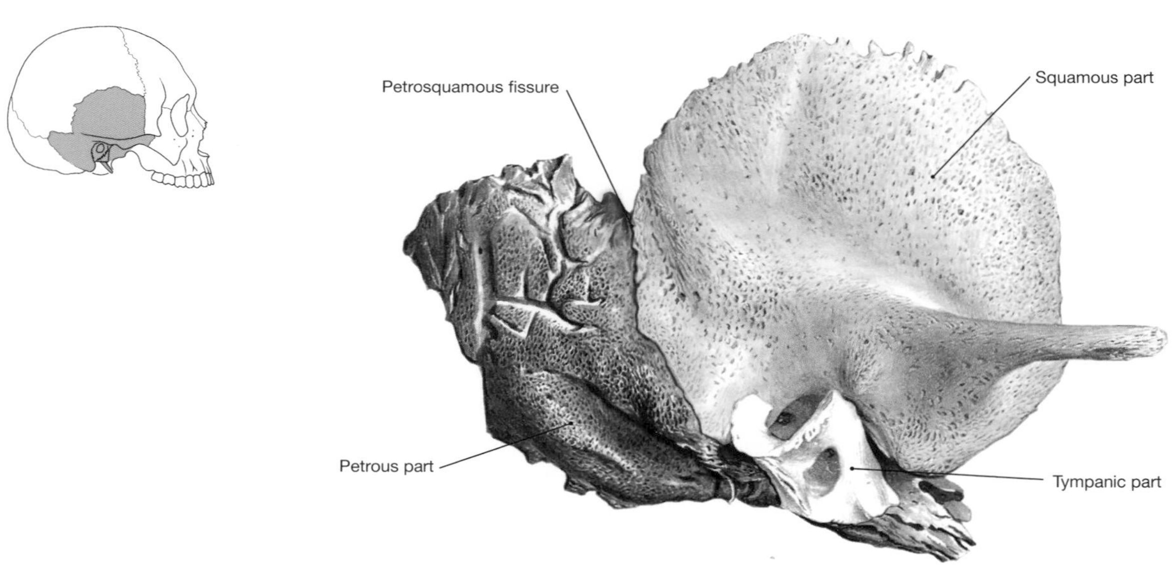
Petrosquamous fissure
Squamous part
Petrous part
Tympanic part

**Fig. 8.42 Temporal bone, of a newborn, right side;** lateral view; schematic drawing; color chart see inside of the back cover of this volume.

The image displays different parts of the temporal bone: squamous part, petrous part, and tympanic part.

## Temporal bone

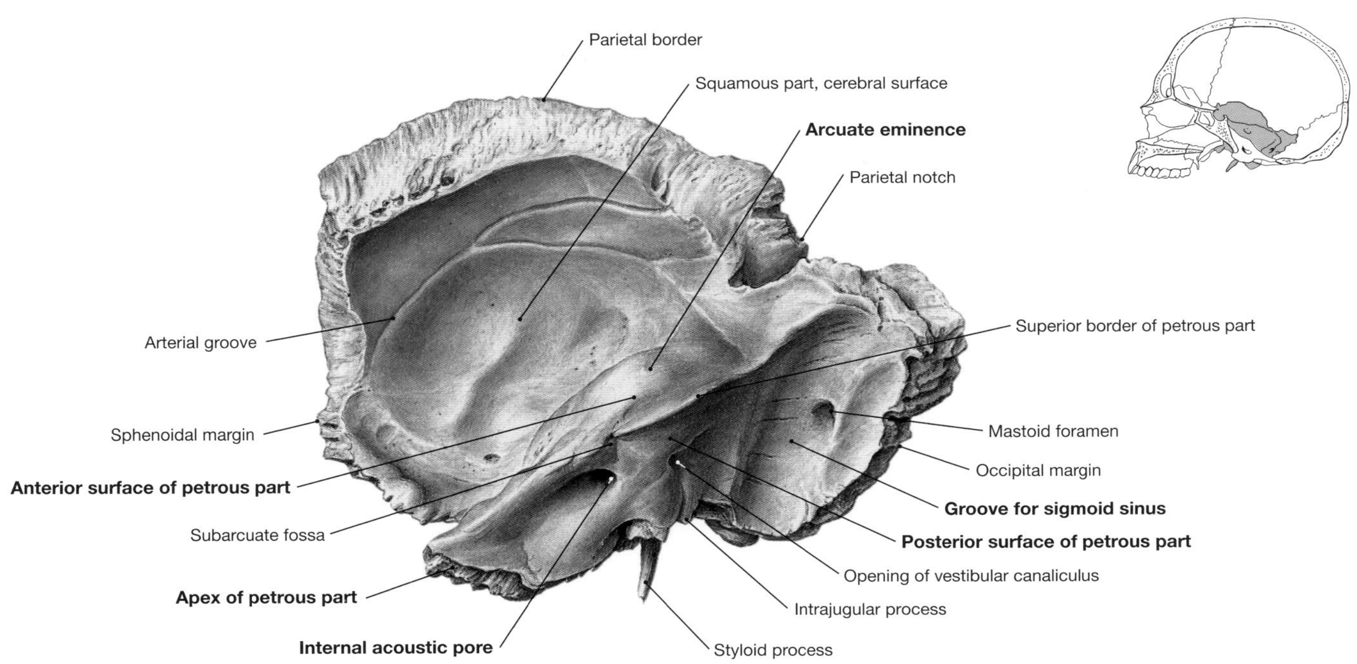
Parietal border
Squamous part, cerebral surface
Arcuate eminence
Parietal notch
Arterial groove
Superior border of petrous part
Sphenoidal margin
Mastoid foramen
Occipital margin
Anterior surface of petrous part
Groove for sigmoid sinus
Subarcuate fossa
Posterior surface of petrous part
Opening of vestibular canaliculus
Apex of petrous part
Intrajugular process
Internal acoustic pore
Styloid process

**Fig. 8.43 Temporal bone, right side;** inner aspect.
The petrous part is shaped like a pyramid with its tip (apex of petrous part) directed anterior medial and its base pointing towards the mastoid process. The anterior surface is part of the middle cranial fossa and contains the protruding arcuate eminence; contained within the posterior surface is the **internal acoustic pore** which constitutes the entrance to the internal acoustic meatus. The posterior surface of the petrous part shows the indentation by the groove of the sigmoid sinus. The **mastoid foramen** is located here as well. On the inner surface (cerebral surface) of the squamous part the grooves for arteries of the medial meningeal artery are visible.

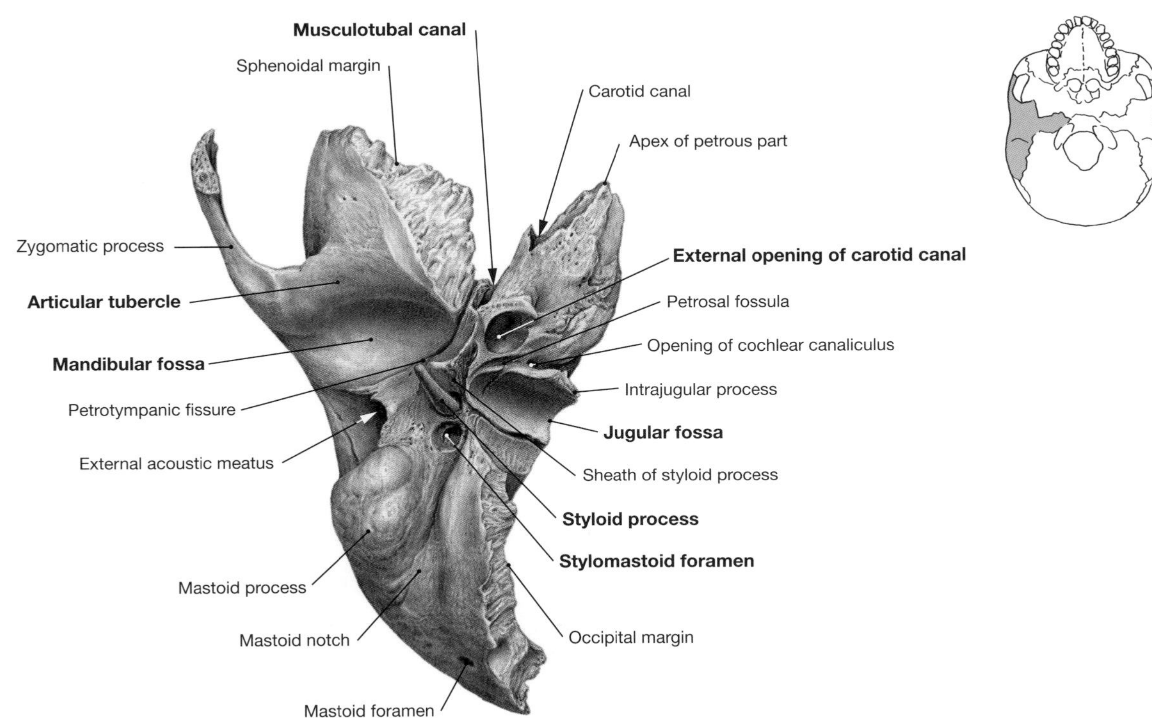
Musculotubal canal
Sphenoidal margin
Carotid canal
Apex of petrous part
Zygomatic process
External opening of carotid canal
Articular tubercle
Petrosal fossula
Opening of cochlear canaliculus
Mandibular fossa
Intrajugular process
Petrotympanic fissure
Jugular fossa
External acoustic meatus
Sheath of styloid process
Styloid process
Stylomastoid foramen
Mastoid process
Mastoid notch
Occipital margin
Mastoid foramen

**Fig. 8.44 Temporal bone, right side;** inferior view.
The inferior surface of the temporal bone depresses to become the **jugular fossa** and, together with the occipital bone, delineates the jugular foramen. The notch at the border between the squamous and petrous part indicates the starting point of the musculotubal canal. In addition, the external opening of the carotid canal and the styloid process are visible. The **stylomastoid foramen** opens to the lateral posterior side. Just in front of the external acoustic meatus, the squamous part contains the **mandibular fossa** which, at its rostral aspect, is demarcated by the articular tubercle.

## Lower jaw

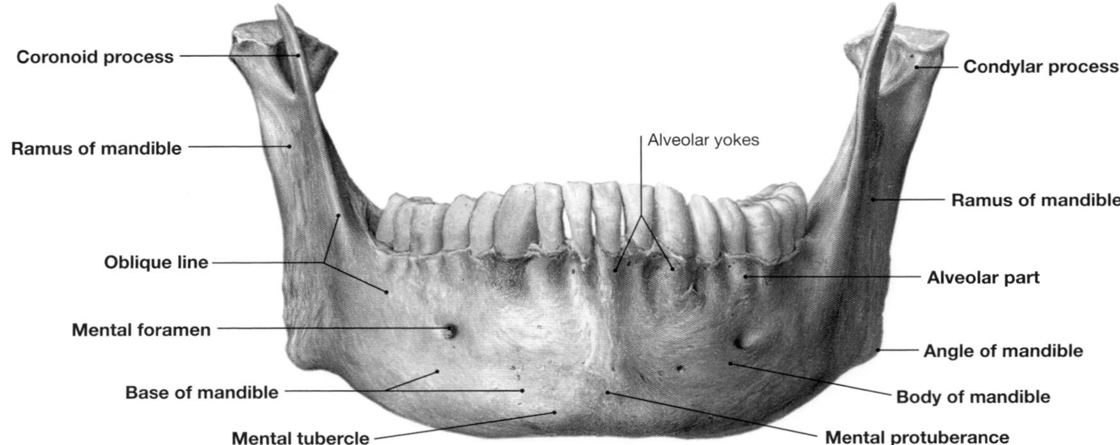
Coronoid process
Condylar process
Ramus of mandible
Alveolar yokes
Ramus of mandible
Oblique line
Alveolar part
Mental foramen
Angle of mandible
Base of mandible
Body of mandible
Mental tubercle
Mental protuberance

**Fig. 8.45 Lower jaw, mandible;** frontal view.
The unpaired mandible consists of a body of the mandible and two rami. Each ramus divides into a **coronoid process** and a **condylar process.** The body of the mandible is composed of the base and the alveolar part separated by the oblique line which descends from the coronoid process in an oblique anterior trajectory. The frontal part of the alveolar part consists of the chin (mentum) with the mental protuberance, the bilateral mental tubercles and the mental foramina.

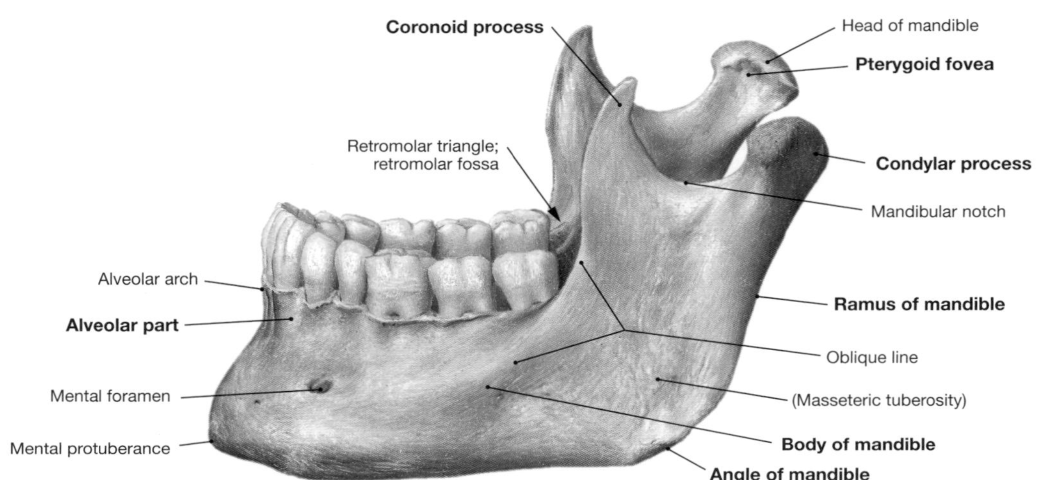
Coronoid process
Head of mandible
Pterygoid fovea
Retromolar triangle; retromolar fossa
Condylar process
Mandibular notch
Alveolar arch
Ramus of mandible
Alveolar part
Oblique line
Mental foramen
(Masseteric tuberosity)
Mental protuberance
Body of mandible
Angle of mandible

**Fig. 8.46 Lower jaw, mandible;** lateral view. Body and ramus of mandible merge at the **angle of mandible.** The **head of mandible** sits on top of the condylary process.

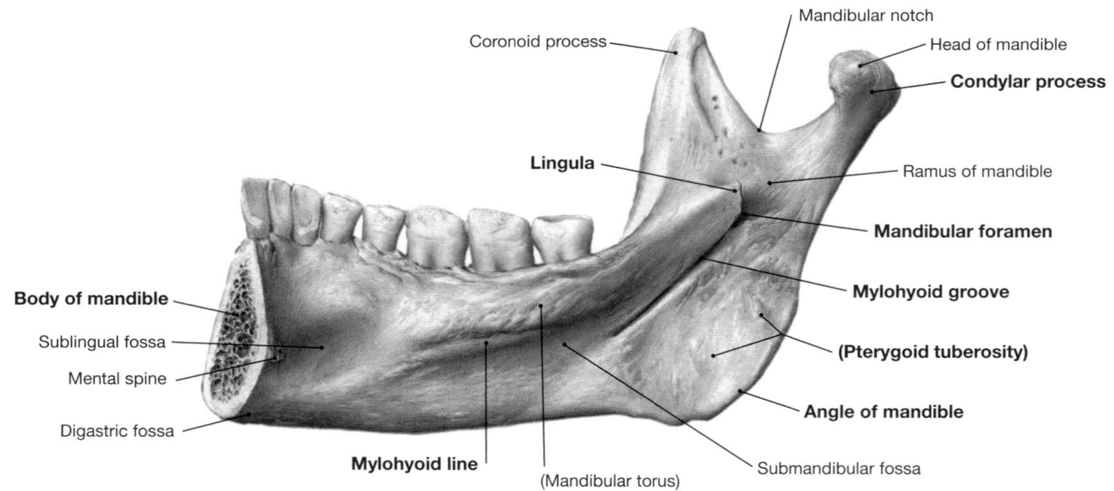
Mandibular notch
Coronoid process
Head of mandible
Condylar process
Lingula
Ramus of mandible
Mandibular foramen
Mylohyoid groove
Body of mandible
Sublingual fossa
(Pterygoid tuberosity)
Mental spine
Angle of mandible
Digastric fossa
Mylohyoid line
Submandibular fossa
(Mandibular torus)

**Fig. 8.47 Lower jaw, mandible;** inner aspect of the mandibular arch. The **mandibular foramen** is located at the inside of the ramus of mandible. In front thereof, the **mylohyoid line** creates a stepwise crest, which serves as an attachment for the mylohyoid muscle and demarcates the level of the floor of the mouth.

## Lower jaw

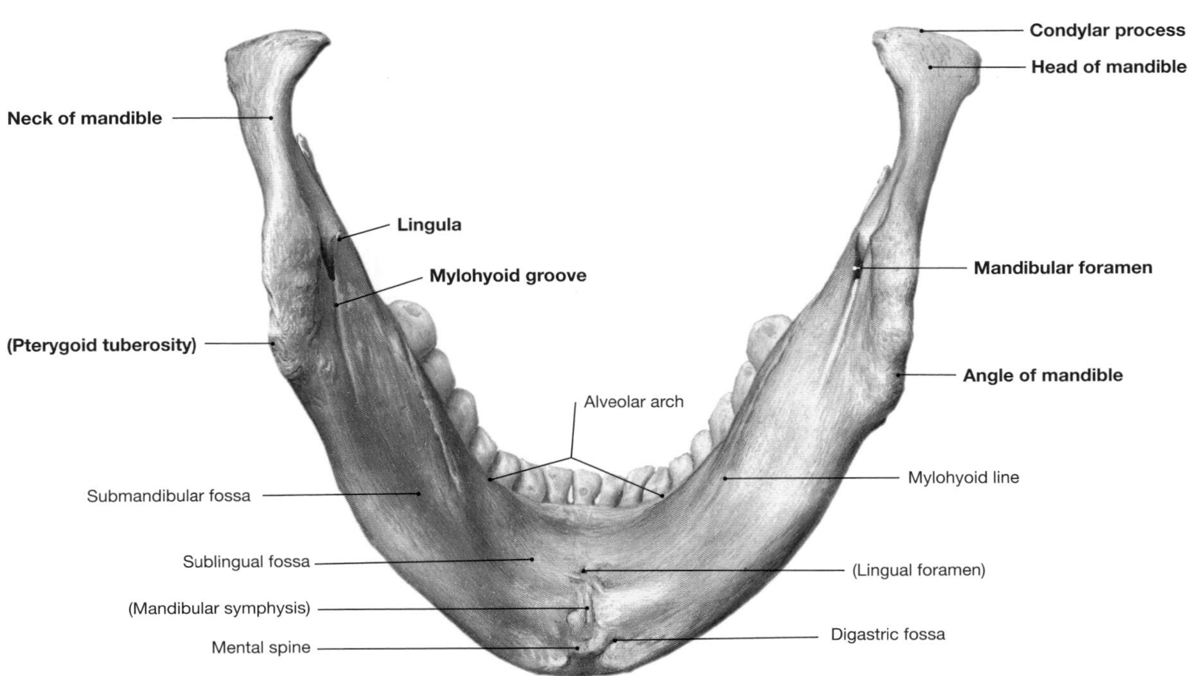
Condylar process
Head of mandible
Neck of mandible
Lingula
Mylohyoid groove
Mandibular foramen
(Pterygoid tuberosity)
Angle of mandible
Alveolar arch
Mylohyoid line
Submandibular fossa
Sublingual fossa
(Lingual foramen)
(Mandibular symphysis)
Digastric fossa
Mental spine

**Fig. 8.48 Lower jaw, mandible;** inferior view.
The mental spine is located at the inside of the mandible close to the midline. Bony depressions represent the digastric fossa below and lateral to the mental spine and the sublingual fossa and submandibular fossa above the mental spine. On the inside of the angle of mandible the **pterygoid tuberosity** is found.

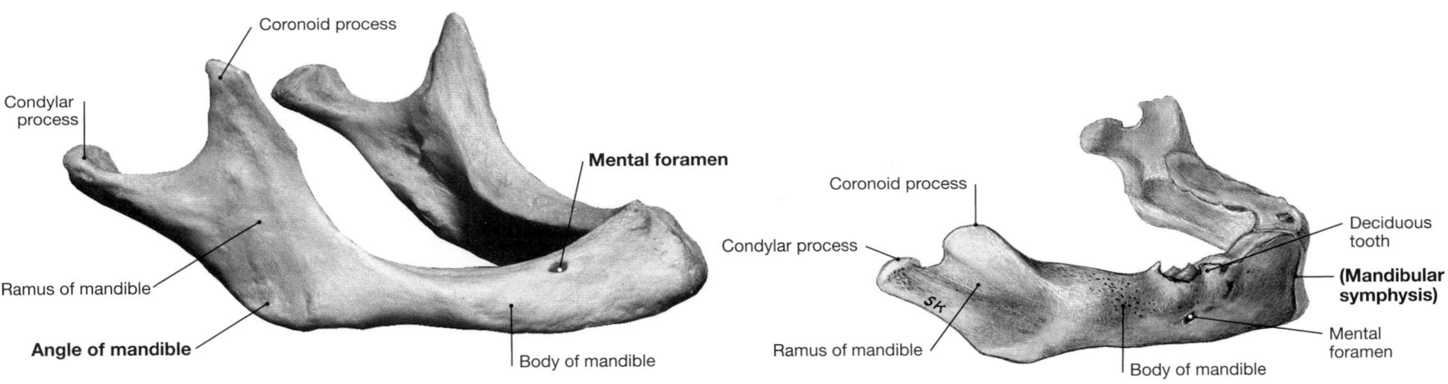
Coronoid process
Condylar process
Mental foramen
Ramus of mandible
Angle of mandible
Body of mandible
Coronoid process
Condylar process
Deciduous tooth
(Mandibular symphysis)
Mental foramen
Ramus of mandible
Body of mandible

**Fig. 8.49 Lower jaw, mandible, of an old person.**
Loss of teeth – particularly at an advanced age – results in a **regression of the alveolar part** of the mandible. This can progress until the mental foramen becomes located at the upper rim of the toothless lower jaw. The **angle of mandible** has a much wider angle than in a mandible with dentition.

**Fig. 8.50 Lower jaw, mandible, of a newborn.**
In a newborn, the **mandibular symphysis** connects the two mandibular segments. The angle between the body and ramus of mandible is still very large.

### Clinical Remarks

Apart from nasal **fractures,** fractures of the mandible are common due to its exposed location in the head region. The U-shaped structure explains the various types of mandibular fractures, in particular at the level of the canines and the third molar teeth. Extravasated blood from the mandible collects in the loose tissue of the floor of the mouth, results in small spotted bleeding under the skin (ekchymoses), and is a typical sign of a mandibular fracture. Without proper prosthetic reconstruction, a **loss of teeth** results in the regression of the alveolar part of mandible in the area of the lost teeth. The fitting of a dental prosthesis onto a largely regressed alveolar part is exceedingly difficult and often requires bone reconstruction.

## Temporomandibular joint

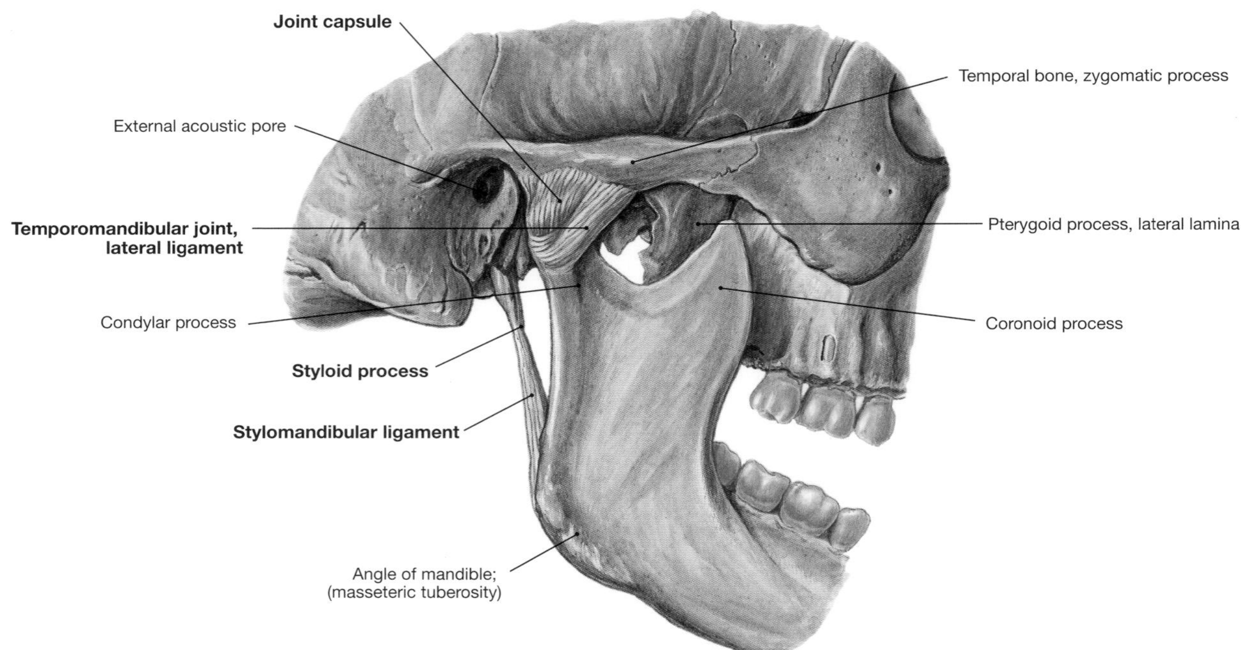
Joint capsule
External acoustic pore
Temporal bone, zygomatic process
Temporomandibular joint, lateral ligament
Pterygoid process, lateral lamina
Condylar process
Coronoid process
Styloid process
Stylomandibular ligament
Angle of mandible; (masseteric tuberosity)

**Fig. 8.51 Temporomandibular joint, right side;** lateral view.
A wide cone-shaped joint capsule stretching from the temporal bone to the condylar process surrounds the mandibular joint. In its frontal and lateral parts, the lateral ligament reinforces the joint capsule and extends from the zygomatic arch in an oblique posterior caudal direction to the head of mandible. At the inside of the joint (not shown), connective tissue generates the variable medial ligament. The lateral and medial ligaments (if present) assist in guiding the joint movements and foremost inhibit posterior movements of the mandibular head. When bite force is applied, the lateral ligament also stabilizes the condyle. The **stylomandibular ligament** projects from the styloid process to the posterior rim of the ramus of mandible. It is usually weak and, together with the **sphenomandibular ligament,** resists further lower jaw movements at a position close to maximal opening of the mouth (→ Fig. 8.52).

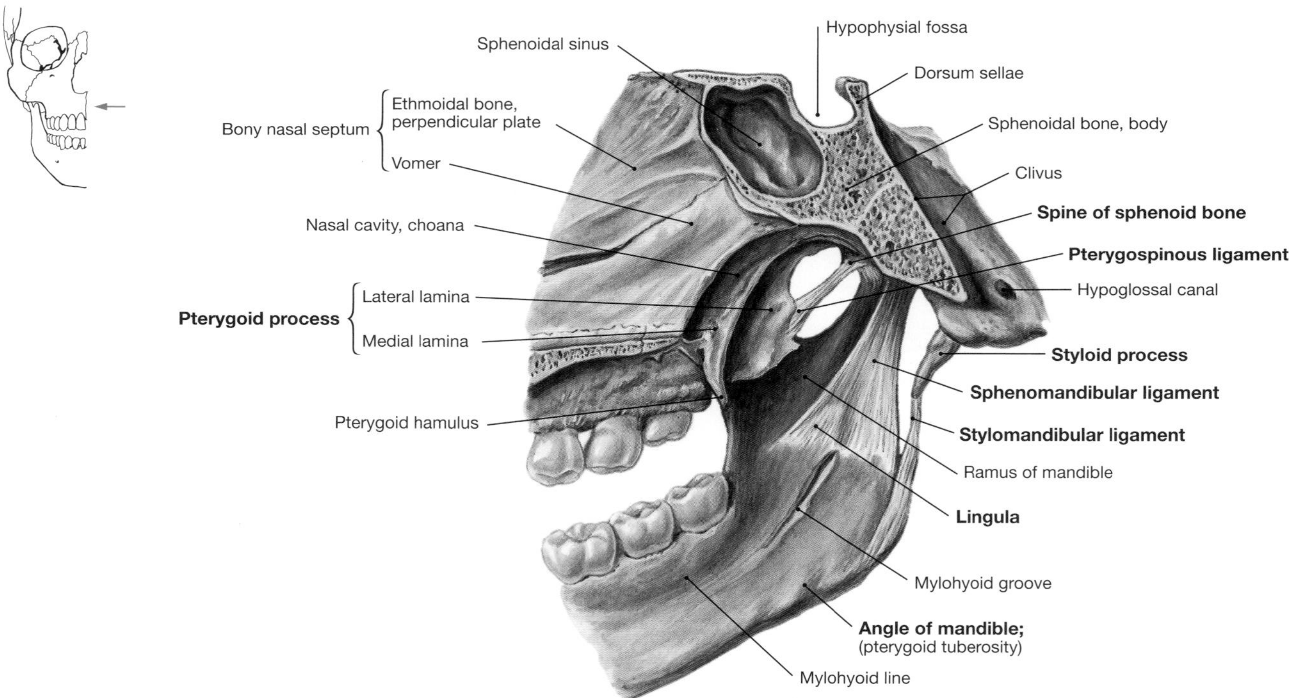
Sphenoidal sinus
Hypophysial fossa
Dorsum sellae
Bony nasal septum
Ethmoidal bone, perpendicular plate
Vomer
Sphenoidal bone, body
Clivus
Spine of sphenoid bone
Nasal cavity, choana
Pterygospinous ligament
Hypoglossal canal
Pterygoid process
Lateral lamina
Medial lamina
Styloid process
Sphenomandibular ligament
Pterygoid hamulus
Stylomandibular ligament
Ramus of mandible
Lingula
Mylohyoid groove
Angle of mandible; (pterygoid tuberosity)
Mylohyoid line

**Fig. 8.52 Stylomandibular ligament and sphenomandibular ligament, right side;** medial view.
Both ligaments affect the kinematics of the temporomandibular joint but are not associated with the joint capsule.
The strong **sphenomandibular ligament** has its origin at the spine of sphenoidal bone and passes between the lateral and medial pterygoid and inserts in a fan-shaped pattern at the lingula of mandible. The **stylomandibular ligament** originates from the styloid process and projects to the angle of mandible. Together, both ligaments inhibit lower jaw movements at a position close to the maximal **opening of the mouth.**
The **pterygospinous ligament** has no relationship to the temporomandibular joint nor does it affect the joint kinematics. It has its origin at the spine of sphenoidal bone and inserts at the lateral lamina of the pterygoid process. This ligament has a **stabilizing** function.

# Temporomandibular joint

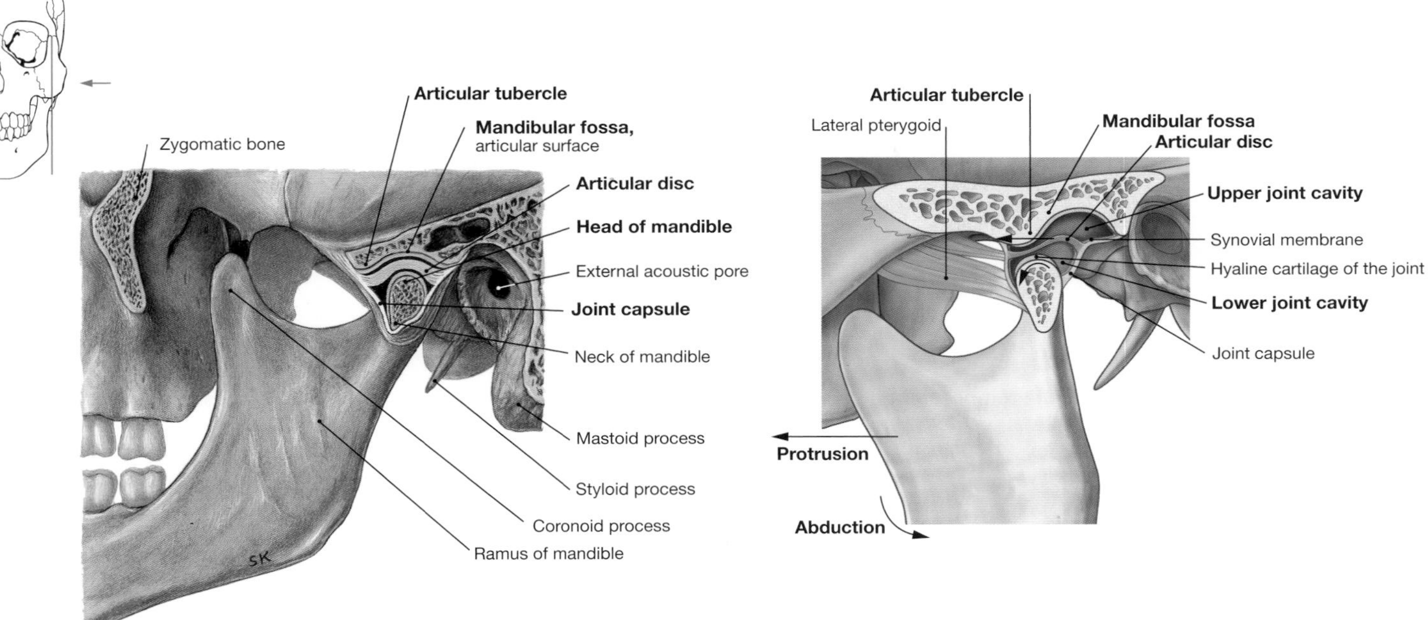
Articular tubercle
Mandibular fossa, articular surface
Zygomatic bone
Articular disc
Head of mandible
External acoustic pore
Joint capsule
Neck of mandible
Mastoid process
Styloid process
Coronoid process
Ramus of mandible
Articular tubercle
Lateral pterygoid
Mandibular fossa
Articular disc
Upper joint cavity
Synovial membrane
Hyaline cartilage of the joint
Lower joint cavity
Joint capsule
Protrusion
Abduction

**Fig. 8.53 Temporomandibular joint, left side;** sagittal section; lateral view; mouth almost closed.
In the temporomandibular joint, the head of mandible, mandibular fossa, and articular tubercle of the temporal bone articulate with each other. Both joint components are separated by an articular disc. The temporomandibular joint is positioned in front of the bony part of the external acoustic pore.

**Fig. 8.54 Temporomandibular joint, left side;** sagittal section; lateral view; mouth opened. [8]
An articular disc completely divides the temporomandibular joint into two separate chambers **(dithalamic joint):**

- The lower chamber permits **hinge-like** opening and closure movements of the mandible.
- The upper chamber allows for the head of mandible to slide forward on the articular tubercle **(protrusion).** This particularly requires the action of the lateral pterygoid. The movement back into the mandibular fossa is called retraction **(retrusion).**

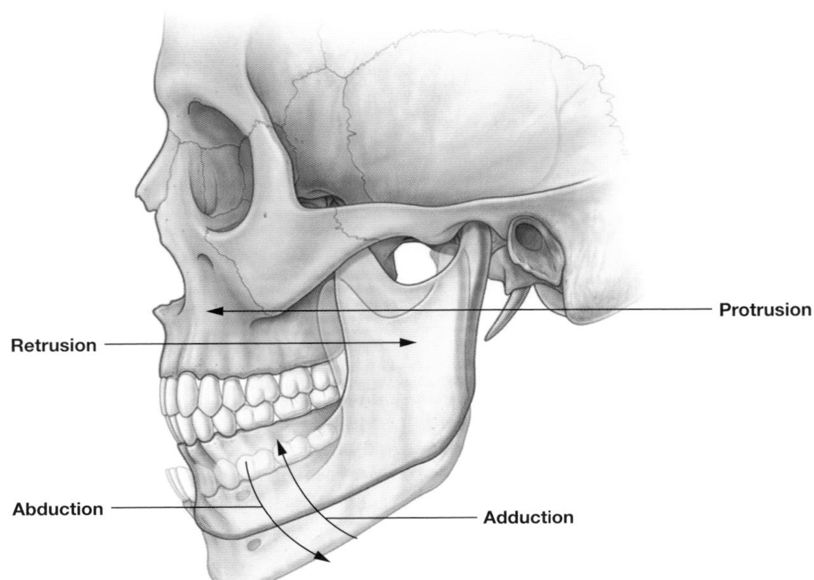
Protrusion
Retrusion
Abduction
Adduction

**Fig. 8.55 Movements of the temporomandibular joint, left side;** lateral view. [8]
Independent movements in one temporomandibular joint are not possible because both temporomandibular joints are joined in the bony mandibular arch. The temporomandibular joints permit two main functions during chewing: elevation **(adduction)** and depression **(abduction)** of the lower jaw as well as grinding movements. Apart from abduction and adduction, the forward **(protrusion)** and backward movement **(retrusion)** as well as grinding (sideways sliding – **laterotrusion** and **mediotrusion**) constitute the movement patterns of the temporomandibular joint. The masticatory muscles contribute in different ways to the mobility of the joint.

## Temporomandibular joint

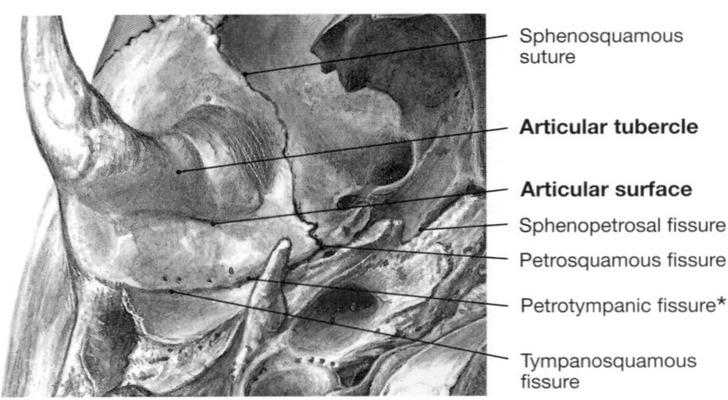
Sphenosquamous suture
Articular tubercle
Articular surface
Sphenopetrosal fissure
Petrosquamous fissure
Petrotympanic fissure*
Tympanosquamous fissure

**Fig. 8.56 Fossa and tubercle of the temporomandibular joint, right side;** inferior view.
View onto the articular surface of the mandibular fossa, which is normally covered with hyaline articular cartilage. Also covered by hyaline cartilage, the articular tubercle is located anterior to the mandibular fossa. In the posterior third of the mandibular fossa, the squamous part connects with the petrous part of the temporal bone, and medially the temporal bone borders at the sphenoidal bone. As a result, this region contains **three fissures:**
- In a lateral position the tympanosquamous fissure is visible.
- In the middle lies the petrotympanic fissure (* GLASERIAN fissure).
- Medially runs the sphenopetrous fissure through which the chorda tympani leaves the cranial basis.

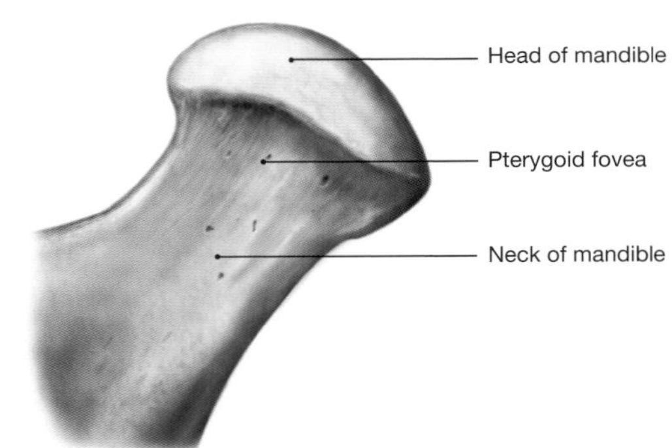
Head of mandible
Pterygoid fovea
Neck of mandible

**Fig. 8.57 Articular process, condylary process, of the lower jaw, right side;** frontal view.
The condylary process is composed of the head and neck of mandible. At the frontal side, it contains the pterygoid fovea. Here, the lateral pterygoid attaches with its inferior head.

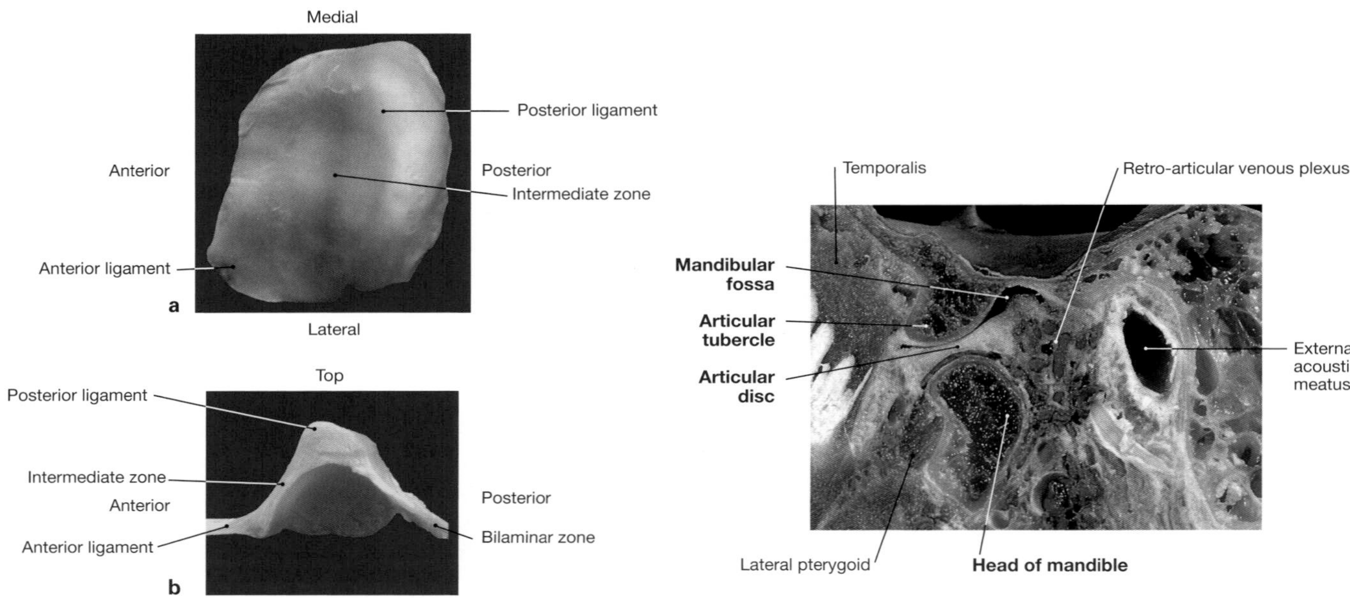
Medial
Posterior ligament
Anterior
Posterior
Intermediate zone
Anterior ligament
a
Lateral
Top
Posterior ligament
Intermediate zone
Anterior
Posterior
Anterior ligament
Bilaminar zone
b
Bottom
Temporalis
Retro-articular venous plexus
Mandibular fossa
Articular tubercle
Articular disc
External acoustic meatus
Lateral pterygoid
Head of mandible

**Figs. 8.58a and b Articular disc of the temporomandibular joint.**
**a** Superior view
**b** Lateral view
From front to back, the articular disc consists of an anterior ligament (connective tissue), an intermediate zone (fibrous cartilage), a posterior ligament (connective tissue), and a bilaminar zone (connective tissue). In its lateral part, the intermediate zone is particularly thin.

**Fig. 8.59 Temporomandibular joint;** sagittal section at the level of the temporomandibular joint region with injected veins (colored); lateral view. [1]
The bilaminar zone between the articular tubercle and head of mandible is visible. The bony septum between the middle cranial fossa and the mandibular fossa is thin. Among the connective tissue of the bilaminar zone lies an extensive **retro-articular venous plexus.** Close proximity exists to the external acoustic meatus.

### Clinical Remarks

Significant external force can result in the fracture of the neck of mandible **(condylar fracture).** An involvement of the joint capsule and the occurence of dislocated bone fragments is possible in such fractures. In addition, bleeding from the retro-articular venous plexus (→ Fig. 8.59) and/or painful sensations from the external acoustic meatus may occur. The temporomandibular joint is a diathrosis. Thus, this joint can be afflicted by the same diseases that also affect the large joints of the limbs, e.g. arthrosis or rheumatoid arthritis. In case of an **arthrosis of the temporomandibular joint,** the lateral part of the articular disc is mostly affected.

## Temporomandibular joint, radiography

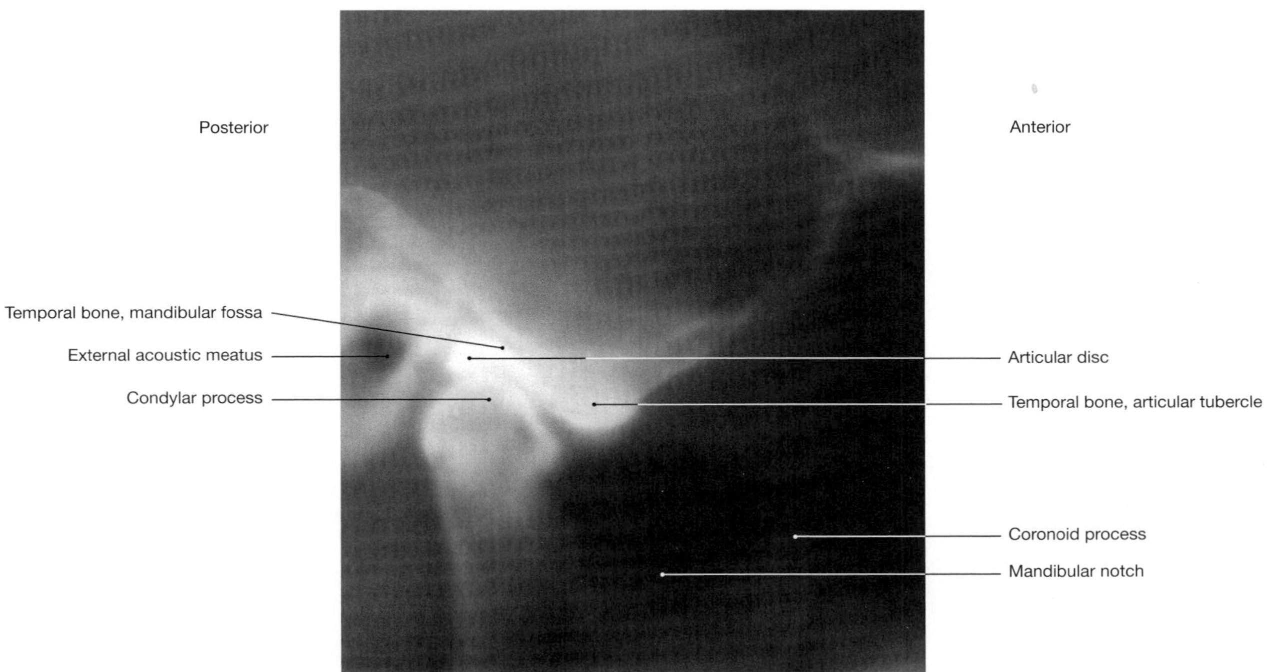
Posterior
Anterior
Temporal bone, mandibular fossa
External acoustic meatus
Condylar process
Articular disc
Temporal bone, articular tubercle
Coronoid process
Mandibular notch

**Fig. 8.60 Temporomandibular joint;** computed tomographic image in lateral beam projection; mouth closed.

With the mouth closed and masticatory muscles relaxed, the condylar process resides in the mandibular fossa.

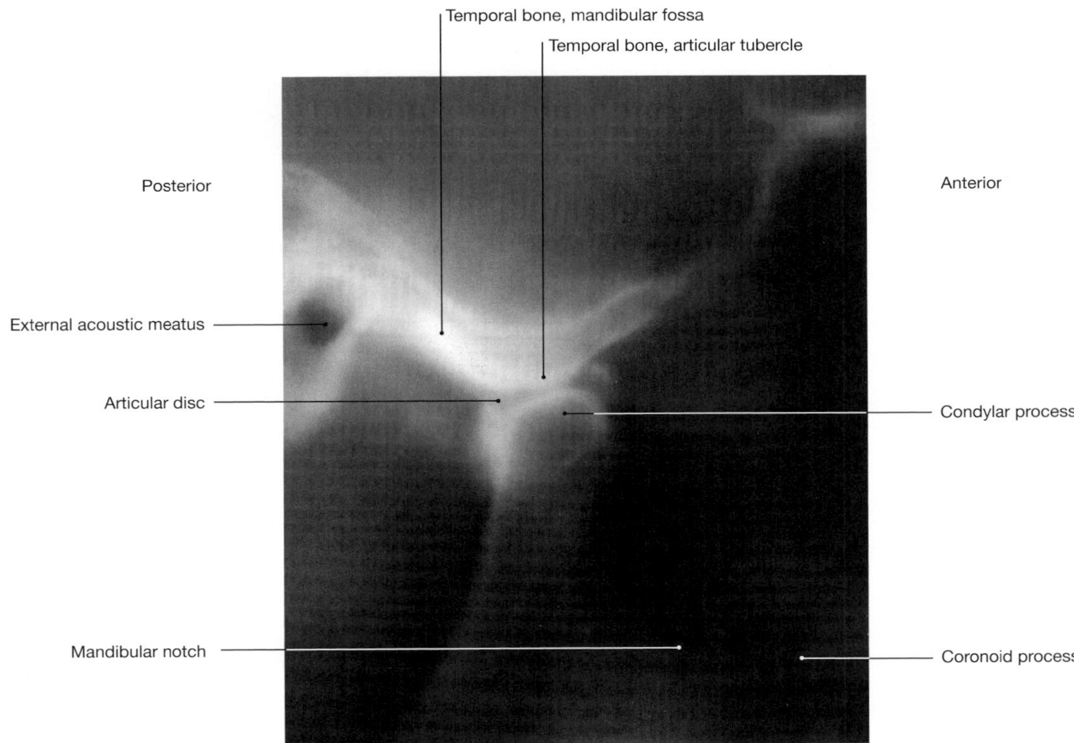
Temporal bone, mandibular fossa
Temporal bone, articular tubercle
Posterior
Anterior
External acoustic meatus
Articular disc
Condylar process
Mandibular notch
Coronoid process

**Fig. 8.61 Temporomandibular joint;** computed tomographic image in lateral beam projection; mouth open.

With the mouth open, the articular disc and the condylar process move forward onto the articular tubercle.

## Facial muscles

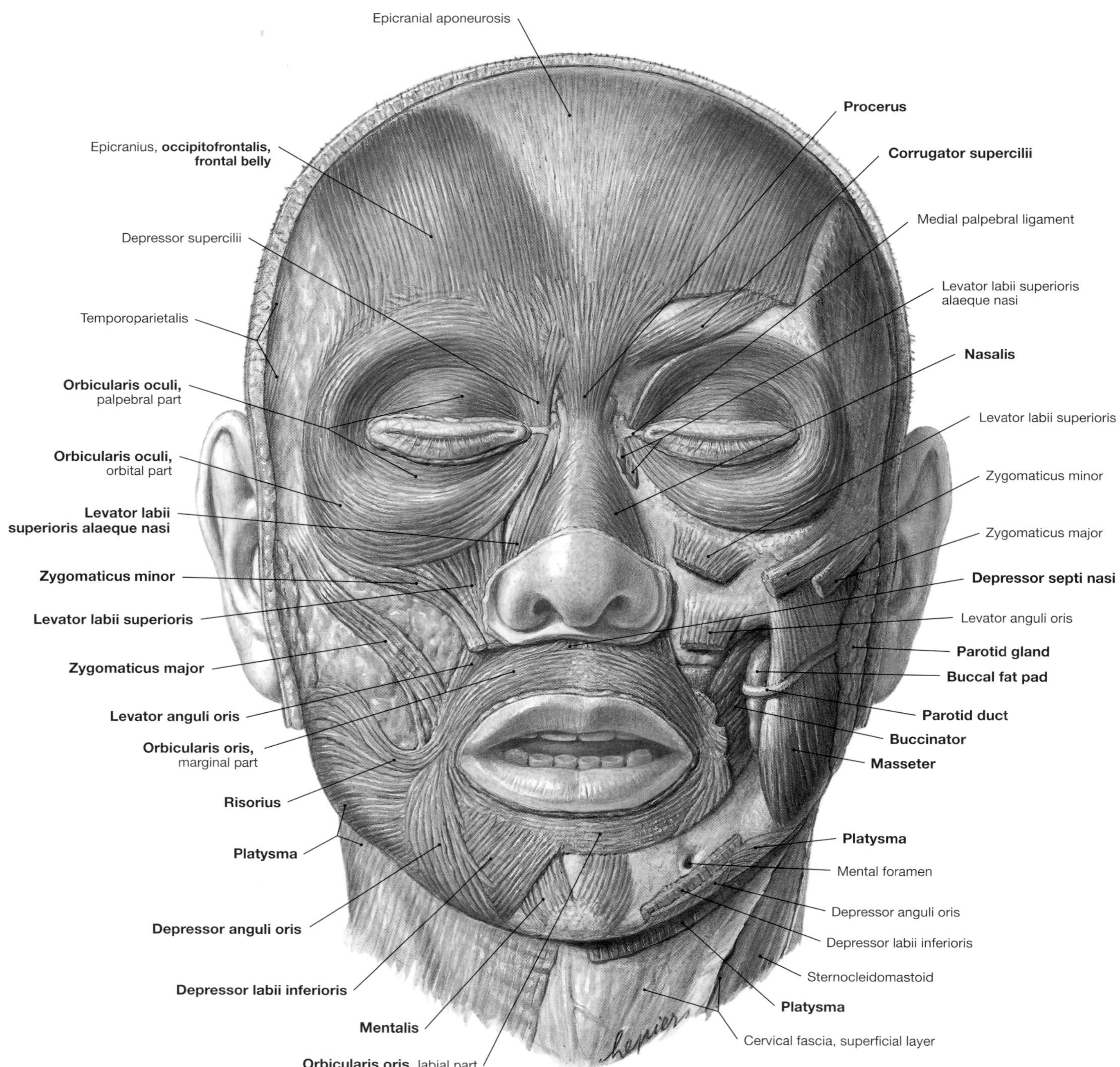
Epicranial aponeurosis
Procerus
Corrugator supercilii
Medial palpebral ligament
Levator labii superioris alaeque nasi
Nasalis
Levator labii superioris
Zygomaticus minor
Zygomaticus major
Depressor septi nasi
Levator anguli oris
Parotid gland
Buccal fat pad
Parotid duct
Buccinator
Masseter
Platysma
Mental foramen
Depressor anguli oris
Depressor labii inferioris
Sternocleidomastoid
Platysma
Cervical fascia, superficial layer
Epicranius, occipitofrontalis, frontal belly
Depressor supercilii
Temporoparietalis
Orbicularis oculi, palpebral part
Orbicularis oculi, orbital part
Levator labii superioris alaeque nasi
Zygomaticus minor
Levator labii superioris
Zygomaticus major
Levator anguli oris
Orbicularis oris, marginal part
Risorius
Platysma
Depressor anguli oris
Depressor labii inferioris
Mentalis
Orbicularis oris, labial part

**Fig. 8.62 Facial muscles and masticatory muscles;** frontal view.
Mimic muscles determine the facial expression and create the individual appearance of a facial physiognomy of a person. The muscles around the eye have important protective functions, while the muscles in the region of the mouth serve in food uptake and articulation.
Visible on both sides of the face are the frontal belly of the occipitofrontalis (epicranius), the orbital and palpebral parts of the orbicularis oculi (lacrimal part → Fig. 9.19), the corrugator supercilii, procerus, nasalis, depressor septi nasi, levator labii superioris alaeque nasi, the orbicularis oris with a labial and marginal part, the buccinator, zygomatici major and minor, risorius, levator labii superioris, levator anguli oris, depressor anguli oris, depressor labii inferioris and mentalis as well as the platysma projecting onto the neck.

Of the masticatory muscles, only the masseter on the left side of the face is shown. The parotid duct (STENSON's duct) of the parotid gland passes across the masseter and bends around its frontal edge in an almost right angle to penetrate the buccinator. A buccal fat pad (BICHAT's fat pad) is located between the masseter and buccinator and contributes to the contour of the region of the cheek. With the exception of the buccinator, the facial muscles do not contain a fascia. The fasciae of the buccinator, the masseter, and the parotid gland have been removed.

→ T 1a, c–f, 4

## Facial muscles

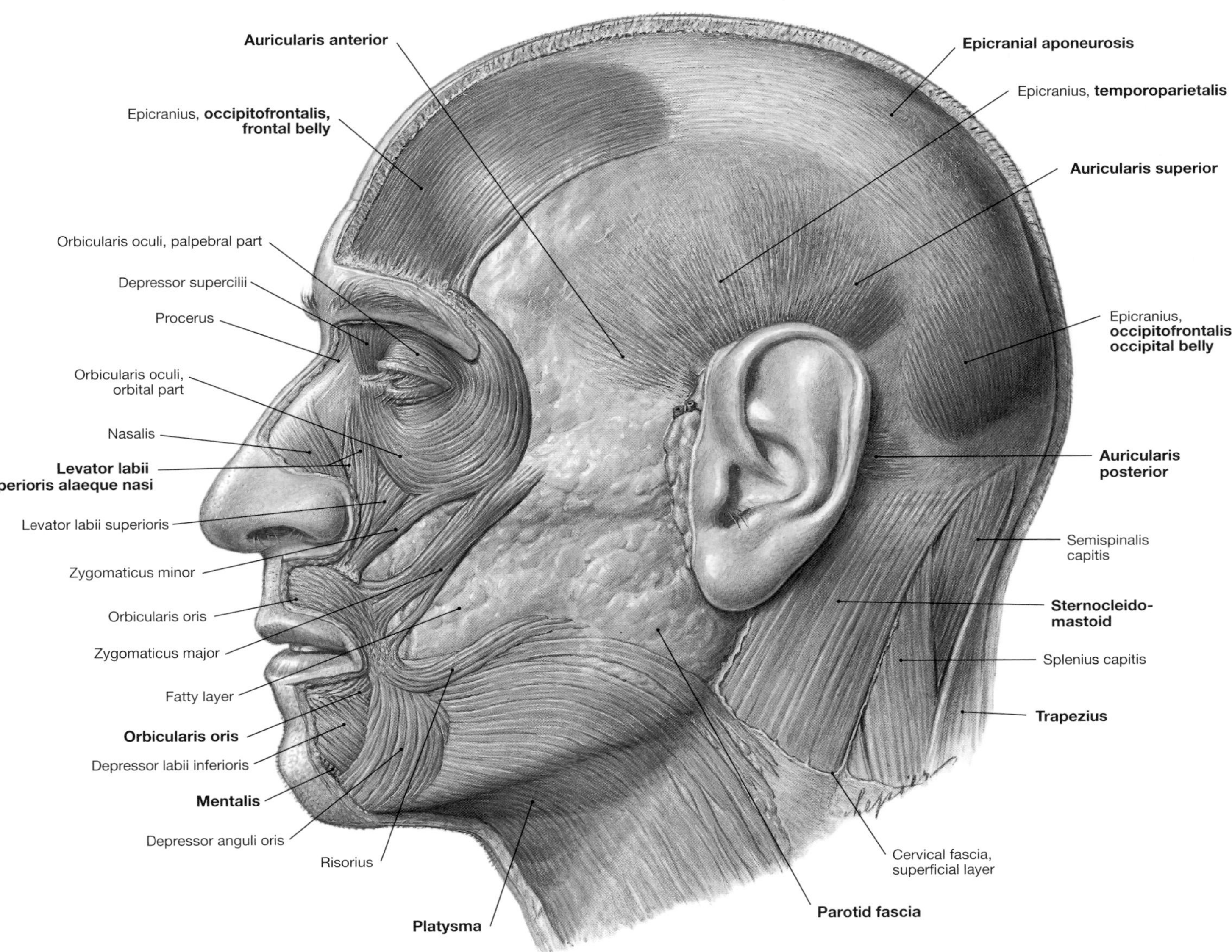
Auricularis anterior
Epicranial aponeurosis
Epicranius, temporoparietalis
Epicranius, occipitofrontalis, frontal belly
Auricularis superior
Orbicularis oculi, palpebral part
Depressor supercilii
Procerus
Epicranius, occipitofrontalis occipital belly
Orbicularis oculi, orbital part
Nasalis
Levator labii superioris alaeque nasi
Auricularis posterior
Levator labii superioris
Semispinalis capitis
Zygomaticus minor
Orbicularis oris
Sternocleido-mastoid
Zygomaticus major
Splenius capitis
Fatty layer
Trapezius
Orbicularis oris
Depressor labii inferioris
Mentalis
Depressor anguli oris
Risorius
Cervical fascia, superficial layer
Platysma
Parotid fascia

**Fig. 8.63 Facial muscles, left side;** lateral view.
In addition to the muscles displayed in → Figure 8.62, this lateral view also shows the occipital belly of the occipitofrontalis (epicranius) with the epicranial aponeurosis extending between the frontal and occipital belly. Located above the ear and also projecting into the epicranial aponeurosis is the temporoparietalis (also a part of the epicranius) which originates from the temporal fascia. Additional mimetic muscles are also shown and include the auriculares anterior, superior, and posterior. In the neck region, parts of the sternocleidomastoid, the trapezius, and some autochthonous muscles of the back are visible.

→T 1

## Clinical Remarks

**Paralysis of the orbicularis oculi** as part of a paresis of the facial nerve [VII] (facial palsy) results in the inability to voluntarily close the eyelid, causing it to stay open even during sleep (paralytic **lagophthalmos,** → Fig. 12.151). Due to lack of tension, the lower eyelid becomes flaccid and hangs down **(paralytic ectropion).** The inferior canaliculus fails to drain the lacrimal fluid from the eye. Instead, the fluid passes over the everted lower eyelid onto the cheek (drooping eye, **epiphora**). The inability to blink the eye causes the cornea to dry out and results in corneal lesions **(keratitis)** and an opaque cornea. The decrease in tension in the lower eyelid at an advanced age can lead to the so-called **senile ectropion.**
**Paralysis of the orbicularis oris** (also in the context of a facial palsy) results in speech disabilities. The corner of the mouth on the paralysed side hangs down and saliva involuntarily droops from the mouth.

## Facial and masticatory muscles

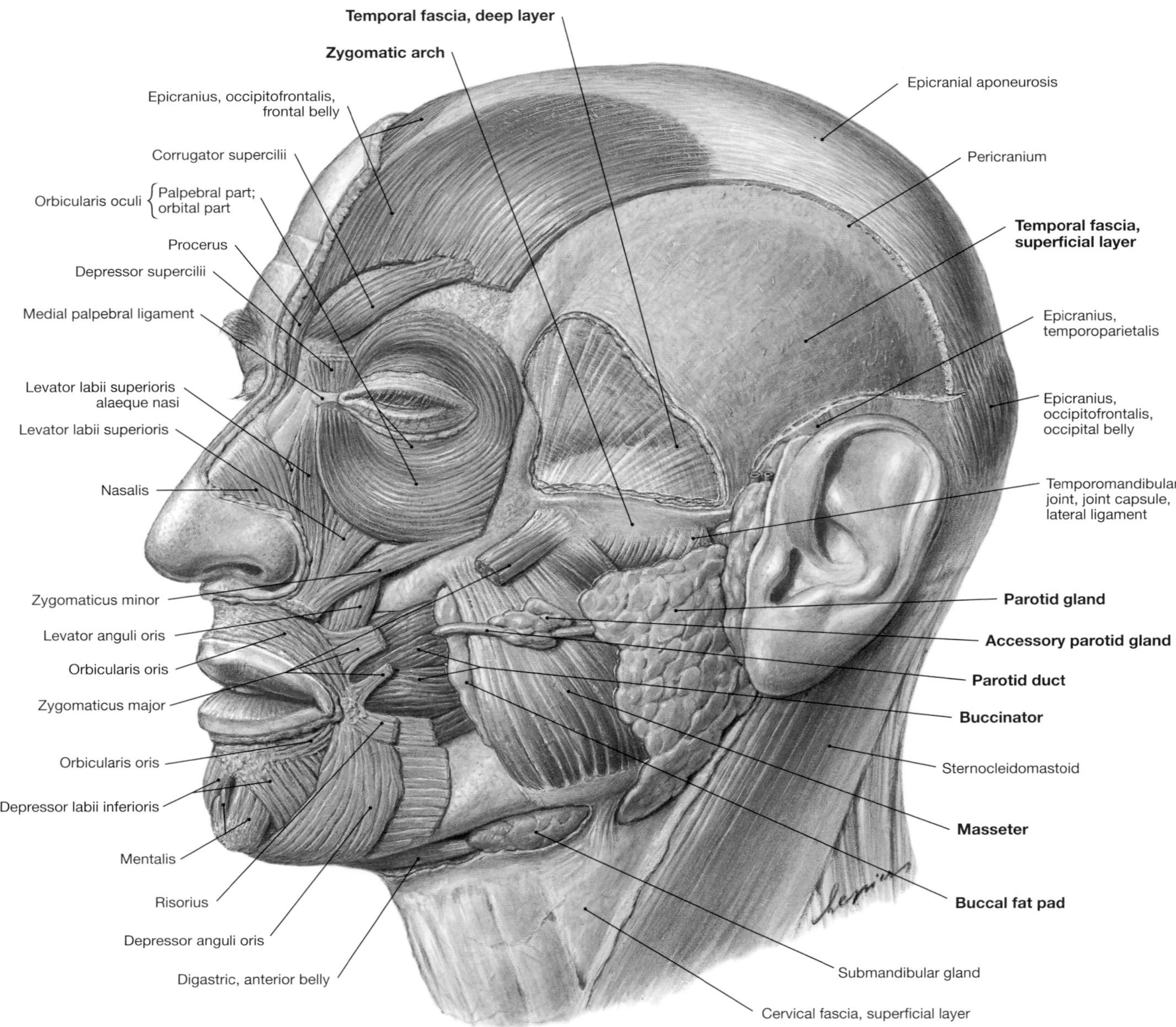
Temporal fascia, deep layer
Zygomatic arch
Epicranius, occipitofrontalis, frontal belly
Corrugator supercilii
Orbicularis oculi {Palpebral part; orbital part
Procerus
Depressor supercilii
Medial palpebral ligament
Levator labii superioris alaeque nasi
Levator labii superioris
Nasalis
Zygomaticus minor
Levator anguli oris
Orbicularis oris
Zygomaticus major
Orbicularis oris
Depressor labii inferioris
Mentalis
Risorius
Depressor anguli oris
Digastric, anterior belly
Epicranial aponeurosis
Pericranium
Temporal fascia, superficial layer
Epicranius, temporoparietalis
Epicranius, occipitofrontalis, occipital belly
Temporomandibular joint, joint capsule, lateral ligament
Parotid gland
Accessory parotid gland
Parotid duct
Buccinator
Sternocleidomastoid
Masseter
Buccal fat pad
Submandibular gland
Cervical fascia, superficial layer

**Fig. 8.64 Facial muscles and masticatory muscles;** lateral view from an oblique angle.
The fascia of the buccinator, the masseter, the parotid gland as well as part of the superficial fascia of the neck were removed. As a result, the corresponding muscles, the parotid gland extending to the neck, and the submandibular gland become visible. The major excretory duct of the parotid gland, the parotid duct (STENSEN's duct), exits the gland at its anterior pole, crosses the **masseter** in a horizontal line from posterior to anterior and, at the anterior margin of the masseter, bends inwards in an almost perfect right angle to penetrate the **buccinator.** Between the buccinator and masseter lies the buccal fat pad (BICHAT's fat pad). Associated with the parotid duct is accessory glandular tissue (accessory parotid gland).
In the temporal region, the parietoparietalis of the epicranius was removed. This allows a clear view onto the superficial lamina of the temporal fascia.
Above the zygomatic arch parts of the superficial lamina and the temporal fat pad underneath were removed to permit a clear view onto the deep lamina of the temporal fascia with the temporalis shining through.

→T 1, 4

## Clinical Remarks

**Swelling of the parotid gland** (e.g. in the case of an epidemic parotitis [mumps], → p. 90) can cause severe pain sensations because of the close proximity of the parotid gland to the masticatory muscles and the fact that the parotid gland and the masseter share a mutual fascia (parotideomasseteric fascia). Often, the pain also involves the external acoustic meatus and is aggravated by palpating the tragus or the auricle (tragus pain).

Patients with a malignant tumor disease **(tumor cachexia)** or suffering from advanced stages of HIV infection are often emaciated. The BICHAT's fat pad which models the typical contour of the cheeks is wasting and gives way to the emaciated cheeks in these patients.

## Facial and masticatory muscles

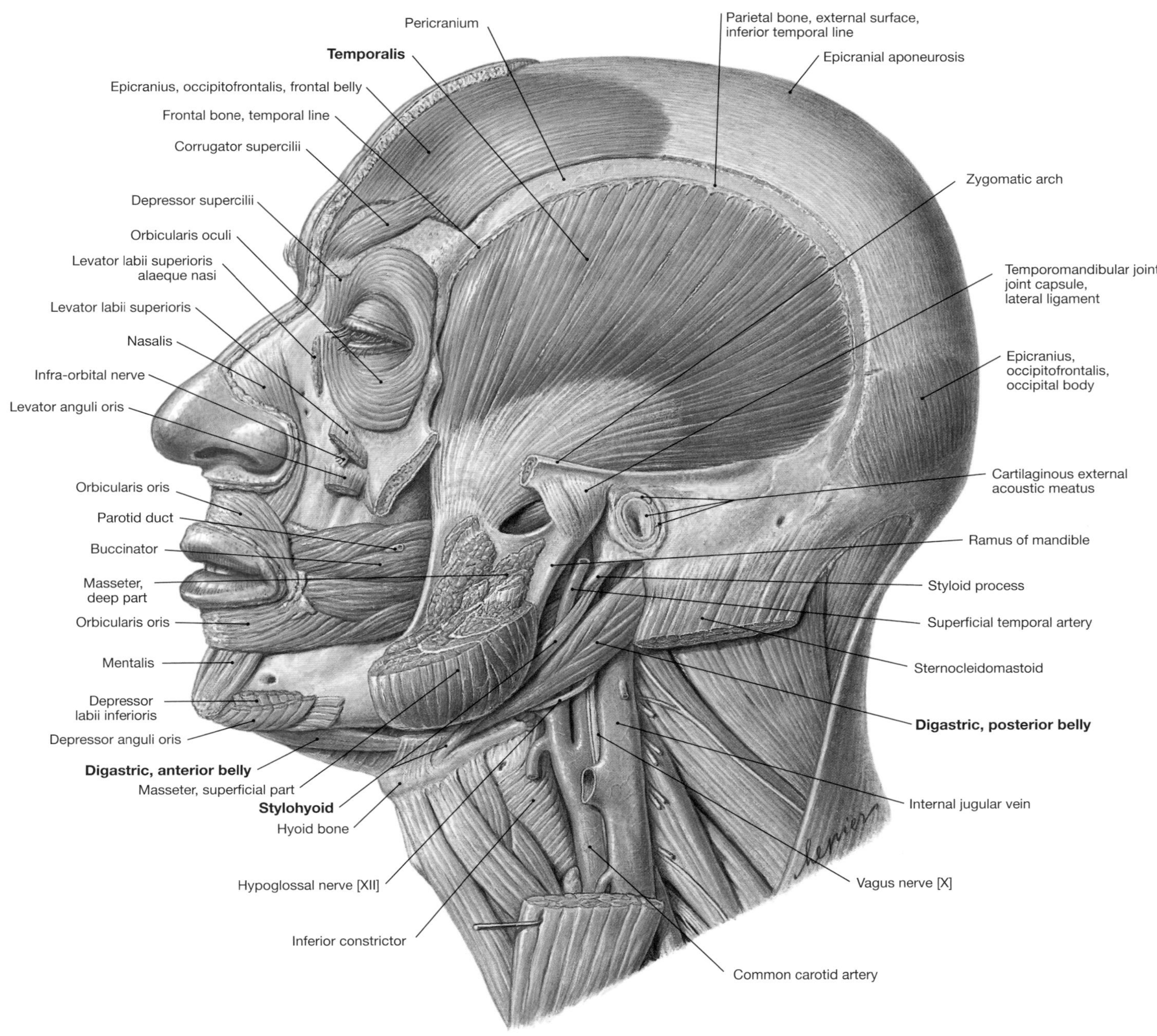
Pericranium
Temporalis
Epicranius, occipitofrontalis, frontal belly
Frontal bone, temporal line
Corrugator supercilii
Depressor supercilii
Orbicularis oculi
Levator labii superioris alaeque nasi
Levator labii superioris
Nasalis
Infra-orbital nerve
Levator anguli oris
Orbicularis oris
Parotid duct
Buccinator
Masseter, deep part
Orbicularis oris
Mentalis
Depressor labii inferioris
Depressor anguli oris
Digastric, anterior belly
Masseter, superficial part
Stylohyoid
Hyoid bone
Hypoglossal nerve [XII]
Inferior constrictor
Parietal bone, external surface, inferior temporal line
Epicranial aponeurosis
Zygomatic arch
Temporomandibular joint, joint capsule, lateral ligament
Epicranius, occipitofrontalis, occipital body
Cartilaginous external acoustic meatus
Ramus of mandible
Styloid process
Superficial temporal artery
Sternocleidomastoid
Digastric, posterior belly
Internal jugular vein
Vagus nerve [X]
Common carotid artery

**Fig. 8.65 Facial muscles and masticatory muscles, left side;** lateral view.
Upon removal of the superficial and the deep laminae of the temporal fascia and the partial removal of the zygomatic arch and parts of the masseter, the **temporalis** becomes visible.
The origin of the temporalis along the inferior temporal line of the external surface of the parietal bone and the temporal line of the frontal bone are shown. The muscle fibers converge into a flat tendon that disappears in the infratemporal fossa behind the zygomatic arch and inserts at the coronoid process.

**Origins of the temporalis:**
- inferior temporal line of the external surface of the parietal bone
- temporal surface of the frontal bone
- temporal surface, squamous part of the temporal bone
- temporal surface of the zygomatic bone
- temporal surface of the sphenoidal bone up to the infratemporal crest

The image also displays a few suprahyal muscles (digastric with anterior belly and posterior belly, stylohyoid).

→T 1, 4

## Masticatory muscles

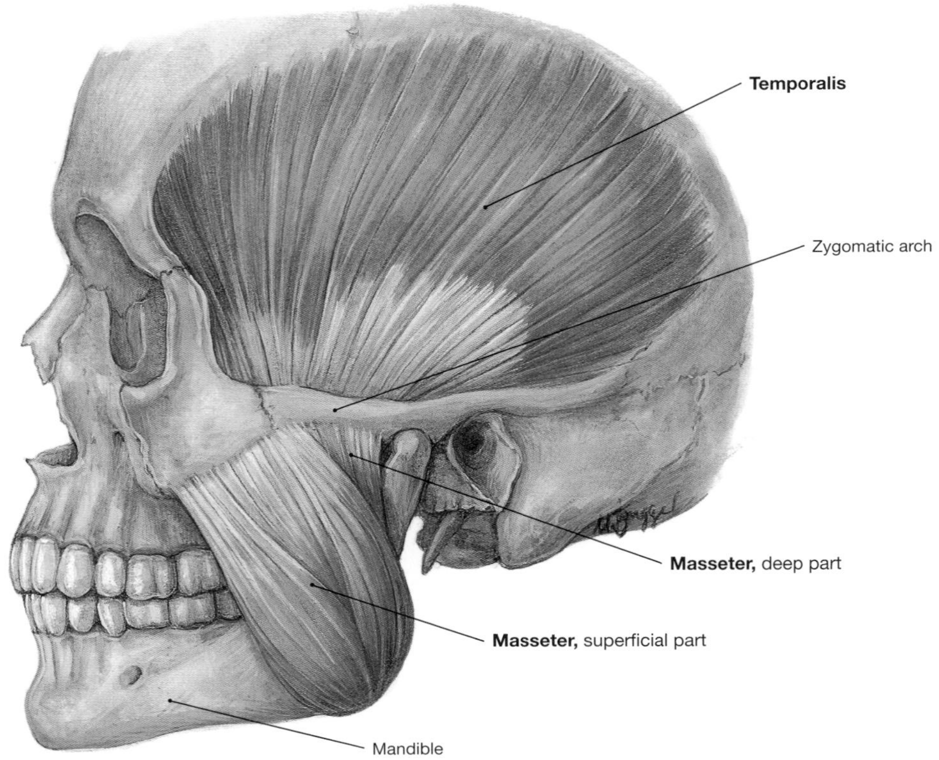
Temporalis
Zygomatic arch
Masseter, deep part
Masseter, superficial part
Mandible

**Fig. 8.66 Masseter and temporalis, left side;** lateral view.
The **masseter** consists of a superficial part and a deep part.

→T 4

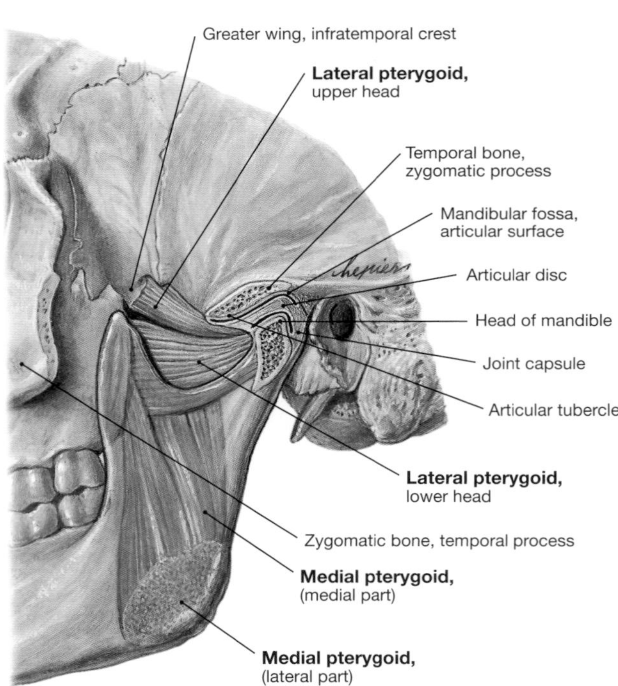
Greater wing, infratemporal crest
Lateral pterygoid, upper head
Temporal bone, zygomatic process
Mandibular fossa, articular surface
Articular disc
Head of mandible
Joint capsule
Articular tubercle
Lateral pterygoid, lower head
Zygomatic bone, temporal process
Medial pterygoid, (medial part)

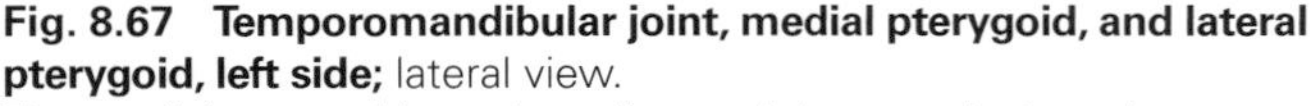
Medial pterygoid, (lateral part)

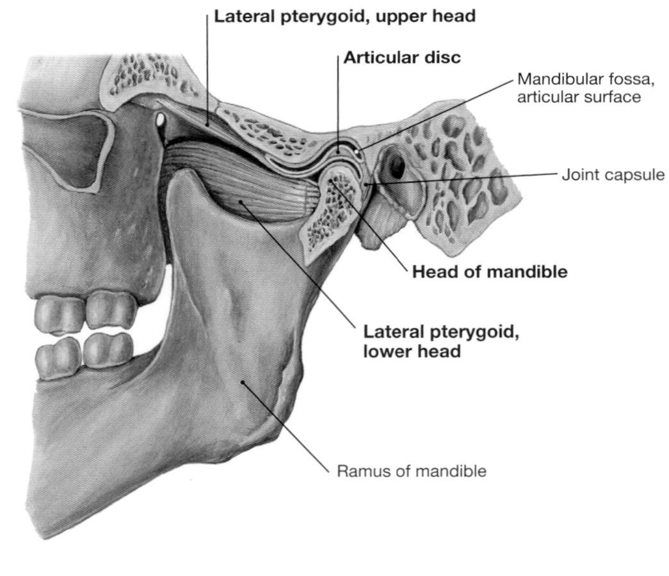
Lateral pterygoid, upper head
Articular disc
Mandibular fossa, articular surface
Joint capsule
Head of mandible
Lateral pterygoid, lower head
Ramus of mandible

**Fig. 8.67 Temporomandibular joint, medial pterygoid, and lateral pterygoid, left side;** lateral view.
The medial pterygoid consists of a medial part and a lateral part.

→T 4

**Fig. 8.68 Temporomandibular joint and relationship to the lateral pterygoid, left side;** lateral view.
The lateral pterygoid consists of an upper head and a lower head (→ Fig. 8.67).

## Masticatory muscles

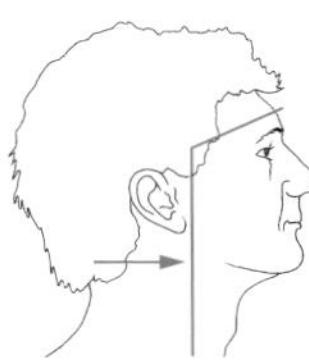

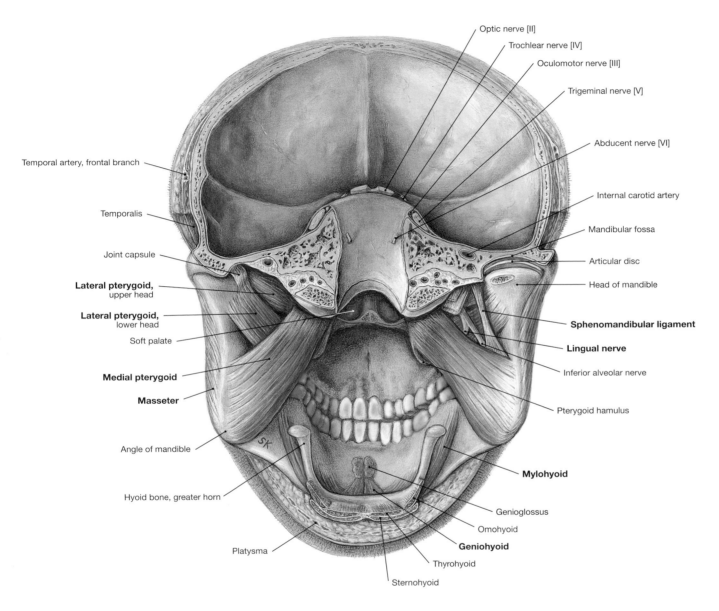

Optic nerve [II]
Trochlear nerve [IV]
Oculomotor nerve [III]
Trigeminal nerve [V]
Abducent nerve [VI]
Internal carotid artery
Mandibular fossa
Articular disc
Head of mandible
**Sphenomandibular ligament**
**Lingual nerve**
Inferior alveolar nerve
Pterygoid hamulus
**Mylohyoid**
Genioglossus
Omohyoid
**Geniohyoid**
Thyrohyoid
Sternohyoid
Temporal artery, frontal branch
Temporalis
Joint capsule
**Lateral pterygoid,** upper head
**Lateral pterygoid,** lower head
Soft palate
**Medial pterygoid**
**Masseter**
Angle of mandible
Hyoid bone, greater horn
Platysma

**Fig. 8.69 Masticatory muscles;** frontal section at the level of the temporomandibular joint and horizontal section of the skull cap; posterior view.
The bilateral insertion sites of the masseter and medial pterygoid at the angle of mandible are shown. The mandible is suspended by these muscles like a swing. On the right side, the sphenomandibular ligament between the lateral pterygoid and the medial pterygoid as well as the lingual nerve are visible.

→T 4

### Clinical Remarks

**Trismus** can make it impossible to open or close the mouth. Abscesses in the facial compartments of the masticatory muscles can result in the mouth being locked in a close position. Excessive yawning movements, extreme mouth opening, or accidents can cause a **lockjaw** with the mouth being locked in the open position.

## Vessels and nerves of head and neck

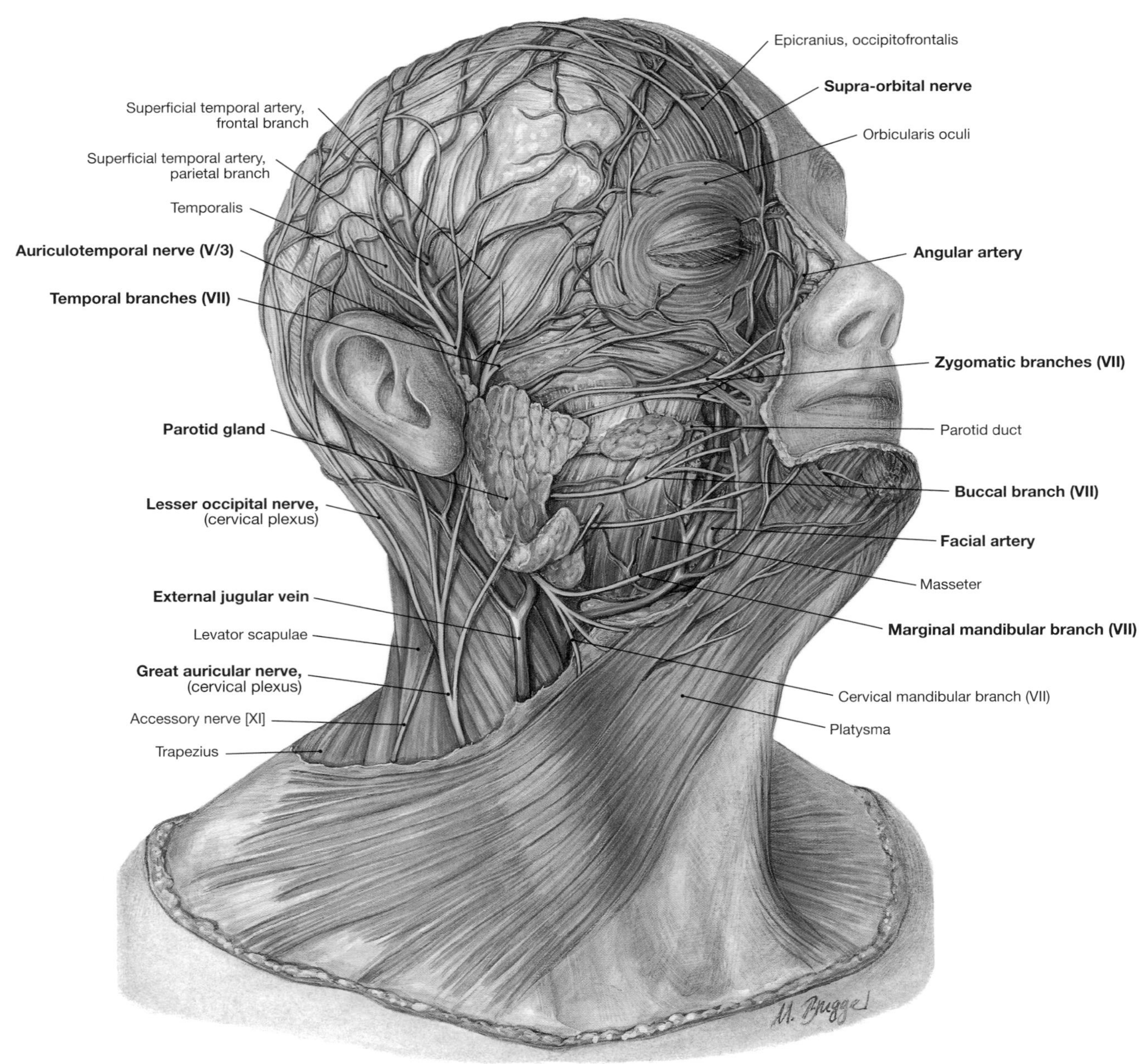
Epicranius, occipitofrontalis
Supra-orbital nerve
Orbicularis oculi
Superficial temporal artery, frontal branch
Superficial temporal artery, parietal branch
Temporalis
Auriculotemporal nerve (V/3)
Temporal branches (VII)
Angular artery
Zygomatic branches (VII)
Parotid gland
Parotid duct
Buccal branch (VII)
Lesser occipital nerve, (cervical plexus)
Facial artery
Masseter
External jugular vein
Marginal mandibular branch (VII)
Levator scapulae
Great auricular nerve, (cervical plexus)
Cervical mandibular branch (VII)
Accessory nerve [XI]
Platysma
Trapezius
M. Brugger

**Fig. 8.70 Vessels and nerves of head and neck, lateral superficial regions, right side;** lateral view.

Superficial arteries in the area of the face are the **facial artery** and its branches and the parietal branch and frontal branch of the **superficial temporal artery,** which originates from the external carotid artery in the lateral head region. The blood drains from here through identically named veins into the **external jugular vein.**

The terminal branches of the **facial nerve [VII]** are the superficial nerves radiating from the intraparotid plexus located within the parotid gland (temporal, zygomatic, buccal branches, marginal mandibular branch, cervical mandibular branch). In front of the auricle the **auriculotemporal nerve,** a branch of the trigeminal nerve [V], ascends. The **supra-orbital nerve,** also a branch of the trigeminal nerve [V], leaves the orbit and pierces the orbicularis oculi.

Neck and occiput receive sensory innervation from branches of the **cervical plexus** which largely derive from the punctum nervosum (ERB's point) at the posterior margin of the sternocleidomastoid: the transverse cervical nerve, greater auricular nerve, lesser occipital nerve, and supraclavicular nerves.

## Vessels and nerves of head and neck

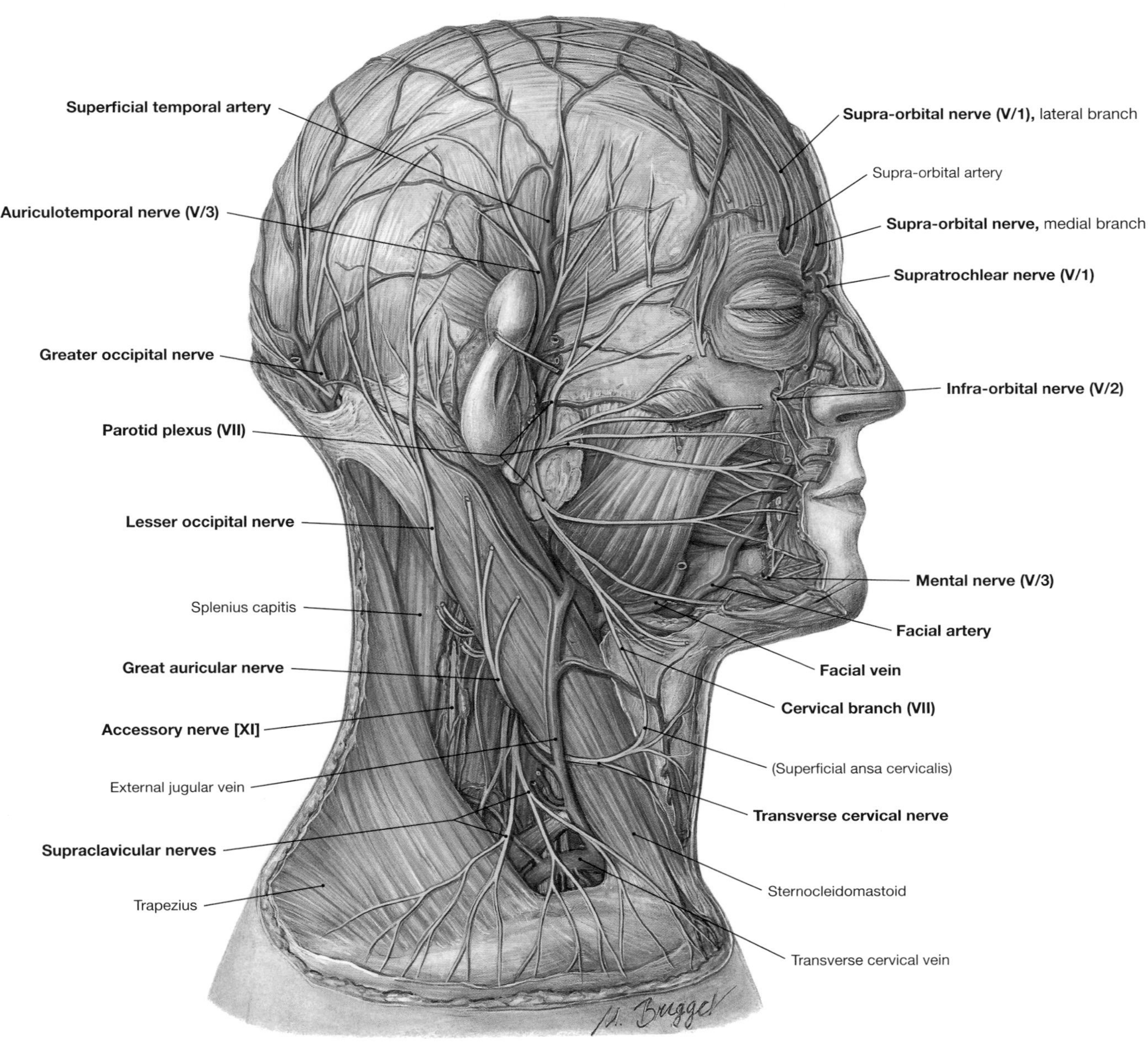
Superficial temporal artery
Auriculotemporal nerve (V/3)
Greater occipital nerve
Parotid plexus (VII)
Lesser occipital nerve
Splenius capitis
Great auricular nerve
Accessory nerve [XI]
External jugular vein
Supraclavicular nerves
Trapezius
Supra-orbital nerve (V/1), lateral branch
Supra-orbital artery
Supra-orbital nerve, medial branch
Supratrochlear nerve (V/1)
Infra-orbital nerve (V/2)
Mental nerve (V/3)
Facial artery
Facial vein
Cervical branch (VII)
(Superficial ansa cervicalis)
Transverse cervical nerve
Sternocleidomastoid
Transverse cervical vein

**Fig. 8.71 Vessels and nerves of the head and neck, lateral deep regions, right side;** lateral view.
Upon removal of the facial muscles and the superficial parts of the parotid gland, the course of the **facial artery** and the origin of the terminal branches of the facial nerve derived from the **infraparotid plexus** become visible. Also shown are the **terminal sensory branches of the trigeminal nerve [V]** which originate from its three parts:
- supraorbital and supratrochlear nerves (from ophthalmic nerve [V/1])
- infraorbital nerve (from maxillary nerve [V/2])
- mental nerve (from mandibular nerve [V/3])

In the lateral triangle of the neck at the posterior side of the sternocleidomastoid, the **four cervical branches** exit at the ERB's point:
- transverse cervical nerve
- great auricular nerve
- lesser occipital nerve
- supraclavicular nerves

The transverse cervical nerve receives motor fibers via the cervical branches of the facial nerve [VII] for the innervation of more distal parts of the platysma. Further, in the lateral triangle of the neck the **accessory nerve [XI]** runs from the posterior border of the sternocleidomastoid to the anterior border of the trapezius. The occiput receives sensory innervation through the **greater occipital nerve** (branch of the cervical plexus) and blood supply through the **occipital artery and vein.**

### Clinical Remarks

Extirpation of lymph nodes in the lateral triangle of the neck can result in **lesions of the accessory nerve [XI]** and partial palsy of the trapezius (almost always the trapezius is also innervated by the cervical plexus – in 6.4% of cases exclusively by this plexus) which results in shoulder dysfunctions.

## Vessels and nerves of the lateral facial region

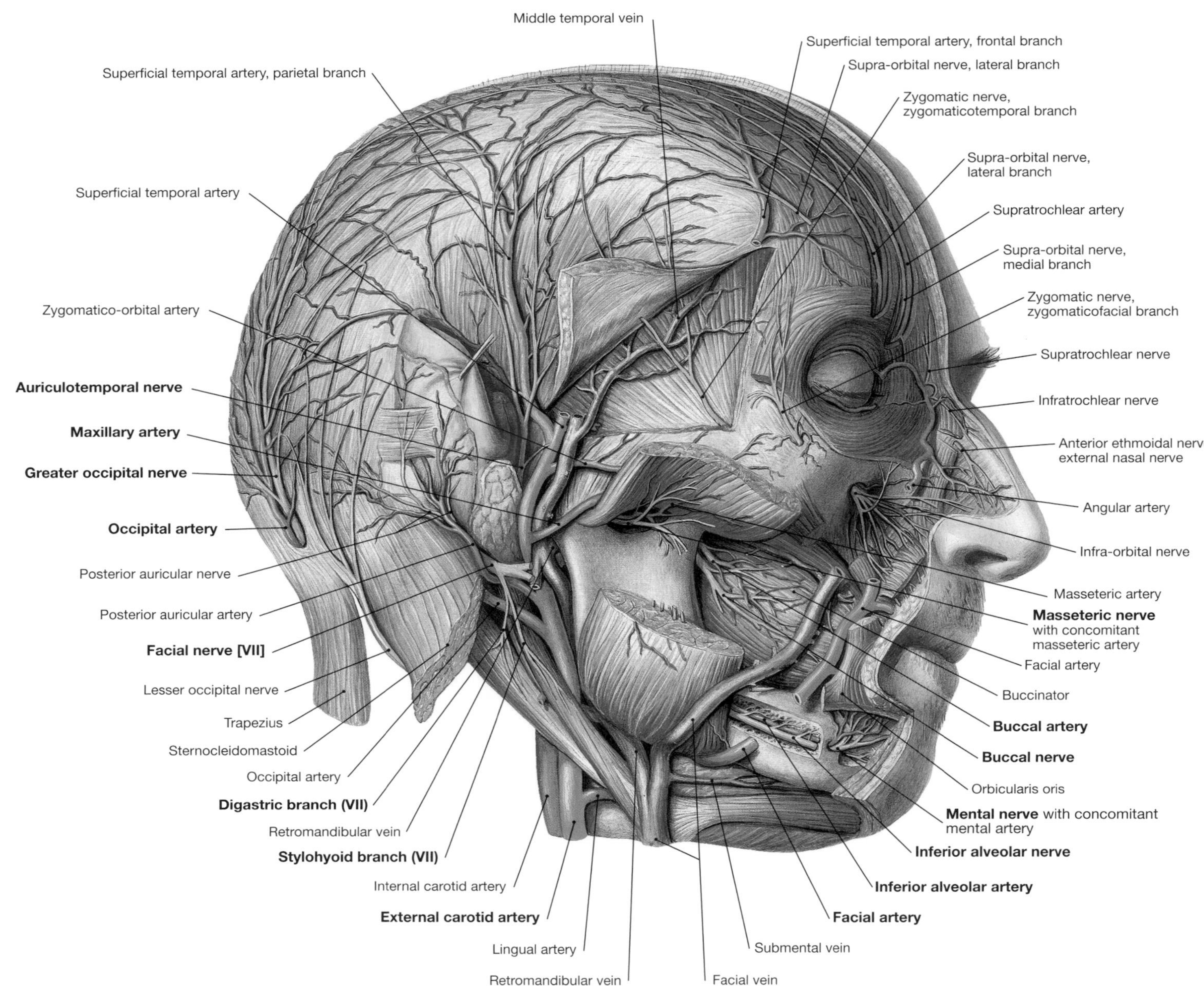
Middle temporal vein
Superficial temporal artery, frontal branch
Supra-orbital nerve, lateral branch
Superficial temporal artery, parietal branch
Zygomatic nerve, zygomaticotemporal branch
Supra-orbital nerve, lateral branch
Superficial temporal artery
Supratrochlear artery
Supra-orbital nerve, medial branch
Zygomatico-orbital artery
Zygomatic nerve, zygomaticofacial branch
Supratrochlear nerve
Auriculotemporal nerve
Infratrochlear nerve
Maxillary artery
Anterior ethmoidal nerve, external nasal nerve
Greater occipital nerve
Angular artery
Occipital artery
Infra-orbital nerve
Posterior auricular nerve
Masseteric artery
Posterior auricular artery
Masseteric nerve with concomitant masseteric artery
Facial nerve [VII]
Facial artery
Lesser occipital nerve
Buccinator
Trapezius
Buccal artery
Sternocleidomastoid
Buccal nerve
Occipital artery
Orbicularis oris
Digastric branch (VII)
Mental nerve with concomitant mental artery
Retromandibular vein
Stylohyoid branch (VII)
Inferior alveolar nerve
Internal carotid artery
Inferior alveolar artery
External carotid artery
Facial artery
Lingual artery
Submental vein
Retromandibular vein
Facial vein

**Fig. 8.72 Vessels and nerves of the head, lateral deep regions, right side;** lateral view.

Upon removal of large parts of the parotid gland, the structures of the **retromandibular fossa** in the deep lateral head region become visible. Below the auricle, the undivided stem of the **facial nerve [VII]** is visible. Shortly after exiting the stylomastoid foramen, the facial nerve [VII] provides branches to the digastric, posterior belly (digastric branch), to the stylohyoid (stylohyoid branch), and to the auricular muscles (posterior auricular nerve).

Beneath the digastric and stylohyoid, the internal and external carotid arteries ascend. Together with the retromandibular vein and the auriculotemporal nerve, the **external carotid artery** runs in the retromandibular fossa and branches into the occipital, posterior auricular, maxillary, and superficial temporal arteries as well as multiple small branches. The masseter was cut and folded backwards to demonstrate its supplying structures located on the back of this muscle (masseteric nerve – branch of the mandibular nerve [V/3]; masseteric artery – branch of the maxillary artery). These supplying structures reach this muscle through the mandibular notch. In the lower facial region, all mimic muscles were removed from the mandible; the mandibular canal, which runs within the bone from the mandibular foramen to the mental foramen, was opened up to display the **inferior alveolar nerve** and the corresponding artery. At the mental foramen, this nerve becomes the **mental nerve.** Below the orbit, the facial artery was partly removed. This artery continues as angular artery below the eye and in the orbit it anastomoses with branches of the ophthalmic artery. On top of the buccinator, the sensory **buccal nerve,** a branch of the mandibular nerve [V/3], is visible.

## Maxillary artery

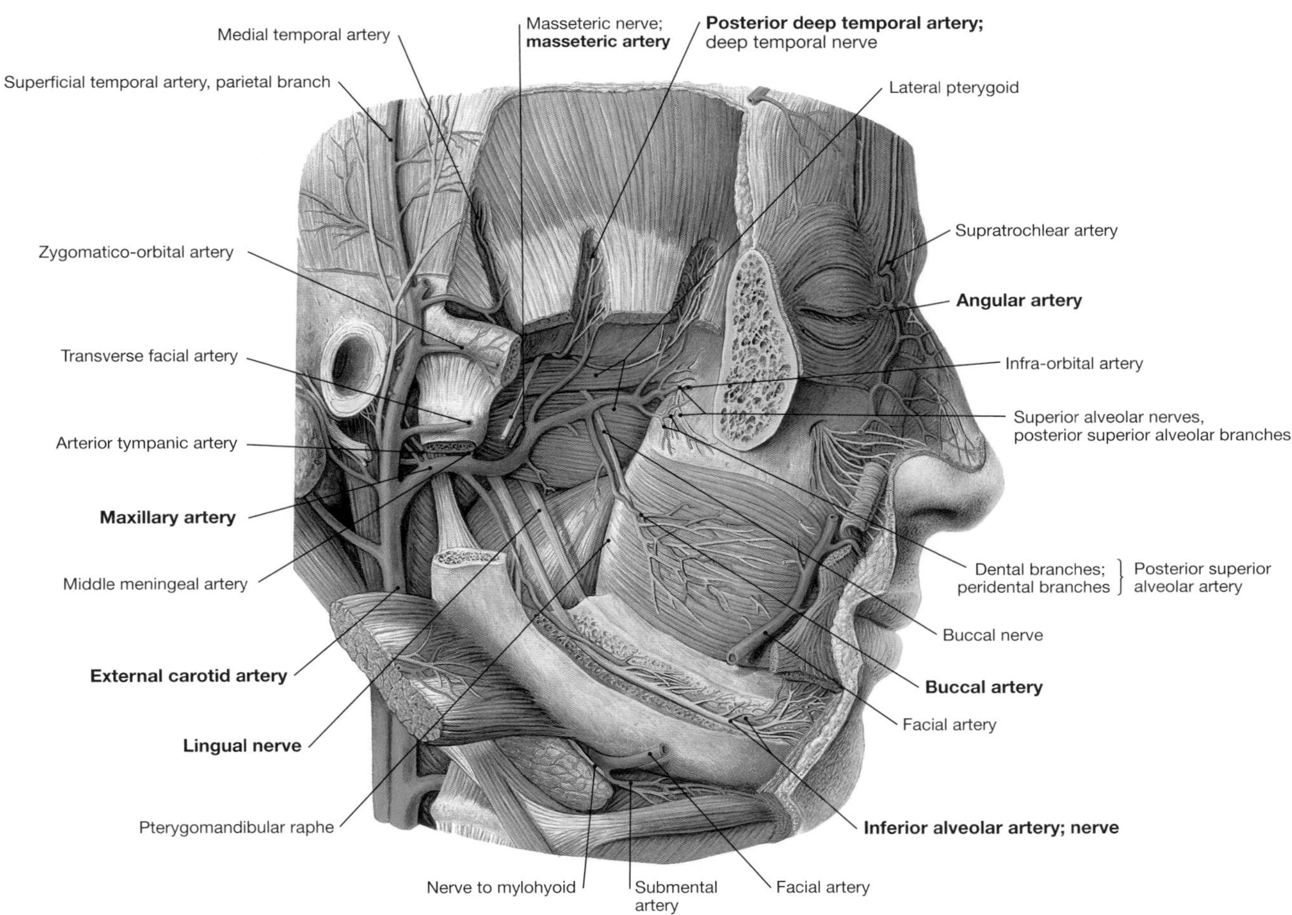
Medial temporal artery
Masseteric nerve; masseteric artery
Posterior deep temporal artery; deep temporal nerve
Superficial temporal artery, parietal branch
Lateral pterygoid
Supratrochlear artery
Zygomatico-orbital artery
Angular artery
Transverse facial artery
Infra-orbital artery
Superior alveolar nerves, posterior superior alveolar branches
Anterior tympanic artery
Maxillary artery
Dental branches; peridental branches
Posterior superior alveolar artery
Middle meningeal artery
Buccal nerve
External carotid artery
Buccal artery
Facial artery
Lingual nerve
Inferior alveolar artery; nerve
Pterygomandibular raphe
Nerve to mylohyoid
Submental artery
Facial artery

**Fig. 8.73 Arteries and nerves of the head, lateral deep regions, right side;** lateral view.
In most cases, the **maxillary artery** courses behind the ramus of mandible. Only rarely does the artery run laterally to the ramus. The maxillary artery continues through the masticatory muscles, supplies these muscles with blood, and provides branches to the buccinator and the mandible. Its terminal branches reach the orbit, nose, maxilla, and palate. The **external carotid artery** and its branches course through the retromandibular fossa. The facial artery was removed at the level of the body of mandible. Normally, the pulse of the facial artery is palpable where it bends around the edge of the mandible.

| Branches of the Maxillary Artery | |
|---|---|
| **Retromandibular part** | • Deep auricular artery<br>• Anterior tympanic artery<br>• Inferior alveolar artery<br>– dental branches<br>– peridental branches<br>– mental branch<br>– mylohyoid branch<br>• Medial meningeal artery<br>• Pterygomeningeal artery |
| **Intermuscular part** | • Masseteric artery<br>• Anterior deep temporal artery<br>• Posterior deep temporal artery<br>• Pterygoid branches<br>• Buccal artery |
| **Sphenopalatine part** | • Posterior superior alveolar artery<br>– dental branches<br>– peridental branches<br>• Infraorbital artery<br>– anterior superior alveolar arteries<br>– dental branches<br>– peridental branches<br>• Artery of pterygoid canal<br>• Descending palatine artery<br>• Sphenopalatine artery |

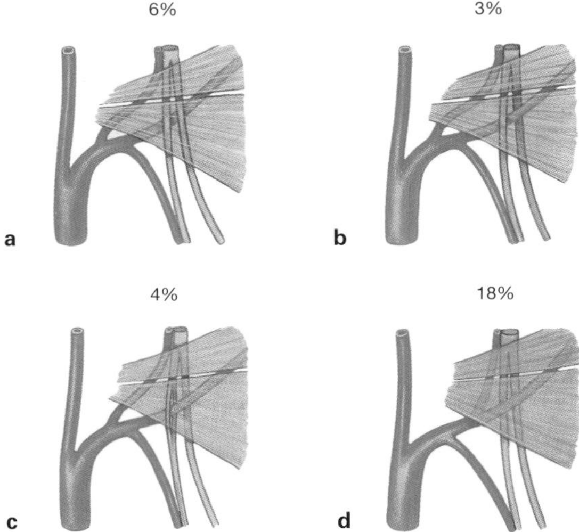
6%
3%
a
b
4%
18%
c
d

**Figs. 8.74a to d Variations of the course of the maxillary artery.**
**a** Course of the maxillary artery medial of the lateral pterygoid and medial to the lingual and inferior alveolar nerve
**b** Course of the maxillary artery between the lingual nerve and the inferior alveolar nerve
**c** Course of the maxillary artery through a loop of the inferior alveolar nerve
**d** Branching of the medial meningeal artery distal of the bifurcation of the inferior alveolar artery

## Pterygoid plexus

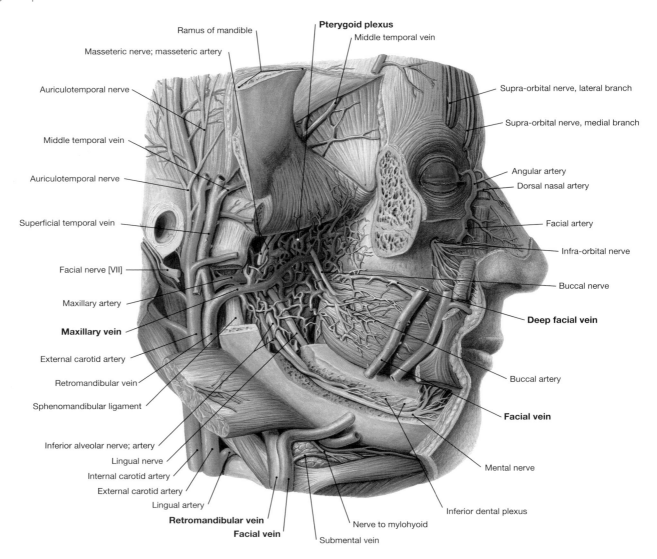

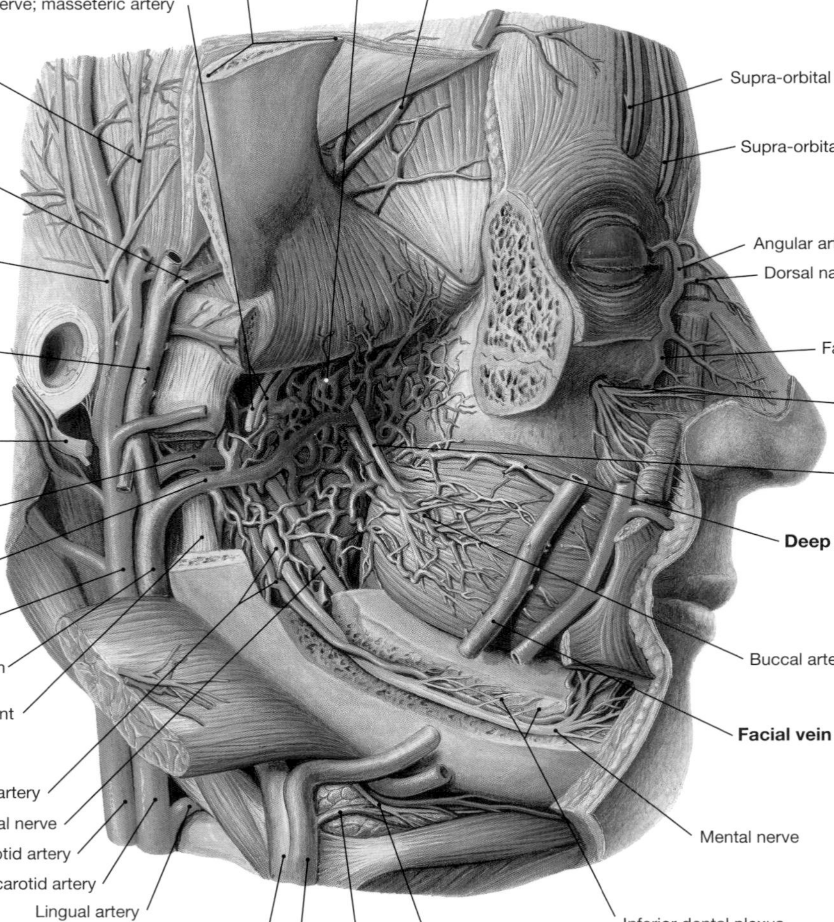

**Fig. 8.75 Vessels and nerves of the head, lateral deep regions, right side;** lateral view.

The **pterygoid plexus** drains the venous blood in the region of the masticatory muscles and releases it mainly into the maxillary vein. The pterygoid plexus also connects with the facial vein via the deep facial vein and with the cavernous sinus via the inferior ophthalmic vein.

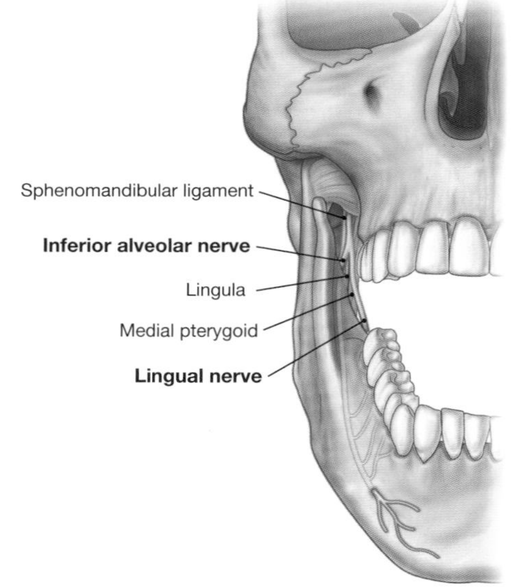
Sphenomandibular ligament
Inferior alveolar nerve
Lingula
Medial pterygoid
Lingual nerve

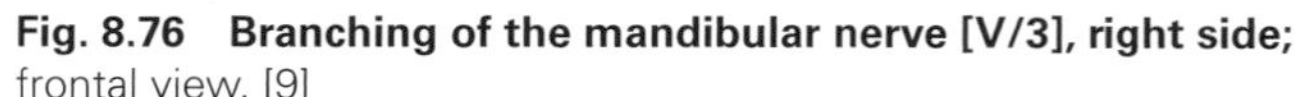

**Fig. 8.76 Branching of the mandibular nerve [V/3], right side;** frontal view. [9]

The branching of the mandibular nerve [V/3] (→ Fig. 12.144) into the **lingual nerve** and **inferior alveolar nerve** normally occurs between the sphenomandibular ligament and the medial part of the medial pterygoid. Then the inferior alveolar nerve turns lateral and enters the mandibular canal lateral of the sphenomandibular ligament.

## Mandibular nerve [V/3]

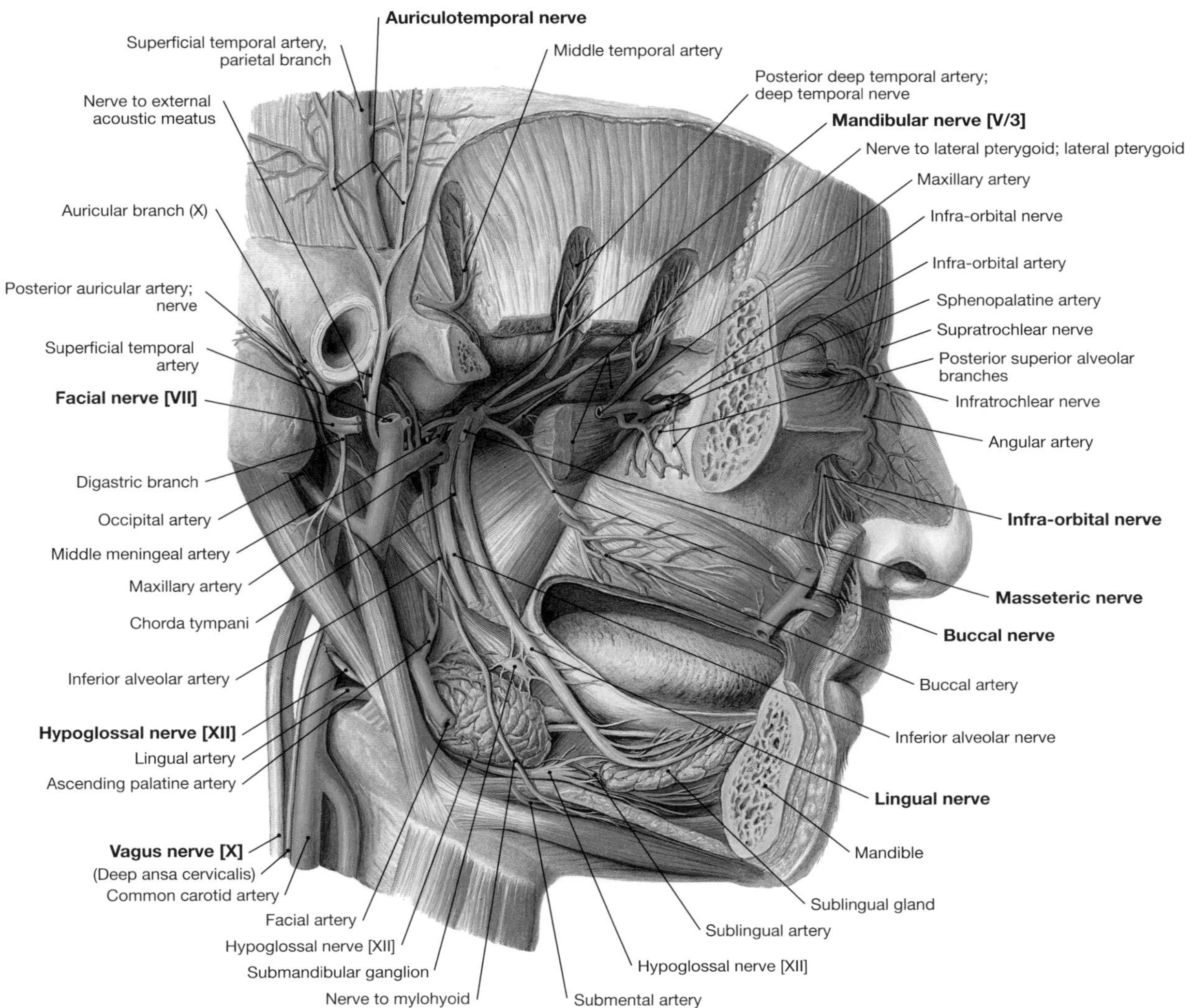
Auriculotemporal nerve
Superficial temporal artery, parietal branch
Middle temporal artery
Nerve to external acoustic meatus
Posterior deep temporal artery; deep temporal nerve
Mandibular nerve [V/3]
Nerve to lateral pterygoid; lateral pterygoid
Maxillary artery
Auricular branch (X)
Infra-orbital nerve
Infra-orbital artery
Posterior auricular artery; nerve
Sphenopalatine artery
Supratrochlear nerve
Superficial temporal artery
Posterior superior alveolar branches
Facial nerve [VII]
Infratrochlear nerve
Angular artery
Digastric branch
Infra-orbital nerve
Occipital artery
Middle meningeal artery
Maxillary artery
Masseteric nerve
Chorda tympani
Buccal nerve
Inferior alveolar artery
Buccal artery
Hypoglossal nerve [XII]
Inferior alveolar nerve
Lingual artery
Ascending palatine artery
Lingual nerve
Vagus nerve [X]
Mandible
(Deep ansa cervicalis)
Common carotid artery
Sublingual gland
Facial artery
Sublingual artery
Hypoglossal nerve [XII]
Submandibular ganglion
Hypoglossal nerve [XII]
Nerve to mylohyoid
Submental artery

**Fig. 8.77 Arteries and nerves of the head, lateral deepest regions, right side;** lateral view.
Upon exiting the Foramen ovale, the mandibular nerve [V/3] divides into the **lingual nerve, inferior alveolar nerve,** buccal nerve, and the auriculotemporal nerve and sends branches to the masticatory muscles.

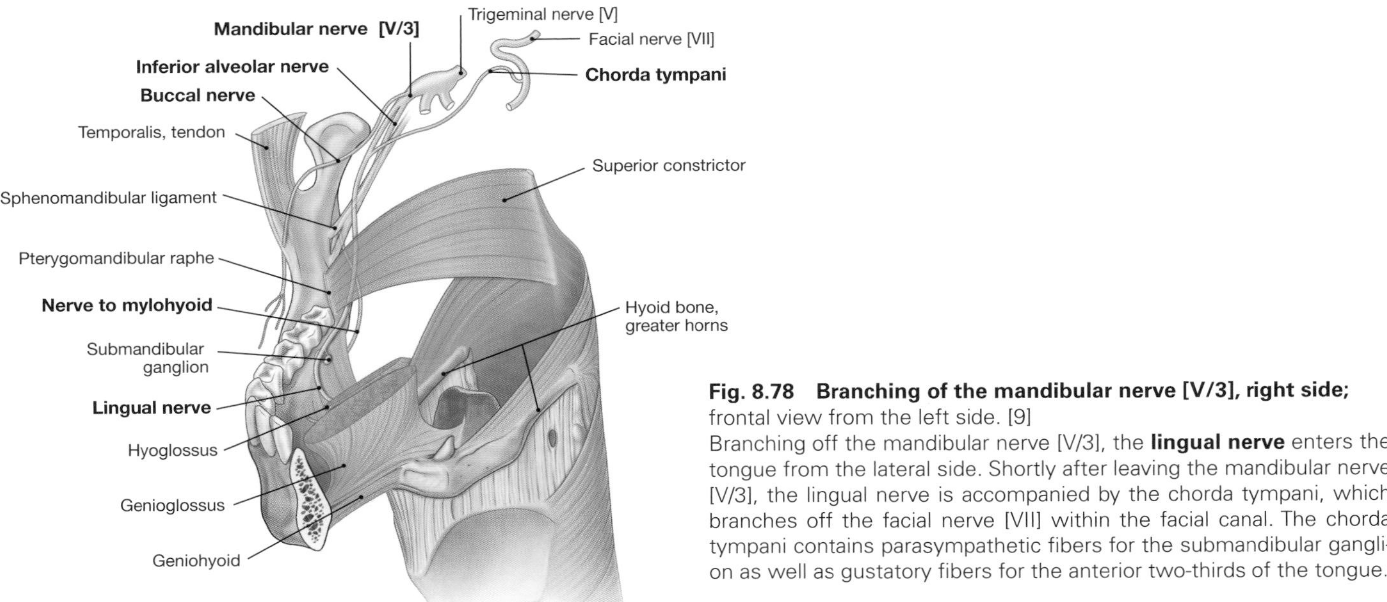
Trigeminal nerve [V]
Mandibular nerve [V/3]
Facial nerve [VII]
Inferior alveolar nerve
Chorda tympani
Buccal nerve
Temporalis, tendon
Superior constrictor
Sphenomandibular ligament
Pterygomandibular raphe
Hyoid bone, greater horns
Nerve to mylohyoid
Submandibular ganglion
Lingual nerve
Hyoglossus
Genioglossus
Geniohyoid

**Fig. 8.78 Branching of the mandibular nerve [V/3], right side;** frontal view from the left side. [9]
Branching off the mandibular nerve [V/3], the **lingual nerve** enters the tongue from the lateral side. Shortly after leaving the mandibular nerve [V/3], the lingual nerve is accompanied by the chorda tympani, which branches off the facial nerve [VII] within the facial canal. The chorda tympani contains parasympathetic fibers for the submandibular ganglion as well as gustatory fibers for the anterior two-thirds of the tongue.

## Arteries of the head

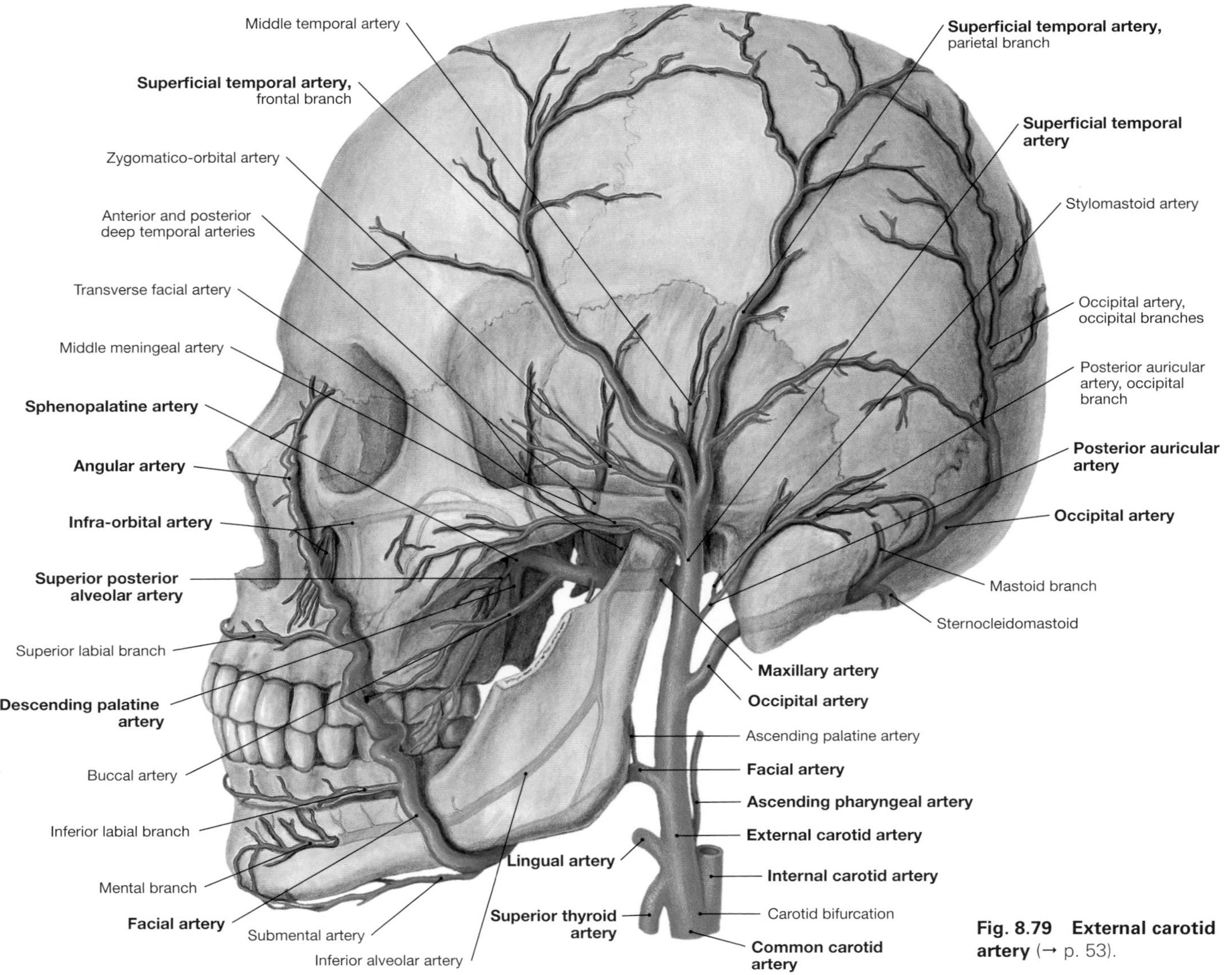
Middle temporal artery
Superficial temporal artery, frontal branch
Zygomatico-orbital artery
Anterior and posterior deep temporal arteries
Transverse facial artery
Middle meningeal artery
Sphenopalatine artery
Angular artery
Infra-orbital artery
Superior posterior alveolar artery
Superior labial branch
Descending palatine artery
Buccal artery
Inferior labial branch
Mental branch
Facial artery
Submental artery
Inferior alveolar artery
Lingual artery
Superior thyroid artery
Superficial temporal artery, parietal branch
Superficial temporal artery
Stylomastoid artery
Occipital artery, occipital branches
Posterior auricular artery, occipital branch
Posterior auricular artery
Occipital artery
Mastoid branch
Sternocleidomastoid
Maxillary artery
Occipital artery
Ascending palatine artery
Facial artery
Ascending pharyngeal artery
External carotid artery
Internal carotid artery
Carotid bifurcation
Common carotid artery

**Fig. 8.79 External carotid artery** (→ p. 53).

### Branches of the External Carotid Artery

1. **Superior thyroid artery**
   - Infrahyoid branch
   - Superior laryngeal artery
   - Cricothyroid branch
   - Sternocleido-mastoid branch
   - Glandular branches

2. **Ascending pharyngeal artery**
   - Pharyngeal branches
   - Inferior tympanic artery
   - Posterior meningeal artery

3. **Lingual artery**
   - Dorsal lingual branches
   - Sublingual artery
   - Deep lingual artery

4. **Facial artery**
   - Ascending palatine artery
   - Tonsillar branch
   - Submental artery
   - Glandular branches
   - Inferior labial artery
   - Superior labial artery
   - Nasal septal branch
   - Lateral nasal branch
   - Angular artery

5. **Occipital artery**
   - Mastoid branch
   - Auricular branch
   - Sternocleido-mastoid branches
   - Occipital branches
   - Meningeal branch
   - Descending branch

6. **Posterior auricular artery**
   - Stylomastoid artery
     - posterior tympanic artery
   - Auricular branch
   - Occipital branch
   - Parotid branch

7. **Superficial temporal artery**
   - Parotid branch
   - Transverse facial artery
   - Anterior auricular branches
   - Zygomatico-orbital artery
   - Medial temporal artery
   - Frontal branch
   - Parietal branch

8. **Maxillary artery**
   - Mandibular part:
     - Inferior alveolar artery
       - mental branch
     - Medial meningeal artery
       - superior tympanic artery
   - Pterygoid part:
       - deep auricular artery
       - anterior tympanic artery
     - Masseteric artery
     - Deep posterior and anterior temporal arteries
   - Pterygoid branches
   - Buccal artery

8. **Maxillary artery** *(continuation)*
   - Pterygo-palatine part:
     - Posterior superior alveolar artery
       - dental branches
       - peridental branches
     - Infraorbital artery
       - anterior superior alveolar arteries
     - Descending palatine artery
       - greater palatine artery
       - lesser palatine arteries
         - pharyngeal branch
     - Sphenopalatine artery
       - posterior lateral nasal arteries
       - posterior septal branches
       - nasopalatine artery

Terminal branches of the maxillary artery are the infraorbital artery, sphenopalatine artery, posterior superior alveolar artery, and descending palatine artery

## Veins of the head

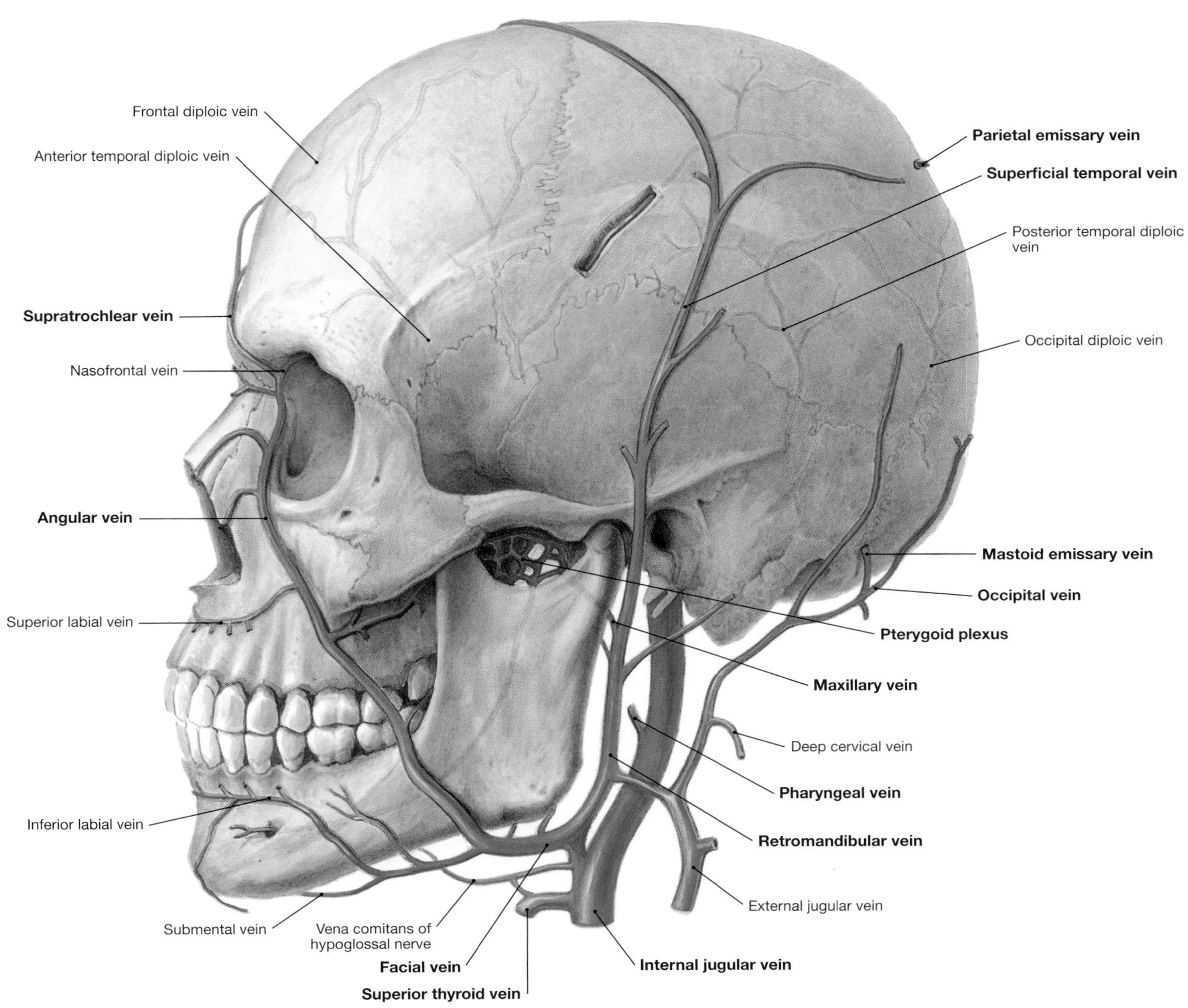
Frontal diploic vein
Anterior temporal diploic vein
Supratrochlear vein
Nasofrontal vein
Angular vein
Superior labial vein
Inferior labial vein
Submental vein
Vena comitans of hypoglossal nerve
Facial vein
Superior thyroid vein
Internal jugular vein
External jugular vein
Retromandibular vein
Pharyngeal vein
Deep cervical vein
Maxillary vein
Pterygoid plexus
Occipital vein
Mastoid emissary vein
Occipital diploic vein
Posterior temporal diploic vein
Superficial temporal vein
Parietal emissary vein

**Fig. 8.79 External carotid artery, left side;** lateral view (→ p. 52).
The branches of the external carotid artery are listed in the table (→ p. 52) in their consecutive branching order.

**Fig. 8.80 Internal jugular vein, left side;** lateral view.
The internal jugular vein starts as a dilated extension of the sigmoid sinus at the cranial base. This vein drains the blood from the regions of the skull, brain, face, and parts of the neck. The facial, lingual, pharyngeal, occipital, superior thyroid, middle thyroid, and emissary veins drain blood from the superficial head region into the internal jugular vein.

## Clinical Remarks

The pulse of the jugular vein **(jugular pulse)** provides useful information on the venous blood pressure and the wave-like characteristic of the jugular pulse reflects the function of the right heart.

In rare cases, **inflammations in the facial area** can spread via the valve-free angular vein to intraorbital veins (superior ophthalmic vein) and eventually from there to the cavernous sinus. This results in a life-threatening phlebitis or even a venous sinus thrombosis.

## Facial nerve [VII]

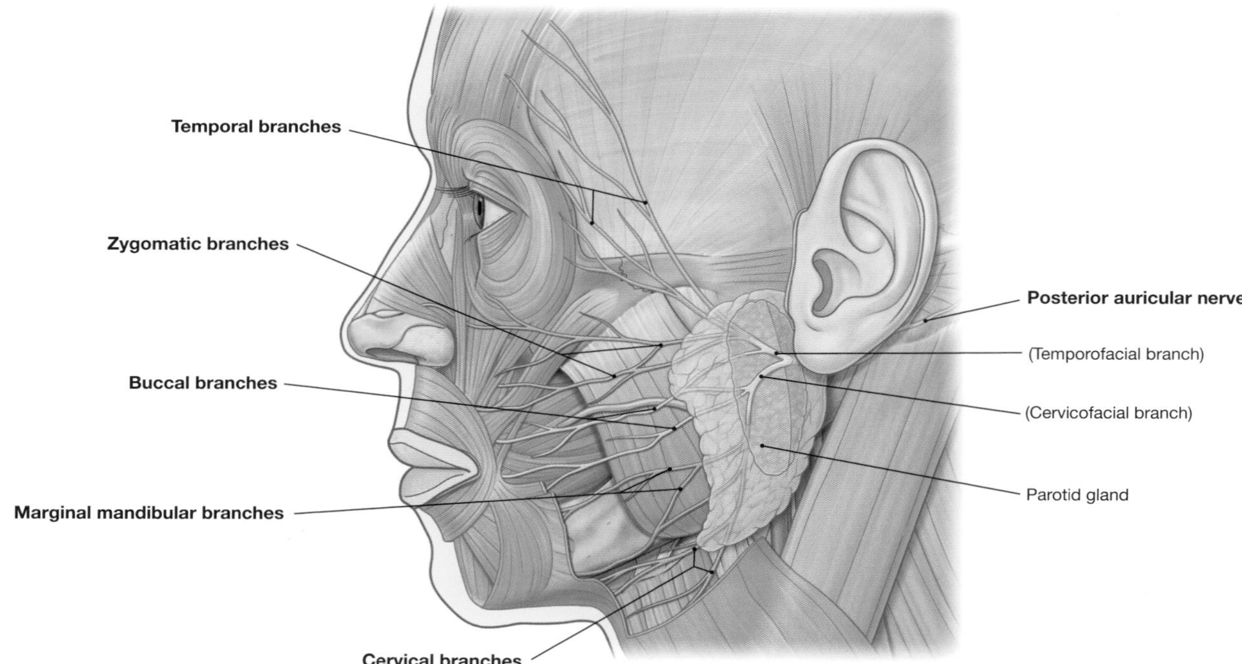
Temporal branches
Zygomatic branches
Buccal branches
Marginal mandibular branches
Cervical branches
Posterior auricular nerve
(Temporofacial branch)
(Cervicofacial branch)
Parotid gland

**Fig. 8.81 Terminal branches of the facial nerve [VII] in the face, left side;** lateral view. [8]
Within the parotid gland, the facial nerve [VII] (→ Fig. 12.149) creates the intraparotid plexus which, for clinical purposes, is divided into a temporofacial (temporofacial part) and a cervicofacial branch (cervicofacial part). These two parts generate the terminal branches of the facial nerve [VII]: temporal, zygomatic, buccal, marginal mandibular, and cervical branches. Projecting dorsally behind the auricle is the posterior auricular nerve, another terminal branch of the facial nerve [VII].

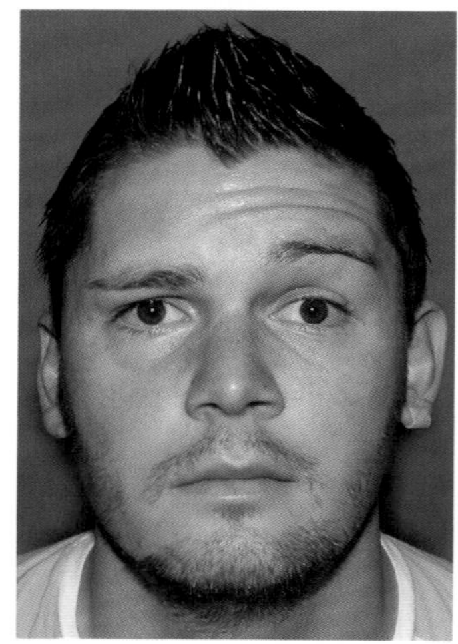

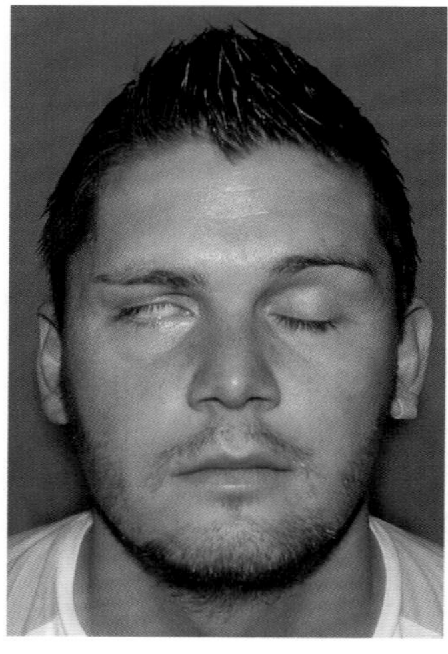

**Figs. 8.82a and b Peripheral palsy of the facial nerve [VII], right side.**

**a** Upon the request to raise the eyebrows, only the left half of the forehead displays wrinkles (loss of function of the occipitofrontalis, sign of peripheral facial nerve palsy).

**b** Upon the request to tightly shut both eyes, the eye on the injured side fails to close properly (lagophthalmos). When closing the eyes, the eyeball automatically turns upwards. Because the eyelid on the affected side fails to close properly, the white sclera becomes visible (BELL's phenomenon).

## Clinical Remarks

A **peripheral facial nerve palsy** (→ Fig. 12.151) involves damage to the 2nd motor neuron; this damage can be located anywhere between the nucleus of facial nerve and its peripheral branches. Causes are most frequently viral infections or nerve injuries during surgery on the parotid gland. The so-called central (supranuclear) lesion of the facial nerve [VII] **(central facial nerve palsy)** is the result of a damage to the 1st motor neuron, mainly caused by bleedings or infarctions in the area of the corticonuclear tract of the inner capsule on the contralateral side. As the temporal branches of the facial nerve [VII] contain fibers derived from the nuclei located on the contra- and ipsilateral side, the muscles of the forehead and the orbicularis oculi in the upper eyelid region can still contract on both sides. However, on the contralateral side the muscles innervated by the zygomatic, buccal, marginal mandibular, and cervival branches are paralysed (so-called lower facial nerve palsy).

## Skin innervation

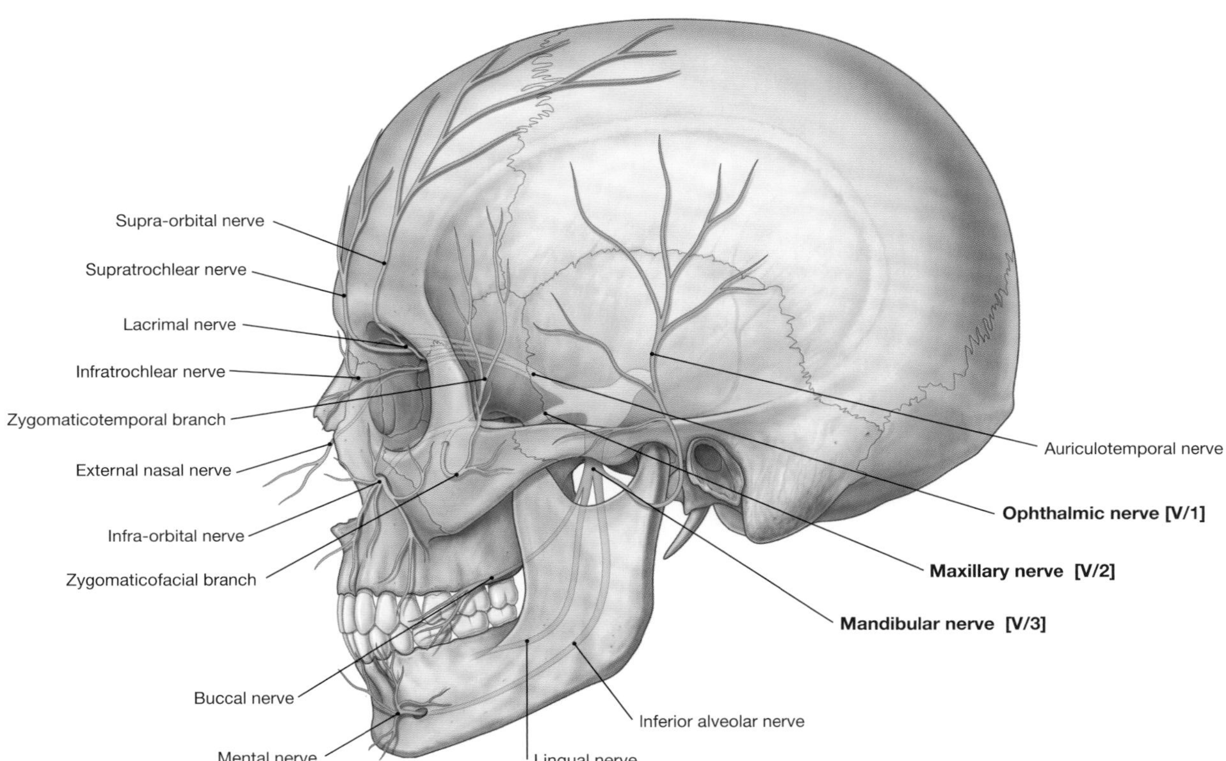
Supra-orbital nerve
Supratrochlear nerve
Lacrimal nerve
Infratrochlear nerve
Zygomaticotemporal branch
External nasal nerve
Infra-orbital nerve
Zygomaticofacial branch
Buccal nerve
Mental nerve
Lingual nerve
Inferior alveolar nerve
Mandibular nerve [V/3]
Maxillary nerve [V/2]
Ophthalmic nerve [V/1]
Auriculotemporal nerve

**Fig. 8.83 Branches of the trigeminal nerve [V], left side;** lateral view. [8]
Upon exit from the cranium, the three major branches of the trigeminal nerve [V], ophthalmic nerve [V/1], maxillary nerve [V/2], and mandibular nerve [V/3], subdivide into smaller branches in a specific topographic order. Visible branches of the **ophthalmic nerve [V/1]** are the supra-orbital, supratrochlear, lacrimal, infratrochlear nerves and the external nasal branches. The **maxillary nerve [V/2]** provides the infraorbital and zygomatic nerves with its zygomaticotemporal and zygomaticofacial branches as shown in the image. Branches of the **mandibular nerve [V/3]** are the buccal, lingual, inferior alveolar, and auriculotemporal nerves. When leaving the mandibular canal, the mental nerve represents the terminal branch of the inferior alveolar nerve.

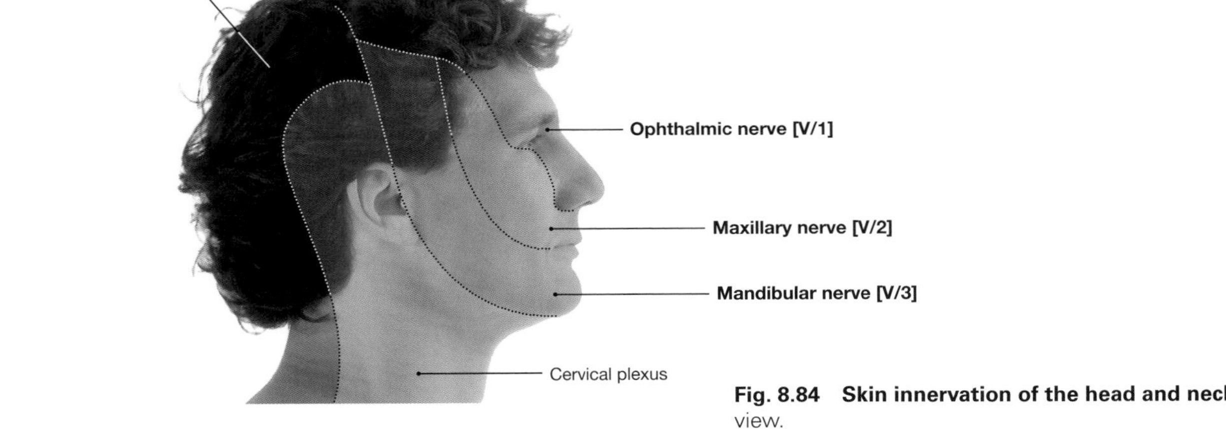
Greater occipital nerve
Ophthalmic nerve [V/1]
Maxillary nerve [V/2]
Mandibular nerve [V/3]
Cervical plexus

**Fig. 8.84 Skin innervation of the head and neck, right side;** lateral view.
The view from ventral is depicted in → Fig. 12.146.

## Clinical Remarks

As part of the physical examination of a patient, the trigeminal nerve [V] is tested by applying pressure on the three exit points **(trigeminal pressure points).** Patients should not show signs of increased sensitivity or pain at the supraorbital foramen/supraorbital notch, infraorbital foramen, or mental foramen.

**Trigeminal neuralgia** (tic douloureux) is a complex and painful dysfunction of the sensory trigeminal root. Typically located in the innervation areas of the mandibular nerve [V/3] and maxillary nerve [V/2], the facial pain can be intense and occur quite suddenly. Touch of the skin in the corresponding facial areas often triggers an attack.

## Lymph vessels and lymph nodes of the head

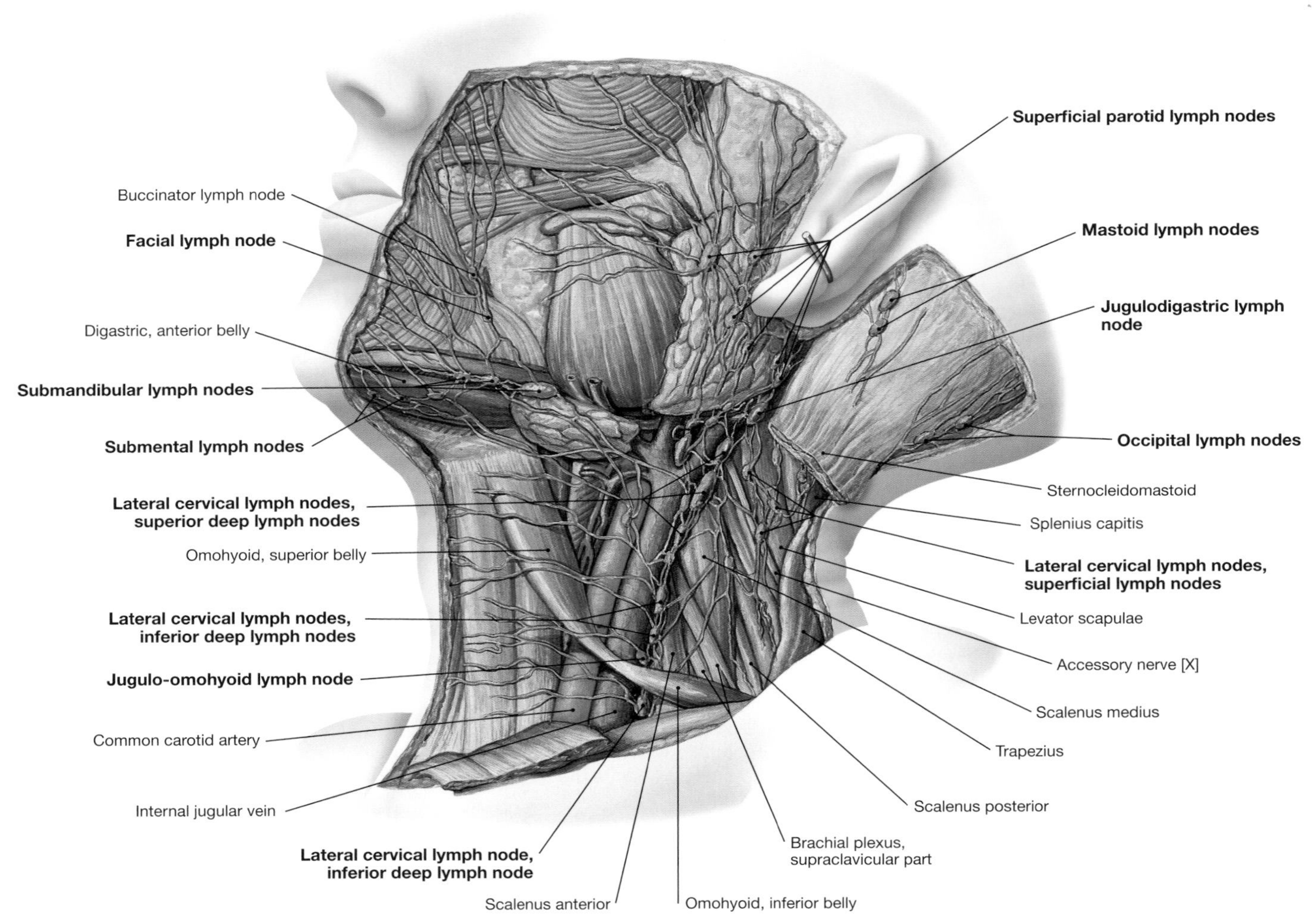
Superficial parotid lymph nodes
Buccinator lymph node
Facial lymph node
Mastoid lymph nodes
Jugulodigastric lymph node
Digastric, anterior belly
Submandibular lymph nodes
Submental lymph nodes
Occipital lymph nodes
Sternocleidomastoid
Lateral cervical lymph nodes, superior deep lymph nodes
Splenius capitis
Omohyoid, superior belly
Lateral cervical lymph nodes, superficial lymph nodes
Lateral cervical lymph nodes, inferior deep lymph nodes
Levator scapulae
Jugulo-omohyoid lymph node
Accessory nerve [X]
Scalenus medius
Common carotid artery
Trapezius
Internal jugular vein
Scalenus posterior
Brachial plexus, supraclavicular part
Lateral cervical lymph node, inferior deep lymph node
Scalenus anterior
Omohyoid, inferior belly

**Fig. 8.85 Superficial lymph vessels and lymph nodes of the head and neck of a child, left side;** lateral view.
The **regional** submental, submandibular, parotid, mastoid, and occipital lymph nodes collect the lymphatic fluid of the face, scalp, and occiput. From here, the lymph is drained into **superficial lateral** and **superior and inferior deep lateral cervical lymph nodes** (→ Fig. 11.75).
An important deep cervical lymph node is the jugulodigastric lymph node located between the anterior margin of the sternocleidomastoid and the mandibular angle at the lower border of the parotid gland.
The **parotid lymph nodes** are divided into **superficial** and **deep** nodes. The latter include the pre-auricular, infra-auricular, and intraglandular lymph nodes. In addition, there are isolated facial lymph nodes (buccinator, nasolabial, mandibular, malar lymph nodes) and lymph nodes of the tongue.

| Lymph Nodes of the Head |
|---|
| • Occipital lymph nodes |
| • Mastoid lymph nodes |
| • Superficial parotid lymph nodes |
| • Deep parotid lymph nodes<br>– preauricular lymph nodes<br>– infraauricular lymph nodes<br>– intraglandular lymph nodes |
| • Facial lymph nodes<br>– buccinator lymph node<br>– nasolabial lymph node<br>– malar lymph node<br>– mandibular lymph node |
| • Submental lymph nodes |
| • Submandibular lymph nodes |
| • Lingual lymph nodes |

## Deep lymph vessels of the neck

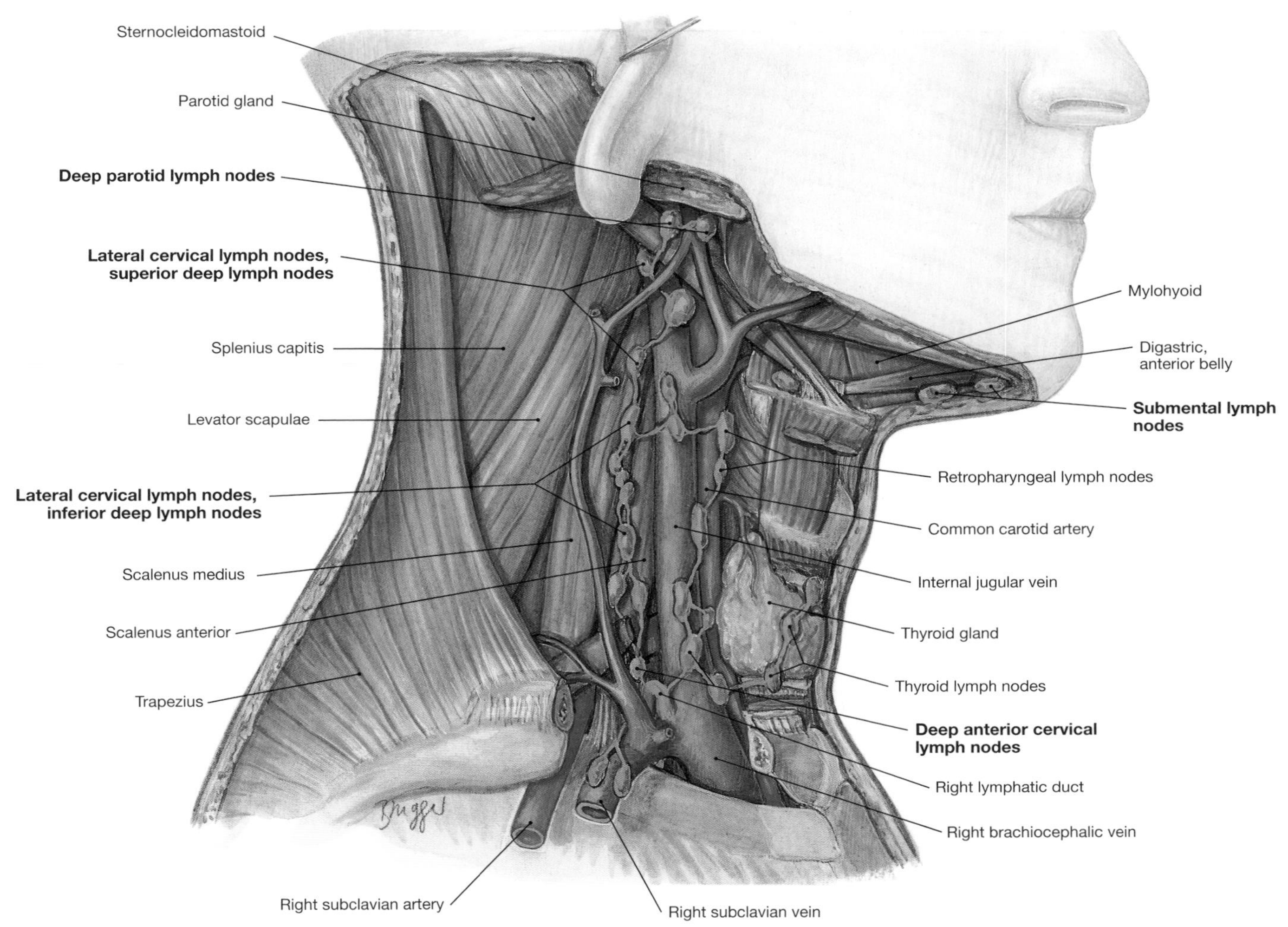
Sternocleidomastoid
Parotid gland
Deep parotid lymph nodes
Lateral cervical lymph nodes, superior deep lymph nodes
Splenius capitis
Levator scapulae
Lateral cervical lymph nodes, inferior deep lymph nodes
Scalenus medius
Scalenus anterior
Trapezius
Right subclavian artery
Right subclavian vein
Mylohyoid
Digastric, anterior belly
Submental lymph nodes
Retropharyngeal lymph nodes
Common carotid artery
Internal jugular vein
Thyroid gland
Thyroid lymph nodes
Deep anterior cervical lymph nodes
Right lymphatic duct
Right brachiocephalic vein

**Fig. 8.86 Deep lymph nodes of the neck, right side;** lateral view. Cervical lymph nodes of both the anterior and lateral aspects of the neck are divided into a superficial and deep lymph node compartment. The infrahyoid lymph nodes with the prelaryngeal, thyroid, pretracheal, paratracheal, and retropharyngeal lymph nodes constitute the **anterior** deep cervical lymph nodes.

The **lateral** deep cervical lymph nodes are divided into an **upper group,** composed of the jugulodigastric, lateral, and anterior lymph node, and a **lower group** with the juguloomohyoid and lateral lymph node and anterior lymph nodes. In addition, there are the supraclavicular and accessory lymph nodes (in association with the accessory nerve [XI]) with the retropharyngeal lymph nodes.

## Nasal skeleton

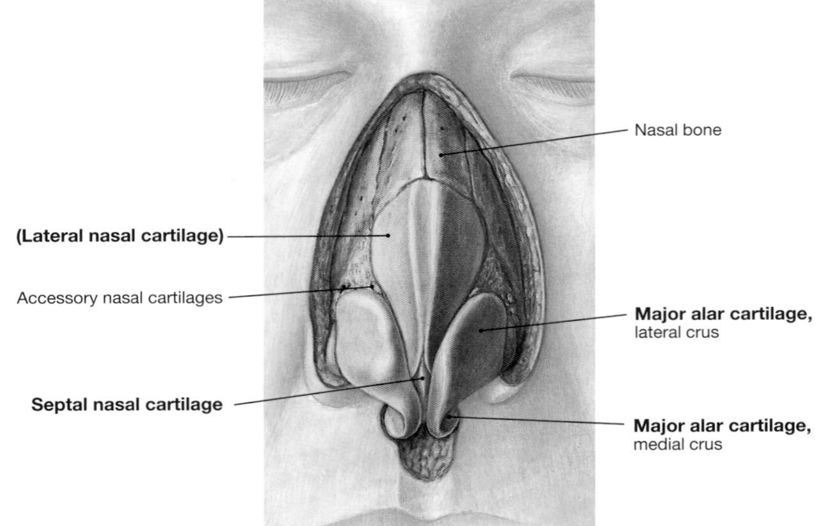
Nasal bone
(Lateral nasal cartilage)
Accessory nasal cartilages
Major alar cartilage, lateral crus
Septal nasal cartilage
Major alar cartilage, medial crus

**Fig. 8.87 Nasal skeleton;** frontal view.
The nasal skeleton consists of a bony and a cartilaginous part. Connective tissue fixes the cartilaginous part to the piriform aperture which is composed of the nasal and maxillary bone. The individual elements consist of hyaline cartilage and are linked by connective tissue. The **upper lateral or triangular nasal cartilage** forms the roof; the **nasal tip or major alar cartilage** with a lateral crus and a medial crus creates the nasal wings. In addition, two smaller **alar cartilages** exist bilaterally. At its bottom and central part, the cartilaginous part of the nasal septum supports the nasal skeleton.

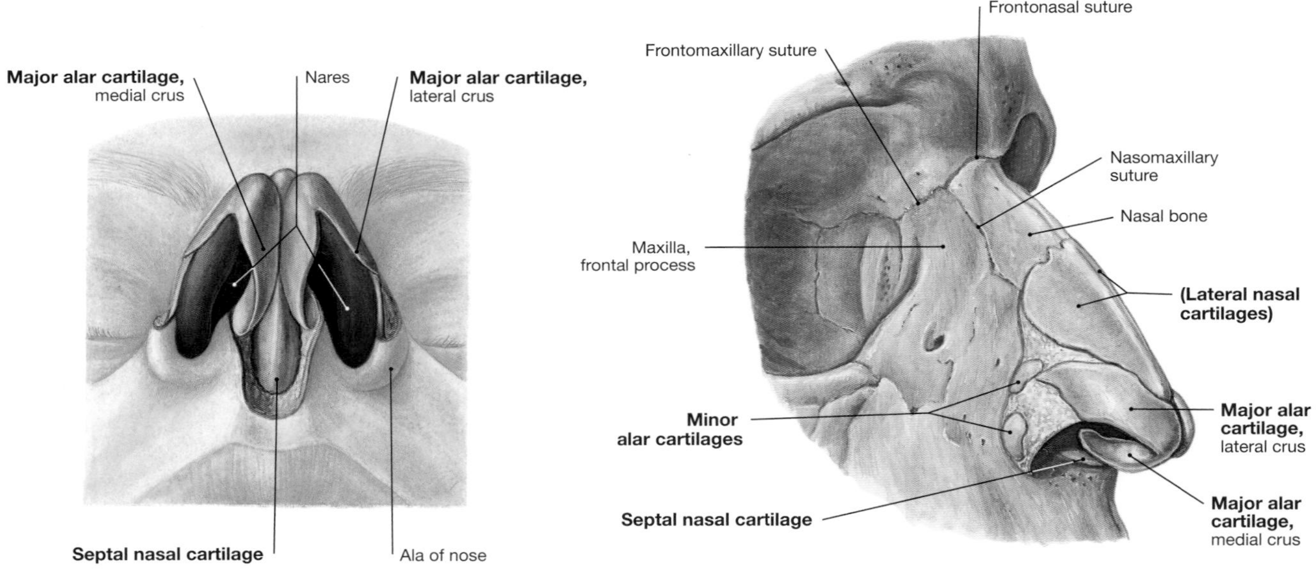
Major alar cartilage, medial crus
Nares
Major alar cartilage, lateral crus
Septal nasal cartilage
Ala of nose
Frontonasal suture
Frontomaxillary suture
Nasomaxillary suture
Nasal bone
Maxilla, frontal process
(Lateral nasal cartilages)
Minor alar cartilages
Major alar cartilage, lateral crus
Septal nasal cartilage
Major alar cartilage, medial crus

**Fig. 8.88 Nasal cartilages;** inferior view.
The view from below shows the nasal orifices (Nares) which are delineated by the two crura of the major alar cartilage (medial and lateral crus). In the central lower region, the cartilaginous part of the nasal septum is visible.

**Fig. 8.89 Nasal skeleton;** frontal view from the right side.
The cartilaginous nasal skeleton attaches to the piriform aperture by connective tissue. The lateral nasal cartilagines, major alar, minor alar and the septal nasal cartilages are visible. There is connective tissue within the non-cartilaginous nasal areas.

### Clinical Remarks

Specific clinical terms are often used: **columella** (anterior part of the nasal septum between the nasal tip and the philtrum), the **"keystone area"** (where the nasal bone overlaps the lateral cartilages), a **soft triangle** (skin area at the upper rim of the nostril, close to the point where the medial crus bends to become the lateral crus; this **cartilage-free area** is composed exclusively of a skin duplication), the **"supratip area"** (on the bridge of the nose just above the tip), and the **weak triangle** (similar to the "supratip area" since here the bridge of the nose is exclusively formed by the septum). These designated areas are important landmarks that require special attention by the rhinoplastic surgeon.
A **hematoma of the nasal septum** (e.g., as a result of a fractured nose) requires an immediate decompression or relieve by puncture or an incision and nasal tamponade as otherwise the cartilage will become necrotic.

## Nasal septum

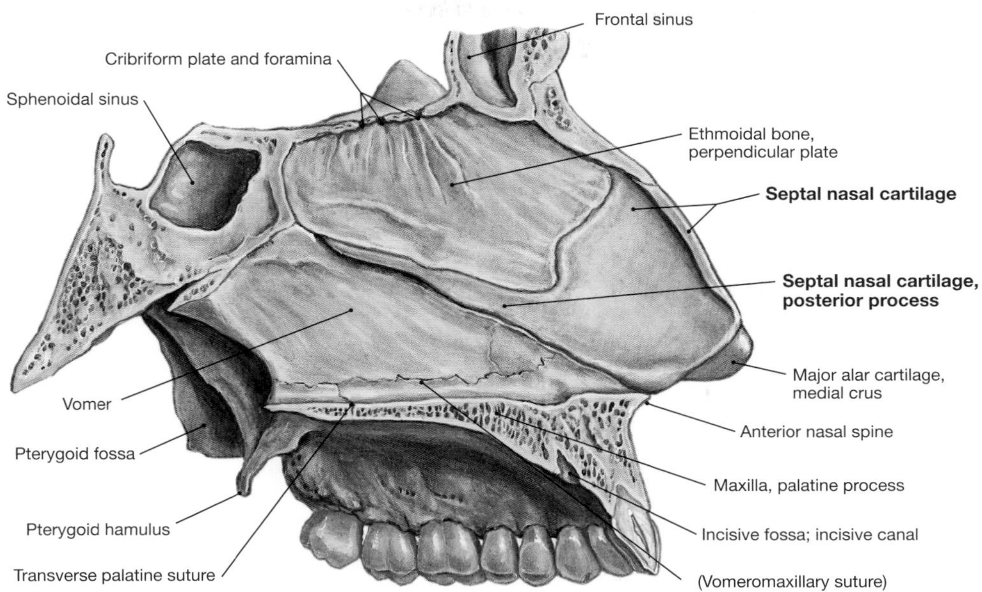
Frontal sinus
Cribriform plate and foramina
Sphenoidal sinus
Ethmoidal bone, perpendicular plate
Septal nasal cartilage
Septal nasal cartilage, posterior process
Major alar cartilage, medial crus
Vomer
Anterior nasal spine
Pterygoid fossa
Maxilla, palatine process
Pterygoid hamulus
Incisive fossa; incisive canal
Transverse palatine suture
(Vomeromaxillary suture)

**Fig. 8.90 Nasal septum;** view from the right side.
The septal nasal cartilage forms the frontal part of the nasal septum and extends as a long cartilaginous posterior process between the bony parts of the nasal septum (top), composed of the perpendicular plate of the ethmoidal bone, and the vomer (bottom).

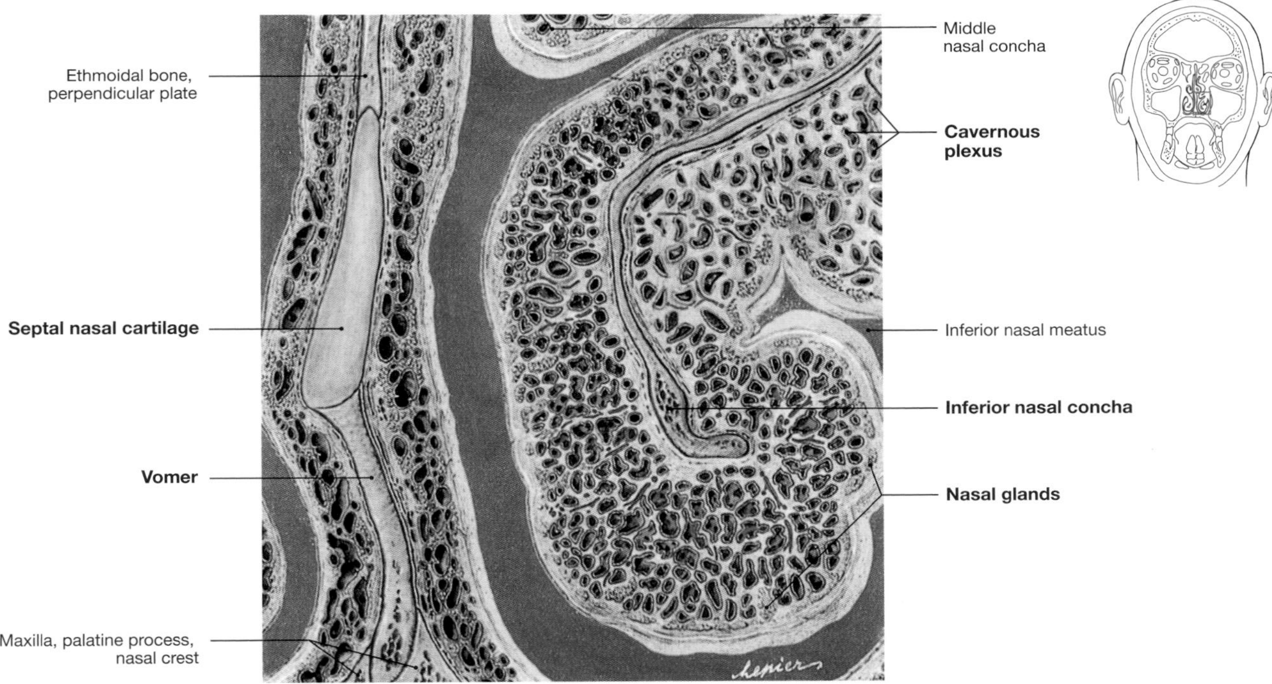
Middle nasal concha
Ethmoidal bone, perpendicular plate
Cavernous plexus
Septal nasal cartilage
Inferior nasal meatus
Inferior nasal concha
Vomer
Nasal glands
Maxilla, palatine process, nasal crest

**Fig. 8.91 Inferior nasal concha, left side;** frontal section at the level of the initial part of the posterior process of the septal nasal cartilage; frontal view.
This section demonstrates the thin bony skeleton of the inferior nasal concha which is covered by a vascular plexus (cavernous plexus) composed of a network of specialized arteries and veins. Ciliated epithelium and interspersed serous glands (nasal glands) cover the surface of the nasal concha.

### Clinical Remarks

A characteristic feature of the nasal mucosa is a dense subepithelial plexus of venous sinusoids. Depending on the particular state of swelling, approximately 35% of the nasal mucosa is composed of vascular plexuses. The highest density of subepithelial venous plexuses is found at the lower and middle nasal conchae and the KIESSELBACH's area of the nasal septum.

Some 80% of all humans display a **nasal cycle:** this refers to spontaneous alternating changes in the swelling of the nasal mucosa in the two nasal passages lasting 2–7 hours. This alternating swelling results in a 3-fold increase of the airway resistance in the particular nasal passage during nasal breathing while the total nasal airway resistance remains unchanged.

## Nasal cavity

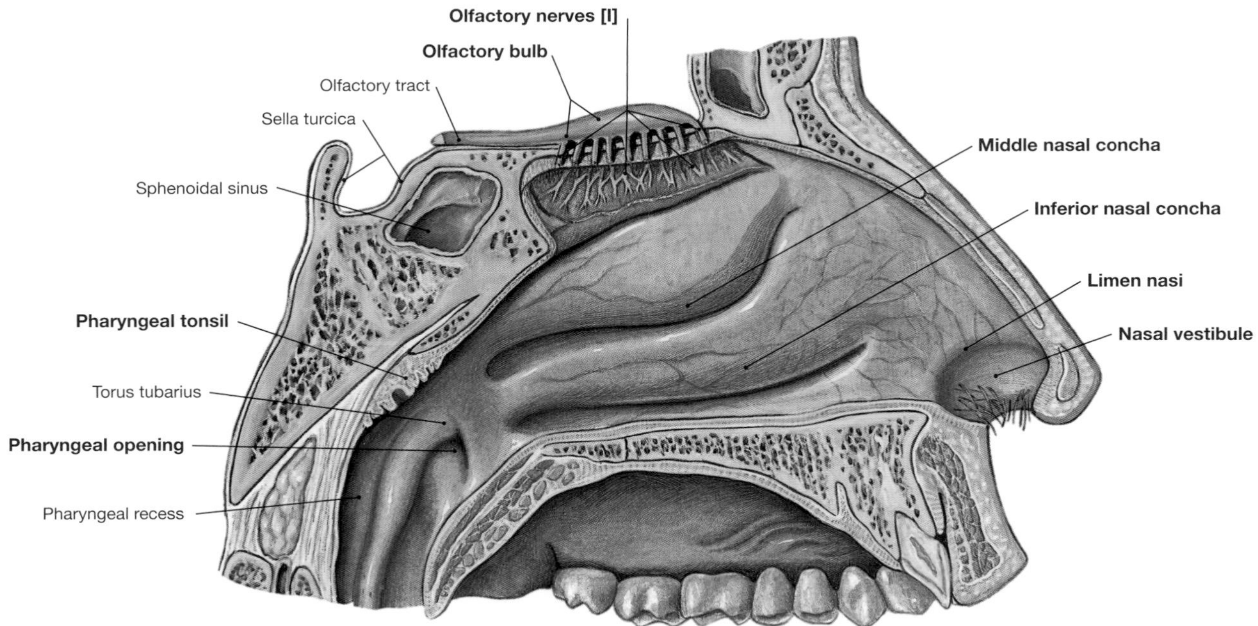
Olfactory nerves [I]
Olfactory bulb
Olfactory tract
Sella turcica
Sphenoidal sinus
Pharyngeal tonsil
Torus tubarius
Pharyngeal opening
Pharyngeal recess
Middle nasal concha
Inferior nasal concha
Limen nasi
Nasal vestibule

**Fig. 8.92 Lateral wall of the nasal cavity, left side;** lateral view.
The lateral wall of the nasal cavity is mainly occupied by the **inferior** and **middle nasal conchae.** The superior nasal concha is small and located in close vicinity to the olfactory region at the nasal roof. Here, the olfactory nerves of the olfactory bulb penetrate the cribriform plate and reach the neighboring mucosa, including the mucosa of the upper nasal concha.

Keratinized stratified squamous epithelium covers the **nasal vestibule.** At the limen nasi, the epithelial layer transforms into non-keratinized stratified squamous epithelium and then into ciliated pseudostratified columnar epithelium. An imaginary line from the inferior nasal concha projects to the pharyngeal opening of the auditory tube (pharyngotympanic tube). Above the pharyngeal opening at the pharyngeal roof lies pharyngeal tonsil.

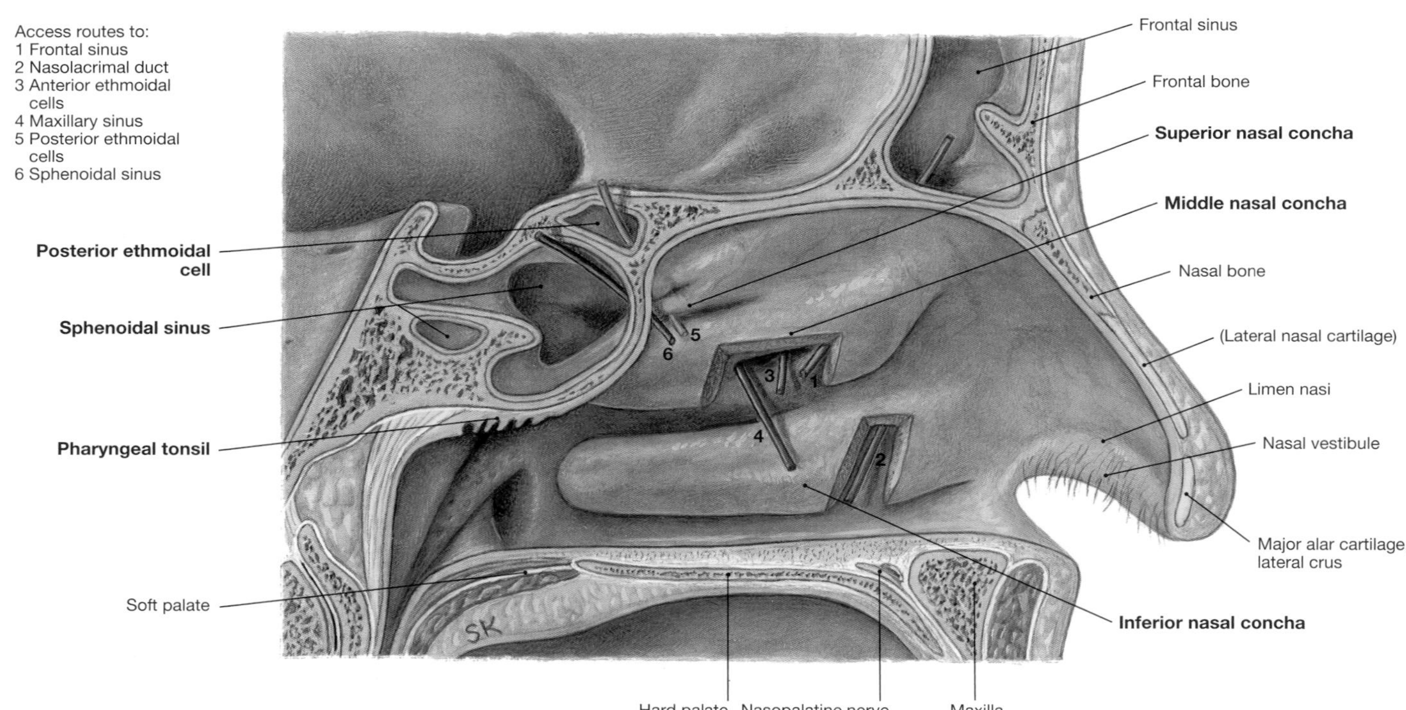
Access routes to:
1 Frontal sinus
2 Nasolacrimal duct
3 Anterior ethmoidal cells
4 Maxillary sinus
5 Posterior ethmoidal cells
6 Sphenoidal sinus
Posterior ethmoidal cell
Sphenoidal sinus
Pharyngeal tonsil
Soft palate
Frontal sinus
Frontal bone
Superior nasal concha
Middle nasal concha
Nasal bone
(Lateral nasal cartilage)
Limen nasi
Nasal vestibule
Major alar cartilage, lateral crus
Inferior nasal concha
Hard palate
Nasopalatine nerve
Maxilla
1
2
3
4
5
6

**Fig. 8.93 Nasal cavity and entrance into the paranasal sinuses, left side;** view from the right side.
Beneath the anterior third of the inferior nasal concha, the nasolacrimal duct opens into the lower nasal meatus (purple probe). Beneath the middle nasal concha, the openings of the **frontal sinus** (green probe), **maxillary sinus** (red probe), and **anterior ethmoidal cells** (blue probe) are located. Beneath and behind the superior nasal concha, the **posterior ethmoidal cells** (yellow probe) and the **sphenoidal sinus** (dark blue probe) open into the nasal cavity.

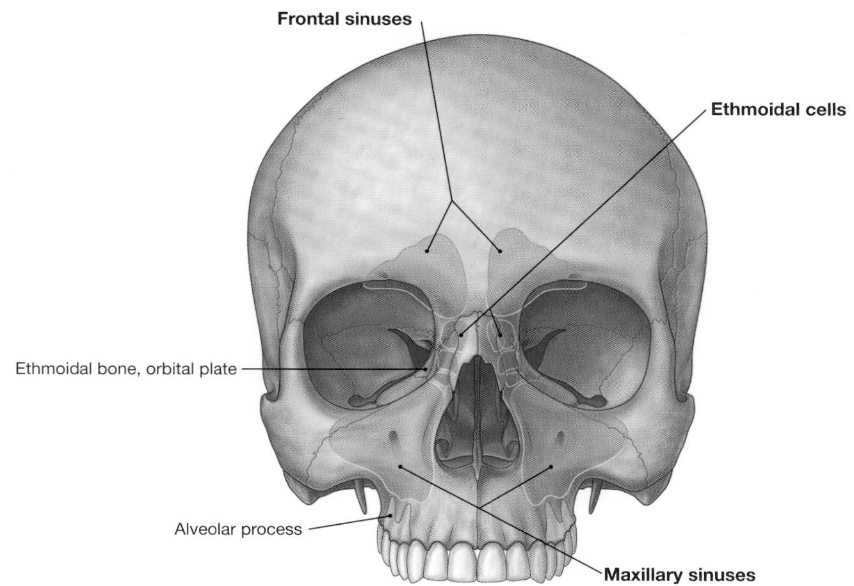
Frontal sinuses
Ethmoidal cells
Ethmoidal bone, orbital plate
Alveolar process
Maxillary sinuses

**Fig. 8.94 Projection of the paranasal sinuses onto the skull;** frontal view. [8]
The projections of the frontal and maxillary sinus as well as the ethmoidal cells are shown.

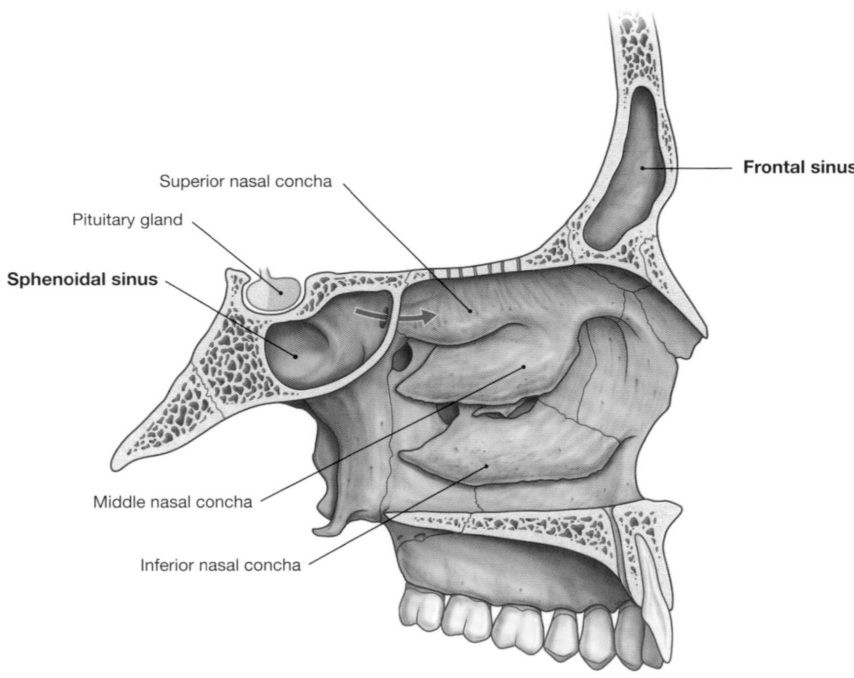
Frontal sinus
Superior nasal concha
Pituitary gland
Sphenoidal sinus
Middle nasal concha
Inferior nasal concha

**Fig. 8.95 Location of the frontal sinus and sphenoidal sinus in the skull, right side;** view from the left side. [8]
The sphenoidal sinus is in close topographic relationship to the pituitary gland.

## Clinical Remarks

The **sphenoidal sinus** can extend into large areas of the sphenoidal bone. During surgical interventions, this extensive pneumatization can endanger the internal carotid artery (internal carotid tubercle) and the optic nerve [II] (optic nerve tubercle) because of their close proximity to the lateral wall of the sinus.

## Paranasal sinuses, radiography

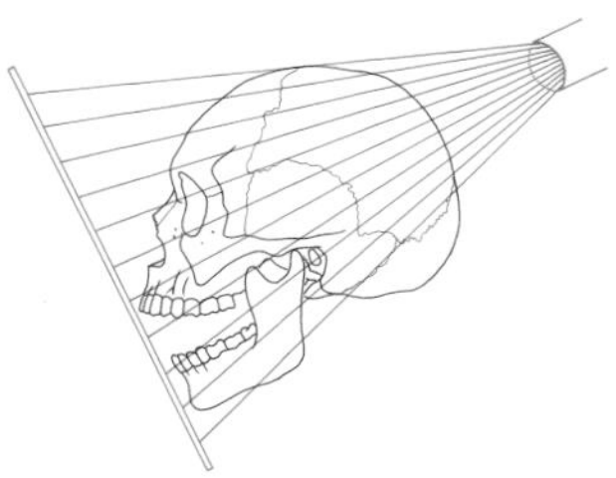

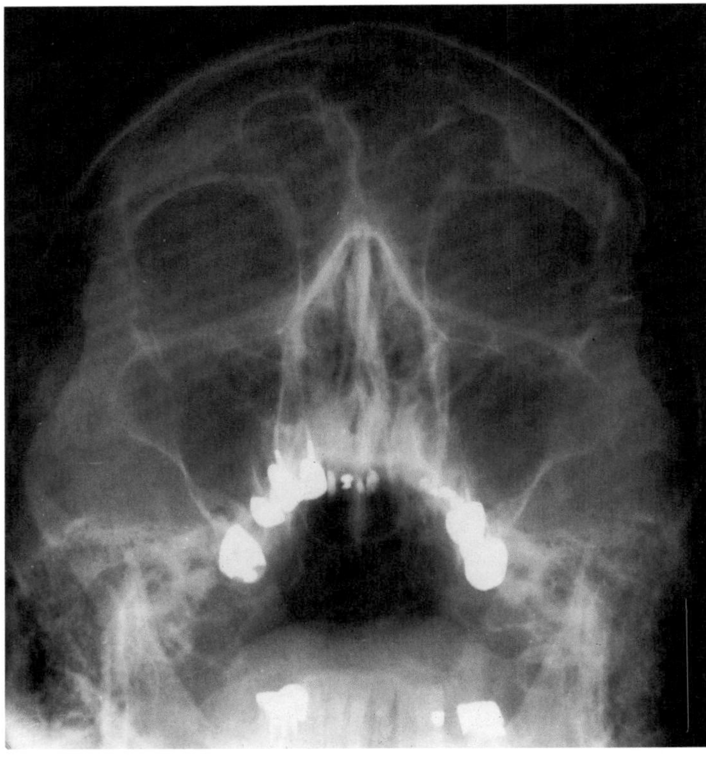

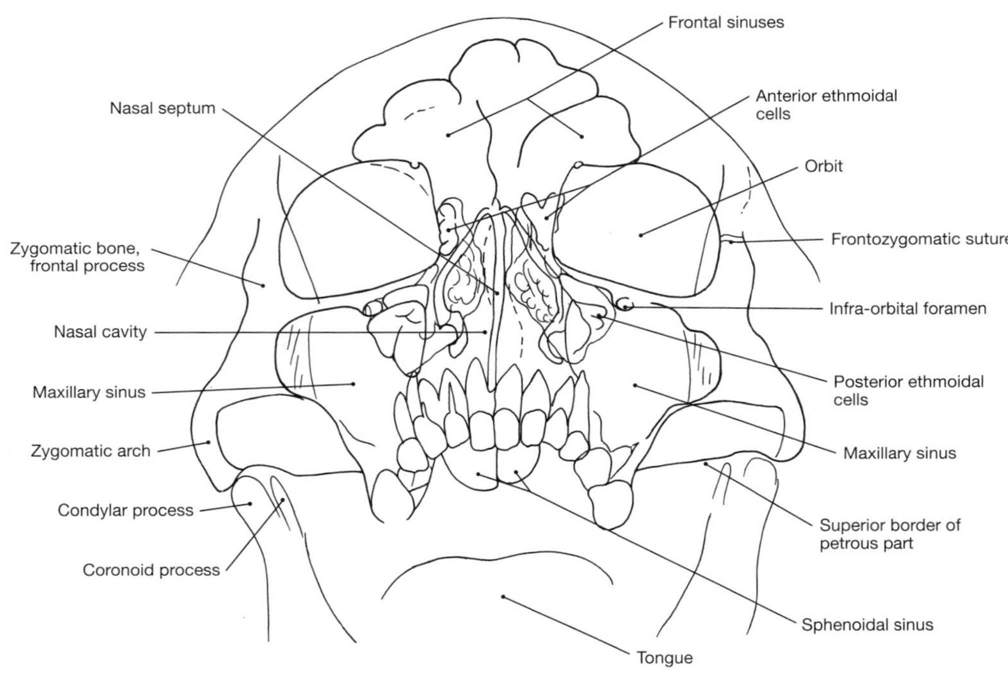
Frontal sinuses
Nasal septum
Anterior ethmoidal cells
Orbit
Frontozygomatic suture
Zygomatic bone, frontal process
Infra-orbital foramen
Nasal cavity
Posterior ethmoidal cells
Maxillary sinus
Maxillary sinus
Zygomatic arch
Condylar process
Superior border of petrous part
Coronoid process
Sphenoidal sinus
Tongue

**Fig. 8.96 Paranasal sinuses;** radiograph of the skull with opened mouth in posterior-anterior (PA) beam projection.

## Clinical Remarks

Conventional radiographs provide a quick overview of the state of the paranasal sinuses. However, computed tomography and magnetic resonance imaging have largely replaced X-ray imaging as the diagnostic tool of choice in determining indications for surgical intervention.

**Sinusitis** is a frequent disease. In children, the ethmoidal sinuses are most frequently affected, whereas in adults an inflammation of the maxillary sinuses is most often observed. Inflammations of the ethmoidal sinuses can break through the thin orbital plate (lamina papyracea) of the ethmoidal bone and spread into the orbit or can reach the optic canal from the posterior ethmoidal sinuses or the sphenoidal sinus and damage the optic nerve.

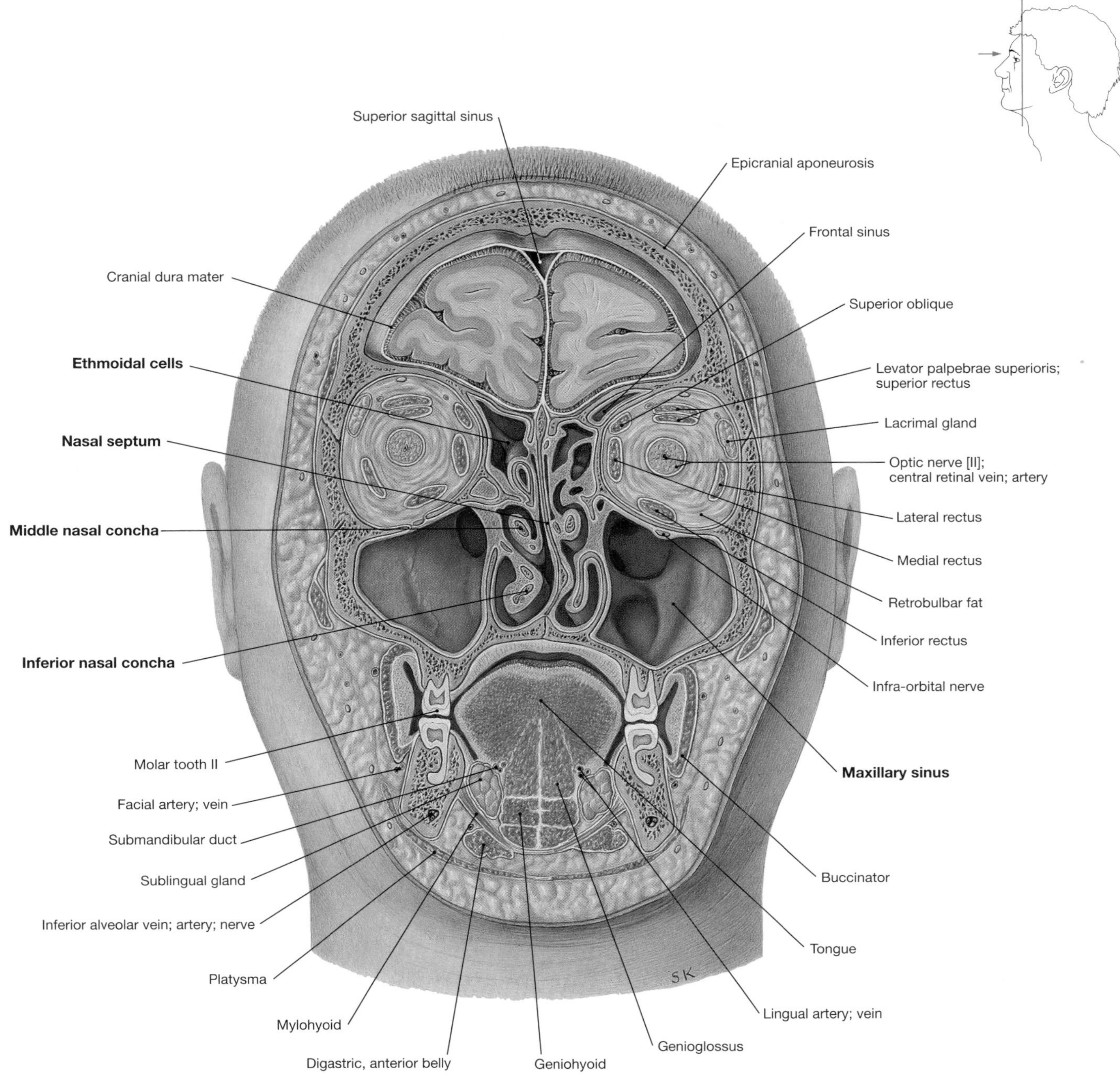
Superior sagittal sinus
Epicranial aponeurosis
Frontal sinus
Cranial dura mater
Superior oblique
Ethmoidal cells
Levator palpebrae superioris; superior rectus
Lacrimal gland
Nasal septum
Optic nerve [II]; central retinal vein; artery
Lateral rectus
Middle nasal concha
Medial rectus
Retrobulbar fat
Inferior rectus
Inferior nasal concha
Infra-orbital nerve
Molar tooth II
Maxillary sinus
Facial artery; vein
Submandibular duct
Sublingual gland
Buccinator
Inferior alveolar vein; artery; nerve
Tongue
Platysma
SK
Lingual artery; vein
Mylohyoid
Genioglossus
Digastric, anterior belly
Geniohyoid

**Fig. 8.97 Frontal section through the head at the level of the second upper molar;** frontal view.
This section emphasizes the individual bilateral differences in the formation of the sectioned paranasal sinuses. On both sides, the differently shaped maxillary sinuses display variable degrees of compartmentalization. The nasal septum deviates to the left side (septum deviation). As a result, the lower and middle nasal conchae on the right side are markedly more developed than on the left side. The ethmoidal cells show differences in shape between the right and left side. In the left supraorbital region, part of the frontal sinus is visible.

## Clinical Remarks

Due to a severe **septum deviation,** nasal breathing can be markedly restricted and as a consequence headache, hyposmia, or even anosmia may occur. The shape and size of the paranasal sinuses is extremely variable. This accounts for interindividual as well as side differences within the same individual and can include the complete lack of individual sinuses **(aplasia).** However, individual sinuses can reach extreme sizes. If the frontal sinus extends in an occipital direction well beyond the orbital roof **(supra-orbital recess),** the clinician refers to it as a dangerous frontal sinus. An inflammatory process of the frontal sinus can overcome the thin bony barrier and can spread into the anterior cranial fossa and lead to meningitis, epidural abscesses, or even brain abscesses.

## Development and clinics of the paranasal sinuses

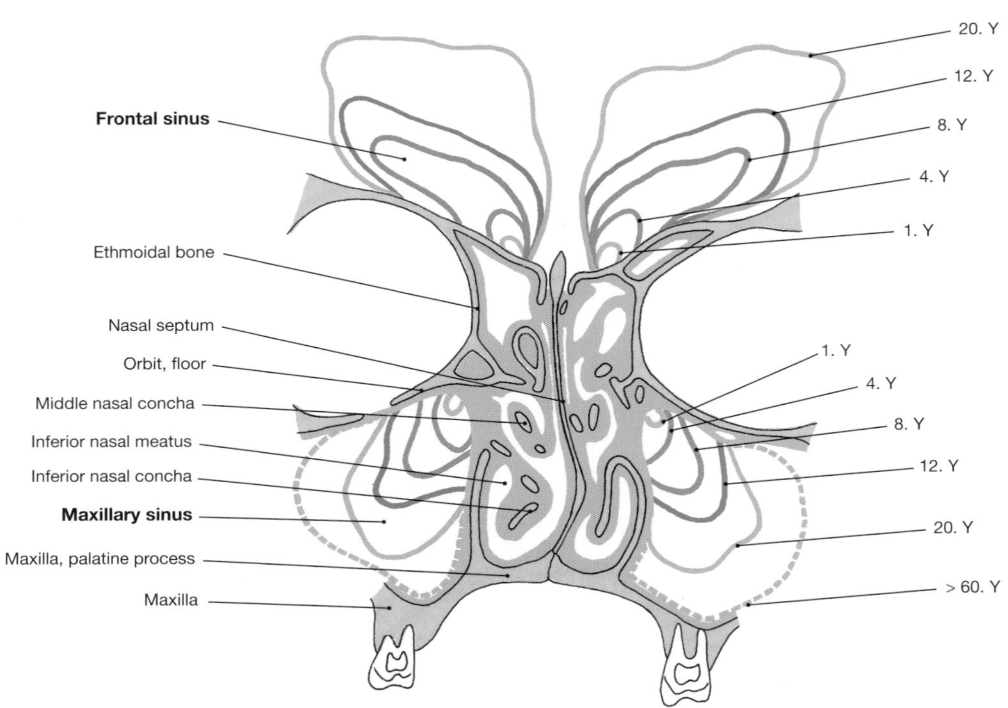
Frontal sinus
Ethmoidal bone
Nasal septum
Orbit, floor
Middle nasal concha
Inferior nasal meatus
Inferior nasal concha
Maxillary sinus
Maxilla, palatine process
Maxilla
20. Y
12. Y
8. Y
4. Y
1. Y
1. Y
4. Y
8. Y
12. Y
20. Y
> 60. Y

**Fig. 8.98 Development of the maxillary and frontal sinuses.**
Y: year of life.
At about 5 years of age, the developing frontal sinus reaches the upper margin of the orbit.

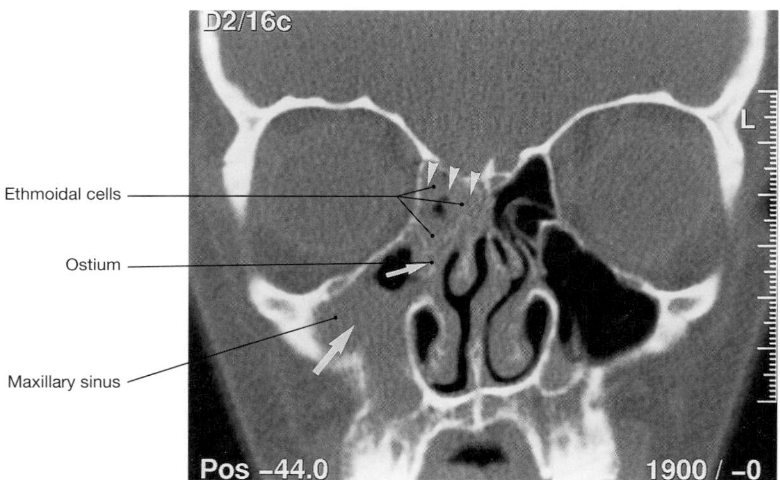
D2/16c
L
Pos -44.0
1900 / -0
Ethmoidal cells
Ostium
Maxillary sinus

**Fig. 8.99 Chronic sinusitis;** coronal computed tomography (CT) of the paranasal sinuses; white arrows indicate a swelling of the inflamed mucosa in the right maxillary sinus and the ostium, while white arrow heads point to a swelling of the ethmoidal cells. [17]

### Clinical Remarks

The middle nasal meatus is the endonasal access route in paranasal surgery for the treatment of a chronic inflammation of the frontal, maxillary, and anterior ethmoidal sinuses. An unilateral **inflammation of the maxillary sinus** often has an odontogenic origin (odontogenic maxillary sinusitis). Commonly, the cause is an inflammation of the second premolar or the first molar (→ Fig. 8.35).

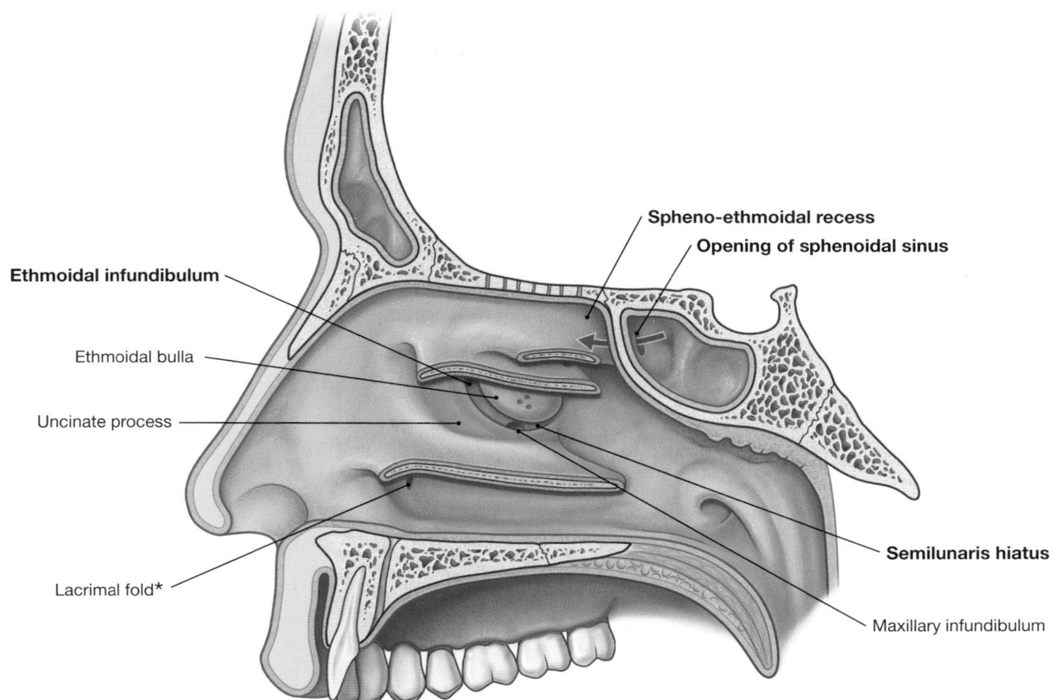
Spheno-ethmoidal recess
Opening of sphenoidal sinus
Ethmoidal infundibulum
Ethmoidal bulla
Uncinate process
Semilunaris hiatus
Lacrimal fold*
Maxillary infundibulum

**Fig. 8.100 Lateral nasal wall, right side;** view from the left side; nasal conchae separated from the wall at the base. [8]
The nasolacrimal duct opens into the lower nasal passage via the lacrimal fold (HASNER's valve). Beneath the middle nasal concha, the semilunaris hiatus is shown. The ethmoidal bulla and the uncinate process are located above and below the semilunaris hiatus, respectively. Posterior to the superior nasal concha the sphenoethmoidal recess with the opening of the sphenoidal sinus (blue arrow) is located.

* HASNER's valve

| Paranasal Sinuses – Common Clinical Terms | |
|---|---|
| **Agger nasi** | An anterior ethmoidal cell in front of and superior to the base of the middle nasal concha |
| **Semilunaris hiatus** | A crescent-shaped and up to 3 cm wide cleft between the ethmoidal bulla and the upper free margin of the uncinate process; the semilunaris hiatus provides access to the ethmoidal infundibulum |
| **Ethmoidal infundibulum** | Space delineated by the uncinate process, the lamina papyracea and the ethmoidal bulla |
| **Ethmoidal bulla** | An anterior ethmoidal cell above the semilunaris hiatus; regularly present but may not be found in all cases |
| **Uncinate process** | A thin lamellar bone of the ethmoidal bone participating in the formation of the medial wall of the maxillary sinus and confining the semilunaris hiatus at its anteroposterior aspect |
| **Basal lamella** | Embryonic residual lamellae present in the ethmoidal bone<br>There are four basal lamellae (BL):<br>• 1. BL: uncinate process<br>• 2. BL: ethmoidal bulla<br>• 3. BL: medial nasal concha<br>• 4. BL: superior nasal concha |
| **Fontanelle** | Accessory opening in the medial wall of the maxillary sinus |
| **Osteomeatal complex** | General term to describe the complex anatomy in the area around the semilunaris hiatus |
| **Frontal recess** | A cleft providing a connection between the frontal sinus and the main nasal cavity (nasofrontal duct, nasofrontal canal) |
| **HALLER's cell** | An ethmoidal cell assuring the pneumatization of the lower orbital wall (infraorbital cell) |
| **ÓNODI's cell (spheno-ethmoidal air cell)** | A posterior ethmoidal cell protruding beyond the sphenoidal sinus |

## Arteries of the nasal cavity

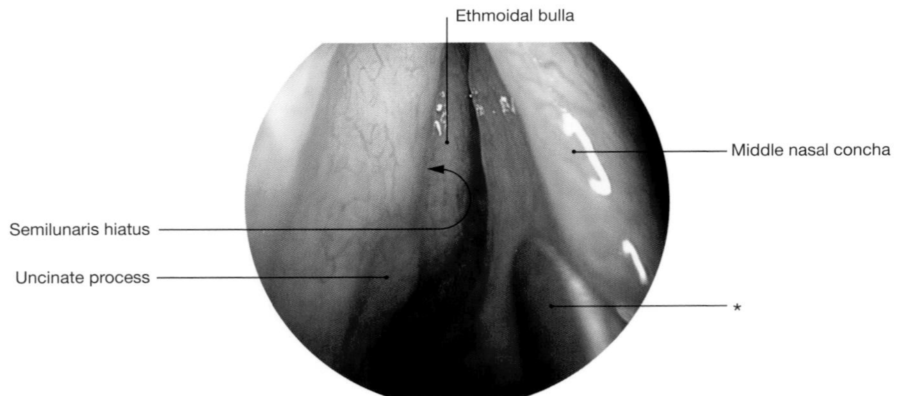
Ethmoidal bulla
Middle nasal concha
Semilunaris hiatus
Uncinate process
*

**Fig. 8.101 Nasal cavity, left side;** transnasal endoscopy with 30° optics.
The examiner views the head of the middle nasal concha.

* spatula

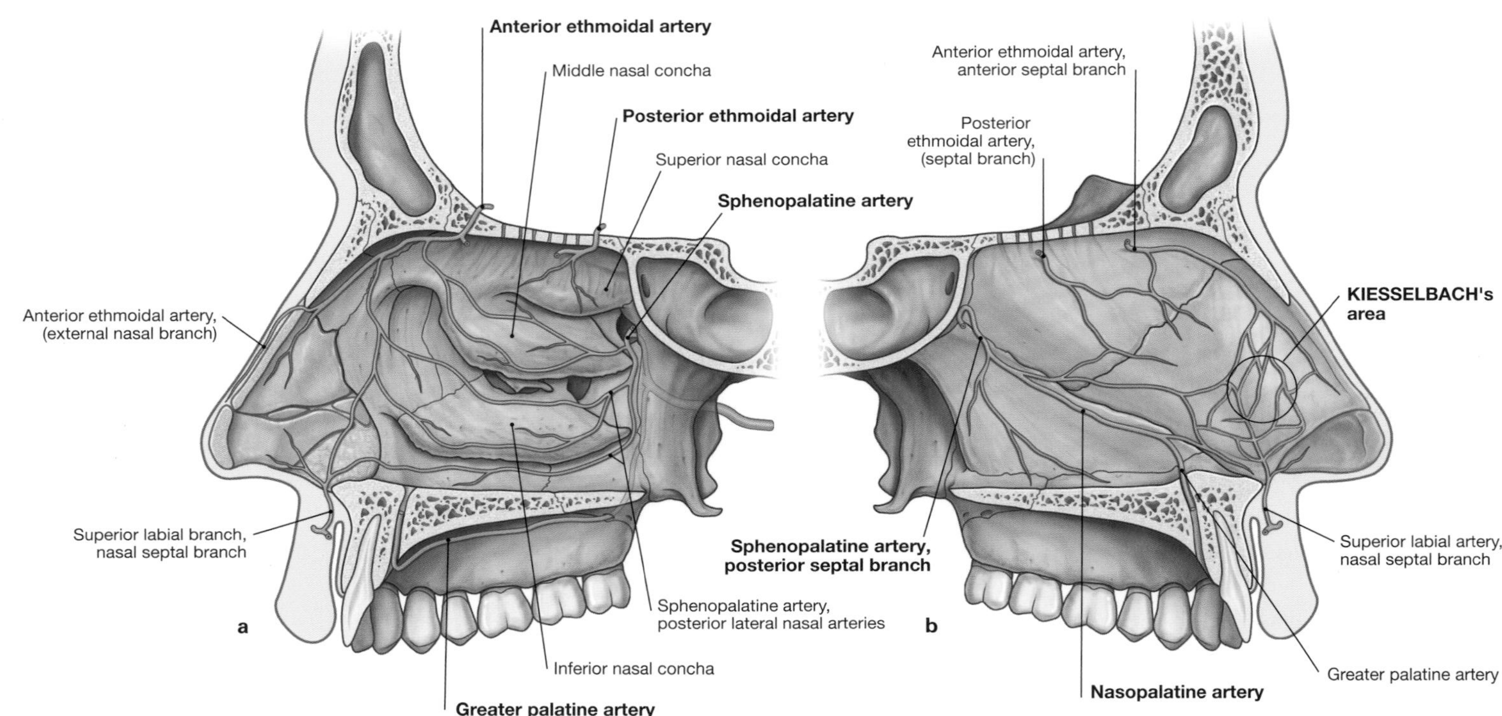
Anterior ethmoidal artery
Middle nasal concha
Posterior ethmoidal artery
Superior nasal concha
Sphenopalatine artery
Anterior ethmoidal artery, (external nasal branch)
Superior labial branch, nasal septal branch
a
Sphenopalatine artery, posterior lateral nasal arteries
Inferior nasal concha
Greater palatine artery
Anterior ethmoidal artery, anterior septal branch
Posterior ethmoidal artery, (septal branch)
KIESSELBACH's area
Sphenopalatine artery, posterior septal branch
b
Superior labial artery, nasal septal branch
Greater palatine artery
Nasopalatine artery

**Figs. 8.102a and b Arteries of the nasal cavity.** [8]
**a** Lateral wall of the right nasal cavity
**b** Nasal septum of the right nasal cavity
The external carotid artery provides the arterial supply to the nose. The **anterior and posterior ethmoidal arteries** from the ophthalmic artery reach the lateral wall of the nose and the nasal septum by traversing through the anterior and posterior part of the ethmoidal bone. As a terminal branch of the maxillary artery, the **sphenopalatine artery** gains access to the nasal cavity through the sphenopalatine foramen. There are anastomoses via arterial vessels of the lip to the facial artery. At the nasal septum, the sphenopalatine artery becomes the **nasopalatine artery** which passes through the incisive canal to reach the oral cavity where it anastomoses with the greater palatine artery. The KIESSELBACH's area, an arteriovenous plexus, is supplied by the nasopalatine artery and the anterior and posterior ethmoidal arteries.

### Clinical Remarks

The most frequent location for a **nasal bleeding** (epistaxis) is the KIESSELBACH's area at the nasal septum.
Basilar skull fractures involving the cribriform plate can lead to the rupture of the anterior and/or posterior ethmoidal arteries with consecutive nasal bleeding.
In those cases of nasal bleeding where a nasal balloon tamponade is unsuccessful, the sphenopalatine artery has to be ligated.

## Veins and nerves of the nasal cavity

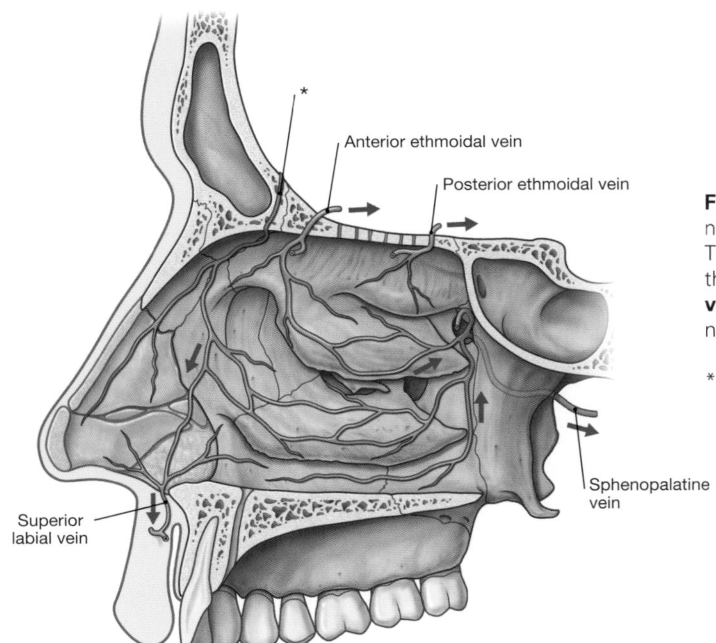
*
Anterior ethmoidal vein
Posterior ethmoidal vein
Sphenopalatine vein
Superior labial vein

**Fig. 8.103 Veins of the nasal cavity, right side;** view onto the lateral nasal wall. [8]
The blood is drained via the **anterior and posterior ethmoidal veins** to the cavernous sinus at the base of the skull, via the **sphenopalatine vein** to the pterygoid plexus in the infratemporal fossa, and via the connection to the **labial veins** to the facial vein.

* connecting vein to the superior sagittal sinus via the foramen cecum (only present during childhood)

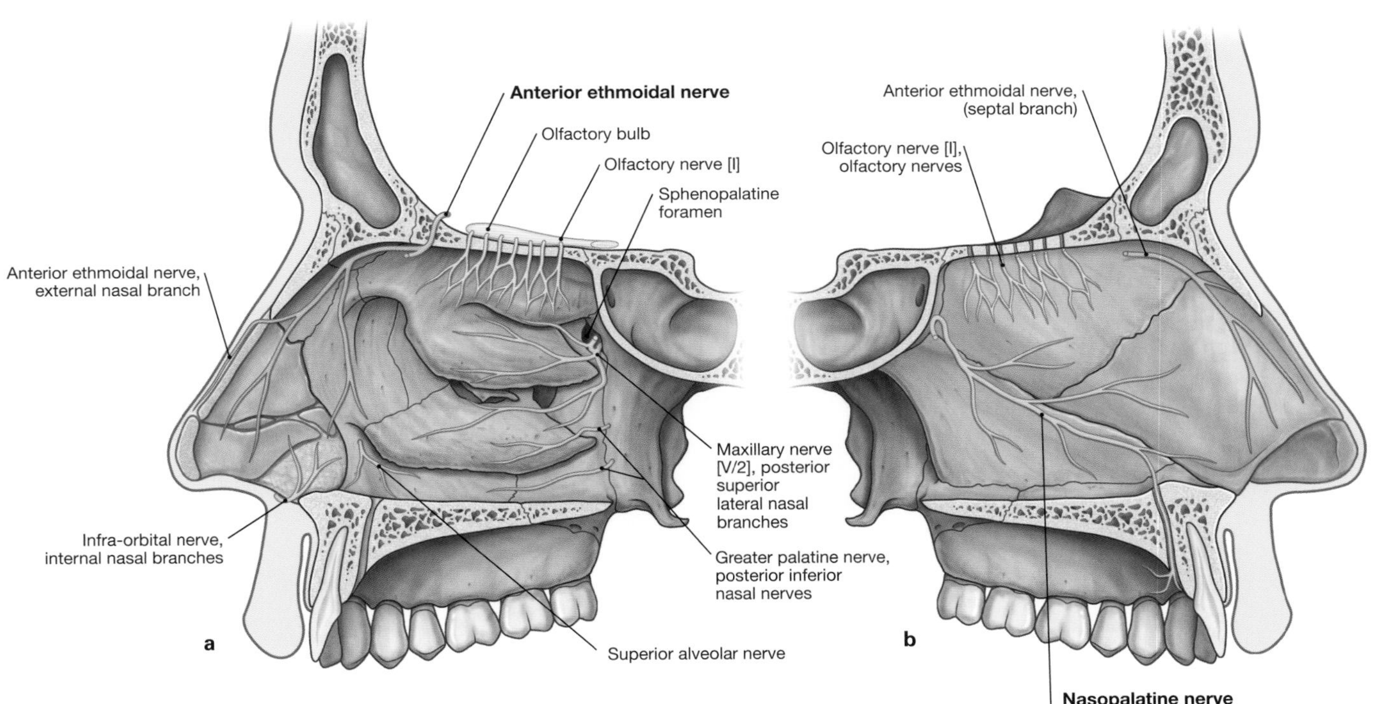
Anterior ethmoidal nerve
Olfactory bulb
Olfactory nerve [I]
Sphenopalatine foramen
Anterior ethmoidal nerve, external nasal branch
Maxillary nerve [V/2], posterior superior lateral nasal branches
Infra-orbital nerve, internal nasal branches
Greater palatine nerve, posterior inferior nasal nerves
Superior alveolar nerve
a
Anterior ethmoidal nerve, (septal branch)
Olfactory nerve [I], olfactory nerves
b
Nasopalatine nerve

**Figs. 8.104a and b Innervation of the nasal cavity.** [8]
**a** Lateral wall of the right nasal cavity
**b** Nasal septum of the right nasal cavity
Sensory innervation of the nasal mucosa is provided by branches of the trigeminal nerve [V]: ophthalmic nerve [V/1] → anterior ethmoidal nerve and maxillary nerve [V/2] → nasal branches, nasopalatine nerve. The **olfactory nerve [I]** innervates the olfactory area. The **nasopalatine nerve** runs alongside the nasal septum through the incisive canal, and innervates the mucosal area of the hard palate that stretches from the backside of the incisors to the canine teeth.

### Clinical Remarks

As the nasal mucosa receives rich sensory innervation, each manipulation in the nose can cause extreme pain sensations. Brain injuries with damage to the olfactory nerves can result in **anosmia** (the patient is unable to smell).
Rupture of the dura mater can cause a **cerebrospinal fluid rhinorrhea.** A clear transparent fluid drops from the nose of the patient. The diagnosis of cerebrospinal fluid is confirmed by the detection of glucose using glucose test strips. A surgical intervention is mandatory to prevent an infection.

## Oral cavity

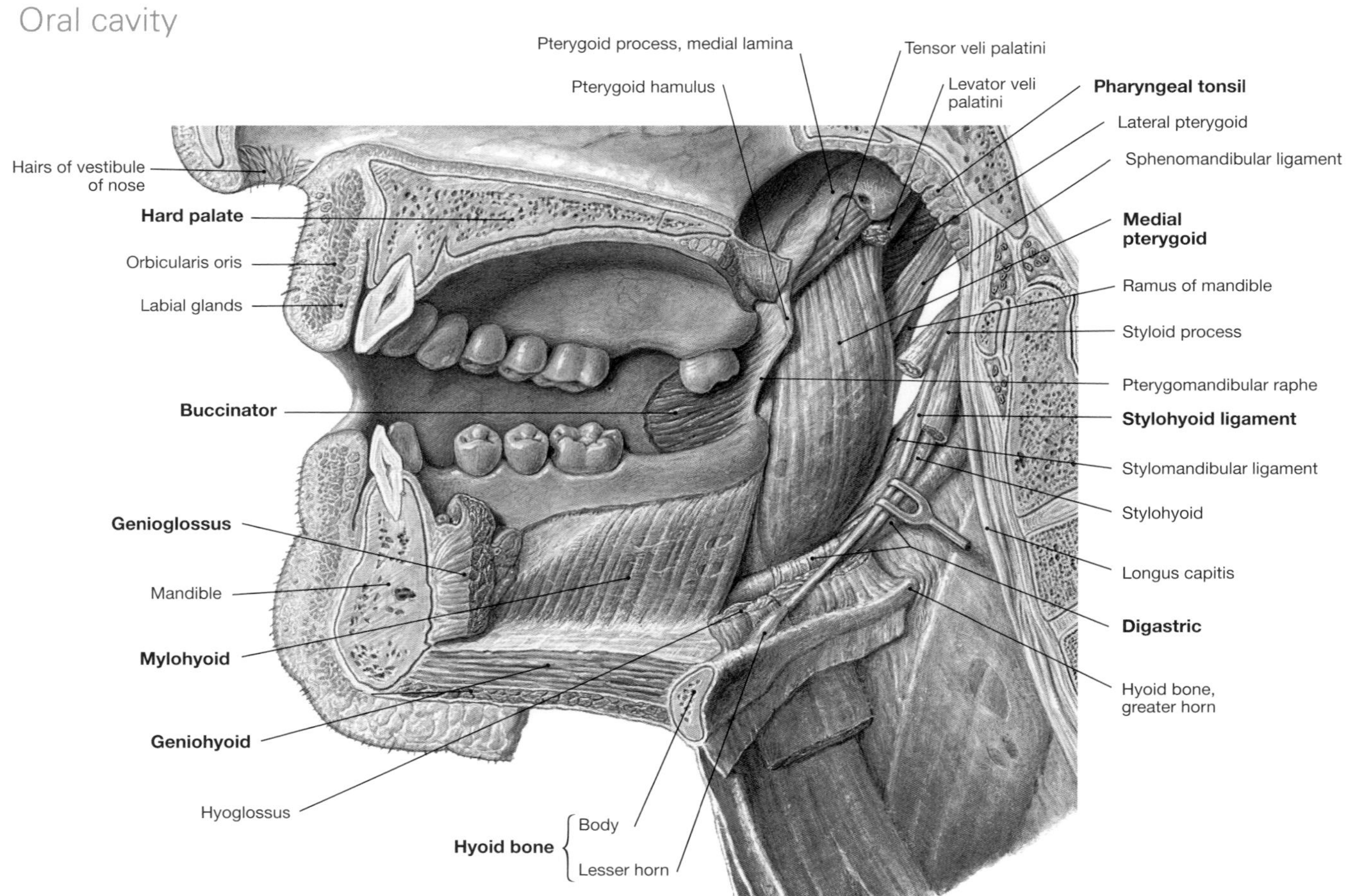

Pterygoid process, medial lamina
Tensor veli palatini
Pterygoid hamulus
Levator veli palatini
Pharyngeal tonsil
Lateral pterygoid
Sphenomandibular ligament
Hairs of vestibule of nose
Hard palate
Medial pterygoid
Orbicularis oris
Labial glands
Ramus of mandible
Styloid process
Pterygomandibular raphe
Buccinator
Stylohyoid ligament
Stylomandibular ligament
Genioglossus
Stylohyoid
Longus capitis
Mandible
Digastric
Mylohyoid
Hyoid bone, greater horn
Geniohyoid
Hyoglossus
Hyoid bone
Body
Lesser horn


**Fig. 8.105 Oral cavity, right side;** view from the left side.
The margins of the oral cavity are the lips (anterior), the cheeks (lateral), the muscular floor of the mouth (bottom, caudal), and the palate (top, cranial).

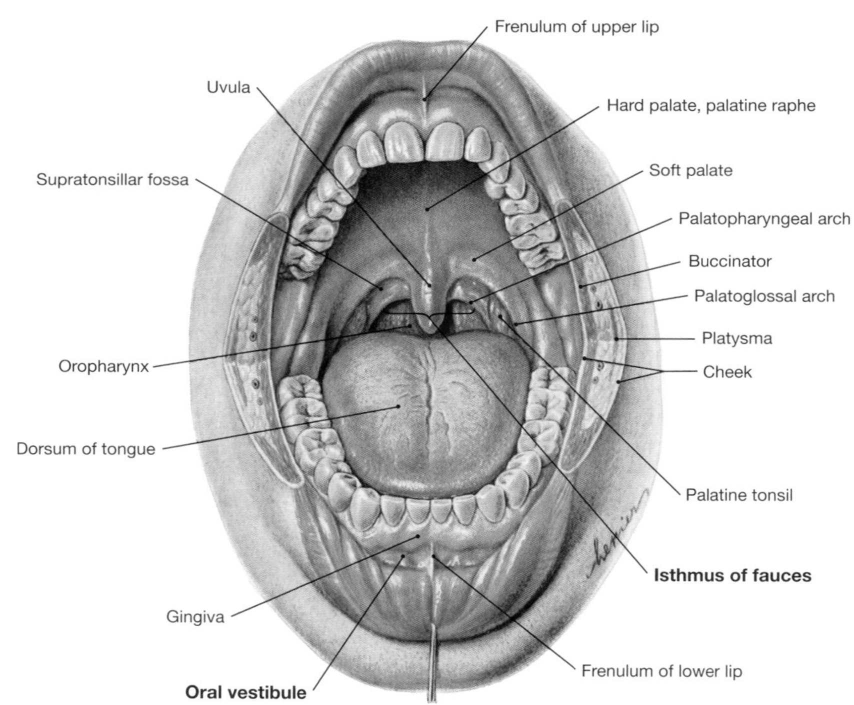

Frenulum of upper lip
Uvula
Hard palate, palatine raphe
Soft palate
Supratonsillar fossa
Palatopharyngeal arch
Buccinator
Palatoglossal arch
Platysma
Oropharynx
Cheek
Dorsum of tongue
Palatine tonsil
Isthmus of fauces
Gingiva
Frenulum of lower lip
Oral vestibule


**Fig. 8.106 Oral cavity;** frontal view; mouth open.
The oral opening (oral fissure) represents the entrance to the digestive tract and the oral cavity. The latter is divided into an oral vestibule and the cavity proper. The borders of the oral vestibule are the lips and cheeks at the outside and the alveolar processes and teeth at the inside. With the occlusion of teeth, a space behind the last molar tooth on each side allows access to the oral cavity. In the region of the oropharyngeal isthmus **(isthmus of fauces)** the oral cavity becomes the oral part of the pharynx (oropharynx). The excretory ducts of numerous smaller salivary glands and those of the three paired large salivary glands all drain into the oral vestibule and the cavity proper. The body of the tongue fills large parts of the inside of the oral cavity.

## Dental arches

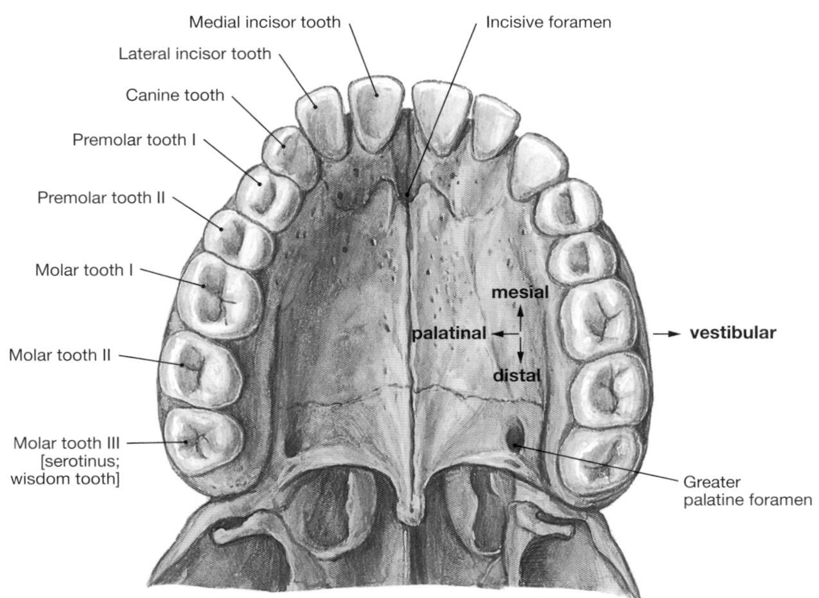
Medial incisor tooth
Incisive foramen
Lateral incisor tooth
Canine tooth
Premolar tooth I
Premolar tooth II
Molar tooth I
mesial
palatinal
vestibular
Molar tooth II
distal
Molar tooth III [serotinus; wisdom tooth]
Greater palatine foramen

**Fig. 8.107 Upper dental arch.**
The teeth are arranged in two dental arches, the upper (maxillary or superior dental arch) and the lower dental arch (mandibular or inferior dental arch), and are anchored in the upper and lower jaw. Dentition in the human is **heterodont;** the teeth come in characteristic shapes as incisors, canines, premolars, and molars. Incisors and canine teeth are also named front teeth, whereas premolars and molars are lateral teeth.

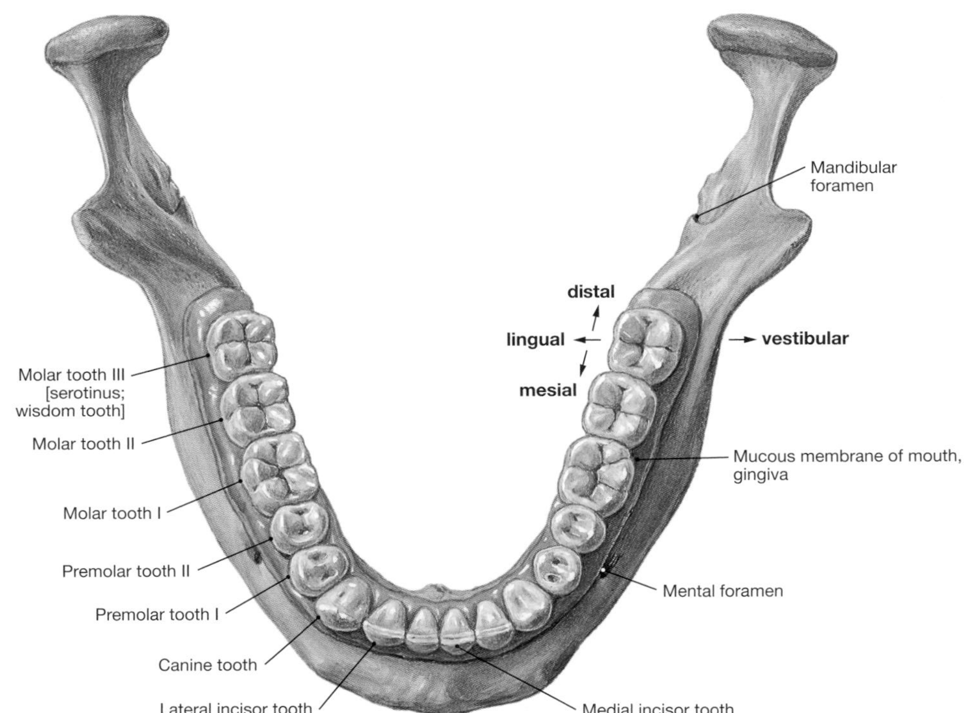
Mandibular foramen
distal
lingual
vestibular
mesial
Molar tooth III [serotinus; wisdom tooth]
Molar tooth II
Mucous membrane of mouth, gingiva
Molar tooth I
Premolar tooth II
Mental foramen
Premolar tooth I
Canine tooth
Lateral incisor tooth
Medial incisor tooth

**Fig. 8.108 Lower dental arch.**
With one exception, the arrangement of teeth in the lower dental arch is similar to that in the upper dental arch. For a precise indication of the "oral" topographic relationships, the terms "palatinal" is used in the upper jaw and "lingual" in the lower jaw. The **gingiva** or gums are the part of the mucosal lining of the mouth which covers the alveolar bony processes and the interdental bony septa, known as gingival embrasure. In addition, it covers the cervical part of the tooth and transitions into the oral mucosal layer at the gingival margin. The gingiva supports the anchorage of the teeth and stabilizes their position in the alveolar bone; as part of the oral mucosa, the marginal gingiva forms the junctional epithelium which is attached to the dental surfaces.

## Teeth, structure

**Fig. 8.109 Incisor tooth.**
Typical features of each tooth are the crown, the cervical part, and the root of the tooth. The **crown** of a tooth is the visible part of a tooth, rising above the gingiva, and is covered with enamel.
The **root** of a tooth sits in the alveolar tooth socket, a cavity in the alveolar process of the maxilla and mandible, and is covered with cement. Periodontal fibers (periodontium, desmodontium) anchor the root of a tooth in the alveolar bone. The cemento-enamel junction (frequently abbreviated as CEJ) locates at the **cervical part** of a tooth. Here, gingival fibers connect the gingiva with the cement of the tooth.
The deepest point in a tooth is the **root apex.** At the apical foramen, the dental papilla is perforated by the root canal which provides an access route for blood vessels and nerves to the dental pulp cavity. The dental **pulp cavity** divides into the radicular pulp and the coronal pulp. The dental pulp consists of connective tissue, containing blood vessels, lymph vessels, and nerves, and thus nourishes the tooth. Similar to the dental pulp cavity, one can distinguish between radicular/root and a coronal/crown pulp. Collectively, the cement, desmodontium, alveolar bone, and parts of the gingiva are referred to as the parodontium.

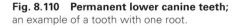

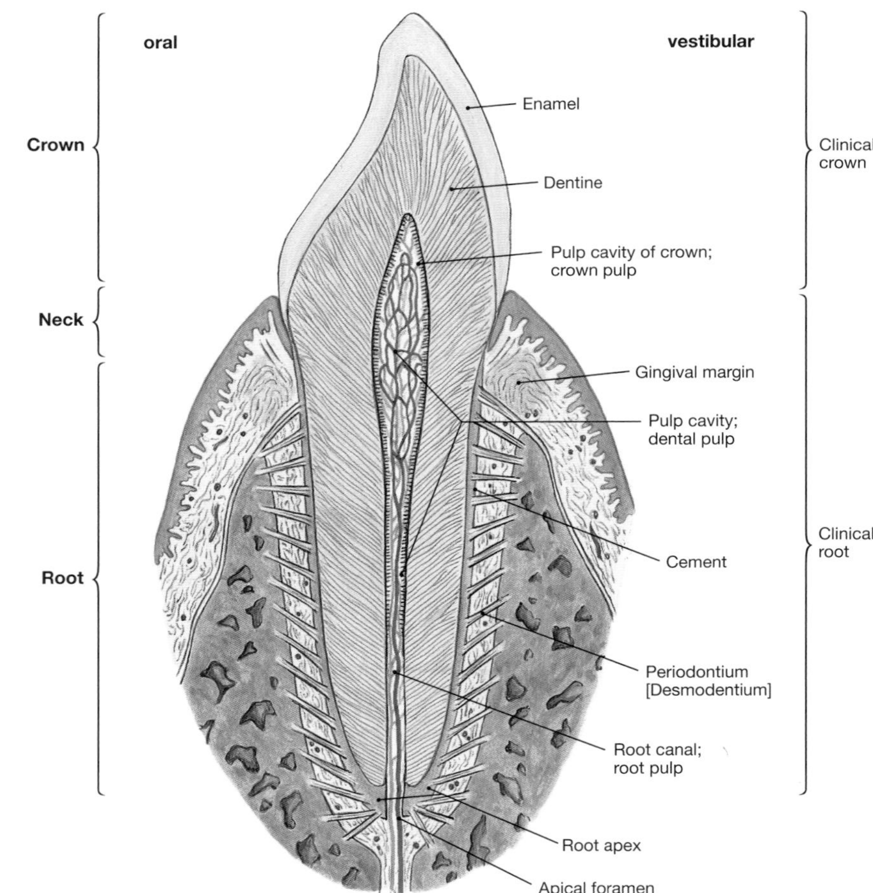
oral
vestibular
Crown
Neck
Root
Enamel
Dentine
Pulp cavity of crown; crown pulp
Clinical crown
Gingival margin
Pulp cavity; dental pulp
Cement
Clinical root
Periodontium [Desmodentium]
Root canal; root pulp
Root apex
Apical foramen

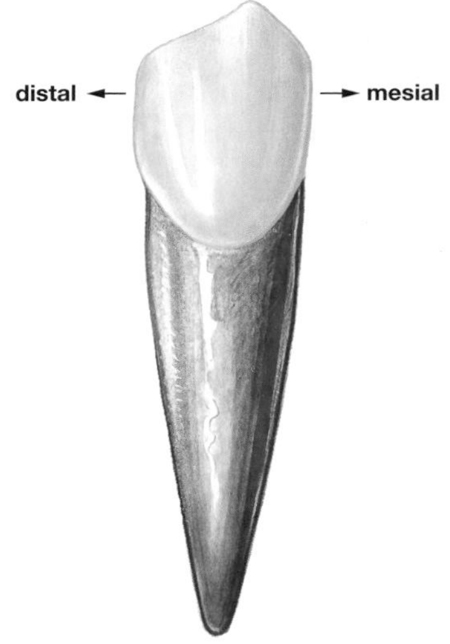
distal
mesial

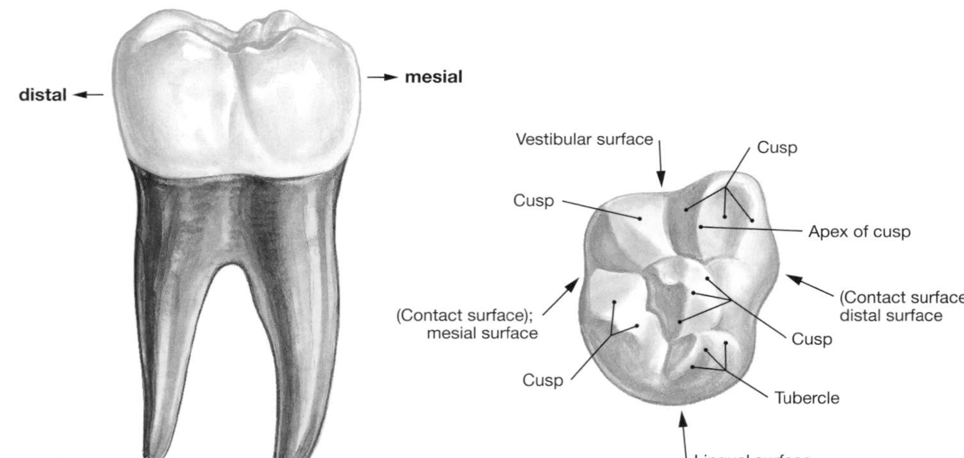
distal
mesial
Vestibular surface
Cusp
Cusp
Apex of cusp
(Contact surface); mesial surface
(Contact surface); distal surface
Cusp
Cusp
Tubercle
Lingual surface

**Fig. 8.110 Permanent lower canine teeth;** an example of a tooth with one root.

**Fig. 8.111 Second deciduous (milk) molar tooth;** an example of a tooth with two roots.

**Fig. 8.112 First permanent upper molar tooth;** occlusal surface of a molar tooth with a detailed description of the individual parts.

## Clinical Remarks

**Form, topography, rules for orientation**
The midline is the reference line when **describing the surface** of a tooth. Dental structures closest to the midline are named mesial, those located away from the midline are named distal. Contact areas to neighboring teeth are defined as surfaces. Number, dimension, and form of the roots are functionally adapted to the dental crown. The morphology of the roots of individual teeth in deciduous and permanent dentition is different and variable. Teeth with a single root are the incisor, canine, and premolar teeth. The upper premolars I and the lower molars have two roots, and the upper molars have three roots.

## Deciduous teeth

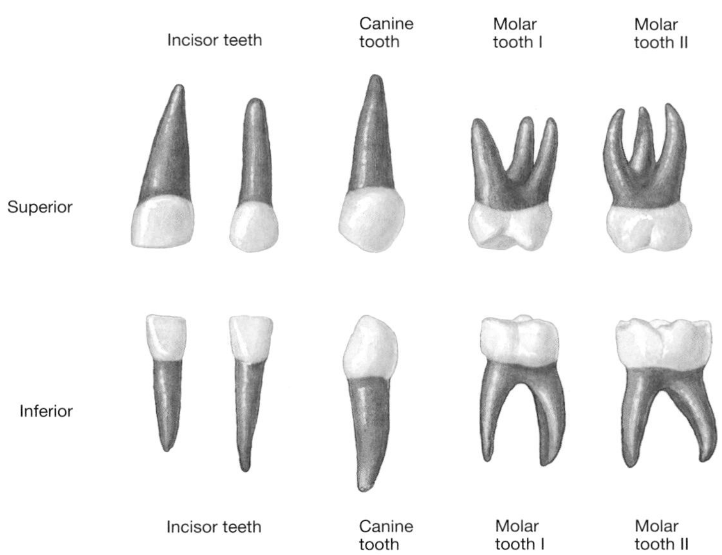
Incisor teeth
Canine tooth
Molar tooth I
Molar tooth II
Superior
Inferior
Incisor teeth
Canine tooth
Molar tooth I
Molar tooth II

**Fig. 8.113 Milk or deciduous teeth of a three year old child;** vestibular view.

A complete set of milk (deciduous) teeth is usually present at 30 months of age.

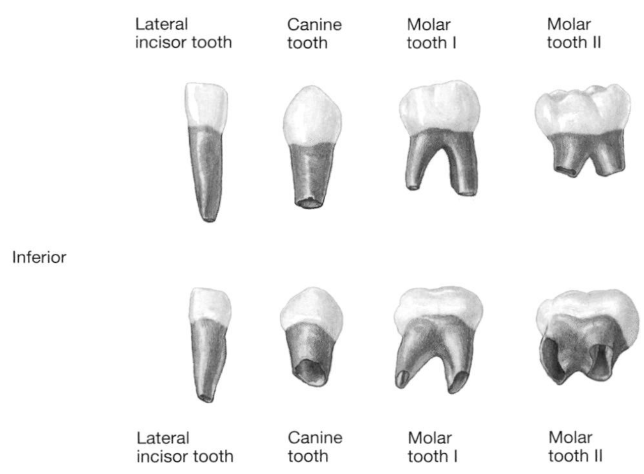
Lateral incisor tooth
Canine tooth
Molar tooth I
Molar tooth II
Inferior
Lateral incisor tooth
Canine tooth
Molar tooth I
Molar tooth II

**Fig. 8.114 Milk or deciduous teeth of a two year old child;** upper row, vestibular view, lower row, inferior view in an oblique angle.
The medial incisors are not shown. In a two year old child, the development of the roots of the teeth is not completed in numerous teeth. This process is only complete after dental eruption.

## Clinical Remarks

**Dental formula**
There is an internationally accepted dental formula which is applied by all disciplines of dental medicine. Each half of a jaw **(quadrant)** is numbered. Starting from the midline, **teeth** of the permanent and deciduous dentition are numbered consecutively from one to eight (permanent dentition) and from one to five (deciduous dentition), respectively. The digit of the quadrant is followed by the digit of the tooth; e.g., the description 11 (pronounced: one one) means the first incisor in the right upper jaw of the permanent dentition; the digits 52 (pronounced: five two) means the second incisor in the right upper jaw of the deciduous dentition.

Dental Formula of the Adult

Upper jaw

| Right | | | | | | | | | | | | | | | | | Left |
|---|---|---|---|---|---|---|---|---|---|---|---|---|---|---|---|---|---|
| | 18 | 17 | 16 | 15 | 14 | 13 | 12 | 11 | 21 | 22 | 23 | 24 | 25 | 26 | 27 | 28 | |
| | 48 | 47 | 46 | 45 | 44 | 43 | 42 | 41 | 31 | 32 | 33 | 34 | 35 | 36 | 37 | 38 | |

Lower jaw

Dental Formula of Deciduous Dentition

Upper jaw

| Right | | | | | | | | | | | Left |
|---|---|---|---|---|---|---|---|---|---|---|---|
| | 55 | 54 | 53 | 52 | 51 | 61 | 62 | 63 | 64 | 65 | |
| | 85 | 84 | 83 | 82 | 81 | 71 | 72 | 73 | 74 | 75 | |

Lower jaw

## Permanent teeth

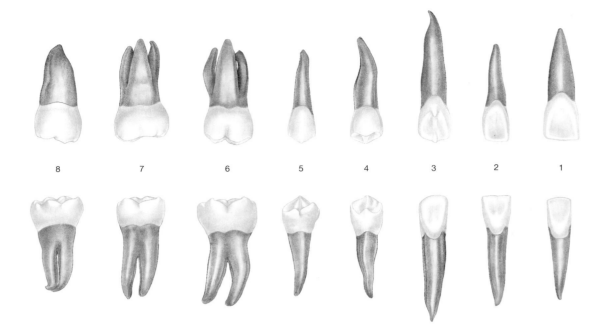

**Fig. 8.115 Permanent teeth;** oral view.

1 Incisor tooth I
2 Incisor tooth II
3 Canine tooth
4 Premolar tooth I
5 Premolar tooth II
6 Molar tooth I
7 Molar tooth II
8 Molar tooth III [serotinus; wisdom tooth]

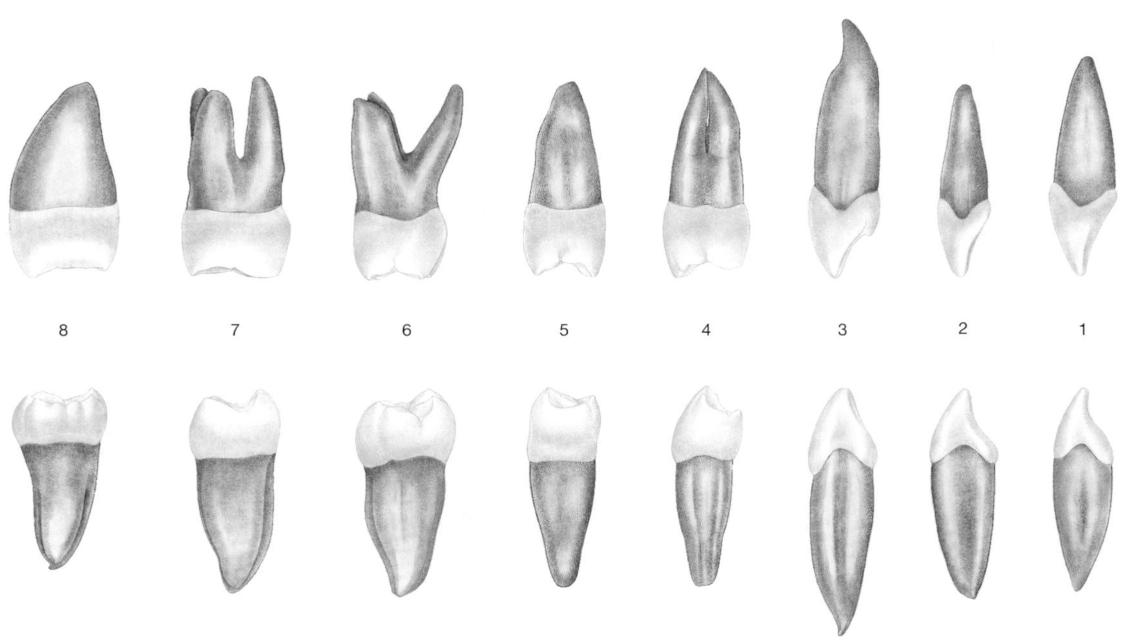
8
7
6
5
4
3
2
1

**Fig. 8.116 Permanent teeth;** distal view.

1 Incisor tooth I
2 Incisor tooth II
3 Canine tooth
4 Premolar tooth I
5 Premolar tooth II
6 Molar tooth I
7 Molar tooth II
8 Molar tooth III [serotinus; wisdom tooth]

### Clinical Remarks

Teeth are the most resistant structures in the body and serve as important evidence in **forensic** medicine for the identification of a victim.

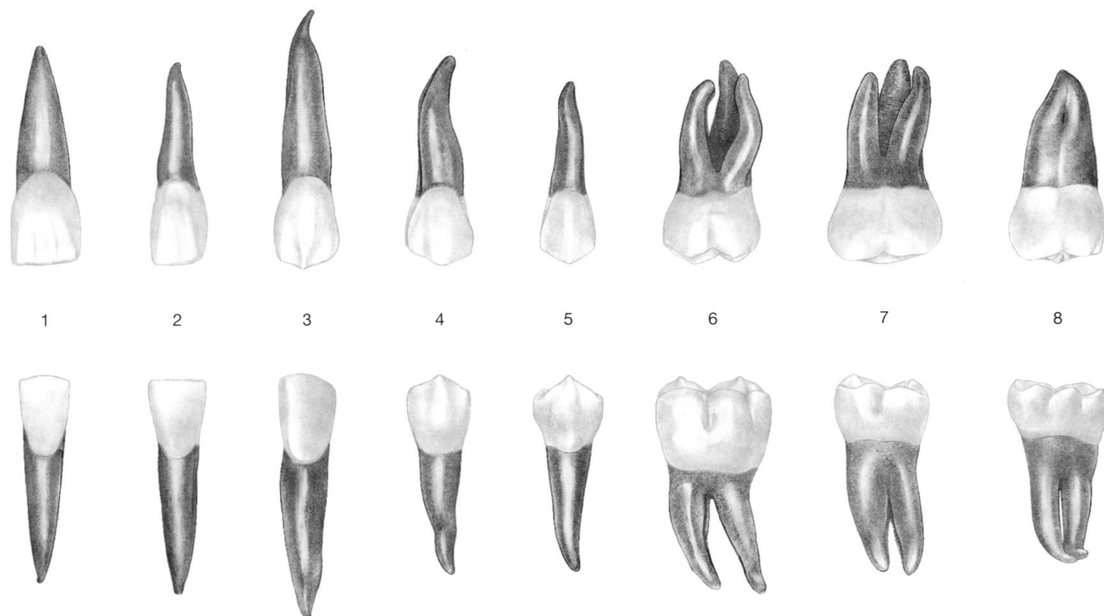
1
2
3
4
5
6
7
8

**Fig. 8.117 Permanent teeth;** vestibular view.

1 Incisor tooth I
2 Incisor tooth II
3 Canine tooth
4 Premolar tooth I
5 Premolar tooth II
6 Molar tooth I
7 Molar tooth II
8 Molar tooth III [serotinus; wisdom tooth]

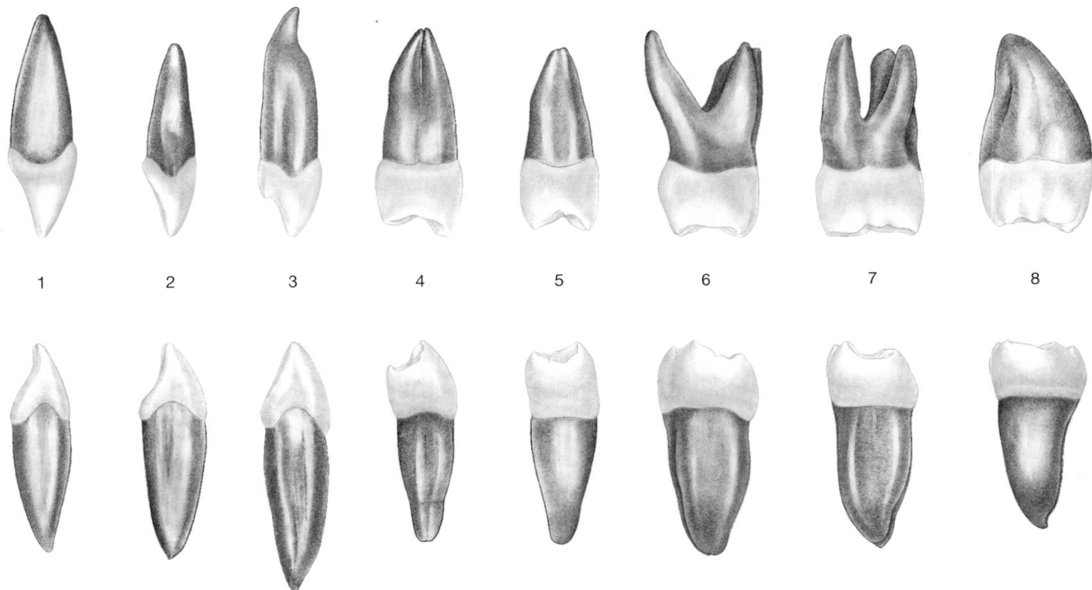
1
2
3
4
5
6
7
8

**Fig. 8.118 Permanent teeth;** mesial view.

1 Incisor tooth I
2 Incisor tooth II
3 Canine tooth
4 Premolar tooth I
5 Premolar tooth II
6 Molar tooth I
7 Molar tooth II
8 Molar tooth III [serotinus; wisdom tooth]

## Clinical Remarks

- Environmental and genetic factors can influence the **dental development.** Resulting dental anomalies affect the size, form, and number of teeth.
- The administration of **tetracyclines** (a member of the family of antibiotics) during the phase of dental development can result in discoloration of teeth and enamel defects.
- Also important are discolorations of teeth and enamel defects caused by high doses of fluorides in form of tablets **(dental fluorosis).**
- Enamel defects can point towards hypovitaminosis D **(rickets).**
- Residual elements of the odontogenic epithelium can remain as SERRE's bodies, remnants of the epithelial root sheath as epithelial cell rests of MALASSEZ, and both can generate cysts.

## Times of tooth eruption

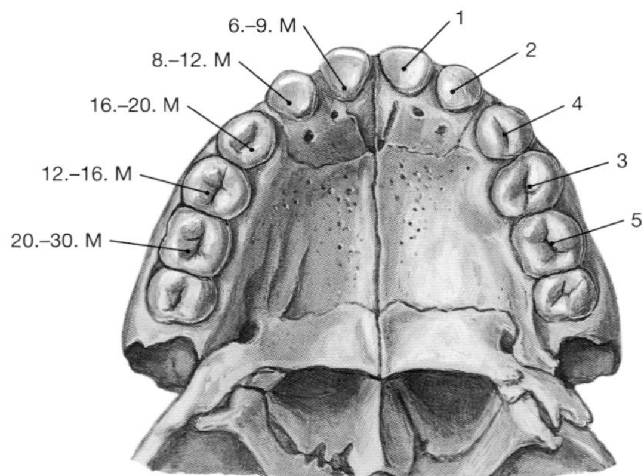
6.–9. M
8.–12. M
16.–20. M
12.–16. M
20.–30. M
1
2
4
3
5

**Fig. 8.119 Upper jaw, maxilla, with deciduous teeth and the first permanent tooth;** left side: average time of tooth eruption in months (M); right side: sequence of tooth eruption.
The development of permanent teeth (replacement teeth) and deciduous (milk) teeth is similar but happens at different times. The time of eruption and the sequence at which milk teeth appear in the oral cavity is subject to significant interindividual differences. However, at 30 months of age the set of deciduous teeth usually will be completed.

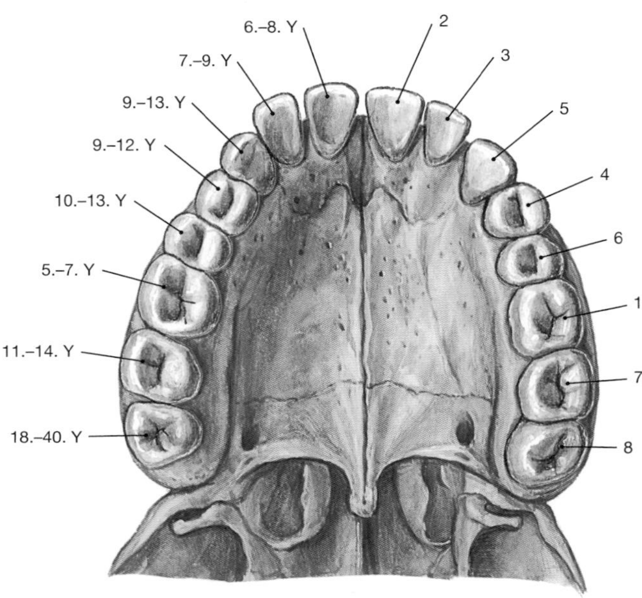
6.–8. Y
7.–9. Y
9.–13. Y
9.–12. Y
10.–13. Y
5.–7. Y
11.–14. Y
18.–40. Y
2
3
5
4
6
1
7
8

**Fig. 8.120 Upper jaw, maxilla, with permanent teeth;** left side: average time of tooth eruption in years (Y); right side: sequence of tooth eruption.
With the exception of the molar teeth, deciduous dentition (first dentition with 20 teeth) is similar to the permanent dentition (second dentition with 32 teeth). The sequence of eruption of the permanent molars is always the same: first molars with six years of age **(6-year molars),** second molars with twelve years of age, and third molars with 18 years of age or later.

## Clinical Remarks

**Periodontopathies** are diseases affecting the supporting structures of the teeth. **Parodontosis** is a chronic degenerative form of periodontal disease and results in an increased tooth mobility and tooth loss with subsequent atrophy of the alveolar process caused by the decline of the periodontal support system.

Systemic administration of fluoride ions during the time of enamel formation of the permanent teeth increases the deposition of **fluorapatite,** instead of hydroxyapatite, resulting in a more durable enamel capable of better resisting dental caries.

## Development of teeth

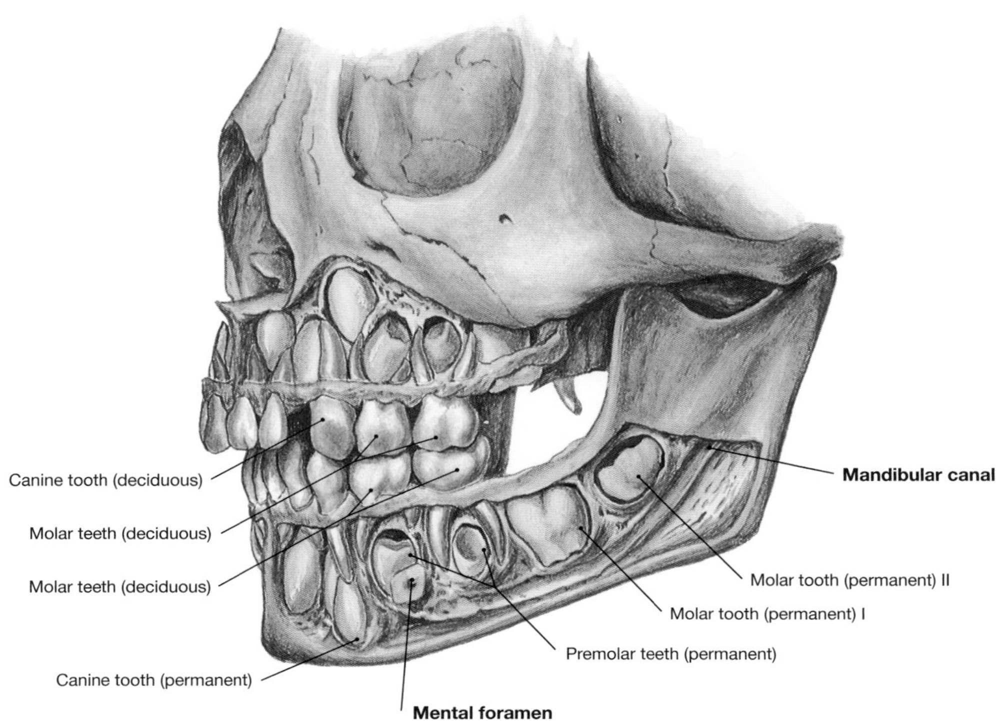
Canine tooth (deciduous)
Molar teeth (deciduous)
Molar teeth (deciduous)
Canine tooth (permanent)
Mental foramen
Mandibular canal
Molar tooth (permanent) II
Molar tooth (permanent) I
Premolar teeth (permanent)

**Fig. 8.121 Upper jaw, maxilla, and lower jaw, mandible, of a five year old child;** deciduous teeth and primordium of the later permanent teeth.
Human dentition is diphyodont; there are two consecutive dentitions, known as deciduous and permanent dentition. First, the 20 milk (deciduous) teeth form in children. Development and eruption of the first and second dentitions and the body growth are synchronized in a timely manner. Resorption of the root of the milk teeth occurs at different time points.

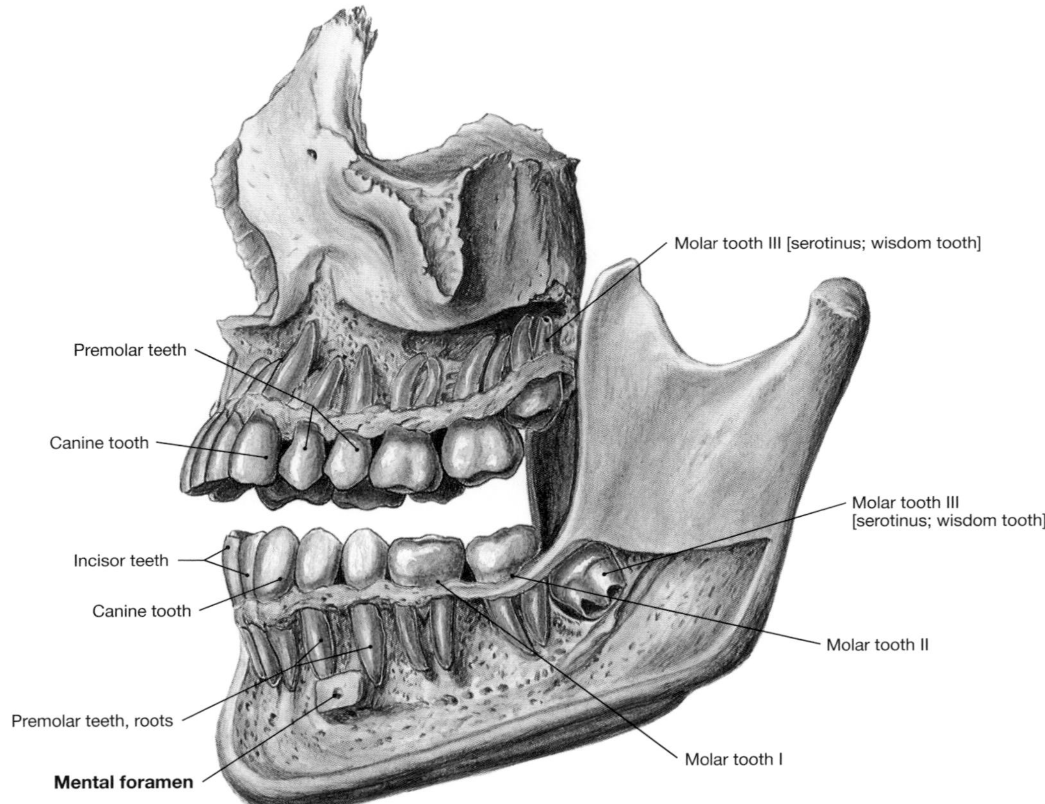
Molar tooth III [serotinus; wisdom tooth]
Premolar teeth
Canine tooth
Incisor teeth
Canine tooth
Premolar teeth, roots
Mental foramen
Molar tooth III
[serotinus; wisdom tooth]
Molar tooth II
Molar tooth I

**Fig. 8.122 Upper jaw, maxilla, and lower jaw, mandible, of a 20 year old person.**
Completion of the permanent dentition results in up to 32 permanent teeth. The third molar (serotinus; wisdom tooth) has not yet erupted in the lower jaw. It can regress or may not have developed at all (aplasia). Usually, the molar teeth erupt approximately seven months earlier in girls than in boys. In both sexes, the molar teeth in the lower jaw erupt earlier than molar teeth in the maxilla. The roots of the deciduous teeth require another 16 to 26 months to develop; the roots of the permanent teeth are fully developed only after another 1.7 to 3.5 years.

## Upper jaw, radiography and blood supply to the teeth

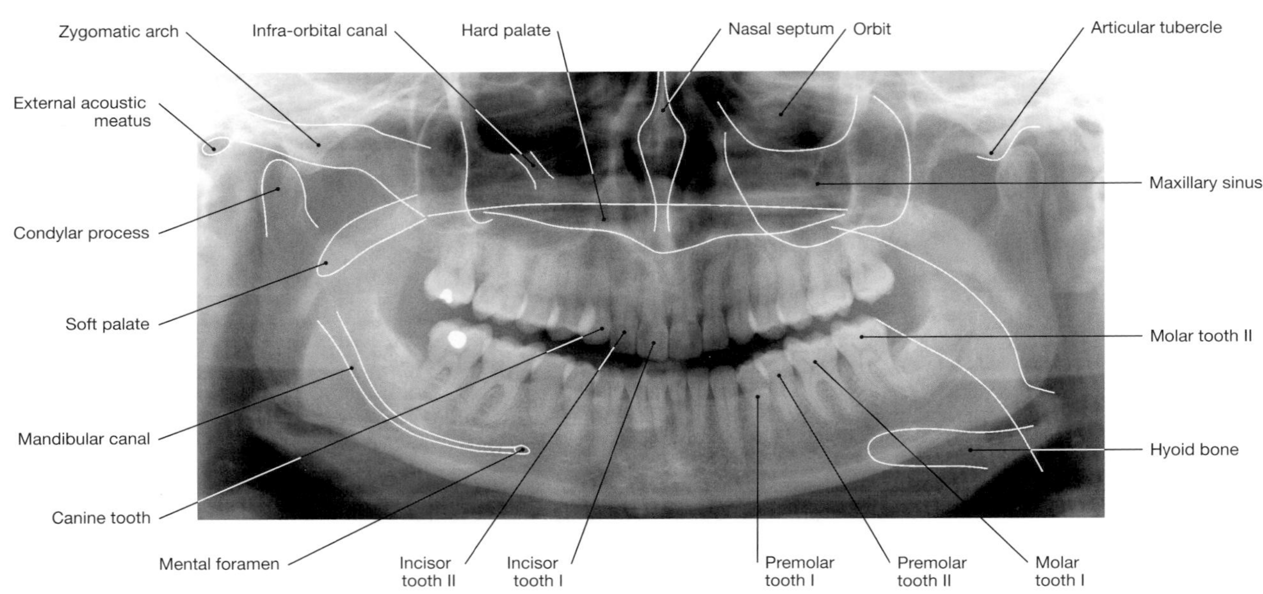
Zygomatic arch
Infra-orbital canal
Hard palate
Nasal septum
Orbit
Articular tubercle
External acoustic meatus
Maxillary sinus
Condylar process
Soft palate
Molar tooth II
Mandibular canal
Hyoid bone
Canine tooth
Mental foramen
Incisor tooth II
Incisor tooth I
Premolar tooth I
Premolar tooth II
Molar tooth I

**Fig. 8.123 Upper jaw, maxilla, and lower jaw, mandible, without wisdom teeth;** panoramic radiograph.

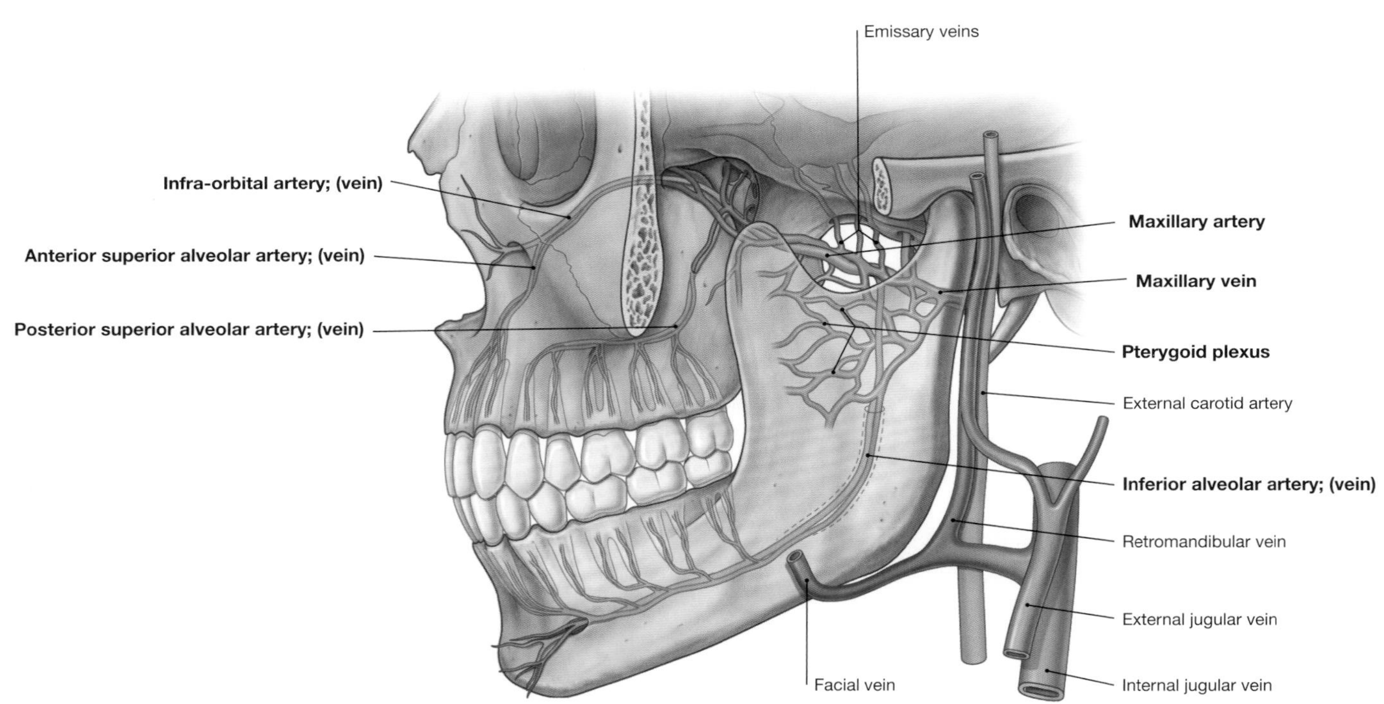
Emissary veins
Infra-orbital artery; (vein)
Anterior superior alveolar artery; (vein)
Posterior superior alveolar artery; (vein)
Maxillary artery
Maxillary vein
Pterygoid plexus
External carotid artery
Inferior alveolar artery; (vein)
Retromandibular vein
External jugular vein
Internal jugular vein
Facial vein

**Fig. 8.124 Blood supply of the teeth.** [8]
The arterial blood supply to the upper lateral teeth comes from the **posterior superior alveolar artery** and to the upper front teeth from the **infraorbital artery,** both branches of the maxillary artery. Teeth and gingiva of the lower jaw are supplied by the **inferior alveolar artery,** which runs in the mandibular canal. Concomitant veins drain the blood into the **pterygoid plexus.**

## Innervation of the teeth and pterygopalatine ganglion

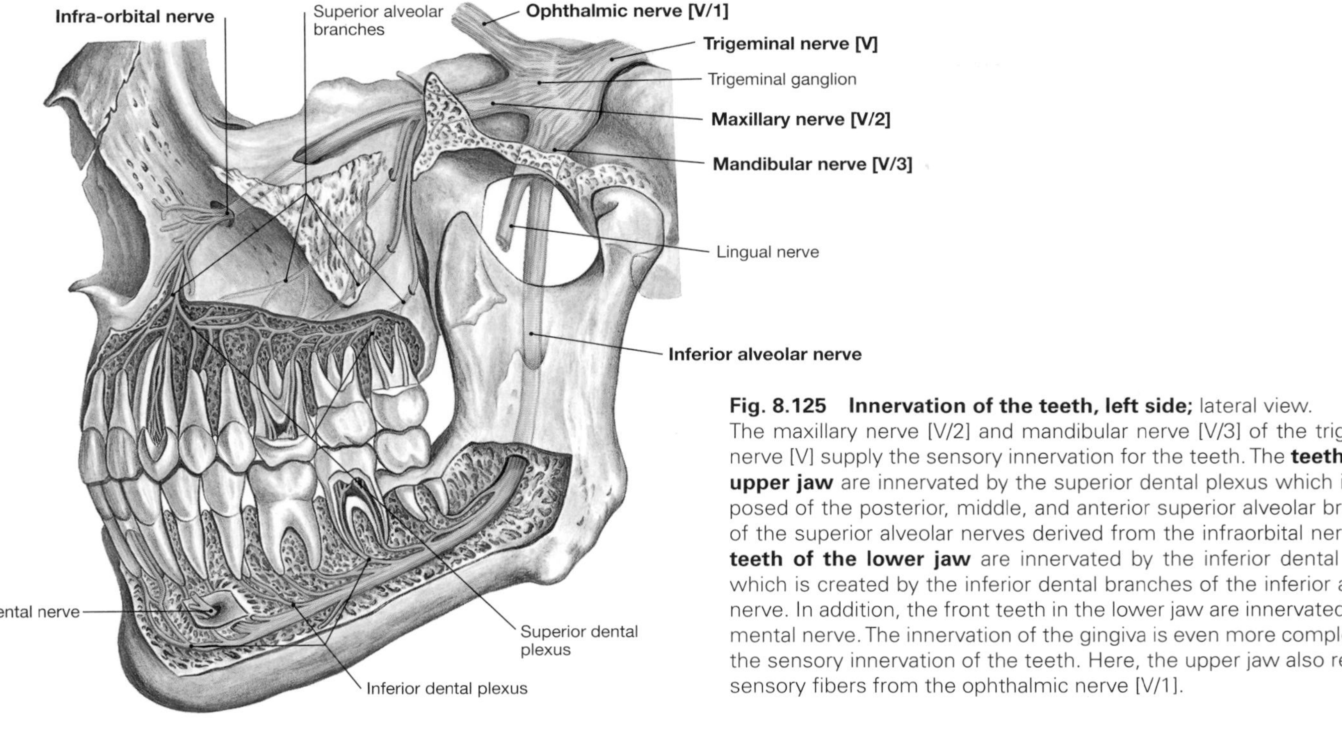
Infra-orbital nerve
Superior alveolar branches
Ophthalmic nerve [V/1]
Trigeminal nerve [V]
Trigeminal ganglion
Maxillary nerve [V/2]
Mandibular nerve [V/3]
Lingual nerve
Inferior alveolar nerve
Mental nerve
Superior dental plexus
Inferior dental plexus

**Fig. 8.125 Innervation of the teeth, left side;** lateral view.
The maxillary nerve [V/2] and mandibular nerve [V/3] of the trigeminal nerve [V] supply the sensory innervation for the teeth. The **teeth of the upper jaw** are innervated by the superior dental plexus which is composed of the posterior, middle, and anterior superior alveolar branches of the superior alveolar nerves derived from the infraorbital nerve. The **teeth of the lower jaw** are innervated by the inferior dental plexus which is created by the inferior dental branches of the inferior alveolar nerve. In addition, the front teeth in the lower jaw are innervated by the mental nerve. The innervation of the gingiva is even more complex than the sensory innervation of the teeth. Here, the upper jaw also receives sensory fibers from the ophthalmic nerve [V/1].

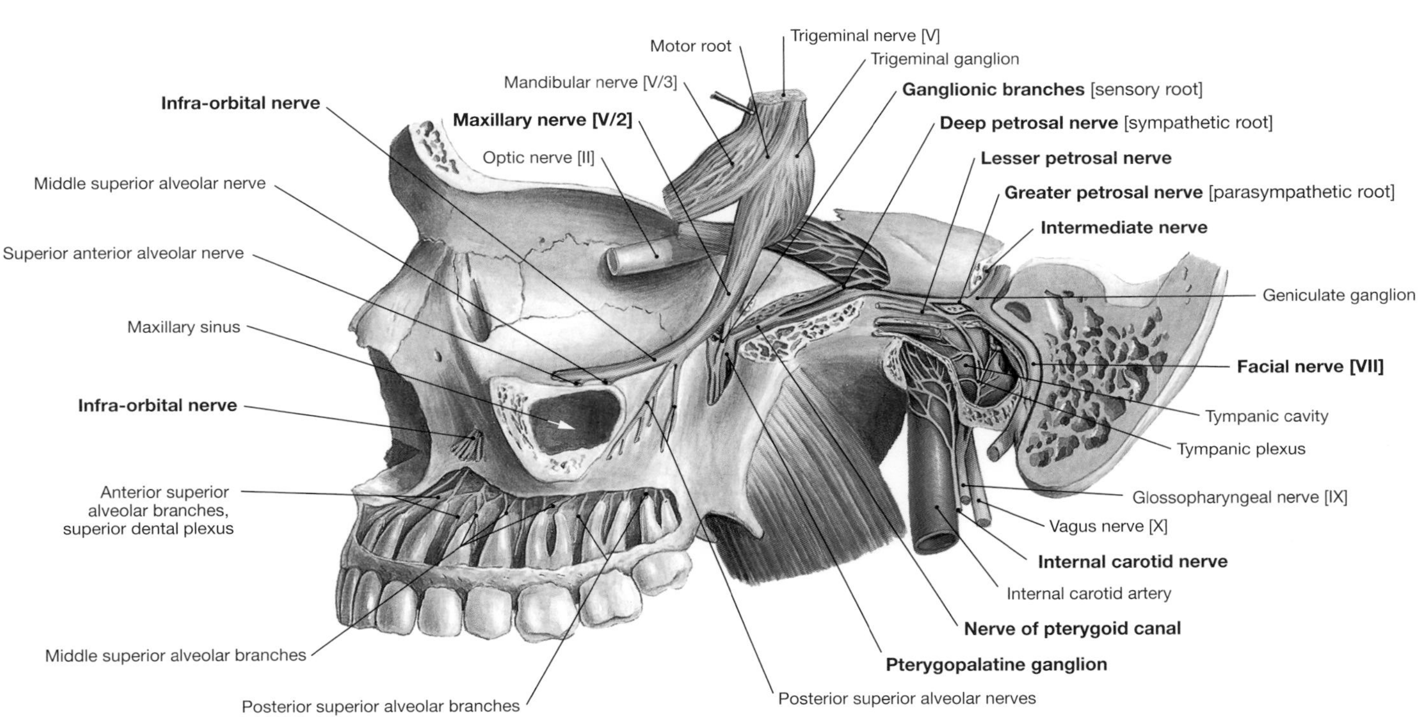
Motor root
Trigeminal nerve [V]
Trigeminal ganglion
Mandibular nerve [V/3]
Infra-orbital nerve
Ganglionic branches [sensory root]
Maxillary nerve [V/2]
Deep petrosal nerve [sympathetic root]
Optic nerve [II]
Lesser petrosal nerve
Middle superior alveolar nerve
Greater petrosal nerve [parasympathetic root]
Intermediate nerve
Superior anterior alveolar nerve
Geniculate ganglion
Maxillary sinus
Facial nerve [VII]
Infra-orbital nerve
Tympanic cavity
Tympanic plexus
Anterior superior alveolar branches, superior dental plexus
Glossopharyngeal nerve [IX]
Vagus nerve [X]
Internal carotid nerve
Internal carotid artery
Nerve of pterygoid canal
Middle superior alveolar branches
Pterygopalatine ganglion
Posterior superior alveolar branches
Posterior superior alveolar nerves

**Fig. 8.126 Pterygopalatine ganglion.**
Sensory nerve fibers run within the ganglionic branches of the maxillary nerve [V/2] via the pterygopalatine ganglion to reach the soft and hard palate. Preganglionic parasympathetic fibers from the superior salivatory nucleus reach the pterygopalatine ganglion via the facial nerve [VII] (intermediate nerve), the greater petrosal nerve, and the nerve of pterygoid canal. In the pterygopalatine ganglion, these preganglionic parasympathetic fibers are synapsed to postganglionic parasympathetic fibers which innervate the lacrimal glands and glands of the nose and oropharynx. These glands receive postganglionic sympathetic fibers from the deep petrosal nerve which runs through the pterygopalatine ganglion and derives from the internal carotid nerve (internal carotid plexus).

## Clinical Remarks

Local **infiltrative anesthesia** is required for teeth in the upper jaw since teeth and gingiva in the upper jaw receive their innervation from different nerve branches. A unilateral branch block anesthetizes the teeth on the ipsilateral half of the mandible by blocking the sensory impulses of the inferior alveolar nerve shortly before it enters the mandibular canal. Because the lingual nerve is also anesthetized in the process, the sensory block extends to the ipsilateral half of the tongue with the exception of the tip of the tongue. Further, the chin and parts of the lower lip are numb since all the terminal branches of the inferior alveolar nerve are also anesthetized.

## Pterygopalatine fossa and pterygopalatine ganglion

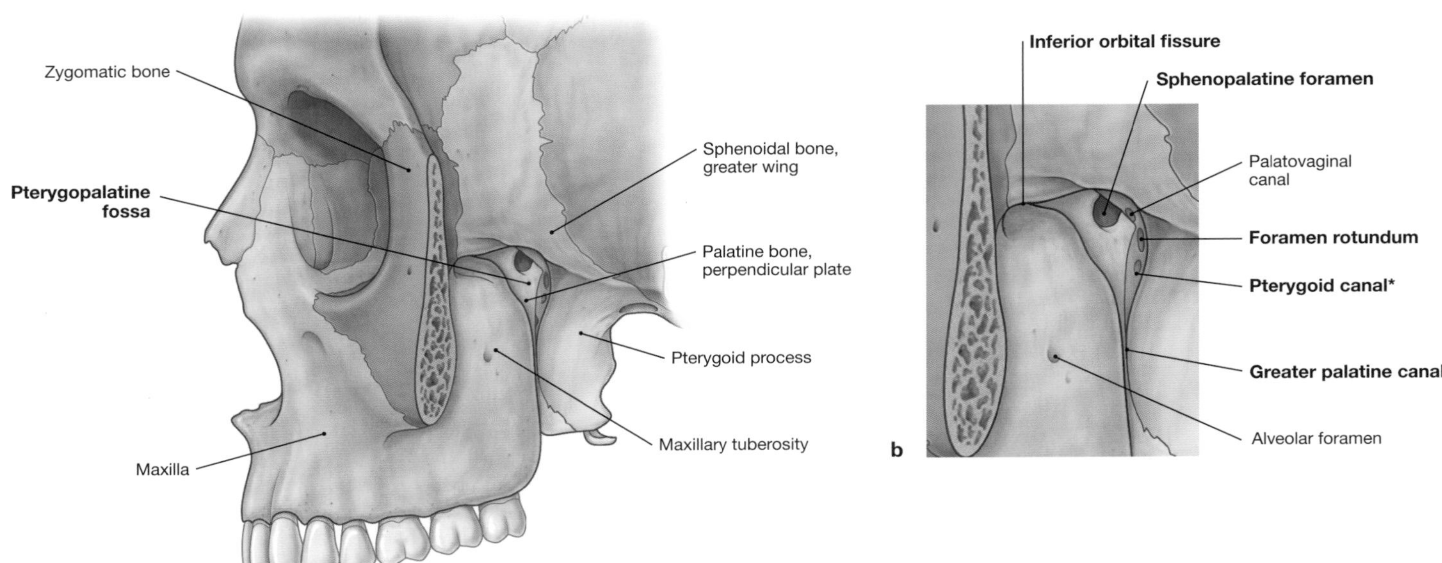

Zygomatic bone
Pterygopalatine fossa
Sphenoidal bone, greater wing
Palatine bone, perpendicular plate
Pterygoid process
Maxillary tuberosity
Maxilla
a
Inferior orbital fissure
Sphenopalatine foramen
Palatovaginal canal
Foramen rotundum
Pterygoid canal*
Greater palatine canal
Alveolar foramen
b


**Figs. 8.127a and b Pterygopalatine fossa, left side;** lateral view; color chart see inside of the back cover of this volume. [8]
**a** Overview
**b** Magnification
The pterygopalatine fossa represents a connecting point for the structures of the nervous system of the middle cranial fossa, the orbit, and the nose. Maxilla, palatine bone, and sphenoidal bone participate in defining the margins of this fossa. The borders of the pterygopalatine fossa are formed by the maxillary tuberosity in its anterior part, posterior by the pterygoid process, medial by the perpendicular plate of the palatine bone, and cranial by the greater wing of the sphenoidal bone. A cranial passage leads to the inferior orbital fissure providing access to the orbit. The posterior part of the pterygopalatine fossa opens into the retropharyngeal space; its lateral opening leads into the infratemporal fossa.

* VIDIAN canal

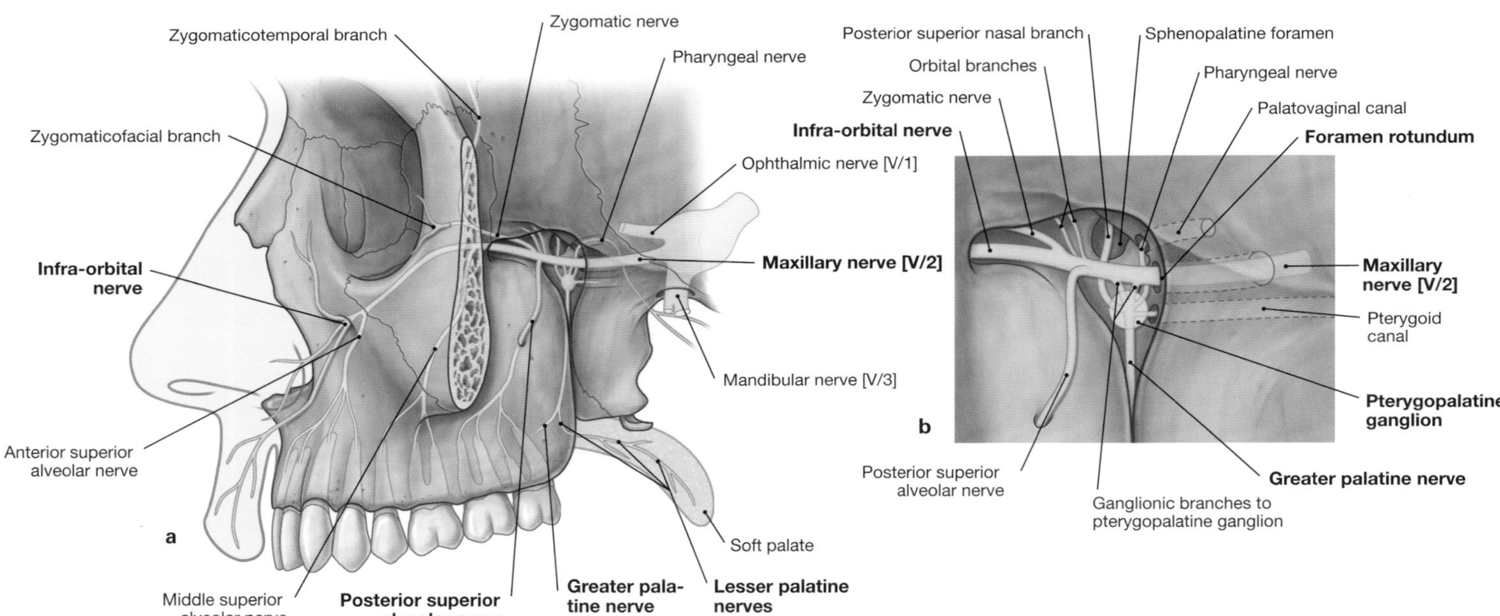

Zygomaticotemporal branch
Zygomatic nerve
Pharyngeal nerve
Zygomaticofacial branch
Infra-orbital nerve
Ophthalmic nerve [V/1]
Maxillary nerve [V/2]
Mandibular nerve [V/3]
Anterior superior alveolar nerve
a
Soft palate
Middle superior alveolar nerve
Posterior superior alveolar nerve
Greater palatine nerve
Lesser palatine nerves
Posterior superior nasal branch
Sphenopalatine foramen
Orbital branches
Pharyngeal nerve
Zygomatic nerve
Palatovaginal canal
Infra-orbital nerve
Foramen rotundum
Maxillary nerve [V/2]
Pterygoid canal
Pterygopalatine ganglion
b
Greater palatine nerve
Posterior superior alveolar nerve
Ganglionic branches to pterygopalatine ganglion


**Figs. 8.128a and b Maxillary nerve [V/2], left side;** lateral view. [8]
**a** Terminal branches
**b** Spacial relationship to the pterygopalatine ganglion
The maxillary nerve [V/2] exits the base of the skull through the **foramen rotundum** to enter the pterygopalatine fossa and exits this fossa through the **infraorbital fissure.** In the pterygopalatine fossa, the maxillary nerve [V/2] provides orbital branches, the zygomatic nerve, the posterior superior alveolar nerve as well as ganglionic branches to the pterygopalatine ganglion.

## Pterygopalatine fossa

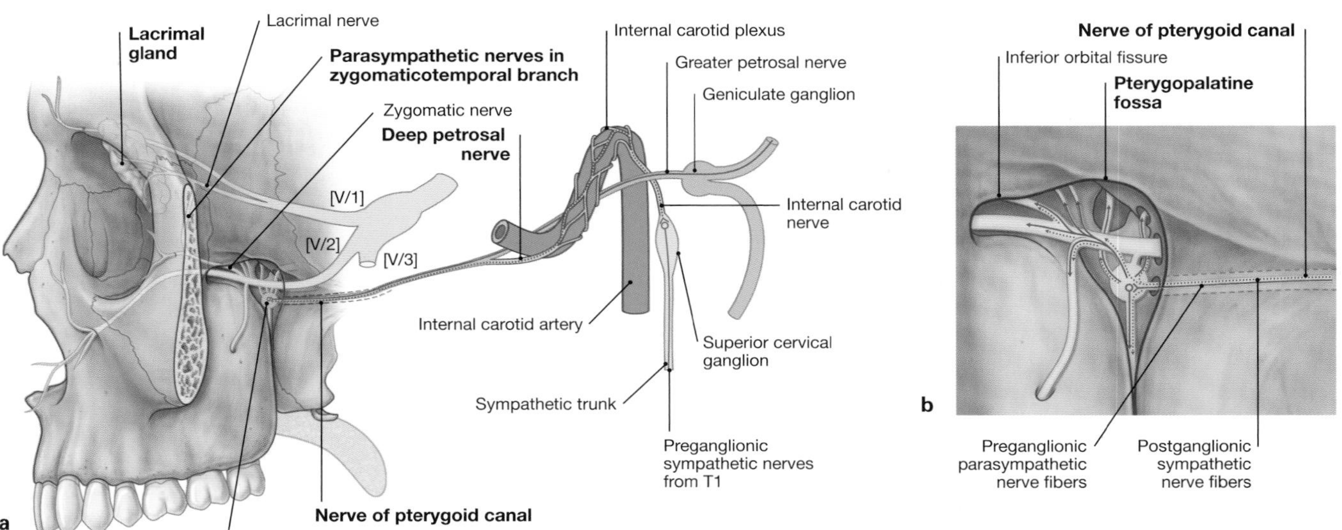
Lacrimal gland
Lacrimal nerve
Parasympathetic nerves in zygomaticotemporal branch
Zygomatic nerve
Deep petrosal nerve
[V/1]
[V/2]
[V/3]
Internal carotid plexus
Greater petrosal nerve
Geniculate ganglion
Internal carotid nerve
Internal carotid artery
Superior cervical ganglion
Sympathetic trunk
Preganglionic sympathetic nerves from T1
Nerve of pterygoid canal
Pterygopalatine ganglion
a
Nerve of pterygoid canal
Inferior orbital fissure
Pterygopalatine fossa
b
Preganglionic parasympathetic nerve fibers
Postganglionic sympathetic nerve fibers

**Figs. 8.129a and b Nerve of pterygoid canal, left side;** lateral view. [8]

**a** Overview

**b** Nerves in the pterygopalatine fossa

**Parasympathetic** fibers of the facial nerve [VII], which form the greater petrosal nerve, reach the pterygopalatine ganglion, synapse here from preganglionic to postganglionic neurons, and run to the lacrimal, nasal, and oropharyngeal glands. **Postganglionic sympathetic** fibers originating from the internal carotid plexus, assemble as the deep petrosal nerve, and run through the pterygopalatine ganglion without synapsing in this parasympathetic ganglion. They also reach the lacrimal, nasal, and oropharyngeal glands.

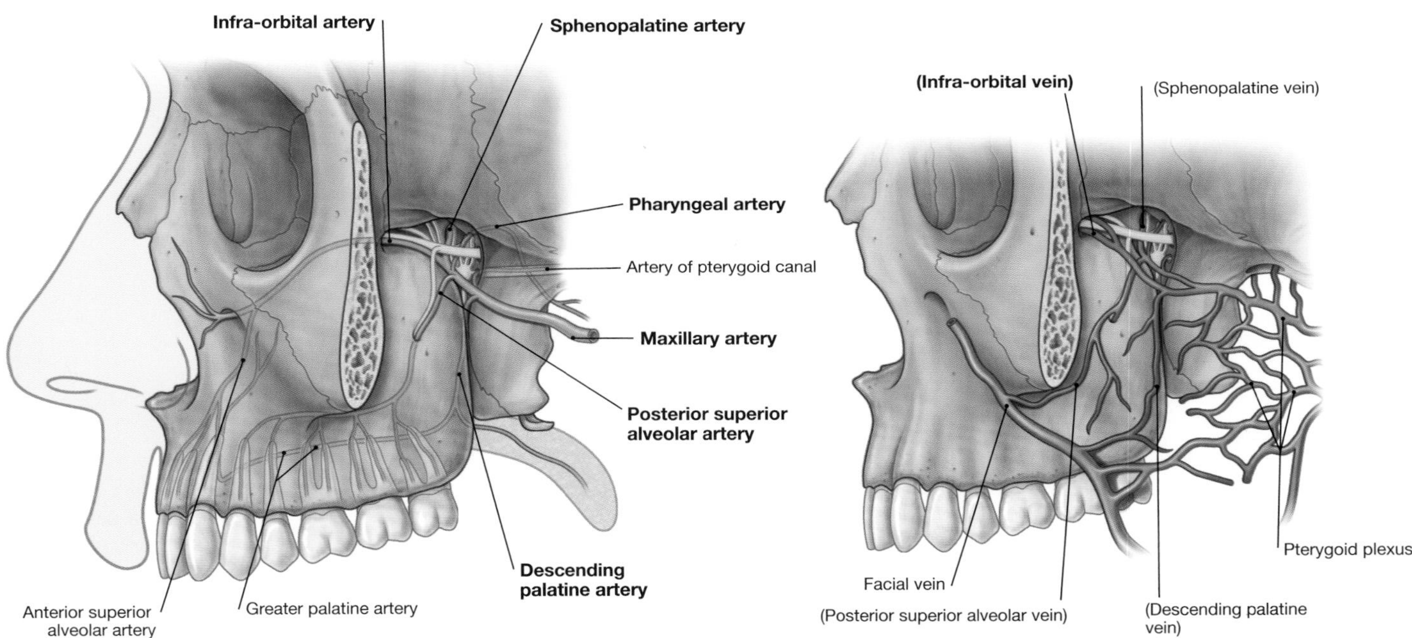
Infra-orbital artery
Sphenopalatine artery
Pharyngeal artery
Artery of pterygoid canal
Maxillary artery
Posterior superior alveolar artery
Descending palatine artery
Anterior superior alveolar artery
Greater palatine artery
(Infra-orbital vein)
(Sphenopalatine vein)
Pterygoid plexus
Facial vein
(Posterior superior alveolar vein)
(Descending palatine vein)

**Fig. 8.130 Maxillary artery in the pterygopalatine fossa, left side;** lateral view. [8]

Within the pterygopalatine fossa, the maxillary artery divides into its **terminal branches:** infraorbital, sphenopalatine, posterior superior alveolar, descending palatine arteries, and pharyngeal branch.

**Fig. 8.131 Veins of the pterygopalatine fossa, left side;** lateral view. [8]

The infraorbital, sphenopalatine, posterior superior alveolar, and descending palatine veins drain into the **pterygoid plexus,** which is located in the infratemporal fossa.

## Clinical Remarks

A lesion of the parasympathetic fibers exiting the brain in association with the facial nerve [VII] and then reaching the lacrimal gland via branches of the ophthalmic nerve [V/1] can result in a reduced production of lacrimal fluid by the lacrimal gland, leading to a **dry eye syndrome** (sicca syndrome).

## Palate and palatine muscles

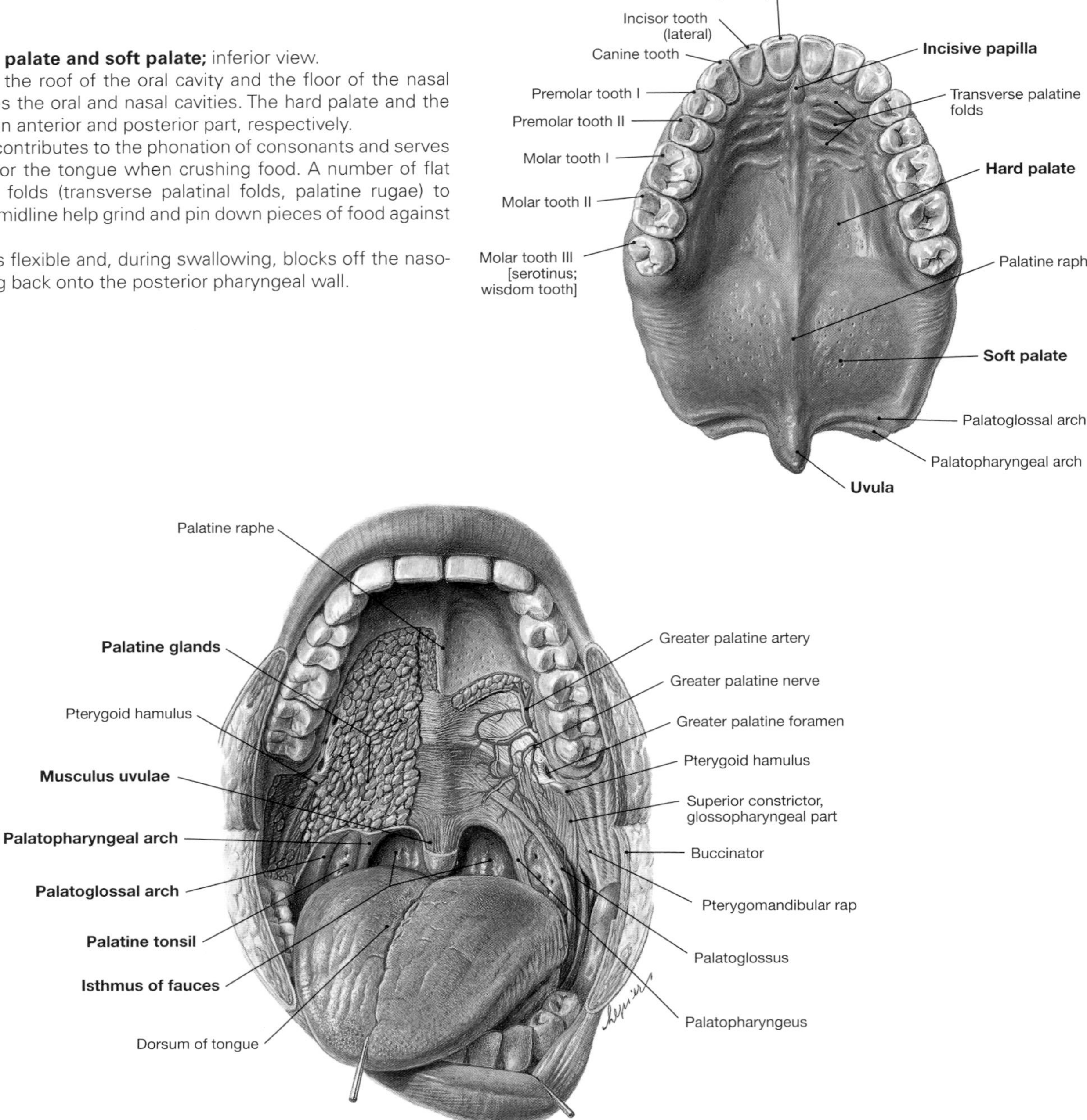
Incisor tooth (medial)
Incisor tooth (lateral)
Canine tooth
Premolar tooth I
Premolar tooth II
Molar tooth I
Molar tooth II
Molar tooth III [serotinus; wisdom tooth]
Incisive papilla
Transverse palatine folds
Hard palate
Palatine raphe
Soft palate
Palatoglossal arch
Palatopharyngeal arch
Uvula
Palatine raphe
Palatine glands
Pterygoid hamulus
Musculus uvulae
Palatopharyngeal arch
Palatoglossal arch
Palatine tonsil
Isthmus of fauces
Dorsum of tongue
Greater palatine artery
Greater palatine nerve
Greater palatine foramen
Pterygoid hamulus
Superior constrictor, glossopharyngeal part
Buccinator
Pterygomandibular rap
Palatoglossus
Palatopharyngeus

**Fig. 8.132 Hard palate and soft palate;** inferior view.
The palate forms the roof of the oral cavity and the floor of the nasal cavity. It separates the oral and nasal cavities. The hard palate and the soft palate form an anterior and posterior part, respectively.
The **hard palate** contributes to the phonation of consonants and serves as an abutment for the tongue when crushing food. A number of flat palatine mucosal folds (transverse palatinal folds, palatine rugae) to both sides of the midline help grind and pin down pieces of food against the hard palate.
The **soft palate** is flexible and, during swallowing, blocks off the nasopharynx by folding back onto the posterior pharyngeal wall.

**Fig. 8.133 Oral cavity and palatine muscles;** frontal view.
The palate is covered by a thick mucosal layer firmly attached to the periosteum. In its subepithelial layer, the palatine mucosa contains packages of small mucosal glands (palatine glands). The flexible soft palate extends posterior of the hard palate and ends in the uvula. The latter consists of a muscle (musculus uvulae) and mucosal glands. From both sides, the **palatine arches** (palatoglossal arch and palatopharyngeal arch), formed by the identically named muscles, project into the soft palate and the palatine uvula. On each side, a palatine arch frames a palatine tonsil. The palatine arches create the **pharyngeal isthmus** (isthmus of fauces), the entrance to the pharynx. The passage through the isthmus of fauces is controlled by muscles.

→T 3

### Clinical Remarks

Varying degrees of **cleft formations of the palate, upper jaw, and face** result from an insufficient mesenchymal tissue proliferation and the subsequent failure of fusion of the maxillary and medial nasal processes. Uni- or bilateral clefting is possible and, in severe cases, a gap extends from the upper lip through the hard and soft palate **(cheilognathopalatoschisis).** It occurs at a frequency of 1 : 2500 births with a preference in females. **Isolated cleft palates** occur if the fusion of the maxillary processes of the secondary palate or the fusion between the primary and secondary palate fails. The mildest form is the split uvula **(bifid uvula).** These clefts are not hereditary but the result of a deficiency in folic acid in the maternal nutrition during pregnancy (→ Clinical Remarks on p. 84).

## Development of the palate and palatine muscles

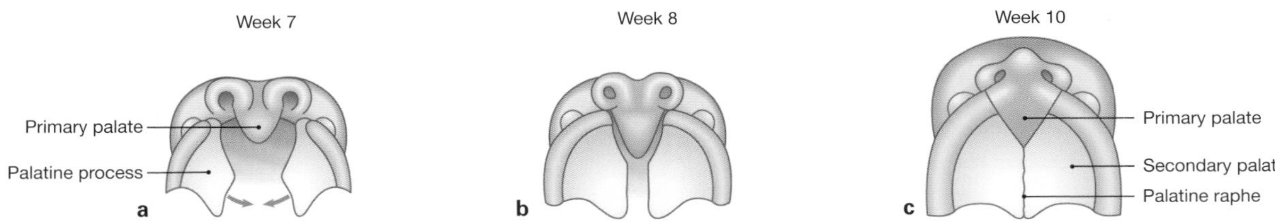
Week 7
Week 8
Week 10
Primary palate
Palatine process
a
b
c
Primary palate
Secondary palate
Palatine raphe

**Figs. 8.134a to c Development of the palate, separation of the nasal and oral cavities.** [20]
The merger of the two medial nasal prominences creates the median palatine process (intermaxillary segment) which is the structural basis for the future philtrum of the upper lip, part of the maxilla (with the four incisors), and the future primary palate. The primary palate extends into the anterior part of the oronasal cavity. The two opposing palatine processes of the maxilla form the major part of the definitive bony palate. By week 7, the tongue moves into a caudal position, the opposing palatine processes assume a horizontal position, start closing the gap between nose and mouth, and finally merge in the midline as secondary palate. In the anterior part, these palatine processes fuse with the primary palate.

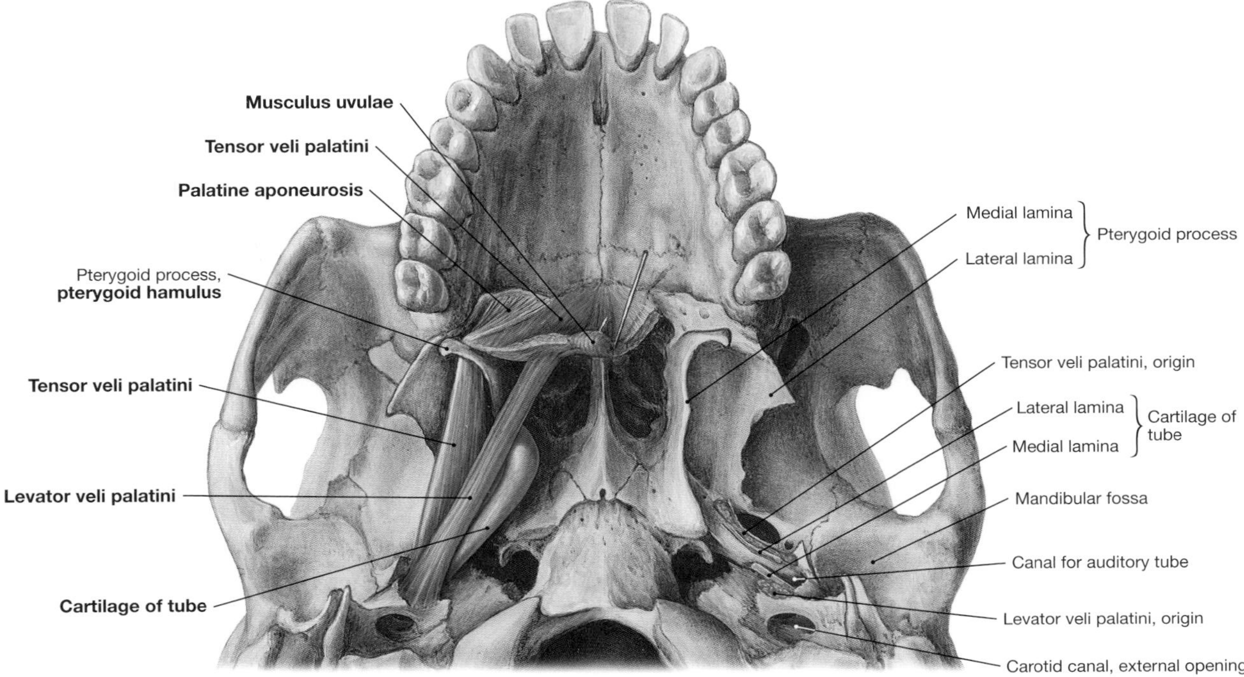
Musculus uvulae
Tensor veli palatini
Palatine aponeurosis
Pterygoid process,
pterygoid hamulus
Tensor veli palatini
Levator veli palatini
Cartilage of tube
Medial lamina
Lateral lamina
Pterygoid process
Tensor veli palatini, origin
Lateral lamina
Medial lamina
Cartilage of tube
Mandibular fossa
Canal for auditory tube
Levator veli palatini, origin
Carotid canal, external opening

**Fig. 8.135 Levator veli palatini, tensor veli palatini, and cartilage of the pharyngotympanic tube, cartilage of tube;** inferior view.
In addition to the palatoglossus and palatopharyngeus (→ Fig. 8.137) which facilitate the depression/pull-down of the soft palate, and the musculus uvulae which helps empty the mucous glands of the uvula, both the tensor veli palatini and the levator veli palatini project into the **palatine aponeurosis.** Both muscles attach at the base of the skull. The pterygoid hamulus serves as a hypomochlion (center of rotation of a joint) for the tensor veli palatini. Upon contraction, this paired muscle pulls the soft palate backwards and upwards and **occludes the nasopharynx against the oropharynx** during swallowing. In addition, this muscle participates in the opening of the auditory tube (→ pp. 149 and 150).

→T 3

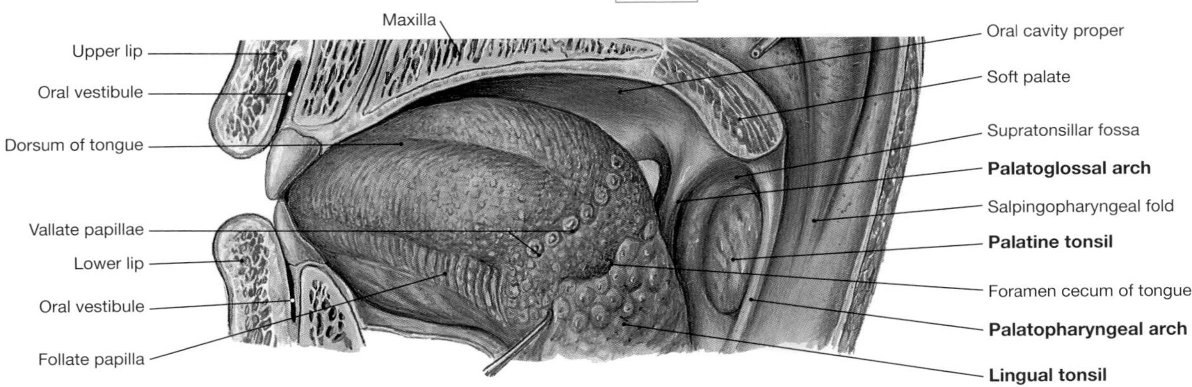
Maxilla
Upper lip
Oral vestibule
Dorsum of tongue
Vallate papillae
Lower lip
Oral vestibule
Follate papilla
Oral cavity proper
Soft palate
Supratonsillar fossa
Palatoglossal arch
Salpingopharyngeal fold
Palatine tonsil
Foramen cecum of tongue
Palatopharyngeal arch
Lingual tonsil

**Fig. 8.136 Tongue in the oral cavity;** posterior lateral view.
Posterior to the sulcus terminalis lies the root of the tongue with the lingual tonsil.
The Tonsilla lingualis is part of the WALDEYER's tonsillar ring, as is the The lingual tonsil is part of the WALDEYER's tonsillar ring, as is the palatine tonsil, which is located between the two palatine arches (palatoglossal and palatopharyngeal arch).

## Tongue

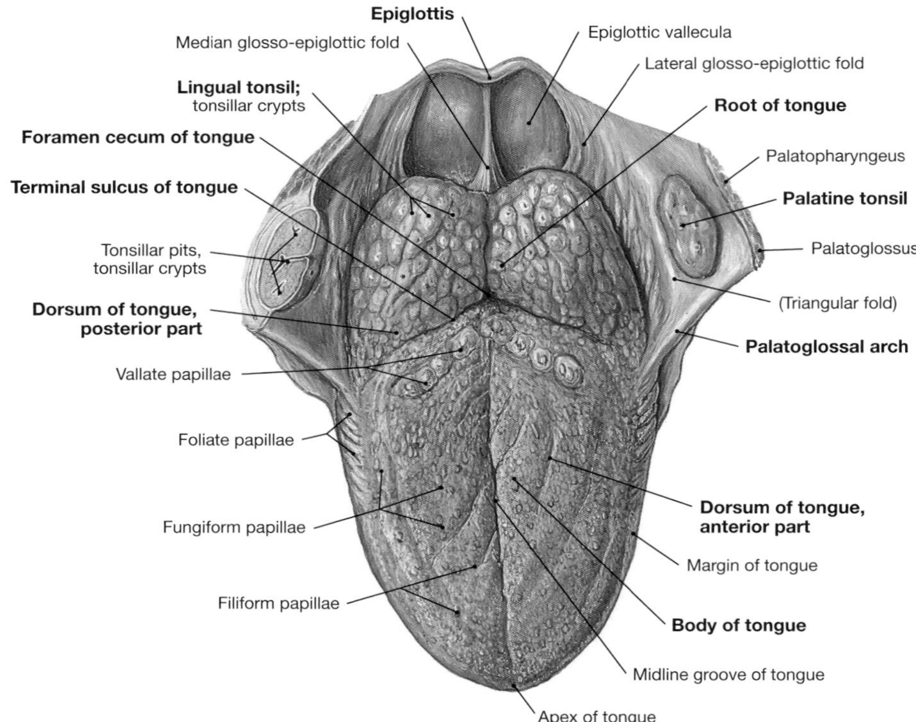
Epiglottis
Median glosso-epiglottic fold
Epiglottic vallecula
Lateral glosso-epiglottic fold
Lingual tonsil;
tonsillar crypts
Root of tongue
Foramen cecum of tongue
Palatopharyngeus
Terminal sulcus of tongue
Palatine tonsil
Tonsillar pits,
tonsillar crypts
Palatoglossus
(Triangular fold)
Dorsum of tongue,
posterior part
Palatoglossal arch
Vallate papillae
Foliate papillae
Dorsum of tongue,
anterior part
Fungiform papillae
Margin of tongue
Filiform papillae
Body of tongue
Midline groove of tongue
Apex of tongue

**Fig. 8.137 Tongue;** superior view.
On the **dorsum of tongue,** the midline groove (median sulcus) of tongue divides the tongue into a right and left half. The terminal sulcus of tongue (a V-shaped groove) delineates the body of tongue from the root of tongue and separates the tongue into an anterior (presulcal) part and a posterior (postsulcal) part. At the tip of the terminal sulcus of tongue, the surface epithelium forms a depression, the **foramen cecum of tongue.** This foramen is the place where the thyroid gland started its descent from the ectoderm of the floor of the mouth to its final destination in front of the larynx (origin of the thyroglossal duct).

The mucosa of the anterior part is rough since it contains multiple small, partially macroscopically visible papillae (lingual, filiform, foliate, fungiform, and vallate papillae) which play a role in the perception of touch and convey the sensory perception of taste.
The **root of tongue** is covered by the lingual tonsil, framed bilaterally by the two palatine arches, palatoglossal and palatopharyngeal arch, and posteriorly by the epiglottis. The singular median glosso-epiglottic fold and the paired lateral glosso-epiglottic fold project from the root of tongue towards the epiglottis and delineate the epiglottic valleculae.

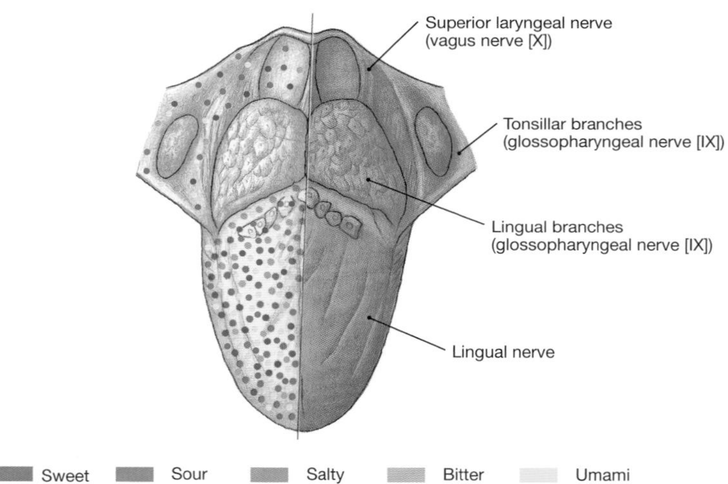
Superior laryngeal nerve
(vagus nerve [X])
Tonsillar branches
(glossopharyngeal nerve [IX])
Lingual branches
(glossopharyngeal nerve [IX])
Lingual nerve
Sweet
Sour
Salty
Bitter
Umami

**Fig. 8.138 Innervation and taste qualities of the dorsum of tongue.**
The lingual nerve, a branch of the mandibular nerve [V/3], supplies the sensory innervation of the anterior part of the tongue, lingual branches of the glossopharyngeal nerve [IX] supply the region of the terminal sulcus of tongue, and the superior laryngeal nerve, a branch of the vagus nerve [X], innervates the root of tongue.
Taste sensations by the **anterior two-thirds** of the tongue are conveyed by branches of the facial nerve [VII] (chorda tympani, intermediate nerve) to the upper part of the solitary tract in the brain stem; the perikarya of these sensory fibers are located in the geniculate ganglion.

Taste sensations by the **posterior third** of the tongue are projected to the lower part of the solitary tract in the brain stem by sensory fibers of the glossopharyngeal nerve [IX] and vagus nerve [X]. The perikarya of these nerve fibers reside in the inferior ganglion of the glossopharyngeal nerve [IX] or the vagus nerve [X].
All regions within in the anterior two-thirds of the tongue are capable of perceiving all five basic qualities of taste, albeit with different intensity. For example, the perception of "sweet" is more intense at the tip of the tongue, whereas the posterior root of the tongue contains receptors that are particularly sensitive to a "bitter" taste.

## Muscles of the tongue

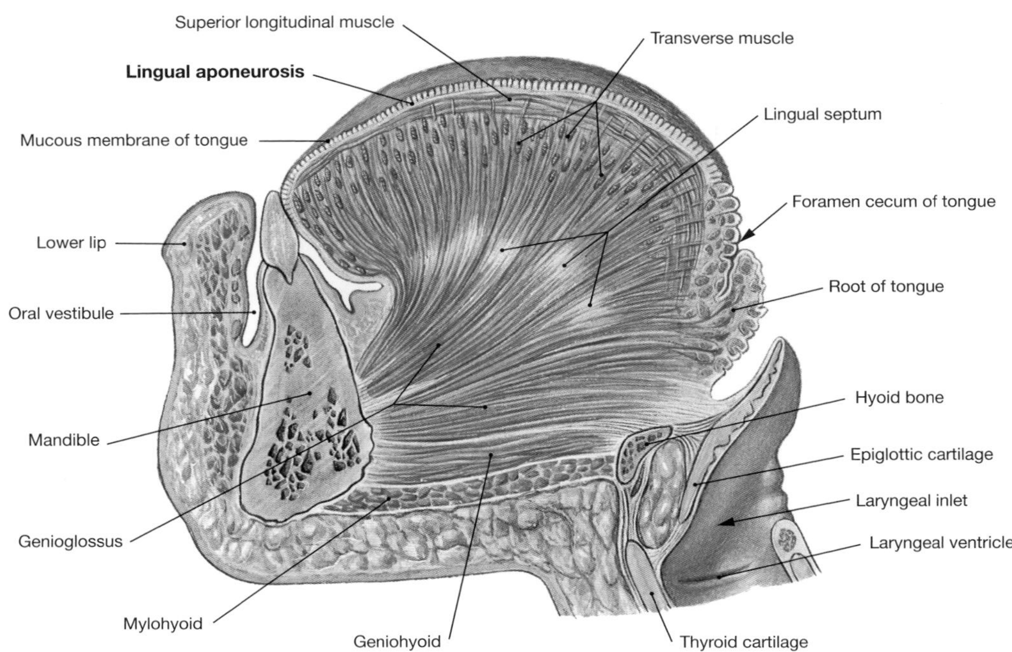
Superior longitudinal muscle
Lingual aponeurosis
Mucous membrane of tongue
Lower lip
Oral vestibule
Mandible
Genioglossus
Mylohyoid
Geniohyoid
Transverse muscle
Lingual septum
Foramen cecum of tongue
Root of tongue
Hyoid bone
Epiglottic cartilage
Laryngeal inlet
Laryngeal ventricle
Thyroid cartilage

**Fig. 8.139 Tongue and muscles of the tongue;** median section.
The tongue is a highly flexible muscular body. It is essential for chewing and swallowing, facilitates sucking, and provides the ability to speak. In addition, the tongue has an acute sense of touch and is the organ of taste sensations. The tongue is composed of intrinsic muscles, making up the body of the tongue, and extrinsic muscles, which have their origin at the skeleton and project into the tongue. The extrinsic muscles of the tongue alter the position of the tongue, whereas the intrinsic muscles change the shape of the tongue. The majority of the tongue muscles insert at the **lingual aponeurosis,** a tough plate of connective tissue beneath the mucosa of the dorsum of tongue.

→T 2a

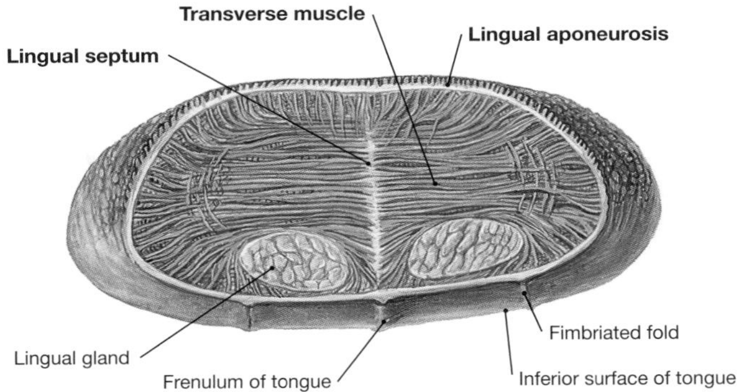
Transverse muscle
Lingual septum
Lingual aponeurosis
Lingual gland
Frenulum of tongue
Fimbriated fold
Inferior surface of tongue

**Fig. 8.140 Tongue and intrinsic muscles of the tongue;** cross-section at the level of the tip of the tongue.
Like a wickerwork, the intrinsic muscles of the tongue are interlaced in all three dimensions. In the median plane, the lingual septum intersects the tongue incompletely into two halves. Agonistic and antagonistic muscle facilitate the flexibility of the tongue. To both sides at the tip of the tongue a mucous gland is present (lingual gland, BLANDIN's gland).

→T 2a

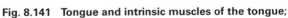

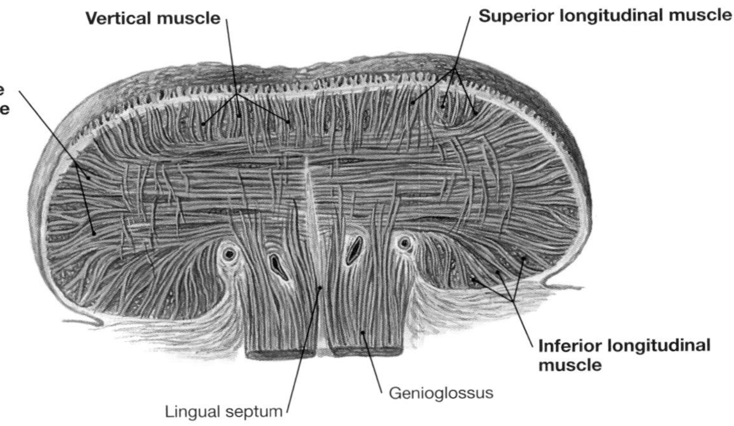
Vertical muscle
Superior longitudinal muscle
Transverse muscle
Inferior longitudinal muscle
Genioglossus
Lingual septum

**Fig. 8.141 Tongue and intrinsic muscles of the tongue;** cross-section at the level of the middle part.
The origin and insertion sites of all intrinsic muscles of the tongue are within the tongue itself. There are the superior longitudinal, inferior longitudinal, transverse, and vertical muscles. These muscles are interlaced and positioned perpendicular to each other in all three dimensions. The ability of the tongue to change its shape helps during chewing, sucking, singing, speaking, and whistling. The genioglossus belongs to the extrinsic muscles of the tongue.

→T 2a

## Hyoid bone and hyoid muscles

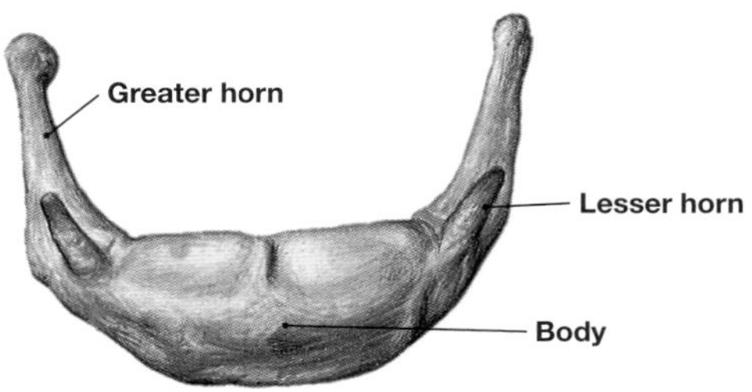
Greater horn
Lesser horn
Body

**Fig. 8.142 Hyoid bone;** anterior superior view.
The horseshoe-shaped hyoid bone consists of a body which holds the paired greater and lesser horns.

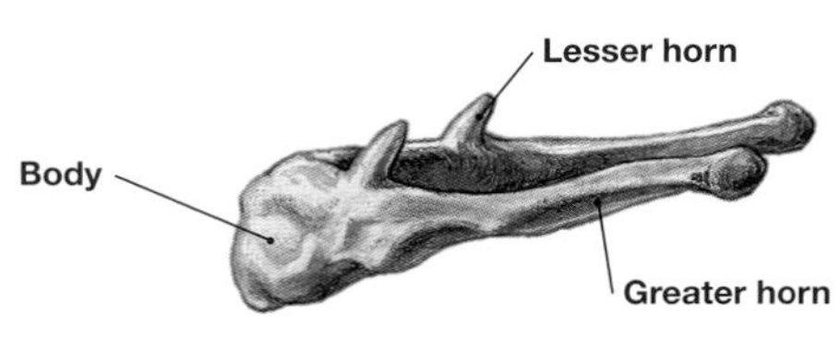
Lesser horn
Body
Greater horn

**Fig. 8.143 Hyoid bone;** lateral view.

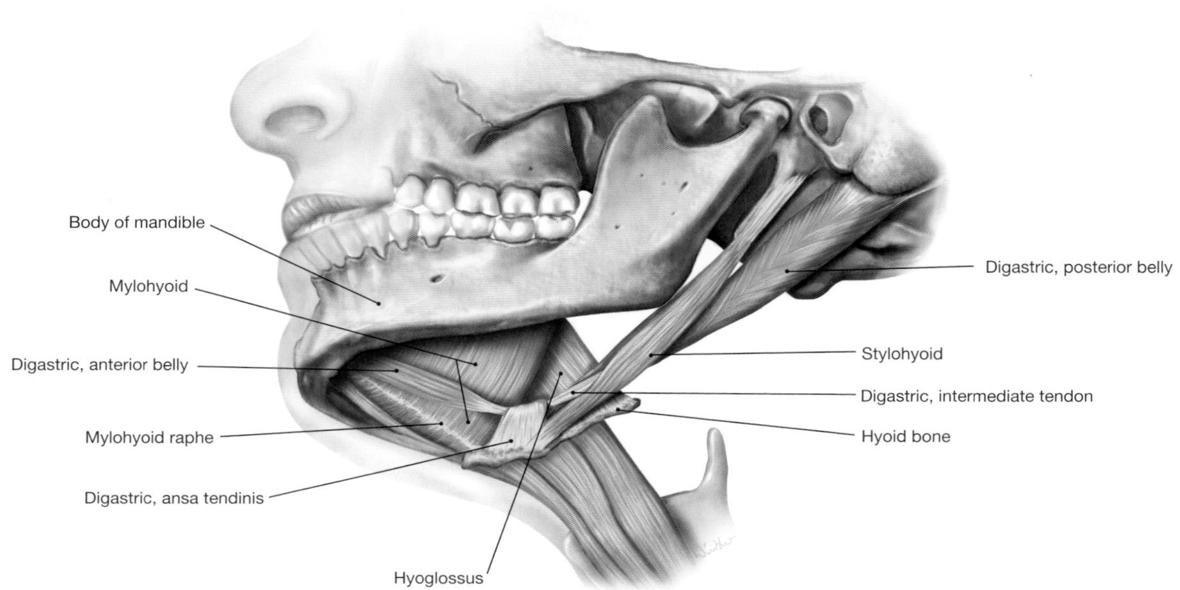
Body of mandible
Mylohyoid
Digastric, anterior belly
Mylohyoid raphe
Digastric, ansa tendinis
Hyoglossus
Digastric, posterior belly
Stylohyoid
Digastric, intermediate tendon
Hyoid bone

**Fig. 8.144 Mouth region;** lateral inferior view.
The muscular **oral diaphragm** consists of the two mylohyoid muscles and forms the floor of the oral cavity. In addition, the geniohyoid (not shown) and digastric muscles participate in the formation of the floor of the mouth. Directly or indirectly, all these muscles are attached to the hyoid bone and, together with the stylohyoid muscles, are collectively referred to as **suprahyoid muscles.** From a functional standpoint, the floor of the mouth represents an adjustable abutment for the tongue.

→ T 2b, 9

### Clinical Remarks

Touching the floor of the mouth, the palatine arches or the back of the throat initiates either the **swallowing** or the **gag reflex.** Muscles of the tongue, pharynx, larynx, and esophagus participate in these reflexes.
**Allergic reactions** can result in a life-threatening swelling of the mucosal lining of the soft palate.
**Inflammations** of the palatine mucosa, here particularly the mucosa of the soft palate, typically evoke severe discomfort during swallowing.

**Impaired blood perfusion of the brain stem** frequently coincides with palatine muscle palsy. This causes difficulties in swallowing and an impaired tubal ventilation of the middle ear. These patients can display a velopalatine palsy (nuclear lesions of the glossopharyngeal nerve [IX] and vagus nerve [X]) resulting in the soft palate hanging down on the side of the paralysed levator veli palatini. The uvula deviates to the other (healthy) side.
Often, the tongue is the first to be injured by **chemical burns and scalding.** At the margins of the tongue, potential **precancerous lesions** can show as hyperkeratosis or leukoplakia.

## Floor of the mouth and muscles of the floor of the mouth

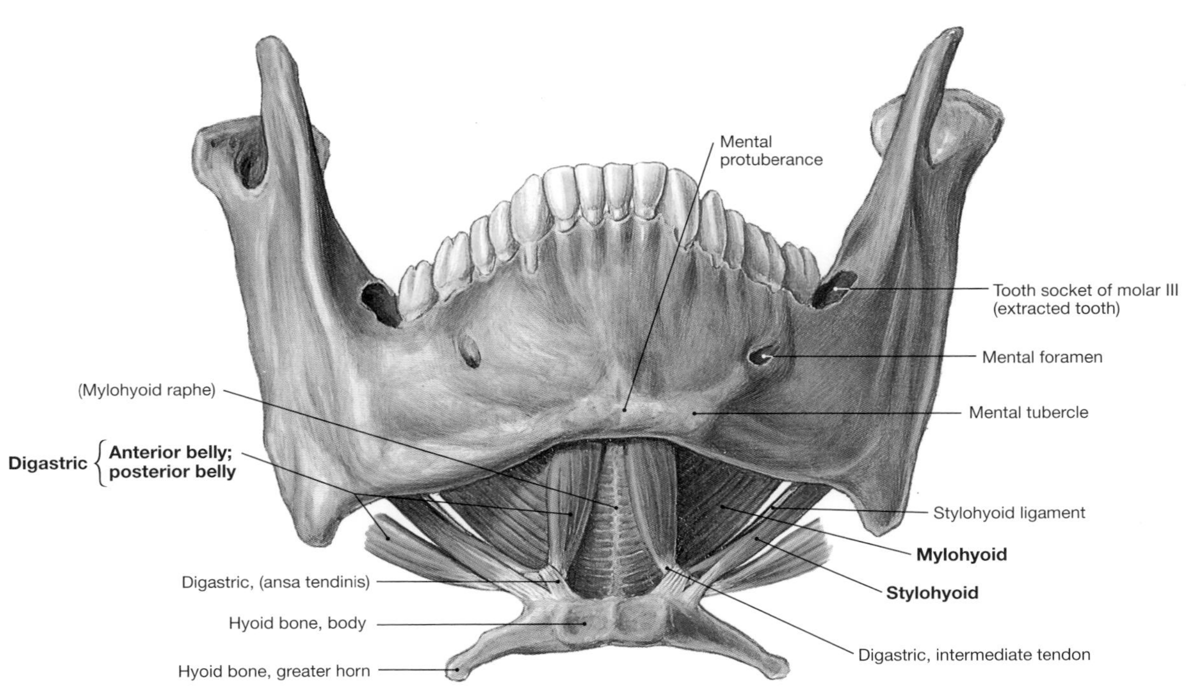
Mental protuberance
Tooth socket of molar III (extracted tooth)
Mental foramen
(Mylohyoid raphe)
Mental tubercle
Digastric { Anterior belly; posterior belly
Stylohyoid ligament
Mylohyoid
Digastric, (ansa tendinis)
Stylohyoid
Hyoid bone, body
Hyoid bone, greater horn
Digastric, intermediate tendon

**Fig. 8.145 Lower jaw, mandible, and muscles of the floor of the mouth, suprahyoid muscles;** frontal view.
The floor of the mouth (oral diaphragm) is a muscular layer created by the suprahyoid group of muscles. The central muscle at the floor of the mouth is the **mylohyoid** which extends between the two rami of mandible to both sides and joins in the midline at the mylohyoid raphe. Beneath this muscle lies the paired anterior belly of the **digastric** which connects with the posterior belly by an intramuscular tendon. This intramuscular tendon passes through a tendinous pulley and attaches the digastric to the hyoid bone. A third suprahyoid muscle coming from the hyoid bone is the **stylohyoid.**

→T 9

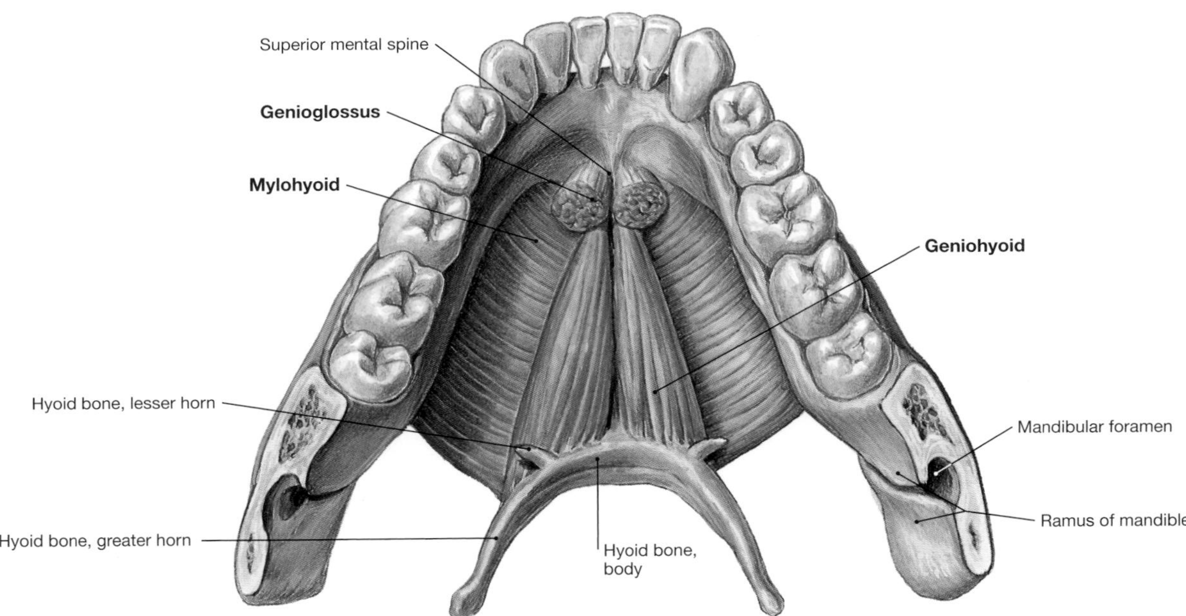
Superior mental spine
Genioglossus
Mylohyoid
Geniohyoid
Hyoid bone, lesser horn
Mandibular foramen
Ramus of mandible
Hyoid bone, greater horn
Hyoid bone, body

**Fig. 8.146 Lower jaw, mandible, muscles of the floor of the mouth, suprahyoid muscles, and hyoid bone;** superior view.
The oral diaphragm, formed by the two mylohyoid and the paired geniohyoid muscles, is shown. The **geniohyoid** belongs to the suprahyoid muscle group and stretches from the inside of the mandible to the hyoid bone. As a member of the extrinsic muscles of the tongue, the overlying genioglossus has been cut at its origin at the superior mental spine of the mandible.

→T 9

## Muscles of the tongue

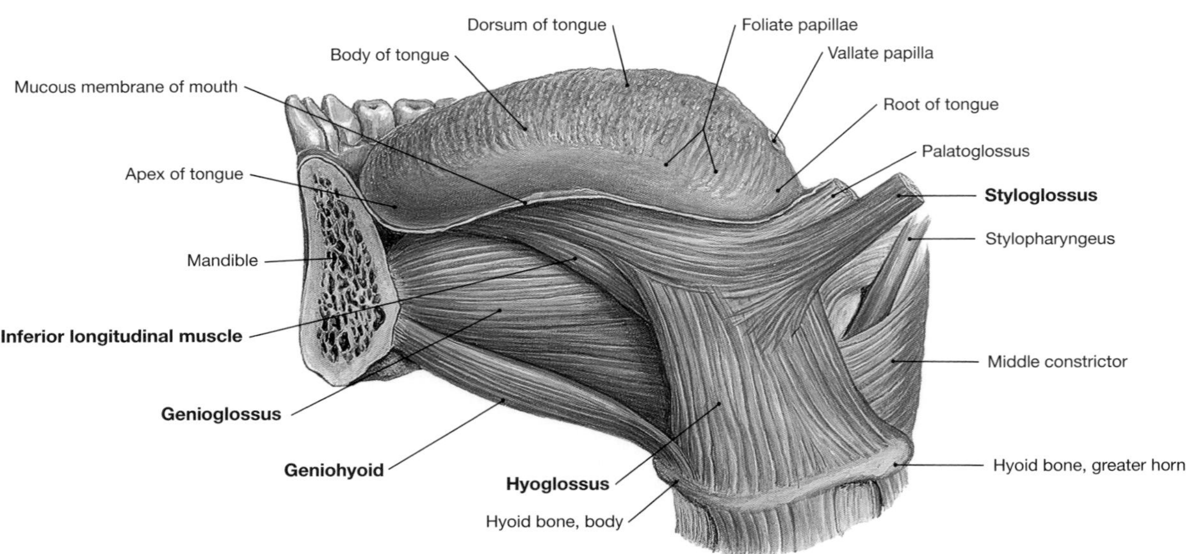
Dorsum of tongue
Foliate papillae
Body of tongue
Vallate papilla
Mucous membrane of mouth
Root of tongue
Palatoglossus
Apex of tongue
Styloglossus
Stylopharyngeus
Mandible
Inferior longitudinal muscle
Middle constrictor
Genioglossus
Geniohyoid
Hyoid bone, greater horn
Hyoglossus
Hyoid bone, body

**Fig. 8.147 Tongue and extrinsic muscles of the tongue;** view from the left side.
The extrinsic muscles of the tongue project into the tongue. They consist of the **genioglossus, hyoglossus,** and **styloglossus.** In addition, the palatoglossus is an extrinsic muscle of the tongue. The hyoglossus can receive functional support by a chondroglossus, which originates from the lesser horn of the hyoid bone (→ Figs. 8.148 and 8.149).

→ T 2b

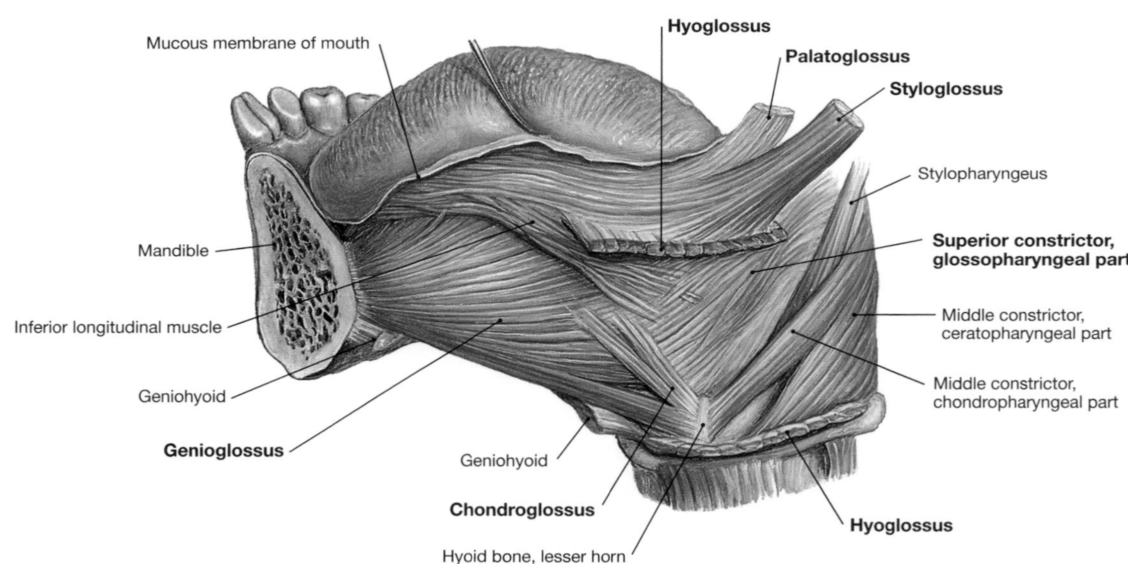
Hyoglossus
Mucous membrane of mouth
Palatoglossus
Styloglossus
Stylopharyngeus
Superior constrictor, glossopharyngeal part
Mandible
Middle constrictor, ceratopharyngeal part
Inferior longitudinal muscle
Middle constrictor, chondropharyngeal part
Geniohyoid
Genioglossus
Geniohyoid
Chondroglossus
Hyoglossus
Hyoid bone, lesser horn

**Fig. 8.148 Tongue and extrinsic muscles of the tongue;** view from the left side.
Beneath the dissected hyoglossus, the small **chondroglossus** is shown originating from the lesser horn of the hyoid bone and functionally assisting the hyoglossus. In addition to the extrinsic muscles of the tongue, the palatoglossus and the glossopharyngeal part of the superior constrictor project into the posterior aspect of the tongue.

→ T 2b

## Clinical Remarks

The protrusion of the tongue requires a functionally intact genioglossus muscle. In a deep **coma,** the genioglossus becomes flaccid. In a supine position, the tongue slides back into the pharynx and can block the airways. Thus, as a precaution unconscious patients should always be placed in the lateral recovery position.

## Muscles of the tongue and pharynx

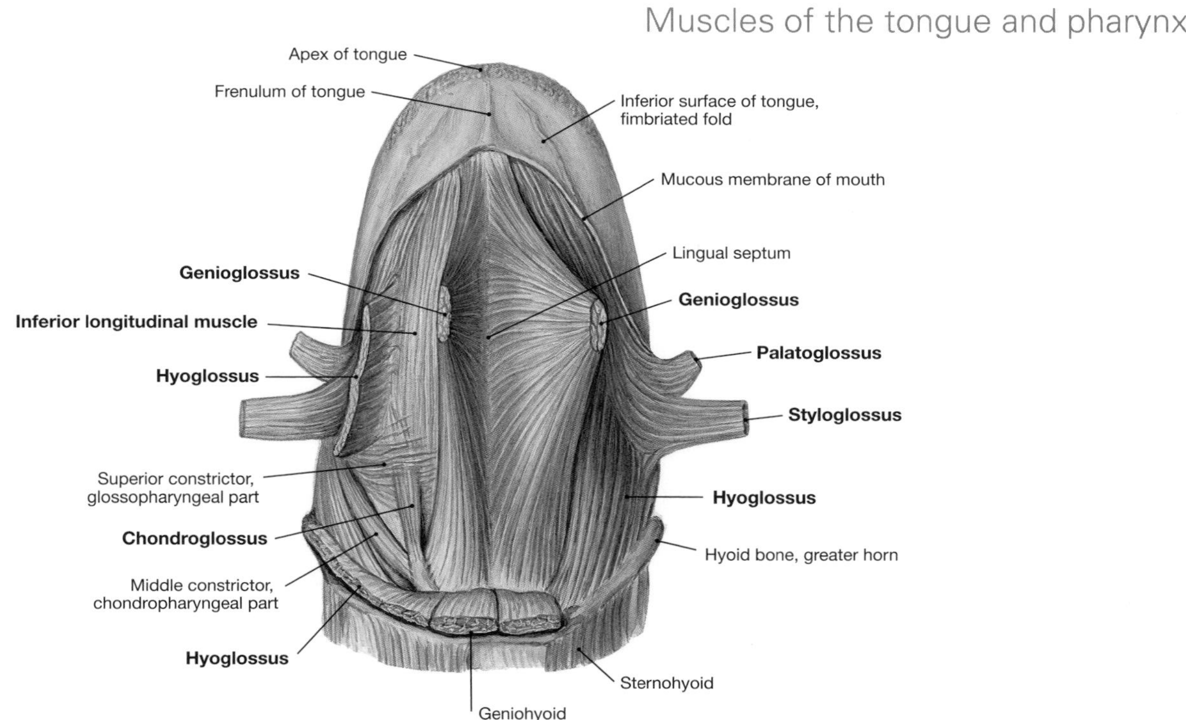
Apex of tongue
Frenulum of tongue
Inferior surface of tongue, fimbriated fold
Mucous membrane of mouth
Lingual septum
Genioglossus
Inferior longitudinal muscle
Genioglossus
Palatoglossus
Hyoglossus
Styloglossus
Superior constrictor, glossopharyngeal part
Hyoglossus
Chondroglossus
Hyoid bone, greater horn
Middle constrictor, chondropharyngeal part
Hyoglossus
Sternohyoid
Geniohyoid

**Fig. 8.149 Muscles of the tongue;** inferior view.
The genioglossus was removed at its mandibular origin. Also, the styloglossus and palatoglossus were removed. At the lateral side, the hyoglossus (cut at the right side of the tongue) and chondroglossus are shown, which are extrinsic muscles of the tongue. As part of the intrinsic muscles of the tongue, the inferior longitudinal muscle stretches out within the inferior aspect of the tongue.

→ T 2b

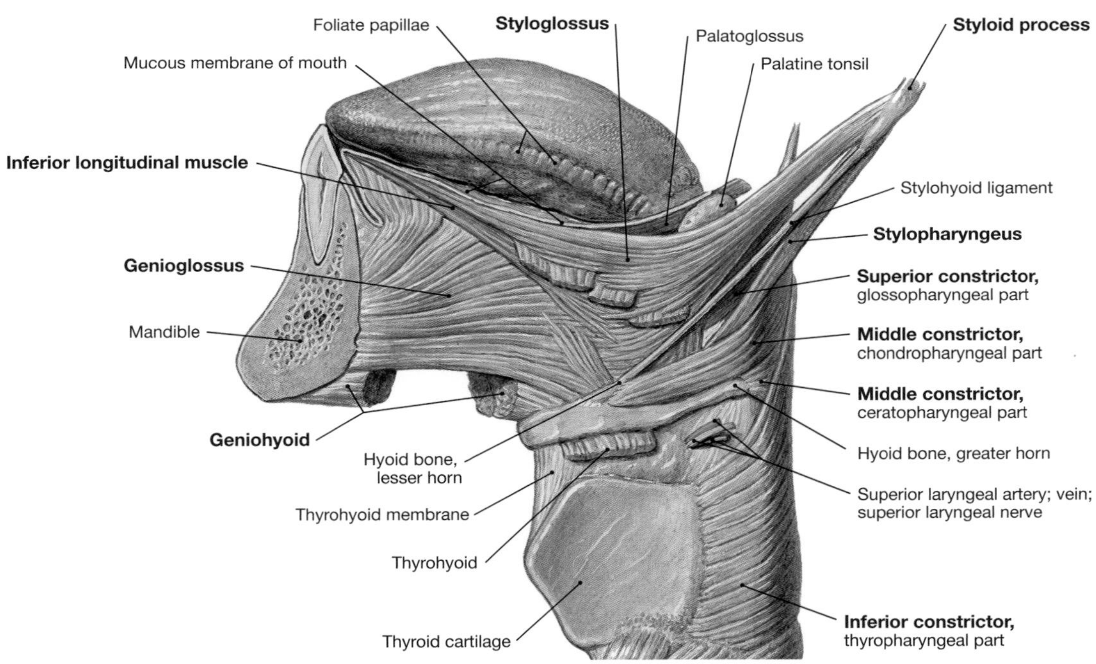
Foliate papillae
Styloglossus
Palatoglossus
Styloid process
Mucous membrane of mouth
Palatine tonsil
Inferior longitudinal muscle
Stylohyoid ligament
Stylopharyngeus
Genioglossus
Superior constrictor, glossopharyngeal part
Mandible
Middle constrictor, chondropharyngeal part
Middle constrictor, ceratopharyngeal part
Geniohyoid
Hyoid bone, lesser horn
Hyoid bone, greater horn
Superior laryngeal artery; vein; superior laryngeal nerve
Thyrohyoid membrane
Thyrohyoid
Inferior constrictor, thyropharyngeal part
Thyroid cartilage

**Fig. 8.150 Extrinsic muscles of the tongue and pharyngeal muscles, constrictor muscles;** lateral view; mandibular arch removed.
The stylohyoid ligament extends between styloglossus and stylopharyngeus. Located below are the pharyngeal muscles: the superior constrictor with the glossopharyngeal parts and the middle constrictor with the chondropharyngeal and ceratopharyngeal parts. The inferior constrictor with the thyropharyngeal part is located below the hyoid bone.

→ T 2b, 5

## Vessels and nerves of the tongue

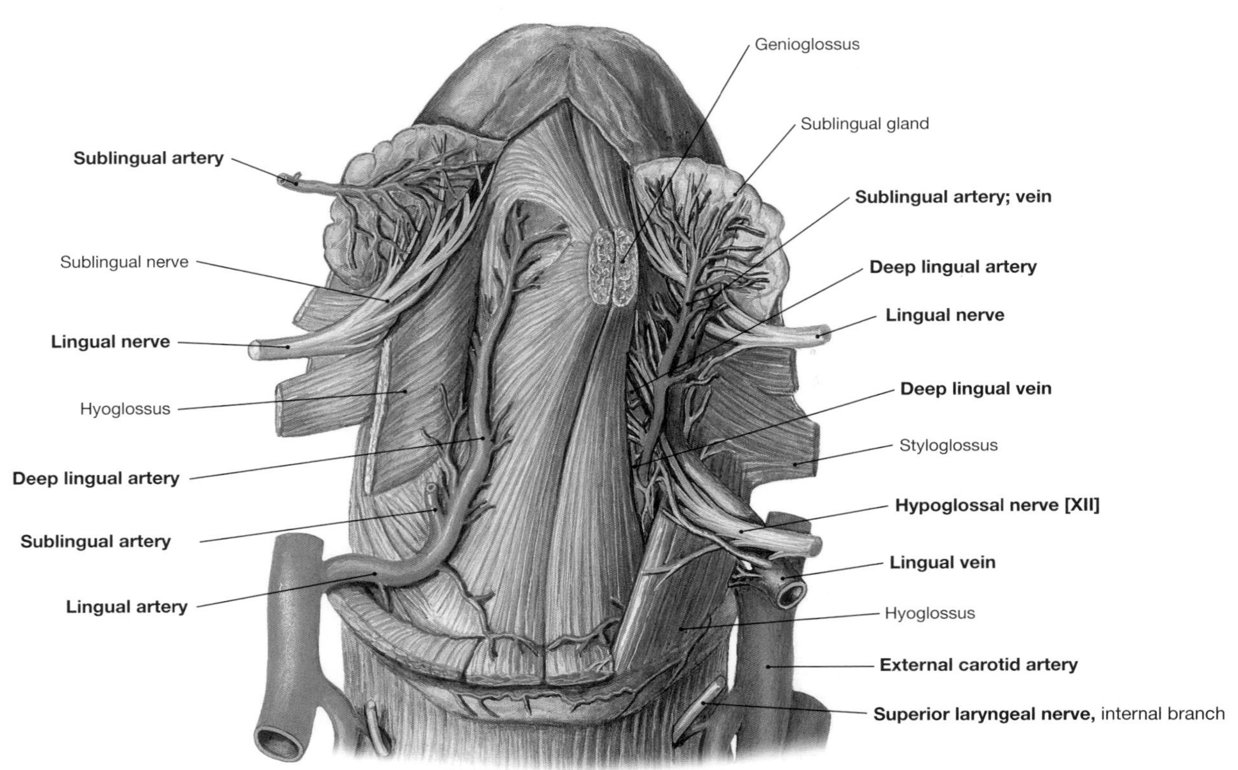
Genioglossus
Sublingual gland
Sublingual artery
Sublingual artery; vein
Sublingual nerve
Deep lingual artery
Lingual nerve
Lingual nerve
Hyoglossus
Deep lingual vein
Styloglossus
Deep lingual artery
Hypoglossal nerve [XII]
Sublingual artery
Lingual vein
Lingual artery
Hyoglossus
External carotid artery
Superior laryngeal nerve, internal branch

**Fig. 8.151 Vessels and nerves of the tongue;** inferior view.
The lingual artery from the external carotid artery provides the **arterial** blood supply of the tongue. Branches of the lingual artery are deep lingual artery, mainly supplying the muscles of the middle and anterior part of the tongue, and the sublingual artery, passing to the sublingual gland and to the floor of the mouth. Projecting backwards, the dorsal lingual branches can communicate with each other, whereas all other branches from each side are separated by the lingual septum and only provide arterial blood to one half of the tongue.
The **venous** drainage is achieved by the lingual vein. The lingual vein runs adjacent to the hyoglossus and drains into the internal jugular vein. The lingual vein collects blood from the sublingual, deep lingual, and dorsal lingual veins as well as from the vena comitans of hypoglossal nerve.

With the exception of the innervation of the palatoglossus by the pharyngeal plexus, the **motor** innervation of the tongue derives from the hypoglossal nerve [XII]. Sensory innervation in the anterior two-thirds of the tongue is provided by the lingual nerve, a branch of the mandibular nerve [V/3], in the region of the terminal sulcus by the glossopharyngeal nerve [IX], and at the base of the tongue by the superior laryngeal nerve (a branch of the vagus nerve [X]).

**Branches of the lingual artery:**
- (hyoid branch)
- dorsal lingual branches
- suprahyoid branch
- sublingual artery
- deep lingual artery

## Clinical Remarks

A **subepithelial venous plexus** is located in the mucosal lining at the underside of the tongue. This facilitates quick resorption of medication placed underneath the tongue.

**Injuries to the hypoglossal nerve [XII]** on one side cause the protruding tongue to deviate to the affected side; muscular atrophy occurs on the ipsilateral side of the hypoglossal nerve palsy.

## Vessels and nerves of the tongue, tonsils

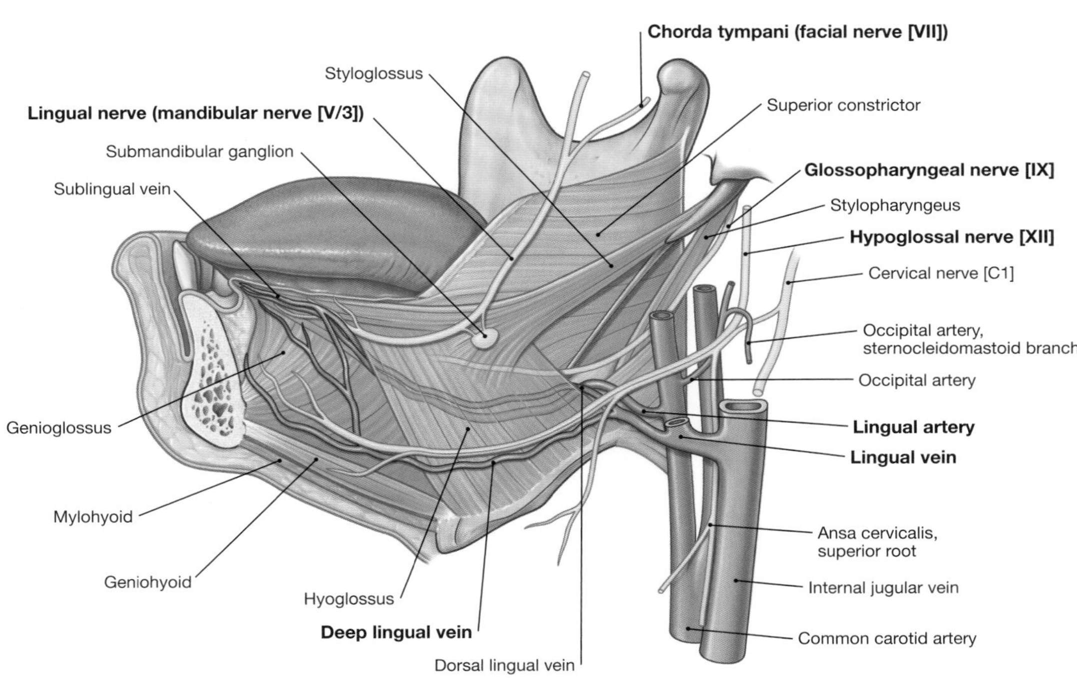
Chorda tympani (facial nerve [VII])
Styloglossus
Lingual nerve (mandibular nerve [V/3])
Submandibular ganglion
Sublingual vein
Superior constrictor
Glossopharyngeal nerve [IX]
Stylopharyngeus
Hypoglossal nerve [XII]
Cervical nerve [C1]
Occipital artery, sternocleidomastoid branch
Occipital artery
Lingual artery
Lingual vein
Genioglossus
Mylohyoid
Geniohyoid
Hyoglossus
Deep lingual vein
Dorsal lingual vein
Ansa cervicalis, superior root
Internal jugular vein
Common carotid artery

**Fig. 8.152 Vessels and nerves of the tongue;** lateral view; mandibular arch removed. [10]

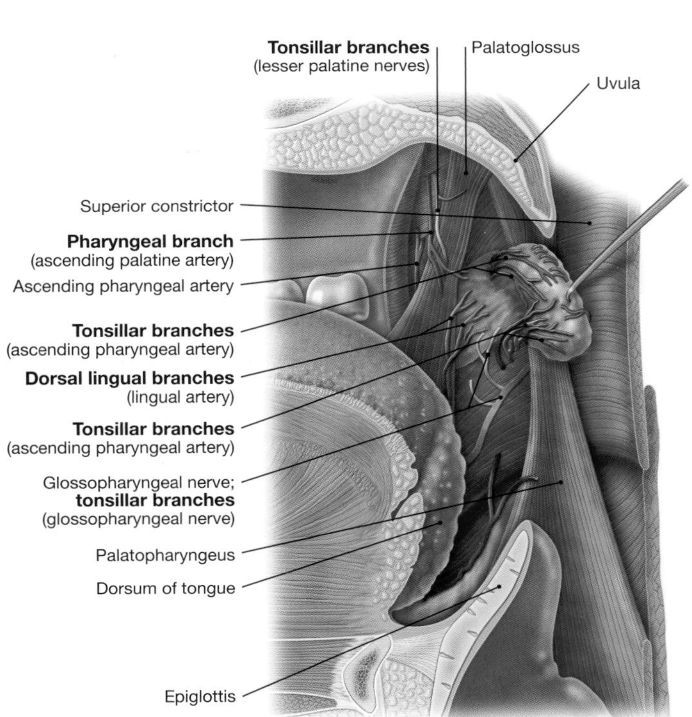
Tonsillar branches (lesser palatine nerves)
Palatoglossus
Uvula
Superior constrictor
Pharyngeal branch (ascending palatine artery)
Ascending pharyngeal artery
Tonsillar branches (ascending pharyngeal artery)
Dorsal lingual branches (lingual artery)
Tonsillar branches (ascending pharyngeal artery)
Glossopharyngeal nerve; tonsillar branches (glossopharyngeal nerve)
Palatopharyngeus
Dorsum of tongue
Epiglottis

| Pharyngeal Lymphoid Ring (WALDEYER's Tonsillar Ring) | | |
|---|---|---|
| **Definition** | A cluster of lympho-epithelial tissues located at the transitional zone between oral and nasal cavity and the pharynx form the pharyngeal lymphoid ring. The pharyngeal lymphoid ring serves in immune responses and is part of the mucosa-associated lymphoid tissue (MALT). | |
| **Components** | • Pharyngeal tonsil<br>• Tubal tonsil<br>• Palatine tonsil<br>• Lingual tonsil<br>• Lateral assortment of MALT | → pp. 60, 68<br><br>→ pp. 80, 82<br>→ pp. 81, 82 |

**Fig. 8.153 Blood and nerve supply of the palatine tonsil, right side;** medial view.
The **tonsillar branches** of the ascending palatine artery, the pharyngeal branch of the descending palatine artery and the pharyngeal branches of the ascending pharyngeal artery as well as the dorsal lingual branches of the lingual artery supply blood to the palatine tonsil. The innervation of the tonsillar bed comes from **tonsillar branches** of the lesser palatine nerves and the glossopharyngeal nerve [IX].

## Clinical Remarks

Frequent recurrent infection of the palatine tonsils is an indication for their surgical removal **(tonsillectomy),** one of the most frequently conducted surgical ENT procedures. Postoperative bleedings can occur up to three weeks after the operation (in rare cases even longer) and can be a serious complication.

## Parotid gland

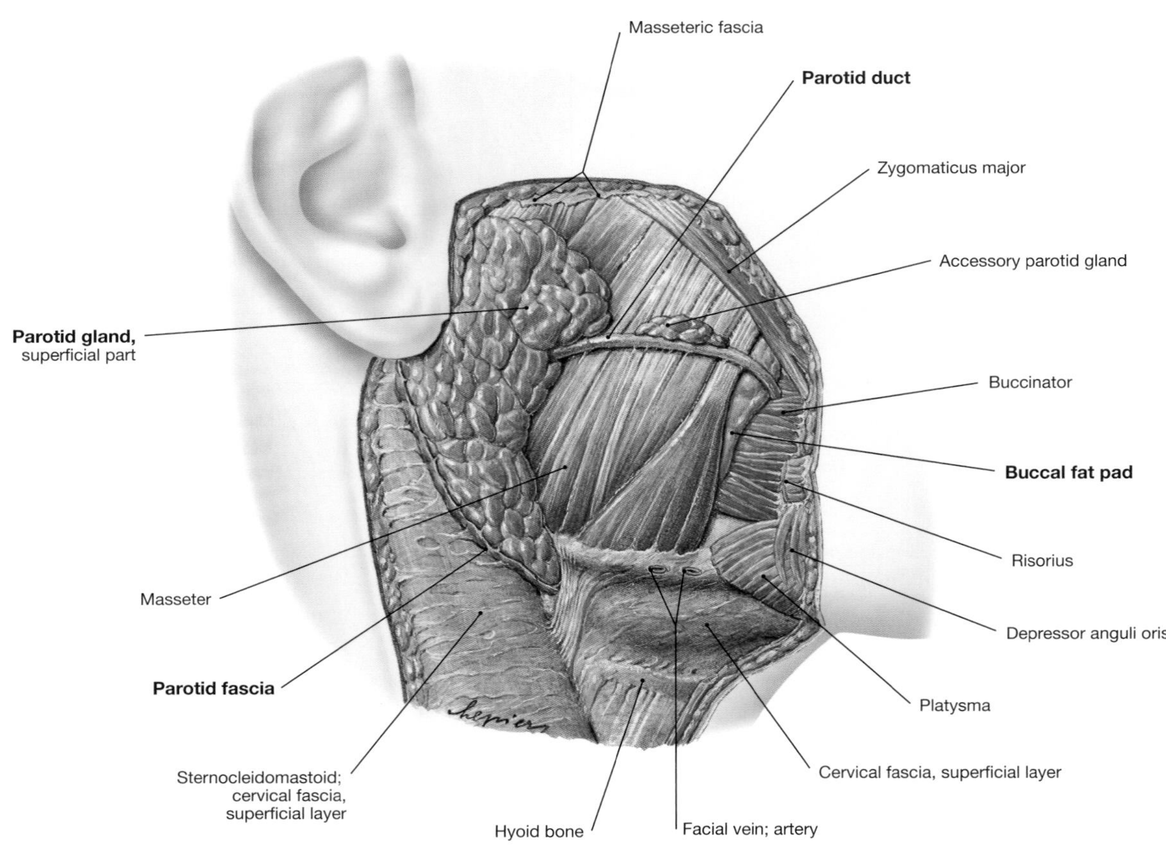
Masseteric fascia
Parotid duct
Zygomaticus major
Accessory parotid gland
Parotid gland, superficial part
Buccinator
Buccal fat pad
Risorius
Masseter
Depressor anguli oris
Parotid fascia
Platysma
Cervical fascia, superficial layer
Sternocleidomastoid; cervical fascia, superficial layer
Hyoid bone
Facial vein; artery

**Fig. 8.154 Parotid gland, right side;** lateral view.
The exclusively serous parotid gland is the largest salivary gland. Size and dimensions are quite variable. The superficial layer of the gland is positioned directly in front of the outer ear and covered by a tough fascia (parotid fascia; cut margins shown).
The parotid fascia is a continuation of the superficial layer of the cervical fascia. At the anterior margin of the gland, the parotid duct exits and runs horizontally across the upper half of the masseter to the buccinator, pierces this muscle, and, in the papilla of parotid duct, opens into the oral vestibule opposite to the second upper molar tooth. Frequently, accessory glandular tissue (accessory parotid gland) is associated with the excretory duct.

### Clinical Remarks

Surgical removal of tumors the parotid gland can result in **gustatory sweating (FREY's syndrome).** During the surgery, damage occurs to the sympathetic and parasympathetic nerve fibers innervating the glandular parenchyma. Postoperative recovery includes the regeneration of parasympathetic fibers and the accidental synapsing of these regenerated fibers with sweat glands of the skin, formerly innervated by sympathetic fibers. Acetylcholine is the neurotransmitter for the sympathetic innervation of sweat glands (as it is in parasympathetic nerve endings). Thus, the formerly sympathetic innervation of sweat glands has now turned into a parasympathetic innervation of the same glands. Activation of the parasympathetic system (e.g. in a hungry person seeing delicious food) results in sweating of the cheek area adjacent to the ear (thus, gustatory sweating).
**Parotitis epidemica** or mumps is very painful because the parotid fascia restricts the expansion of the swollen glandular tissue.
Malignant **tumors of the parotid gland** can result in a lesion of the facial nerve [VII]; by contrast, benign parotid gland tumors are the most common tumors of the parotid gland and rarely damage the facial nerve [VII].

## Parotid gland, horizontal section

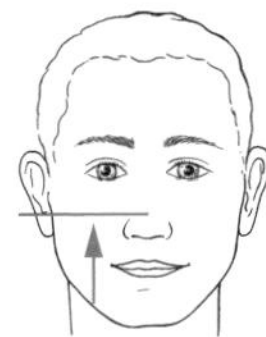

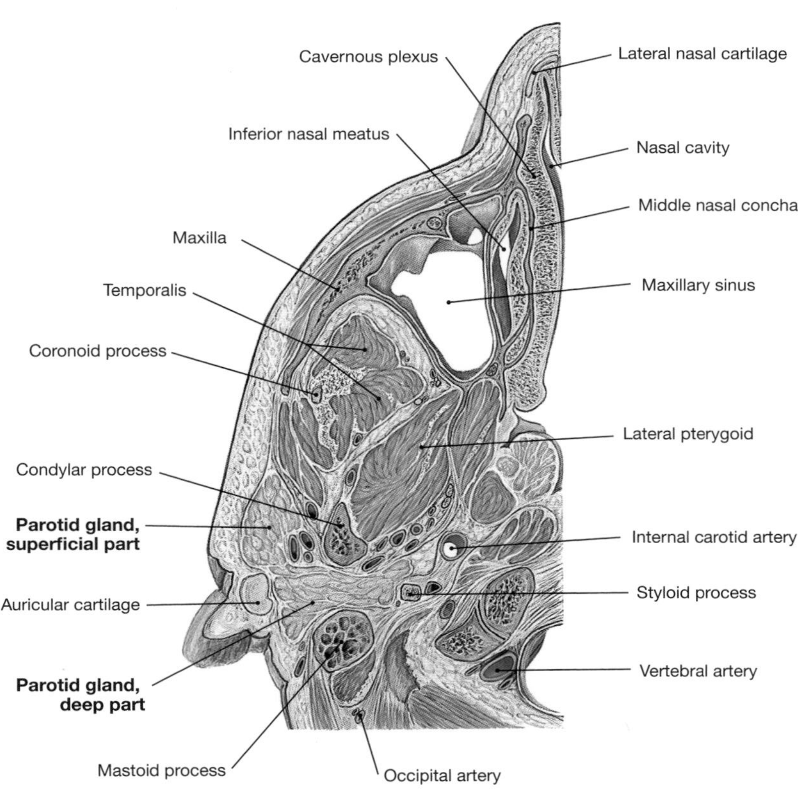

Cavernous plexus
Lateral nasal cartilage
Inferior nasal meatus
Nasal cavity
Middle nasal concha
Maxilla
Maxillary sinus
Temporalis
Coronoid process
Lateral pterygoid
Condylar process
Parotid gland, superficial part
Internal carotid artery
Auricular cartilage
Styloid process
Vertebral artery
Parotid gland, deep part
Mastoid process
Occipital artery


**Fig. 8.155 Parotid gland and masticatory muscles;** horizontal section; inferior view.
The parotid gland consists of two parts. The **superficial part** is located immediately in front of the outer ear. Projecting deep into the retromandibular fossa is the larger **deep part** of the gland which is devoid of a fascia. This section shows the temporalis and lateral pterygoid positioned between the parotid gland and the maxillary sinus.

| **Salivary Glands** | | |
|---|---|---|
| Three bilateral large salivary glands and multiple small salivary glands supply saliva to the oral cavity. | | |
| **Large salivary glands** | • Parotid gland<br>• Submandibular gland<br>• Sublingual gland | → pp. 40, 42, 46, 54, 90, 96<br>→ pp. 42, 92–96<br>→ pp. 63, 88, 93–96 |
| **Small salivary glands** | • Lip (labial glands)<br>• Cheek (buccal glands)<br>• Tongue (lingual glands)<br>• Palate (palatine glands)<br>• Around molars (molar glands) | → p. 68<br><br>→ pp. 83, 95, 96<br>→ pp. 80, 96 |

## Openings of the salivary glands

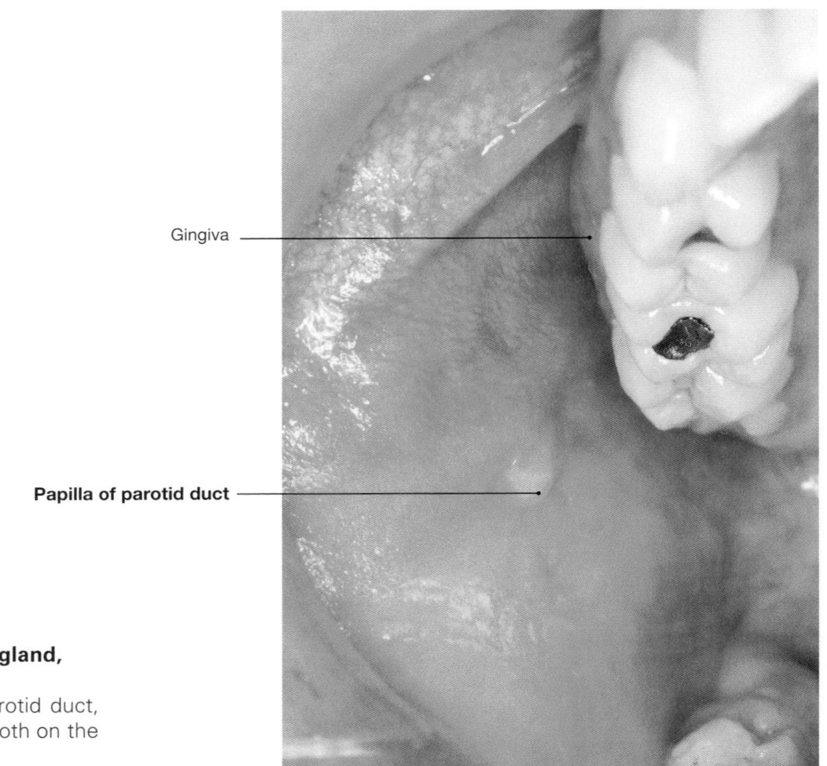
Gingiva
Papilla of parotid duct

**Fig. 8.156 Opening of the excretory duct of the parotid gland, right side;** inferior view from an oblique angle.
The opening of the excretory duct of the parotid gland (parotid duct, STENSEN's duct) is located opposite to the second molar tooth on the papilla of parotid duct in the oral vestibule.

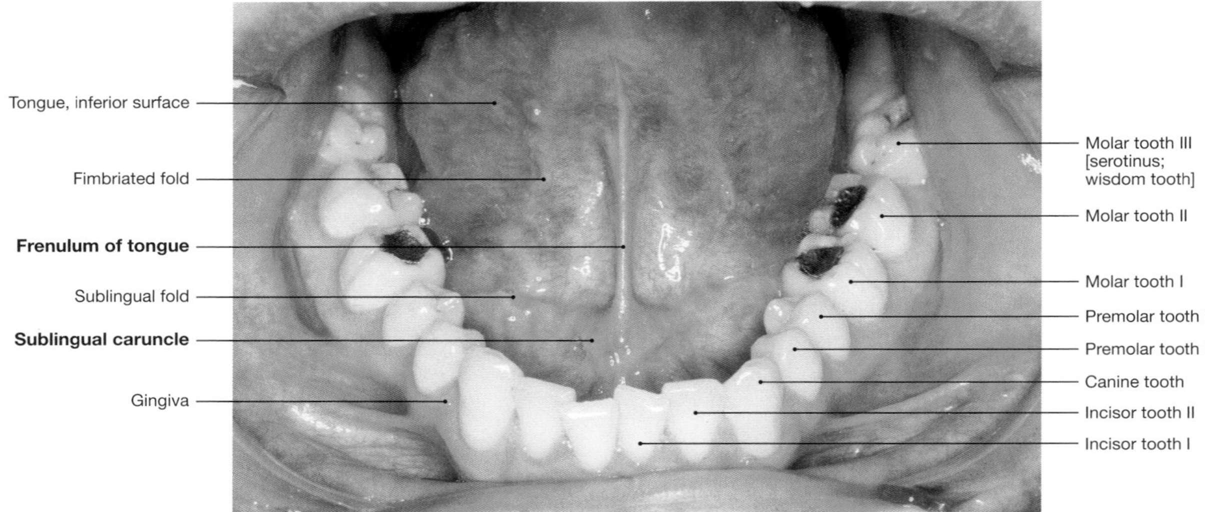
Tongue, inferior surface
Fimbriated fold
Frenulum of tongue
Sublingual fold
Sublingual caruncle
Gingiva
Molar tooth III [serotinus; wisdom tooth]
Molar tooth II
Molar tooth I
Premolar tooth II
Premolar tooth I
Canine tooth
Incisor tooth II
Incisor tooth I

**Fig. 8.157 Opening of the excretory duct of the submandibular gland, sublingual caruncle;** frontal superior view.
The excretory duct of the submandibular gland (submandibular duct, WHARTON's duct) runs at the floor of the mouth (→ Figs. 8.160 and 8.161), merges with the main excretory duct of the sublingual gland (greater sublingual duct), and opens at the sublingual caruncle on both sides of the frenulum of tongue and behind the incisors into the oral cavity proper.

### Clinical Remarks

**Anomalies of the excretory duct system,** in particular the submandibular duct, can result in the formation of a **ranula** (retention cyst filled with saliva).
In kidney disease, increased levels of renally cleared substances can be detected in the saliva. Salt (calcium phosphate as main component) deposition from the saliva can cause calculus or tartar, particularly at the lingual side of the lower incisors, or can lead to salivary glandular stones **(sialoliths)** within the excretory ducts of salivary glands. This can cause the obstruction of the duct with episodes of salivary "colics" and swelling of the gland (so-called) salivary tumor. Radiation therapy of head and neck tumors can lead to the **dry mouth syndrome** with difficulties in swallowing and speaking. **Inflammations** of the salivary glands can be acute or show a chronic progression.

## Submandibular gland

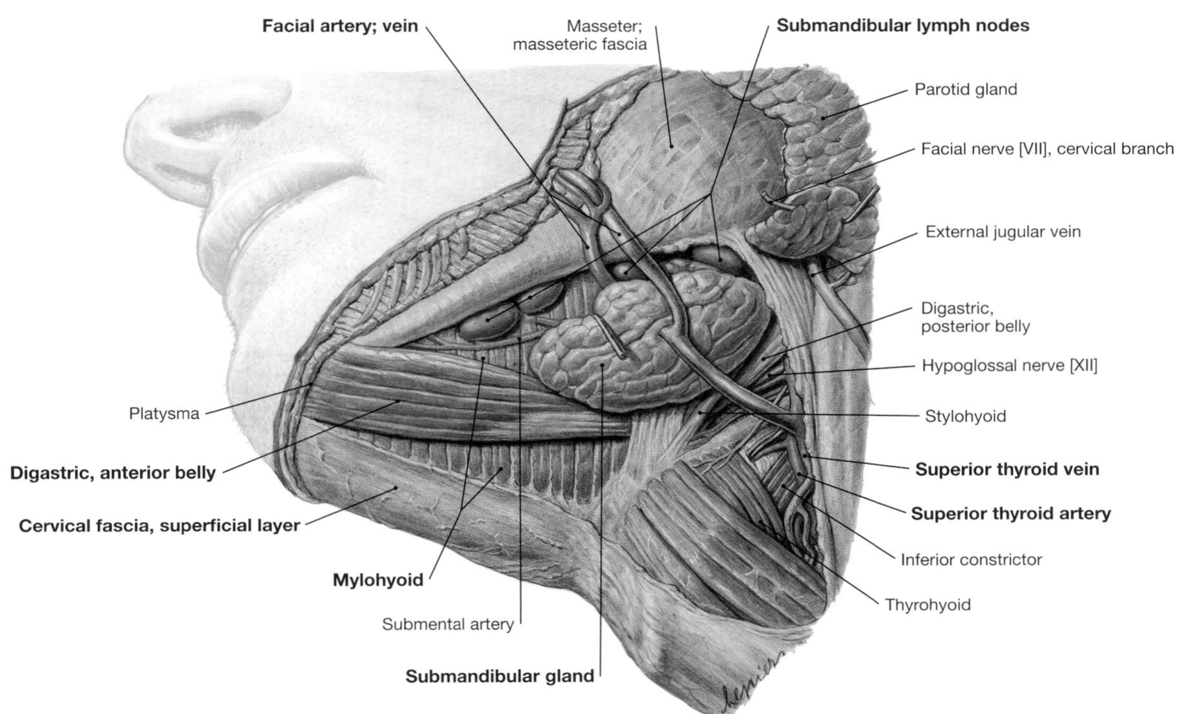
Facial artery; vein
Masseter; masseteric fascia
Submandibular lymph nodes
Parotid gland
Facial nerve [VII], cervical branch
External jugular vein
Digastric, posterior belly
Hypoglossal nerve [XII]
Stylohyoid
Superior thyroid vein
Superior thyroid artery
Inferior constrictor
Thyrohyoid
Platysma
Digastric, anterior belly
Cervical fascia, superficial layer
Mylohyoid
Submental artery
Submandibular gland

**Fig. 8.158 Submandibular gland, left side;** inferior view from an oblique lateral angle.
The submandibular gland is located in the submandibular triangle. The gland has its own fascia enclosed within the superficial cervical compartment as delineated by the superficial layer of the cervical fascia (→ p. 169). This gland has a direct topographic relationship to the facial artery and vein.

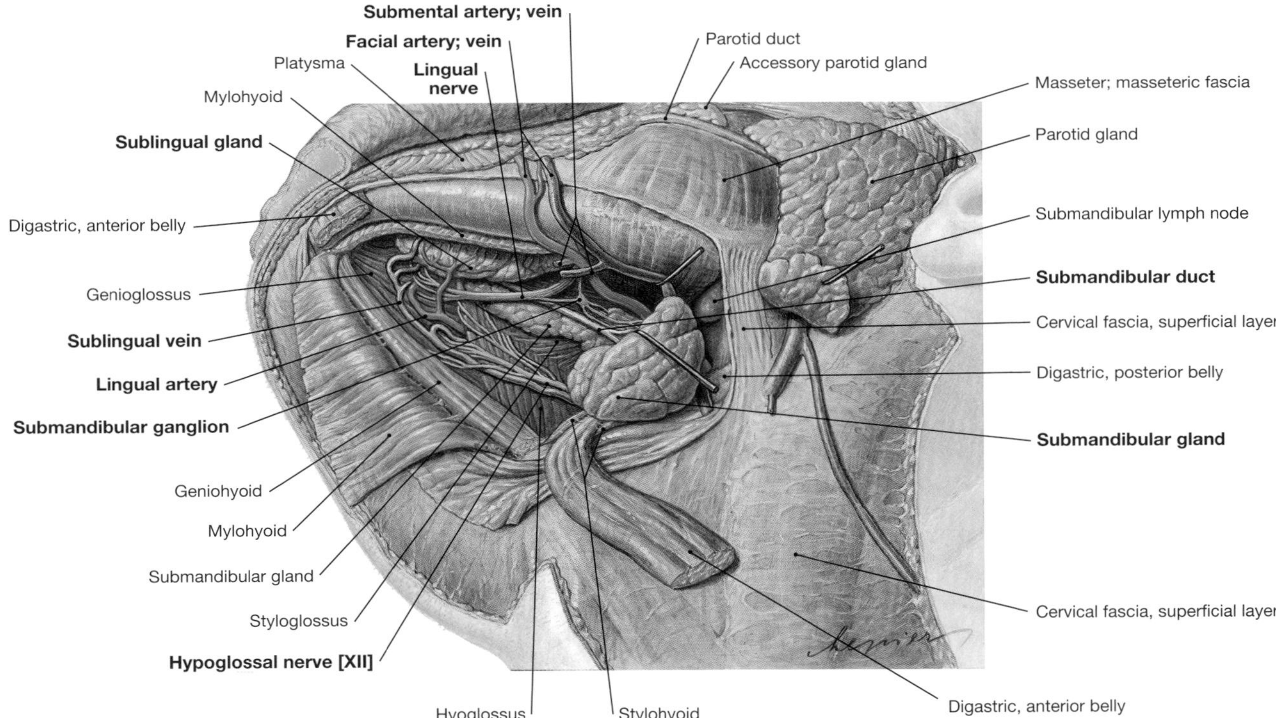
Submental artery; vein
Facial artery; vein
Platysma
Lingual nerve
Mylohyoid
Sublingual gland
Digastric, anterior belly
Genioglossus
Sublingual vein
Lingual artery
Submandibular ganglion
Geniohyoid
Mylohyoid
Submandibular gland
Styloglossus
Hypoglossal nerve [XII]
Hyoglossus
Stylohyoid
Parotid duct
Accessory parotid gland
Masseter; masseteric fascia
Parotid gland
Submandibular lymph node
Submandibular duct
Cervical fascia, superficial layer
Digastric, posterior belly
Submandibular gland
Cervical fascia, superficial layer
Digastric, anterior belly

**Fig. 8.159 Submandibular gland and sublingual gland, left side;** lateral inferior view.
The superficial glandular portion of the submandibular gland is bent backward, the mylohyoid is separated from the mandible and folded medially. Beneath the removed muscle, the deep glandular portion of the submandibular gland and the lingual gland, positioned parallel to the body of mandible, become visible.

**Arterial** supply to the glands comes from the facial, submental, and lingual arteries. The **venous** blood is drained by the sublingual and submental veins into the facial vein or directly into the internal jugular vein. **Regional lymph nodes** are the submental and submandibular lymph nodes.

## Submandibular and sublingual glands

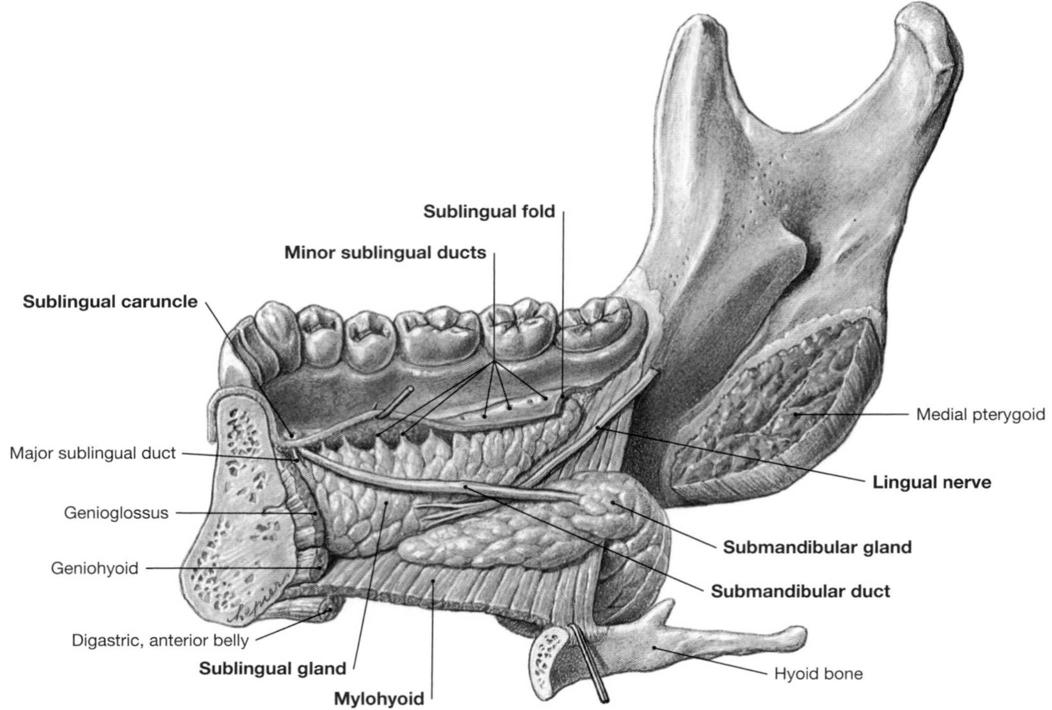
Sublingual fold
Minor sublingual ducts
Sublingual caruncle
Medial pterygoid
Major sublingual duct
Lingual nerve
Genioglossus
Submandibular gland
Geniohyoid
Submandibular duct
Digastric, anterior belly
Sublingual gland
Hyoid bone
Mylohyoid

**Fig. 8.160 Submandibular gland and sublingual gland, right side;** medial view.
The sublingual gland is located above the mylohyoid and lateral to the genioglossus. The gland sometimes perforates the floor of the mouth. The glandular body bulges out the mucosa at the floor of the mouth creating the sublingual fold which contains multiple openings of smaller excretory ducts (minor sublingual ducts) derived from the posterior glandular part. The lower part of the submandibular gland embraces the posterior margin of the mylohyoid in a hook-shaped manner and extends as submandibular duct above this muscle. The lingual nerve courses between the submandibular gland and the sublingual gland and below the submandibular duct to the tongue.

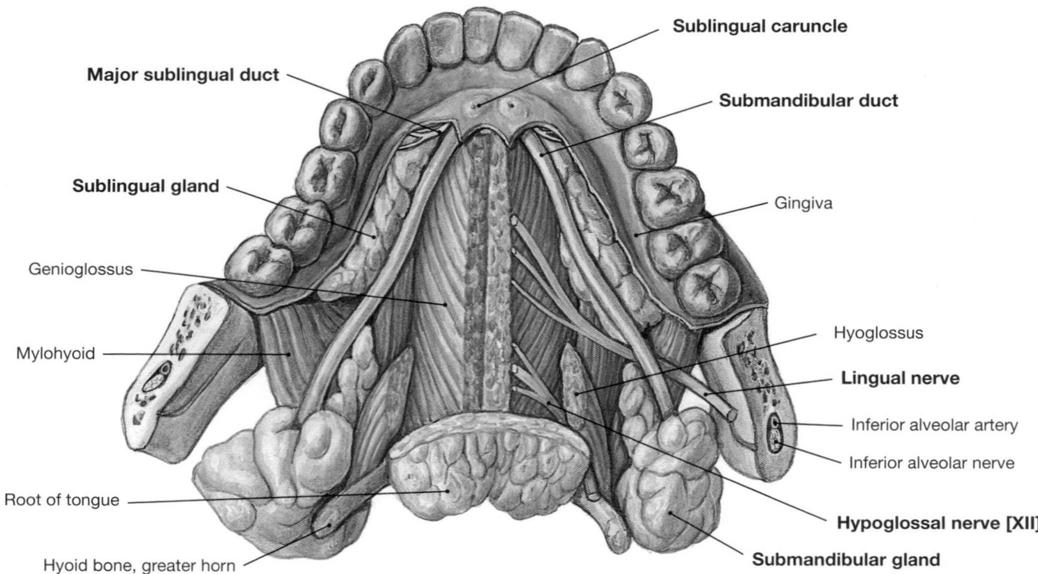
Sublingual caruncle
Major sublingual duct
Submandibular duct
Sublingual gland
Gingiva
Genioglossus
Hyoglossus
Mylohyoid
Lingual nerve
Inferior alveolar artery
Inferior alveolar nerve
Root of tongue
Hypoglossal nerve [XII]
Hyoid bone, greater horn
Submandibular gland

**Fig. 8.161 Sublingual gland and submandibular gland;** superior view.
The anterior portion of the sublingual gland contains a single larger excretory duct **(major sublingual duct)** which merges with the submandibular duct superior to the hyoglossus. The merged excretory ducts open at the sublingual caruncle. The hypoglossal nerve [XII] reaches the tongue between the hyoglossus and genioglossus.

### Clinical Remarks

**Sialoliths** are most frequently observed in the excretory duct of the submandibular gland. In a concentrated saliva, salts form crystals that create a sialolith which can block the excretory duct. During meals, the gland quickly increases in size and becomes painful (→ p. 92).

## Submandibular and sublingual glands

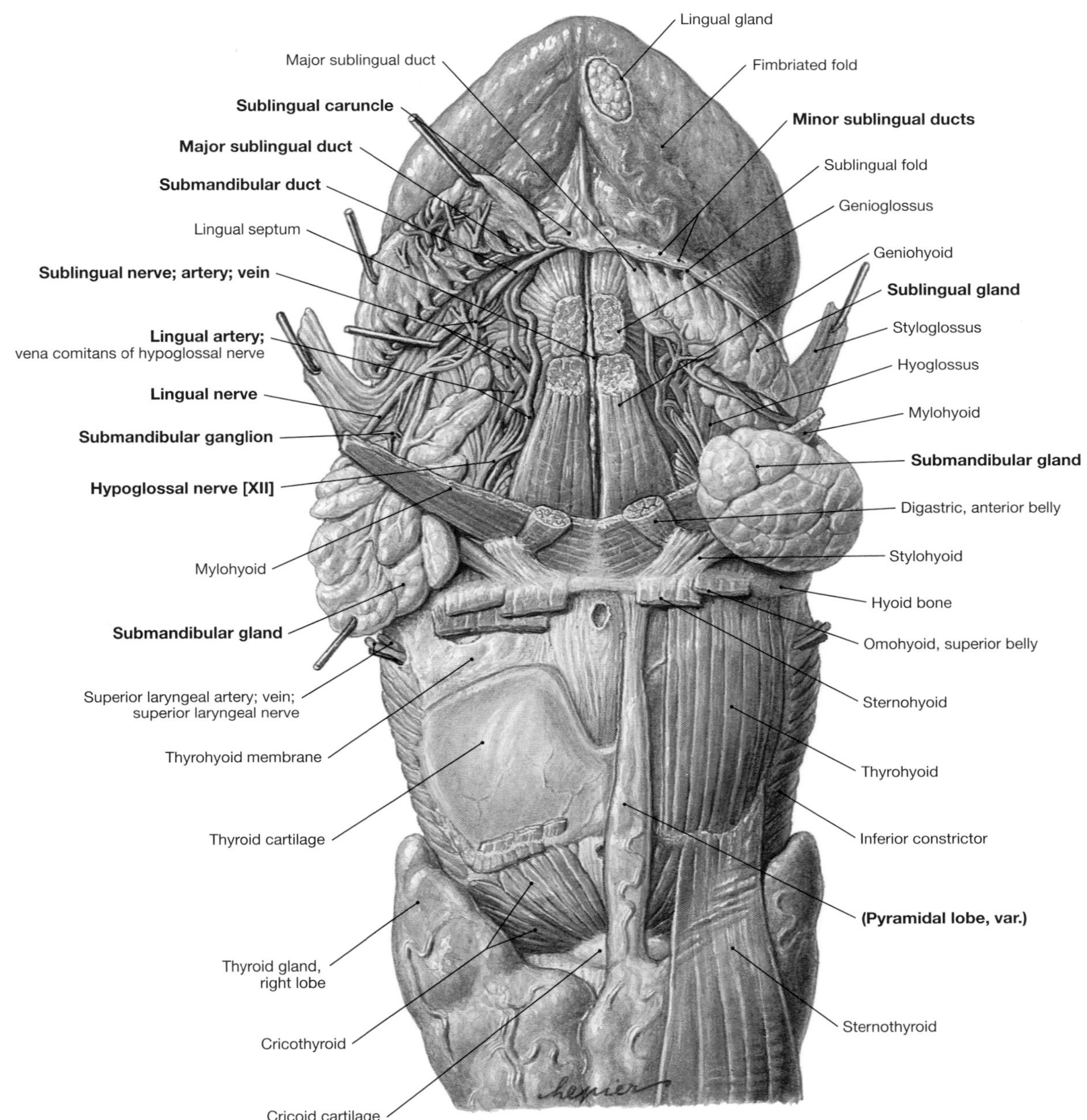
Lingual gland
Major sublingual duct
Fimbriated fold
Sublingual caruncle
Minor sublingual ducts
Major sublingual duct
Sublingual fold
Submandibular duct
Genioglossus
Lingual septum
Geniohyoid
Sublingual nerve; artery; vein
Sublingual gland
Styloglossus
Lingual artery;
vena comitans of hypoglossal nerve
Hyoglossus
Lingual nerve
Mylohyoid
Submandibular ganglion
Submandibular gland
Hypoglossal nerve [XII]
Digastric, anterior belly
Stylohyoid
Mylohyoid
Hyoid bone
Submandibular gland
Omohyoid, superior belly
Superior laryngeal artery; vein;
superior laryngeal nerve
Sternohyoid
Thyrohyoid membrane
Thyrohyoid
Thyroid cartilage
Inferior constrictor
(Pyramidal lobe, var.)
Thyroid gland,
right lobe
Sternothyroid
Cricothyroid
Cricoid cartilage

**Fig. 8.162 Vessels and nerves of the tongue and large salivary glands;** frontal inferior view.
A frontal view onto the elevated tongue displays a subepithelial venous plexus on the underside of the tongue. On the right side, the sublingual gland was reflected upwards to allow an unperturbed view of the lingual nerve and the submandibular duct (WHARTON's duct) beneath. The hypoglossal nerve [XII] enters the tongue slightly deeper. As a frequent remnant of the thyroid development, a pyramidal lobe, located in front of the larynx, can extend up to the hyoid bone.

## Parasympathetic innervation of the glands of the head

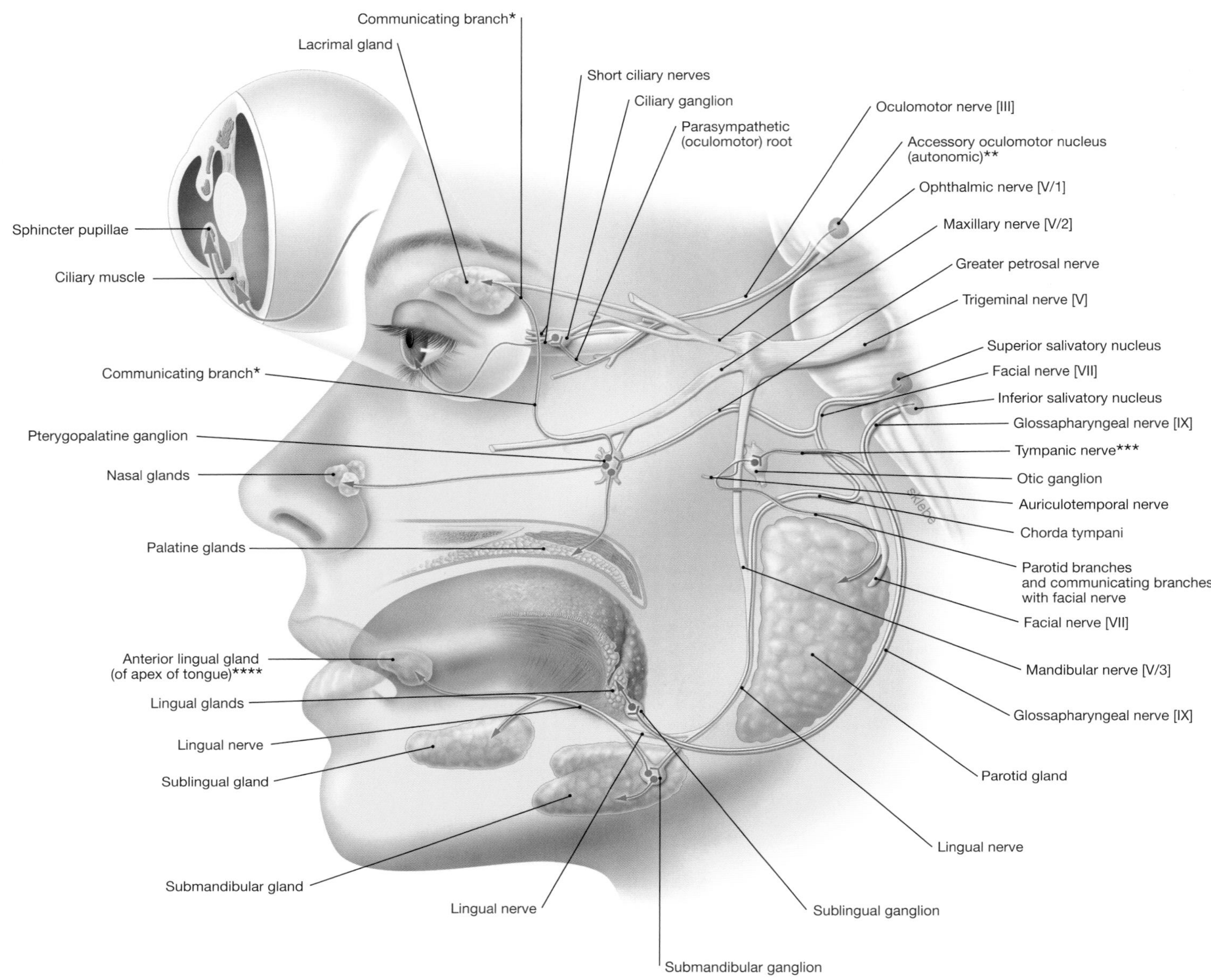
Communicating branch*
Lacrimal gland
Short ciliary nerves
Ciliary ganglion
Parasympathetic (oculomotor) root
Oculomotor nerve [III]
Accessory oculomotor nucleus (autonomic)**
Ophthalmic nerve [V/1]
Maxillary nerve [V/2]
Greater petrosal nerve
Trigeminal nerve [V]
Superior salivatory nucleus
Facial nerve [VII]
Inferior salivatory nucleus
Glossapharyngeal nerve [IX]
Tympanic nerve***
Otic ganglion
Auriculotemporal nerve
Chorda tympani
Parotid branches and communicating branches with facial nerve
Facial nerve [VII]
Mandibular nerve [V/3]
Glossapharyngeal nerve [IX]
Parotid gland
Lingual nerve
Sublingual ganglion
Submandibular ganglion
Lingual nerve
Submandibular gland
Sublingual gland
Lingual nerve
Lingual glands
Anterior lingual gland (of apex of tongue)****
Palatine glands
Nasal glands
Pterygopalatine ganglion
Communicating branch*
Ciliary muscle
Sphincter pupillae

**Fig. 8.163 Parasympathetic innervation of the glands of the head by autonomic ganglia of the head;** schematic drawing.
Parasympathetic fibers originate from the superior and inferior salivatory nuclei. **Preganglionic parasympathetic** fibers associate with various nerves to reach the parasympathetic ganglia of the head (otic, submandibular, sublingual, pterygopalatine, ciliary ganglia). Here, these fibers synapse and, as short postganglionic fibers, reach their target structures (glands). **Preganglionic sympathetic** fibers for the head derive from the lateral horn of the spinal cord. For the most part, these fibers synapse in the superior cervical ganglion (upper ganglion of the sympathetic chain). Postganglionic fibers create sympathetic plexus around arteries (e.g. internal carotid artery) and reach their destinations via blood vessels or by associating with local nerves.

* lacrimal gland anastomosis of parasympathetic secretory fibers from the intermediate nerve of the facial nerve [VII] with the lacrimal branch of the ophthalmic nerve [V/1] to the lacrimal gland

** EDINGER-WESTPHAL nucleus

*** JACOBSON's nerve

**** BLANDIN's gland

# Eye



9

# The Eye –
# a Window to the World

When anatomists discuss the visual organ, firstly they mean the eyeball and, secondly, the auxiliary structures in its immediate surroundings (accessory visual structures). Except for the eyelids, all auxiliary structures – including the eyeball – are enclosed within the orbit.

## Orbit

"Orbit" is certainly one of the least appropriate anatomical terms. The word is derived from the word "orbis" (circle), but a quick look at the skull confirms immediately that the outer opening of the orbit is not completely circular but its contour is rather oval to round. At the nasal margin of the orbital opening, the bony structures of the nasolacrimal canal open towards the orbit. The walls of the orbit form a steep pyramid towards the inside of the orbit, with its upper and lower wall perforated by two large fissures (superior and inferior orbital fissure) to allow many nerves and vessels to pass through. The canal for the optic nerve is located at the tip of this pyramid.

## Eyeball

The eyeball (bulbus) resembles an onion more than a ball. One can imagine a multi-layered onion sprouting at one pole and rooting at the opposite pole. Made up of multiple layers, the eyeball contains a watch-glass-curved transparent cornea and the optic nerve [II] at its anterior and posterior pole, respectively.

The **outer (fibrous) layer of the eyeball** is composed of the sclera and cornea and consists of firm collagenous connective tissue. The extra-ocular muscles (see below) are anchored in what one perceives as "the white of the eye", which is the sclera. The sclera turns into the avascular and transparent cornea which consists also mainly of collagen.

The **middle (vascular) layer of the eyeball** consists of choroid, ciliary body and iris. It is very rich in vasculature (branches of ciliary arteries) and strongly pigmented. This vascular layer of the eye also contains the intra-ocular muscles which are not subject to voluntary control. From the outside, the iris, the anterior portion of the vascular layer, along with the pupil are visible. Muscles located within the iris can constrict or dilate the pupil (adaptation). Along and beyond the outer margin of the iris, the vascular layer forms a circular bulge known as the ciliary body. The ciliary muscle is anchored within the ciliary body. The ciliary body received its name because of the radial zonular fibers which radiate towards the middle to secure the lens in its position immediately behind the pupil. Normally, the lens is transparent and elastic. The effect of the zonular fibers and the ciliary body on the shape of the lens changes the refractive power of the lens and leads to focussing of the eye (accommodation). The actual vascular layer separates the sclera and retina and covers the posterior half of the eyeball.

The **inner layer of the eyeball** (syn. with retina) consists of a photoreceptor-free non-optic part of retina and a photoreceptor-containing optic part of retina. The non-optic part of retina is a thin, heavily pigmented epithelium that covers the posterior part of the iris and the ciliary body. Along the serrated edge (ora serrata), just behind the ciliary body, it transforms into the much thicker optic part of retina. However, this "seeing" optic part of retina has a blind spot (optic disc), where the optic nerve leaves the retina and the branches of the central retinal artery penetrate the retina.

All layers of the eyeball and their differentiations surround the gelatinous, totally transparent interior of the eye, the **vitreous body** It stabilizes the entire membranous structure of the eye by its swelling pressure (intra-ocular pressure) – similar to the air bubble inside a football ball stabilizing its leathery coat.

## Auxiliary Structures

The auxiliary structures of the eye consist of the eyelids, the conjunctiva, the lacrimal apparatus, the six extra-ocular muscles and their three motor (cranial) nerves, numerous blood vessels, and a considerable orbital fat body.

The **eyelids** are not only responsible for the protection of the eyeball but distribute the tear film across the surface of the eye while constantly blinking. This prevents the surface of the eye from drying out. Located in the eyelids, numerous specialized sebaceous glands (MEIBOMIAN glands; tarsal glands) contribute a fatty secretion to the tear film.

The **conjunctiva** is a thin, transparent epithelial layer and covers the inner side of the eyelids and the visible part of the sclera. Its mucous secretions are a component of the tear film. At the corneal limbus (corneoscleral junction) the conjunctiva transitions into the corneal epithelium.

The **lacrimal gland,** positioned at the upper outer (lateral) corner of the orbit, and numerous accessory lacrimal glands located in the eyelids, produce the watery constituent of the tears. During eyelid closure the tear film is wiped towards the medial (nasal) angle of eye (nasal palpebral commissure) which contains the lacrimal caruncle, where the collected tears accumulate to create a lacrimal lake. The lacrimal puncta, one opening above and the other below the caruncle, are connected to two lacrimal canaliculi. These small canals drain the tears into the lacrimal sac, which opens into the nasolacrimal duct and empties the tears into the nasal cavity.

All six **extra-ocular muscles** insert at the eyeball and move it in different directions. Most of them arise from a common tendinous ring which surrounds the optic nerve [II] at its entry into the orbit. An exception is the inferior oblique eye muscle which lies on the floor of the orbit and originates directly lateral to the opening of the nasolacrimal canal. The extra-ocular muscles form a muscle cone behind the eyeball with its tip pointing towards the optic canal. Located in the center of the optic canal, the ophthalmic artery and the optic nerve [II] reach the posterior pole of the eyeball. The three nerves innervating the extra-ocular muscles, various branches of the ophthalmic nerve [V/1], as well as the branches of the ophthalmic vein are positioned within or adjacent to the cone. The remaining gaps between the structures are filled by adipose tissue, the **orbital fat body** (retrobulbar fat).

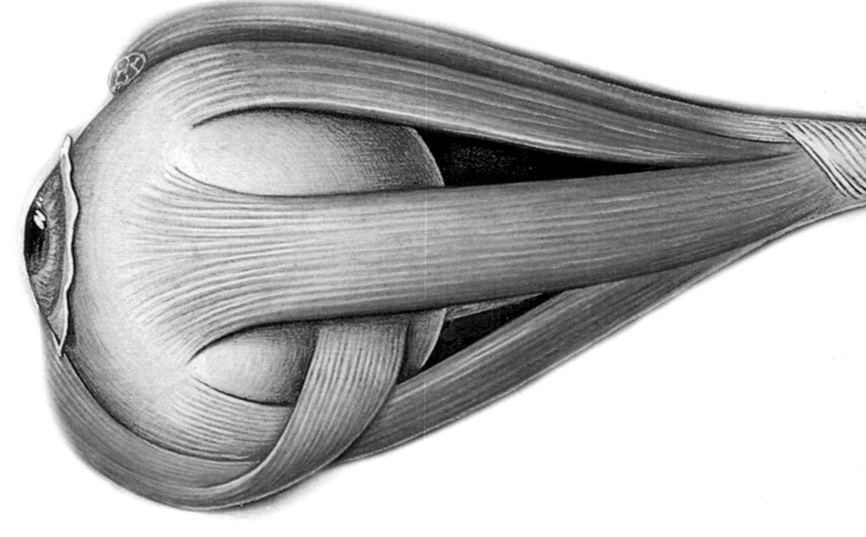

## Clinical Remarks

The **dry eye syndrome** (keratoconjunctivitis sicca complex) is one of the most frequent chronic diseases affecting the surface of the eye. Every second patient consulting an ophthalmologist in Western industrial countries suffers from this disease.
The age-dependent **macular degeneration** (AMD) is the most frequent cause of blindness in the industrialized world, followed by diabetic retinopathy and glaucoma. While AMD mostly affects elderly people, **diabetic retinopathy** mostly affects individuals during the prime of their life (approx. 2000 new cases of blindness per year). Similar incidence rates as reported for diabetic retinopathy apply to **glaucoma.**
Despite the fact that **cataract** is a common disease, it is not a frequent cause of blindness in Western industrial countries since prompt surgical intervention is an effective remedy in symptomatic cataract patients. However, cataract is the main cause of blindness worldwide. According to the World Health Organization (WHO), cataract is responsible for 48% of all cases of blindness (approx. 17 million patients) worldwide. The main reason is a poor healthcare system in large parts of the world.
In Africa, Southeast Asia, Central and Latin (South) America, and in the Middle East, approximately 84 million patients suffer from **trachoma infection** and 1.3 million of those infected cannot be cured (costs for treatment approx. US$ 20/person!). Trachoma infection is a classical disease of developing countries with poor sanitation and contaminated drinking water. Another cause of blindness during childhood in developing countries is **vitamin A deficiency** (costs of treatment approx. US$ 1.5/child!).

→ ***Dissection Link***

For the **dissection of the orbit,** the orbital part of the orbicularis oculi together with the palpebral parts of the upper and the lower lid are removed from the underlying connective tissue and turned over medially. The structures should not be detached at the medial angle of eye. Orbital septum, superior and inferior tarsus, and the medial and lateral palpebral ligaments are presented. For **cranial access to the orbit,** skin and muscles covering the frontal bone and the dura mater in the anterior cranial fossa are removed. The **opening of the orbital roof** should be carried out carefully to avoid damage to the periorbita and other structures passing through the superior orbital fissure. Upon **opening of the periorbita,** the levator palpebrae superioris with attached eyelid is dissected towards the tendinous ring (do not detach the trochlear nerve and the superior branch of the oculomotor nerve). Next, all the structures of the orbit are dissected from top to bottom by removing the orbital fat body. Careful blunt removal of the orbital fat body should be performed to preserve the ciliary ganglion.

## EXAM-CHECK LIST

• Orbit: bony margins, openings, structure, topographic relationships • clinical remarks (e.g. blow-out fracture, orbital phlegmon) • blood vessels (thrombosis of cavernous sinus) • cranial nerves [II–VI] (including nuclei of the cerebral trunk, trigeminal ganglion) • lacrimal gland • ciliary ganglion • retro-orbital fat body (GRAVES' disease, MERSEBURG triad, endocrine orbitopathy) • extra-ocular muscles: location, innervation, function, paralysis • eyeball: blood supply and innervation • intra-ocular muscles: innervation, function, paralysis, HORNER's syndrome • supportive structures and eye surface: eyelids, tear film, conjunctiva, cornea, draining lacrimal ducts

## Development

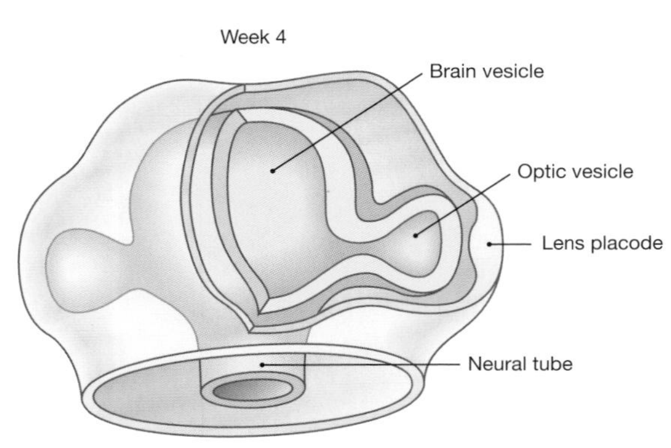

Week 4
Brain vesicle
Optic vesicle
Lens placode
Neural tube


**Fig. 9.1 Development of the eye, week 4.** [21]
At week 4, the optic vesicle bulges out of the diencephalic area of the prosencephalon. As the optic vesicle grows, its distal part gets in contact with the surrounding surface ectoderm and induces the formation of the lens placode.

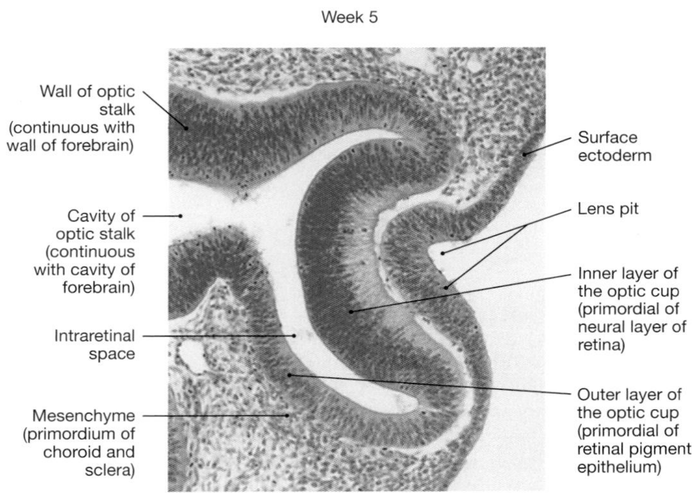

Week 5
Wall of optic stalk (continuous with wall of forebrain)
Cavity of optic stalk (continuous with cavity of forebrain)
Intraretinal space
Mesenchyme (primordium of choroid and sclera)
Surface ectoderm
Lens pit
Inner layer of the optic cup (primordial of neural layer of retina)
Outer layer of the optic cup (primordial of retinal pigment epithelium)


**Fig. 9.2 Development of the eye, week 5;** photomicrograph of a sagittal section. [20]
This image displays an invaginated double-walled optic vesicle with optic cup formation in close connection with the lens placode. Located between the two layers of the optic cup (primordium of the retina) and in the optic stalk (primordium of the optic nerve [II]), the intraretinal space is still relatively wide.

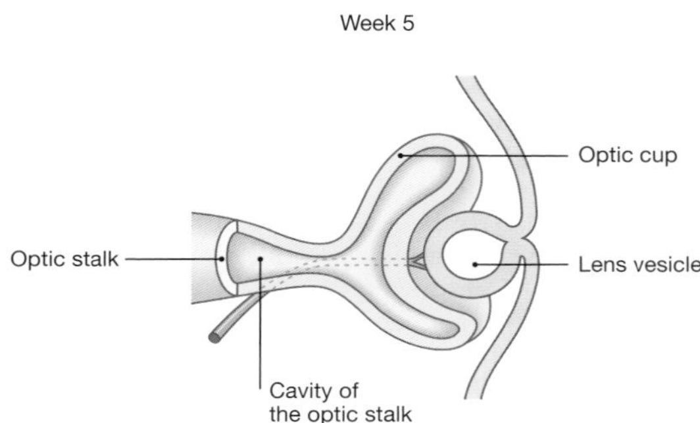

Week 5
Optic cup
Optic stalk
Lens vesicle
Cavity of the optic stalk


**Fig. 9.3 Development of the eye, week 5.** [21]
The spherical lens vesicle separates from the surface ectoderm and the rim of the optic cup infolds on the lens vesicle. The optic cup remains connected with the diencephalon by a small optic stalk, the former optic sulcus.

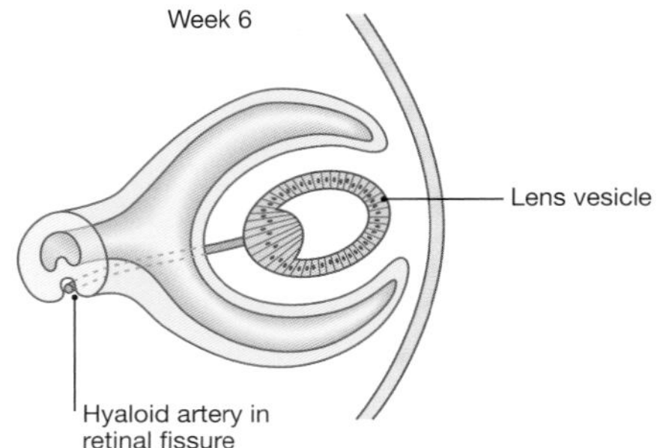

Week 6
Lens vesicle
Hyaloid artery in retinal fissure


**Fig. 9.4 Development of the eye, week 6.** [21]
At the deepest point in the optic cup, a longitudinal groove, the optic fissure, becomes visible. This optic fissure contains blood vessels and the first nerve fibers of the later optic nerve [II]. The inside of the optic cup is supplied by the hyaloid artery and vein. At 7 months, distal parts of the hyaloid blood vessels degenerate, whereas the proximal parts persist as central retinal artery and vein in close connection with the optic nerve [II].

### Development of the Eye

Eye development starts at the beginning of week 4 with the formation of the optic vesicle in the prosencephalic area that gives rise to the diencephalon. Early on, the anterior pole folds inwards to form a primitive optic cup. The retinal pigment epithelium derives from the posterior section of the outer layer of the optic cup, whereas its anterior section gives rise to the ciliary body and iris. The inner layer of the optic cup develops to become the retina. At the contact zone between the optic cup and the surface epithelium, the lens vesicle forms as part of the epithelial layer overlying the optic cup. The lens vesicle translocates beneath this epithelial layer. The ectoderm is also the origin for the cornea and conjunctiva. Most of the other components of the middle and outer eye are of mesenchymal origin. A web of blood vessels (with contribution by the hyaloid artery) initially surrounds the primordium of the lens which disappears later on. The proximal stump of the hyaloid artery becomes the central retinal artery.

## Development

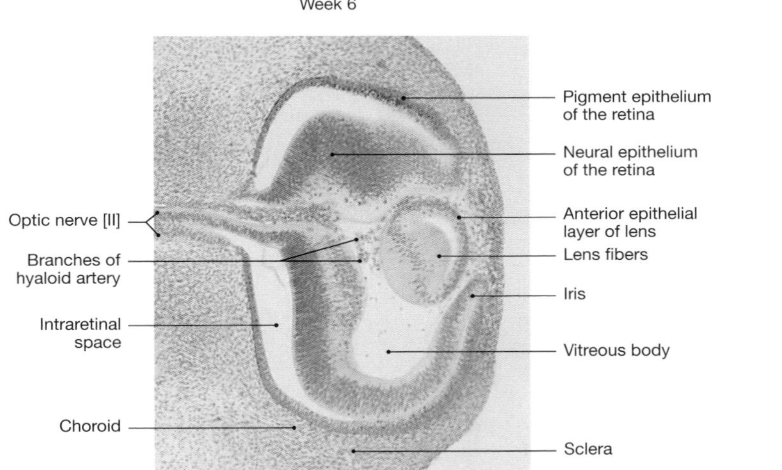
Week 6
Pigment epithelium of the retina
Neural epithelium of the retina
Optic nerve [II]
Anterior epithelial layer of lens
Branches of hyaloid artery
Lens fibers
Iris
Intraretinal space
Vitreous body
Choroid
Sclera

**Fig. 9.5 Development of the eye, week 6;** photomicrograph of a sagittal section. [20]
At week 7, lens fibers form as an elongation of epithelial cells at the posterior wall of the lens vesicle.

Week 8
Choroid
Vitreous body
Cornea
Lens with lens fibers
Hyaloid artery

**Fig. 9.6 Development of the eye, week 8.** [21]
Mesenchymal cells migrate into the optic cup and form the vitreous body that is composed of vitreous humor, a gelatinous substance with tiny fibers embedded. The vitreous body gives the eyeball its firm shape.

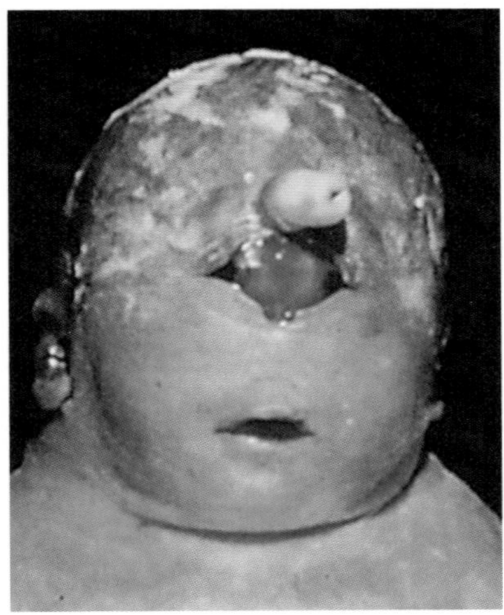

**Fig. 9.7 Male newborn with cyclopia.** [20]
Cyclopia is an anomaly of the face and eye associated with a proboscis-shaped nasal appendage above a single medially located eye.

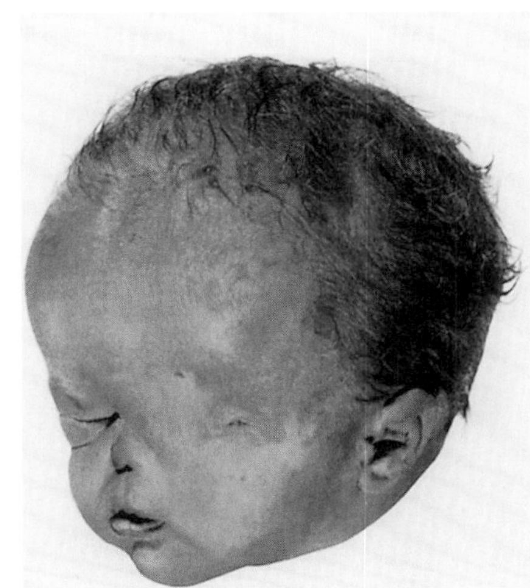

**Fig. 9.8 Male newborn with anophthalmia.** [20]
Congenital absence of all components of the eye and a single right nostril, with left nostril not formed. Although eyelids are formed, the upper and lower eyelids remain largely fused.

### Clinical Remarks

**Developmental defects** of the eye are relatively rare. Inherited blindness has an incidence of 20 per 100 000 live births and in most cases coincides with other (mental) disabilities. In some cases, remnants of the hyaloid artery can persist and project from the papilla of the optic nerve into the vitreous body and even into the lens. As a result, opacity of the lens can occur; however, often a **persistent hyaloid artery** is of no clinical significance. **Cyclopia** refers to the partial or complete merger of both eyes in the middle of the face (→ Fig. 9.7). Complete lack of eye development is referred to as **anophthalmia** (→ Fig. 9.8).

## Bony orbit

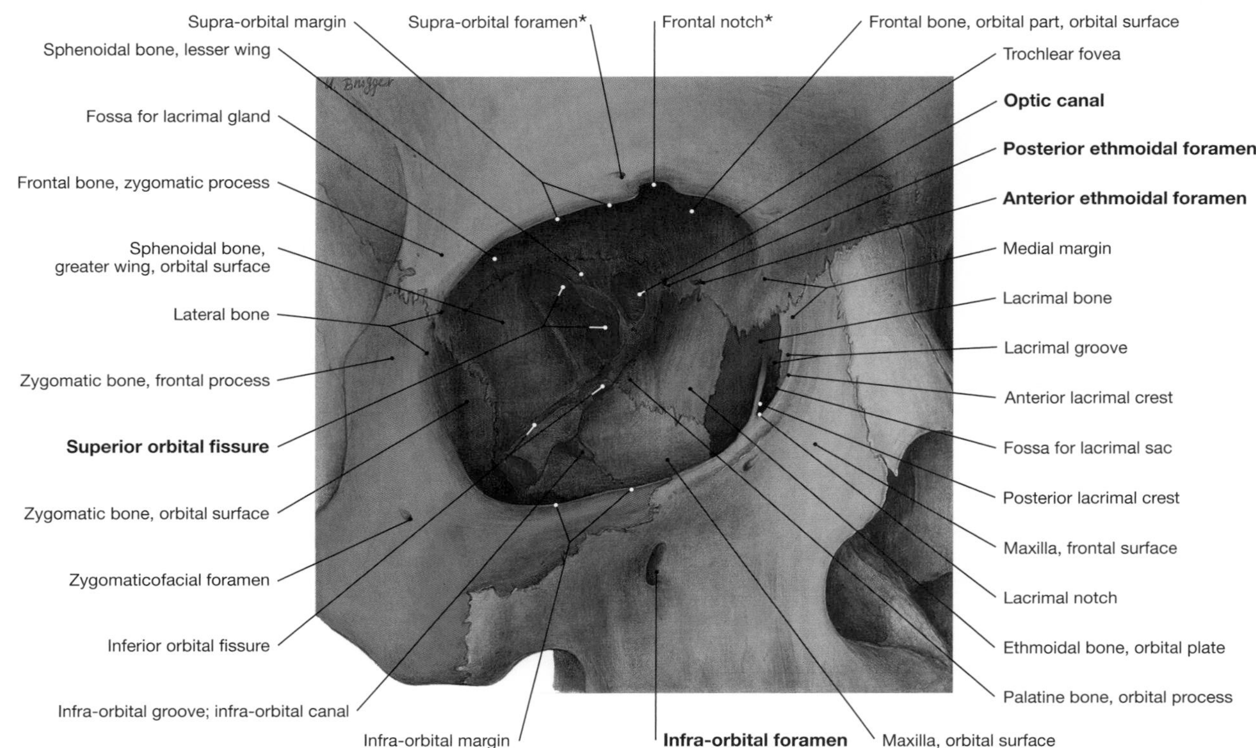
Supra-orbital margin
Supra-orbital foramen*
Frontal notch*
Frontal bone, orbital part, orbital surface
Sphenoidal bone, lesser wing
Trochlear fovea
Fossa for lacrimal gland
Optic canal
Posterior ethmoidal foramen
Frontal bone, zygomatic process
Anterior ethmoidal foramen
Sphenoidal bone, greater wing, orbital surface
Medial margin
Lateral bone
Lacrimal bone
Lacrimal groove
Zygomatic bone, frontal process
Anterior lacrimal crest
Superior orbital fissure
Fossa for lacrimal sac
Posterior lacrimal crest
Zygomatic bone, orbital surface
Maxilla, frontal surface
Zygomaticofacial foramen
Lacrimal notch
Inferior orbital fissure
Ethmoidal bone, orbital plate
Palatine bone, orbital process
Infra-orbital groove; infra-orbital canal
Infra-orbital margin
Infra-orbital foramen
Maxilla, orbital surface

**Fig. 9.9 Orbit, right side;** frontal view from an oblique angle; color chart see inside of the back cover of this volume.

Seven bones form the walls of the orbit (frontal, ethmoidal, lacrimal, palatine, maxillary, sphenoidal, and zygomatic bones). The lateral wall borders on the temporal fossa, the medial wall is located close to the ethmoidal cells and the nasal cavity. At its posterior aspect, the orbit is in topographic proximity to the middle cranial fossa, the optic canal, and the pterygopalatine fossa.

* These structures can be present as foramen or notch.

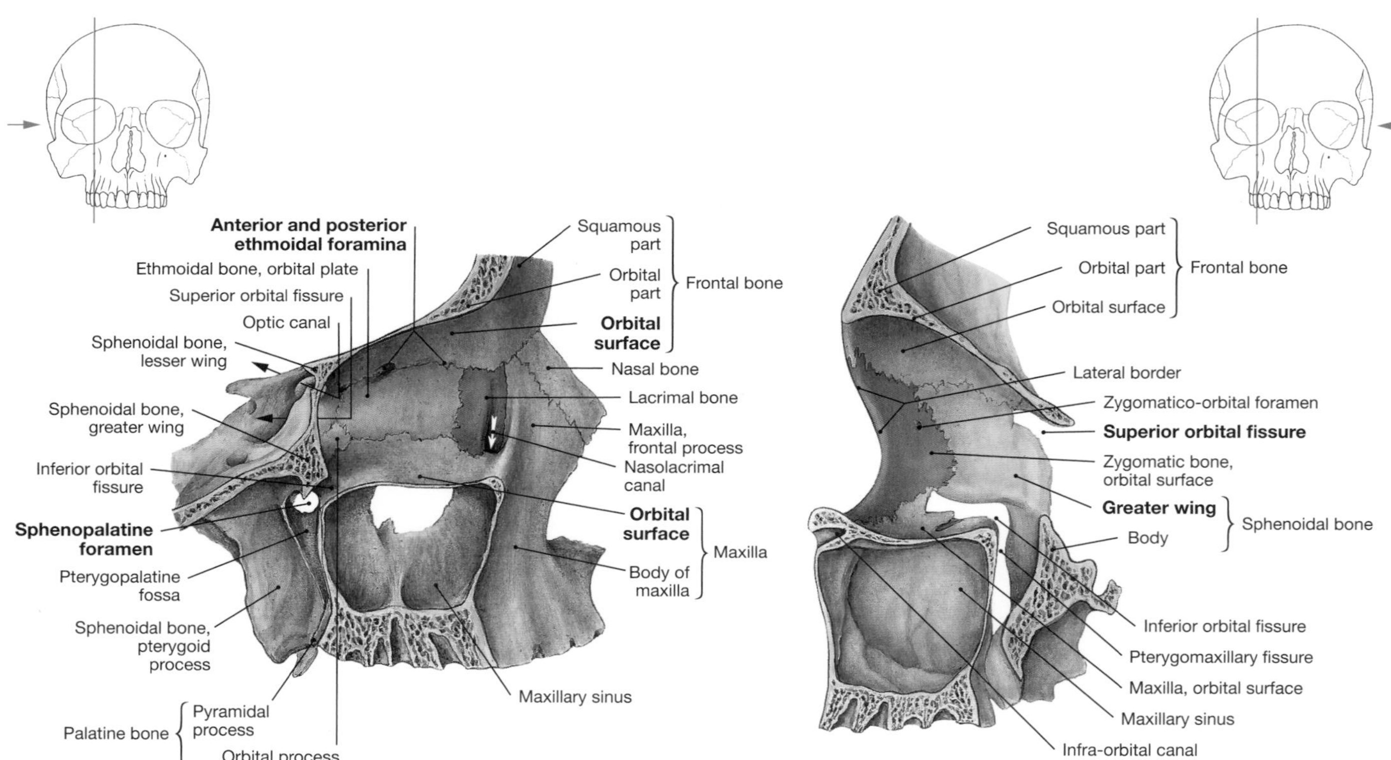
Anterior and posterior ethmoidal foramina
Ethmoidal bone, orbital plate
Superior orbital fissure
Optic canal
Sphenoidal bone, lesser wing
Sphenoidal bone, greater wing
Inferior orbital fissure
Sphenopalatine foramen
Pterygopalatine fossa
Sphenoidal bone, pterygoid process
Palatine bone
Pyramidal process
Orbital process
Squamous part
Orbital part
Orbital surface
Frontal bone
Nasal bone
Lacrimal bone
Maxilla, frontal process
Nasolacrimal canal
Orbital surface
Body of maxilla
Maxilla
Maxillary sinus
Squamous part
Orbital part
Orbital surface
Frontal bone
Lateral border
Zygomatico-orbital foramen
Superior orbital fissure
Zygomatic bone, orbital surface
Greater wing
Body
Sphenoidal bone
Inferior orbital fissure
Pterygomaxillary fissure
Maxilla, orbital surface
Maxillary sinus
Infra-orbital canal

**Fig. 9.10 Medial wall of the orbit, right side;** lateral view; color chart see inside of the back cover of this volume.

**Fig. 9.11 Lateral wall of the orbit, right side;** medial view; color chart see inside of the back cover of this volume.

## Bony orbit

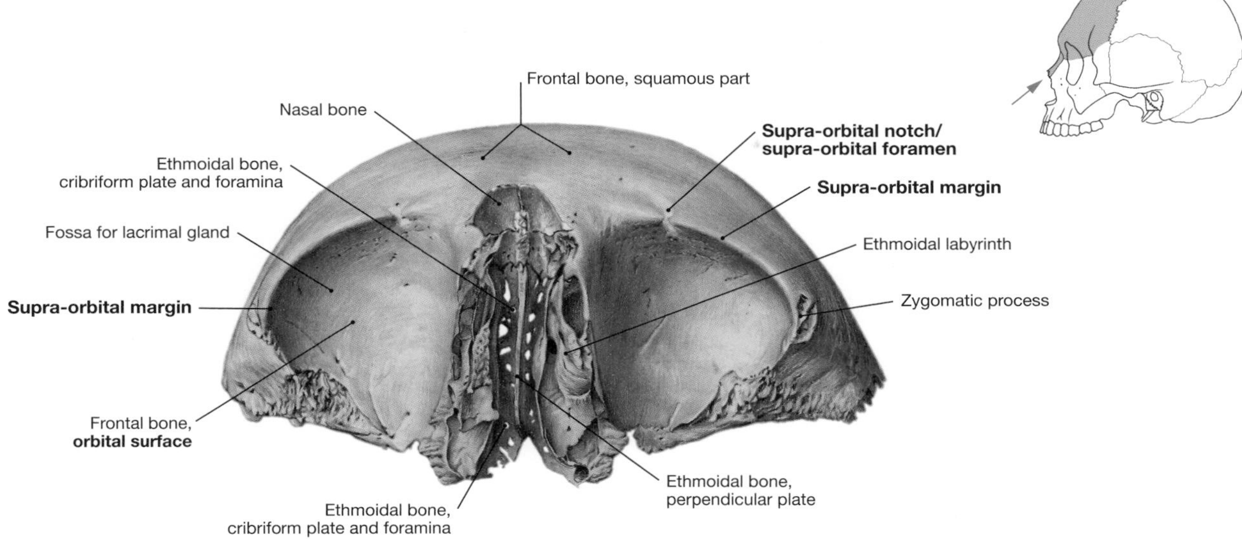
Frontal bone, squamous part
Nasal bone
Supra-orbital notch/ supra-orbital foramen
Ethmoidal bone, cribriform plate and foramina
Supra-orbital margin
Fossa for lacrimal gland
Ethmoidal labyrinth
Supra-orbital margin
Zygomatic process
Frontal bone, orbital surface
Ethmoidal bone, perpendicular plate
Ethmoidal bone, cribriform plate and foramina

**Fig. 9.12 Roof of the orbit;** inferior view; color chart see inside of the back cover of this volume.

The roof of the orbit is also the floor of the anterior cranial fossa and of parts of the frontal sinus. All bones of the ethmoidal labyrinth are extremely thin and are easily fractured during surgical procedures.

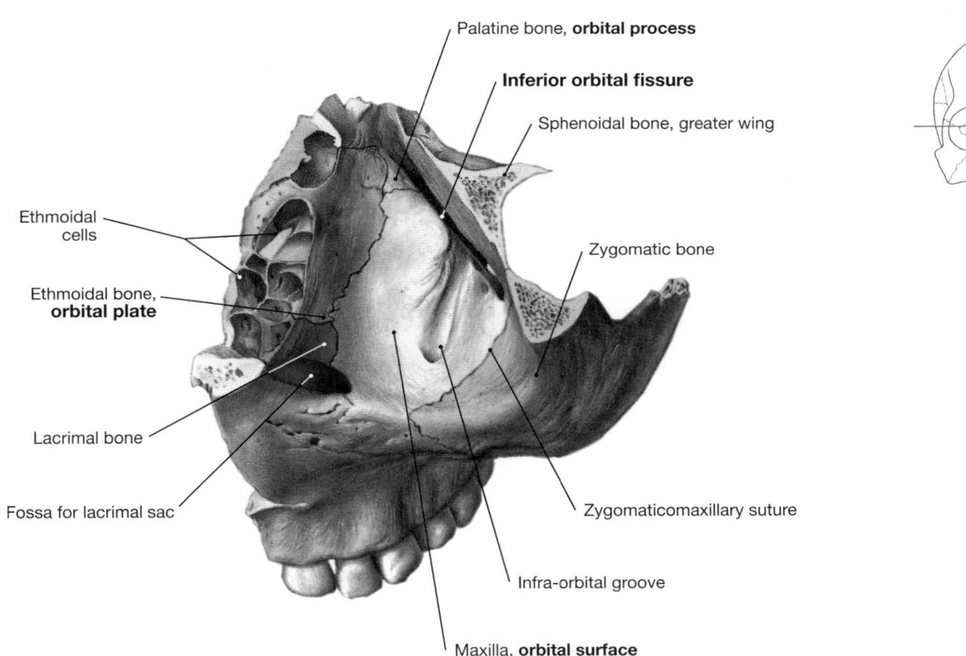
Palatine bone, orbital process
Inferior orbital fissure
Sphenoidal bone, greater wing
Ethmoidal cells
Zygomatic bone
Ethmoidal bone, orbital plate
Lacrimal bone
Fossa for lacrimal sac
Zygomaticomaxillary suture
Infra-orbital groove
Maxilla, orbital surface

**Fig. 9.13 Floor of the orbit, left side;** superior view; color chart see inside of the back cover of this volume.
The floor of the orbit is also the roof of the maxillary sinus. The infra-orbital groove is located in the posterior aspect of the orbit and turns into a bony canal midway through the orbit. This infra-orbital canal penetrates the maxilla and terminates at the infra-orbital foramen (not visible) located below the orbit.

### Clinical Remarks

Despite the fact that the medial wall of the orbit is paper-thin (thus, the name lamina papyracea), blunt force to the eyeball (e.g. center blow to the orbit by a tennis ball) usually results in a fracture of the base of the orbit (so-called **blow-out fracture**). As a result, intra-orbital structures (inferior rectus and inferior oblique) can be trapped in the fracture gap or be translocated into the maxillary sinus entirely **(orbital hernia).** Reduced mobility of the eyeball can cause double vision, enophthalmos, and/or the inability of this eye to look upwards. Involvement of the infra-orbital nerve, which runs in the floor of the orbit, is likely if **sensory dysfunction** in the dermal region of the upper jaw occurs.

## Eyelids

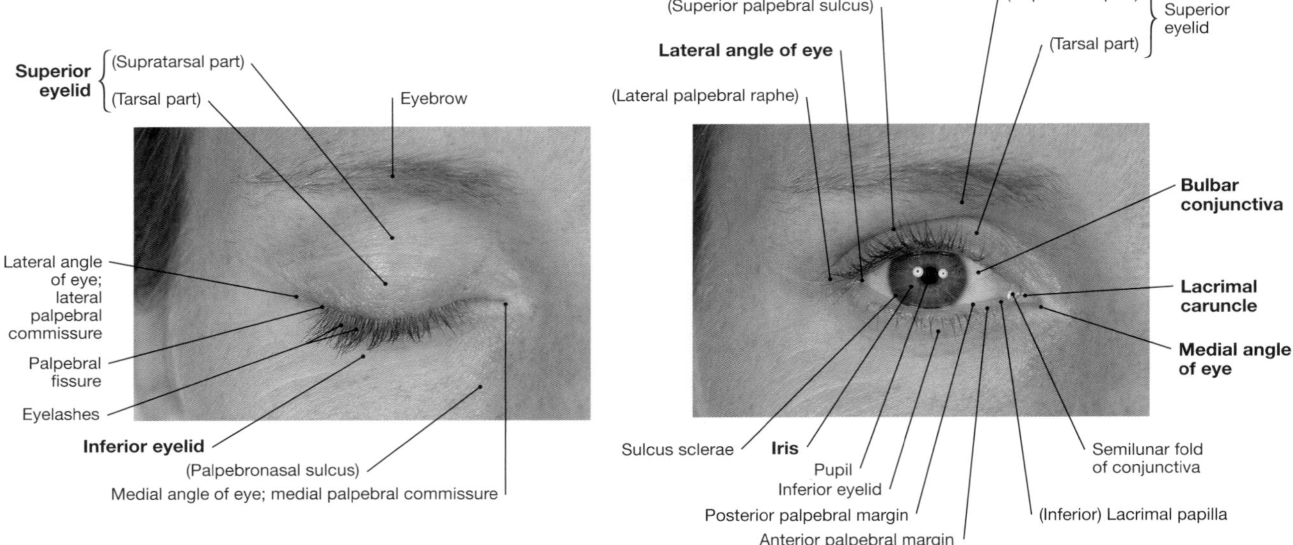
Superior eyelid
(Supratarsal part)
(Tarsal part)
Eyebrow
Lateral angle of eye; lateral palpebral commissure
Palpebral fissure
Eyelashes
Inferior eyelid
(Palpebronasal sulcus)
Medial angle of eye; medial palpebral commissure
(Superior palpebral sulcus)
Lateral angle of eye
(Lateral palpebral raphe)
(Supratarsal part)
(Tarsal part)
Superior eyelid
Bulbar conjunctiva
Lacrimal caruncle
Medial angle of eye
Sulcus sclerae
Iris
Pupil
Inferior eyelid
Posterior palpebral margin
Anterior palpebral margin
Semilunar fold of conjunctiva
(Inferior) Lacrimal papilla

**Fig. 9.14 Eye, right side, with eyelids closed.**
On average, a human eye blinks 20 to 30 times per minute. Each eyelid movement distributes a tear film across the surface of the eye. Blinking involves a consecutive contraction of the orbicularis oculi from temporal to nasal and results in a wiping motion in the direction of the medial angle of eye. Mechanical irritations (e.g. sudden draft, dust particle, fly) activate the blink reflex (also known as corneal reflex) to protect the surface of the eye.

**Fig. 9.15 Eye, right side, with eyelids open.**
In an adult with eyelids open, the width between the upper and lower eyelid ranges between 6–10 mm, and the distance between the temporal and medial angle of eye is 28–30 mm.

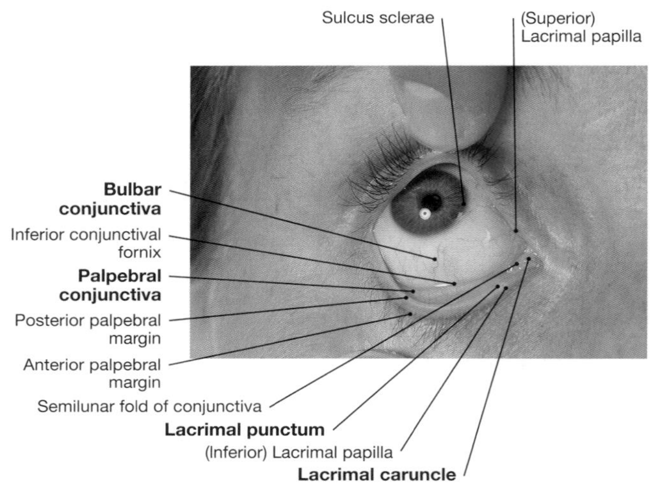
Sulcus sclerae
(Superior) Lacrimal papilla
Bulbar conjunctiva
Inferior conjunctival fornix
Palpebral conjunctiva
Posterior palpebral margin
Anterior palpebral margin
Semilunar fold of conjunctiva
Lacrimal punctum
(Inferior) Lacrimal papilla
Lacrimal caruncle

**Fig. 9.16 Eye, right side, with upper and lower eyelid everted.**
With the exception of the cornea, the conjunctiva, a translucent thin layer of mucosa with blood vessels, covers the part of the eyeball creating the eye surface, and the side of the eyelids in contact with the eye surface.

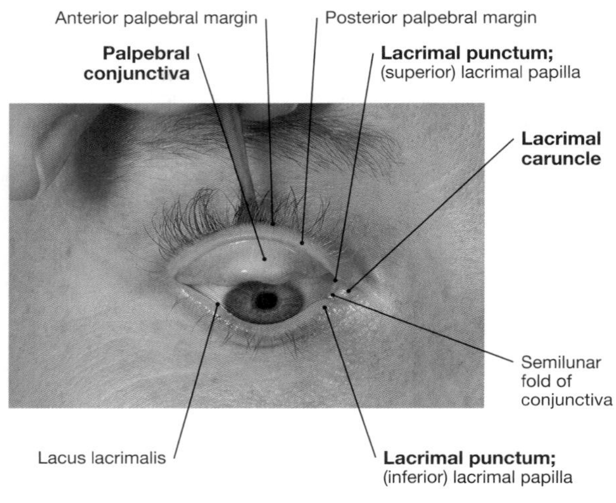
Anterior palpebral margin
Posterior palpebral margin
Palpebral conjunctiva
Lacrimal punctum; (superior) lacrimal papilla
Lacrimal caruncle
Semilunar fold of conjunctiva
Lacus lacrimalis
Lacrimal punctum; (inferior) lacrimal papilla

**Fig. 9.17 Eye, right side, with assisted ectropionized upper eyelid.**
The palpebral and ocular conjunctiva cover the rear side of the eyelid and the eyeball, respectively. Both conjunctival parts merge at the superior (upper) and inferior (lower) conjunctival fornix. The latter being the so-called conjunctival sac. Eyedrop medication is administered into the lower conjunctival sac.

### Clinical Remarks

A number of diseases involve the **narrowing** or **widening** of the **palpebral fissure.** Lesions of sympathetic fibers can result in palsy of the superior tarsal muscle in the upper eyelid, resulting in the palpebral fissure becoming narrower. Paralysis of the oculomotor nerve causes ptosis of the upper eyelid (which hangs down) due to the paralysis of the levator palpebrae superioris. By contrast, a facial nerve palsy results in impaired function of the orbicularis oculi and a widening of the palpebral fissure.

**Inflammation** of the conjunctiva (conjunctivitis) is encountered frequently in individuals wearing contact lenses. Anemic patients display a whitish pale conjunctiva because the low erythrocyte count in these patients prevents a normal filling of conjunctival blood vessels with red blood cells. Eversion of the lower eyelid and inspection of the conjunctival sac is a simple diagnostic test to identify this condition.

## Facial muscles

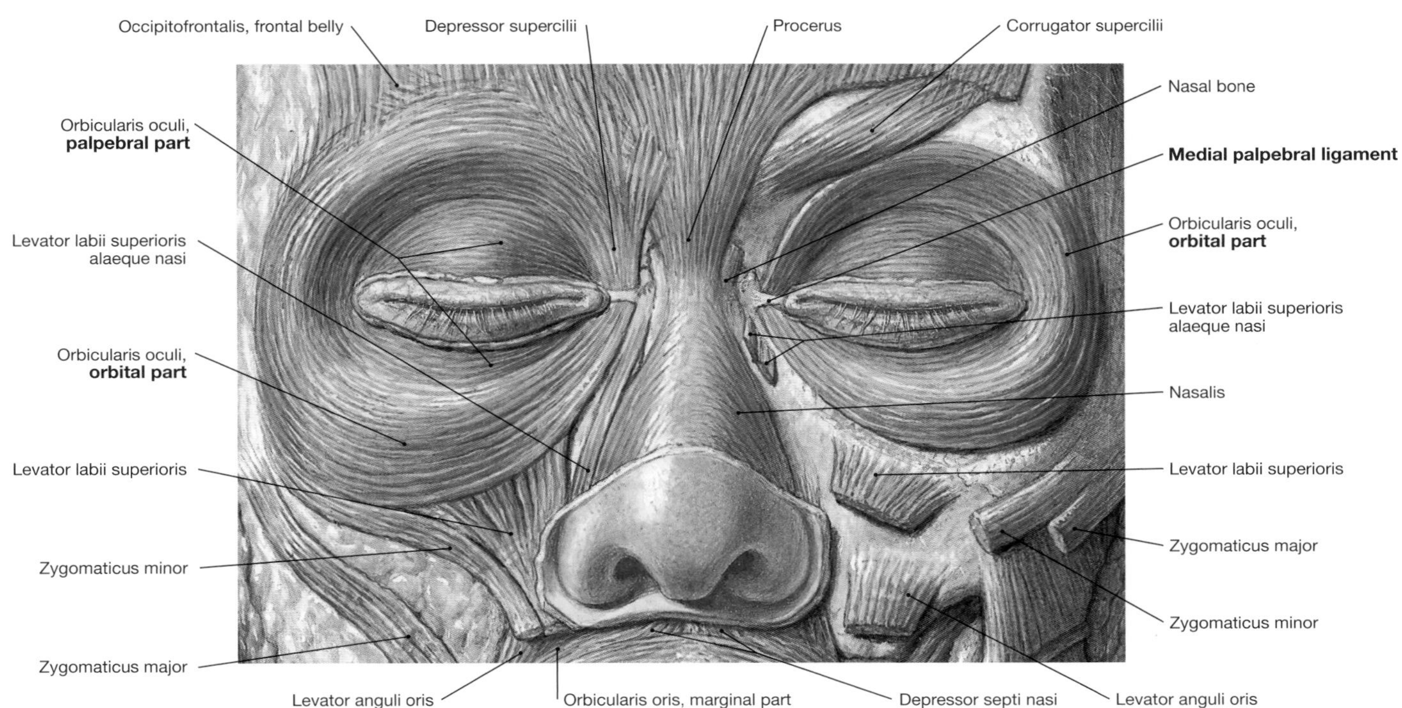
Occipitofrontalis, frontal belly
Depressor supercilii
Procerus
Corrugator supercilii
Nasal bone
Orbicularis oculi, palpebral part
Medial palpebral ligament
Orbicularis oculi, orbital part
Levator labii superioris alaeque nasi
Levator labii superioris alaeque nasi
Orbicularis oculi, orbital part
Nasalis
Levator labii superioris
Levator labii superioris
Zygomaticus major
Zygomaticus minor
Zygomaticus minor
Zygomaticus major
Levator anguli oris
Orbicularis oris, marginal part
Depressor septi nasi
Levator anguli oris

**Fig. 9.18 Facial muscles in the orbital region;** frontal view.
The orbital part of the orbicularis oculi encircles the anterior opening of the orbit. The palpebral part of this muscle projects into the eyelids.

→ T 1a, c, d, e

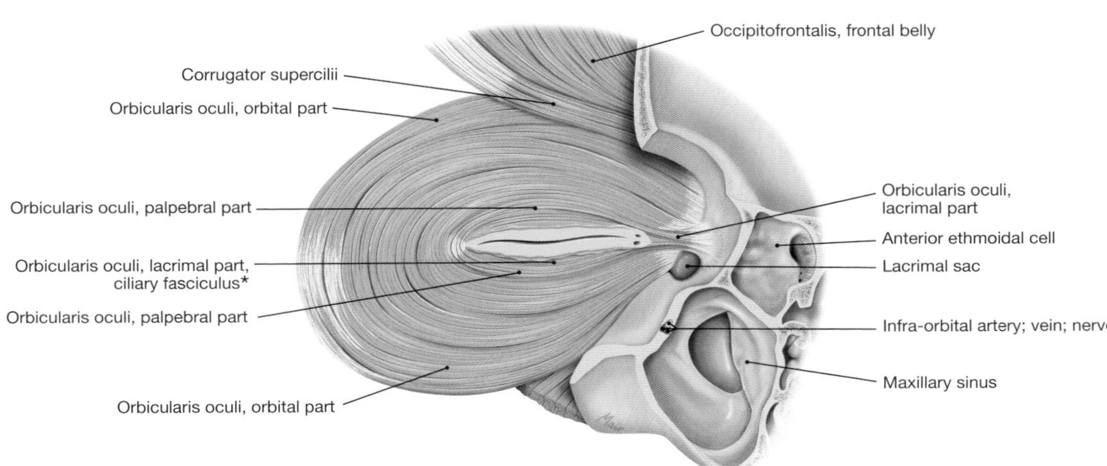
Occipitofrontalis, frontal belly
Corrugator supercilii
Orbicularis oculi, orbital part
Orbicularis oculi, palpebral part
Orbicularis oculi, lacrimal part
Anterior ethmoidal cell
Orbicularis oculi, lacrimal part, ciliary fasciculus*
Lacrimal sac
Orbicularis oculi, palpebral part
Infra-orbital artery; vein; nerve
Maxillary sinus
Orbicularis oculi, orbital part

**Fig. 9.19 Orbicularis oculi, left side;** posterior view.
At the medial angle of eye the lacrimal part of the muscle (HORNER's muscle), which assists in draining the tear fluid, is visible.
The orbicularis oculi consists of three parts. The **orbital part** is responsible for the voluntary firm occlusion of the eyelids. Contraction of the **palpebral part** results in blinking of the eye, which can occur voluntarily but usually happens involuntarily. Placed around the lacrimal canaliculi, the **lacrimal part** (HORNER's muscle) is essential for the drainage of the tear fluid. During blinking, the superior and inferior **lacrimal puncta** in the nasal third of the medial angle of eye dip into the lacrimal lake. It is assumed is that the contraction of the lacrimal part results in a suction effect (pressure-suction pump mechanism). Channeled via the lacrimal puncta, the tear fluid is sucked through the upper and lower lacrimal canaliculi into the lacrimal sac. The lower lacrimal canaliculus transports most of the tear fluid.

* muscle of RIOLAN

→ T 1c

## Clinical Remarks

**Injuries to the facial nerve** can result in the paralysis of the orbicularis oculi with the inability to close the eye **(lagophthalmos).** When the patient is asked to close his/her eyes, the eyeball rolls upwards as usual (the outer extra-ocular muscles are intact) and the white sclera becomes the only visible part of the eye (**BELL's phenomenon;** → Fig. 12.151). The inability to close the eyes prevents the even distribution of the tear film across the eye surface. As the tear film becomes discontinuous, the cornea starts to become dry and loses transparency shortly thereafter. The patient is unable to see with this eye. The missing eyelid closure represents the greatest challenge in the treatment of patients with facial nerve palsy.

## Eyelids, structure

**Fig. 9.20 Upper eyelid;** photograph of a histological specimen; azan stain; sagittal section, magnified. [26]
The eyelid can be divided into an outer and inner lamina. The outer lamina is composed of the striated orbicularis oculi with its palpebral part. The inner lamina consists of the conjunctiva, the tarsus with integrated MEIBOMIAN glands (tarsal glands, modified sebaceous glands) and, close to the rim of the eyelid, muscle fibers (muscle of RIOLAN, ciliary fasciculi) derived from the orbital part of the orbicularis oculi projecting into the tarsus.

* MEIBOMIAN glands
** muscle of RIOLAN

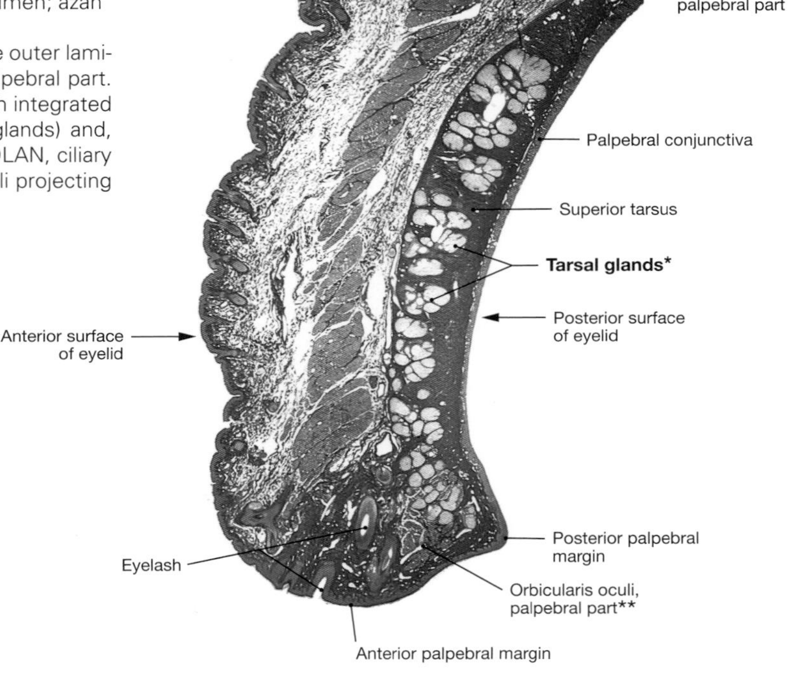
Orbicularis oculi, palpebral part
Palpebral conjunctiva
Superior tarsus
Tarsal glands*
Posterior surface of eyelid
Anterior surface of eyelid
Posterior palpebral margin
Eyelash
Orbicularis oculi, palpebral part**
Anterior palpebral margin

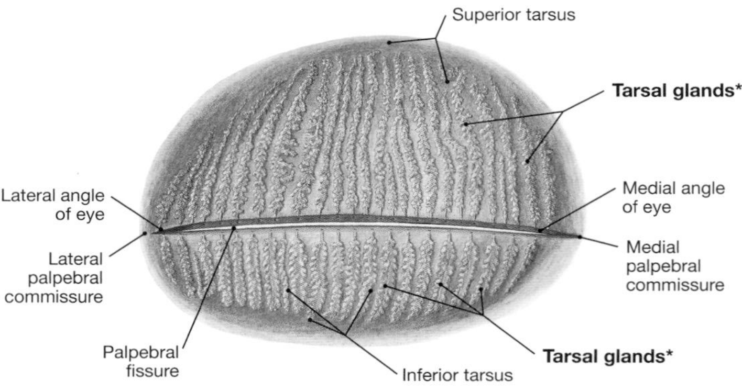
Superior tarsus
Tarsal glands*
Lateral angle of eye
Lateral palpebral commissure
Medial angle of eye
Medial palpebral commissure
Palpebral fissure
Inferior tarsus
Tarsal glands*

**Fig. 9.21 Eyelids, right side;** posterior view; translucent specimen illustrating the small excretory ducts (ductules) of the tarsal glands. Each eyelid contains approximately 25 to 30 individual glands with their excretory ductules opening into the rim of the eyelid (palpebral fissure).

* MEIBOMIAN glands

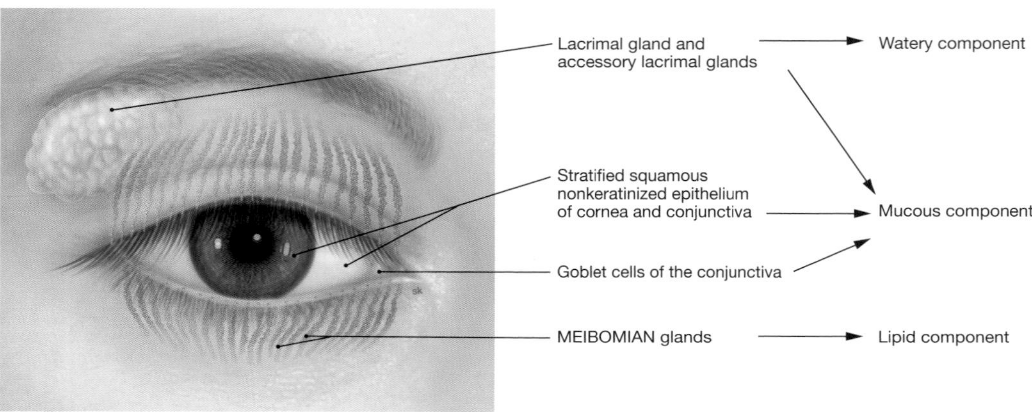
Lacrimal gland and accessory lacrimal glands
Watery component
Stratified squamous nonkeratinized epithelium of cornea and conjunctiva
Mucous component
Goblet cells of the conjunctiva
MEIBOMIAN glands
Lipid component

**Fig. 9.22 Structures of the eye surface** involved in the formation of the three components of the tear film; schematic drawing.

## Blood supply and innervation of the lacrimal gland and eyelids

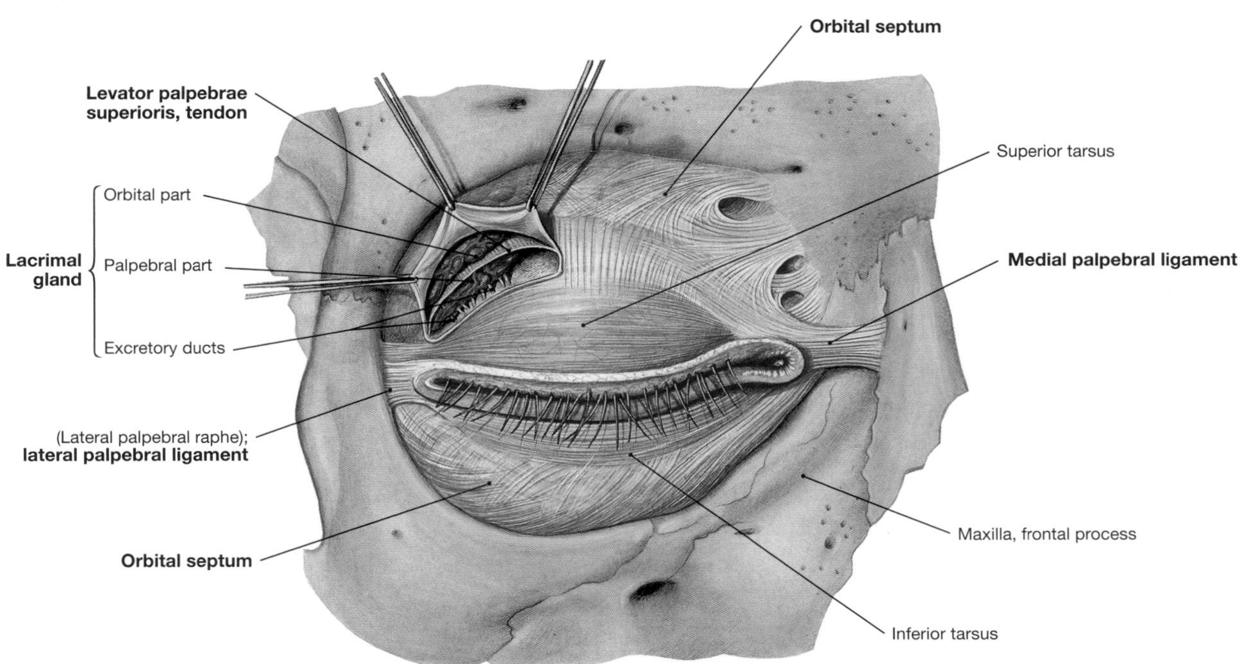
Orbital septum
Levator palpebrae superioris, tendon
Superior tarsus
Orbital part
Lacrimal gland
Palpebral part
Medial palpebral ligament
Excretory ducts
(Lateral palpebral raphe); lateral palpebral ligament
Maxilla, frontal process
Orbital septum
Inferior tarsus

**Fig. 9.23 Orbital opening, right side, with orbital septum, tarsal plates, and palpebral ligaments;** frontal view.
Dissection of the orbital septum and of the inserting tendon of the levator palpebrae superioris displays the lacrimal gland. The tendon of the levator palpebrae superioris divides the lacrimal gland located in the temporal upper quadrant of the bulbus into an orbital part and a palpebral part.

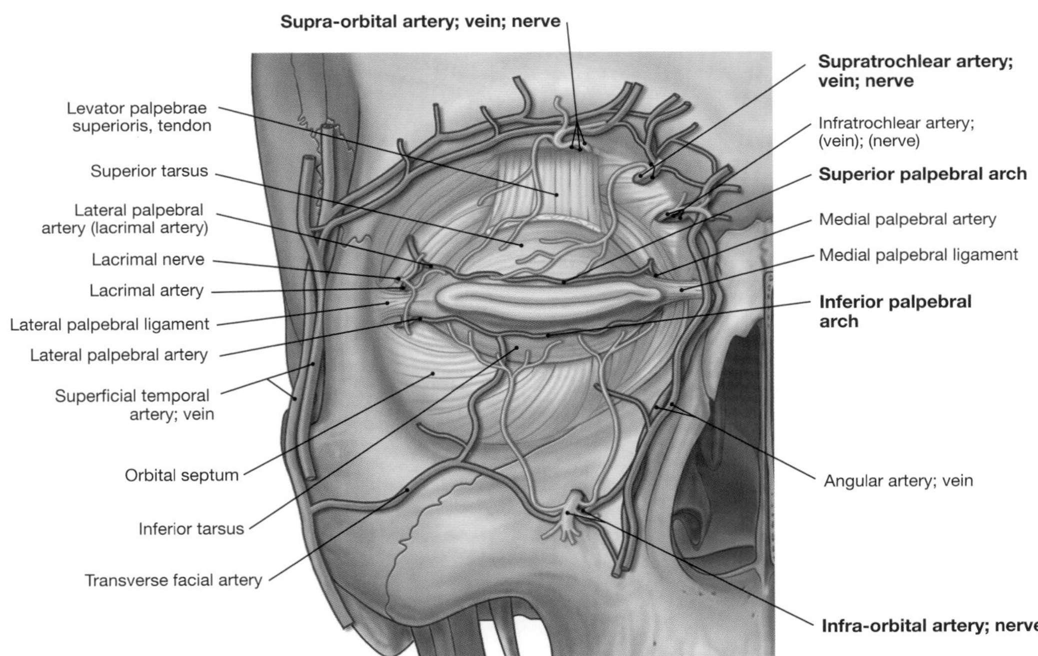
Supra-orbital artery; vein; nerve
Supratrochlear artery; vein; nerve
Levator palpebrae superioris, tendon
Infratrochlear artery; (vein); (nerve)
Superior tarsus
Superior palpebral arch
Lateral palpebral artery (lacrimal artery)
Medial palpebral artery
Medial palpebral ligament
Lacrimal nerve
Lacrimal artery
Inferior palpebral arch
Lateral palpebral ligament
Lateral palpebral artery
Superficial temporal artery; vein
Angular artery; vein
Orbital septum
Inferior tarsus
Transverse facial artery
Infra-orbital artery; nerve

**Fig. 9.24 Arteries, veins, and nerves at the orbital opening and in the periorbital region, right side;** frontal view. [10]
The superior and inferior palpebral arch create an arterial circle located above the orbital septum and surrounding the orbit. This arterial circle is supplied by numerous arteries derived from the **internal carotid artery** (supra-orbital artery, lateral palpebral arteries of the lacrimal artery, medial palpebral arteries) and the **external carotid artery** (facial artery, angular artery, infra-orbital artery, superficial temporal artery, zygomatico-orbital artery). The supra-orbital and infra-orbital nerves are branches of the ophthalmic nerve [V/1] and maxillary nerve [V/2], respectively, and exit the orbit through the identically named foramina (the supra-orbital nerve may exit the orbit through the supra-orbital notch). The sensory perception of the ophthalmic nerve [V/1] and maxillary nerve [V/2] can be tested at both nerve exit points.

## Clinics

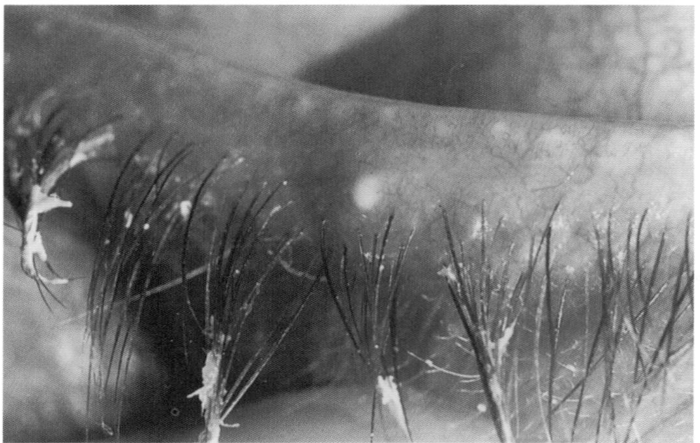

Fig. 9.25 **Inflammation at the rim of the eyelids, seborrheic blepharitis.** [15]

### Clinical Remarks

A **chalazion** is a granulomatous inflammation of a MEIBOMIAN gland, usually as a result of an occluded opening of the excretory duct. Located just below the rim of the eyelid, a chalazion can be palpated as painless, non-movable mass with the size of a grape seed up to a hazelnut. A stye **(hordeolum)** is a frequently putrid inflammation of individual glands of the eyelids (usually caused by bacteria and painful). Inflammations of the rim of the eyelid often result in **blepharitis** (→ Fig. 9.25) with typical signs of dry eye, including burning. Sensation of foreign object in the eye, mild photophobia, and reddening of the eyelid rim.

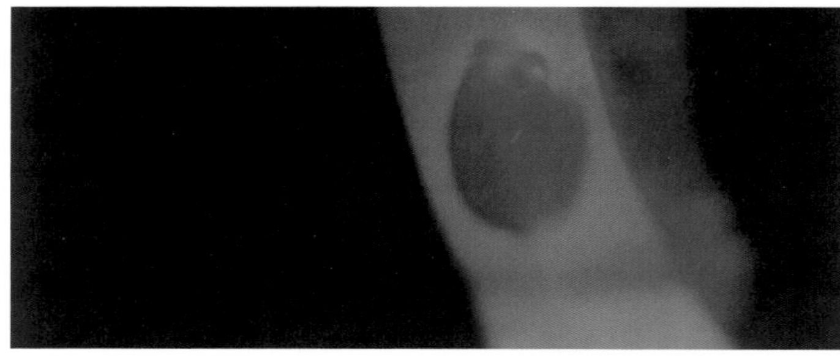

**Fig. 9.26 Tear film of the eye, right side;** frontal view; slit lamp examination with fluorescent dye in blue light. [15]
The spot represents a dry corneal area resulting from the disrupted tear film.

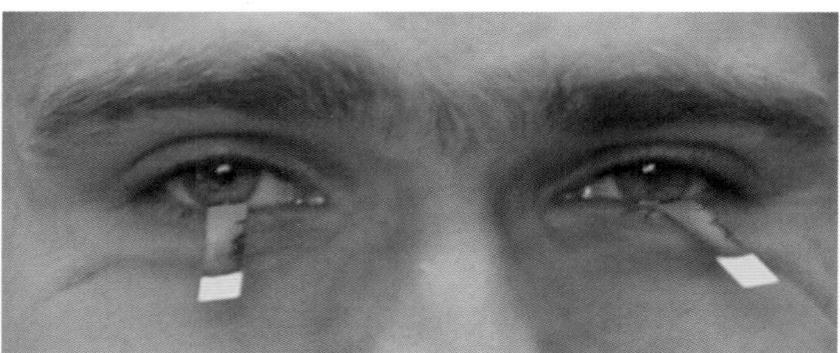

**Fig. 9.27 SCHIRMER's test performed on a healthy person.**
The two paper strips display a clear purple coloration of the yellow SCHIRMER's paper strip. Within 5 minutes, the paper strips are completely purple.

### Clinical Remarks

If an impaired function of the lacrimal gland is suspected, e.g. as part of a facial nerve palsy, the **SCHIRMER's test** is performed. A filter paper strip of standardized length, bent at one end, is hooked into the conjunctival sac. Absorbed tear fluid causes a change in color (→ Fig. 9.27). At a normal rate of tear production, more than two thirds of the paper strip should be colored within 5 minutes. A shorter length of the moisturized (colored) paper strip suggests a reduced tear production.

Another test of the tear film examines its ability to maintain a continuous film across the entire eye surface by measuring the time it takes for the tear film to break up **(tear break-up time).** A normal tear break-up time is approximately 20–30 seconds but break-up times below 10 seconds can cause the dry eye syndrome.

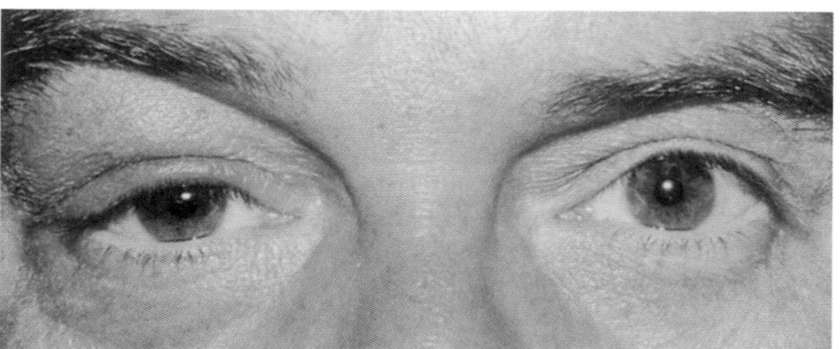

**Fig. 9.28 Reduced eyelid opening, right side; in the case of an acute dacryoadenitis (inflammation of the lacrimal gland).** [15]

### Clinical Remarks

The angular vein located in the medial (nasal) angle of eye transitions into the intra-orbital ophthalmic vein and connects a part of the facial venous drainage system (facial vein) with the cavernous sinus. Infections in the outer facial area (e.g. improper squeezing of pimples on the cheek) can lead to a spread of bacteria reaching the cavernous sinus and causing a **cavernous sinus thrombosis** (→ p. 223). At the first signs of ascending infection, the angular vein should be ligated at the medial angle of eye to prevent a potentially life-threatening thrombosis of the sinus. **Inflammation** of the **lacrimal gland** (dacryoadenitis; → Fig. 9.28) causes protrusion of the orbital septum and reduced eyelid opening.

## Lacrimal apparatus, innervation

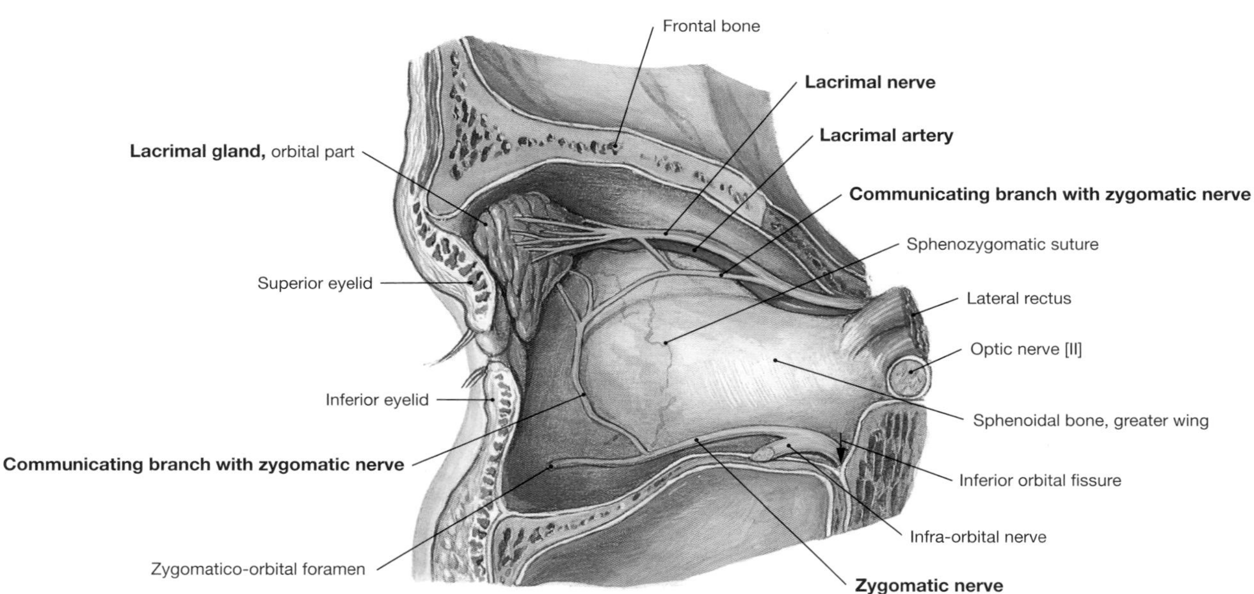
Frontal bone
Lacrimal nerve
Lacrimal artery
Lacrimal gland, orbital part
Communicating branch with zygomatic nerve
Sphenozygomatic suture
Superior eyelid
Lateral rectus
Optic nerve [II]
Inferior eyelid
Sphenoidal bone, greater wing
Communicating branch with zygomatic nerve
Inferior orbital fissure
Infra-orbital nerve
Zygomatico-orbital foramen
Zygomatic nerve

**Fig. 9.29 Innervation of the lacrimal gland, right side;** medial view onto the lateral wall of the orbit.
Presentation of the lacrimal gland, the lacrimal artery and nerve and the connection between the zygomatic nerve and lacrimal nerve via the communicating branch with zygomatic nerve.

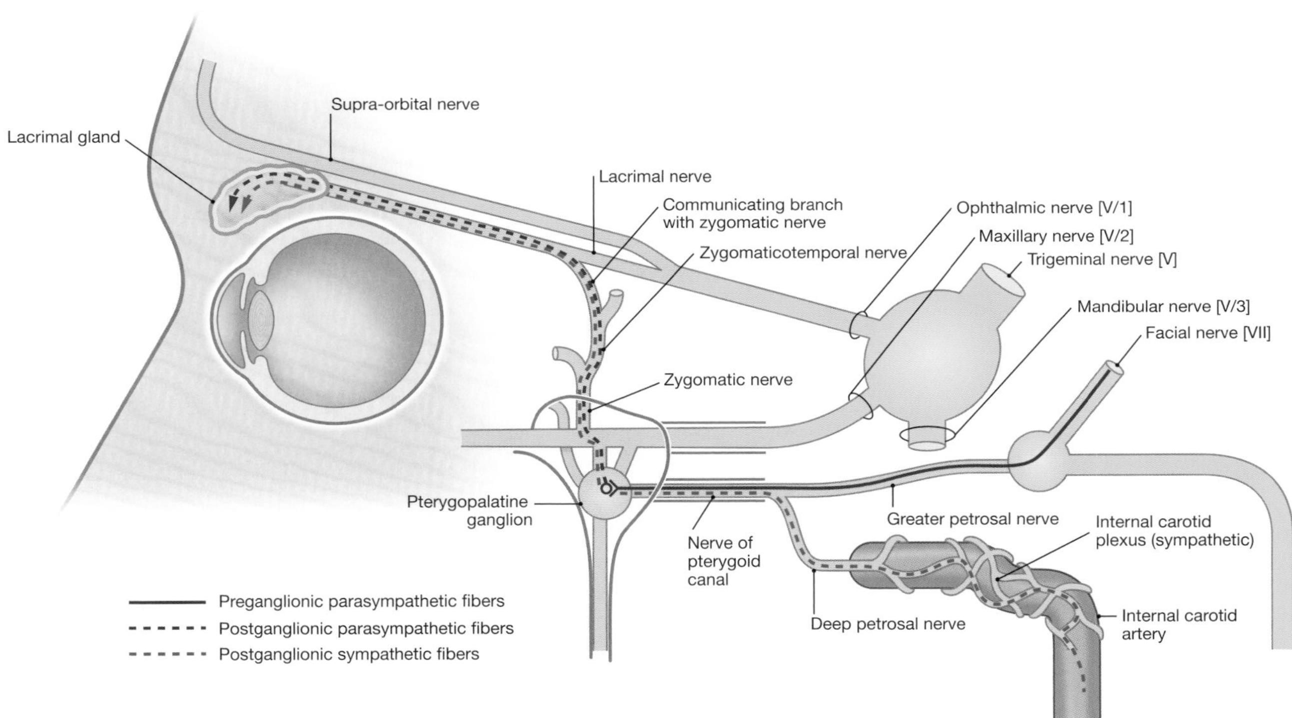
Supra-orbital nerve
Lacrimal gland
Lacrimal nerve
Communicating branch with zygomatic nerve
Zygomaticotemporal nerve
Ophthalmic nerve [V/1]
Maxillary nerve [V/2]
Trigeminal nerve [V]
Mandibular nerve [V/3]
Facial nerve [VII]
Zygomatic nerve
Pterygopalatine ganglion
Greater petrosal nerve
Internal carotid plexus (sympathetic)
Nerve of pterygoid canal
Deep petrosal nerve
Internal carotid artery
Preganglionic parasympathetic fibers
Postganglionic parasympathetic fibers
Postganglionic sympathetic fibers

**Fig. 9.30 Sympathetic and parasympathetic innervation of the lacrimal gland;** schematic drawing. [10]
Preganglionic sympathetic nerve fibers synapse in the superior cervical ganglion and postganglionic sympathetic fibers leave this ganglion to reach the lacrimal gland either by accompanying the internal carotid, ophthalmic, and lacrimal arteries, or by parting already from the internal carotid artery at the foramen lacerum and joining the parasympathetic fibers on their way to the lacrimal gland. Preganglionic parasympathetic nerve fibers run with the intermediate nerve of the facial nerve [VII], pass through the geniculate ganglion without synapsing and reach the pterygopalatine ganglion via the greater petrosal nerve. Upon synapsing, postganglionic parasympathetic fibers associate with the zygomatic nerve and reach the lacrimal nerve and the lacrimal gland via the communicating branch with zygomatic nerve.

## Lacrimal apparatus

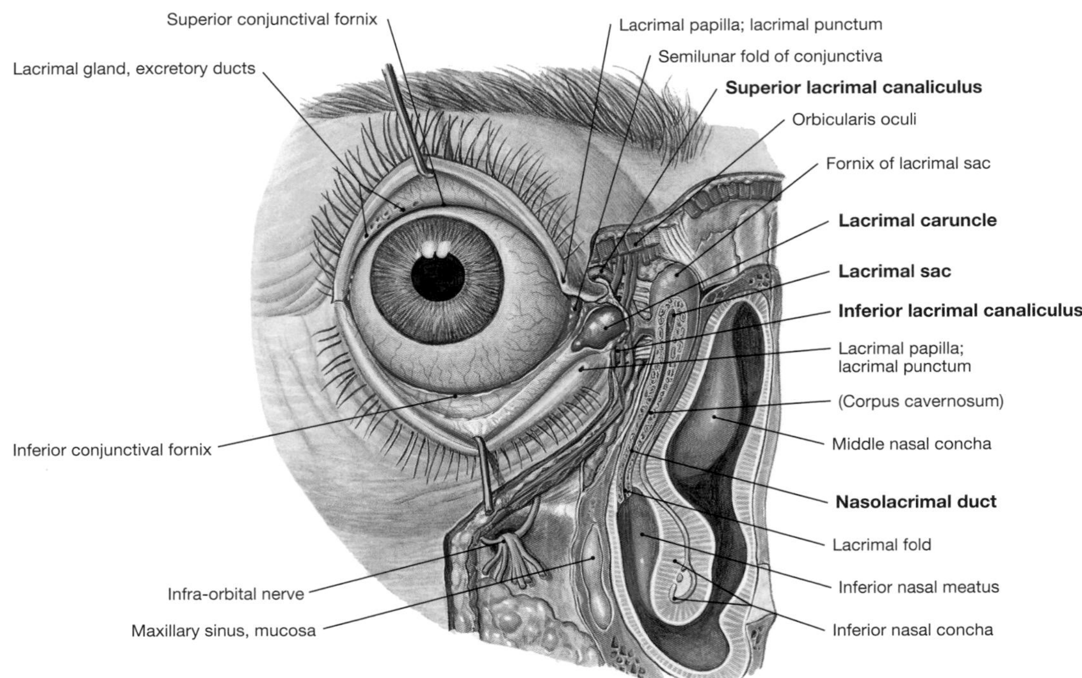
Superior conjunctival fornix
Lacrimal gland, excretory ducts
Lacrimal papilla; lacrimal punctum
Semilunar fold of conjunctiva
Superior lacrimal canaliculus
Orbicularis oculi
Fornix of lacrimal sac
Lacrimal caruncle
Lacrimal sac
Inferior lacrimal canaliculus
Lacrimal papilla; lacrimal punctum
(Corpus cavernosum)
Middle nasal concha
Inferior conjunctival fornix
Nasolacrimal duct
Lacrimal fold
Infra-orbital nerve
Inferior nasal meatus
Maxillary sinus, mucosa
Inferior nasal concha

**Fig. 9.31 Lacrimal apparatus, right side;** frontal view; the eyelids have been pulled away from the eyeball providing a view into the upper and lower conjunctival sac; the nasolacrimal duct has been opened up to the inferior nasal meatus.

The draining nasolacrimal duct is composed of the upper and lower lacrimal canaliculi, the lacrimal sac, and the nasolacrimal duct. The nasolacrimal duct exits into the inferior nasal meatus beneath the inferior nasal concha.

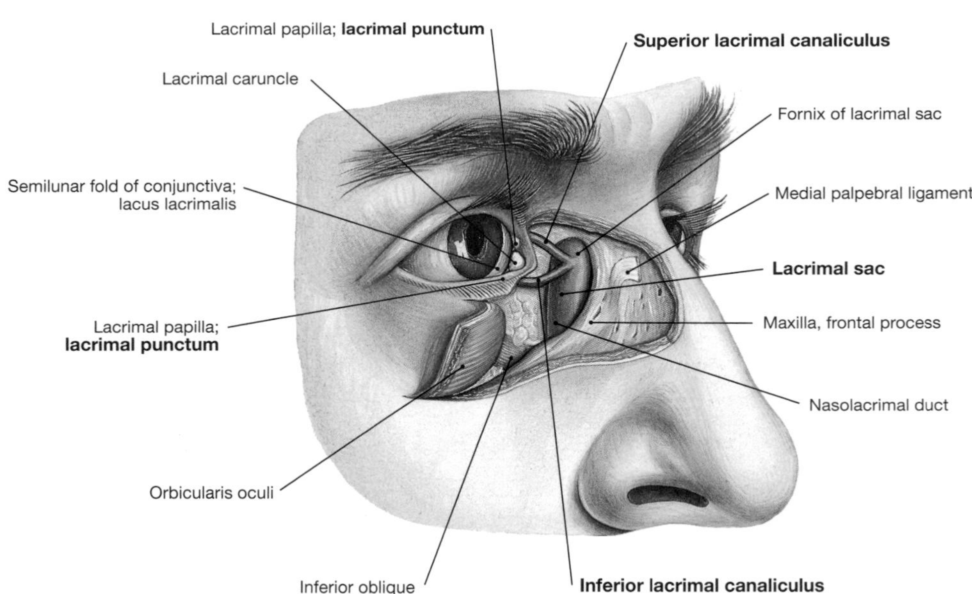
Lacrimal papilla; lacrimal punctum
Superior lacrimal canaliculus
Lacrimal caruncle
Fornix of lacrimal sac
Semilunar fold of conjunctiva; lacus lacrimalis
Medial palpebral ligament
Lacrimal sac
Lacrimal papilla; lacrimal punctum
Maxilla, frontal process
Nasolacrimal duct
Orbicularis oculi
Inferior oblique
Inferior lacrimal canaliculus

**Fig. 9.32 Lacrimal apparatus, right side;** frontolateral view; after removal of skin, muscles, and orbital septum in the medial angle of eye. The lacrimal sac is located in the fossa for lacrimal sac and continues caudally as nasolacrimal duct in a bony enclosure formed by the maxilla and the lacrimal bone in its anterior and posterior section, respectively. Each canaliculus originates as a 0.25 mm (upper) to 0.3 mm (lower) wide, round, oval or slit-shaped lacrimal punctum which continues as an approximately 2 mm long vertical tube. Then, each canaliculus bends in an almost right angle and proceeds as an approximately 8 mm long horizontal segment. In the majority of cases (65–70%), both canaliculi merge to form a common tube approximately 1–2 mm long that opens into the lacrimal sac about 2–3 mm below the fornix of lacrimal sac.

## Lacrimal apparatus

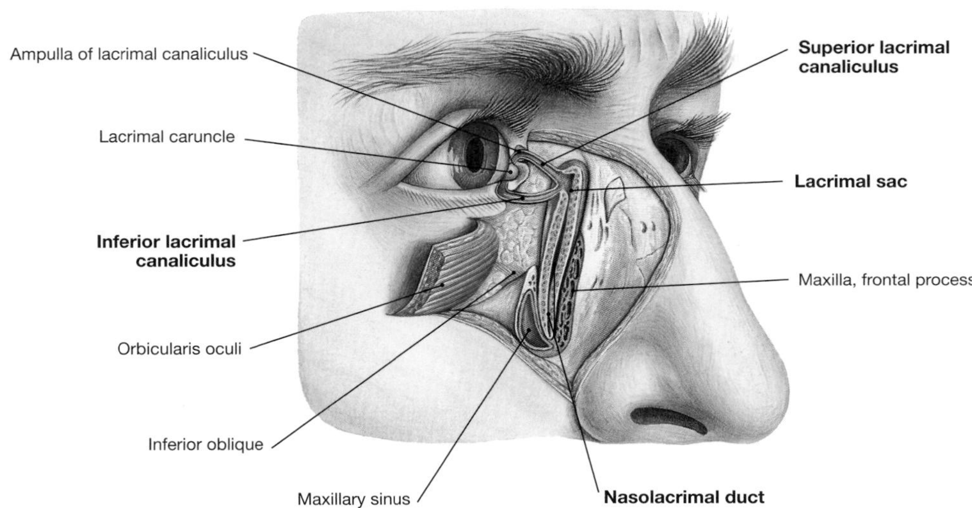
Ampulla of lacrimal canaliculus
Lacrimal caruncle
Inferior lacrimal canaliculus
Orbicularis oculi
Inferior oblique
Maxillary sinus
Nasolacrimal duct
Superior lacrimal canaliculus
Lacrimal sac
Maxilla, frontal process

**Fig. 9.33 Lacrimal apparatus, right side;** horizontal section at the level of the lacrimal sac.
A cavernous body of tissue functionally supporting the transport of the tear fluid surrounds the lumen of the lacrimal sac. Swelling of this cavernous tissue reduces or blocks the transport of fluid and tears run down the cheek (crying). The blood vessels of the cavernous tissue dilate when a foreign particle enters the conjunctival sac or during strong emotions (e.g. intense happiness or sadness).

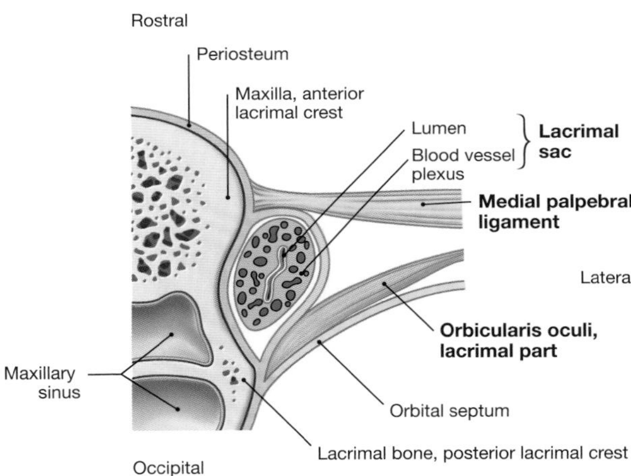
Rostral
Periosteum
Maxilla, anterior lacrimal crest
Lumen
Blood vessel plexus
Lacrimal sac
Medial palpebral ligament
Lateral
Orbicularis oculi, lacrimal part
Orbital septum
Lacrimal bone, posterior lacrimal crest
Maxillary sinus
Occipital

**Fig. 9.34 Lacrimal apparatus, right side;** horizontal section at the level of the lacrimal sac. [8]
The vertical diameter of the lacrimal sac measures approximately 12 mm, the sagittal diameter 5–6 mm, and the transverse diameter 4–5 mm. The nasolacrimal duct of an adult is about 12.4 mm long. The surrounding bony canal is approximately 10 mm long and has a diameter of 4.6 mm.
Notice the close topographic proximity to the maxillary sinus.

### Clinical Remarks

Inflammation **(dacryocystitis),** stenosis **(dacryostenosis),** and concrement formation **(dacryolithiasis)** are the most frequent ailments afflicting the nasolacrimal drainage system, causing tears to overflow and drip out onto the face **(epiphora).** There is an inherited form of dacryostenosis. In most cases, this is the result of a persistent HASNER's valve, a thin membrane of connective tissue at the entrance of the inferior nasal meatus. This valve usually ruptures shortly after birth but needs to be perforated by a physician if it persists.

## Extra-ocular muscles

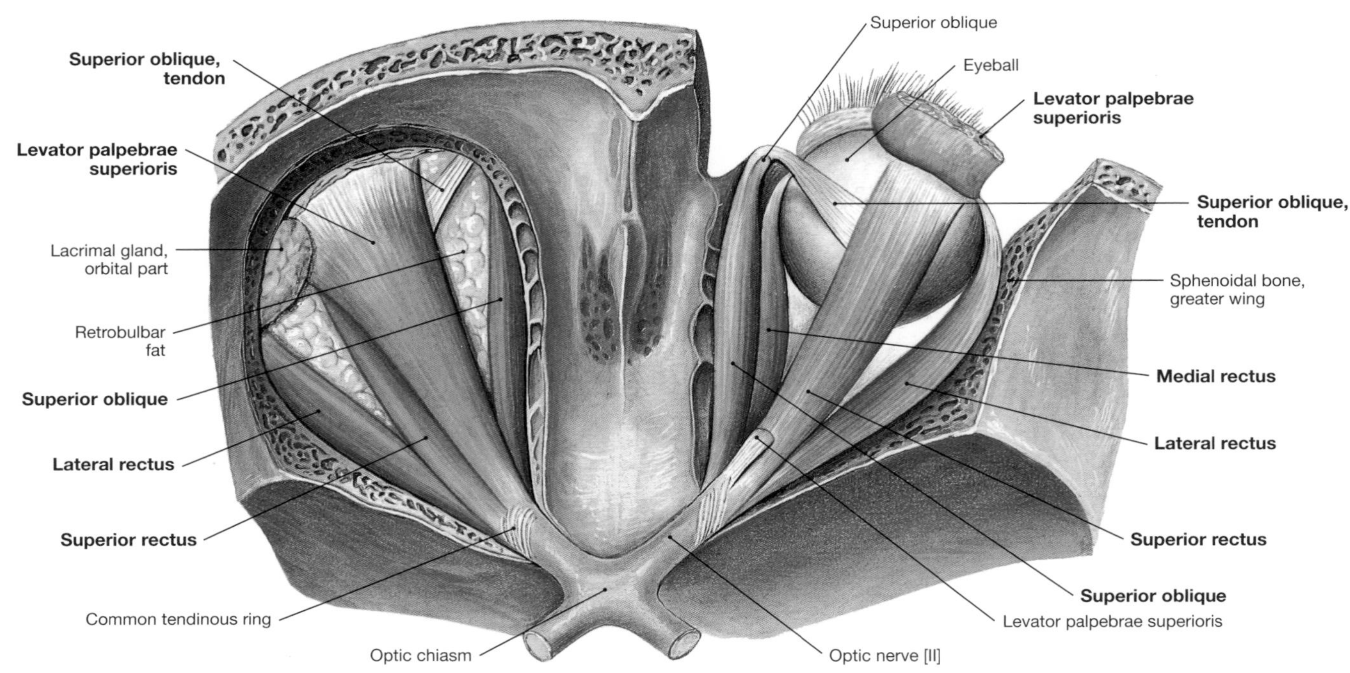
Superior oblique, tendon
Levator palpebrae superioris
Lacrimal gland, orbital part
Retrobulbar fat
Superior oblique
Lateral rectus
Superior rectus
Common tendinous ring
Optic chiasm
Superior oblique
Eyeball
Levator palpebrae superioris
Superior oblique, tendon
Sphenoidal bone, greater wing
Medial rectus
Lateral rectus
Superior rectus
Superior oblique
Levator palpebrae superioris
Optic nerve [II]

**Fig. 9.35 Extra-ocular muscles;** superior view; upon removal of the roof of the orbit on both sides, and removal of the major part of the levator palpebrae superioris and of the orbital fat body on the right side.

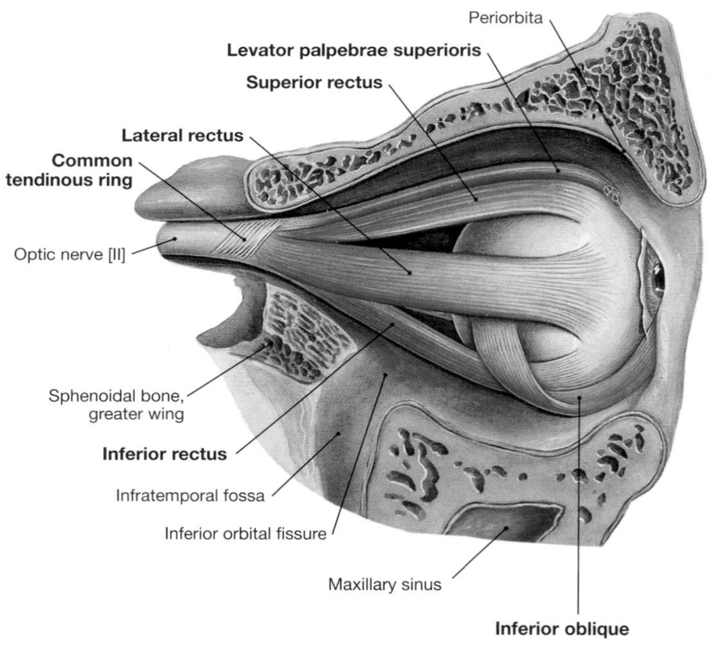
Periorbita
Levator palpebrae superioris
Superior rectus
Lateral rectus
Common tendinous ring
Optic nerve [II]
Sphenoidal bone, greater wing
Inferior rectus
Infratemporal fossa
Inferior orbital fissure
Maxillary sinus
Inferior oblique

**Fig. 9.36 Extra-ocular muscles, right side;** lateral view; upon removal of the lateral wall of the orbit.
The movement of the eyeball is controlled by six extra-ocular muscles in the orbit (four rectus muscles: superior, inferior, medial, and lateral rectus; two oblique muscles: superior and inferior oblique). With the exception of the inferior oblique (origin at the orbital surface of the maxilla lateral of the lacrimal notch in the anterior medial region of the orbit) and the superior oblique (origin at the body of sphenoidal bone medial of the common tendinous ring and the dural sheath of the optic nerve [II]), all other extra-ocular muscles originate from the **common tendinous ring (tendinous anulus of ZINN).**
All six muscles insert at the sclera. All four extra-ocular rectus muscles insert anterior to the equator of the eyeball, whereas the oblique muscles of the orbit insert posterior to the equator. A tendinous pulley-like structure (trochlea), which attaches to the anterior upper area of the frontal bone and acts as a hypomochlion for the superior oblique, redirects this muscle backwards to its insertion area at the top of the eyeball posterior to its equator. The tendinous anulus of ZINN is also the origin of the levator palpebrae superioris which projects into the upper eyelid.

## Clinical Remarks

**Paralysis of the levator palpebrae superioris** (resulting from damage to the oculomotor nerve[III]) causes **ptosis** (drooping upper eyelid). The patient does not experience double vision (diplopia) because the affected eye is closed. However, upon lifting the eyelid manually, double vision occurs since the superior, inferior, and medial rectus are paralysed as well. Palsy of the abducent nerve and trochlear nerve can also cause paralytic strabism with diplopia.

## Extra-ocular muscles

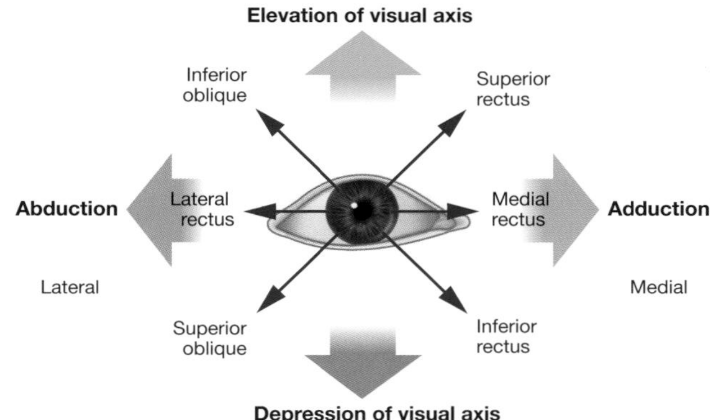
Elevation of visual axis
Inferior oblique
Superior rectus
Abduction
Lateral rectus
Medial rectus
Adduction
Lateral
Medial
Superior oblique
Inferior rectus
Depression of visual axis

**Fig. 9.37 Function of the extra-ocular muscles.** [8]
Testing the ability of the eyeball to move into the **four main directions of the visual axis** is part of a proper physical exam. Shown are the activated muscles during the movement of each eyeball into the four directions of the visual axis. The coordination of the synchronous movement of both eyeballs is very complex since the various extra-ocular muscles are innervated by different cranial nerves (oculomotor, trochlear, and abducent nerves). The extra-ocular muscles receive very rich innervations and are distinct in fine structure from the normal striated muscles.

| Muscle | Function | Innervation |
|---|---|---|
| Right Eye (Lateral / Medial)<br>Superior rectus | Elevation of the visual axis<br>Adduction and medial rotation of the eyeball | Oculomotor nerve [III], superior branch |
| Inferior rectus | Depression of the visual axis<br>Adduction and lateral rotation of the eyeball | Oculomotor nerve [III], inferior branch |
| Lateral rectus | Abduction of the eyeball | Abducent nerve [VI] |
| Medial rectus | Adduction of the eyeball | Oculomotor nerve [III], inferior branch |
| Inferior oblique | Elevation of the visual axis<br>Abduction and lateral rotation of the eyeball | Oculomotor nerve [III], inferior branch |
| Superior oblique | Depression of the visual axis<br>Abduction and medial rotation of the eyeball | Trochlear nerve [IV] |

**Fig. 9.38 Function and innervation of the extra-ocular muscles inserting at the eyeball.**
The respective muscle is colored in dark red.

## Clinical Remarks

**Palsy of the oculomotor nerve** [III] results in the paralysis of all extra-ocular muscles, except for the lateral rectus (abducent nerve [VI]) and the superior oblique (trochlear nerve [IV]). The non-paralysed muscles pull the eye downward and outward **(down-and-out).** At the same time, paralysis of the levator palpebrae superioris results in ptosis and the inability of the patient to see with this eye. Only when the drooping eyelid is pulled up manually, the patient complains about double vision (diplopia).

## Extra-ocular muscles

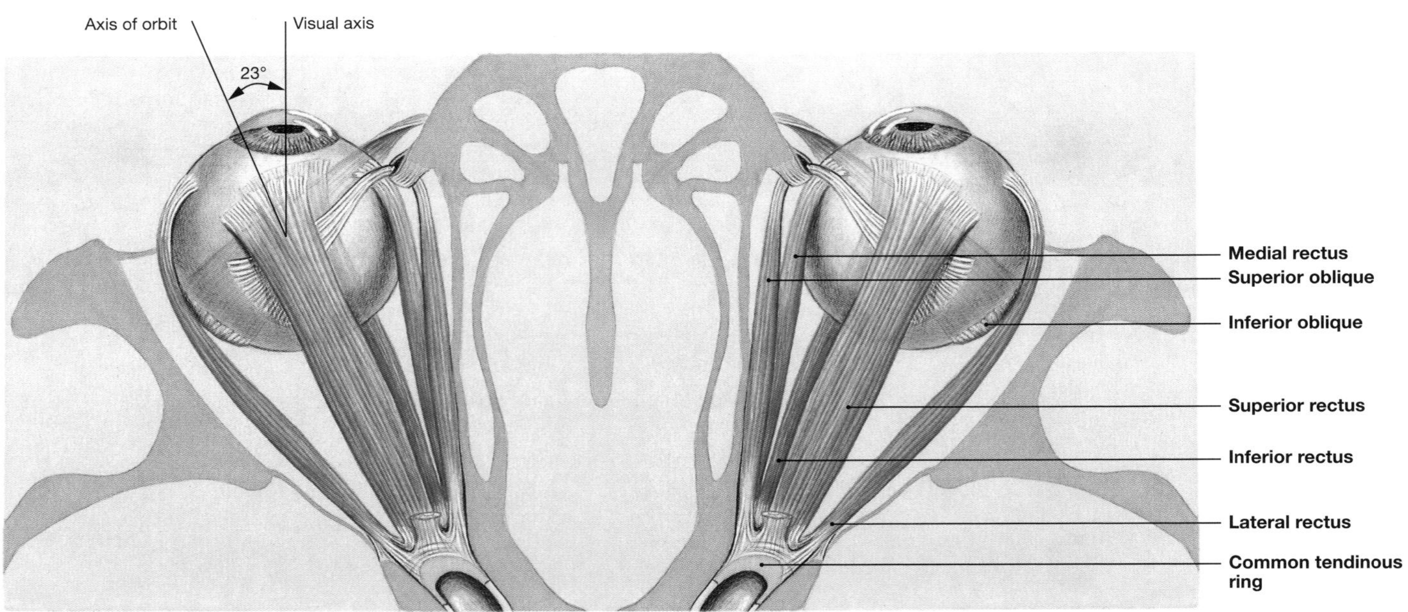
Axis of orbit
Visual axis
23°
Medial rectus
Superior oblique
Inferior oblique
Superior rectus
Inferior rectus
Lateral rectus
Common tendinous ring

**Fig. 9.39 Extra-ocular muscles;** superior view.
Shown are the common tendinous ring (tendinous anulus of ZINN) and the insertion sites of the muscles at the eyeball.
The visual axis (imaginary line from the midpoint of the visual field to the fovea centralis) and the axis of the orbit (imaginary line through the center of the lens) differ by an angle of 23°. This is the reason why the fovea centralis (retinal location of focused central vision) is located lateral to the optic disc (blind spot).

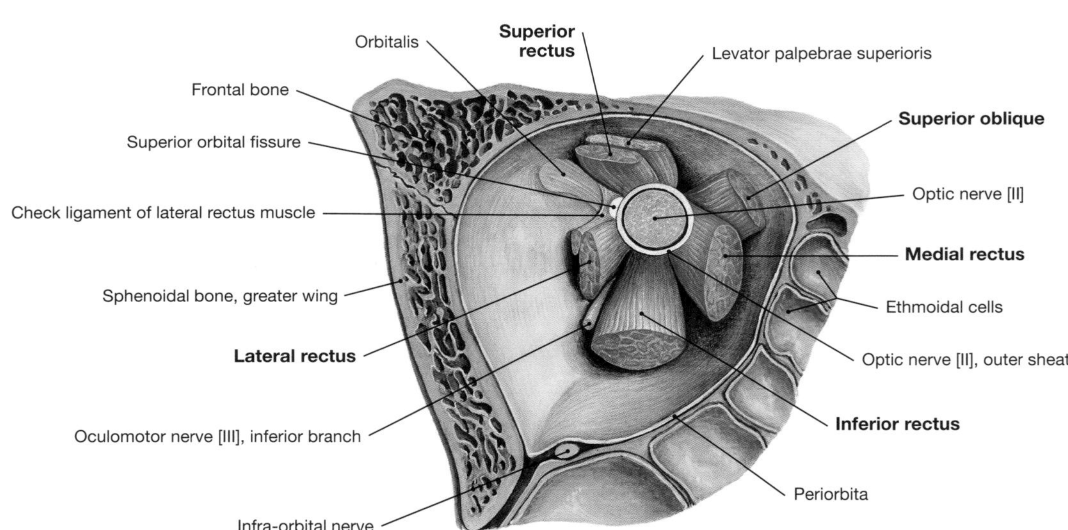
Orbitalis
Superior rectus
Levator palpebrae superioris
Frontal bone
Superior oblique
Superior orbital fissure
Optic nerve [II]
Check ligament of lateral rectus muscle
Medial rectus
Sphenoidal bone, greater wing
Ethmoidal cells
Lateral rectus
Optic nerve [II], outer sheath
Inferior rectus
Oculomotor nerve [III], inferior branch
Periorbita
Infra-orbital nerve

**Fig. 9.40 Extra-ocular muscles, right side;** frontal view onto the posterior wall of the orbit. The periorbital space near the superior orbital fissure contains muscle fibers with sympathetic nerve innervation; collectively, these form the orbital muscle.

## Clinical Remarks

Damage to the trochlear nerve [IV] can cause **palsy of the trochlear nerve.** Paralysis of the superior oblique causes the optic axis to point medially (nasal) and upward because the normal abduction and downward movement of the eyeball by the superior oblique muscle is absent. **Abducent nerve palsies** are the most frequent palsies of the extra-ocular muscles (in part, because the abducent nerve [VI] [→ Fig. 9.41] runs through the center of the cavernous sinus and can be damaged more easily here than in the peripheral zone of the sinus where the oculomotor nerve [III] and the trochlear nerve [IV] are located). Paralysis of the lateral rectus shifts the optic axis medially (nasally).

## Extra-ocular muscles

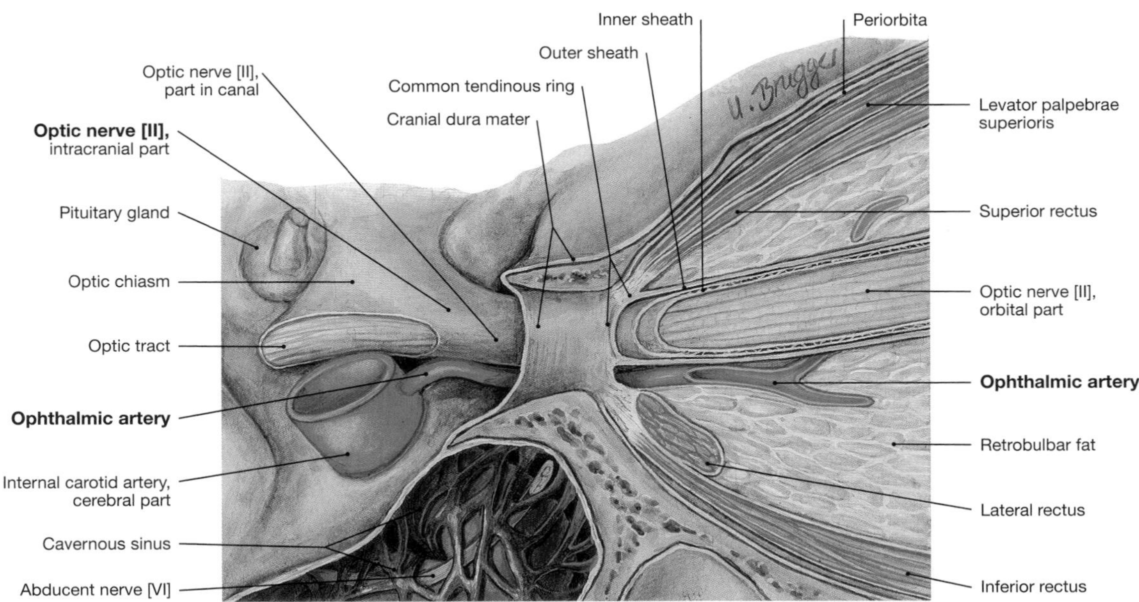
Inner sheath
Periorbita
Outer sheath
Optic nerve [II], part in canal
Common tendinous ring
Cranial dura mater
Optic nerve [II], intracranial part
Levator palpebrae superioris
Pituitary gland
Superior rectus
Optic chiasm
Optic nerve [II], orbital part
Optic tract
Ophthalmic artery
Ophthalmic artery
Retrobulbar fat
Internal carotid artery, cerebral part
Lateral rectus
Cavernous sinus
Abducent nerve [VI]
Inferior rectus

**Fig. 9.41 Optic nerve [II]; right side;** lateral view upon opening of the optic canal.
Both, the optic nerve [II] and the ophthalmic artery (branch of the internal carotid artery) course through the optic canal and the common tendinous ring (tendinous anulus of ZINN) into the orbit.

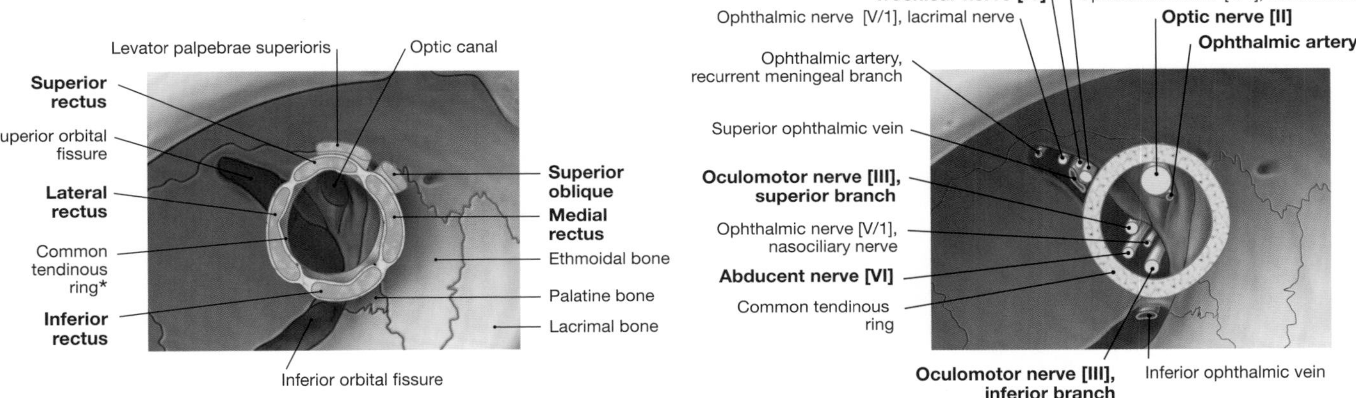
Levator palpebrae superioris
Optic canal
Superior rectus
Superior orbital fissure
Superior oblique
Lateral rectus
Medial rectus
Common tendinous ring*
Ethmoidal bone
Palatine bone
Inferior rectus
Lacrimal bone
Inferior orbital fissure
Trochlear nerve [IV]
Ophthalmic nerve [V/1], frontal nerve
Ophthalmic nerve [V/1], lacrimal nerve
Optic nerve [II]
Ophthalmic artery
Ophthalmic artery, recurrent meningeal branch
Superior ophthalmic vein
Oculomotor nerve [III], superior branch
Ophthalmic nerve [V/1], nasociliary nerve
Abducent nerve [VI]
Common tendinous ring
Oculomotor nerve [III], inferior branch
Inferior ophthalmic vein

**Fig. 9.42 Muscular origins at the common tendinous ring (tendinous anulus of ZINN), right side;** frontal view. [10]
The common tendinous ring is the origin for the superior rectus, medial rectus, inferior rectus, and lateral rectus. A neurovascular bundle not depicted in this image passes through the anulus of ZINN (→ Fig. 9.43). Also shown is the levator palpebrae superioris which originates at the tip of the orbit from the lesser wing of the sphenoidal bone. The superior oblique has its origin at the body of sphenoidal bone medial to the common tendinous ring at the dural sheath.

* tendinous anulus of ZINN

**Fig. 9.43 Neurovascular structures passing through the optic canal, and the superior orbital fissure, right side;** frontal view. [10]
The oculomotor nerve [III], nasociliary nerve, abducent nerve [VI], and the sympathetic root of ciliary ganglion pass through the superior orbital fissure and the common tendinous ring (tendinous anulus of ZINN). The superior ophthalmic vein, lacrimal nerve, frontal nerve, and trochlear nerve [IV] also pass through the superior orbital fissure into the orbit. However, these neurovascular structures run outside of the common tendinous ring. Not shown are the inferior ophthalmic vein, infra-orbital artery, infra-orbital nerve, and zygomatic nerve which enter the orbit through the inferior orbital fissure. Centrally within the optic nerve [II] courses the central retinal artery as the first branch of the ophthalmic artery.

## Clinical Remarks

Incomplete or complete **ophthalmoplegia** (ophthalmoparesis) refers to the paralysis of one or more extra-ocular muscles due to different neurological illnesses or caused by chronic inflammations and tumors at the tip of the orbit. **Embolic occlusion of the central retinal artery** is a frequent vascular cause of acute blindness.

## Blood vessels of the orbit

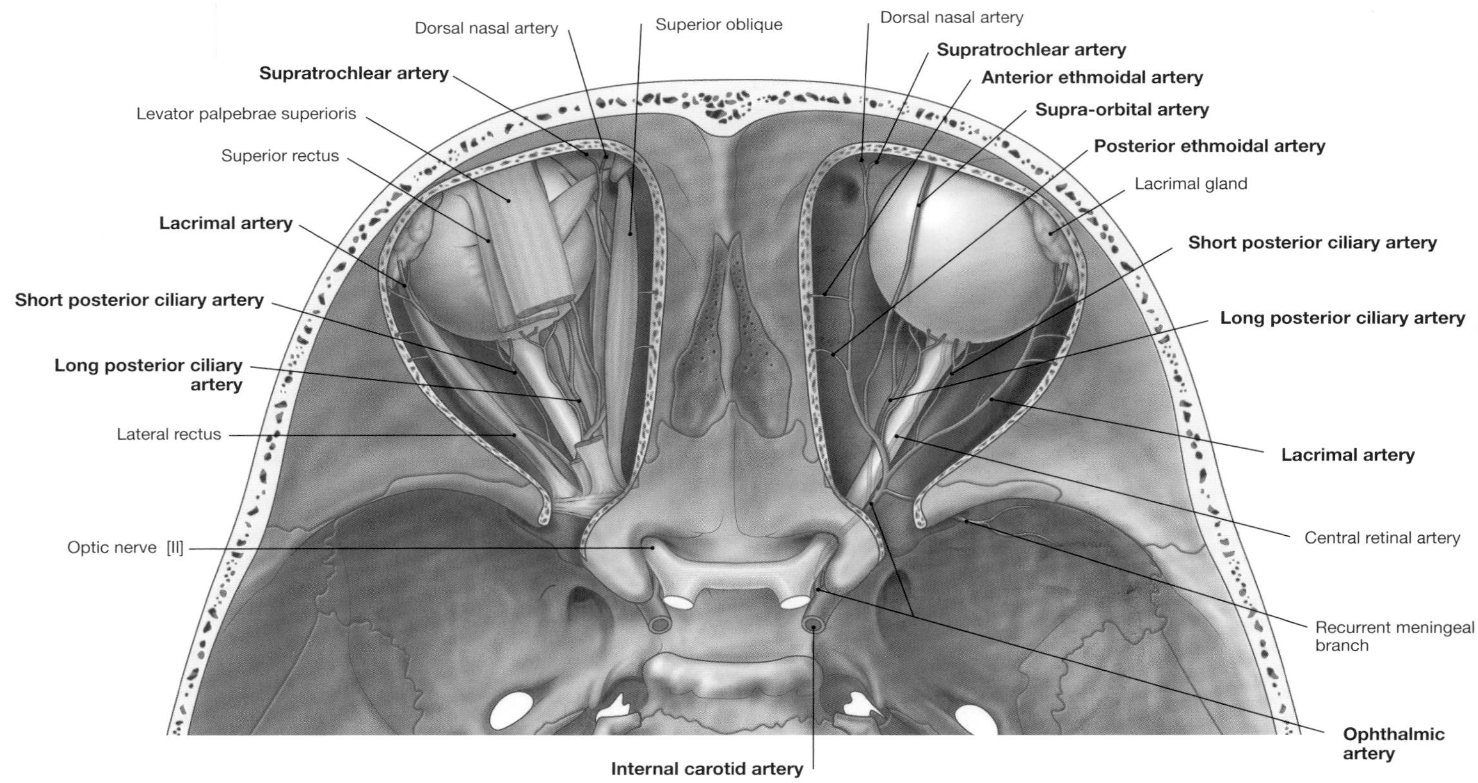
Dorsal nasal artery
Superior oblique
Dorsal nasal artery
Supratrochlear artery
Supratrochlear artery
Anterior ethmoidal artery
Levator palpebrae superioris
Supra-orbital artery
Superior rectus
Posterior ethmoidal artery
Lacrimal gland
Lacrimal artery
Short posterior ciliary artery
Short posterior ciliary artery
Long posterior ciliary artery
Long posterior ciliary artery
Lateral rectus
Lacrimal artery
Central retinal artery
Optic nerve [II]
Recurrent meningeal branch
Ophthalmic artery
Internal carotid artery

**Fig. 9.44 Arteries of the eye and of the orbit;** superior view onto the openend orbits; left side: content of the orbit with extra-ocular muscles, right side: without extra-ocular muscles. [10]
The ophthalmic artery is the main artery of the orbit and branches off the cerebral part of the internal carotid artery. The ophthalmic artery normally courses below the optic nerve [II] through the optic canal into the orbit. Here, the artery divides into many branches which supply the eyeball and the structures of the orbit with blood. Anastomoses exist via an orbital branch to the medial meningeal artery, via the anterior and posterior ethmoidal arteries to blood vessels in the nose, and via blood vessels penetrating the orbital septum or the bone to the facial arteries (supra-orbital, supratrochlear, medial and lateral palpebral, dorsal nasal artery).

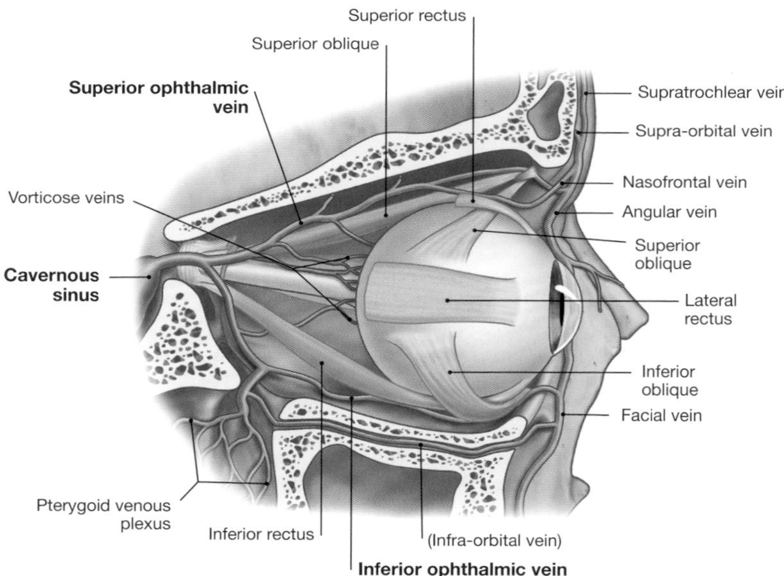
Superior rectus
Superior oblique
Superior ophthalmic vein
Supratrochlear vein
Supra-orbital vein
Nasofrontal vein
Vorticose veins
Angular vein
Superior oblique
Cavernous sinus
Lateral rectus
Inferior oblique
Facial vein
Pterygoid venous plexus
Inferior rectus
(Infra-orbital vein)
Inferior ophthalmic vein

**Fig. 9.45 Veins of the eye and of the orbit; right side;** lateral view into the orbit; after removal of the lateral wall of the orbit. [10]
The superior and inferior ophthalmic veins drain the venous blood. The latter is usually smaller than the superior ophthalmic artery. Venous anastomoses exist to the veins of the superficial and deep facial regions (pterygoid plexus) and the cavernous sinus.

## Clinical Remarks

An ascending **transmission of germs from the facial region** via the facial vein, the angular vein in the nasal part of the orbit, and the inferior ophthalmic vein can cause a thrombosis of the cavernous sinus (→ p. 223). In turn, this can result in the damage of the abducent nerve [VI] (often the first cranial nerve affected because of its central location within the sinus), oculomotor nerve [III], trochlear nerve [IV], and the first and second trigeminal branch (ophthalmic [V/1] and maxillary [V/2] nerves) with corresponding deficiencies (paralysis of extra-ocular muscles, sensory deficits etc.).

## Arteries and nerves of the orbit

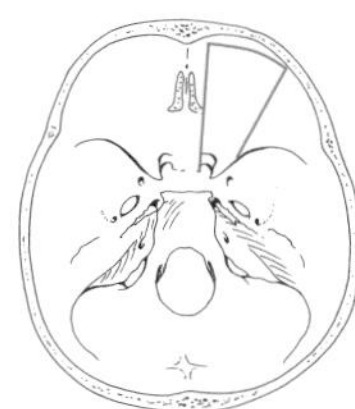

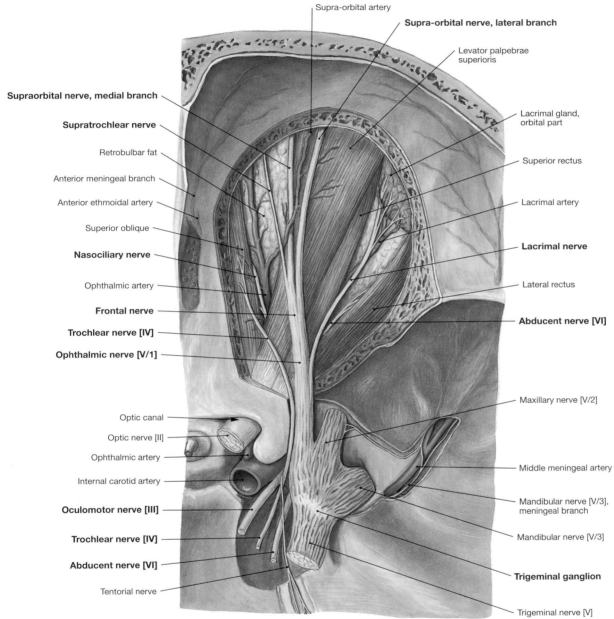

Supra-orbital artery
Supra-orbital nerve, lateral branch
Levator palpebrae superioris
Supraorbital nerve, medial branch
Supratrochlear nerve
Lacrimal gland, orbital part
Retrobulbar fat
Superior rectus
Anterior meningeal branch
Anterior ethmoidal artery
Lacrimal artery
Superior oblique
Lacrimal nerve
Nasociliary nerve
Ophthalmic artery
Lateral rectus
Frontal nerve
Abducent nerve [VI]
Trochlear nerve [IV]
Ophthalmic nerve [V/1]
Maxillary nerve [V/2]
Optic canal
Optic nerve [II]
Ophthalmic artery
Middle meningeal artery
Internal carotid artery
Mandibular nerve [V/3], meningeal branch
Oculomotor nerve [III]
Mandibular nerve [V/3]
Trochlear nerve [IV]
Abducent nerve [VI]
Trigeminal ganglion
Tentorial nerve
Trigeminal nerve [V]

**Fig. 9.46 Arteries and nerves of the orbit, right side;** superior view onto the openend orbit (upper level of the orbit); demonstration of the trigeminal ganglion (semilunar ganglion, ganglion GASSERI); bony roof of the orbit, periorbita, and orbital fat body were partially removed. Shown is the **course of the ophthalmic nerve** [V/1] through the opened superior orbital fissure and its branching into the lacrimal and frontal nerve (incl. consecutive branching) and, running more deeply, the nasociliary nerve. In addition, the gracile trochlear nerve [IV] for the motor innervation of the superior oblique and the more deeply located abducent nerve [VI] for the innervation of the lateral rectus are depicted.

## Arteries and nerves of the orbit

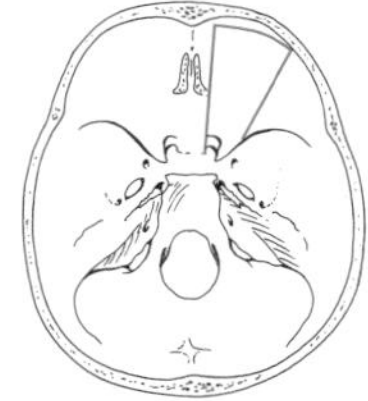

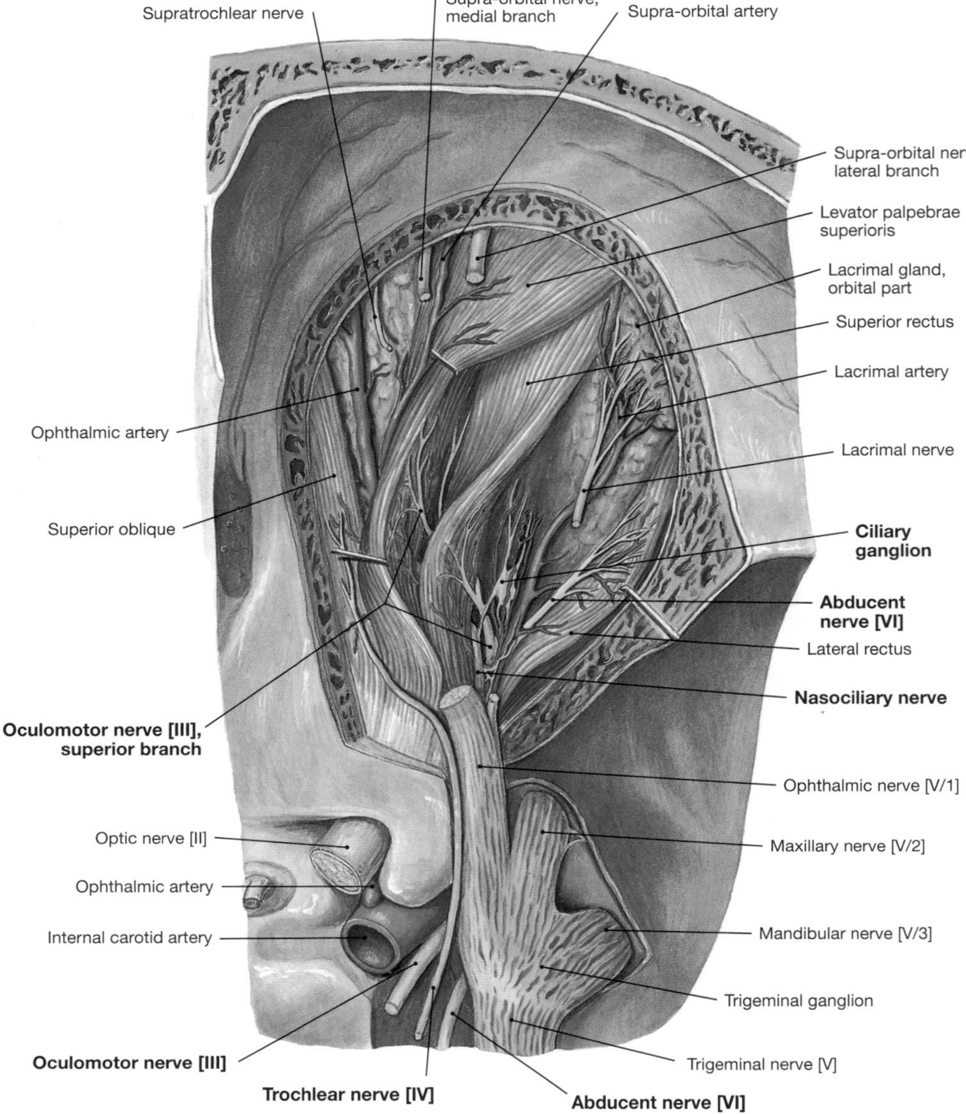
Supratrochlear nerve
Supra-orbital nerve, medial branch
Supra-orbital artery
Supra-orbital nerve, lateral branch
Levator palpebrae superioris
Lacrimal gland, orbital part
Superior rectus
Lacrimal artery
Lacrimal nerve
Ciliary ganglion
Abducent nerve [VI]
Lateral rectus
Nasociliary nerve
Ophthalmic nerve [V/1]
Maxillary nerve [V/2]
Mandibular nerve [V/3]
Trigeminal ganglion
Trigeminal nerve [V]
Abducent nerve [VI]
Trochlear nerve [IV]
Oculomotor nerve [III]
Internal carotid artery
Ophthalmic artery
Optic nerve [II]
Oculomotor nerve [III], superior branch
Superior oblique
Ophthalmic artery

**Branches of the Ophthalmic Artery**

- Central retinal artery
- Lacrimal artery
  - Anastomotic branch with middle meningeal artery
  - Lateral palpebral arteries
- Recurrent meningeal branch
- Long posterior ciliary arteries
- Muscular arteries
  - Anterior ciliary arteries
  - Anterior conjunctival arteries
  - Episcleral arteries
- Supra-orbital artery
  - Diploic branch
- Anterior ethmoidal artery
  - Anterior meningeal branch
  - Anterior septal branches
  - Anterior lateral nasal branches
- Posterior ethmoidal artery
- Medial palpebral artery
  - Posterior conjunctival arteries
  - Superior palpebral arch
  - Inferior palpebral arch
- Supratrochlear artery
- Dorsal nasal artery

**Fig. 9.47 Arteries and nerves of the orbit, right side;** superior view; after removal of the roof of the orbit; presentation of the ciliary ganglion; the levator palpebrae superioris and superior rectus were folded back. Shown are nerve branches of the oculomotor nerve [III] entering beneath the muscles. Upon removal of the orbital fat body beneath the muscles, the **ciliary ganglion,** approximately 2 mm in size, becomes visible. Positioned approximately 2 cm lateral to the optic nerve [II] behind the eyeball, the ciliary ganglion is embedded in the orbital fat body. The ciliary ganglion contains perikarya of postganglionic parasympathetic neurons which synapse with the axons of preganglionic parasympathetic neurons located in the accessory oculomotor nucleus (autonomicus, EDINGER-WESTPHAL nucleus).
These parasympathetic fibers innervate the inner muscles of the eye (ciliary und sphincter pupillae muscle, → Fig. 8.163). Having switched earlier from preganglionic to postganglionic fibers in the superior cervical ganglion, postganglionic sympathetic fibers for the dilatator pupillae simply pass through the ciliary ganglion.

## Arteries and nerves of the orbit

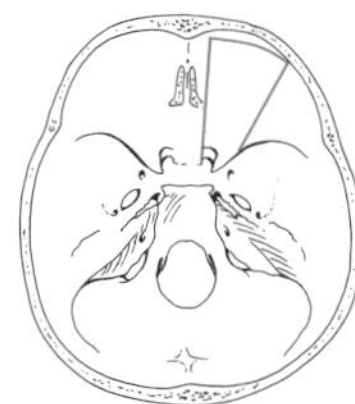

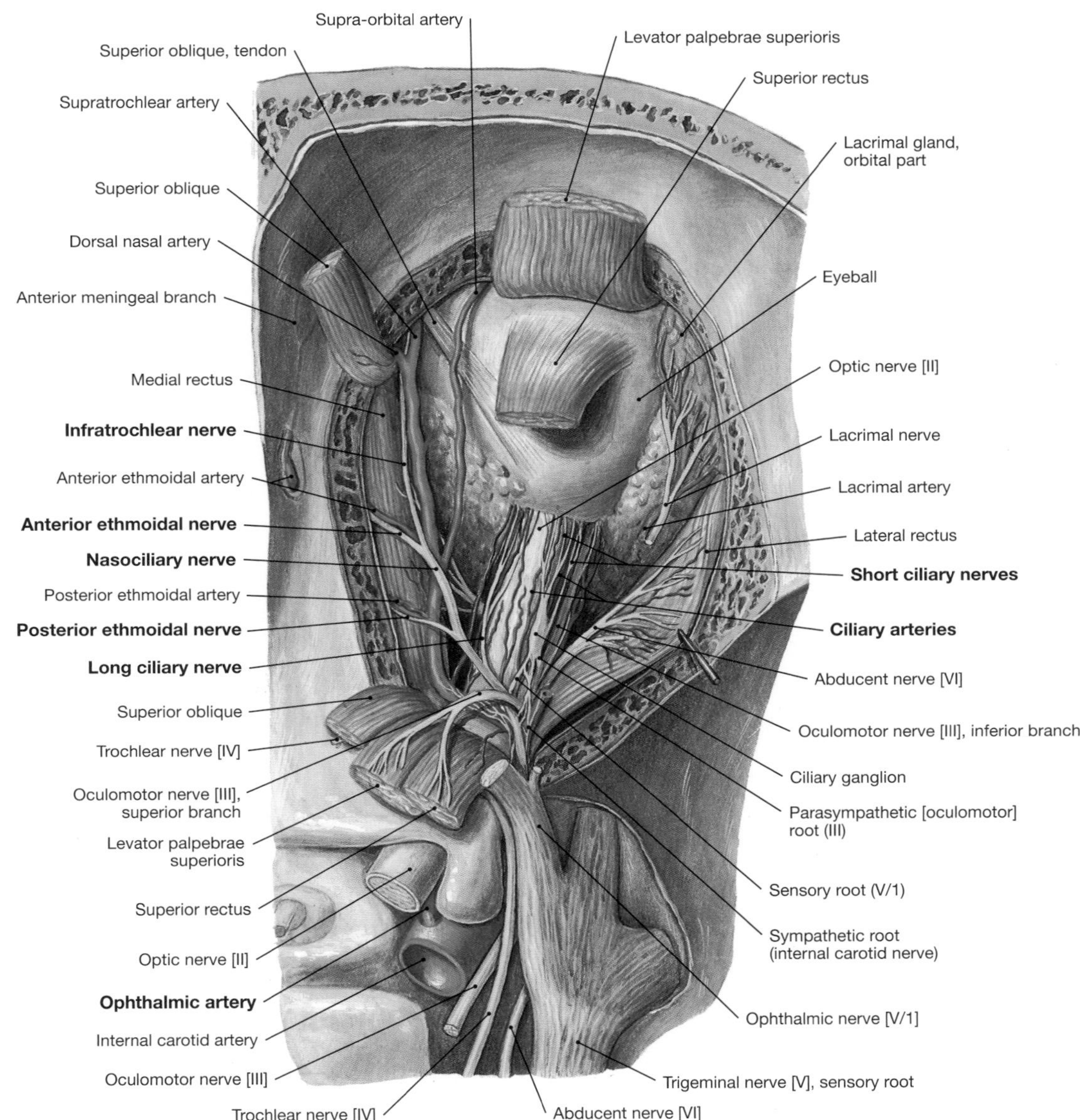
Supra-orbital artery
Superior oblique, tendon
Levator palpebrae superioris
Superior rectus
Supratrochlear artery
Lacrimal gland, orbital part
Superior oblique
Dorsal nasal artery
Eyeball
Anterior meningeal branch
Optic nerve [II]
Medial rectus
Infratrochlear nerve
Lacrimal nerve
Anterior ethmoidal artery
Lacrimal artery
Anterior ethmoidal nerve
Lateral rectus
Nasociliary nerve
Short ciliary nerves
Posterior ethmoidal artery
Posterior ethmoidal nerve
Ciliary arteries
Long ciliary nerve
Abducent nerve [VI]
Superior oblique
Oculomotor nerve [III], inferior branch
Trochlear nerve [IV]
Ciliary ganglion
Oculomotor nerve [III], superior branch
Parasympathetic [oculomotor] root (III)
Levator palpebrae superioris
Sensory root (V/1)
Superior rectus
Sympathetic root (internal carotid nerve)
Optic nerve [II]
Ophthalmic artery
Ophthalmic nerve [V/1]
Internal carotid artery
Oculomotor nerve [III]
Trigeminal nerve [V], sensory root
Trochlear nerve [IV]
Abducent nerve [VI]

**Fig. 9.48 Arteries and nerves of the orbit, right side;** superior view; upon partial removal of the levator palpebrae superioris, superior rectus, and superior oblique.
The **middle level of the orbit** is depicted. Shown are the optic nerve [II] with supplying network of arteries (ciliary arteries) branching off the ophthalmic artery, which is running through the orbit, as well as the long and short ciliary nerves, the ciliary ganglion, and the terminal branching of the nasociliary nerve.

## Arteries and nerves of the orbit

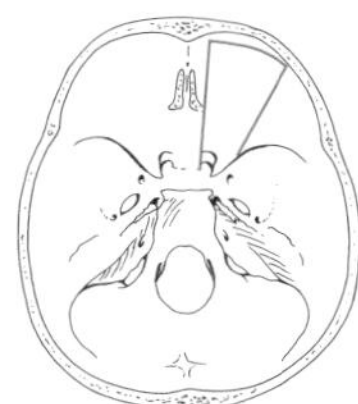

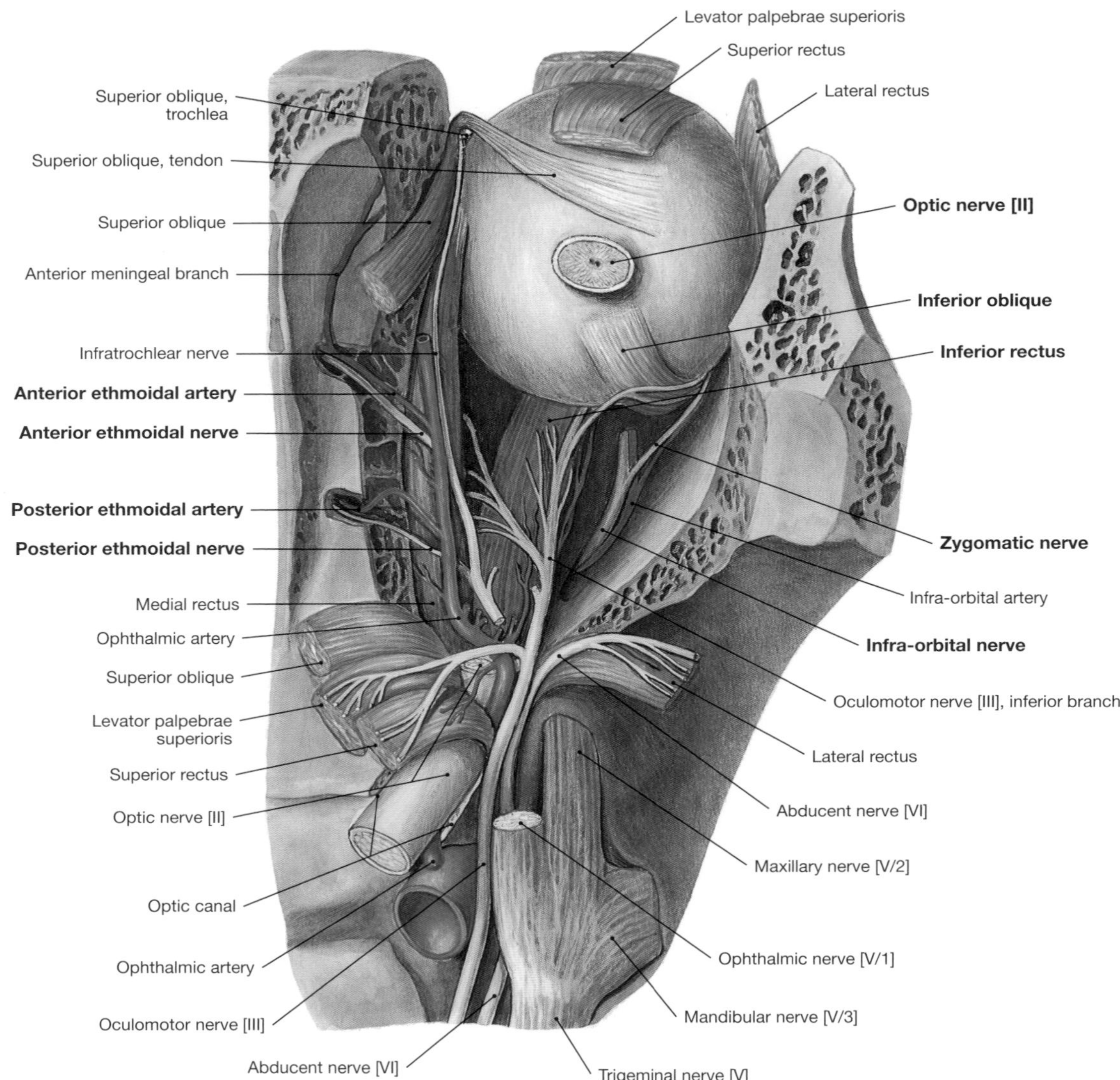
Levator palpebrae superioris
Superior rectus
Lateral rectus
Superior oblique, trochlea
Superior oblique, tendon
Superior oblique
Anterior meningeal branch
Optic nerve [II]
Inferior oblique
Inferior rectus
Infratrochlear nerve
Anterior ethmoidal artery
Anterior ethmoidal nerve
Posterior ethmoidal artery
Posterior ethmoidal nerve
Zygomatic nerve
Infra-orbital artery
Medial rectus
Ophthalmic artery
Infra-orbital nerve
Superior oblique
Oculomotor nerve [III], inferior branch
Levator palpebrae superioris
Lateral rectus
Superior rectus
Abducent nerve [VI]
Optic nerve [II]
Maxillary nerve [V/2]
Optic canal
Ophthalmic nerve [V/1]
Ophthalmic artery
Mandibular nerve [V/3]
Oculomotor nerve [III]
Abducent nerve [VI]
Trigeminal nerve [V]

**Fig. 9.49 Arteries and nerves of the orbit, right side;** superior view; the optic nerve [II] has been cut.
After dissecting additional structures and upon removal of the entire orbital fat body, the inferior rectus and the **lower level of the orbit** become visible. The eyeball is rotated in such a way that the insertion site of the inferior oblique close to the entry site of the cut optic nerve [II] can be seen. The ethmoidal cells at the medial side have been opened up to demonstrate the course of the anterior and posterior ethmoidal nerves as well as the anterior and posterior ethmoidal arteries from the orbit into the ethmoidal bone. The infra-orbital artery and nerve are located in the lower level of the orbit. In addition to sensory fibers, the zygomatic nerve, a branch of the infra-orbital nerve, also contains postganglionic parasympathetic fibers for the autonomic innervation of the lacrimal gland.

### Clinical Remarks

The optic nerve [II] has a close topographic relationship to the sphenoidal sinus. **Disease processes involving the sphenoidal sinus** (sinusitis, tumors) can affect the optic nerve [II] separated from the sphenoidal sinus by only a thin bony wall that may sometimes not be present. During surgery of the sphenoidal sinus, great care is required not to damage the optic nerve.

## Nerves of the orbit

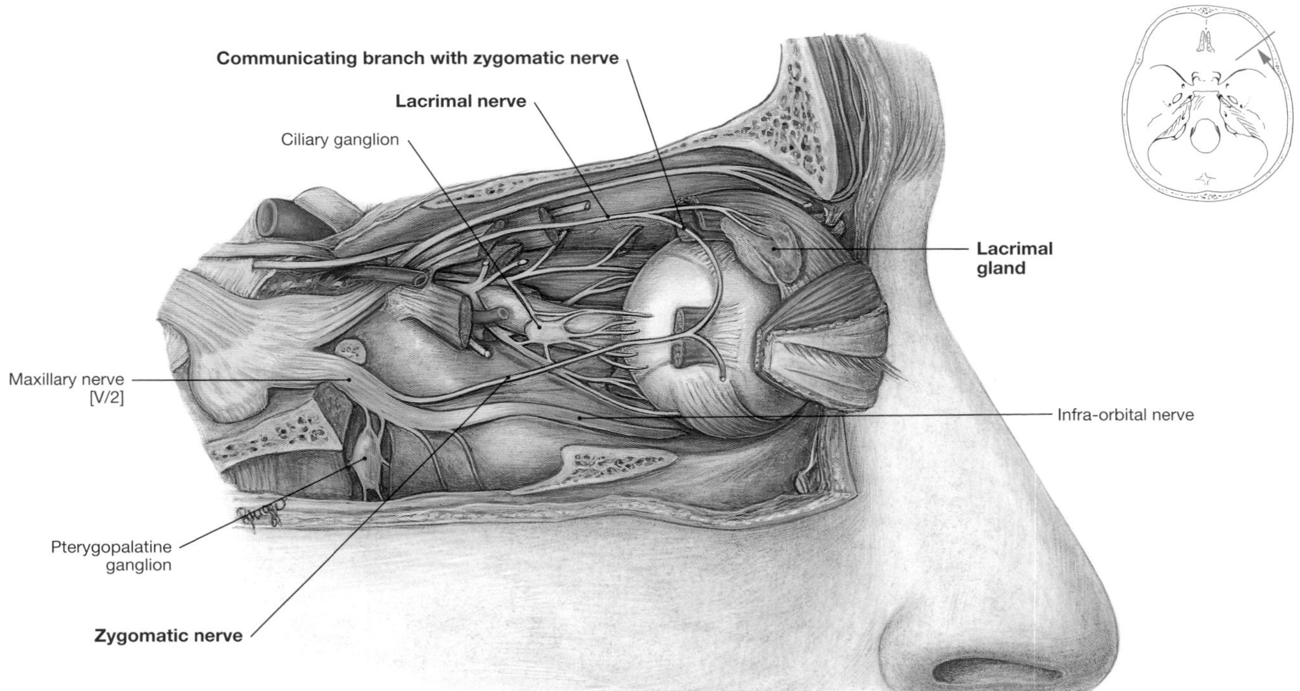
Communicating branch with zygomatic nerve
Lacrimal nerve
Ciliary ganglion
Lacrimal gland
Maxillary nerve [V/2]
Infra-orbital nerve
Pterygopalatine ganglion
Zygomatic nerve

**Fig. 9.50 Nerves of the orbit and the eye, innervation of the lacrimal gland, and demonstration of the ciliary ganglion, right side;** lateral view; after removal of the temporal wall and orbital fat body.

Sympathetic, parasympathetic, and sensory fibers innervate the lacrimal gland. **Postganglionic parasympathetic fibers** derive from the pterygopalatine ganglion to stimulate excretion by this gland. The fibers leave the pterygopalatine ganglion, associate with the zygomatic nerve (a branch of the maxillary nerve [V/2]), and separate as communicating branch with zygomatic nerve (→ Figs. 8.163 and 9.30) ) to anastomose with the lacrimal nerve and reach the lacrimal gland. The lacrimal nerve (a branch of the ophthalmic nerve [V/1]) provides the **sensory** innervation of the lacrimal gland. The sympathetic fibers inhibit glandular secretion. **Postganglionic sympathetic fibers** derive from the superior cervical ganglion. These fibers pass through the pterygopalatine ganglion without synapsing and, by taking the same route as the parasympathetic fibers, reach the lacrimal gland (→ Fig. 9.30).

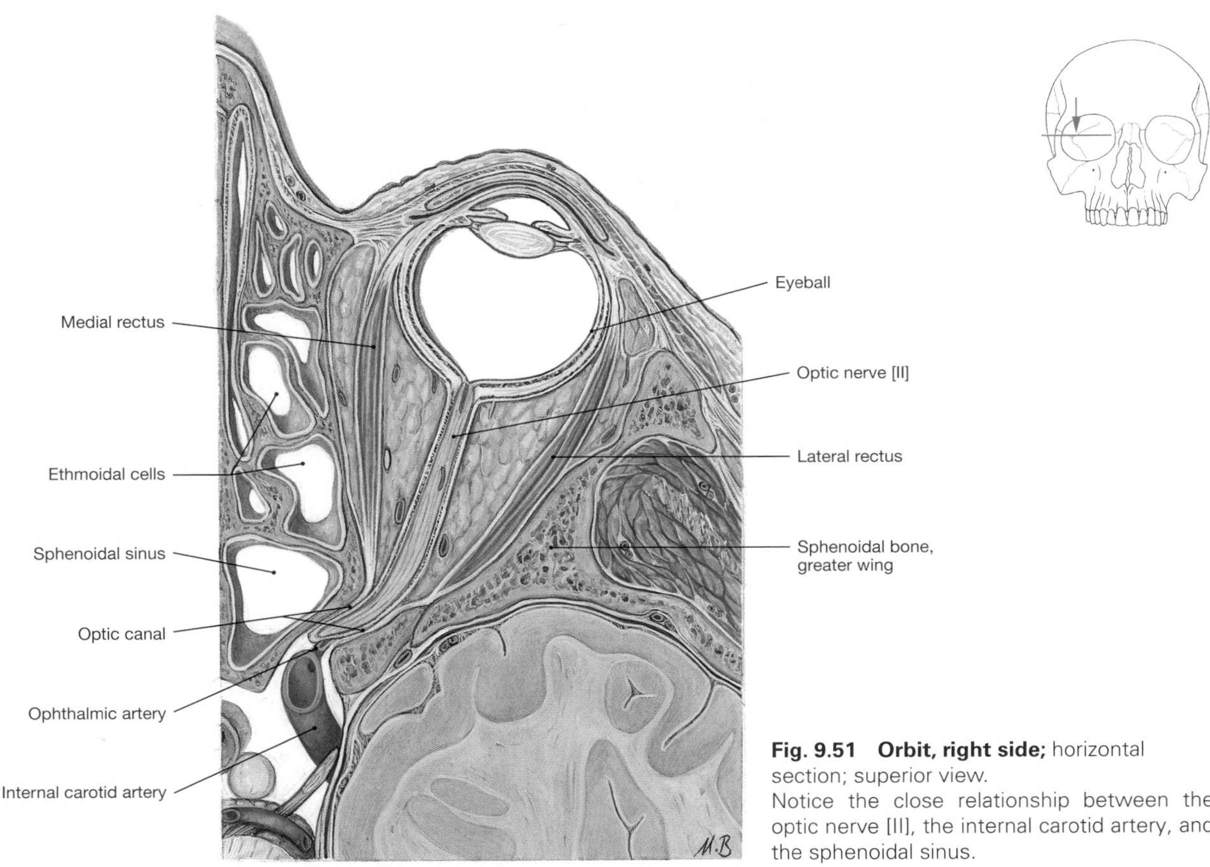
Medial rectus
Ethmoidal cells
Sphenoidal sinus
Optic canal
Ophthalmic artery
Internal carotid artery
Eyeball
Optic nerve [II]
Lateral rectus
Sphenoidal bone, greater wing

**Fig. 9.51 Orbit, right side;** horizontal section; superior view.

Notice the close relationship between the optic nerve [II], the internal carotid artery, and the sphenoidal sinus.

## Orbit, topography

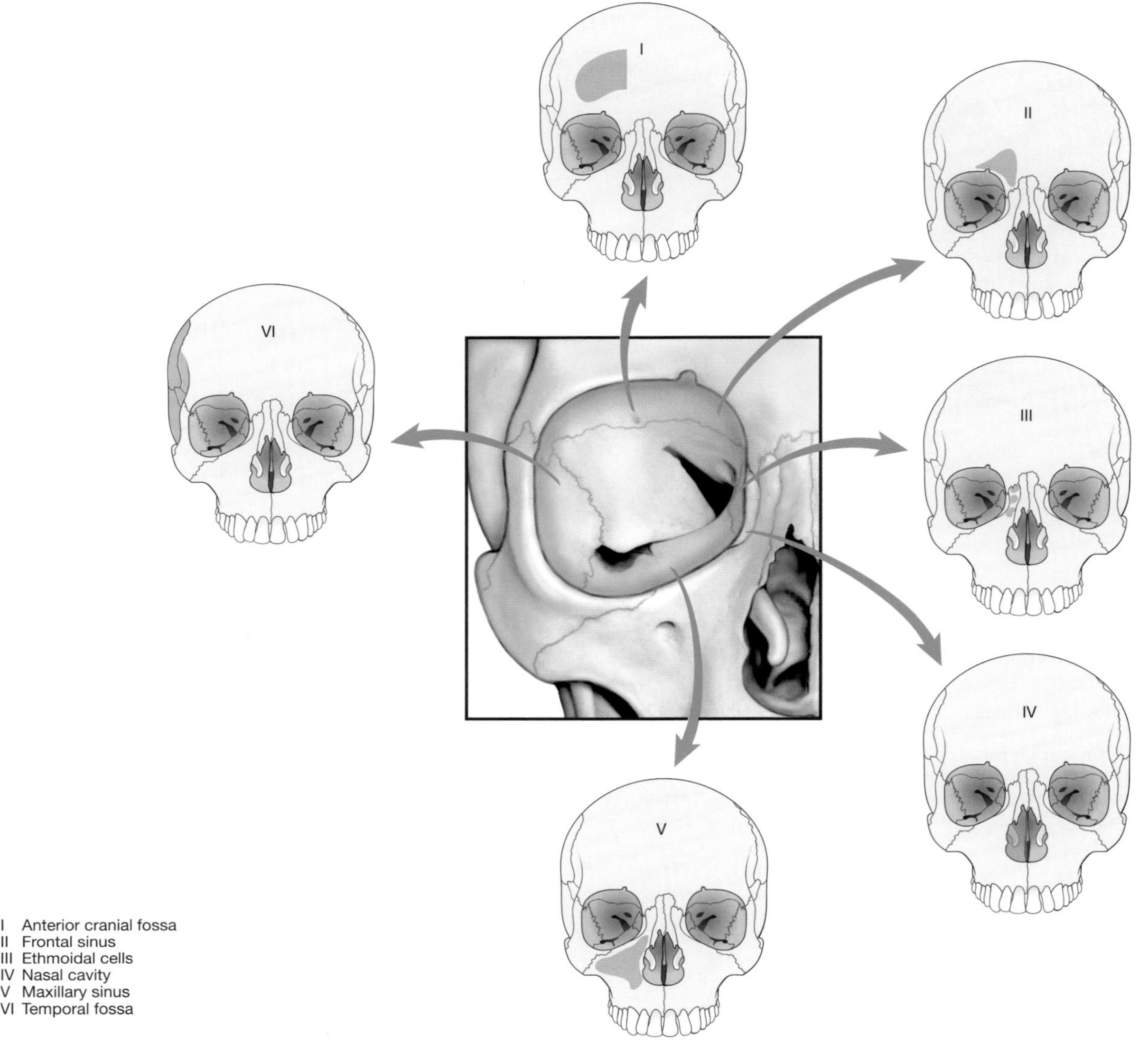
I
II
III
IV
V
VI
I Anterior cranial fossa
II Frontal sinus
III Ethmoidal cells
IV Nasal cavity
V Maxillary sinus
VI Temporal fossa

**Fig. 9.52 Topographical relationships of the orbit and neighboring regions, right side;** frontal view.
The orbit has a close topographical relationship with neighboring regions. This includes the anterior cranial fossa, the frontal sinus, the ethmoidal cells, the nasal cavity, the maxillary sinus, and the temporal fossa.

### Clinical Remarks

The treatment of diseases, particularly those affecting facial structures, requires an interdisciplinary approach including specialists from ophthalmology, otolaryngology, radiology, neurology, head/neck/cosmetic surgery, neurosurgery, and potentially other disciplines (e.g. pediatrics, anesthesia, nuclear medicine, and others). An inflammation or tumor in the orbit can spread to neighboring areas (and partially vice versa) and may require an interdisciplinary therapeutic intervention.

## Orbit, topography

### Clinical Remarks

**Endocrine orbitopathy** is an inflammation of the orbit as part of GRAVES' disease. The latter is an autoimmune disease which is believed to result from autoantibodies directed against the thyroid gland and some tissues in the orbit (e.g. extra-ocular muscles and orbital fat body). However, the details of this disease mechanism are not entirely clear. The disease phenotype involves hyperfunction of the thyroid gland (hyperthyroidism) and exophthalmos (bulging out of the eyes, → Fig. 9.53). Exophthalmos coincides with widening of the palpebral fissure, retraction of the eyelid, and distorted eye movements.

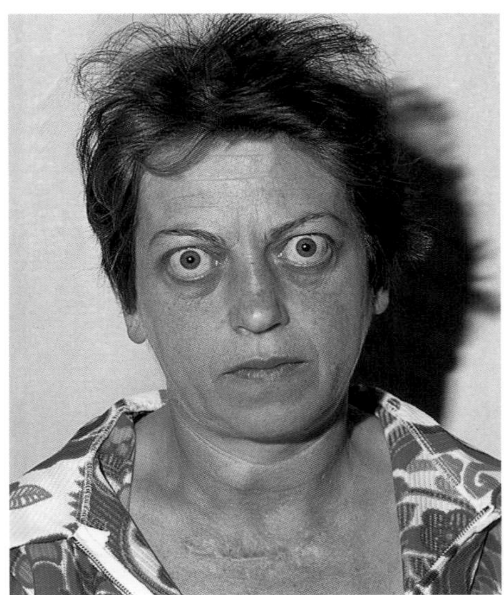

**Fig. 9.53 Patient suffering from endocrine orbitopathy.** [18]
Shown is the pronounced exophthalmos as well as a scar in the neck region (condition after thyroidectomy).

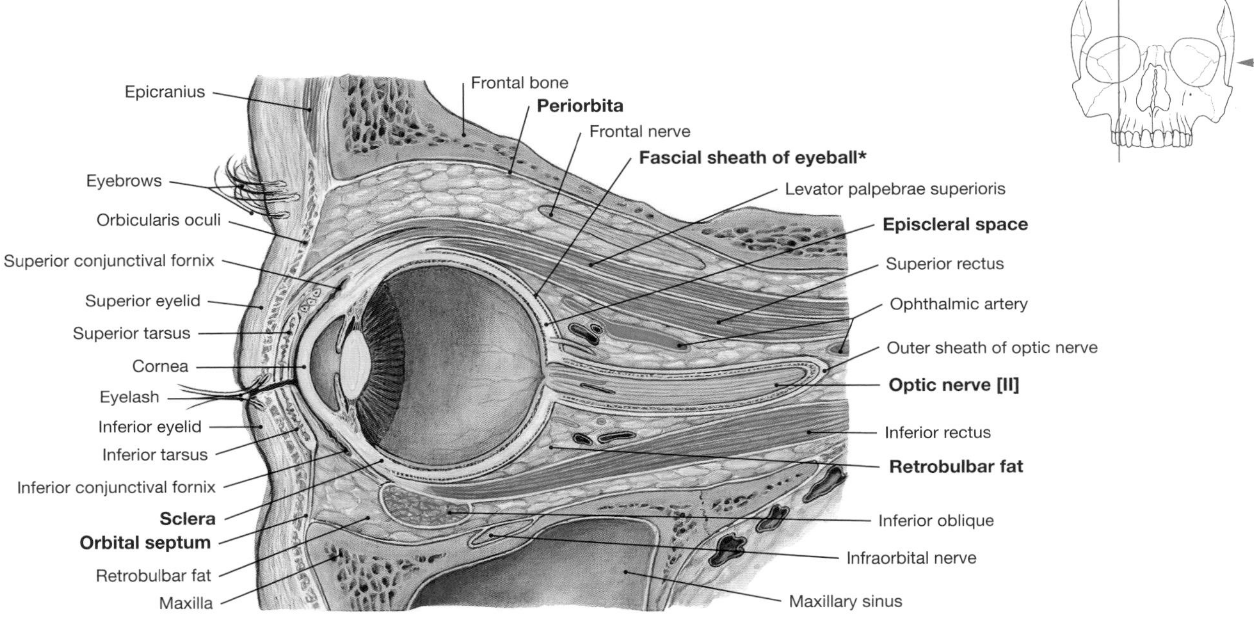
Epicranius
Eyebrows
Orbicularis oculi
Superior conjunctival fornix
Superior eyelid
Superior tarsus
Cornea
Eyelash
Inferior eyelid
Inferior tarsus
Inferior conjunctival fornix
Sclera
Orbital septum
Retrobulbar fat
Maxilla
Frontal bone
Periorbita
Frontal nerve
Fascial sheath of eyeball*
Levator palpebrae superioris
Episcleral space
Superior rectus
Ophthalmic artery
Outer sheath of optic nerve
Optic nerve [II]
Inferior rectus
Retrobulbar fat
Inferior oblique
Infraorbital nerve
Maxillary sinus

**Fig. 9.54 Orbit, right side;** medial view; vertical midline section.
The periorbita (periosteum) covers the inside of the orbit. All structures of the orbit are embedded in adipose tissue (orbital fat body). The orbital septum delineates the entrance to the orbit; a thin layer of connective tissue (fascial sheath of eyeball or TENON's capsule) surrounds the eyeball. A narrow gap (episcleral space) separates the fascial sheath of eyeball and the sclera of the eyeball.

* TENON's capsule

### Clinical Remarks

To describe the optimal surgical access route, the orbit is divided into parts according to different clinical criteria:

- bulbar part (eyeball) – retrobulbar part
- central or intraconal (delineated by the cone-shaped arrangement of the extra-ocular rectus muscles) part – peripheral or extra-conal part
- upper level – middle level – lower level of the orbit:
  - The **upper level** of the orbit is the space between the orbital roof and the levator palpebrae superioris. It contains: frontal nerve, trochlear nerve, lacrimal nerve, supra-orbital artery, supratrochlear artery, lacrimal artery and vein, and superior ophthalmic vein (→ Fig. 9.46).
  - The **middle level** of the orbit extends between the extra-ocular rectus muscles and, thus, includes the intraconal space (→ Fig. 9.48). It contains: oculomotor nerve, nasociliary nerve, abducent nerve, zygomatic nerve, ciliary ganglion, ophthalmic artery, superior ophthalmic vein, short and long posterior ciliary arteries.
  - The **lower level** of the orbit extends from the inferior rectus and inferior oblique to the orbital floor (→ Fig. 9.49). It contains: infra-orbital nerve, infra-orbital artery and inferior ophthalmic vein.

## Orbit, frontal sections

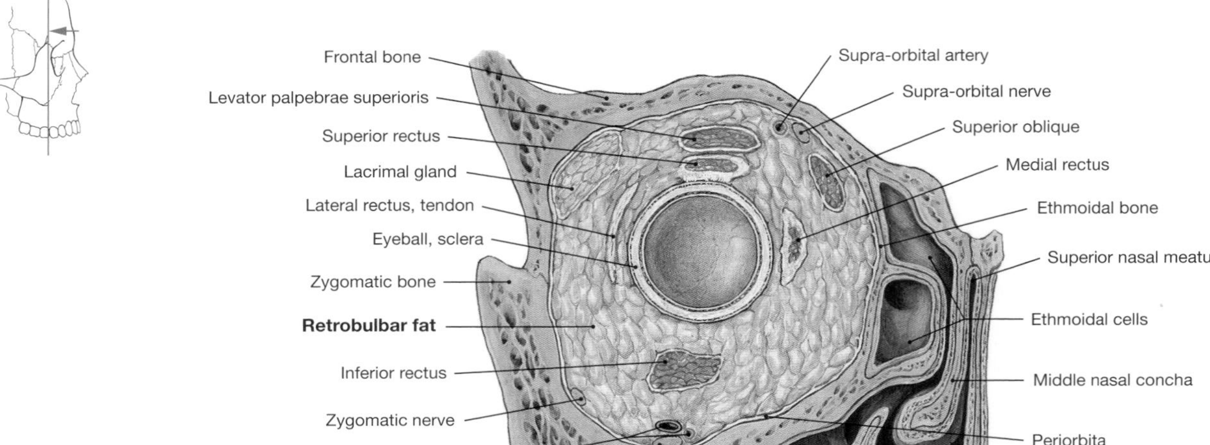
Frontal bone
Levator palpebrae superioris
Superior rectus
Lacrimal gland
Lateral rectus, tendon
Eyeball, sclera
Zygomatic bone
Retrobulbar fat
Inferior rectus
Zygomatic nerve
Infra-orbital (vein); artery
Infra-orbital nerve
Supra-orbital artery
Supra-orbital nerve
Superior oblique
Medial rectus
Ethmoidal bone
Superior nasal meatus
Ethmoidal cells
Middle nasal concha
Periorbita
Maxillary sinus

**Fig. 9.55 Orbit, right side;** frontal section through the orbit at the level of the posterior aspect of the eyeball; frontal view.

The orbital fat body surrounds and buffers all structures within the orbit.

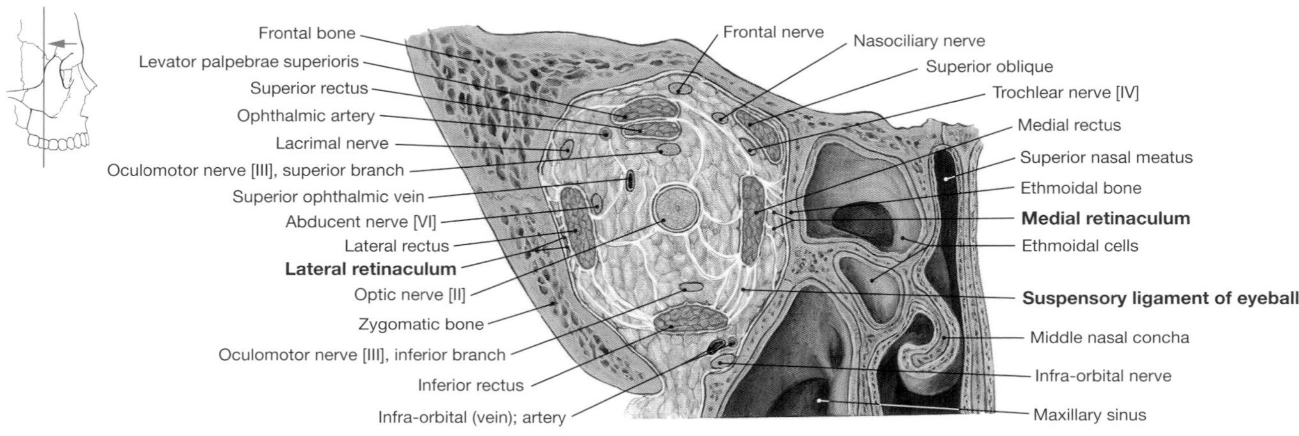
Frontal bone
Levator palpebrae superioris
Superior rectus
Ophthalmic artery
Lacrimal nerve
Oculomotor nerve [III], superior branch
Superior ophthalmic vein
Abducent nerve [VI]
Lateral rectus
Lateral retinaculum
Optic nerve [II]
Zygomatic bone
Oculomotor nerve [III], inferior branch
Inferior rectus
Infra-orbital (vein); artery
Frontal nerve
Nasociliary nerve
Superior oblique
Trochlear nerve [IV]
Medial rectus
Superior nasal meatus
Ethmoidal bone
Medial retinaculum
Ethmoidal cells
Suspensory ligament of eyeball
Middle nasal concha
Infra-orbital nerve
Maxillary sinus

**Fig. 9.56 Orbit, right side;** frontal section through the retrobulbar region of the orbit; frontal view.

The eyeball and the structures of the retrobulbar space connect to the periorbita and among each other through thin ligaments. Stronger ligaments are the medial retinaculum (between the medial rectus and the periorbita), the lateral retinaculum (between lateral rectus and the periorbita), and the suspensory ligament of eyeball (LOCKWOOD's ligament, between the medial rectus, inferior rectus and the periorbita).

## Clinical Remarks

Thrombosis of the central retinal vein **(central venous thrombosis)** is a relatively frequent retinal disease associated with significant reduction in vision. Diabetic patients often develop microvascular changes also involving the retinal blood vessels which can rupture resulting in bleeding into the vitreous body and impairment of vision. If remnants of such bleeding into the vitreous body fail to resolve after 2–3 months and impairment in vision continues, removal of the vitreous body (vitrectomy) is often performed.

Various conditions (e.g. keratitis = corneal inflammation, degenerative keratoconus or chemical irritation) may require the surgical replacement of the cornea to restore proper vision **(corneal transplantation).** Due to the lack of vascularization of the cornea, the risk of an immunological rejection is much lower than with vascularized organs. Therefore, corneal transplantation is the most frequently performed tissue transplantation procedure worldwide.

## Eyeball

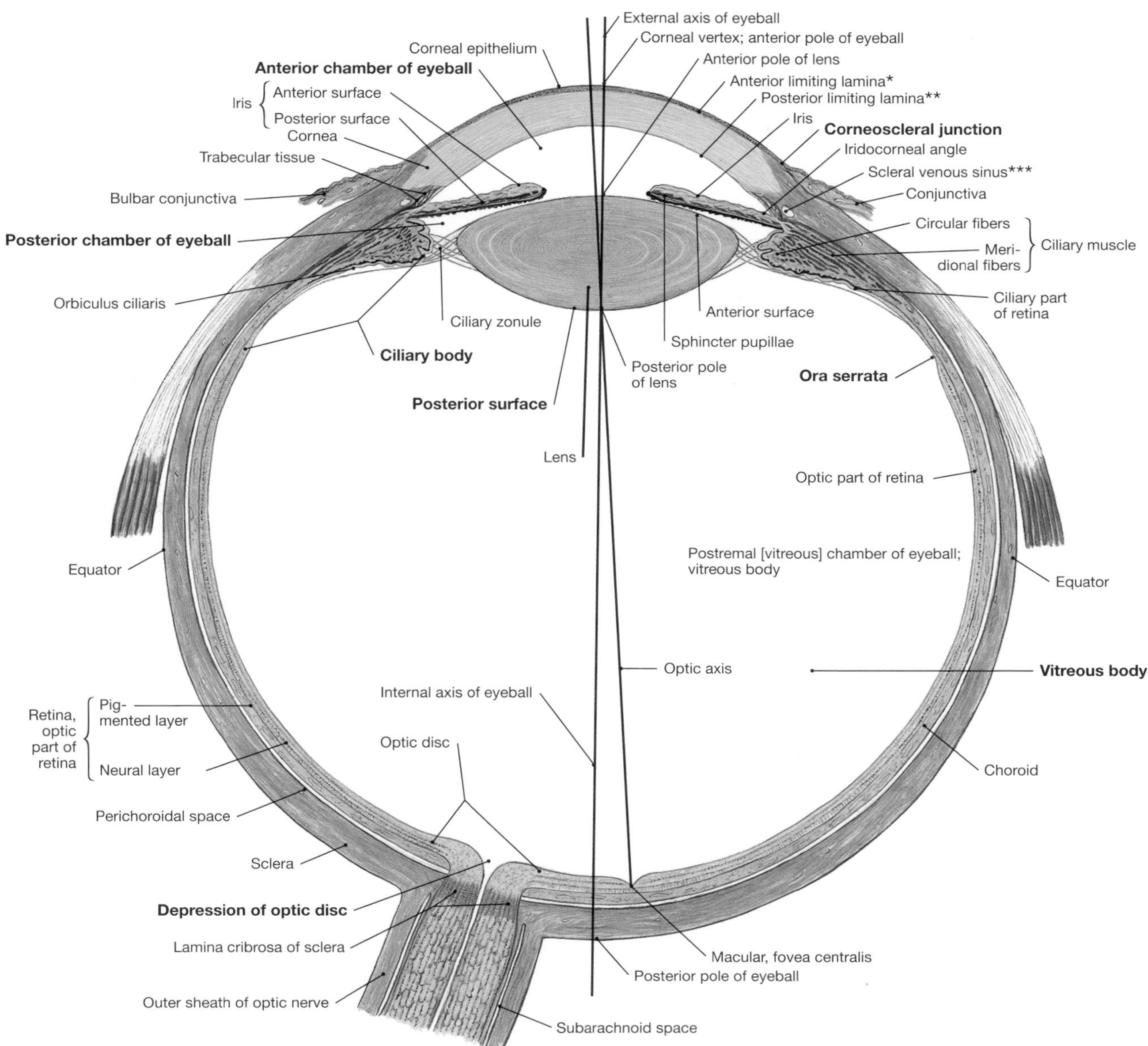
External axis of eyeball
Corneal vertex; anterior pole of eyeball
Corneal epithelium
Anterior pole of lens
Anterior chamber of eyeball
Anterior limiting lamina*
Iris
Anterior surface
Posterior surface
Posterior limiting lamina**
Iris
Cornea
Corneoscleral junction
Trabecular tissue
Iridocorneal angle
Scleral venous sinus***
Bulbar conjunctiva
Conjunctiva
Circular fibers
Posterior chamber of eyeball
Meri-
dional fibers
Ciliary muscle
Orbiculus ciliaris
Ciliary part
of retina
Anterior surface
Ciliary zonule
Sphincter pupillae
Ciliary body
Posterior pole
of lens
Ora serrata
Posterior surface
Lens
Optic part of retina
Postremal [vitreous] chamber of eyeball;
vitreous body
Equator
Equator
Optic axis
Vitreous body
Internal axis of eyeball
Retina,
optic
part of
retina
Pig-
mented layer
Neural layer
Optic disc
Choroid
Perichoroidal space
Sclera
Depression of optic disc
Lamina cribrosa of sclera
Macular, fovea centralis
Posterior pole of eyeball
Outer sheath of optic nerve
Subarachnoid space

**Fig. 9.57 Eyeball, right side;** schematic horizontal part at the level of the exit of the optic nerve.

In the anterior part of the eye, the **cornea** forms the outer cover of the eyeball. Shaped like a convex disc, the cornea bulges out from the rest of the eyeball. At the corneal limbus (corneoscleral junction), the cornea merges into the less curved **sclera** which forms the fibrous layer of the eyeball in the posterior part of the eye. The extra-ocular muscles insert from outside at the sclera. The vascular layer of the eyeball (uvea) lies beneath the sclera. Its anterior part consists of the **iris** and the ciliary body, while the choroid forms the posterior part. At the ora serrata, the ciliary body and the choroid meet. The choroid represents the most highly vascularized structure in the body. Its blood supply provides nutrients and oxygen to the adjacent retinal layer and is involved in thermoregulation of the eyeball. The **retina** is the innermost layer of the eyeball. It contains the neural layer (photoreceptive cells) and the pigmented layer (pigment cells), and in the anterior part the pigmented layer of the ciliary body and the epithelium of the iris. The inner space of the eyeball consists of the vitreous body.

* clinical term: BOWMAN's membrane
** clinical term: DESCEMET's membrane
*** clinical term: canal of SCHLEMM

## Clinical Remarks

**Retinal ablation** describes the detachment of the inner parts of the retina (neural layer, neuroretina) from its supplying retinal pigment epithelial layer (pigmented layer). Symptoms include the sensation of flashes or colored spots. This may not occur if the macula (point of central vision) is unaffected. However, if the macula is detached from its supplying pigment epithelium for more than 48 hours, a permanent the loss of function of the corresponding retinal part will occur. After a successful reattachment of the retina to the pigment epithelium, the retina may partially recover, depending on the duration of the retinal ablation. In the case of a continued complete retinal ablation, blindness is inevitable.

## Blood vessels of the eyeball

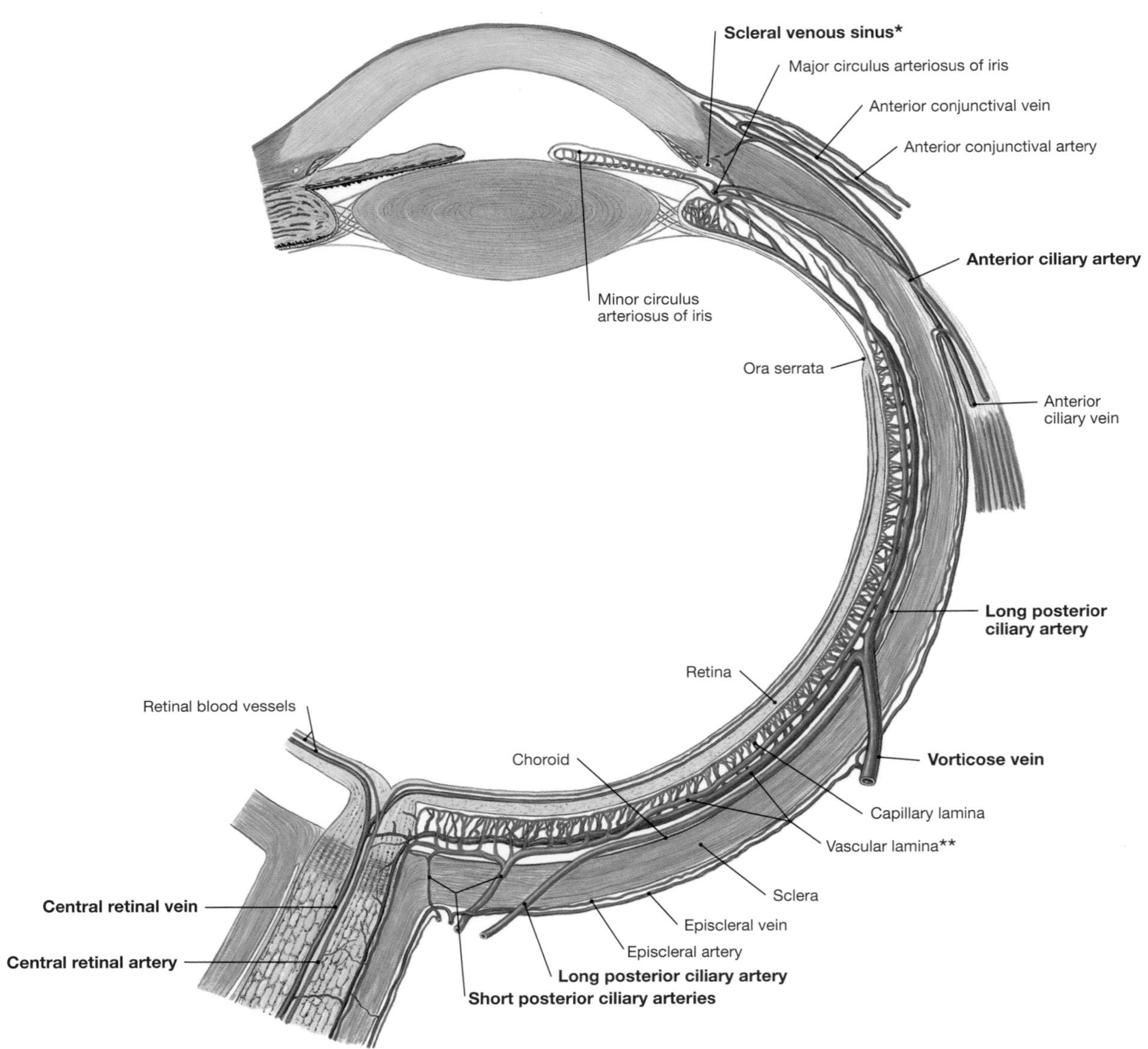
Scleral venous sinus*
Major circulus arteriosus of iris
Anterior conjunctival vein
Anterior conjunctival artery
Anterior ciliary artery
Minor circulus arteriosus of iris
Ora serrata
Anterior ciliary vein
Long posterior ciliary artery
Retina
Retinal blood vessels
Choroid
Vorticose vein
Capillary lamina
Vascular lamina**
Sclera
Central retinal vein
Episcleral vein
Central retinal artery
Episcleral artery
Long posterior ciliary artery
Short posterior ciliary arteries

**Fig. 9.58 Blood vessels of the eyeball, right side;** horizontal section at the level of the optic nerve [II]; superior view.
Arterial blood supply (→ Fig. 9.44). Venous drainage is through the central retinal vein and four to eight vorticose veins (→ Fig. 9.45). The latter pierce the sclera posterior to the equator of the eyeball and join the superior and inferior ophthalmic veins.
* clinical term: canal of SCHLEMM
** clinical term: Uvea

| **Dimensions of the Eyeball** (average values according to the anatomic and ophthalmologic literature) | | | |
|---|---|---|---|
| External bulbar axis | 24.0 mm | Radius of curvature of the sclera | 13.0 mm |
| Internal bulbar axis | 22.5 mm | Radius of curvature of the cornea | 7.8 mm |
| Thickness of the cornea | 0.5 mm | Refractive index of the entire eye (distance vision) | 59 dioptres |
| Depth of the anterior chamber | 3.6 mm | Refractive index of the cornea | 43 dioptres |
| Thickness of the lens | 3.6 mm | Refractive index of the lens (distance vision) | 19 dioptres |
| Distance between lens and retina | 15.6 mm | Interpupillary distance | 61–69 mm |
| Thickness of the retina | 0.3 mm | | |

## Iris and ciliary body

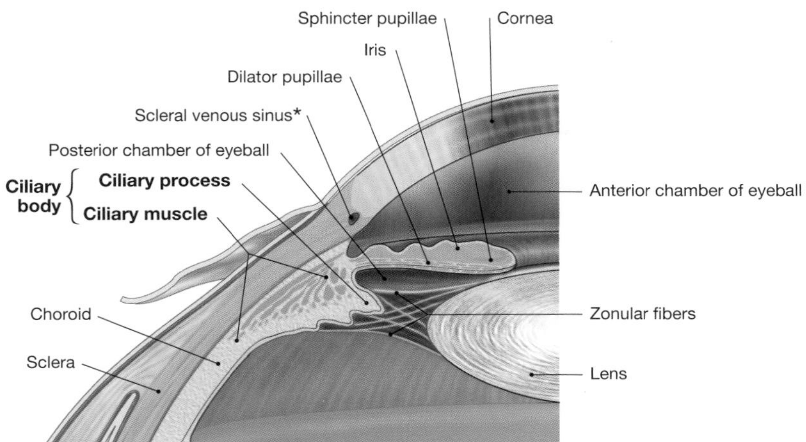
Sphincter pupillae
Cornea
Iris
Dilator pupillae
Scleral venous sinus*
Posterior chamber of eyeball
Ciliary body
Ciliary process
Ciliary muscle
Choroid
Sclera
Anterior chamber of eyeball
Zonular fibers
Lens

**Fig. 9.59 Iridocorneal angle and adjacent structures.** [8]
The cornea, iris, and sclera provide the borders for the iridocorneal angle. The epithelial layer of the ciliary body produces the aqueous humor that flows from the posterior to the anterior chamber of the eye. When it reaches the trabecular meshwork at the iridocorneal angle, the fluid is collected in the canal of SCHLEMM (*) and drained into episcleral veins. The ciliary muscle is the major component of the ciliary body and important for accommodation. It consists of meridional (longitudinal, BRÜCKE's muscle), radial, and circular (MÜLLER's muscle) muscle cells.

### Clinical Remarks

Insufficient drainage of the aqueous humor from the iridocorneal angle leads to an increased intra-ocular pressure (normal 15 mmHg) and results in **glaucoma.** Damage occurs primarily to the papilla of the optic nerve with the risk of blindness. Causes include blockage of the iridocorneal angle, for example by adhesion of the iris to the cornea (closed-angle glaucoma; rare), or the impaired drainage through the trabecular meshwork of the canal of SCHLEMM in open-angle glaucoma (frequent).
The inherited genetic deficiency in the synthesis of the connecting protein fibrillin-1 **(MARFAN's syndrome)** results in the insufficiency of the zonular fibers with luxation of the lens and permanent ball-shaped lens (impaired lens accommodation).

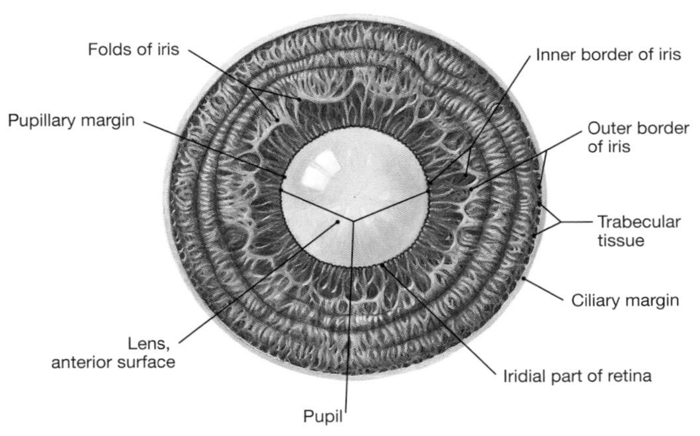
Folds of iris
Inner border of iris
Pupillary margin
Outer border of iris
Trabecular tissue
Ciliary margin
Lens, anterior surface
Iridial part of retina
Pupil

**Fig. 9.60 Iris and lens;** frontal view.

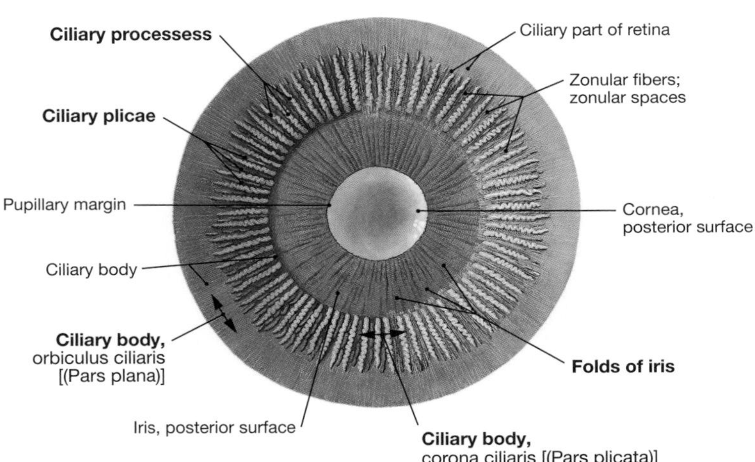
Ciliary processess
Ciliary part of retina
Zonular fibers; zonular spaces
Ciliary plicae
Pupillary margin
Cornea, posterior surface
Ciliary body
Ciliary body, orbiculus ciliaris [(Pars plana)]
Folds of iris
Iris, posterior surface
Ciliary body, corona ciliaris [(Pars plicata)]

**Fig. 9.61 Iris and ciliary body;** posterior view; after removal of the lens.
The ciliary body is divided into a plane and a raised part. The latter serves as origin for approximately 70 ciliary processes. The ciliary body is covered with ciliary epithelium, which, in the area of the raised part, secretes the aqueous humour for the iridocorneal angle. Zonular fibers (suspensory ligaments of the lens) traverse the distance between the ciliary epithelium and the lens capsule.

## Lens

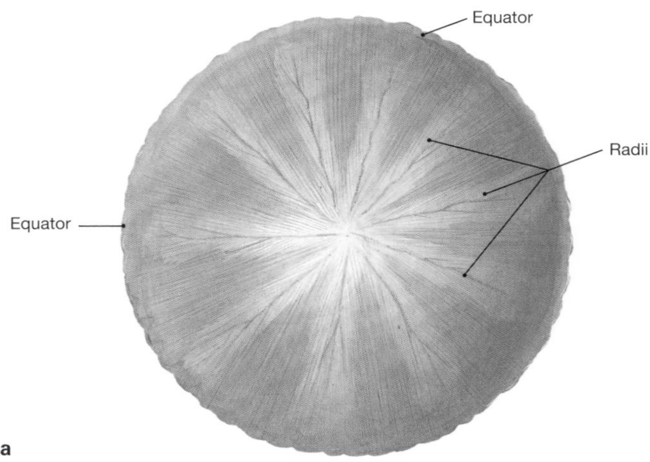
Equator
Radii
Equator
a

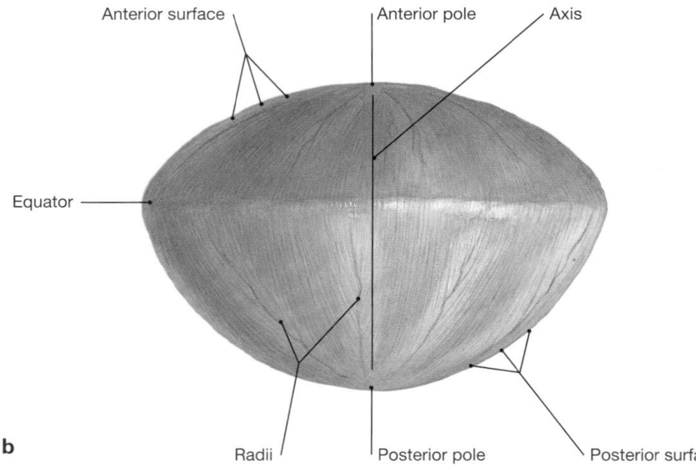
Anterior surface
Anterior pole
Axis
Equator
b
Radii
Posterior pole
Posterior surface

**Figs. 9.62a and b Lens.**
**a** Frontal view
**b** Viewed from the equator

Depending on its particular level of accommodation, the refractive index of the lens varies between 10–20 dioptres (for comparison, the refractive index of the cornea is 43 dioptres but cannot be modified).

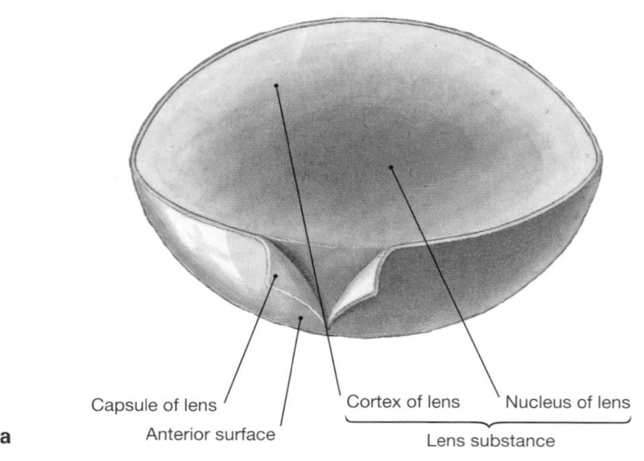
Capsule of lens
Anterior surface
Cortex of lens
Nucleus of lens
Lens substance
a

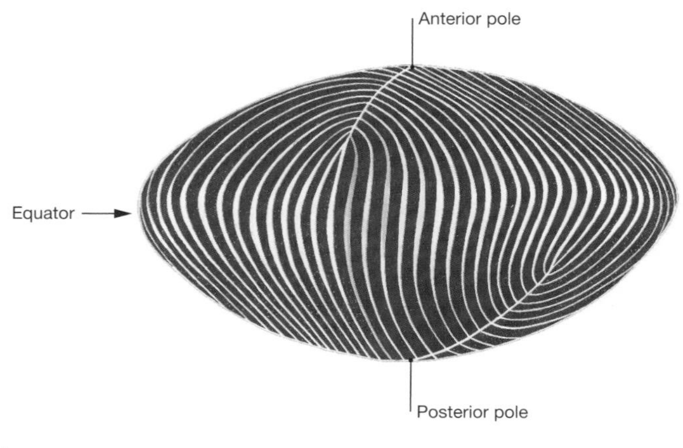
Anterior pole
Equator
Posterior pole
b

**Figs. 9.63a and b Lens.**
**a** Anterior oblique view; after meridional cut and partial detachment of the anterior capsule of lens.

**b** Lens fibers of a neonate; schematic drawing; view from the equator. The centers of the planes are the anterior and posterior pole.

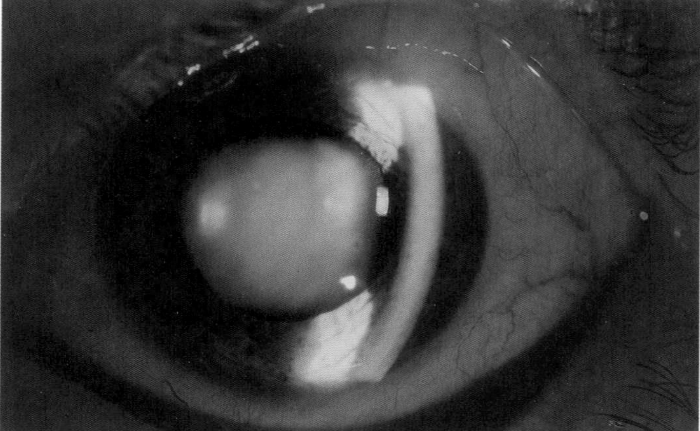

**Fig. 9.64 Senile cataract, right side;** slit lamp examination.
Shown is a condition of progressive cataract with milky white opacity of the lens. The white curved bar on the right side of the image constitutes the reflection of the cornea.

### Clinical Remarks

The continuous apposition of lens fibers reduces the elasticity of the lens (starting at about 40 years of age) which results in a diminished accommodation of the lens, i.e. the inability to properly focusing on objects at various distances **(presbyopia).** Reduction in intracellular water content causes alterations in proteins (crystallines) important for maintaining transparency of the lens. The resulting increase in opacity of the lens **(senile cataract)** represents the most common eye disease and can be diagnosed early by slit lamp examination (→ Fig. 9.64). Cataract surgery is one of the most frequently performed surgical procedures in Western industrialized countries (approx. 10% of all 80 year old patients suffer from advanced cataract).

## Retina

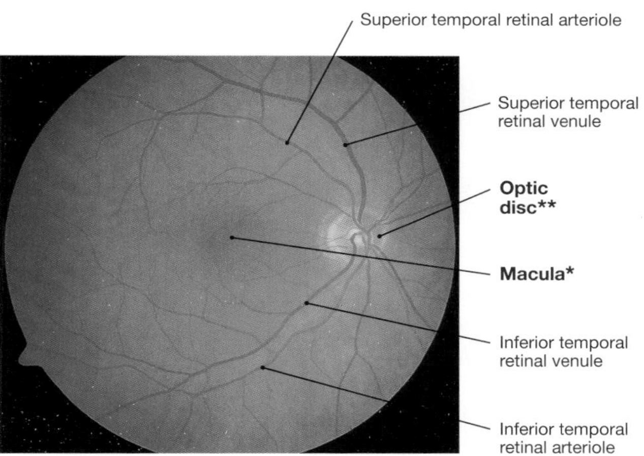
Superior temporal retinal arteriole
Superior temporal retinal venule
Optic disc**
Macula*
Inferior temporal retinal venule
Inferior temporal retinal arteriole

**Fig. 9.65 Ocular fundus, right side;** frontal view; ophthalmoscopic image of the central region.

The examination of the ocular fundus by direct ophthalmoscopy (funduscopy or fundoscopy) allows the clinical assessment of the condition of the retina, its blood vessels (in particular the central retinal artery and vein), the optic disc, as well as the macula and fovea centralis (point of central vision). The blood vessels of the retina (central retinal artery and vein and their branches) can be examined and distinguished according to their diameter. Normally, the optic disc has a sharply delineated margin, a yellow to orange color, and contains a central depression (physiological cup). At 3–4 mm to the temporal side of the optic disc lies the macula (contains the highest concentration of cone cells for color vision). Numerous branches of the central retinal blood vessels converge in a radial fashion onto the macula, but fail to reach the center (fovea centralis). The latter is supplied by the choroid.

* clinical term
** clinical term: blind spot

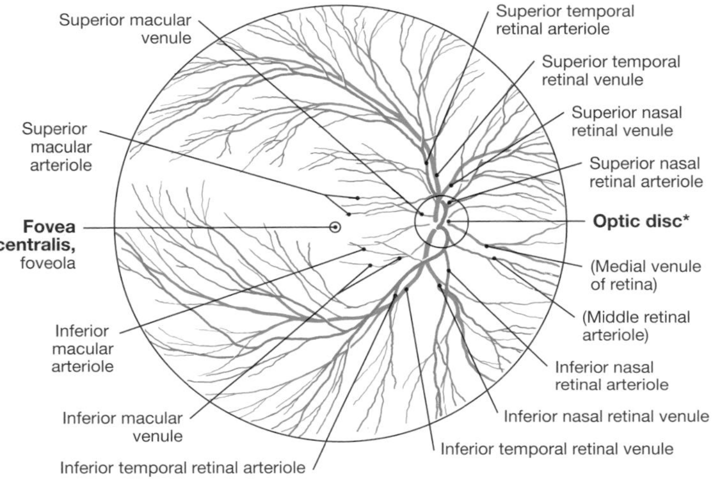
Superior macular venule
Superior temporal retinal arteriole
Superior temporal retinal venule
Superior macular arteriole
Superior nasal retinal venule
Superior nasal retinal arteriole
Fovea centralis, foveola
Optic disc*
(Medial venule of retina)
(Middle retinal arteriole)
Inferior macular arteriole
Inferior nasal retinal arteriole
Inferior macular venule
Inferior nasal retinal venule
Inferior temporal retinal venule
Inferior temporal retinal arteriole

**Fig. 9.66 Ocular fundus and retinal blood vessels, right side;** frontal view; schematic drawing of the course of the blood vessels.

* clinical term: blind spot

**Fig. 9.67 Ocular fundus, right side;** frontal view; fluorescence angiography during the arteriovenous phase with anatomic landmarks: macula (blue circle); fovea (yellow circle). [15]

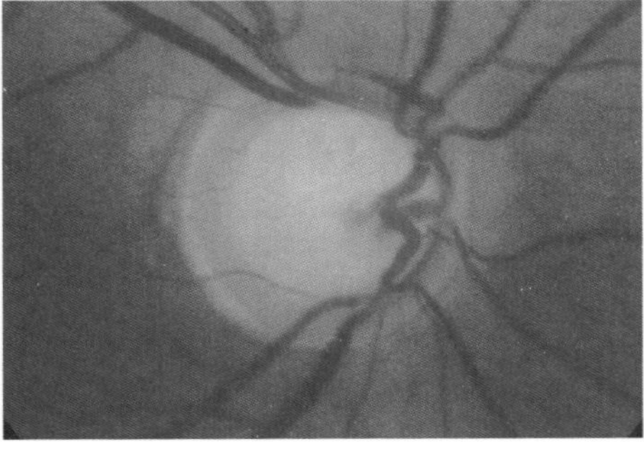

**Fig. 9.68 Concentric enlargement of the optic disc due to glaucoma.** [15]

### Clinical Remarks

After **retinal ablation** the retina takes on a whitish-yellow color. Alterations of the retinal blood vessels, as commonly observed with diabetic retinopathy or hypertension, are visualized early by fundoscopy. Advanced diagnostic procedures include fluorescence angiography (→ Fig. 9.67). Increased intracranial pressure makes the optic disc protrude into the eyeball and its margins appear less well defined **(optic disc edema).** Glaucoma also causes characteristic alterations to the optic disc (→ Fig. 9.68). Pathological alterations to the macula are often age-dependent. The most frequent cause of blindness in Western industrialized nations is **age-dependent macular degeneration** (AMD).

## Orbit, MRI

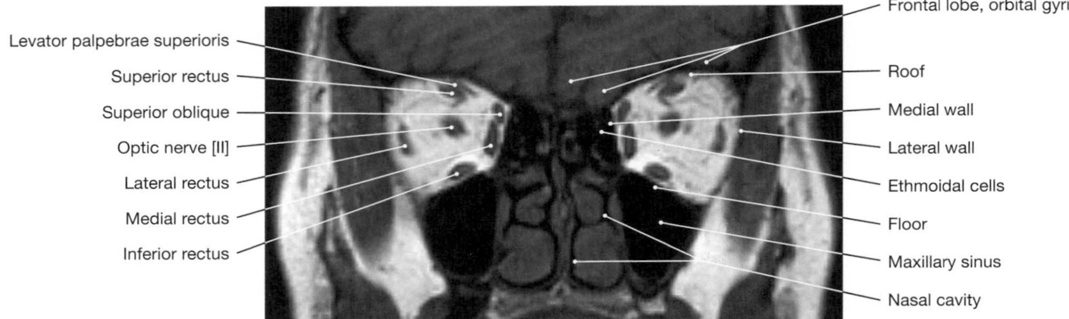
Levator palpebrae superioris
Superior rectus
Superior oblique
Optic nerve [II]
Lateral rectus
Medial rectus
Inferior rectus
Frontal lobe, orbital gyri
Roof
Medial wall
Lateral wall
Ethmoidal cells
Floor
Maxillary sinus
Nasal cavity

**Fig. 9.69 Extra-ocular muscles;** magnetic resonance tomographic image (MRI), frontal section of a healthy individual at the level of the orbital center; frontal view.

The close topographical relationships of the orbit with the maxillary sinus, frontal lobe, ethmoidal cells, and temporalis muscle (not indicated) are clearly visible.

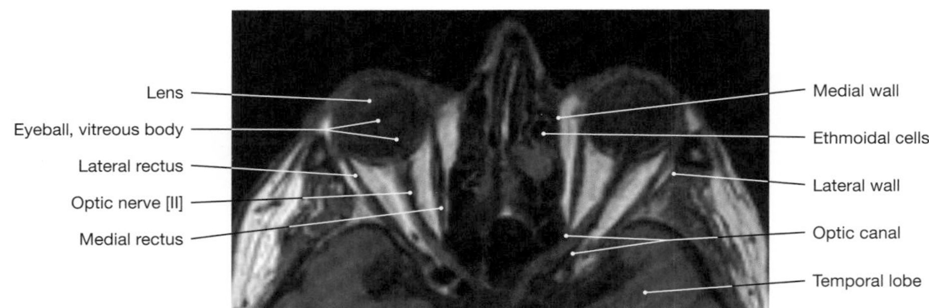
Lens
Eyeball, vitreous body
Lateral rectus
Optic nerve [II]
Medial rectus
Medial wall
Ethmoidal cells
Lateral wall
Optic canal
Temporal lobe

**Fig. 9.70 Eyeball and extra-ocular muscles;** magnetic resonance tomographic image (MRI), transverse section of a healthy individual at the level of the optic nerve [II]; superior view.

This sectional plane displays the slightly contorted course of the optic nerve [II]. The extra length of the nerve serves as reserve during the movements of the eyeball.

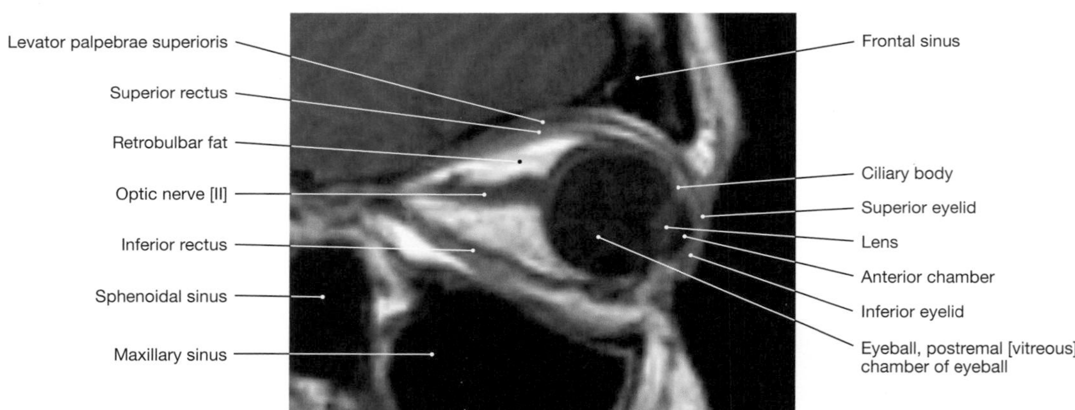
Levator palpebrae superioris
Superior rectus
Retrobulbar fat
Optic nerve [II]
Inferior rectus
Sphenoidal sinus
Maxillary sinus
Frontal sinus
Ciliary body
Superior eyelid
Lens
Anterior chamber
Inferior eyelid
Eyeball, postremal [vitreous] chamber of eyeball

**Fig. 9.71 Eyeball and extra-ocular muscles;** magnetic resonance tomographic image (MRI), sagittal section of a healthy individual at the level of the optic nerve [II]; lateral view.

MRI is an imaging technique ideally suited for the visualization of the bulbar and retrobulbar space because the tissues of both regions provide distinctly different contrast ratios.

### Examination Procedures

Most visible structures of the eye can be examined in vivo with special optic instruments (e.g. magnifying glass, ophthalmoscope, slit lamp), such as cornea, aqueous humour, iridocorneal angle, iris, vitreous body, retina with optic disc and macula.
Imaging techniques assist in the diagnosis of chronic processes and tumors located in parts of the orbit not accessible by visual inspection (outside of the eyeball, retrobulbar space). Among the most frequently used imaging techniques for the examination of intra-orbital structures and their topographic relationships are **computed tomography** (CT) and **magnetic resonance imaging** (MRI). In combination with the intravenous administration of contrast enhancing agents, these imaging techniques can reveal additional clinically relevant information.
In cases where fundoscopy is impossible (e.g. due to pathological alterations of optic media of the eye, like corneal opacity, cataract, bleeding into the vitreous body), **ultrasound** examination (sonography) of the eye can be performed.

## Visual pathway and blood vessels

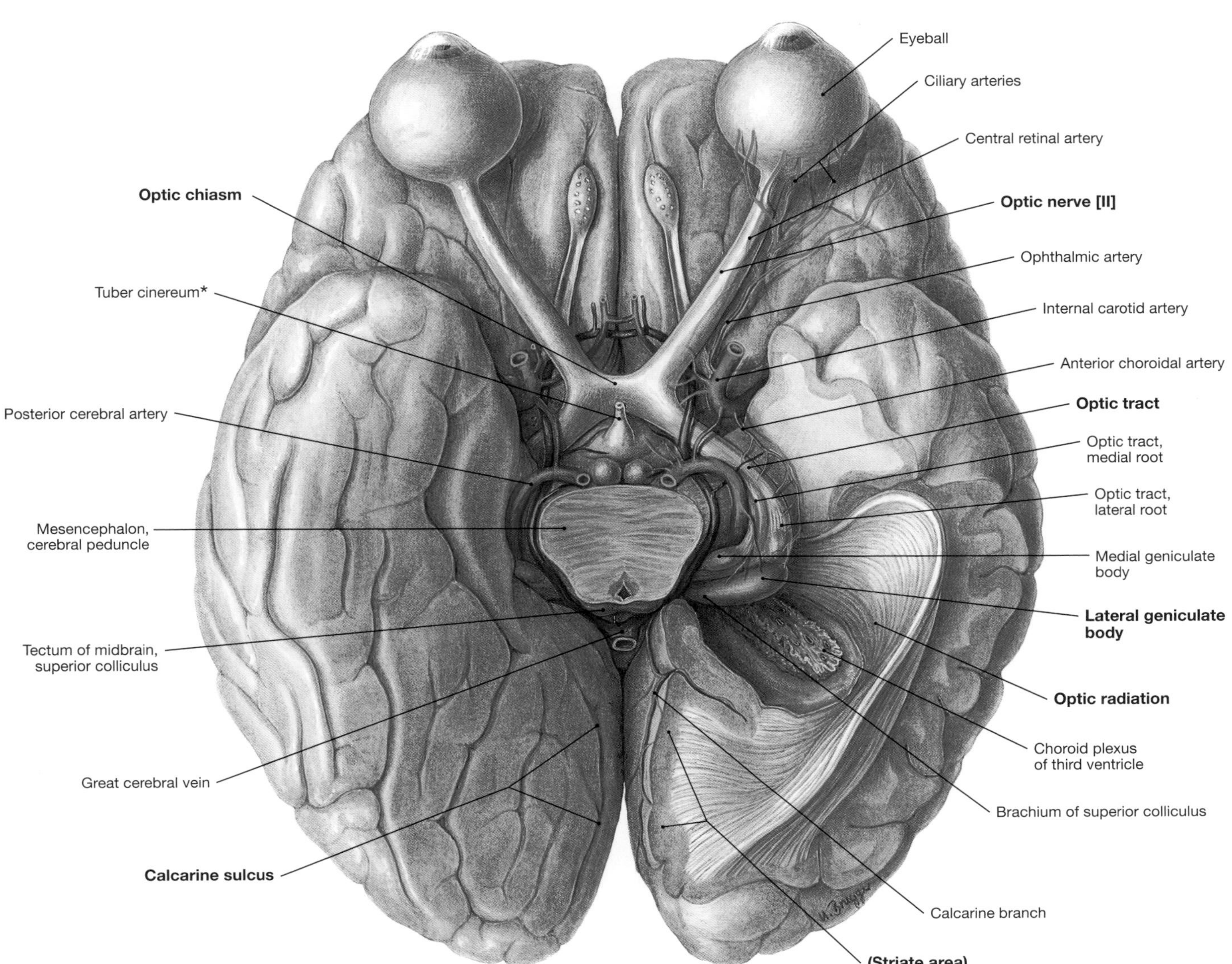
Eyeball
Ciliary arteries
Central retinal artery
Optic chiasm
Optic nerve [II]
Ophthalmic artery
Tuber cinereum*
Internal carotid artery
Anterior choroidal artery
Posterior cerebral artery
Optic tract
Optic tract, medial root
Optic tract, lateral root
Mesencephalon, cerebral peduncle
Medial geniculate body
Lateral geniculate body
Tectum of midbrain, superior colliculus
Optic radiation
Choroid plexus of third ventricle
Great cerebral vein
Brachium of superior colliculus
Calcarine sulcus
Calcarine branch
(Striate area)

**Fig. 9.72 Brain, Cerebrum, and blood supply of the visual pathway;** inferior view. The pituitary gland has been removed at its infundibulum (*). The pituitary gland lies in close proximity to the optic chiasm. The visual pathway originates within the retina and contains the first three neurons and interneurons (horizontal cells, amacrine cells). The different cell layers are (from outside to inside):
**1st Neuron:** photoreceptor cells of the retina (cone and rod cells)
**2nd Neuron:** bipolar ganglion cells of the retina (perikarya in the retinal ganglion) which receive signals from the photoreceptor cells and transmit these signals to a multipolar ganglionic cell (3rd Neuron)
**3rd Neuron:** multipolar ganglion cells of the retina (perikarya in the optic ganglion).
This principle network structure of three neurons forming an intra-retinal chain only applies to the cone cells. Up to 40 rod cells converge their signals onto one bipolar cell and this cell will then transmit these signals indirectly, with the help of amacrine cells (20–50 different types of these cells are described in the literature), to one multipolar ganglionic cell.
The axons of the optic ganglion extend primarily to the lateral geniculate body (lateral root) although several fibers also extend into the pretectal area and into the superior colliculus (medial root) as well as to the hypothalamus. The fibers run within the optic nerve [II] to the optic chiasm, where the fibers from the nasal part of the retina cross to the opposite side. The fibers from the temporal part of the retina do not cross. Each optic tract contains fibers which transmit information from the contralateral half of the visual field.
**4th Neuron:** Its axons travel primarily from the lateral geniculate body to the areas 17 and 18 of the cerebral cortex (striatal area) in the region surrounding the calcarine sulcus.

## Clinical Remarks

Prior to activating the light-sensitive parts of the photoreceptors, light must penetrate through all the other layers of the retina (3rd neuron, 2nd neuron); this is called the inversion of the retina. The outer segments of the photoreceptors (1st neuron) are in close contact with the pigment epithelial cell layer, without developing actual adhesion structures between pigment epithelium and photoreceptors. It is in this region that **retinal ablation** can occur, which, if left untreated, can result in blindness.

## Visual pathway

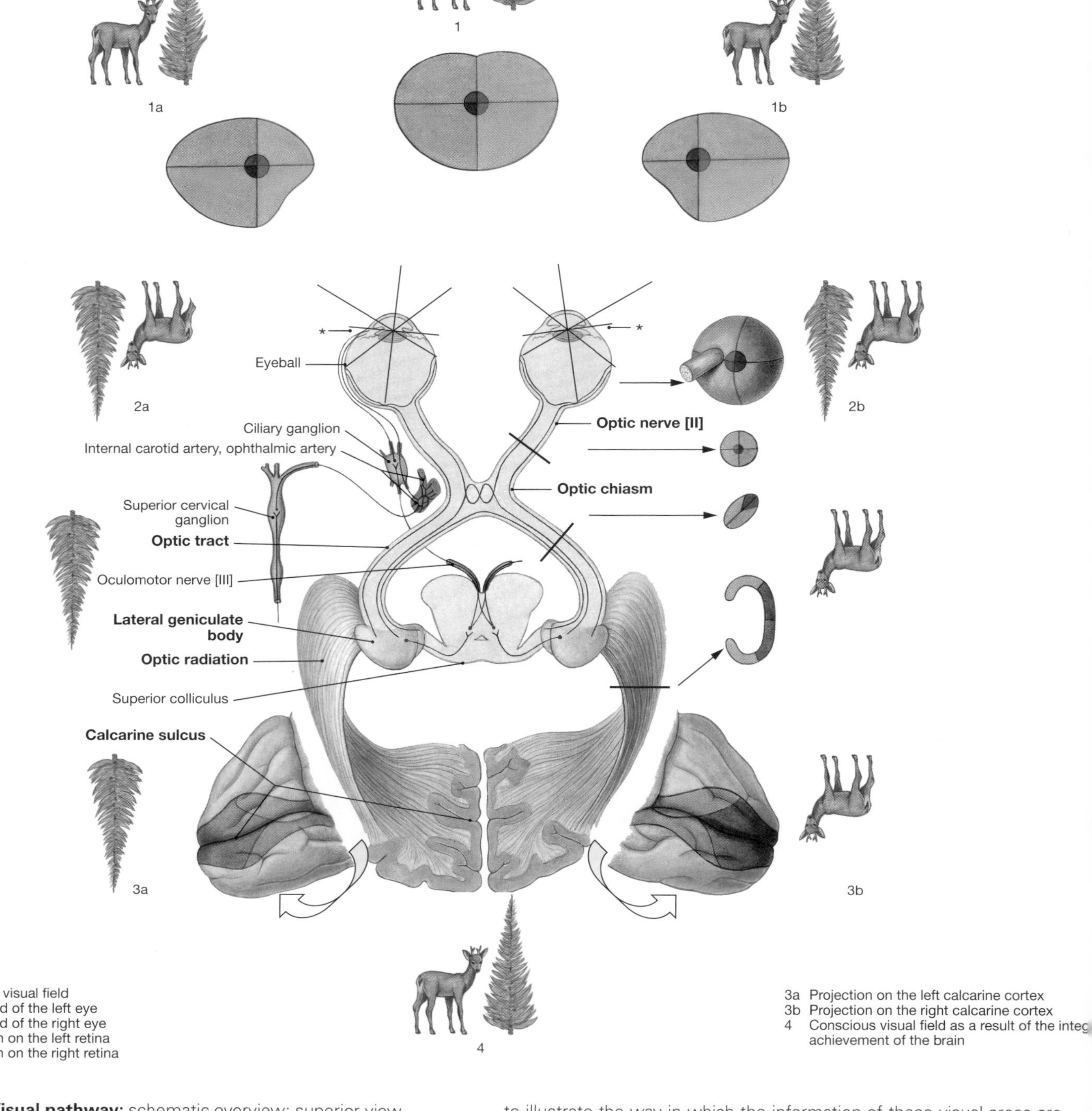
1
1a
1b
Eyeball
Ciliary ganglion
Internal carotid artery, ophthalmic artery
Superior cervical ganglion
Optic tract
Oculomotor nerve [III]
Lateral geniculate body
Optic radiation
Superior colliculus
Calcarine sulcus
Optic nerve [II]
Optic chiasm
2a
2b
3a
3b
4
1 Common visual field
1a Visual field of the left eye
1b Visual field of the right eye
2a Projection on the left retina
2b Projection on the right retina
3a Projection on the left calcarine cortex
3b Projection on the right calcarine cortex
4 Conscious visual field as a result of the integ
achievement of the brain

**Fig. 9.73 Visual pathway;** schematic overview; superior view.
The central vision field has a disproportionately large projection field. The deer and the fir tree demonstrate how images are transmitted from one part of the visual pathway to the next. It is only at the level of the visual association cortices, that the image is perceived as it presents in front of our eyes. The different coloration of the visual quadrants serves to illustrate the way in which the information of these visual areas are transmitted and presented in the visual pathway and on the visual cortex.

* plane of refraction of light

## Clinical Remarks

Due to their close topographical relationship to the optic chiasm, growing pituitary tumors can cause a **bitemporal hemianopsia.** Postchiasmatic and intracerebral lesions along the visual pathway result in **homonymous hemianopsia.** For example, a lesion in the right optic tract causes left-sided homonymous hemianopsia. Injury to the left optic radiation (GRATIOLET's optic radiation) results in a homonymous hemianopsia on the right side. Additional symptoms include a hemianoptic pupillary immobility a pale appearance of the affected pupil after months, or optic papilla edema. Underlying causes can be tumors, basal meningitis, aneurysm, ischemia and bleedings. Loss of function in both visual cortices causes a **cortical amaurosis** (cortical blindness; → Fig. 12.140).

# Ear



10

# The Ear – Tiny Yet Complex Like a Maze

The ear contains the sensory apparatus and nerve cells of two sensory systems that arise from a common embryonic system (the otic placode), but serve very different purposes: hearing and equilibrium or balance. The small, delicate, membranous, convoluted organs, which carry the sensory cells of both modalities, are located in the membranous labyrinth (see below). In turn, the labyrinth is positioned inside the petrous part of the temporal bone, the bony pyramid that separates the posterior and medial cranial fossa. The sensory nerve, the vestibulocochlear nerve [VIII], emerges from the inner ear.
In humans (as in terrestrial vertebrates) a former (the first) pharyngeal groove (also named bronchial groove, pharyngeal cleft, or bronchial cleft) plus surrounding bones and muscles are part of the construction of the acoustic part of the ear – this includes the sound-conducting apparatus, the middle ear and the outer ear. In fish, a pharyngeal groove is a typical "breathing hole"; water "inhaled" through the mouth is expelled from the pharynx via the branchial hole. The "ear-branchial cleft" of terrestrial animals does not longer open, since a very thin membrane, the tympanic membrane, closes it off. If the tympanic membrane had a hole, one could theoretically breathe "through the ears", since a continuous opening would exist that connects the external acoustic (auditory) meatus to the pharynx. Practically, this is not possible because the ducts are too narrow. However, divers with ruptured tympanic membranes can experience difficulties due to influx of water into the pharynx.

## Outer Ear

The outer ear (auricle, pinna) extends from the auricle to the external acoustic (auditory) meatus up to the tympanic membrane. In other words, it is the "outer part" of the former branchial cleft.

**Auricles** of rabbits or horses are flexible, foldable, and are used for directional hearing. In humans, only some flexibility is conserved, whereas folding and motility of the outer ear are lost. Despite the presence of remnants of these ear muscles, they are usually too weak to support significant movement of the auricle. Nevertheless, the concha, made of elastic cartilage, assists in directional hearing in humans.

The **external acoustic (auditory) meatus** is 3–4 cm in length and S-shaped. It consists of a distal cartilaginous component, which continues as an osseous canal in the petrous part of the temporal bone. The osseous canal ends at the tympanic membrane. Immediately above and below to the external acoustic meatus is the temporomandibular joint. One can feel the deformation of the cartilaginous component when chewing, especially if one inserts the fifth finger into the external acoustic meatus.

## Middle Ear

The tympanic membrane marks the lateral margin of the middle ear, which is located inside the petrous part of the temporal bone. The middle ear is a contorted mucosal space connected to other cavities. Various nerve pathways run within the walls and the cavity of the middle ear, where the three auditory ossicles are attached. The "inner part" of the above-mentioned former branchial cleft is connected through the auditory (EUSTACHIAN) tube (pharyngotympanic tube) with the pharynx.

The **auditory tube** is lined by a mucous membrane, descending inferiorly and anteriorly of the tympanic cavity. The auditory tube is located in an osseous meatus in the petrous part of the temporal bone and is supported by elastic cartilage towards the pharynx, where its pharyngeal orifice is shaped like a trumpet bell. The auditory tube serves to equalize the air pressure between the middle ear and the surroundings, which is particularly evident during flying and mountain climbing.

The actual **tympanic cavity** in the petrous part of the temporal bone contains the three auditory ossicles, malleus, incus, and stapes. These ossicles are connected by flexible joints and are mounted to the wall of the tympanic cavity by ligaments to form a V-shaped lever that transmits the vibrations of the tympanic membrane (to which the malleus is attached) to the oval window (which holds the base of the stapes, see below). In addition, two muscles, tensor tympani and stapedius, are attached to the malleus and the stapes, respectively. They regulate the "tension level" of the bony chain and, thus, the efficiency of sound transmission. The branches of the two cranial nerves, the facial nerve [VII] and the glossopharyngeal nerve [IX], run within the mucosal layer of the walls of the tympanic cavity; the chorda tympani, a branch of the facial nerve [VII], descends through the tympanic cavity. These nerve branches are not directly associated with hearing and balance – they supply other regions by passing through the tympanic cavity and petrous part of the temporal bone. A branch of the facial nerve [VII] innervates the stapedius (see above); the branches of the glossopharyngeal nerve [IX] (tympanic plexus) supply the mucous membranes of the tympanic cavity.

The air-filled tympanic cavity extends in an interior and posterior direction into the multi-chambered, also air-filled **mastoid cells** in the mastoid process of the occipital bone (which is palpable just behind and below the auricle).

## Inner Ear

The inner ear is referred to as the labyrinth and is also located in the petrous part of the temporal bone, just superior (vestibular apparatus) and medial (cochlea) of the tympanic cavity. A membranous and bony labyrinth can be distinguished.

The **membranous labyrinth** is a closed tube system. It is filled with a liquid, the endolymph, and contains the sensory organs. Its complex structure consists of three semicircular canals which contain sensory modalities registering accelerated rotation. Sensory modalities (saccule and utricle) of linear acceleration and static position are located in the region of the vestibule.

The **bony labyrinth** is a cavity in the petrous part of the temporal bone. It surrounds the membranous labyrinth and its shape is identical, but bigger in size. Thus, the resulting space between the two labyrinths is filled with a liquid called perilymph. This perilymphatic space opens via two membranous windows towards the middle ear: the oval window and the round window. The stapes is secured in the oval window and the vibrations of the stapedial foot cause the perilymph to oscillate.

The cochlea records the vibrations of the lymph, which are conferred by the sound-conducting apparatus of the ear. The cochlea is the actual auditory organ. The action potentials arising from the sensory modalities of the equilibrium and the auditory organ are conducted via the vestibulocochlear nerve [VIII] which enters the labyrinth from the posterior cranial fossa via the internal acoustic meatus.

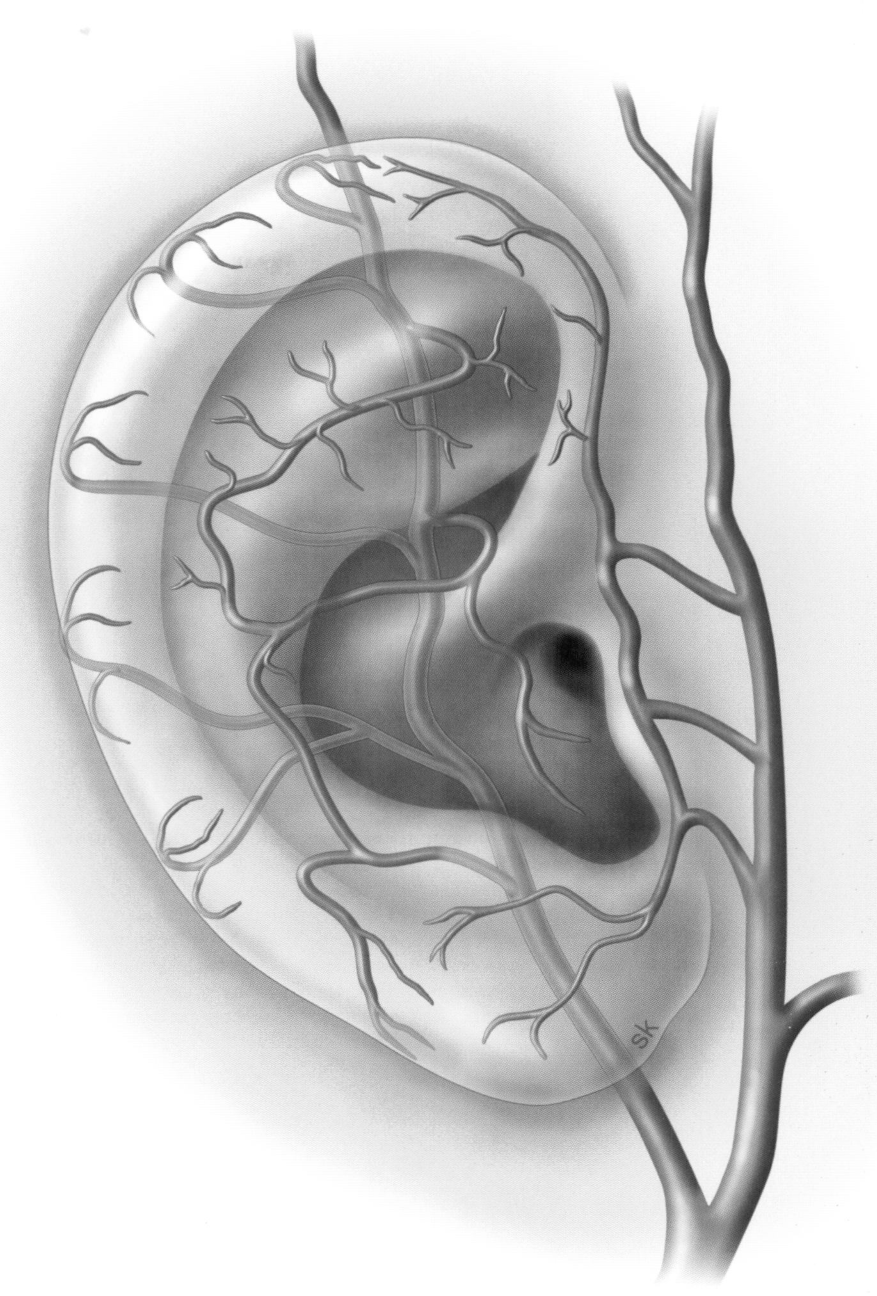
SK

## Clinical Remarks

The most common acute ear diseases affect the inner ear. Permanent **tinnitus,** the perception of sound without real external sound, is experienced by approximately 10–20% of the population. **Sudden sensorineural hearing loss** (SSHL) is an idiopathic disease usually affecting one ear only with variable degree of hearing impairment. In most cases, recovery from SSHL is spontaneous. A frequent disease is **presbyacusis** which occurs after many years of exposure to higher noise levels. **Hearing impairment** (hypacusis) generally describes a reduction in hearing ability. Worldwide, the population over 14 years old frequently have a reduced hearing threshold. There is a wide range of hearing impairment from light reduction in hearing to complete deafness. **Conductive hearing impairment** and **sensorineural causes of hearing impairment** can be distinguished. Common causes of conductive hearing impairment are cerumen (earwax plugging the external acoustic meatus → p. 141), foreign bodies in the external acoustic meatus, inflammation of the external acoustic meatus (→ p. 138), occlusion of the auditory tube (→ p. 143), inflammation of the auditory tube (→ p. 149), middle ear infections (→ p. 144), cholesteatoma (→ p. 147), or otosclerosis (→ p. 142). Sensorineural hearing impairment is frequently caused by aging (see above), genetic syndromes (→ p. 137), infectious diseases, trauma to the head, tumours (→ p. 152), and sudden sensorineural hearing loss. **Vertigo** is the sensation of perceived motion when one is stationary. Vertigo most frequently results from contradictory positional information generated during dysfunction of the vestibular system of the inner ear. There are vestibular causes (inner ear, vestibulocochlear nerve, brain) and non-vestibular causes (e.g. low blood pressure).

*→ Dissection Link*

Auricle (pinna), external acoustic meatus, and tympanic membrane are usually not dissected. The anterior and posterior semicircular canals are displayed by chipping open the bone with a chisel. Both semicircular canals are, in part, deeply embedded in the petrous bone. Usually, the horizontal semicircular canal is only demonstrated. The external acoustic meatus is exposed along the course of the facial nerve [VI] and the vestibulocochlar nerve [VIII] up to the geniculate ganglion, to the cochlea and vestibular system, respectively. Next the branching of the greater petrosal nerve from the geniculate ganglion is visualized. For illustration of the cochlea, the anterior surface of the petrous bone, located medially to the internal acoustic meatus, is removed with a chisel approximately 1–2 mm parallel to the bone surface. The roof of tympanic cavity is now opened. The malleus and incus become visible. For visualization of the stapes, special preparations are required (and therefore this is usually only demonstrated). Starting at the geniculate ganglion, the facial nerve [VII] is traced with care and attention must be paid to the chorda tympani, which runs in the opposite direction in between malleus and incus.

## **EXAM-**CHECK LIST

• Ear development • auricule • external acoustic meatus • ceruminous glands • blood supply • lymph drainage • innervation • otic zoster (RAMSAY HUNT syndrome, geniculate zoster) • middle ear with tympanic membrane and auditory ossicles • walls of the tympanic cavity • topographical relationships • clinical relevance • cholesteatoma • temporal bone • muscles: function and innervation • tympanic plexus • chorda tympani • facial nerve [VII] and vestibulocochlear nerve [VIII] with nuclei • function of the auditory (EUSTACHIAN) tube • cochlea • vestibular labyrinth • semicircular ducts with anatomical position • topography: internal ear in relation to facial nerve [VII] and vestibulocochlear nerve [VIII] • internal acoustic meatus • acoustic neurinoma • petrous part • longitudinal and horizontal fractures of the petrous part • course of the greater and lesser petrosal nerve • geniculate ganglion • vascularization • labyrinthine artery

## Development

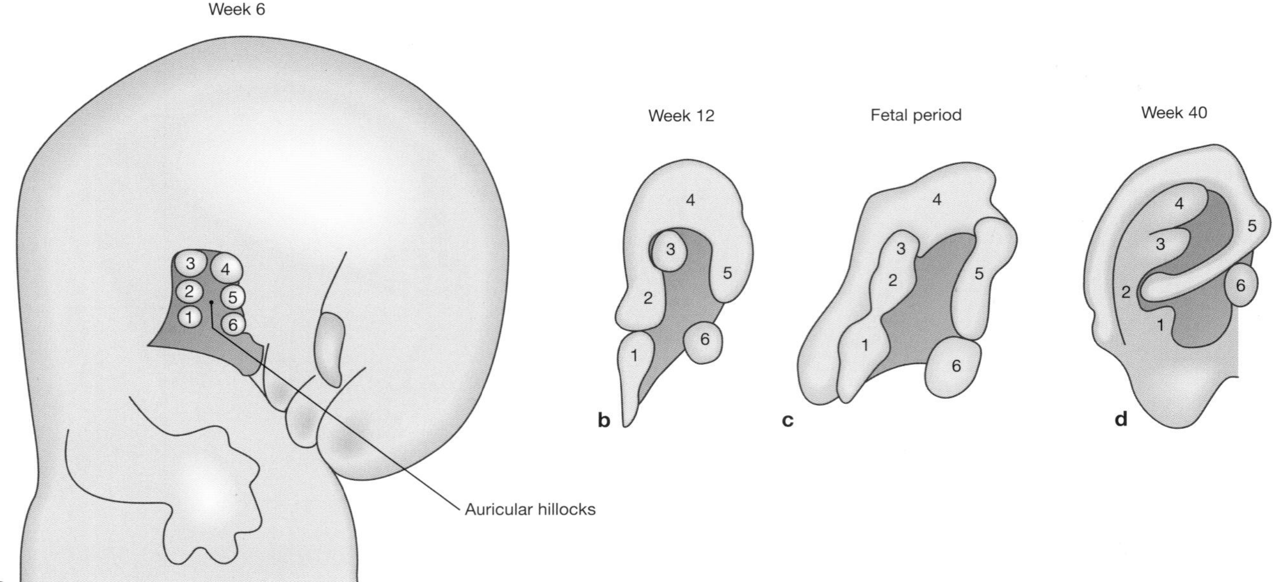
Week 6
Week 12
Fetal period
Week 40
Auricular hillocks
a
b
c
d

**Figs. 10.1a to d Development of the auricle from the six auricular hillocks, right side.** [21]
The merger of the auricular hillocks (1–6) is a complex process and, thus, developmental abnormalities are not infrequent. The primordial auricles start to develop at the base of the neck. As the mandible develops, the auricles move cranially to reach their normal position on both sides of the head at the level of the eyes. Ears positioned deeper in the head frequently are associated with (often chromosomal) developmental abnormalities. The external acoustic canal derives from the posterior part of the first pharyngeal groove which extends inwards as a cone-shaped tube to reach the entodermal epithelial lining of the tympanic cavity (tubotympanic recess). At the beginning of week 9, epithelial cells located at the floor of the external acoustic meatus proliferate to generate a cellular plate, the meatal plug, which normally degenerates by 7 months of fetal development. A persistent plate in the external acoustic meatus is a cause of congenital deafness.

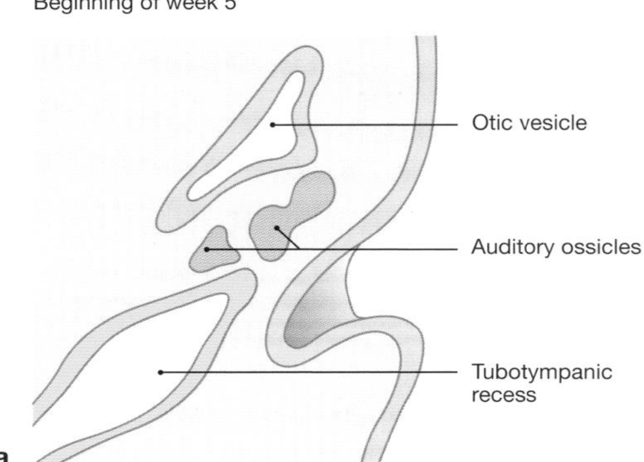
Beginning of week 5
Otic vesicle
Auditory ossicles
Tubotympanic recess
a

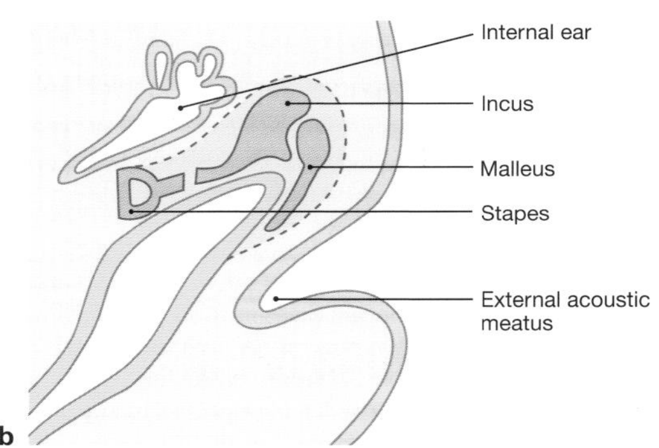
End of week 5
Internal ear
Incus
Malleus
Stapes
External acoustic meatus
b

**Figs. 10.2a and b Differentiation of the auditory ossicles.** [21]
At the beginning of week 5, mesenchymal tissue of the first and second branchial (pharyngeal) arches initiates the formation of auditory ossicles. The first branchial arch (also named manchibular arch) generates the malleus and incus as derivatives of MECKEL's cartilage as well as the tensor tympani which is innervated by the first branchial nerve, the mandibular nerve [V/3]. The second branchial arch generates the stapes, a derivative of REICHERT's cartilage. The stapes can be moved by the stapedius which is innervated by the second branchial nerve, the facial nerve [VII].

### Ear Development

At approximately day 22, a thickening of the **surface ectoderm** occurs on each side of the rhombencephalon. These cellular condensations, the **otic placodes,** invaginate to form the otic or auditory pit which gives rise to the **otic vesicles** (otocyst). Each otic vesicle divides into a **ventral (rostral) part** that gives rise to the saccule and the cochlear ducts and a **dorsal (occipital) part** giving rise to the utricle, semicircular canals, and the endolymphatic ducts. Rostral and occipital parts remain connected through a small duct. The epithelial structures formed in this way are collectively named as the **membranous labyrinth.**
The first pharyngeal groove and the first pharyngeal pouch grow and come in close contact with each other. The external acoustic meatus develops from the ectoderm of the first pharyngeal groove; the **middle ear** derives from the entoderm of the distal part of the first pharyngeal pouch. The proximal part of the first pharyngeal pouch remains narrow and gradually forms the **auditory tube** (EUSTACHIAN tube). The latter has a very narrow connection with the part of the foregut which later becomes the nasopharynx. The distal part of the first pharyngeal pouch develops into the **tympanic cavity.**
In the lateral wall of the tympanic cavity the tubotympanic recess forms and gradually extends towards the invaginating pharyngeal groove. At the site of contact, a thin membrane persists – the **tympanic membrane** (ear drum).
At the beginning of week 5, the **chain of auditory ossicles** develops from mesenchyme derived from the first and second branchial arch. At week 6, six **auricular hillocks** develop at the dorsal end of the first pharyngeal groove and, in a complex progressive process, form the adult auricle.

## Development

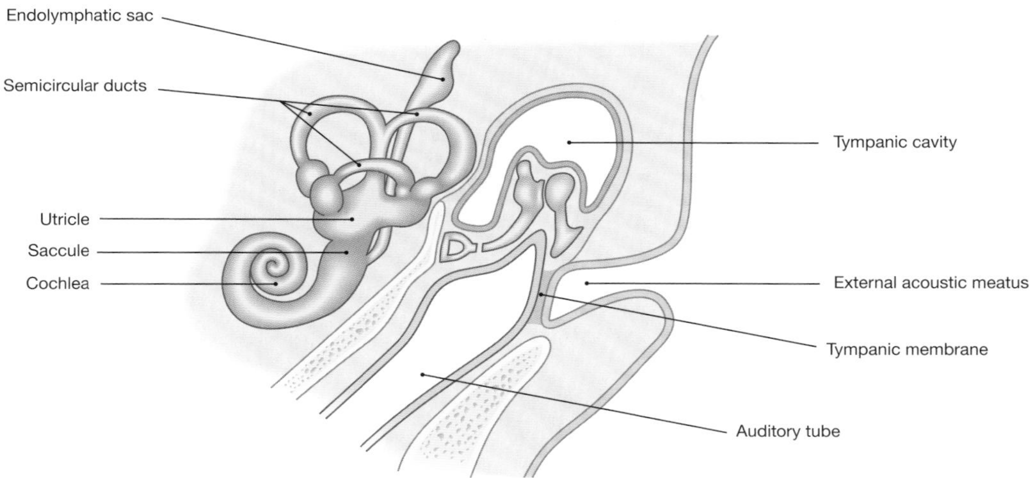
Endolymphatic sac
Semicircular ducts
Utricle
Saccule
Cochlea
Tympanic cavity
External acoustic meatus
Tympanic membrane
Auditory tube

**Fig. 10.3 Structures of the inner, middle, and outer ear at the time of birth.** [21]
Up to 8 months of pregnancy, the initially cartilaginous auditory ossicles are embedded in mesenchyme. Gradually, this mesenchyme is replaced by an entoderm-derived mucosal lining which covers the complete tympanic cavity.

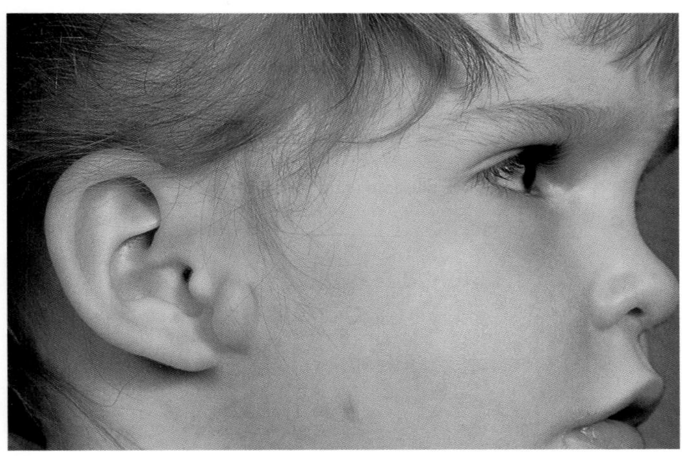

**Fig. 10.4 Child with a pre-auricular skin tag.** [20]
A first degree auricular dysplasia.

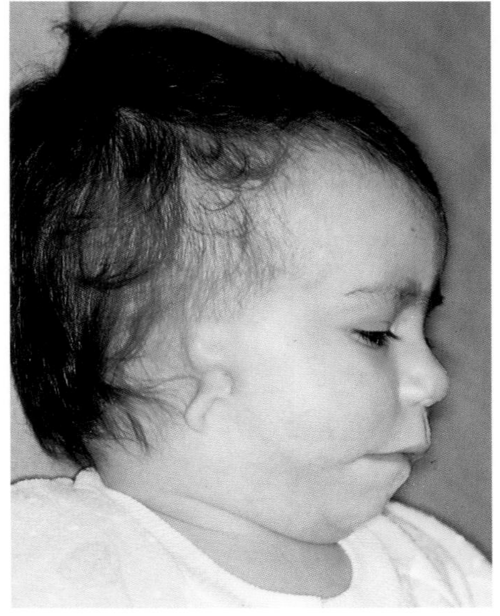

**Fig. 10.5 Child with a small rudimentary auricle (microtia).** [20]
Second degree auricular dysplasia. The auricle is small and severely disfigured. This often includes the external acoustic meatus.

## Clinical Remarks

**Congenital deafness** occurs in 2 of 1000 newborns. One third of these cases have underlying genetic defects. Other causes are infections during pregnancy, chronic diseases of the mother, medication, alcohol, and nicotine. The inability to hear significantly impairs the ability to speak and to develop structured thought processes and communication skills. Thus, early diagnosis and treatment are essential. **External ear defects** are common. These abnormalities are divided into grades 1 to 3 (→ Figs. 10.4 and 10.5). Dominantly inherited FRANCESCHETTI's syndrome (mandibulofacial dysostosis) is an example of a grade 3 dysplasia. Here, a dysplastic first branchial arch and first pharyngeal groove result in defects of the external ear and zygomatic bone, recessed chin, and cleft palate.

## Ear, overview

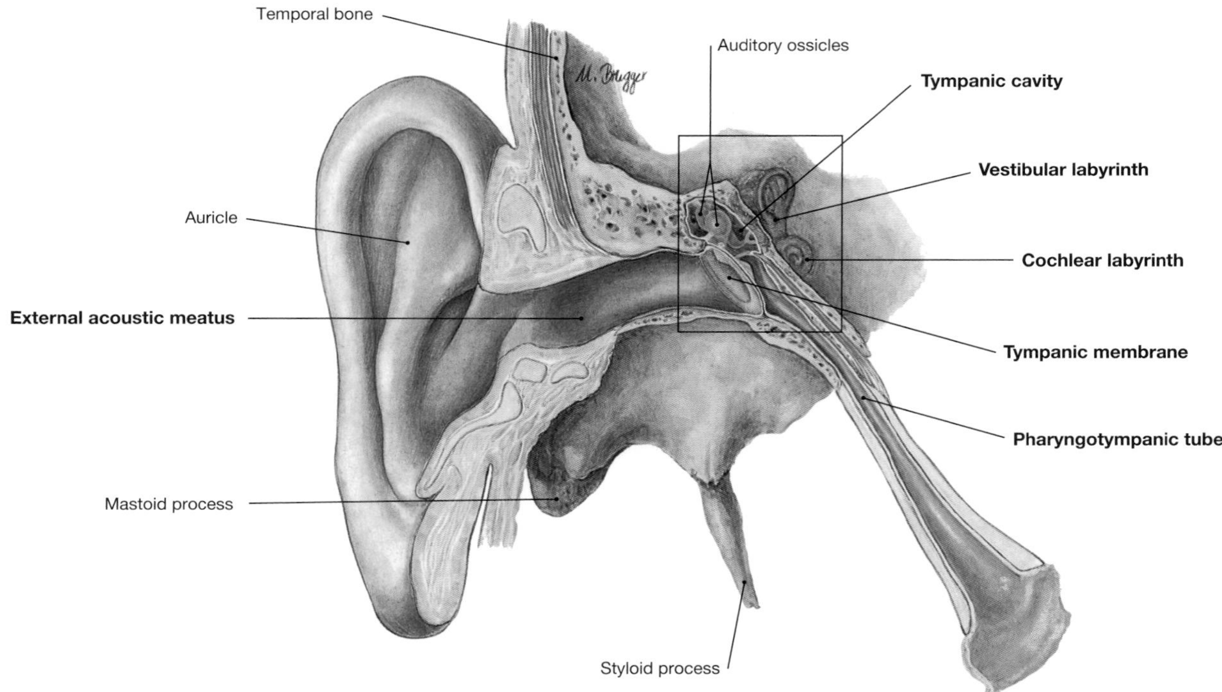
Temporal bone
Auditory ossicles
Tympanic cavity
Vestibular labyrinth
Auricle
Cochlear labyrinth
External acoustic meatus
Tympanic membrane
Pharyngotympanic tube
Mastoid process
Styloid process

**Fig. 10.6 Parts of the ear, right side;** longitudinal section through the acoustic meatus, middle ear, and auditory tube; frontal view.
Presentation of the auricle, external acoustic meatus, tympanic membrane (ear drum), tympanic cavity, auditory ossicles, cochlear labyrinth, and vestibular labyrinth.
Sound waves initiate oscillation of the tympanic membrane **(aerotympanal conduction).** The auditory ossicles transmit the vibrations to the oval window of the inner ear (→ Fig. 10.27) and match the low air impedance (→ Fig. 10.17) with the high fluid impedance of the liquid-filled inner ear (impedance matching). In addition, the inner ear can also sense vibrations of skull bones **(bone conduction).** Within the inner ear, the sound energy propels as a wave (migrating wave). Sensory cells of the inner ear convert the sound energy into **electric impulses** which are transmitted via the cochlear nerve to specific regions of the brain. The vestibular organ serves the perception of rotational and linear accelerations. Motion of the endolymph contained within the vestibular organ results in the deflection of cilia on the surface of sensory cells which are in contact with afferent fibers of the vestibular nerve.

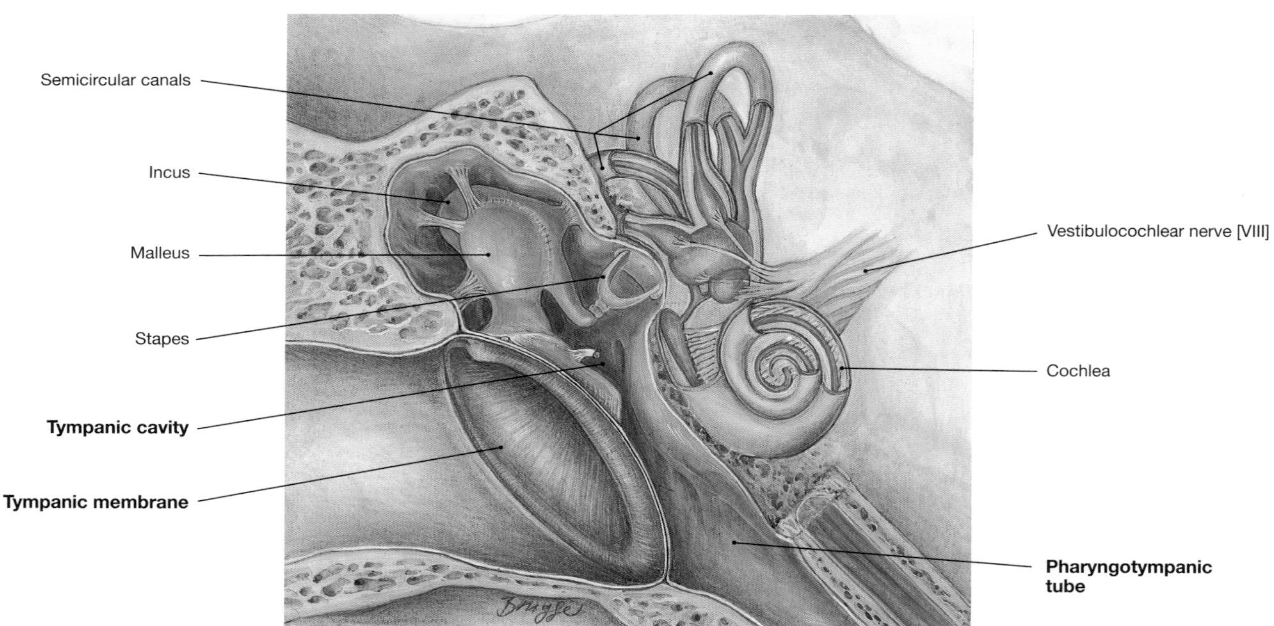
Semicircular canals
Incus
Malleus
Stapes
Tympanic cavity
Tympanic membrane
Vestibulocochlear nerve [VIII]
Cochlea
Pharyngotympanic tube

**Fig. 10.7 Middle and inner ear, right side;** enlarged section of → Figure 10.6; frontal view.
Depicted are the tympanic membrane, the three auditory ossicles in the tympanic cavity: hammer-shaped malleus, anvil-shaped incus, and stirrup-like stapes as well as parts of the membranous labyrinth (blue).

### Clinical Remarks

Mechanical manipulations (e.g., cleaning of the external acoustic meatus) or injury often result in inflammations in the region of the auricle and the external acoustic meatus **(external otitis).**

## Auricle

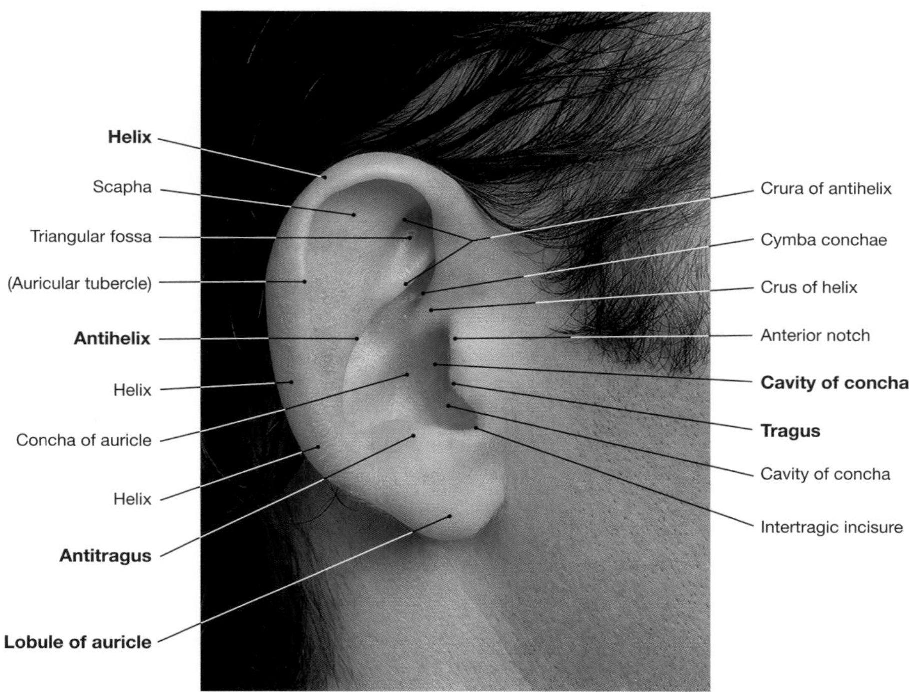
Helix
Scapha
Triangular fossa
(Auricular tubercle)
Antihelix
Helix
Concha of auricle
Helix
Antitragus
Lobule of auricle
Crura of antihelix
Cymba conchae
Crus of helix
Anterior notch
Cavity of concha
Tragus
Cavity of concha
Intertragic incisure

**Fig. 10.8 Auricle, right side;** lateral view.
The basic framework of the auricle consists of elastic cartilage. The skin on the lateral surface of the auricle is fixed to the perichondrium and cannot be moved; on the rear side of the auricle, the skin is movable. Subcutaneous fat tissue is lacking. The earlobe is free of cartilage.

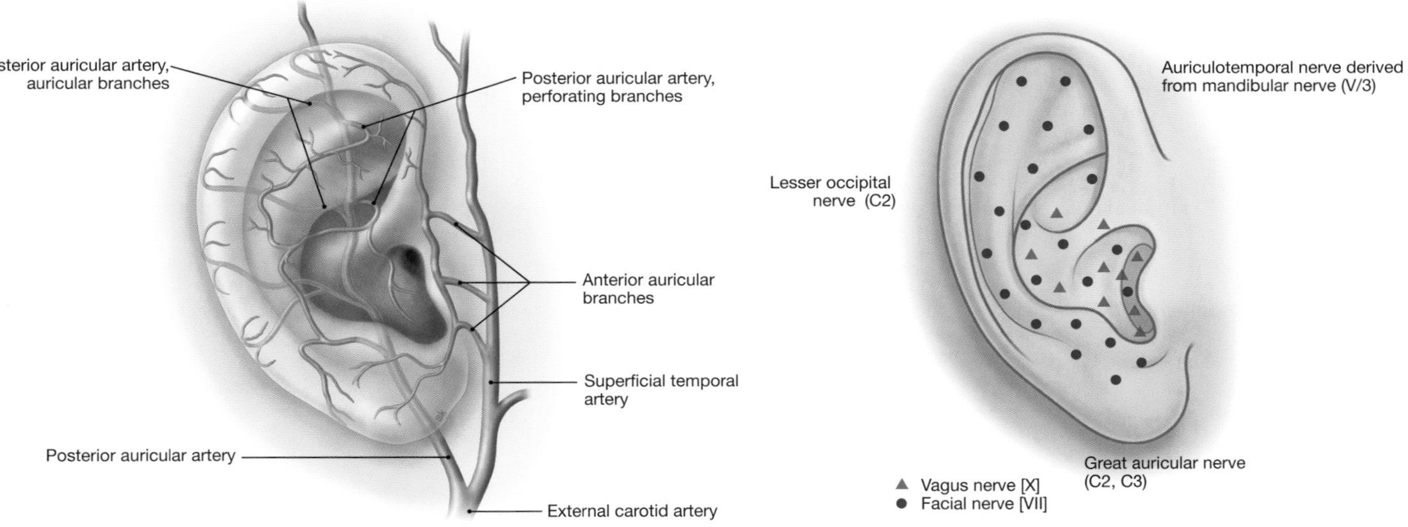
Posterior auricular artery, auricular branches
Posterior auricular artery, perforating branches
Anterior auricular branches
Superficial temporal artery
Posterior auricular artery
External carotid artery
Auriculotemporal nerve derived from mandibular nerve (V/3)
Lesser occipital nerve (C2)
Great auricular nerve (C2, C3)
▲ Vagus nerve [X]
● Facial nerve [VII]

**Fig. 10.9 Arteries of the auricle, right side;** lateral view. [8]
Due to its exposed location, the auricle is highly vascularized (protection against freezing, suitable for heat convection). The supplying arteries are **branches of the external carotid artery** (posterior auricular artery, superficial temporal artery).

**Fig. 10.10 Sensory innervation of the auricle, right side;** lateral view. [8]
The sensory innervation of the auricle is supplied by the **auriculotemporal nerve** (from the mandibular nerve [V/3]) in front of the ear, the **cervical plexus** (great auricular nerve, lesser occipital nerve) for the region behind and below the ear, the **facial nerve** [VII] for the auricle itself (what part of the facial nerve [VII] exactly is involved is not entirely clear), and the **vagus nerve** [X] for the entrance to the external acoustic meatus.

## Auricle and external acoustic meatus

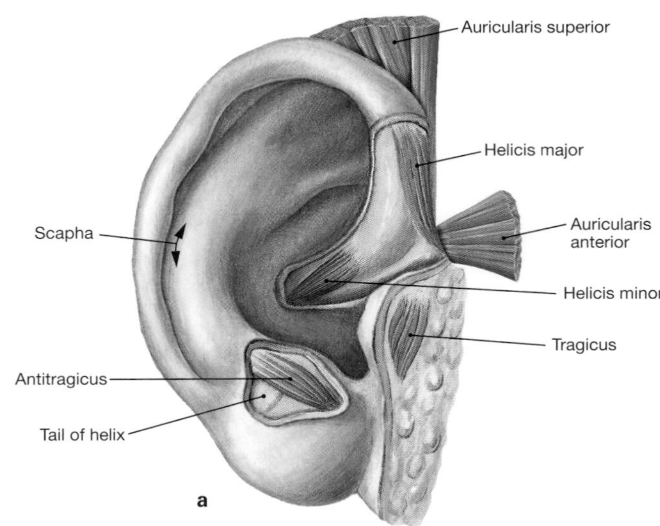
Auricularis superior
Helicis major
Scapha
Auricularis anterior
Helicis minor
Tragicus
Antitragicus
Tail of helix
a

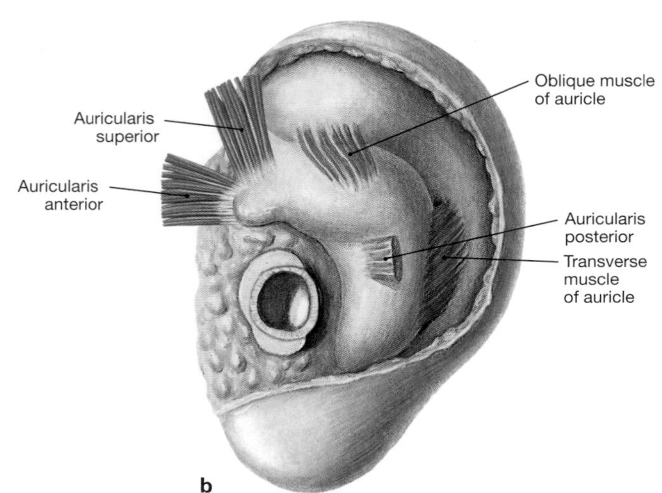
Oblique muscle of auricle
Auricularis superior
Auricularis anterior
Auricularis posterior
Transverse muscle of auricle
b

**Figs. 10.11a and b Muscles and cartilage of the auricle, right side.**
**a** Lateral view
**b** Dorsal view
Rudimentary muscles can sometimes be found attached to the auricle (some people manage to wag their ears). These are facial muscles (innervation by the posterior auricular nerve off the facial nerve [VII]) which are part of a rudimentary sphincter system still found in many animals. Horses, for example, move the auricle such that the external acoustic meatus faces the sound waves. During hibernation, hedgehogs and bears use this sphincter function to occlude the external acoustic meatus and block out unwanted noise.

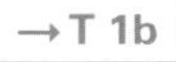
→ T 1b

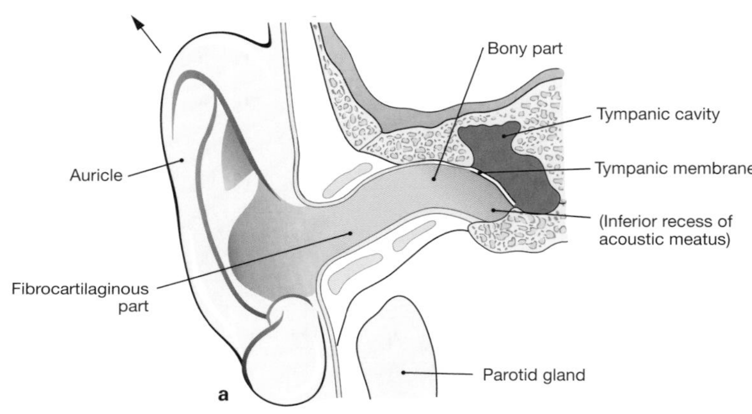
Bony part
Tympanic cavity
Tympanic membrane
(Inferior recess of acoustic meatus)
Auricle
Fibrocartilaginous part
Parotid gland
a

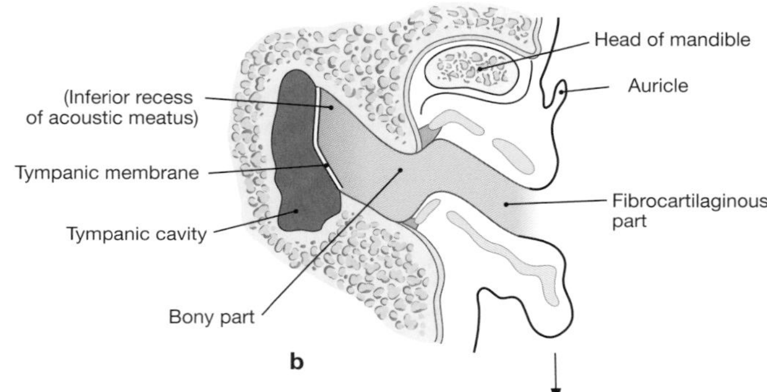
Head of mandible
Auricle
(Inferior recess of acoustic meatus)
Tympanic membrane
Tympanic cavity
Fibrocartilaginous part
Bony part
b

**Figs. 10.12a and b External acoustic meatus, right side;** schematic drawing.
**a** Frontal section
**b** Horizontal section
The external acoustic meatus is S-shaped and is formed by the tympanic part of the temporal bone. The auricle has to be pulled up and backwards in order to inspect the tympanic membrane with a reflecting otoscopic mirror or a microscope (otoscopy). This will straighten the cartilaginous part of the external acoustic meatus and allow the (at least partial) view at the tympanic membrane. **Innervation** of the external acoustic meatus (not shown) is through the nerve to external acoustic meatus of the auriculotemporal nerve (anterior and superior wall), the auricular branch of the vagus nerve [X] (posterior and partially inferior wall), and via the auricular branches of the facial nerve [VII] and the glossopharyngeal nerve [IX] (posterior wall and tympanic membrane).

Arrows: direction of pull on the auricle by the examiner to straighten the external acoustic meatus and allow a view at the tympanic membrane.

## Clinical Remarks

- Inflammation of the elastic cartilage of the auricle **(auricular perichondritis)** can occur as a result of injuries and insect stings. The treatment includes topical application of disinfecting agents as well as local and systemic application of glucocorticoids and antibiotics.
- The earlobes are rich in vascularization, do not contain elastic cartilage, and are easily accessible and, therefore, are often chosen to draw small amounts of blood, e.g. for measuring the blood glucose levels of diabetic patients.
- Abnormalities of the outer ear often require plastic-reconstructive surgery.
- The vagus nerve [X] supplies sensory innervation to the external acoustic meatus. Manipulation in the external acoustic meatus (e.g. removal of cerumen or foreign objects) regularly initiates a cough reflex with the respective person (ARNOLD's reflex). In severe cases, the person can show signs of nausea or collapses.

## Tympanic membrane

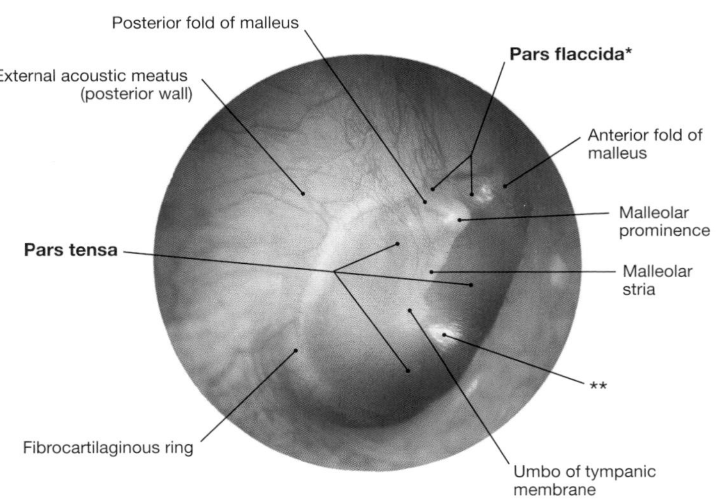
Posterior fold of malleus
Pars flaccida*
External acoustic meatus (posterior wall)
Anterior fold of malleus
Malleolar prominence
Pars tensa
Malleolar stria
**
Fibrocartilaginous ring
Umbo of tympanic membrane

**Fig. 10.13 Tympanic membrane, right side;** lateral view; otoscopic image.
In its anterior, inferior, and posterior aspects, the external acoustic meatus is demarcated by the tympanic part of the temporal bone. In its superior aspect, the bony ring is interrupted by the tympanic notch (attachment point for the pars flaccida of the tympanic membrane). With the exception of the tympanic notch, the otherwise circular tympanic sulcus is located within the tympanic part (the pars tensa of the tympanic membrane is attached here through the fibrocartilaginous ring).

* clinical term: SHRAPNELL's membrane
** typically positioned light reflex

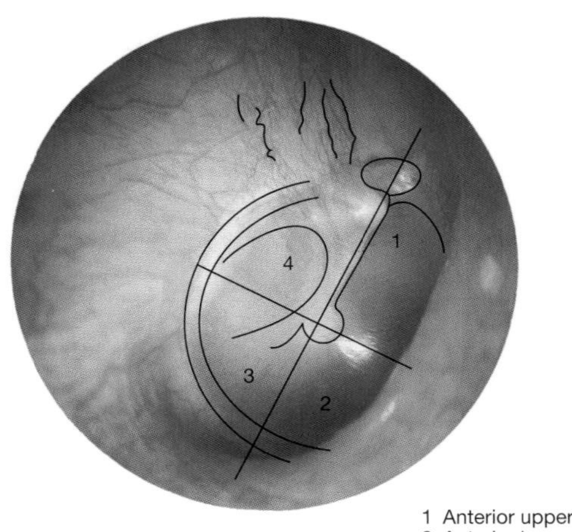
1
2
3
4
1 Anterior upper quadrant
2 Anterior lower quadrant
3 Posterior lower quadrant
4 Posterior upper quadrant

**Fig. 10.14 Tympanic membrane, right side, quadrant scheme.** Lateral view.
Illumination of the pearl-colored tympanic membrane usually results in a triangular light reflex in the anterior lower quadrant, which allows conclusions on the tension of the tympanic membrane.

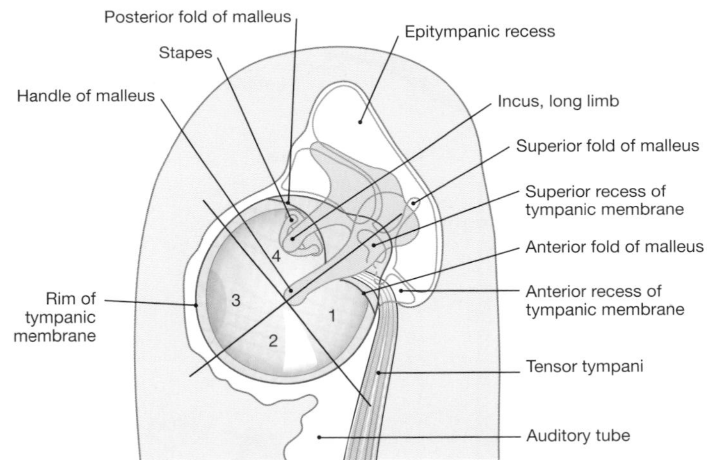
Posterior fold of malleus
Epitympanic recess
Stapes
Handle of malleus
Incus, long limb
Superior fold of malleus
Superior recess of tympanic membrane
Anterior fold of malleus
Rim of tympanic membrane
Anterior recess of tympanic membrane
Tensor tympani
Auditory tube
1
2
3
4

**Fig. 10.15 Tympanic membrane and recess of the tympanic cavity, right side, quadrant scheme;** lateral view; schematic drawing.
The quadrant scheme is of practical clinical relevance. The auditory ossicles are located in the upper quadrants. In addition, the chorda tympani and the attaching tendon of the tensor tympani are localized here (→ Fig. 12.148).

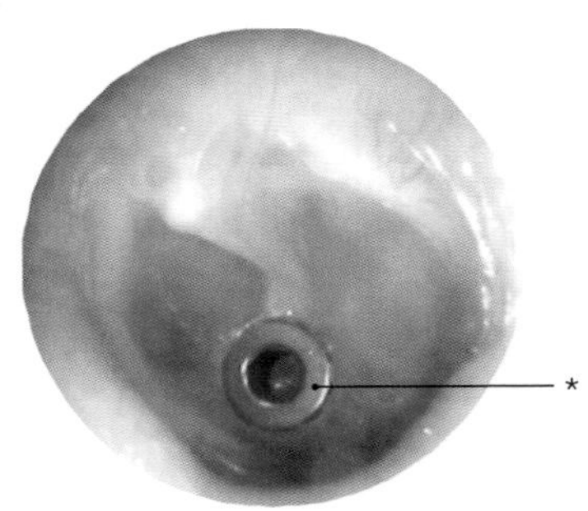
*

**Fig. 10.16 Tympanostomy tube (grommet) in the anterior lower quadrant.**
To avoid injury of structures of the middle ear, a paracentesis (myringotomy; small surgical incision of the tympanic membrane) is performed in the anterior or posterior lower quadrant, respectively. Longer-term ventilation of the tympanic cavity is ensured by inserting a grommet into the incision.

* grommet

## Clinical Remarks

As the pars flaccida is thinner than the pars tensa, spontaneous perforation of the tympanic membrane during **putrid middle ear infection** (otitis media) tends to occur in this part of the tympanic membrane. Serous effusion collecting in the middle ear is visible through the tympanic membrane. This effusion can be drained by myringotomy. Grommets inserted into the opening of the tympanic membrane ensure longer-term drainage and aeration of the middle ear (→ Fig. 10.16). Excessive production of cerumen (earwax) can cause blockage of the external acoustic meatus and conductive hearing loss. Cerumen contains bitter substances that provide some protection against insects and microorganisms.

## Auditory ossicles

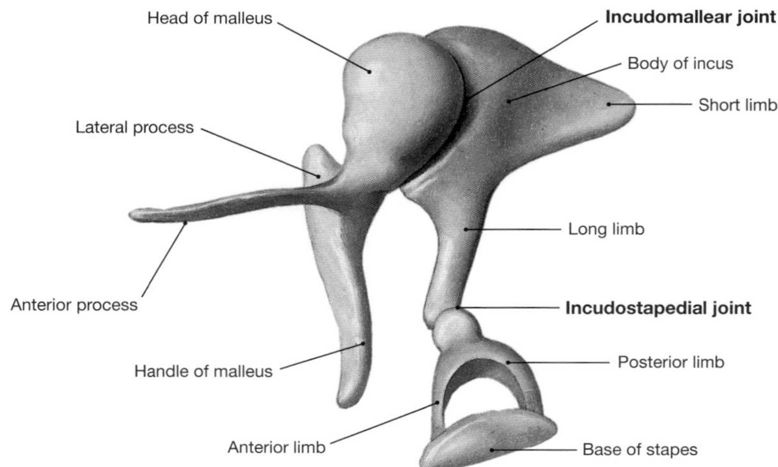
Head of malleus
Incudomallear joint
Body of incus
Short limb
Lateral process
Long limb
Anterior process
Incudostapedial joint
Handle of malleus
Posterior limb
Anterior limb
Base of stapes

**Fig. 10.17 Auditory ossicles, right side;** superomedial view.
The auditory bones of the auditory ossicular chain are connected in series. They are linked by true joints (incudomallear joint– a saddle joint – and incudostapedial joint– a spheroidal joint). The chain of auditory ossicles transmits the energy of the sound waves from the tympanic membrane to the perilymph of the inner ear. This involves the transformation from lower air impedance to the much higher fluid impedance of the inner ear lymph. This requires the amplification of the sound waves (impedance matching), which is accomplished by the size difference between the tympanic membrane (55 mm$^2$) and the oval window (3.2 mm$^2$; 17-times) and the lever action of the auditory ossicles (1.3-times). Thus, the acoustic pressure amplifies by 22-fold.

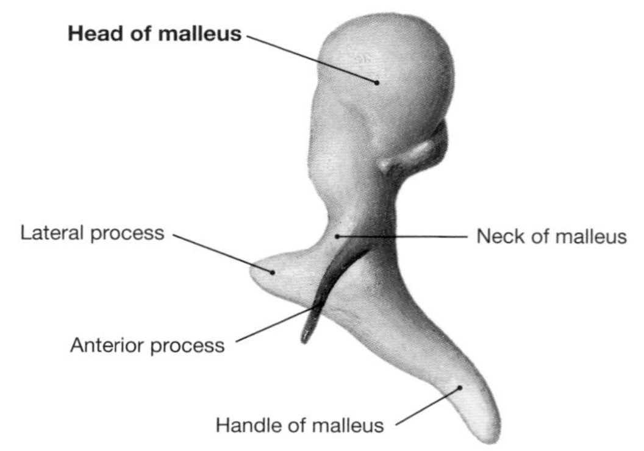
Head of malleus
Lateral process
Neck of malleus
Anterior process
Handle of malleus

**Fig. 10.18 Malleus, right side;** frontal view.

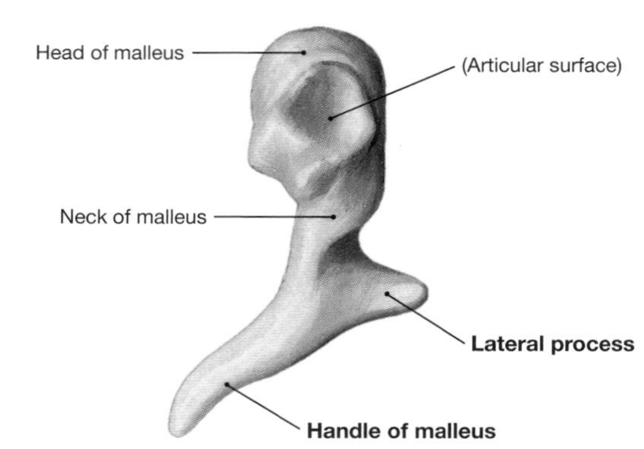
Head of malleus
(Articular surface)
Neck of malleus
Lateral process
Handle of malleus

**Fig. 10.19 Malleus, right side;** posterior view.

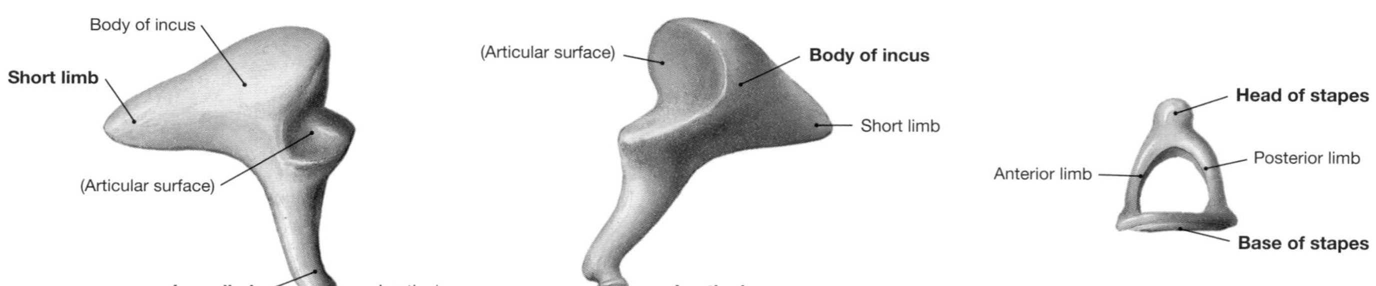
Body of incus
Short limb
(Articular surface)
Long limb
Lenticular process
(Articular surface)
Body of incus
Short limb
Lenticular process
Head of stapes
Posterior limb
Anterior limb
Base of stapes

**Fig. 10.20 Incus, right side;** lateral view.

**Fig. 10.21 Incus, right side;** medial view.

**Fig. 10.22 Stapes, right side;** superior view.

### Clinical Remarks

Defects in the conductive chain (tympanic membrane, auditory ossicles) result in **conductive hearing loss.** Complete loss of transformation of sound pressure results in a reduction of hearing by approximately 20 dB. A typical disease causing such hearing loss is **otosclerosis,** a disease localized in the petrous part of the temporal bone. The base of the stapes progressively fixes to the oval window through ossification of the anular ligament of stapes causing slowly increasing conductive hearing loss. Also noted in some patients is a cochlear contribution with sensorineural hearing loss. Women at 20–40 years of age are affected two times more frequently than men. In 70% of cases, otosclerosis affects both ears.

## Tympanic cavity

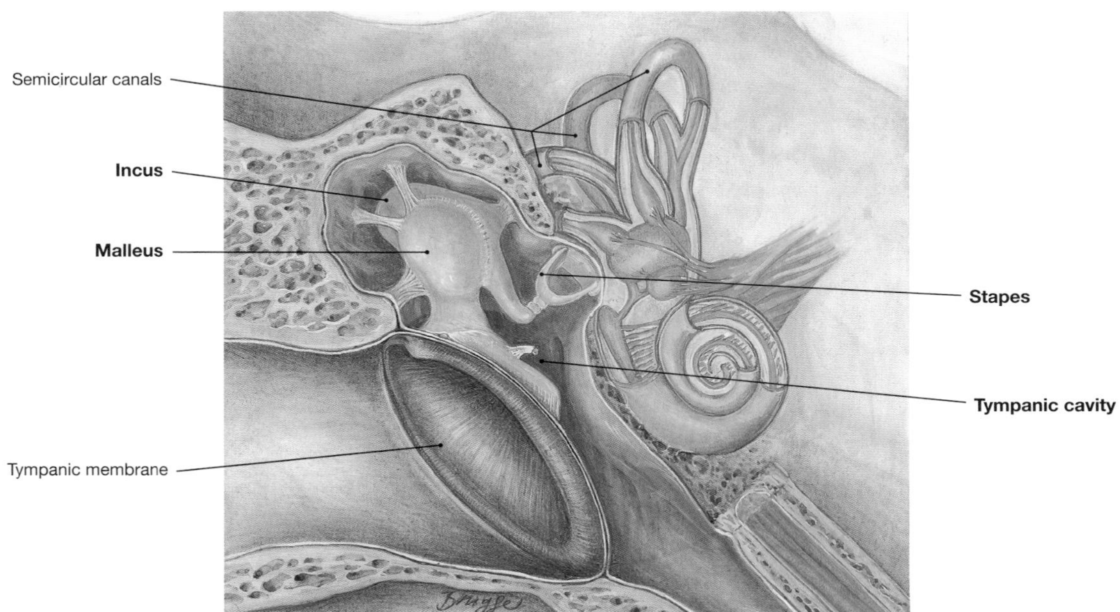
Semicircular canals
Incus
Malleus
Stapes
Tympanic cavity
Tympanic membrane

**Fig. 10.23 Different levels of the tympanic cavity, right side;** frontal view.
From a clinical standpoint, the tympanic cavity divides into three sections named according to their topographic relationship to the tympanic membrane:
- The **epitympanum** (red; epitympanic recess, attic), contains the suspension apparatus and the majority of the ossicles and, through the mastoid antrum, connects with the mastoid cells.
- The **mesotympanum** (blue) contains the handle of malleus, the lenticular process of the incus, and the tendon of the tensor tympani.
- The **hypotympanum** (green; hypotympanic recess) leads into the auditory tube.

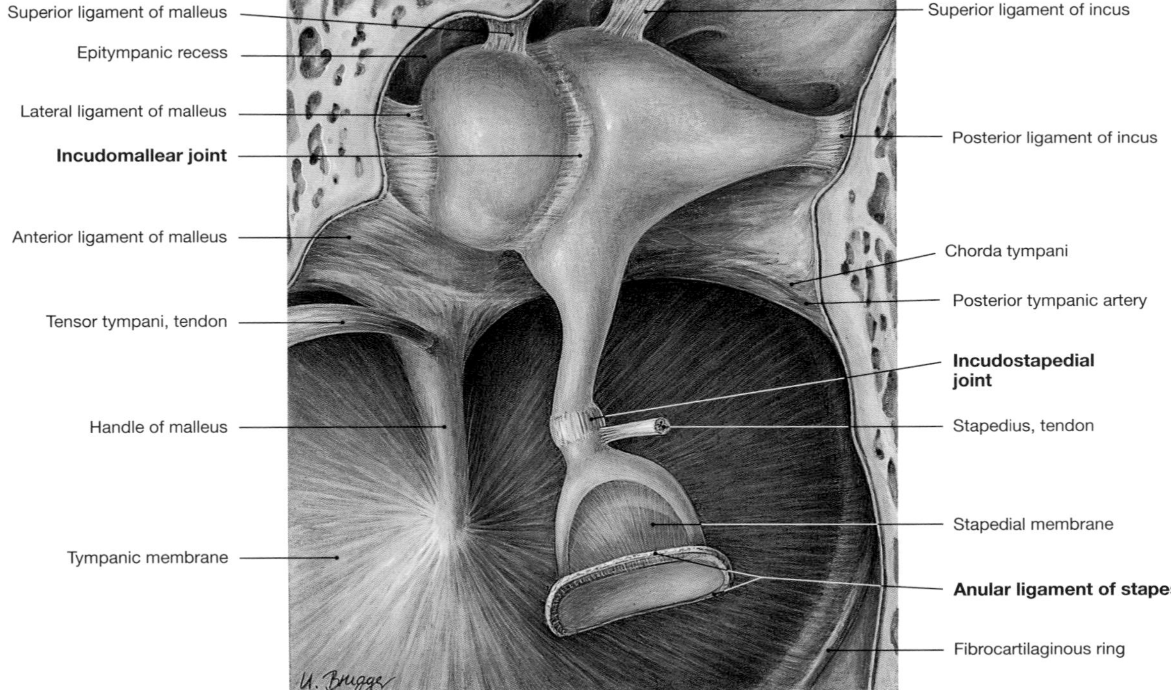
Superior ligament of malleus
Epitympanic recess
Lateral ligament of malleus
Incudomallear joint
Anterior ligament of malleus
Tensor tympani, tendon
Handle of malleus
Tympanic membrane
Superior ligament of incus
Posterior ligament of incus
Chorda tympani
Posterior tympanic artery
Incudostapedial joint
Stapedius, tendon
Stapedial membrane
Anular ligament of stapes
Fibrocartilaginous ring

**Fig. 10.24 Joints and ligaments of the auditory ossicles, right side;** superomedial view.
Ligaments fasten the malleus and incus in the epitympanum. The incudomallear joint (saddle joint) connects both auditory ossicles. The incudostapedial joint (spheroidal joint) connects the stapes with the incus. The base of the stapes is secured to the oval window by the anular ligament of stapes (syndesmosis). All structures in the tympanic cavity, including the chorda tympani, are lined with mucosa of the middle ear.

## Clinical Remarks

In children, one of the most common causes of conductive hearing loss is the **occlusion of the auditory tube** caused by an inflammation of the tube or restricted nasal breathing due to enlarged pharyngeal tonsils (adenoids). With continued functional impairment of the auditory tube, the mucosa of the middle ear starts to secret a seromucous fluid that collects in the tympanic cavity **(seromucous otitis media).**

## Tympanic cavity

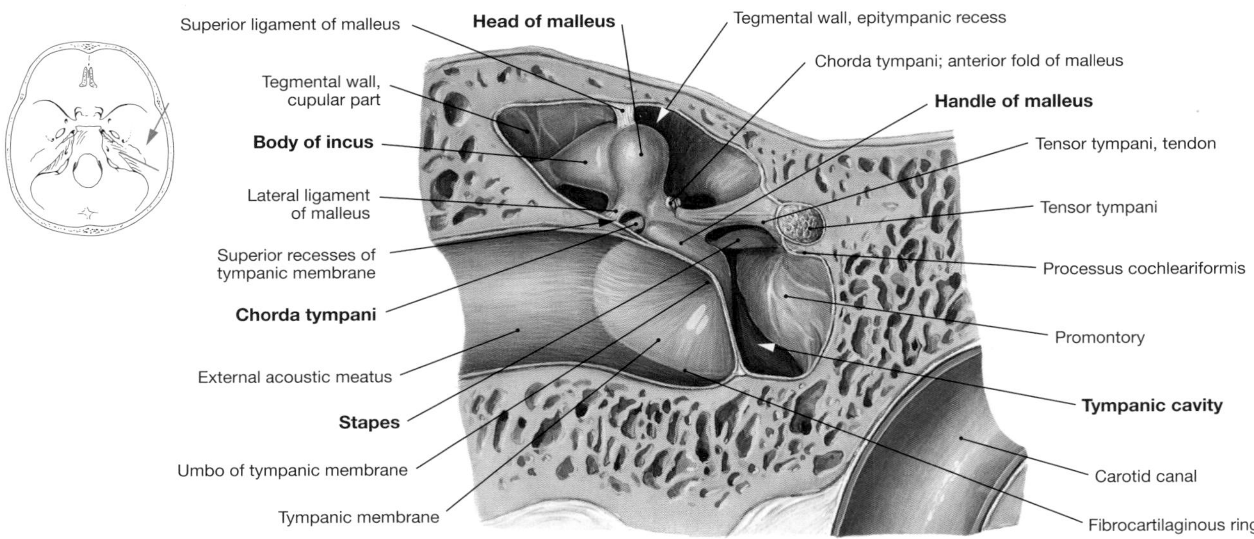
Superior ligament of malleus
Head of malleus
Tegmental wall, epitympanic recess
Chorda tympani; anterior fold of malleus
Tegmental wall, cupular part
Handle of malleus
Body of incus
Tensor tympani, tendon
Lateral ligament of malleus
Tensor tympani
Superior recesses of tympanic membrane
Processus cochleariformis
Chorda tympani
Promontory
External acoustic meatus
Tympanic cavity
Stapes
Umbo of tympanic membrane
Carotid canal
Tympanic membrane
Fibrocartilaginous ring

**Fig. 10.25 Tympanic cavity, right side;** frontal section; frontal view.
The tympanic cavity is an air-filled hollow space within the middle ear and contains the auditory ossicles. The tympanic cavity is located directly behind the tympanic membrane and is aerated and drained by the auditory tube (EUSTACHIAN tube) which also serves in pressure equalization. The spatial distance between the epitympanum and hypotympanum is 12–15 mm and the depth is 3–7 mm, with an inner volume of approximately 1 $cm^3$.

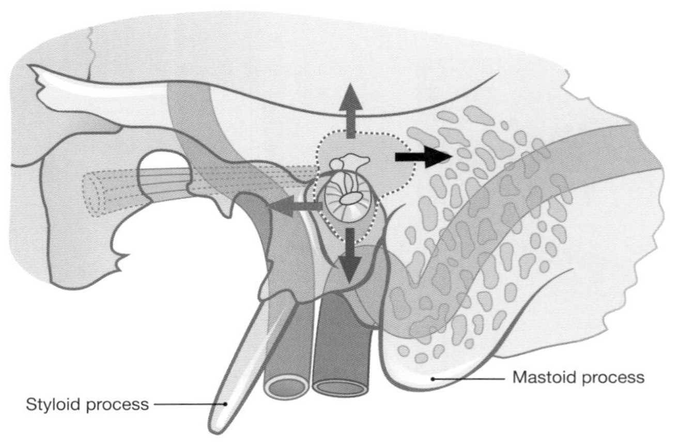
Styloid process
Mastoid process

| Tympanic Cavity | | |
|---|---|---|
| Mastoid process (mastoid wall) | Posterior wall (mastoid process) | → |
| Internal jugular vein (jugular wall) | Inferior wall (jugular fossa) | ↓ |
| Internal carotid artery (carotid wall) | Anterior wall (carotid canal) | ← |
| Middle cranial fossa (tegmental wall) | Superior wall (middle cranial fossa) | ↑ |
| Oval window (labyrinthine wall) | Medial wall (labyrinth) | ⬭ |
| Tympanic membrane (membranous wall) | Lateral wall (tympanic membrane) | |

**Fig. 10.26 Topographical relationships between the tympanic cavity and adjacent structures, right side;** lateral view; schematic drawing.
A thin bony plate (tegmen tympani, **tegmental wall**) separates the epitympanum cranially from the middle cranial fossa. The anterior wall of the mesotympanum **(carotid wall)** is in close proximity to the internal carotid artery. The tympanic membrane makes up the entire lateral wall **(membranous wall).** The auditory tube enters the tympanic cavity in the inferior wall section. The posterior wall (mastoid wall) borders the **mastoid process.** In its posterior upper section, a direct connection exists to the pneumatic spaces of the mastoid (aditus to mastoid antrum). The medial wall (**labyrinthine wall;** → Figs. 10.27 and 10.28) separates the cochlea from the tympanic cavity. The inferior wall of the tympanic cavity **(jungular wall)** belongs to the hypotympanum and separates the tympanic cavity from the internal jugular vein. Here, the bone is very thin and partially air-filled.

## Clinical Remarks

The acute **infection of the middle ear** (otitis media) is one of the most common diseases during childhood. The most frequent cause are bacteria and viruses which reach the middle ear through the auditory tube during or after an infection of the nasopharynx. This inflammation involves increased vascularization (red color), edema, granulocyte infiltration, and pus production. Because the inflammation blocks drainage of pus through the auditory tube, the inflammation can spread to adjacent structures and result in severe **complications,** such as:

- rupture of the tympanic membrane (most frequent case, via membranous wall)
- mastoiditis (via mastoid wall, mastoid antrum, → p. 134)
- thrombophlebitis and thrombosis of the internal jugular vein (via jugular wall)
- septicemia (distribution of pathogenic organisms from the otitis media site through the blood via carotid wall)
- brain abscesses and/or meningitis (via tegmental wall)
- labyrinthitis (with vertigo and hearing impairment via labyrinthine wall)

## Tympanic cavity

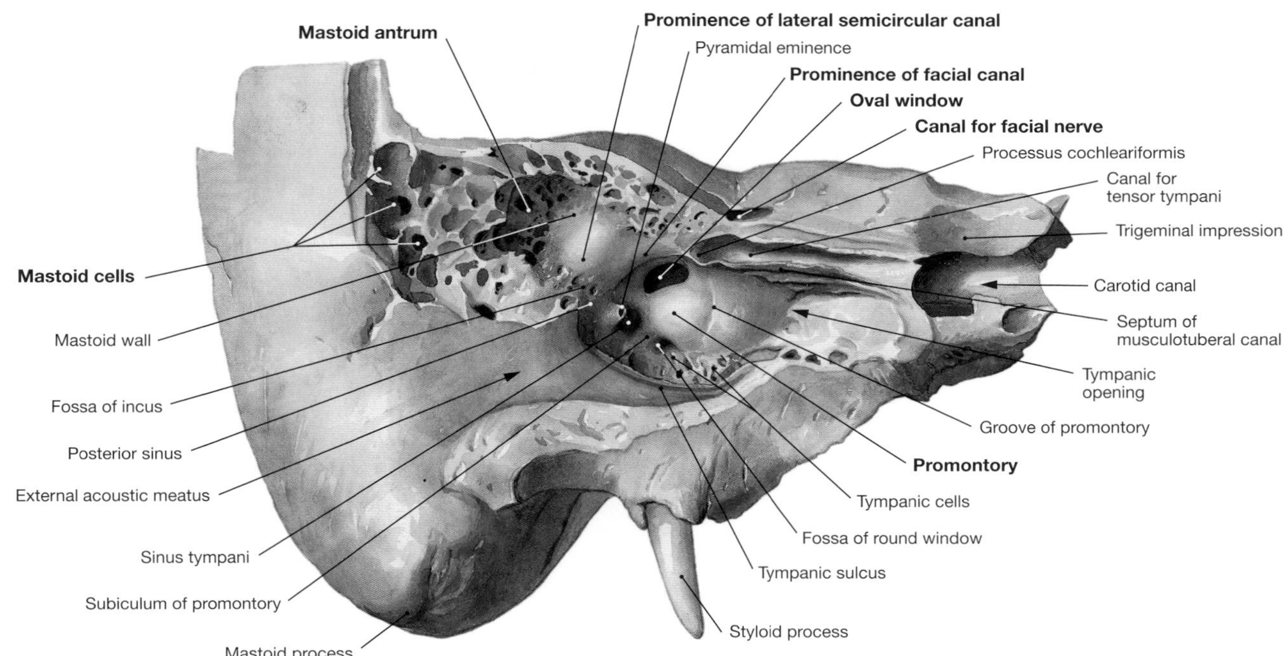
Mastoid antrum
Prominence of lateral semicircular canal
Pyramidal eminence
Prominence of facial canal
Oval window
Canal for facial nerve
Processus cochleariformis
Canal for tensor tympani
Trigeminal impression
Carotid canal
Septum of musculotuberal canal
Tympanic opening
Groove of promontory
Promontory
Tympanic cells
Fossa of round window
Tympanic sulcus
Styloid process
Mastoid cells
Mastoid wall
Fossa of incus
Posterior sinus
External acoustic meatus
Sinus tympani
Subiculum of promontory
Mastoid process

**Fig. 10.27 Medial wall (labyrinthine wall) of the tympanic cavity, right side;** vertical section in the longitudinal axis of the petrous part of the temporal bone; frontolateral view.

Above the oval window, the lateral semicircular canal bulges out the wall of the tympanic cavity to form the prominence of lateral semicircular canal. The facial nerve [VII] passes through the facial canal which is located within the medial wall. This canal creates the horizontal prominence of facial canal in the medial wall. The auditory tube initiates at the tympanic opening. Located along the superior aspect of the auditory tube, the septum of musculotubal canal separates the auditory tube from the canal for tensor tympani. Typically pneumatized (mastoid cells), the mastoid process connects with the tympanic cavity through the mastoid antrum.

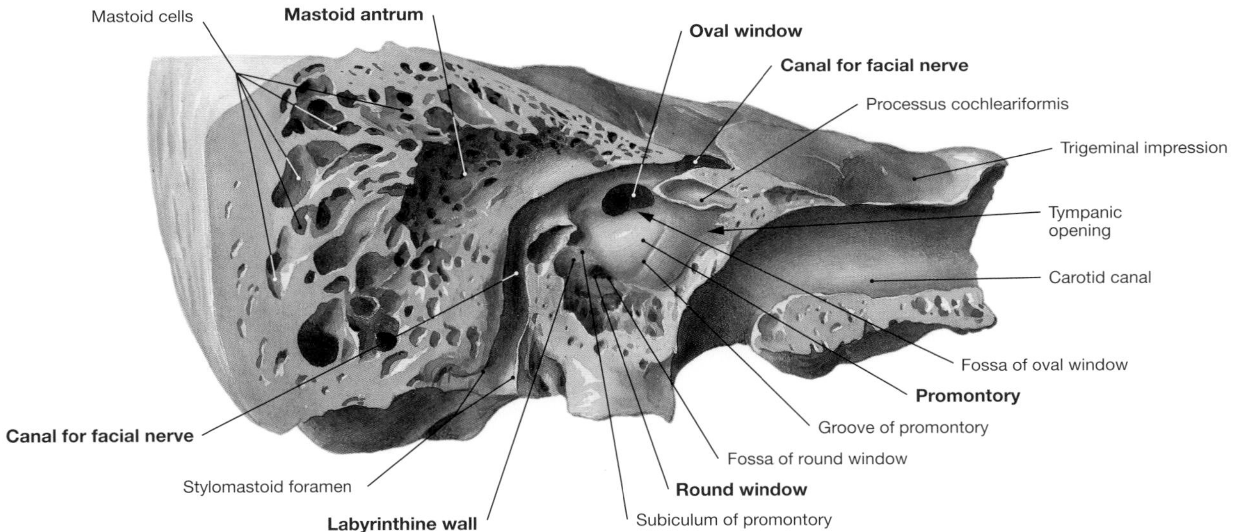
Mastoid cells
Mastoid antrum
Oval window
Canal for facial nerve
Processus cochleariformis
Trigeminal impression
Tympanic opening
Carotid canal
Fossa of oval window
Promontory
Groove of promontory
Fossa of round window
Round window
Subiculum of promontory
Canal for facial nerve
Stylomastoid foramen
Labyrinthine wall

**Fig. 10.28 Medial wall (labyrinthine wall) of the tympanic cavity, right side;** anterolateral view; after removal of the lateral wall and the adjacent parts of the anterior and superior walls; facial canal and carotid canal opened.

The medial walls separates the tympanic cavity from the inner ear (labyrinth) and has two openings:

- the **oval (vestibular) window** with the base of the stapes affixed to it by the anular stapedial ligament
- located more inferiorly, the **round (cochlear) window** occluded by the secundary tympanic membrane.

In the space between oval and round window, the basal cochlear turn creates a prominent bulge in the medial wall of the tympanic cavity, named the promontory.

### Clinical Remarks

Inflammation of the mastoid cells **(mastoiditis)** caused by an inflammatory process in the tympanic cavity is a frequent complication of otitis media. The inflammation can spread from the mastoid and affect the soft tissue behind and in front of the outer ear, the sternocleidomastoid, the inner ear, the sigmoid sinus, the meninges, and the facial nerve [VII].

## Tympanic cavity, topography

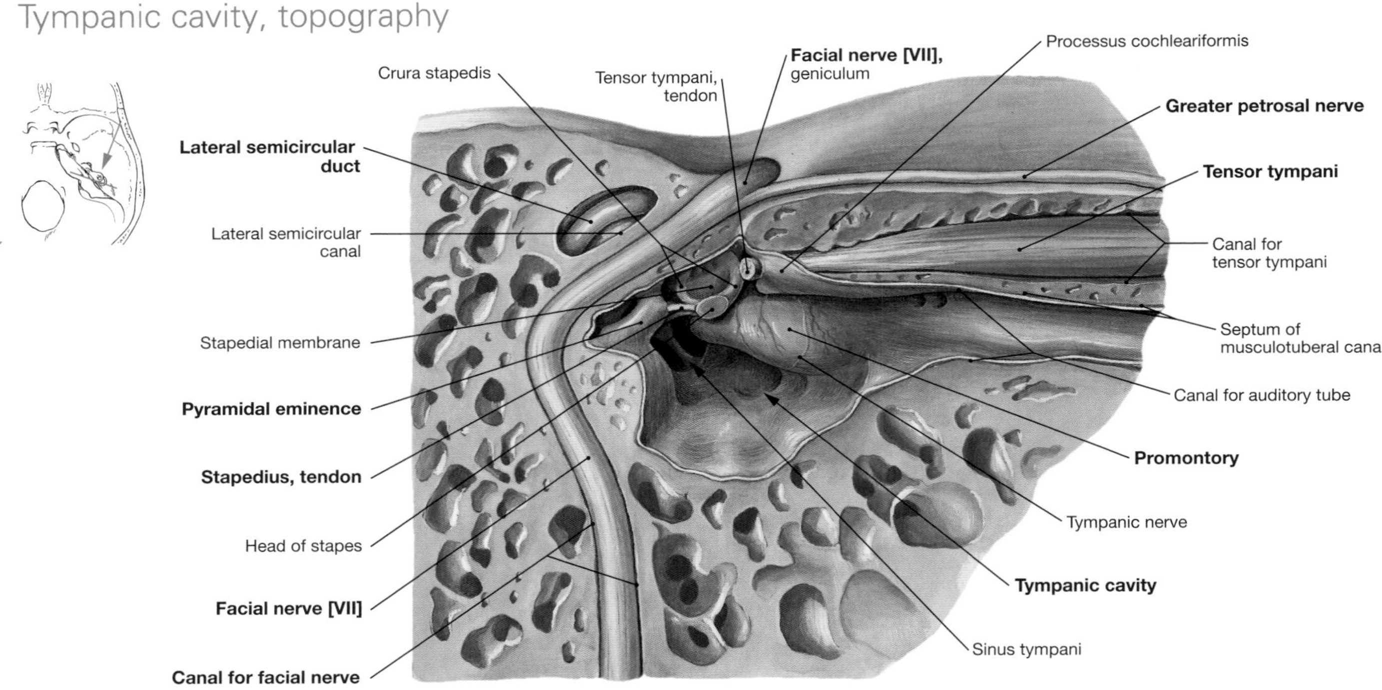
Crura stapedis
Tensor tympani, tendon
Facial nerve [VII], geniculum
Processus cochleariformis
Greater petrosal nerve
Tensor tympani
Canal for tensor tympani
Septum of musculotuberal canal
Canal for auditory tube
Promontory
Tympanic nerve
Tympanic cavity
Sinus tympani
Lateral semicircular duct
Lateral semicircular canal
Stapedial membrane
Pyramidal eminence
Stapedius, tendon
Head of stapes
Facial nerve [VII]
Canal for facial nerve

**Fig. 10.29 Facial nerve [VII], tympanic cavity, and auditory tube, right side;** vertical section in the longitudinal axis of the petrous part of the temporal bone; frontal view; facial canal opened.

The facial nerve [VII] is composed of two branches, the actual facial nerve and the intermediate nerve. Both branches combine deep in the facial canal to form the intermediofacial nerve (henceforth referred to as facial nerve [VII]). It arches around the tympanic cavity and generates the prominence of facial canal in the medial wall of the tympanic cavity. Beneath thereof, the pyramidal eminence protrudes into the cavity. It houses the stapedius muscle innervated by the facial nerve (→ Fig. 12.152). The tendon of the stapedius exits the pyramidal eminence and inserts at the inferior lateral aspect of the stapedial head.

**Function of the stapedius:** It attenuates vibrations at the oval window by slightly tilting the stapes, thus, decreasing the transmission of sound waves and protecting the sensory cells of the inner ear from excessive noise.

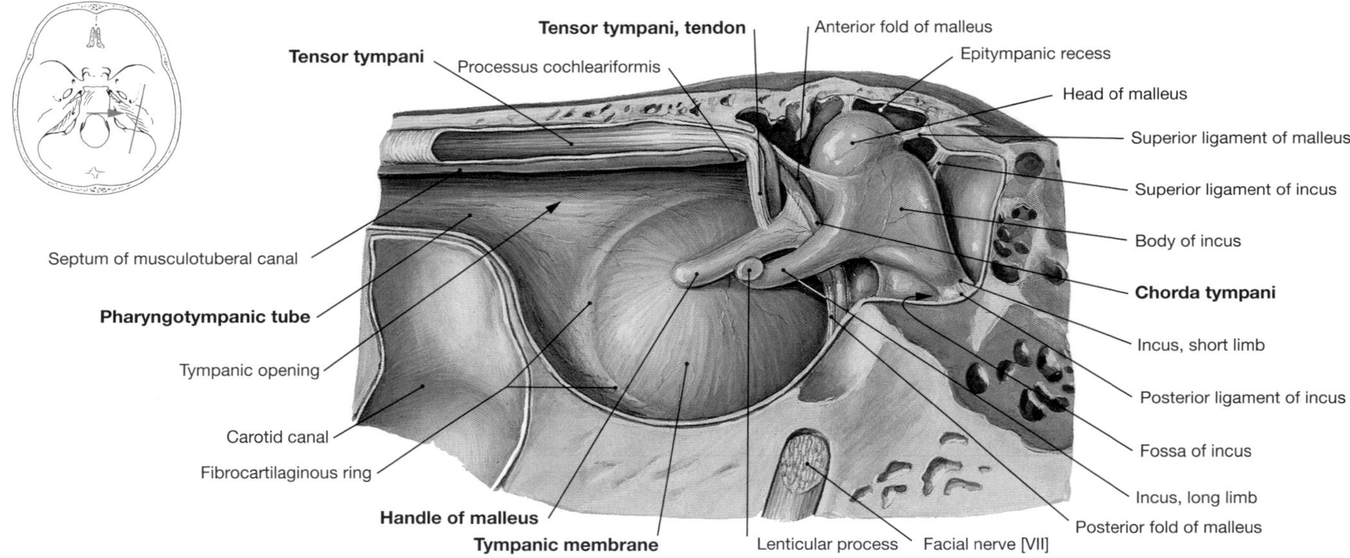
Tensor tympani, tendon
Anterior fold of malleus
Tensor tympani
Processus cochleariformis
Epitympanic recess
Head of malleus
Superior ligament of malleus
Superior ligament of incus
Body of incus
Chorda tympani
Incus, short limb
Posterior ligament of incus
Fossa of incus
Incus, long limb
Posterior fold of malleus
Septum of musculotuberal canal
Pharyngotympanic tube
Tympanic opening
Carotid canal
Fibrocartilaginous ring
Handle of malleus
Tympanic membrane
Lenticular process
Facial nerve [VII]

**Fig. 10.30 Lateral wall (membranous wall) of the tympanic cavity, right side;** medial view.

The musculotubal canal enters the tympanic cavity from the front. It is composed of two bony semicanals, separated by a bony septum, and contains the tensor tympani and the auditory tube. At the processus cochleariformis, the tendon of the tensor tympani makes a right angle turn and inserts at the handle of malleus.

**Function of the tensor tympani:** It increases the tension of the tympanic membrane by pulling at the handle of malleus. This results in the chain of auditory ossicles to become more rigid and this improves their ability to transmit high-frequency sound waves. Shortly before the end of the facial canal, the chorda tympani leaves the facial nerve [VII], runs backwards through its own bony canal into the tympanic cavity and, embedded in mucosa, courses through the center of the tympanic cavity between malleus and long limb of the incus. The chorda tympani exits the cranial base through the sphenopetrosal fissure (or petrotympanic fissure).

### Clinical Remarks

Paralysis of the nerve of stapedius in the case of facial nerve palsy alters the auditory sensation. Normal sounds are perceived as unpleasantly loud **(hyperacusis)** due to the insufficient dampening action of the stapedius muscle (no tilting of the base of the stapes in the oval window).

## Facial nerve [VII], topography

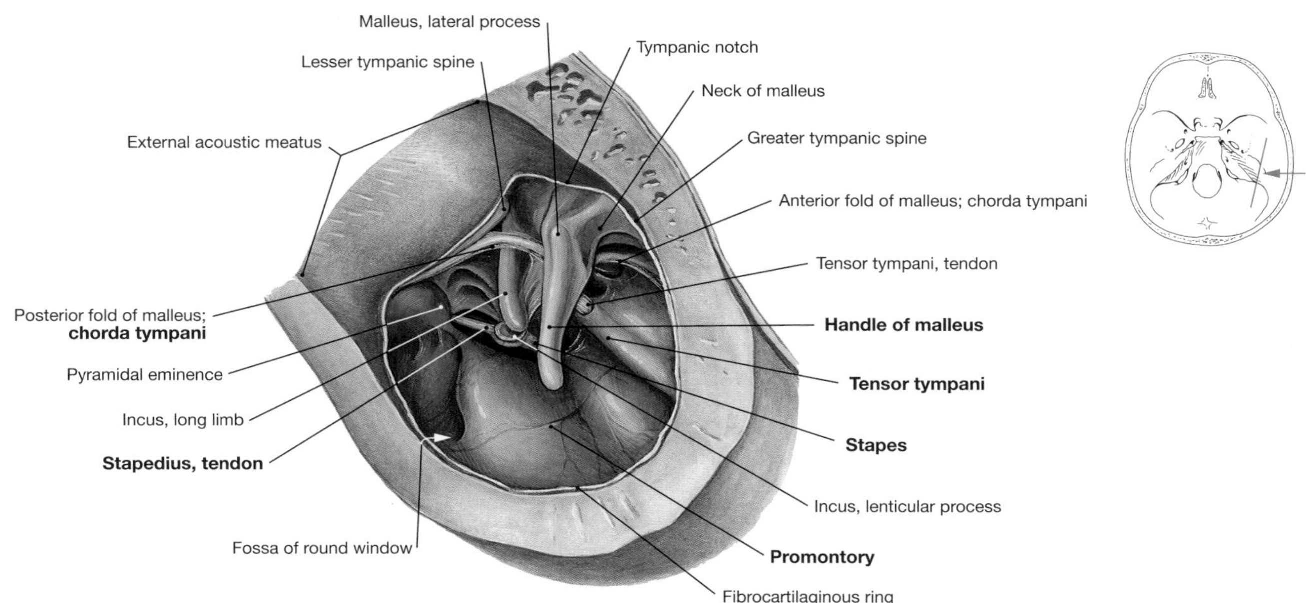
Malleus, lateral process
Lesser tympanic spine
Tympanic notch
Neck of malleus
External acoustic meatus
Greater tympanic spine
Anterior fold of malleus; chorda tympani
Tensor tympani, tendon
Posterior fold of malleus; chorda tympani
Handle of malleus
Pyramidal eminence
Tensor tympani
Incus, long limb
Stapes
Stapedius, tendon
Incus, lenticular process
Fossa of round window
Promontory
Fibrocartilaginous ring

**Fig. 10.31 Tympanic cavity, right side;** lateral view after removal of the tympanic membrane and the mucosal layer around the chorda tympani.
The structures of the tympanic cavity covered by mucosa are shown.

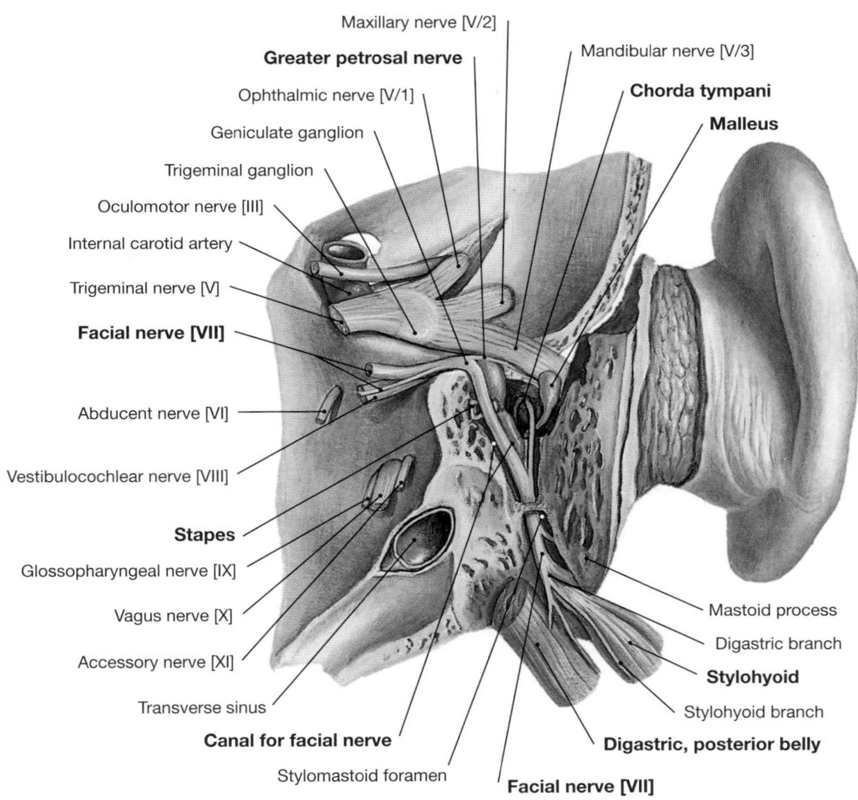
Maxillary nerve [V/2]
Greater petrosal nerve
Mandibular nerve [V/3]
Ophthalmic nerve [V/1]
Chorda tympani
Geniculate ganglion
Malleus
Trigeminal ganglion
Oculomotor nerve [III]
Internal carotid artery
Trigeminal nerve [V]
Facial nerve [VII]
Abducent nerve [VI]
Vestibulocochlear nerve [VIII]
Stapes
Glossopharyngeal nerve [IX]
Vagus nerve [X]
Mastoid process
Digastric branch
Accessory nerve [XI]
Stylohyoid
Transverse sinus
Stylohyoid branch
Canal for facial nerve
Digastric, posterior belly
Stylomastoid foramen
Facial nerve [VII]

**Fig. 10.32 Facial nerve [VII] in the petrous part of the temporal bone, right side;** posterior view; petrous bone partially removed; facial canal and tympanic cavity opened.
After removal of the mastoid process and opening of the facial canal and the tympanic cavity, the entire course of the facial nerve [VII] and its branches in the bony canal become visible (→ Fig. 12.148).

## Clinical Remarks

Injuries to the facial nerve [VII] can occur during fractures of the petrous bone, inflammation of the middle ear or mastoid process, and surgical intervention in response to these scenarios. For proper **diagnosis** of the location of a lesion and follow-up examinations of facial nerve palsy, a variety of tests are employed: SCHIRMER's test (function of the lacrimal gland), stapedius reflex, testing of taste and sometimes sialometry (testing the function of the salivary glands) to examine the chorda tympani as well as electromyography (EMG) and electroneuronography (ENoG) for the testing of the mimic muscles. The chorda tympani courses through the middle ear and is vulnerable to injuries during operations in the middle ear. An isolated **functional loss of the chorda tympani** with dry mouth and loss of taste sensation on the affected side is common during middle ear infections.

## Facial nerve [VII], topography

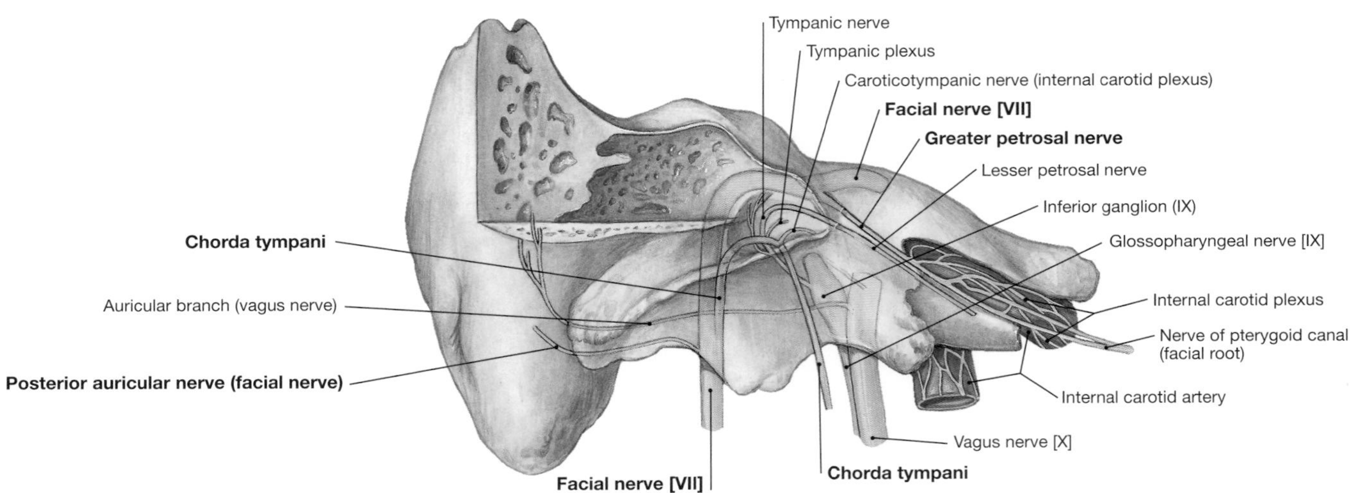
Tympanic nerve
Tympanic plexus
Caroticotympanic nerve (internal carotid plexus)
Facial nerve [VII]
Greater petrosal nerve
Lesser petrosal nerve
Inferior ganglion (IX)
Glossopharyngeal nerve [IX]
Internal carotid plexus
Nerve of pterygoid canal (facial root)
Internal carotid artery
Vagus nerve [X]
Chorda tympani
Facial nerve [VII]
Posterior auricular nerve (facial nerve)
Auricular branch (vagus nerve)
Chorda tympani

**Fig. 10.33 Facial nerve [VII], glossopharyngeal nerve [IX], and vagus nerve [X], right side;** frontal view; petrous bone partially removed; nerves are shown transparently.

The **greater petrosal nerve** is the first branch to leave the facial nerve [VII] at the geniculate ganglion. The greater petrosal nerve projects frontomedially and exits the temporal bone at the hiatus for greater petrosal nerve below the dura mater on the anterior surface of the petrous part of the temporal bone. This nerve provides preganglionic parasympathetic fibers to the pterygopalatine ganglion for the innervation of lacrimal and nasal glands. Shortly after passing through the stylomastoid foramen, the facial nerve [VII] releases the **posterior auricular nerve** for the innervation of the auricle. Shown are also the auricular branch of the vagus nerve [X] for the sensory innervation of the external acoustic meatus and the tympanic nerve which branches off the glossopharyngeal nerve shortly before this cranial nerve passes through the jugular foramen. Together with branches derived from a sympathetic network (internal carotid plexus, caroticotympanic nerves) surrounding the internal carotid artery, the tympanic nerve participates in the formation of a neuronal plexus in the mucosal layer of the promontory. This tympanic plexus innervates the entire mucosa of the middle ear as well as the mucosal layer of the auditory tube and the mastoid process.

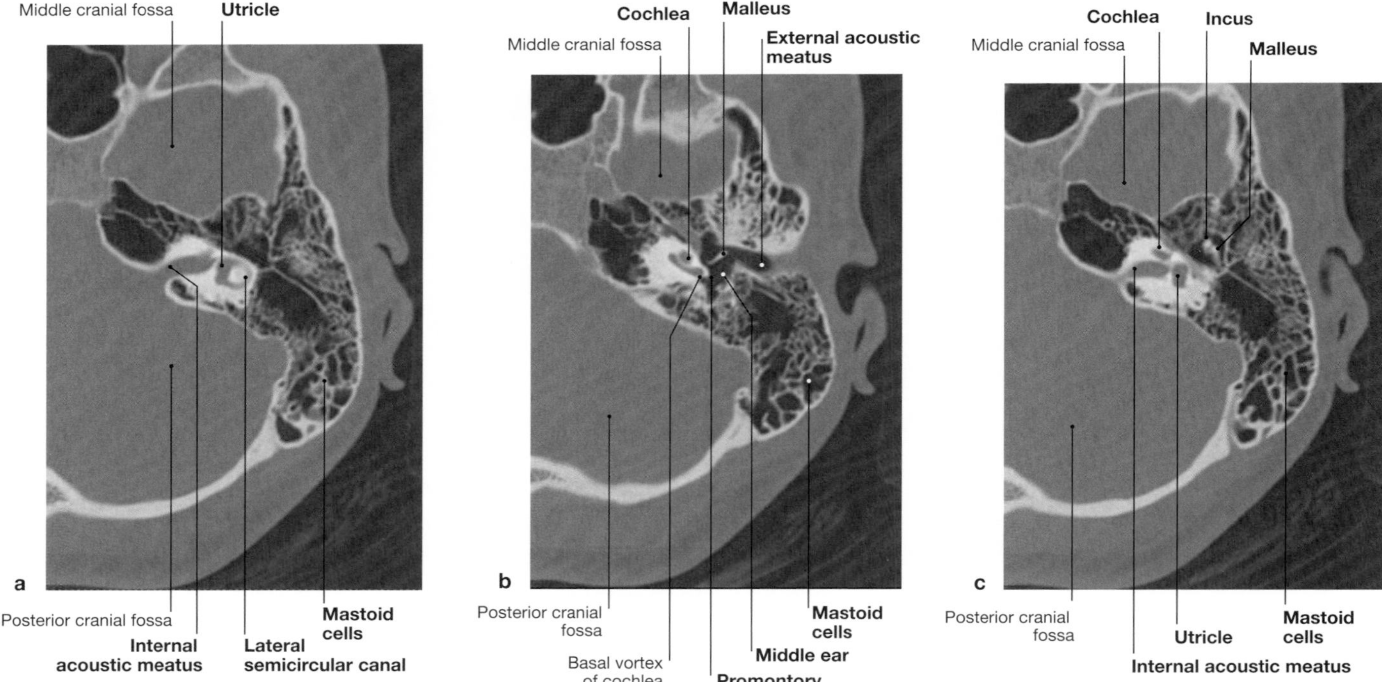
Middle cranial fossa
Utricle
a
Posterior cranial fossa
Internal acoustic meatus
Lateral semicircular canal
Mastoid cells
Cochlea
Malleus
Middle cranial fossa
External acoustic meatus
b
Posterior cranial fossa
Basal vortex of cochlea
Promontory
Middle ear
Mastoid cells
Cochlea
Incus
Middle cranial fossa
Malleus
c
Posterior cranial fossa
Utricle
Internal acoustic meatus
Mastoid cells

**Figs. 10.34a to c Temporal bone with middle and inner ear, left ear;** computed tomographic section (CT), inferior view. [10]

High-resolution CT is able to visualize in detail all structures of the middle and inner ear. For example, this imaging technique allows for the evaluation of the internal acoustic meatus, the pneumatization of the mastoid process, the positioning of the auditory ossicles, and the labyrinth.

### Clinical Remarks

The facial nerve [VII] can be accessed surgically through the mastoid process, for example to provide relief for an inflamed and swollen facial nerve. Upon careful removal of the mastoid bone, the posterior section of the facial canal is exposed.

## Auditory tube

**Fig. 10.35 Cartilage of the auditory tube, right side;** inferior view; exposed at the base of the skull.
Projecting in an oblique angle from a cranial posterolateral to a frontomedial caudal position, the approximately 4 cm long auditory tube, EUSTACHIAN tube) connects the tympanic cavity with the nasopharynx (nasal part of the pharynx). It serves in pressure equalization. The requirement for optimal transmission of sound waves is equal air pressure in both the tympanic cavity (the tympanic membrane is impermeable to air) and the external acoustic meatus compartment. If this is not the case, e.g. during the ascent or descent flight of a plane, impaired hearing results.

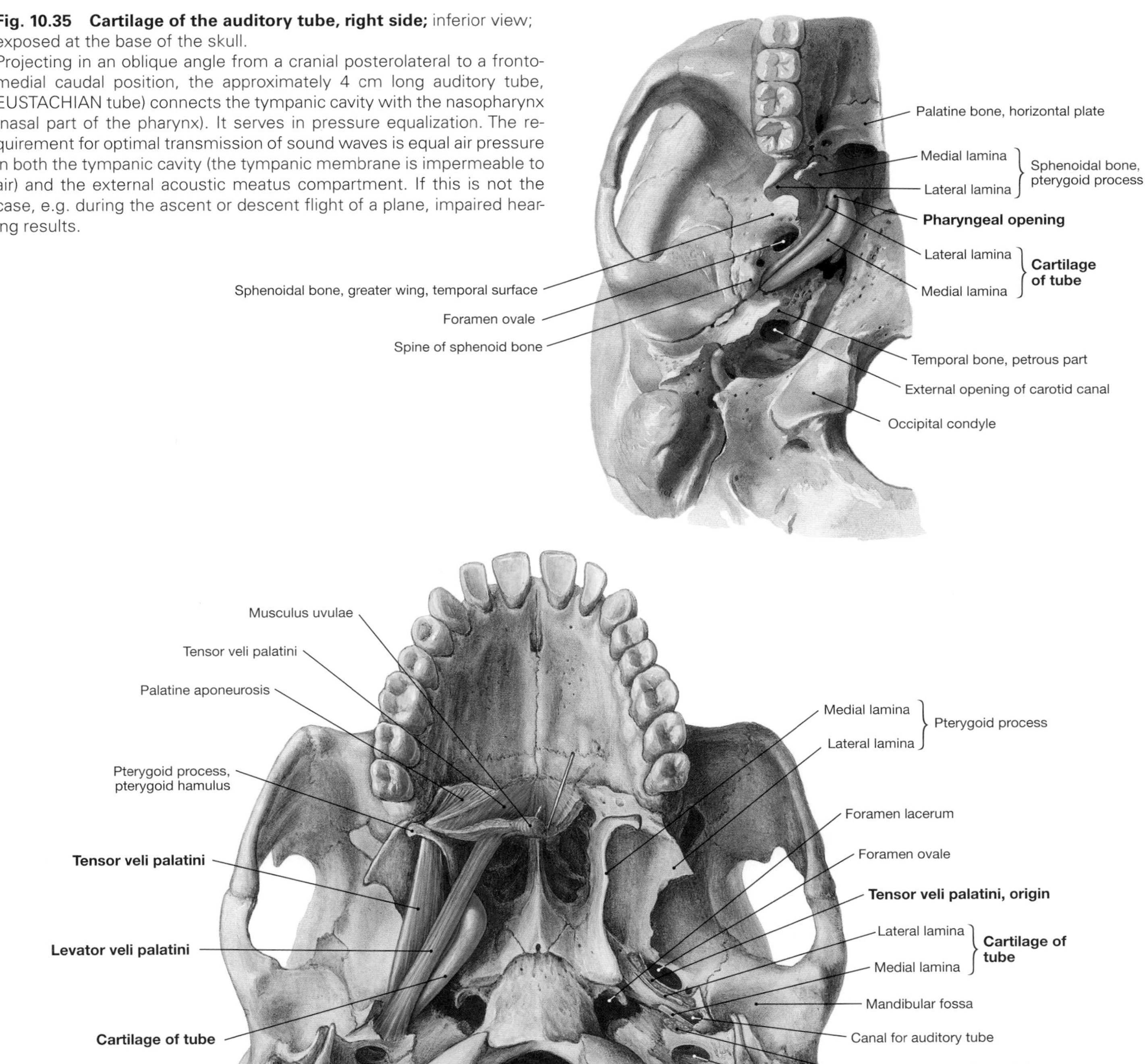
Palatine bone, horizontal plate
Medial lamina
Lateral lamina
Sphenoidal bone, pterygoid process
Pharyngeal opening
Lateral lamina
Medial lamina
Cartilage of tube
Sphenoidal bone, greater wing, temporal surface
Foramen ovale
Spine of sphenoid bone
Temporal bone, petrous part
External opening of carotid canal
Occipital condyle
Musculus uvulae
Tensor veli palatini
Palatine aponeurosis
Pterygoid process, pterygoid hamulus
Tensor veli palatini
Levator veli palatini
Cartilage of tube
Medial lamina
Lateral lamina
Pterygoid process
Foramen lacerum
Foramen ovale
Tensor veli palatini, origin
Lateral lamina
Medial lamina
Cartilage of tube
Mandibular fossa
Canal for auditory tube
Levator veli palatini, origin
Carotid canal, external opening

**Fig. 10.36 Levator veli palatini, tensor veli palatini, and cartilage of the auditory tube;** inferior view.
The auditory tube (bony part not shown) initiates at the opening of the tympanic opening of the anterior wall of the tympanic cavity (carotid wall) and ends at the pharyngeal opening which protrudes in the posterior lateral aspect of the nasopharynx. One can distinguish a bony part and a cartilaginous part which is twice the length of the bony part. The latter consists of a trough-shaped elastic cartilage in an upside-down position with connective tissue (membranous lamina) on its medial side, thus creating a slit-like canal. Contractions of the tensor und levator veli palatini during swallowing result in the opening of the auditory tube.

→T 3

## Clinical Remarks

The epithelial lining of the auditory tube is composed of respiratory pseudostratified ciliated epithelium and goblet cells. The cilia beat in the direction of the nasopharynx (mucociliary escalator). When the protective mechanisms of the tube fail, ascending infections can cause an **inflammation of the auditory tube** and the middle ear. Similar to swallowing, yawning, and chewing, the moderately forceful exhalation with the mouth closed and the nose pinched shut (VALSALVA's maneuver) can open a blocked auditory tube and restore proper aeration of the middle ear.

## Auditory tube

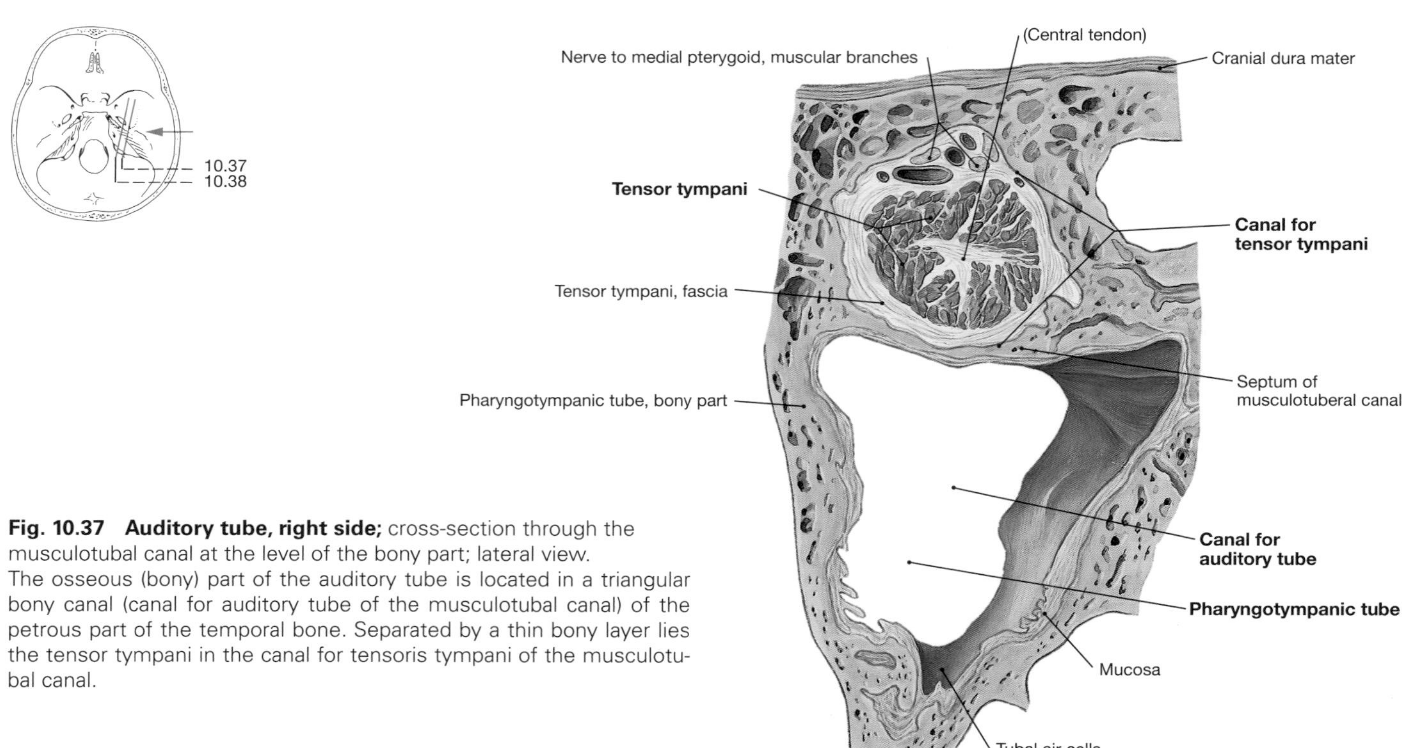
10.37
10.38
Nerve to medial pterygoid, muscular branches
(Central tendon)
Cranial dura mater
Tensor tympani
Canal for tensor tympani
Tensor tympani, fascia
Septum of musculotuberal canal
Pharyngotympanic tube, bony part
Canal for auditory tube
Pharyngotympanic tube
Mucosa
Tubal air cells

**Fig. 10.37 Auditory tube, right side;** cross-section through the musculotubal canal at the level of the bony part; lateral view.
The osseous (bony) part of the auditory tube is located in a triangular bony canal (canal for auditory tube of the musculotubal canal) of the petrous part of the temporal bone. Separated by a thin bony layer lies the tensor tympani in the canal for tensoris tympani of the musculotubal canal.

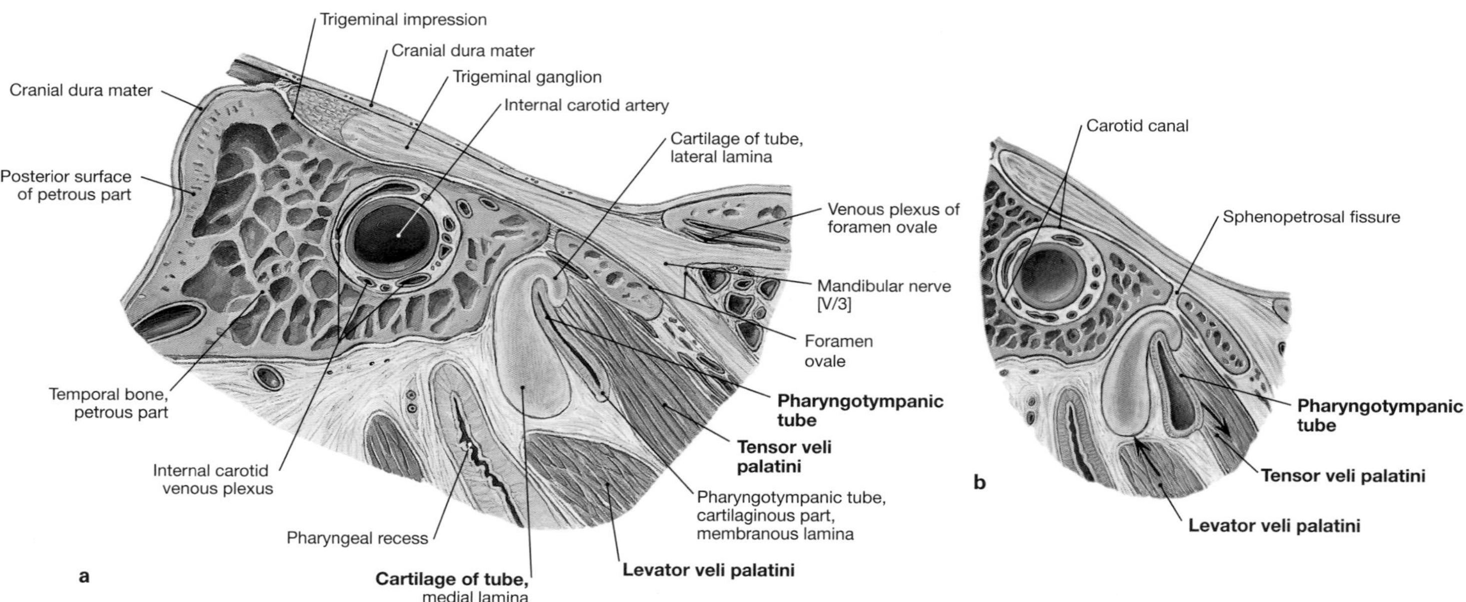
Trigeminal impression
Cranial dura mater
Trigeminal ganglion
Internal carotid artery
Cranial dura mater
Posterior surface of petrous part
Cartilage of tube, lateral lamina
Venous plexus of foramen ovale
Mandibular nerve [V/3]
Foramen ovale
Temporal bone, petrous part
Pharyngotympanic tube
Tensor veli palatini
Internal carotid venous plexus
Pharyngotympanic tube, cartilaginous part, membranous lamina
Pharyngeal recess
a
Cartilage of tube, medial lamina
Levator veli palatini
Carotid canal
Sphenopetrosal fissure
Pharyngotympanic tube
Tensor veli palatini
b
Levator veli palatini

**Figs. 10.38a and b Auditory tube, right side;** cross-section at the level of the lateral part of the cartilaginous part; lateral view.

**a** Closed tube
**b** Opened tube; arrows indicate the effect of muscle contraction on the auditory tube

Swallowing involves the contraction of the tensor and levator veli palatini. **Contraction of the tensor veli palatini** causes a pull at the membranous part and the upper rim of the cartilaginous part of the auditory tube resulting in a dilation of the tube lumen. **Contraction of the levator veli palatini** causes the muscle to bulge out and this muscle belly pushes against the cartilaginous part of the tube from below. As a result, the slit-shaped lumen bends such that it causes the lumen of the auditory tube to dilate. Occlusion of the auditory tube involves the salpingopharyngeus muscle (not shown).

## Clinical Remarks

**Cleft palate** coincides with a loss of function of the tensor and levator veli palatini, as these muscles have lost their attachment point (fixed end) at the hard and soft palate, respectively (→ Fig. 10.36). Thus, the contraction of both muscles fails to open the auditory tube. In patients with cleft palate and no treatment, the middle ear is not aerated and mucosal adhesion processes occur. These children usually have major impairments in hearing and speech.

## Bony labyrinth

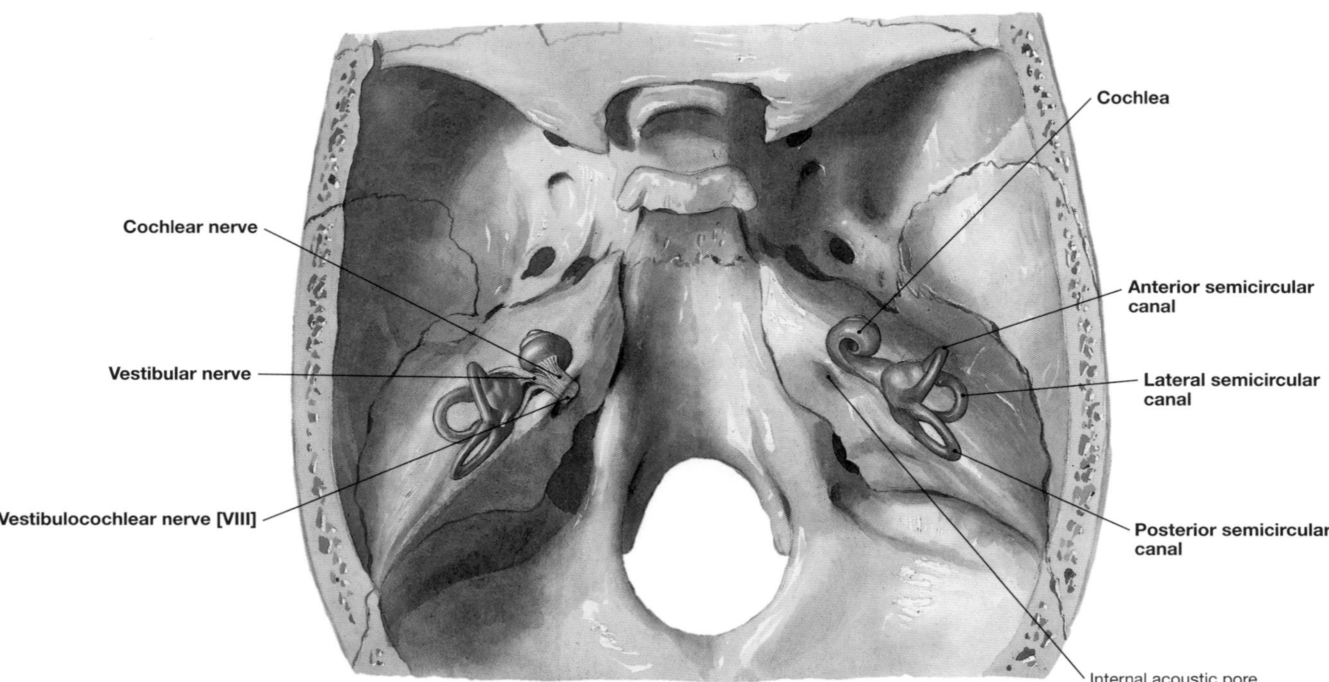
Cochlea
Cochlear nerve
Anterior semicircular canal
Vestibular nerve
Lateral semicircular canal
Vestibulocochlear nerve [VIII]
Posterior semicircular canal
Internal acoustic pore

**Fig. 10.39 Inner ear and vestibulocochlear nerve [VIII];** superior view; inner ear projected onto the petrous part of the temporal bone illustrating its natural position.

The tip of the cochlea is pointed anterolateral. The semicircular canals position in a 45° angle in relation to the main planes of the skull (frontal, sagittal, and horizontal planes). This is important information to know when examining CT scans of the skull.

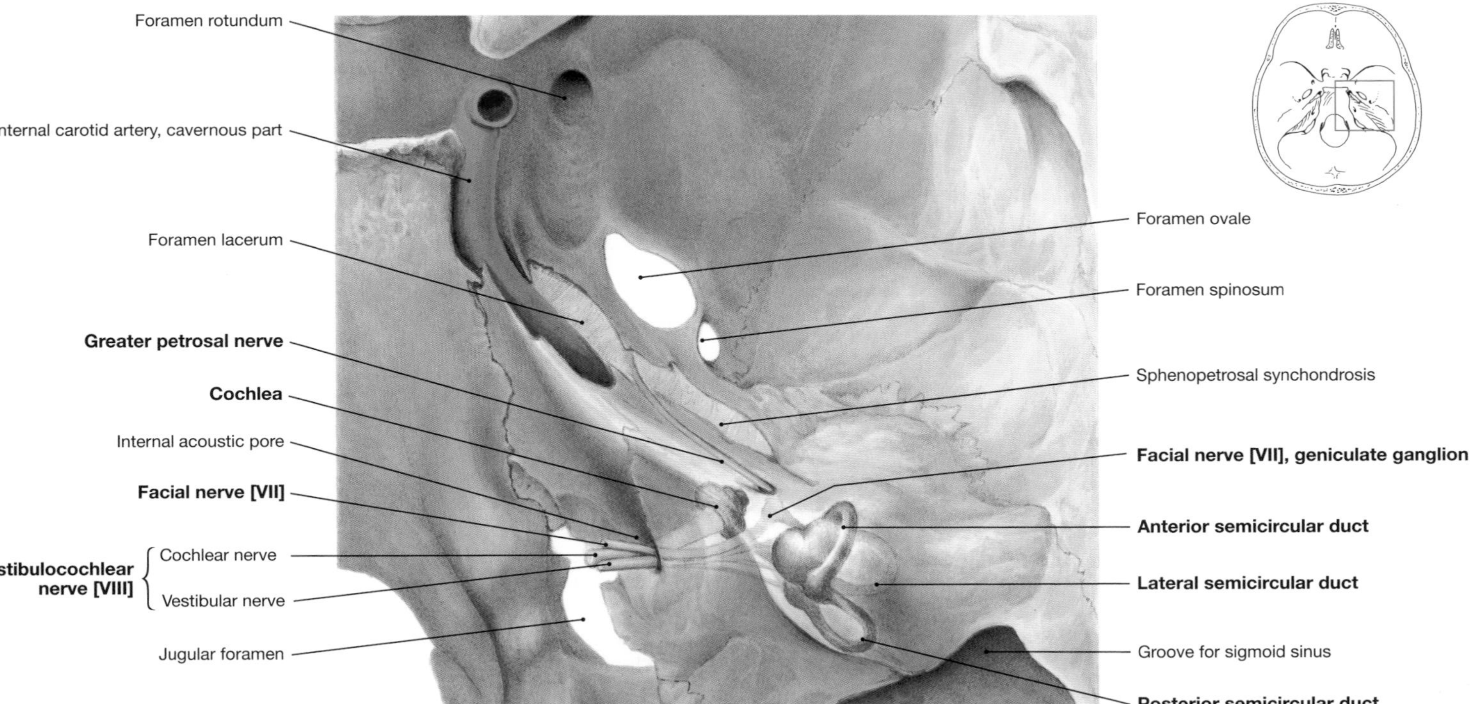
Foramen rotundum
Internal carotid artery, cavernous part
Foramen lacerum
Greater petrosal nerve
Cochlea
Internal acoustic pore
Facial nerve [VII]
Cochlear nerve
estibulocochlear nerve [VIII]
Vestibular nerve
Jugular foramen
Foramen ovale
Foramen spinosum
Sphenopetrosal synchondrosis
Facial nerve [VII], geniculate ganglion
Anterior semicircular duct
Lateral semicircular duct
Groove for sigmoid sinus
Posterior semicircular duct

**Fig. 10.40 Inner ear with facial nerve [VII] and vestibulocochlear nerve [VIII], right side;** superior view onto the petrous part of the temporal bone.

When entering the internal acoustic pore, the facial nerve [VII] and its intermediate part position on top of the vestibulocochlear nerve [VIII] (in clinical terms often referred to as stato-acoustic nerve), which is composed of the cochlear and vestibular nerves. The nerves distribute within the petrous bone. The **cochlear nerve** arches forward to the cochlea. The **vestibular nerve** arches backward and, just before reaching the labyrinth, divides into a superior part for the anterior and lateral semicircular canals and the saccule as well as into an inferior part for the utricle and the posterior semicircular canal. The perikarya of the neurons of both parts are jointly located in the **vestibular ganglion.** The facial nerve [VII] runs above and in between the cochlea and vestibular organ in the facial canal. At the outer facial knee, the facial nerve bends downward in an almost 90° angle. The **greater petrosal nerve** branches off the facial nerve [VII] at the geniculate ganglion. The nerve runs in a duplication of the dura on top of the petrous bone towards the foramen lacerum and contains preganglionic parasympathetic fibers for the innervation of lacrimal and nasal glands.

## Bony labyrinth

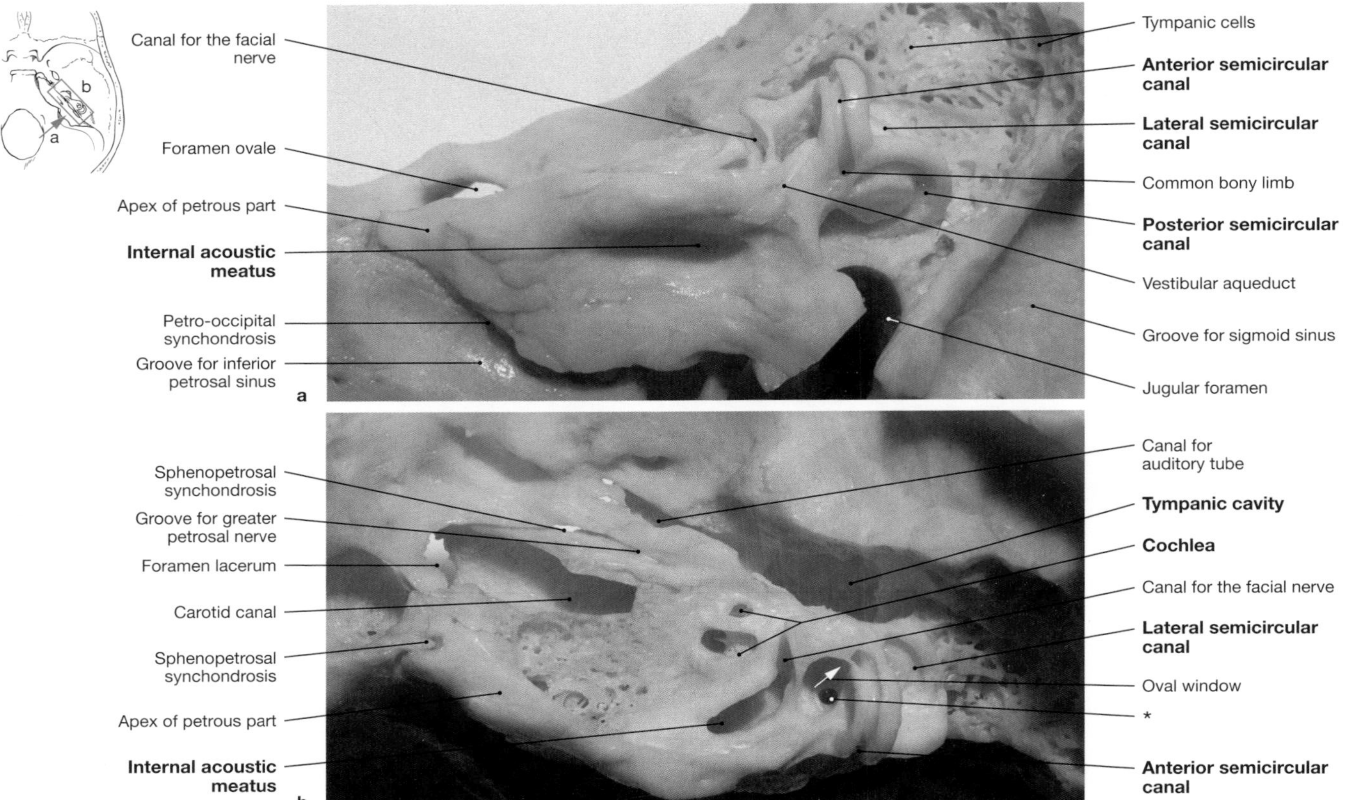
Canal for the facial nerve
Foramen ovale
Apex of petrous part
Internal acoustic meatus
Petro-occipital synchondrosis
Groove for inferior petrosal sinus
a
Tympanic cells
Anterior semicircular canal
Lateral semicircular canal
Common bony limb
Posterior semicircular canal
Vestibular aqueduct
Groove for sigmoid sinus
Jugular foramen
Sphenopetrosal synchondrosis
Groove for greater petrosal nerve
Foramen lacerum
Carotid canal
Sphenopetrosal synchondrosis
Apex of petrous part
Internal acoustic meatus
b
Canal for auditory tube
Tympanic cavity
Cochlea
Canal for the facial nerve
Lateral semicircular canal
Oval window
*
Anterior semicircular canal

**Figs. 10.41a and b Bony labyrinth, right side;** hollowed out of the petrous part of the temporal bone; posterior and superior view (**a**), superior view (**b**).
The inner ear is a complex of bony canals and ampullary extensions in the petrous part of the temporal bone (bony labyrinth). Contained within it is a system of membranous tubes and sacs, known as membranous labyrinth. It harbors the vestibular and cochlear organ (vestibulocochlear organ).

* opening of the posterior canaliculus

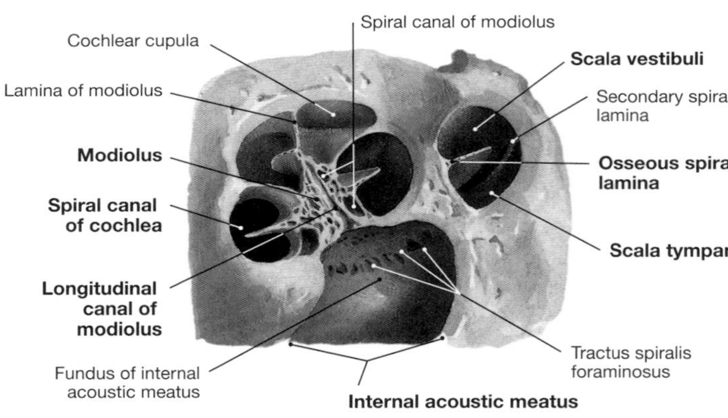
Cochlear cupula
Spiral canal of modiolus
Lamina of modiolus
Scala vestibuli
Secondary spiral lamina
Modiolus
Osseous spiral lamina
Spiral canal of cochlea
Scala tympani
Longitudinal canal of modiolus
Fundus of internal acoustic meatus
Tractus spiralis foraminosus
Internal acoustic meatus

**Fig. 10.42 Spiral canal of the cochlea, right side;** superior view; opened along the axis of the modiolus.
The cochlea consists of a spiral canal of 2½ turns around a central modiolus. The spiral ganglion of cochlea, containing the perikarya of the bipolar neurons of the cochlear nerve, is located within the spiral canals and longitudinal modioli. Originating from the modiolus, the osseus spiral lamina protrudes into the cochlear canal.

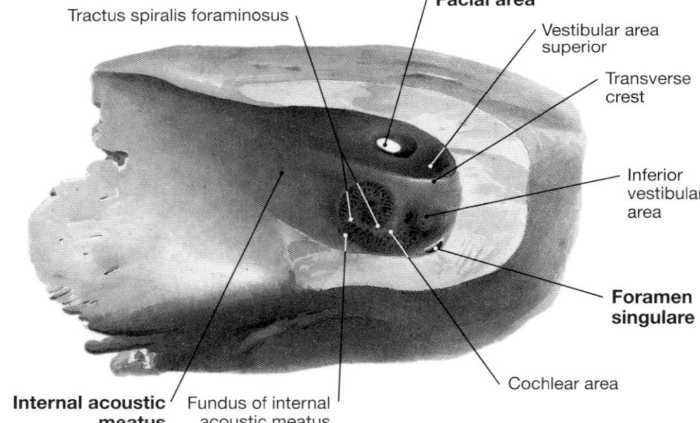
Tractus spiralis foraminosus
Facial area
Vestibular area superior
Transverse crest
Inferior vestibular area
Foramen singulare
Cochlear area
Internal acoustic meatus
Fundus of internal acoustic meatus

**Fig. 10.43 Internal acoustic meatus and fundus of the internal acoustic meatus, right side;** medial view; after partial removal of the posterior wall.
The internal acoustic meatus initiates at the internal acoustic pore and projects laterally for approximately 1 cm. Here it ends in a perforated bony plate. The facial nerve [VII] and vestibulocochlear nerve [VIII] run in this 1 cm long segment.

### Clinical Remarks

The **acoustic neurinoma** (also known as vestibular schwannoma, acoustic neuroma, acoustic neurilemmoma, acoustic neurofibroma) is a benign tumor of the SCHWANN's cells and most frequently affects the vestibular nerve. As it originates in the internal acoustic meatus and grows into the posterior cranial fossa, it presses on adjacent structures (cerebellopontine angle tumor). Early symptoms include asymmetric hearing impairment, dizziness, and loss of balance.

## Bony labyrinth

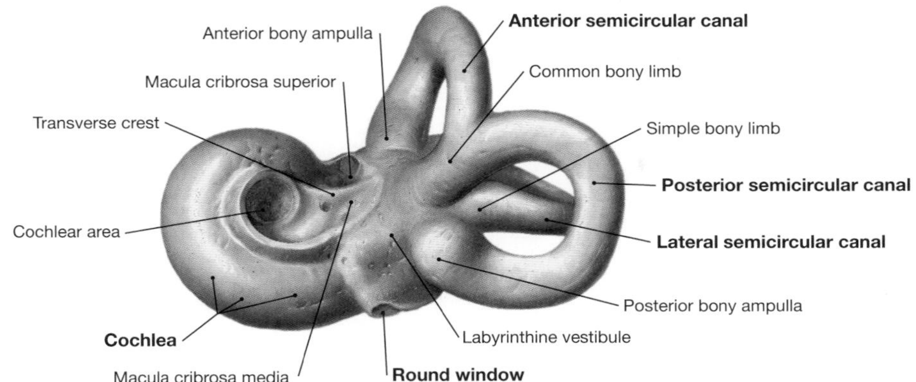
Anterior bony ampulla
Anterior semicircular canal
Macula cribrosa superior
Common bony limb
Transverse crest
Simple bony limb
Posterior semicircular canal
Cochlear area
Lateral semicircular canal
Posterior bony ampulla
Cochlea
Labyrinthine vestibule
Macula cribrosa media
Round window

**Fig. 10.44 Bony labyrinth, right side;** view from an oblique posterior angle; the osseous lining of the membranous labyrinth has been hollowed out of the petrous part of the temporal bone.

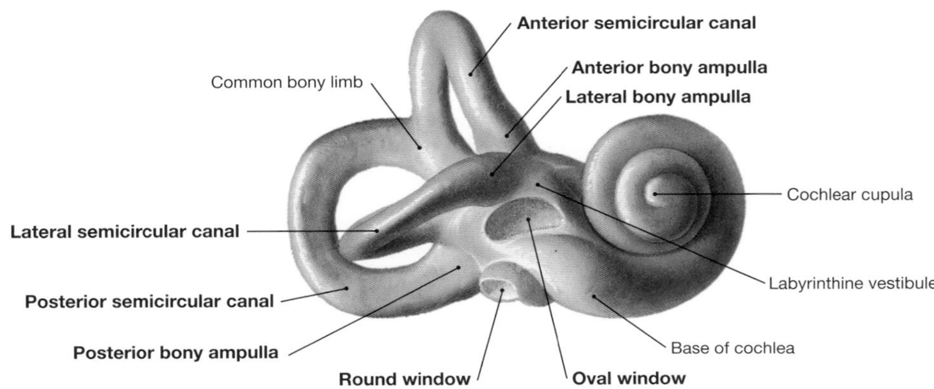
Anterior semicircular canal
Anterior bony ampulla
Common bony limb
Lateral bony ampulla
Cochlear cupula
Lateral semicircular canal
Labyrinthine vestibule
Posterior semicircular canal
Base of cochlea
Posterior bony ampulla
Round window
Oval window

**Fig. 10.45 Bony labyrinth, right side;** lateral view; the osseous lining of the membranous labyrinth has been hollowed out of the petrous part of the temporal bone.

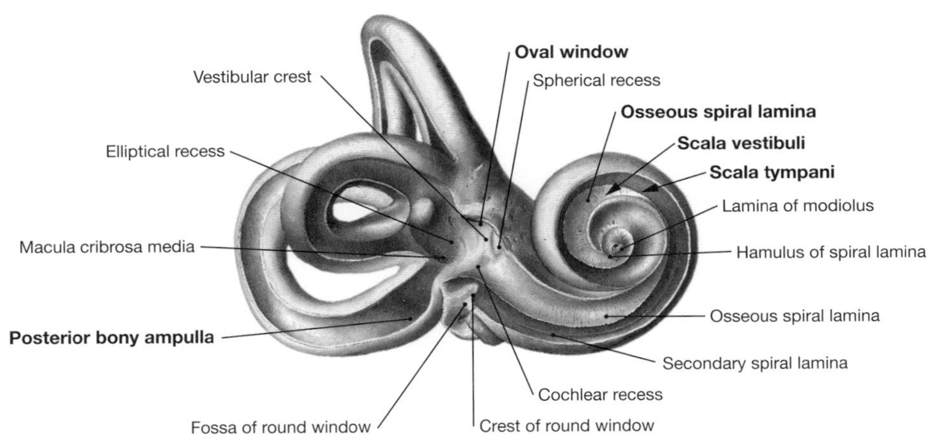
Oval window
Vestibular crest
Spherical recess
Osseous spiral lamina
Scala vestibuli
Elliptical recess
Scala tympani
Lamina of modiolus
Macula cribrosa media
Hamulus of spiral lamina
Osseous spiral lamina
Posterior bony ampulla
Secondary spiral lamina
Cochlear recess
Fossa of round window
Crest of round window

**Fig. 10.46 Bony labyrinth, right side;** anterolateral view; cavities have been hollowed out.
The bony labyrinth consists of the vestibule, three bony semicircular canals, the bony cochlea, and the internal acoustic meatus. Cochlea and semicircular canals originate from the vestibule which connects with the tympanic cavity through the oval window.

## Membranous labyrinth

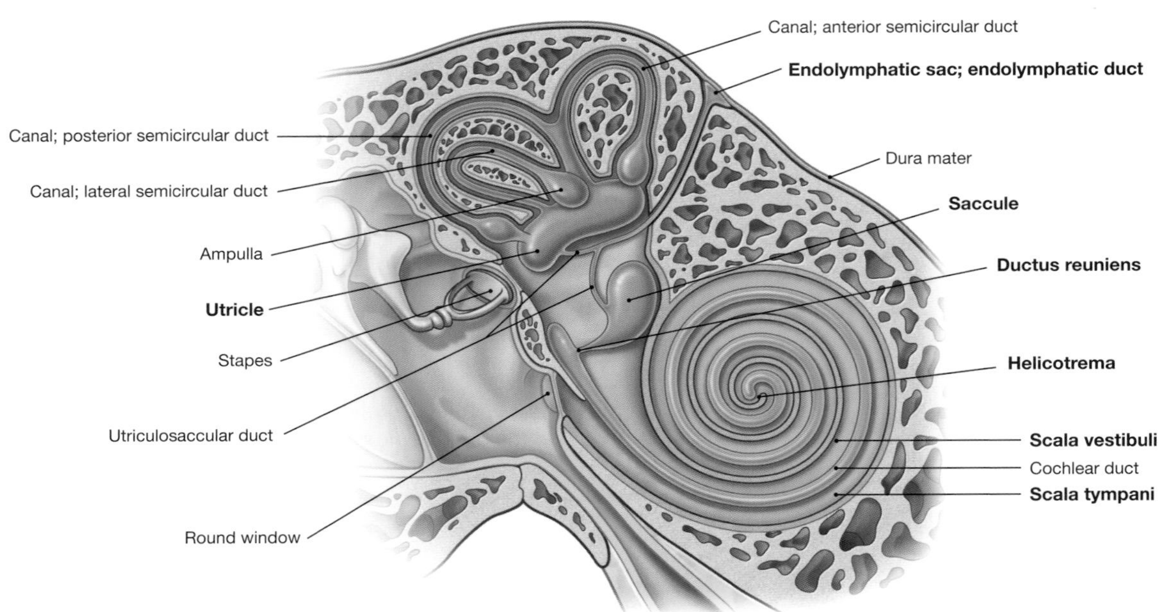
Canal; anterior semicircular duct
Endolymphatic sac; endolymphatic duct
Canal; posterior semicircular duct
Dura mater
Canal; lateral semicircular duct
Saccule
Ampulla
Ductus reuniens
Utricle
Stapes
Helicotrema
Utriculosaccular duct
Scala vestibuli
Cochlear duct
Scala tympani
Round window

**Fig. 10.47 Membranous labyrinth, right side;** longitudinal section through the petrous part of the temporal bone; frontal view, schematic drawing. [8]

The membranous labyrinth contains potassium rich and sodium poor endolymph. A perilymphatic space filled with perilymph separates the membranous labyrinth from the bony labyrinth. According to its function, the membranous labyrinth divides into a vestibular and cochlear compartment. The **vestibular labyrinth** includes the saccule and utricle located in the vestibule, the utriculosaccular duct, the three semicircular canals, and the endolymphatic duct with the endolymphatic sac. The latter is located on the rear side of the petrous bone and represents an epidural sac for the resorption of the endolymph. The **cochlear labyrinth** forms the cochlear duct. The ductus reuniens connects the vestibular and cochlear labyrinths.

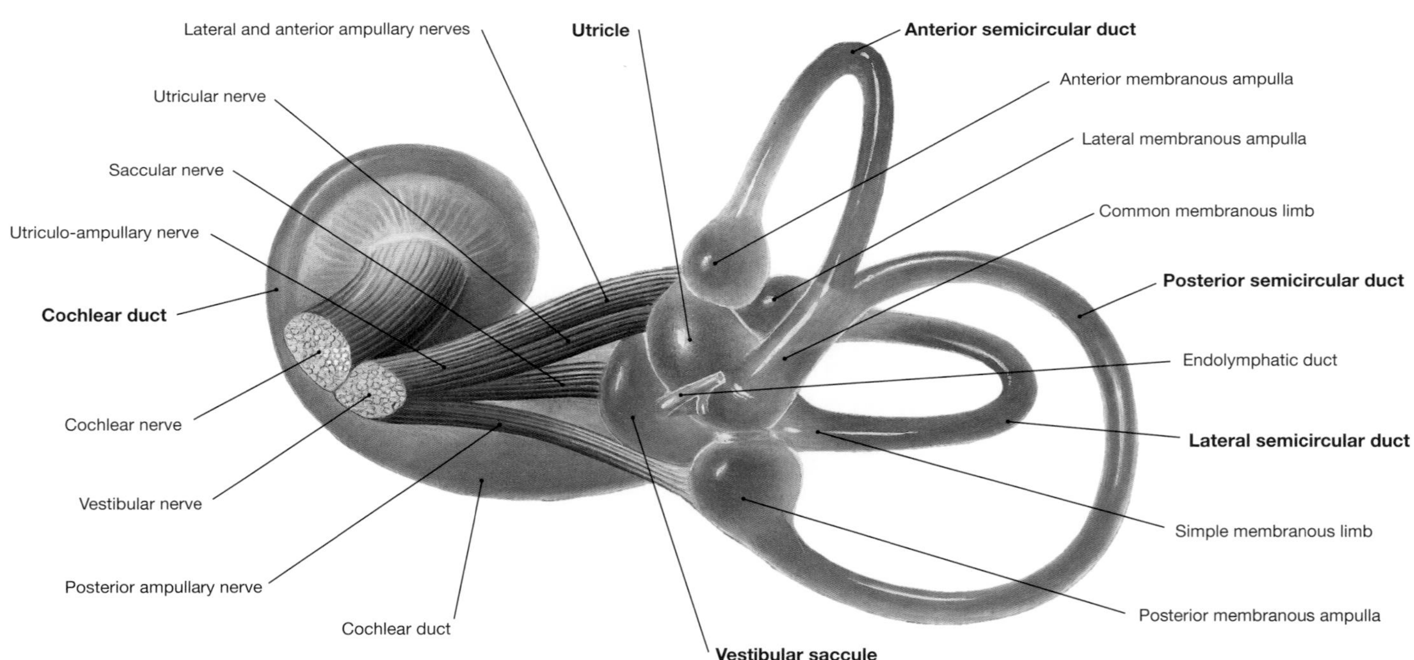
Lateral and anterior ampullary nerves
Utricle
Anterior semicircular duct
Anterior membranous ampulla
Utricular nerve
Lateral membranous ampulla
Saccular nerve
Common membranous limb
Utriculo-ampullary nerve
Posterior semicircular duct
Cochlear duct
Endolymphatic duct
Cochlear nerve
Lateral semicircular duct
Vestibular nerve
Simple membranous limb
Posterior ampullary nerve
Posterior membranous ampulla
Cochlear duct
Vestibular saccule

**Fig. 10.48 Vestibulocochlear nerve [VIII] and membranous labyrinth;** semi-schematic overview, dorsal view.

The membranous labyrinth includes the cochlear duct, the saccule, the utricle as well as the three membranous semicircular canals (semicircular ducts). The latter ones connect with the utricle. At the border to the utricle, each semicircular duct develops an ampulla-shaped dilation (membranous ampulla). At one end, the superior and posterior semicircular canals unite to form one common canal (common limb). Each ampulla contains sensory epithelium (ampullary crest, not shown).

## Blood supply and innervation of the membranous labyrinth

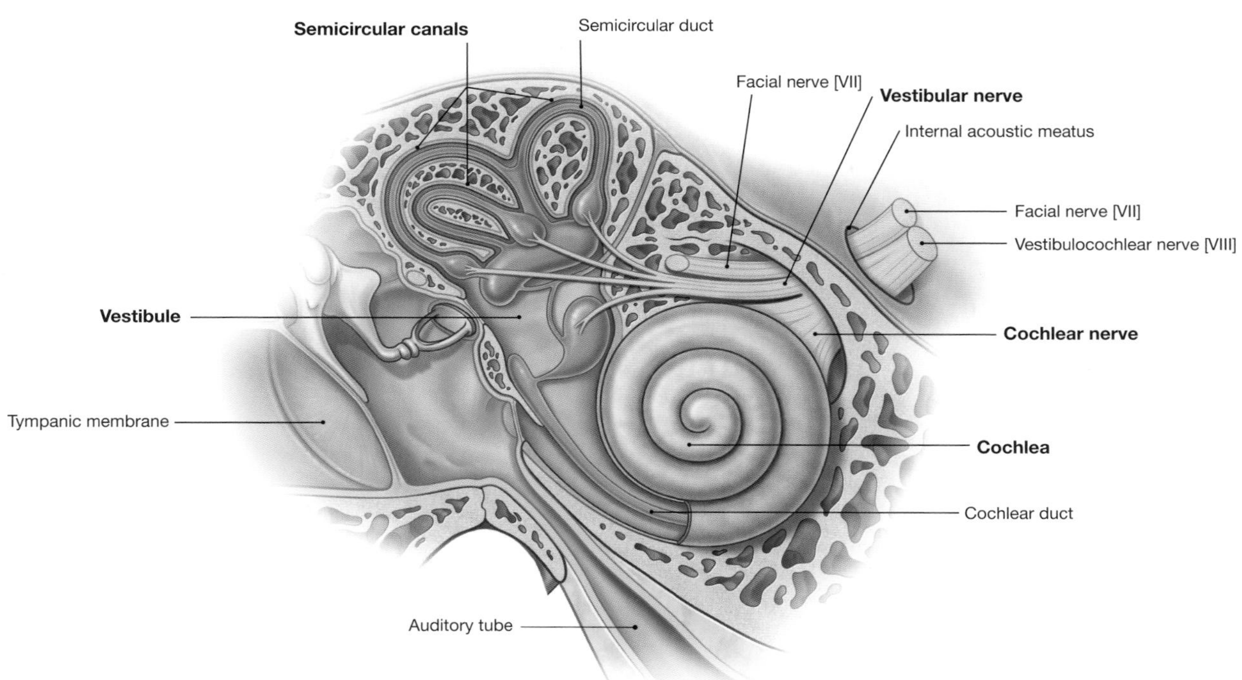
Semicircular canals
Semicircular duct
Facial nerve [VII]
Vestibular nerve
Internal acoustic meatus
Facial nerve [VII]
Vestibulocochlear nerve [VIII]
Vestibule
Cochlear nerve
Tympanic membrane
Cochlea
Cochlear duct
Auditory tube

**Fig. 10.49 Innervation of the inner ear, right side;** longitudinal section through the petrous part of the temporal bone; frontal view, schematic drawing. [8]

The inner ear is composed of the compact bone of the petrous bone surrounding the **bony labyrinth** and, enclosed within it, the **membranous labyrinth,** which resembles a system of membranous tubes.

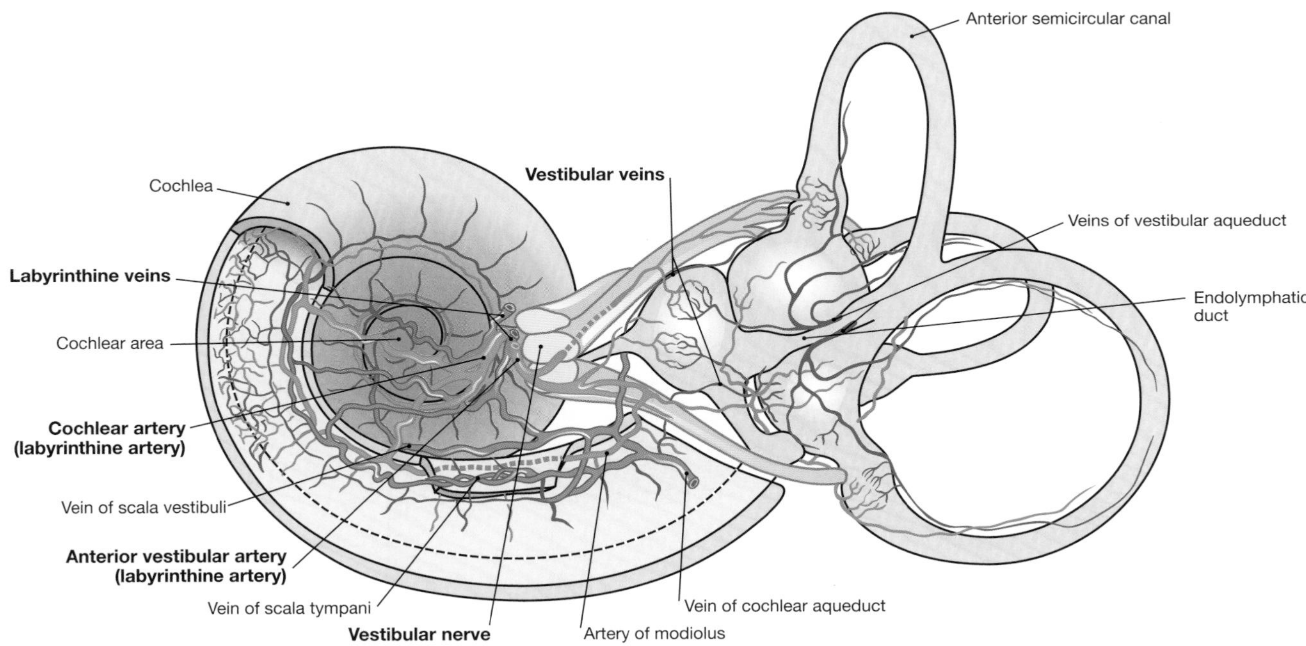
Anterior semicircular canal
Cochlea
Vestibular veins
Veins of vestibular aqueduct
Labyrinthine veins
Endolymphatic duct
Cochlear area
Cochlear artery (labyrinthine artery)
Vein of scala vestibuli
Anterior vestibular artery (labyrinthine artery)
Vein of scala tympani
Vestibular nerve
Artery of modiolus
Vein of cochlear aqueduct

**Fig. 10.50 Blood supply and innervation of the inner ear of the right side;** medial view. (according to [2])
The branches of the **labyrinthine artery** (→ Fig. 12.96) provide the complete blood supply to the inner ear; the labyrinthine veins drain the venous blood. The anterior inferior cerebellar artery and vein project into the internal acoustic meatus for a few millimeters (not shown) before the labyrinthine artery and labyrinthine veins branch off to provide blood supply to the labyrinth (**caveat:** the labyrinthine artery is a terminal artery).

## Clinical Remarks

Being a terminal artery, **thrombotic occlusion of the labyrinthine artery** or its contributing branches causes a loss of balance and hearing impairment.
Attacks of vertigo, unilateral hearing loss, and unilateral tinnitus constitute the triad of symptoms characterizing **MENIÈRE's disease.** Its etiology is not clear, but a hydropic swelling of the membranous labyrinth due to impaired resorption of endolymph (cochlear hydrops) is discussed. The pressure imposed by the increased volume of endolymph damages the sensory cells of the vestibulocochlear system.

## Cochlea

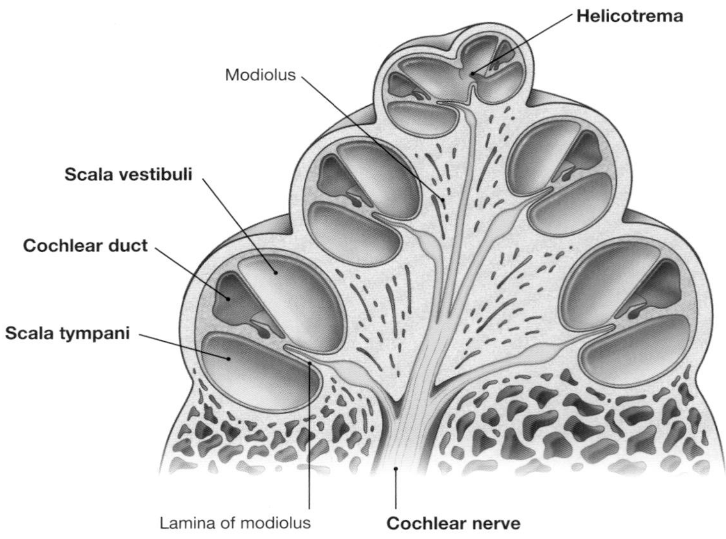
Helicotrema
Modiolus
Scala vestibuli
Cochlear duct
Scala tympani
Lamina of modiolus
Cochlear nerve

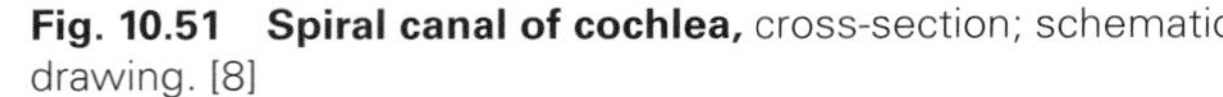

**Fig. 10.51 Spiral canal of cochlea,** cross-section; schematic drawing. [8]
The REISSNER's membrane and the basilar membrane divide the spinal canal of cochlea into three spaces:
- The **scala vestibuli** stretches from the vestibule to the helicotrema and is filled with perilymph.
- The **cochlear duct** is filled with endolymph.
- The **scala tympani** extends from the helicotrema to the round window in the medial wall of the tympanic cavity and is filled with perilymph. Scala vestibuli and scala tympani join at the helicotrema.

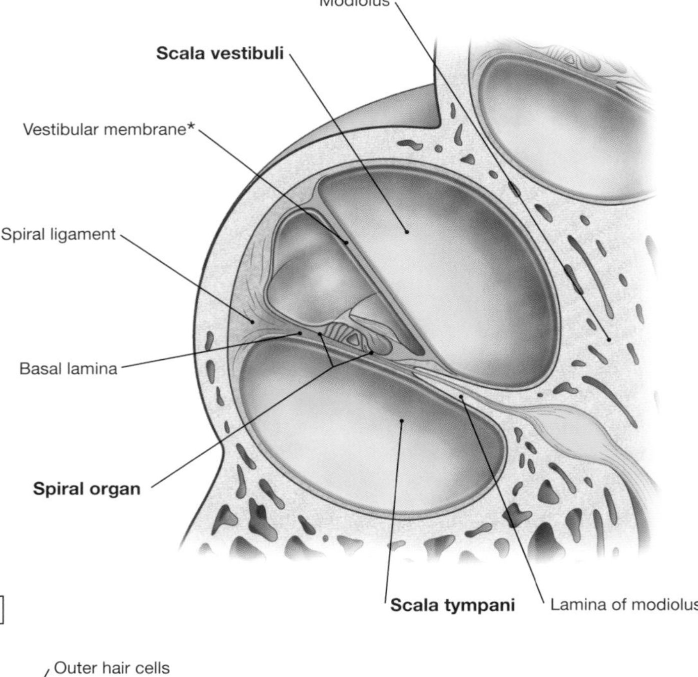
Modiolus
Scala vestibuli
Vestibular membrane*
Spiral ligament
Basal lamina
Spiral organ
Scala tympani
Lamina of modiolus

**Fig. 10.52 Spiral canal of cochlea;** cross-section through a turn of the spiral organ; schematic drawing. [8]
The basilar membrane forms the base of the cochlear duct and supports the cochlear organ (Organ of CORTI or CORTI's organ). The stria vascularis at the lateral bony wall of the cochlea produces the endolymph.

* REISSNER's membrane

Cochlear duct
Inner hair cells
Interdental cells
Inner phalangeal cell
NUEL's space
Outer hair cells
Outer tunnel
Tectorial membrane
Inner border cell
Outer border cell
HENSEN's cells
CLAUDIUS's cells
Spiral limbus
Inner spiral sulcus
Canal of CORTI
Basal lamina
Spiral ligament
Nerve fiber
Vas spirale
Inner pillar cell
Basilar membrane
BOETTCHER's cells
Epithelium of the scala tympani
Outer pillar cell
Outer phalangeal cells
Tympanic amorphous substance
Osseous spiral lamina
Scala tympani

**Fig. 10.53 Spiral organ (Organ of CORTI);** schematic drawing. [24]
This is a simplified presentation of the complex afferent and efferent innervation of the hair cells.

The organ of CORTI represents the actual cochlear organ. Cochlear sensory cells (hair cells) together with different supporting cell types rest on the basilar membrane and a gelatinous membrane (tectorial membrane) covers their apical cell surface. The organ of CORTI stretches along the whole length of the cochlear duct.

### Clinical Remarks

**Tinnitus** is frequently the consequence of damage to the hair cells, e.g. after exposure to loud music or an explosion. Tinnitus aurium, or tinnitus for short ("ringing of the ears"), is a symptom where the affected individual perceives sounds in the absence of real sounds.

## Mechanoelectrical sound conduction and equilibrium (balance) organ

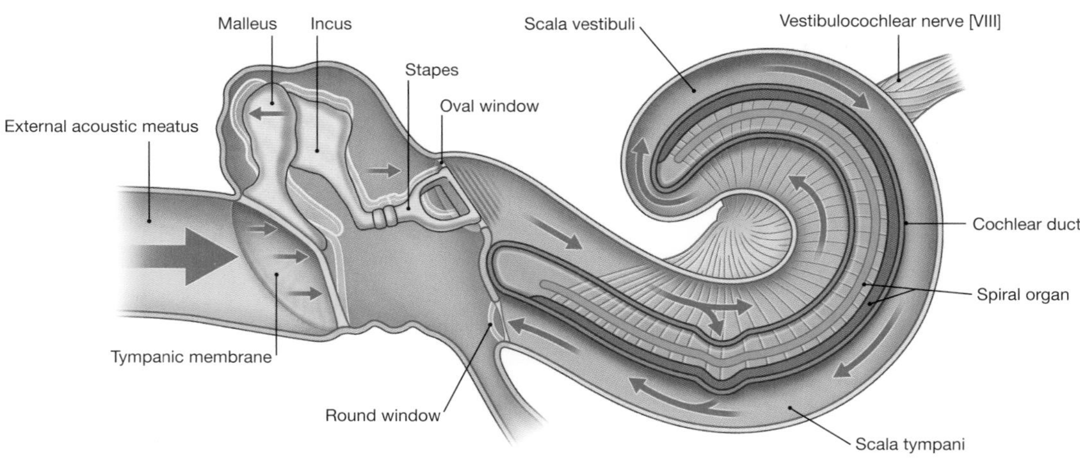
Malleus
Incus
Scala vestibuli
Vestibulocochlear nerve [VIII]
Stapes
Oval window
External acoustic meatus
Cochlear duct
Spiral organ
Tympanic membrane
Round window
Scala tympani

**Fig. 10.54 Mechano-electrical sound conduction.** [8]
Sound propagates by sound waves which reach the outer ear (auricle and external acoustic meatus) and are transmitted by the tympanic membrane and the chain of auditory ossicles through the base of the stapes to the perilymph. Vibrations at the oval window initiate movements of perilymph causing **migrating waves** running along the walls of the cochlear duct (particularly the basilar membrane). These waves cause a deflection of the basilar membrane and the organ of CORTI. Consequently, stereocilia of the inner hair cells deflect. The sensory cells transduce this biomechanic event into a receptor potential (mechanoelectrical transduction).

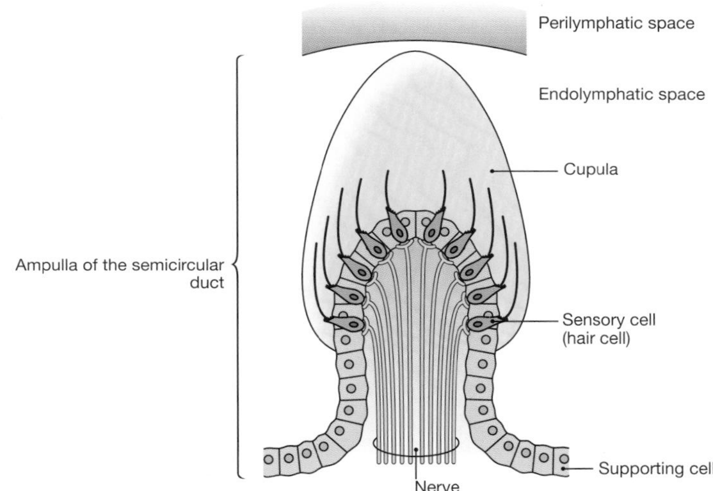
Perilymphatic space
Endolymphatic space
Cupula
Ampulla of the semicircular duct
Sensory cell (hair cell)
Supporting cell
Nerve

**Fig. 10.55 Structure of the ampullary crest.** (according to [25])
The vestibular labyrinth is filled with endolymph and consists of the **saccule** (macula of saccule – vertical linear acceleration), **utricle** (macula of utricle – horizontal linear acceleration), and the **three semicircular canals** (ampullary crests with their cupula – rotational acceleration). The sensory cells of the vestibular organ possess a long kinocilium and stereocilia which extend into a gelatinous substance located within the cupula. Movements of the cupula result in the deflection of these cellular processes on the surface of the sensory cells. This presents a stimulus for the synaptic activation of afferent fibers of the vestibular nerve.

### Clinical Remarks

**Labyrinthitis** with dysequilibrium and/or dizziness, nystagmus, nausea, and anxiety can accompany cholesteatoma (destructive and expanding growth of keratinizing squamous epithelium dislodged from the outer side of the tympanic membrane into the middle ear with chronic putrid inflammation of the middle ear), acute otitis media, mastoiditis, and trauma to the skull. Entry ports for infectious agents are the round and oval window, breaches in the bony labyrinth (caused by trauma and bone erosion due to infected pneumatic spaces), or ascending inflammation of the meninges by nerves and vessels, cochlear duct or vestibular ducts. The result is **sensorineural hearing impairment** with hearing loss and destruction of the vestibular organ.

## Hearing and equilibrium

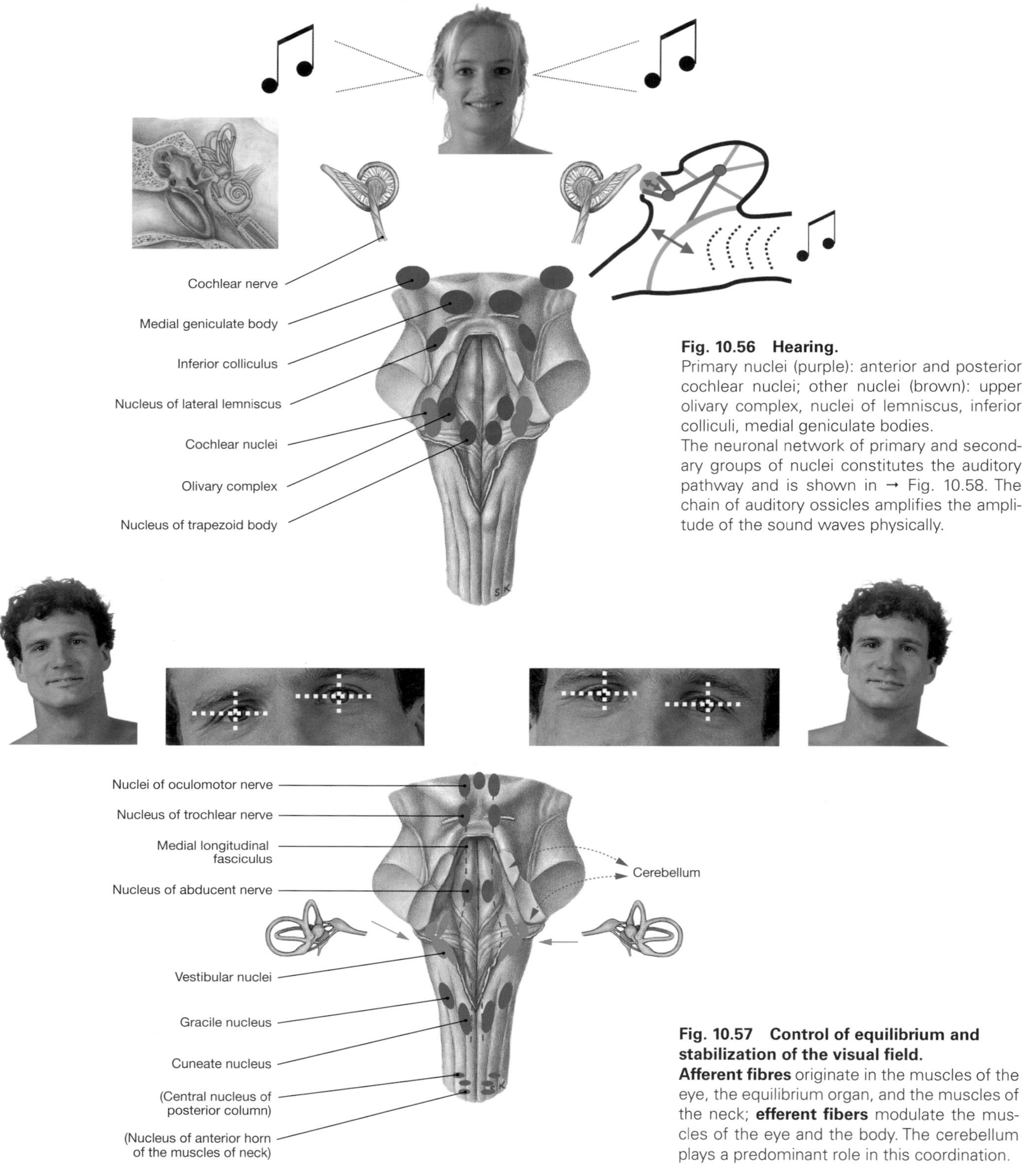
Cochlear nerve
Medial geniculate body
Inferior colliculus
Nucleus of lateral lemniscus
Cochlear nuclei
Olivary complex
Nucleus of trapezoid body
Nuclei of oculomotor nerve
Nucleus of trochlear nerve
Medial longitudinal fasciculus
Nucleus of abducent nerve
Cerebellum
Vestibular nuclei
Gracile nucleus
Cuneate nucleus
(Central nucleus of posterior column)
(Nucleus of anterior horn of the muscles of neck)

**Fig. 10.56 Hearing.**
Primary nuclei (purple): anterior and posterior cochlear nuclei; other nuclei (brown): upper olivary complex, nuclei of lemniscus, inferior colliculi, medial geniculate bodies.
The neuronal network of primary and secondary groups of nuclei constitutes the auditory pathway and is shown in → Fig. 10.58. The chain of auditory ossicles amplifies the amplitude of the sound waves physically.

**Fig. 10.57 Control of equilibrium and stabilization of the visual field.**
**Afferent fibres** originate in the muscles of the eye, the equilibrium organ, and the muscles of the neck; **efferent fibers** modulate the muscles of the eye and the body. The cerebellum plays a predominant role in this coordination.

### Clinical Remarks

Objectively assessing a patient's **vertigo** and localizing the lesion within the vestibular system requires testing of the equilibrium (balance) system as an important part of a physical exam. Commonly used tests are the **ROMBERG's test** (patient stands upright with feet together, eyes closed, and arms stretched forward) and the **UNTERBERGER's stepping test** (patient is asked to walk on the spot with eyes closed) when assessing the body's sense of positioning or a tendency to fall for that matter. Another method is the nystagmus test (nystagmus = involuntary rapid eye movements) using FRENZEL's lenses (FRENZEL's glasses). Rapid shaking of the patient's head provokes a nystagmus. This test is performed with the patient holding the head in different positions. This examination will also reveal any latent nystagmus. A **caloric nystagmus test** examines the responses by the labyrinth on one side. The patient is lying in a supine position (elevated head) in a room with dimmed light and the ear on each side is irrigated with cold and warm water. Cold water will initiate a physiological nystagmus to the opposite side, whereas warm water will stimulate a nystagmus to the same side of the labyrinth tested. A reduced or lacking nystagmus is pathological and suggests a peripheral functional impairment.

## Auditory pathway

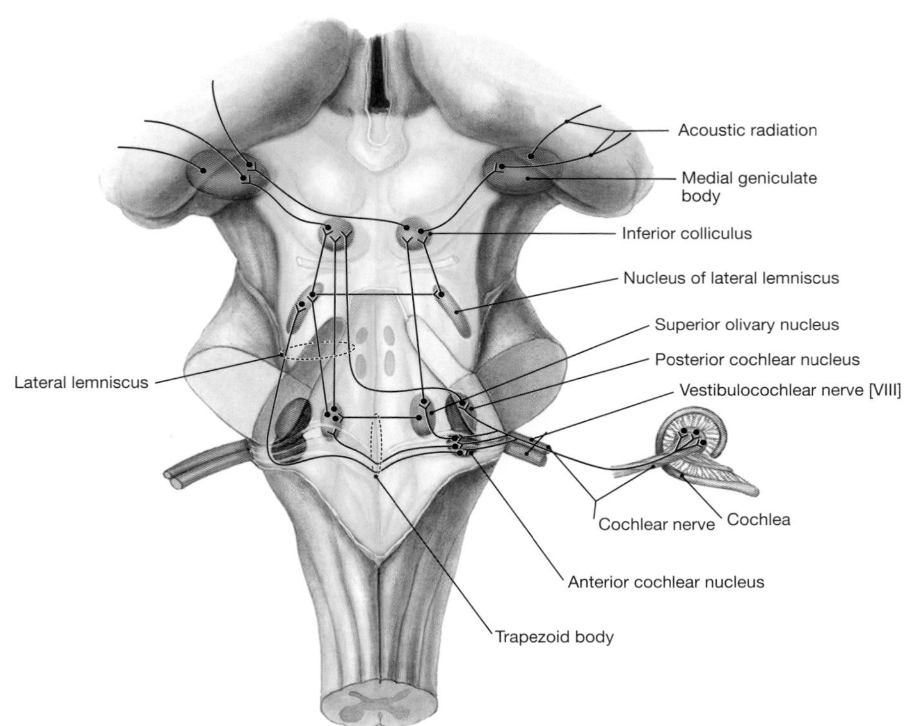
Acoustic radiation
Medial geniculate body
Inferior colliculus
Nucleus of lateral lemniscus
Superior olivary nucleus
Posterior cochlear nucleus
Vestibulocochlear nerve [VIII]
Lateral lemniscus
Cochlear nerve
Cochlea
Anterior cochlear nucleus
Trapezoid body

**Fig. 10.58 Auditory pathway;** overview.
The function of the ascending auditory pathway is to transmit acoustic signals to the brain, to process this information centrally, and to create an acoustic awareness.

**1st neuron: bipolar cells in the spiral ganglion of cochlea**

- After exiting the small apertures of the tractus spiralis foraminosus deep within the internal acoustic meatus, the fibers form the cochlear nerve unite with the vestibular nerve at the floor of the internal acoustic meatus to form the vestibulocochlear nerve [VIII].
- Fibers from the basal cochlear part traverse to the posterior cochlear nucleus and those from the apical parts terminate in the anterior cochlear nucleus.

**2nd neuron: multipolar cells of the cochlear nuclei**

- The fibers from the anterior cochlear nerve pass mainly to the olivary complex on the same or opposite side.
- A part of the fibers crosses to the opposite side and, without synapsing, run in the lateral lemniscus to the inferior colliculus.
- Fibers that reach the olivary complex on the same side, either ascend to the nucleus of lateral lemniscus, synapse, cross to the opposite side, synapse again, and then reach the inferior colliculus or they ascend directly in the lateral lemniscus to reach the inferior colliculus.

**3rd or 4th neuron:** From the inferior colliculus connections are made to the medial geniculate body.

**4th or 5th neuron:** The acoustic radiation connects the medial geniculate body with the transverse temporal HESCHL's gyri or convolutions and the WERNICKE's center in the temporal lobe.

## Equilibrium (balance) pathway

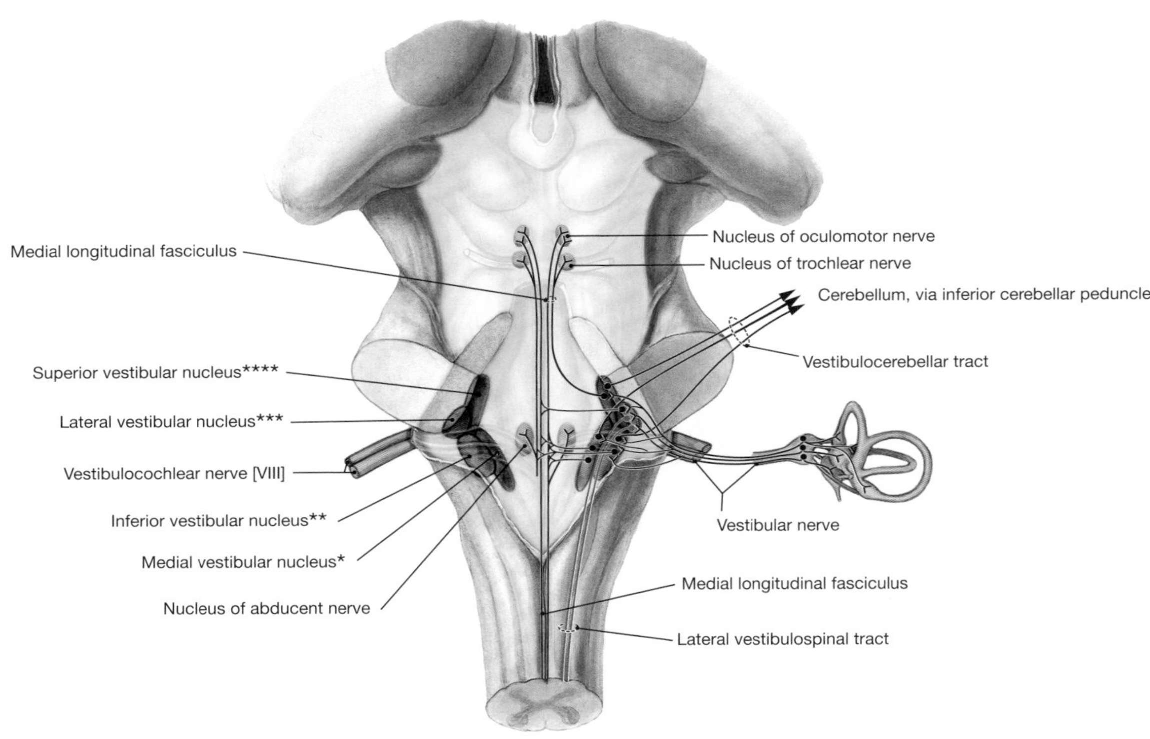
Medial longitudinal fasciculus
Nucleus of oculomotor nerve
Nucleus of trochlear nerve
Cerebellum, via inferior cerebellar peduncle
Vestibulocerebellar tract
Superior vestibular nucleus****
Lateral vestibular nucleus***
Vestibulocochlear nerve [VIII]
Inferior vestibular nucleus**
Medial vestibular nucleus*
Nucleus of abducent nerve
Vestibular nerve
Medial longitudinal fasciculus
Lateral vestibulospinal tract

**Fig. 10.59 Equilibrium (balance) pathway;** overview.
The equilibrium (balance) pathway coordinates eye movements and movements of the torso, neck, and extremities.

**1st neuron:**
- The afferent fibers of the vestibular ganglion mainly project into the medial vestibular nucleus (SCHWALBE's nucleus), the superior vestibular nucleus (nucleus of BEKHTEREV), and the inferior vestibular nucleus (ROLLER's nucleus).
- Afferent fibers of the ampullary crests of the semicircular canals mainly course to the nucleus of BEKHTEREV and SCHWALBE's nucleus as well as into the vestibulocerebellum via the direct sensory cerebellar pathway.
- Afferent fibers of the utricle project into the medial vestibular nucleus, afferent fibers of the saccule project into the lateral vestibular nucleus.
- The lateral vestibular nucleus (DEITERS' nucleus) also receives collateral fibers from the vestibular pathways and, in particular, connections from the cerebellum.

**2nd neuron:** from the vestibular nuclei efferent fibers project
- to the cerebellum (vestibulocerebellar tract)
- to the spinal cord (vestibulospinal tract)
- to the nuclei controlling the extra-ocular muscles (medial longitudinal fasciculus)
- to the thalamus (via the vestibulothalamic tract to the inferior posterior ventral nucleus and from there via the thalamic radiation to the postcentral gyrus)

* SCHWALBE's nucleus
** ROLLER's nucleus
*** DEITERS' nucleus
**** nucleus of BEKHTEREV

# Neck



11

# The Neck – Seamless Connectivity

## Boundaries

The boundaries of the neck (collum/cervix) towards the head, trunk, and shoulder girdle are diffuse. Fish have no necks; their heads adjoin to the trunk and shoulder girdle. Terrestrial animals possess necks, however, the neck is not a fundamental novelty, rather the head-trunk-boundary was stretched or protracted, so to speak. This explains many features such as the fact that cranial nerves participate in the innervation of the shoulder muscles and that the arm is innervated by nerves which emerge from the cervical vertebral column (see below).

If not the soft tissues but the bony structures are used to determine the boundaries of the neck, the upper borders of the neck are defined by the mandible and occipital bone and the lower borders by the clavicle and superior margin of the scapula. Towards the center of the chest, the neck transitions into the thoracic aperture (i.e. through the bony ring comprising of the first rib, the first thoracic vertebra, and sternum) into the mediastinum of the thorax.

## Nape

If one touches the back of the neck, the nape (posterior cervical region), one palpates almost nothing but muscles: below the thin muscular layers of the trapezius on both sides of the vertebral column the powerful strands of the autochthonous (intrinsic) back muscles (→ p. 76, vol. 1) are located. They act as muscles of the neck and insert at the base of the occiput. The spinous processes of the upper six cervical vertebrae cannot be palpated as they lie below a dense sagittal tendon sheath, the nuchal ligament. However, the spinous process of the 7th cervical vertebra is visible and palpable, hence its name vertebra prominens.

## Anterior Cervical Region

If one applied the same force to grab the anterior cervical region (anterior triangle) as is possible for the nape, this would result in very unpleasant and painful sensations. As much as muscles determine the appearance of the nape, sensitive organs such as the viscera of the mediastinum extend into the anterior aspect of the neck. The lateral borders of the anterior cervical region are marked by sternocleidomastoid muscles which turn the head. Turning the head to either side causes the slim, actively flexed muscle belly of the sternocleidomastoid of the opposite side to protrude.

The **jugular fossa** is located at the base of the anterior cervical region between the clavicles and immediately above the sternum. Applying pressure with one's finger directly at the jugular fossa compresses the trachea and causes a feeling of being strangled. The esophagus is located posteriorly to the trachea and extends towards the larynx. The esophagus is impalpable, but one feels its posterior proximity to the trachea when swallowing an overly large and hard-edged bolus. The bolus presses ventrally on the trachea, since the extensibility of the esophagus is limited dorsally by the proximity of the esophagus to the cervical vertebral column.

Palpating along the trachea from the jugular fossa towards the head, one reaches the skeleton of the **larynx;** in men, the Adam's apple (laryngeal prominence) projects prominently. At about the level of the Adam's apple, the larynx separates the airways (anterior) and the alimentary passage (dorsal). The larynx is very mobile, and is held only by muscle loops. When swallowing, it moves cranially by as much as one entire cervical vertebra. The thyroid gland, located next to the trachea and the lower part of the larynx, consists of two large right and left lobes, which are hardly palpable – except in case of a goitre, an abnormal enlargement of the thyroid gland.

The cavity located cranially to the larynx is named the **pharynx.** Airways and alimentary passage cross at this point. Mouth and nasal cavities also open into the pharynx. Pressing the thumb and index finger on both sides of the larynx and moving them upward along the side of the neck towards the mandible while applying pressure causes major discomfort. This area is referred to as the **carotid triangle,** where the pulse of the common carotid artery is palpable very easily. This is where the common carotid artery divides into its two terminal branches, the external carotid artery and the internal carotid artery. If one slightly increases the external pressure, a bone is palpable in this region: the greater horn of the hyoid bone. Provided one has the courage to swallow while applying pressure, one notices the upward movement of the hyoid bone and larynx. In fact, the hyoid bone is a "tension rod" of the larynx, where some pharyngeal muscles attach and engage when swallowing. With further increased firm pressure the carotid artery is pressed against the hyoid bone (and the thyroid cartilage) – which can result in fainting (syncope) – or the hyoid bone can fracture, and in this case the blocking of the passage to the larynx leads to suffocation. Therefore medical examiners investigate the hyoid bone meticulously in doubtful causes of death.

Ensheathed in a common fascia (carotid sheath), the common carotid artery, the internal jugular vein, and the vagus nerve [X] descend bilaterally along the continuum of the trachea, the esophagus, the larynx, and the pharynx. The common carotid artery arises from the aortic arch on the left-hand side or the brachiocephalic trunc on the right-hand side. The internal jugular vein collects blood from the intracranial sinuses and the viscerocranium. The vagus nerve [X], a cranial nerve, descends towards the mediastinum and into the abdominal cavity. In the lower part of the anterior cervical region and in close proximity to the clavicle the sternocleidomastoid largely overlies this neurovascular bundle.

## The Lateral Cervical Region

The lateral cervical region (lateral triangle) is confined caudally by the clavicle, medially by the sternocleidomastoid and dorsally by the trapezius. The broadly defined inner space of the triangle extends – without sharp margins – under the clavicle and into the armpit (axilla). The lateral cervical region contains the large neural pathways descending steeply from the cervical vertebral column to the arm. Most nerves supplying the arm (brachial plexus) emerge from the cervical vertebral column. The lateral triangle also encompasses the great vessels of the arm (subclavian artery and vein), which come from the mediastinum, through the superior thoracic aperture, and descend behind the clavicle first into the lateral triangle and then into the axilla. There is hardly anything palpable, not even the pulse of the subclavian artery, because it lies deep in the lateral triangle, slightly behind the clavicle. There is also hardly anything visible as in a slim neck the skin covering the triangle over the clavicle forms the greater supraclavicular fossa. Sometimes, the large cutaneous vein of the neck, the external jugular vein, is visible through the skin; if one grimaces, the great cervical cutaneous muscle (platysma) stretches the thin skin of the neck.

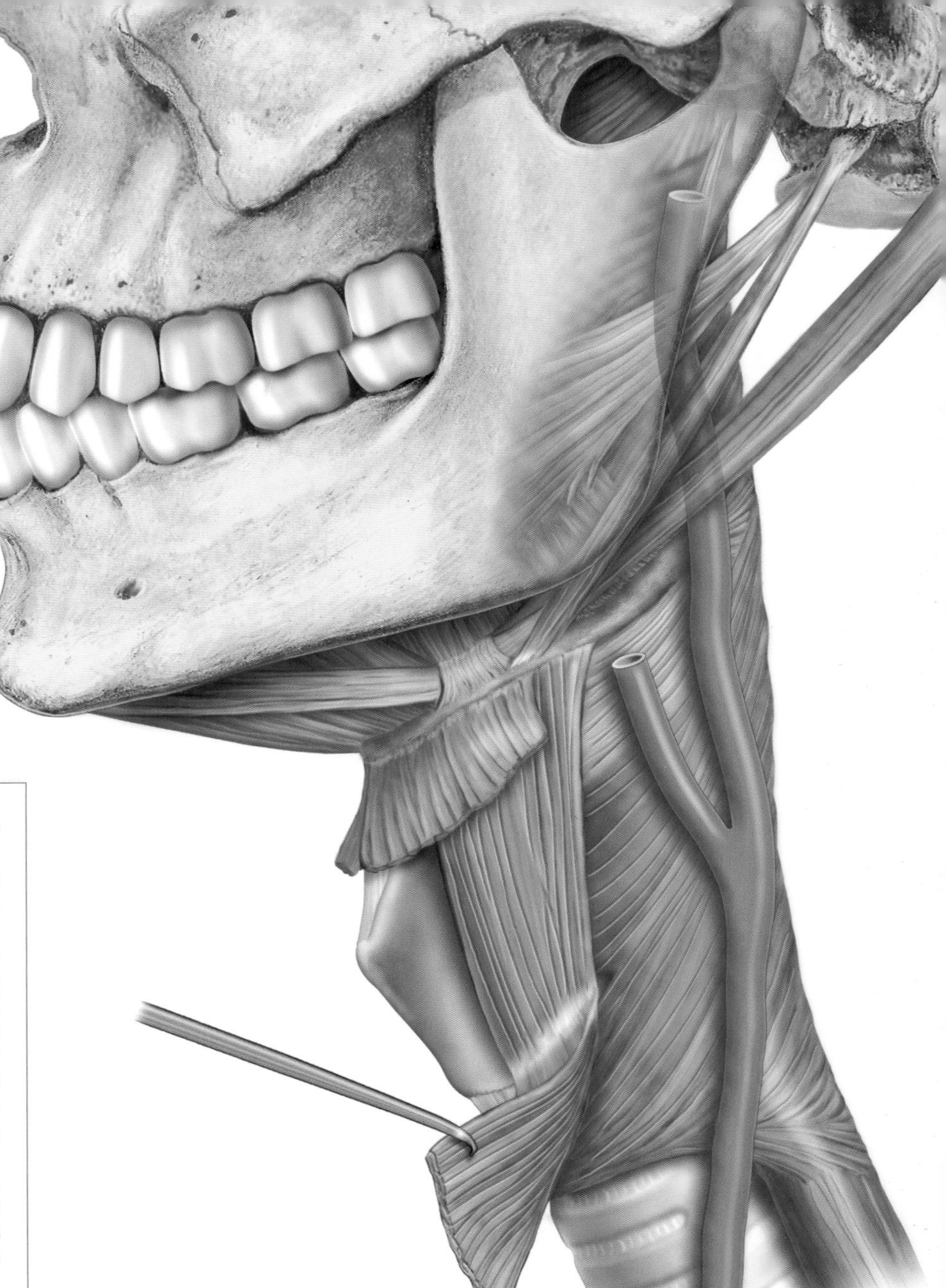

## Clinical Remarks

**Neck injuries** are usually dangerous because the neck acts as conduit between head and torso. With the exception of the cervical part of the vertebral column, all important soft structures of the neck are easily accessible, including major blood vessels, nerves, trachea, and esophagus.
The neck contains approximately 200 to 300 lymph nodes which receive lymph fluid from the entire head and partially also from the torso. Tumors of the head can metastasize to the cervical lymph nodes. Due to their exposed location, swelling of these lymph nodes can be a more obvious sign than the primary tumor itself. Also, the large number of lymph nodes in the neck is the reason why generalised **diseases of the lymphatic system,** like Hodgkin's disease, often become symptomatic in the neck region first.
Diseases affecting the thyroid gland can usually be spotted easily. The neck and its viscera are also important for the physician. The blood vessels can be used for venous puncture or as an **access route,** the anesthetist inserts the intubation tube through the nose or mouth, throat, and larynx into the trachea.
The larynx represents the tightest narrowing of all the airways. Diseases of the larynx or the aspiration of foreign bodies coincide with shortness of breath and in severe cases this can require a tracheotomy or an emergency coniotomy.

*→ Dissection Link*

**Dissection of the neck from ventral:** After exposing and reflecting the platysma superiorly, the epifascial nerves of the cervical plexus are demonstrated. Subsequently, the superficial fascia of the neck is removed, followed by dissection of the sternocleidomastoid, the anterior border of the trapezius and the accessory nerve [XI] in the lateral triangle of the neck. Upon removal of the middle fascia of the neck and exposure of the infrahyoid muscles, the carotid sheath is exposed together with the common, external, and internal caroid arteries, the internal jugular vein, and the vagus nerve [X]. The sternocleidomastoid is severed at the clavicle and deflected superiorly. The bilateral exarticulation of the clavicle is followed by the complete representation of the infrahyoid muscles with ansa cervicalis, by the detachment of the infrahyoid muscles which insert at the sternum, the visualization of the thyroid gland and its ventral blood supply as well as the dissection of the large vessels between head and arm, and of scalene muscles, brachial plexus, phrenic nerve, submandibular gland and its adjacent vessels, and the larynx from ventral and lateral. Subsequently, after the presentation of the sympathetic trunk on the cervical vertebral column, the head is exarticulated at the atlanto-occipital joint of the cervical vertebral column and, together with attached cervical structures, removed from the torso. After preparation of the pharynx from the dorsal side and illustration of the cerebral nerves, the pharynx is opened dorsally in the median line. This is followed by the dissection of the larynx from the dorsal side with a presentation of the vocal folds and the laryngeal muscles. Finally, the ventral aspect of the larynx is dissected.

## EXAM CHECK LIST

• Development of the thyroid gland (thyroglossal duct), the parathyroid gland, larynx, and pharynx • fasciae of the neck, buccopharyngeal fascia • infrahyoid muscles, neck muscles (platysma, sternocleidomastoid, trapezius, scalenus), prevertebral muscles, short neck muscles • vertebral triangle • pharynx • cervical section of the esophagus • larynx • cervical section of the trachea • thyroid gland, epithelial bodies • carotid body • cranial nerves (glossopharyngeal nerve [IX], vagus nerve [X], accessory nerve [XI], hypoglossal nerve [XII]), cervical nerves (dorsal branches, ventral branches, cervical plexus) • autonomic innervation (sympathetic part, parasympathetic part) of vessels • common carotid artery, internal carotid artery, external carotid artery, internal jugular vein, venous angle • superficial and deep cervical lymph nodes, confluence of major lymphatic collector systems • surface anatomy of the neck • peripharyngeal space • regions of the neck • imaging techniques

## Regions of the neck

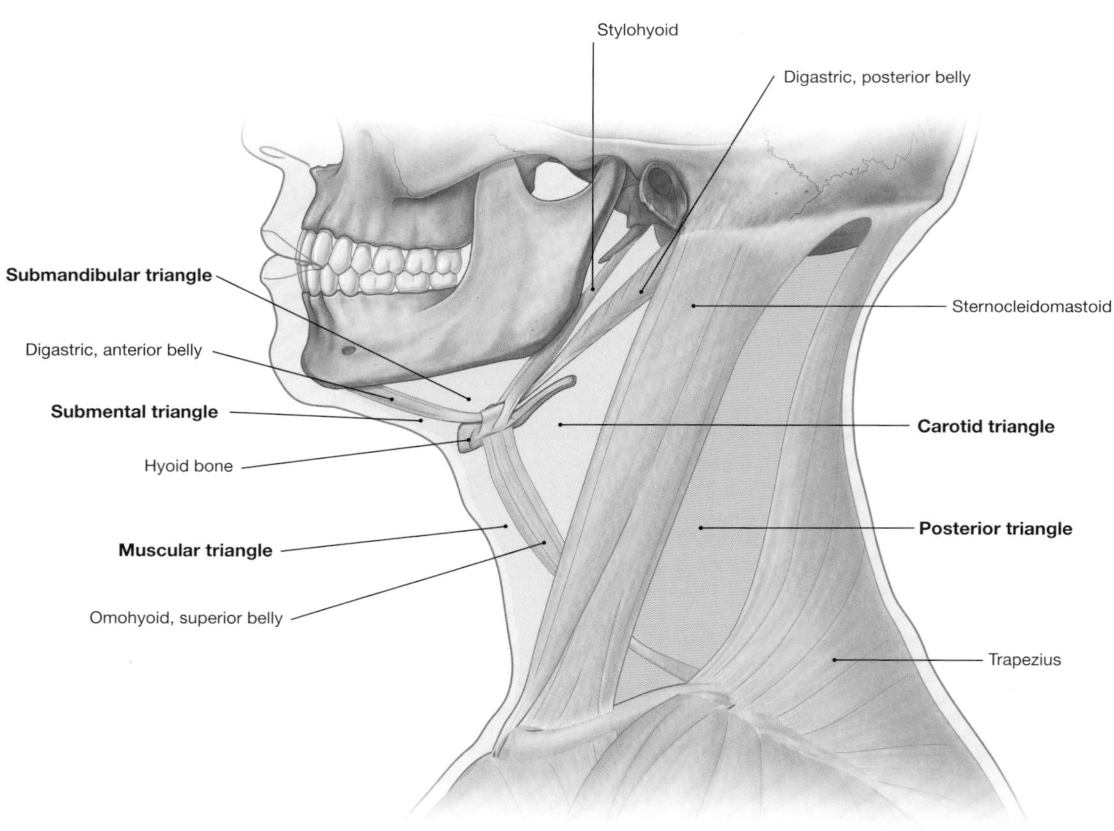
Stylohyoid
Digastric, posterior belly
Submandibular triangle
Sternocleidomastoid
Digastric, anterior belly
Submental triangle
Carotid triangle
Hyoid bone
Muscular triangle
Posterior triangle
Omohyoid, superior belly
Trapezius

**Fig. 11.1 Anterior and lateral regions of the neck, left side;** lateral view. [8]

Boundaries of the **anterior triangle of the neck** (anterior cervical region) are the lower rim of the mandible, the anterior border of the sternocleidomastoid, and the median cervical line (midline of the neck). Located within the anterior triangle of the neck are the submandibular triangle (margins: lower rim of the mandible, anterior belly and posterior belly of the digastric), the submental triangle (margins: hyoid bone, anterior belly of the digastric, median cervical line), the muscular triangle (margins: hyoid bone, superior belly of the omohyoid, sternocleidomastoid, median cervical line), and the carotid triangle (margins: superior belly of the omohyoid, the lowest part of the stylohyoid, posterior belly of the digastric, sternocleidomastoid).

Boundaries of the **posterior triangle of the neck** (posterior cervical region) are the posterior border of the sternocleidomastoid, the anterior border of the trapezius, the upper border of the clavicle and the occipital bone.

## Neck muscles

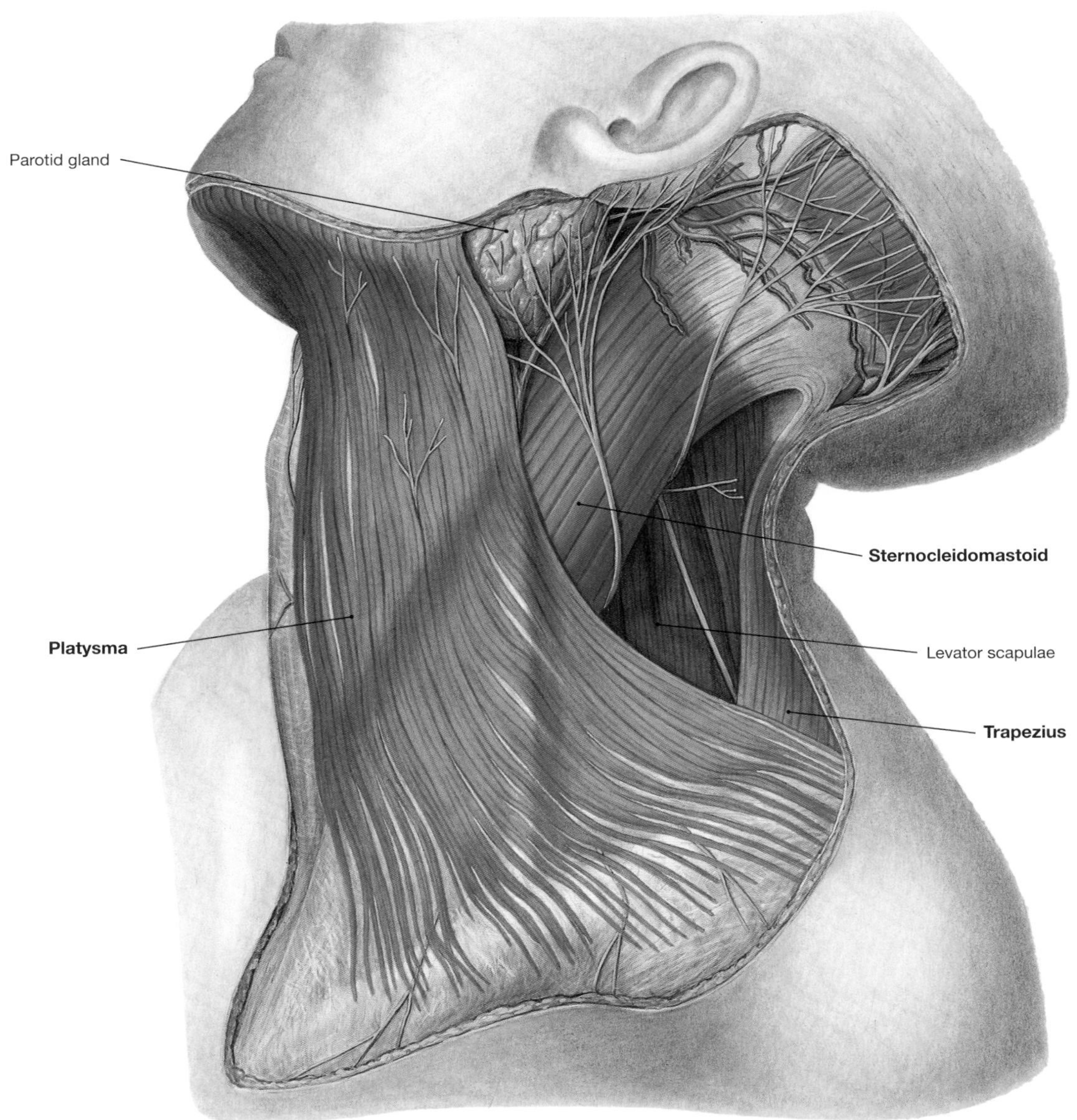
Parotid gland
Sternocleidomastoid
Platysma
Levator scapulae
Trapezius

**Fig. 11.2 Muscles of the anterior and lateral neck regions, superficial layer; left side;** lateral view.

The platysma (a mimetic muscle without fascia) is a thin muscular plate and locates superficially directly under the skin. It extends from the mandible, across the clavicle, and onto the thorax. The posterolateral part of the superficial neck fascia has been removed. The upper part of the sternocleidomastoid is a reference point during surgical interventions. Located further posterior and inferior, the anterior rim of the trapezius becomes visible. The lower pole of the parotid gland lies between the platysma and the sternocleidomastoid and can extend into the neck region to a variable degree. The levator scapulae is visible deep in the posterior triangle of the neck.

→T 1f, 8

## Neck muscles and tracheotomy

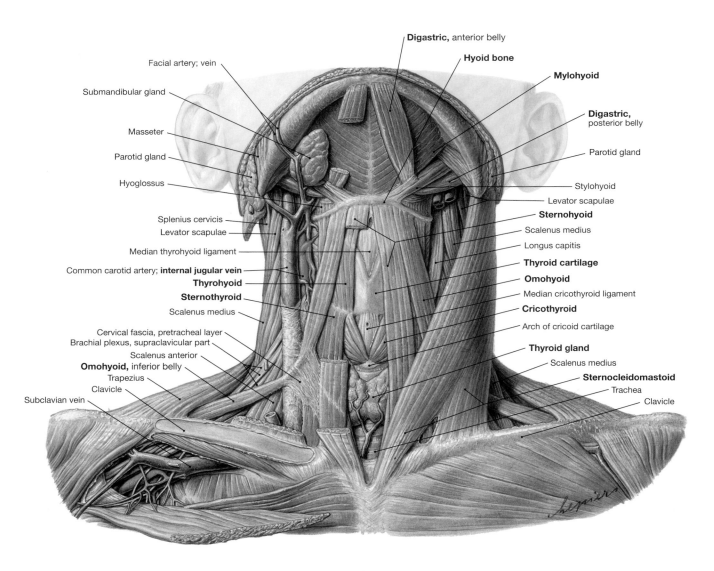

Digastric, anterior belly
Hyoid bone
Facial artery; vein
Mylohyoid
Submandibular gland
Digastric, posterior belly
Masseter
Parotid gland
Parotid gland
Hyoglossus
Stylohyoid
Levator scapulae
Splenius cervicis
Sternohyoid
Levator scapulae
Scalenus medius
Median thyrohyoid ligament
Longus capitis
Common carotid artery; internal jugular vein
Thyroid cartilage
Thyrohyoid
Omohyoid
Sternothyroid
Median cricothyroid ligament
Scalenus medius
Cricothyroid
Arch of cricoid cartilage
Cervical fascia, pretracheal layer
Brachial plexus, supraclavicular part
Thyroid gland
Scalenus anterior
Scalenus medius
Omohyoid, inferior belly
Sternocleidomastoid
Trapezius
Trachea
Clavicle
Clavicle
Subclavian vein

**Fig. 11.3 Neck muscles;** ventral view; chin elevated.
The **superficial** sternocleidomastoid has two origins (sternal head and clavicular head) and extends to the mastoid process. Its caudal section covers the origin of the **infrahyoid muscles** with the sternohyoid, sternothyroid, thyrohyoid and omohyoid, which stretch between the sternum, thyroid cartilage, hyoid bone, and scapula (omohyoid). The omohyoid is composed of two bellies separated by an intermediate tendon affixed to the connective tissue of the carotid sheath and serves to keep the lumen of the jugular vein open. The isthmus of the thyroid gland, the paired cricothyroid (an outer laryngeal muscle), the thyroid cartilage, and the hyoid bone are located beneath the infrahyoid muscles (from caudal to cranial). Above the hyoid bone, the mylohyoid forms the floor of the mouth.

→ T 8–11

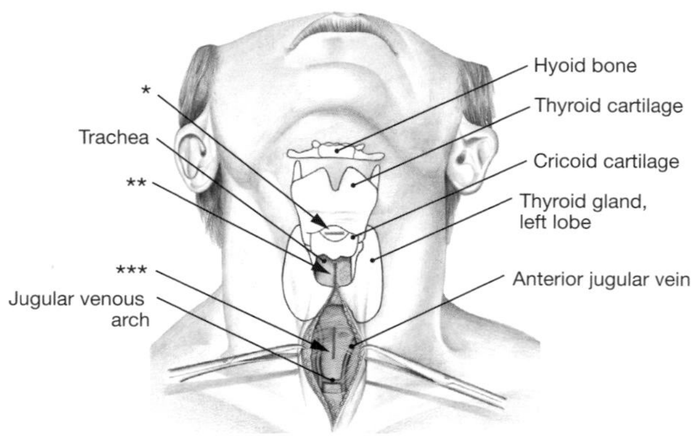
Hyoid bone
*
Thyroid cartilage
Trachea
Cricoid cartilage
**
Thyroid gland, left lobe
***
Anterior jugular vein
Jugular venous arch

**Fig. 11.4 Surgical access to the trachea;** ventral view; with the neck hyperextended dorsally.
During **coniotomy,** an incision or puncture through the median cricothyroid ligament (ligamentum conicum, → Fig. 11.28) in between the thyroid and cricoid cartilages is performed to access the laryngeal lumen shortly beneath the vocal folds.
Performing a **tracheotomy,** there are three possible access routes: (i) an upper access above the isthmus of the thyroid gland, (ii) a middle access route by cutting through the isthmus, and (iii) a lower access below the isthmus of the thyroid gland (→ Fig. 11.50).

* coniotomy
** upper tracheotomy
*** lower tracheotomy

## Neck muscles

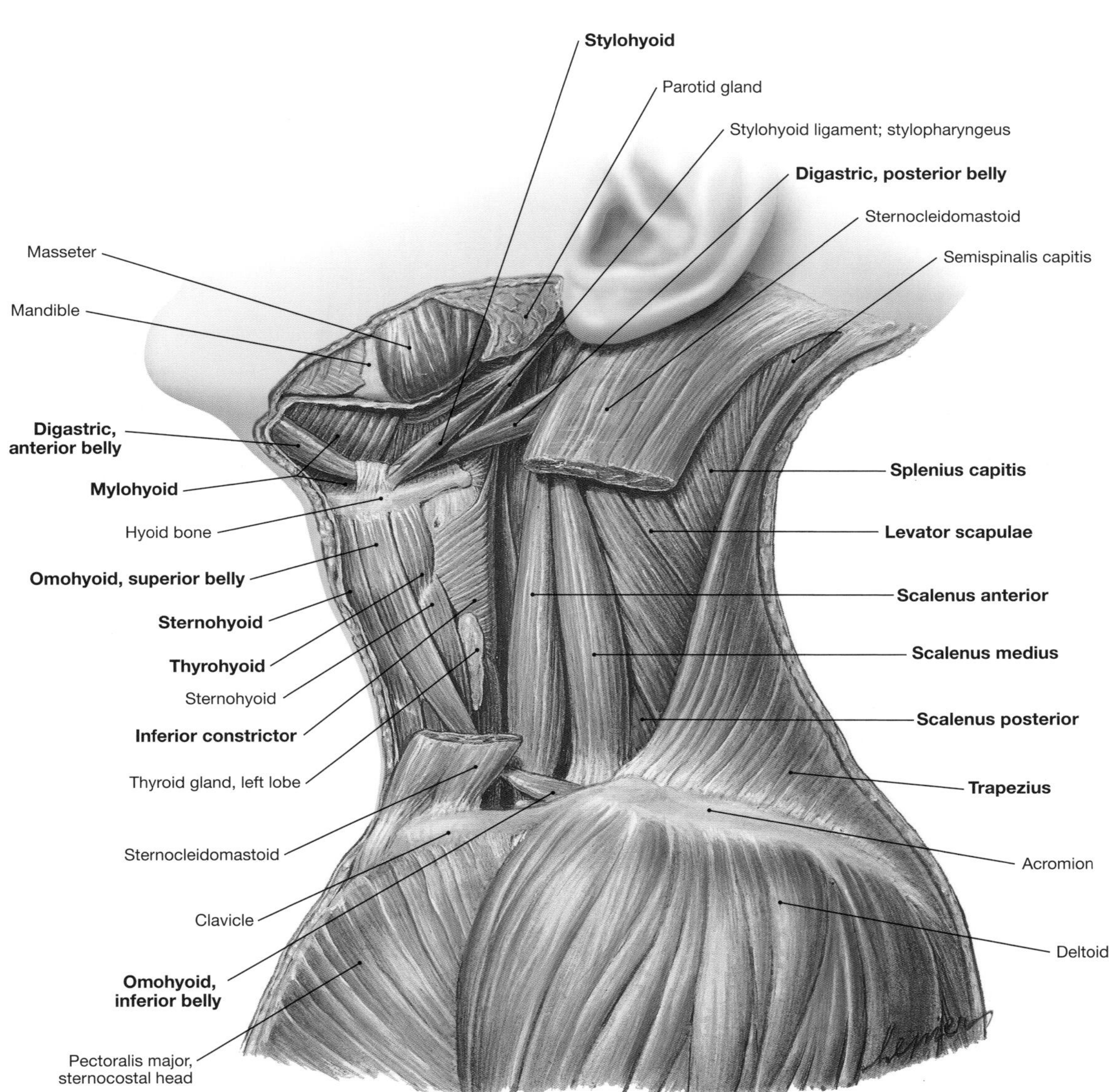
Stylohyoid
Parotid gland
Stylohyoid ligament; stylopharyngeus
Digastric, posterior belly
Sternocleidomastoid
Semispinalis capitis
Masseter
Mandible
Digastric, anterior belly
Mylohyoid
Hyoid bone
Omohyoid, superior belly
Sternohyoid
Thyrohyoid
Sternohyoid
Inferior constrictor
Thyroid gland, left lobe
Sternocleidomastoid
Clavicle
Omohyoid, inferior belly
Pectoralis major, sternocostal head
Splenius capitis
Levator scapulae
Scalenus anterior
Scalenus medius
Scalenus posterior
Trapezius
Acromion
Deltoid

**Fig. 11.5 Neck muscles;** lateral view.
All muscle fascias, the platysma, and the middle portion of the sternocleidomastoid were resected. From anterior to posterior the following structures can be seen: the **infrahyoid muscles** with the sternohyoid, omohyoid (superior belly; the inferior belly runs above the clavicle in the lateral triangle of the neck), thyrohyoid and sternothyroid, parts of the pharyngeal muscles (inferior constrictor), the scalene muscles (anterior, middle, and posterior), the levator scapulae, the splenius capitis, and the trapezius. Above the hyoid bone, three **suprahyoid muscles** (digastric with anterior belly and posterior belly, mylohyoid, and stylohyoid) are visible.

→T 8–11

## Prevertebral muscles

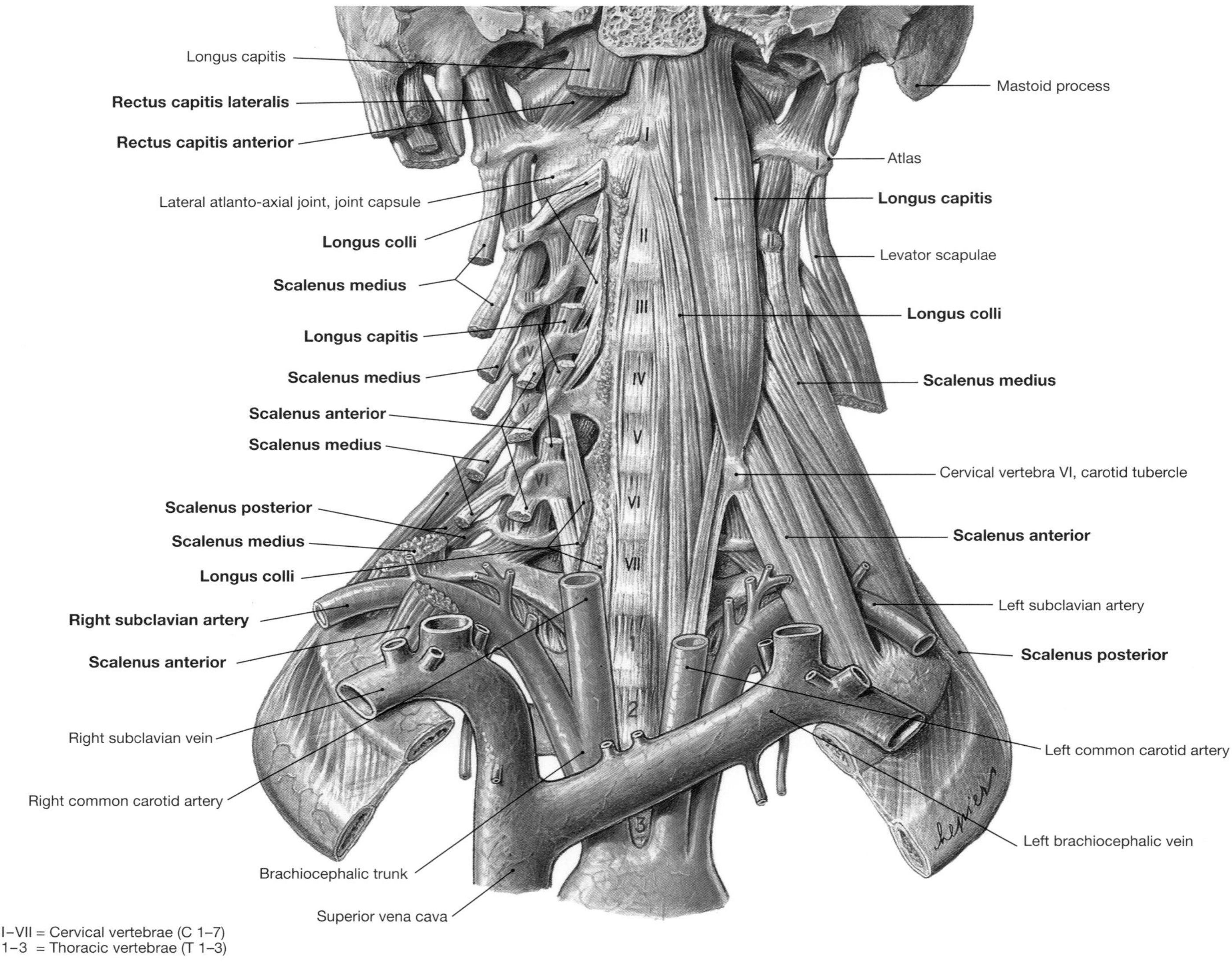
Longus capitis
Rectus capitis lateralis
Rectus capitis anterior
Lateral atlanto-axial joint, joint capsule
Longus colli
Scalenus medius
Longus capitis
Scalenus medius
Scalenus anterior
Scalenus medius
Scalenus posterior
Scalenus medius
Longus colli
Right subclavian artery
Scalenus anterior
Right subclavian vein
Right common carotid artery
Brachiocephalic trunk
Superior vena cava
Mastoid process
Atlas
Longus capitis
Levator scapulae
Longus colli
Scalenus medius
Cervical vertebra VI, carotid tubercle
Scalenus anterior
Left subclavian artery
Scalenus posterior
Left common carotid artery
Left brachiocephalic vein
I–VII = Cervical vertebrae (C 1–7)
1–3 = Thoracic vertebrae (T 1–3)

**Fig. 11.6 Prevertebral muscles and scalene muscles;** ventral view.
The **prevertebral muscles** are located on both sides of the vertebral bodies of the cervical and upper thoracic vertebral column and are covered by the prevertebral lamina of the cervical fascia. The rectus capitis anterior stretches between the anterolateral parts of the atlas and the axis. In addition to the rectus capitis anterior, the longus capitis and the longus colli are prevertebral muscles. As part of the ventrolateral muscle group, the rectus capitis lateralis has migrated into the prevertebral region.
The anterior, middle, and posterior **scalene muscles** insert at the first ribs and form a triangular-shaped muscle plate in the lateral region of the cervical vertebral column. Together with the upper rim of the rib I, the scalenus anterior and scalenus medius create the **scalene hiatus.** The subclavian artery and the brachial plexus pass through the scalene hiatus (not shown).
Some authors distinguish between an anterior and posterior scalene hiatus. The anterior scalene hiatus represents the course of the subclavian vein in front of the scalenus anterior across rib I, while the posterior scalene hiatus marks the space between the scalenus anterior and medius for the subclavian artery and the brachial plexus to cross rib I. Since the anterior scalene hiatus is not a true gap, the term scalene hiatus should only be used for the space between the scalenus anterior and scalenus medius.

→ T 11, 12

## Fasciae of the neck

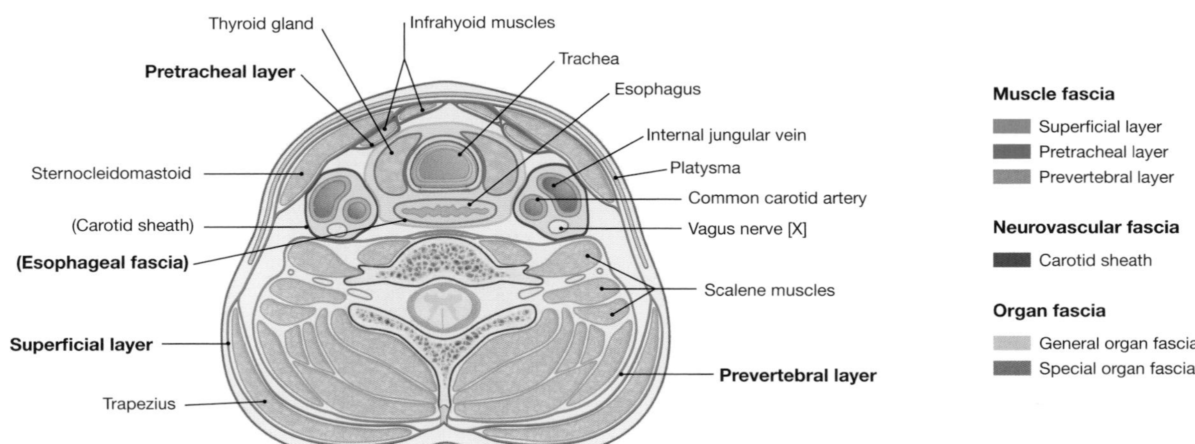
Thyroid gland
Infrahyoid muscles
Pretracheal layer
Trachea
Esophagus
Internal jungular vein
Sternocleidomastoid
Platysma
Common carotid artery
(Carotid sheath)
Vagus nerve [X]
(Esophageal fascia)
Scalene muscles
Superficial layer
Prevertebral layer
Trapezius
Muscle fascia
Superficial layer
Pretracheal layer
Prevertebral layer
Neurovascular fascia
Carotid sheath
Organ fascia
General organ fascia
Special organ fascia

**Fig. 11.7 Cervical fascia;** transverse section through the neck. [8]
A muscle fascia with three layers can be distinguished from a neurovascular fascia, and an organ fascia with two layers.

**Muscle fascia:**
- superficial layer (encases the whole neck and ensheathes the sternocleidomastoid as well as the levator scapulae and trapezius in the neck region)
- pretracheal layer (middle lamina, ensheathes the infrahyoid muscles)
- prevertebral layer (deep lamina, enwraps the scalene muscles, prevertebral muscles, the rectus capitis lateralis, and merges with the fascia of the intrinsic [autochthonous] muscles of the back)

**Neurovascular fascia:**
- carotid sheath (ensheathes the common, internal and external carotid arteries, internal jugular vein, vagus nerve [X])

**Organ fascia:**
- general organ fascia (encases all neck structures like pharynx, larynx, thyroid gland, parathyroid gland, upper part of the trachea, cervical part of the esophagus)
- special organ fascia = organ capsule (ensheathes each of the organs of the neck, e.g. esophageal fascia)

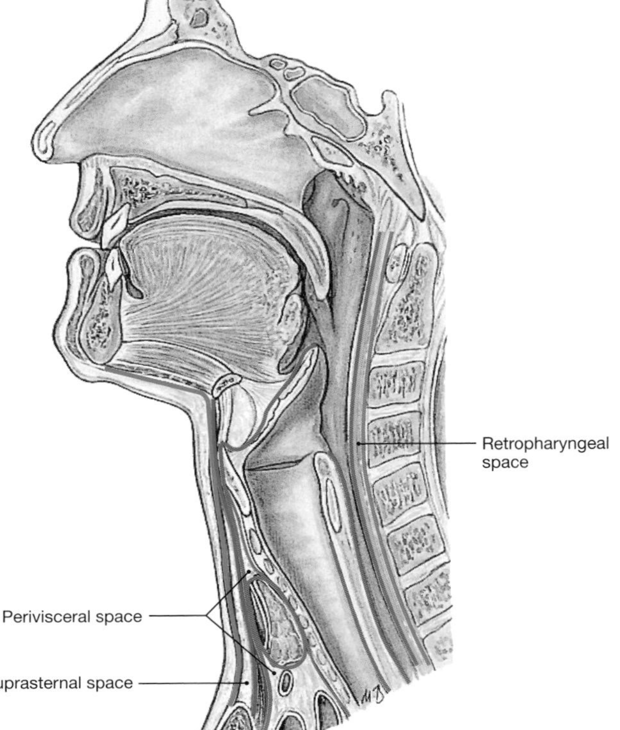
Retropharyngeal space
Perivisceral space
Suprasternal space

**Fig. 11.8 Schematic drawing of the cervical fascia;** sagittal section through the neck at the level of the larynx.
Above the sternum, the suprasternal space is formed between the superficial and middle cervical fascia. The perivisceral space is located in front of the trachea and in between the middle cervical fascia and the general organ fascia. The retropharyngeal space lies in a prevertebral space delineated by the middle cervical fascia and the general organ fascia (→ Fig. 11.17).

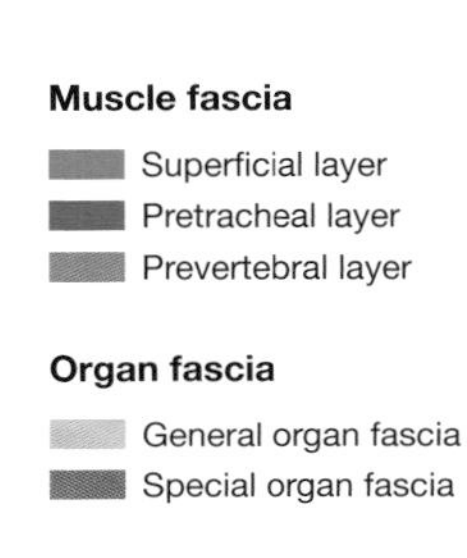
Muscle fascia
Superficial layer
Pretracheal layer
Prevertebral layer
Organ fascia
General organ fascia
Special organ fascia

## Fasciae of the neck

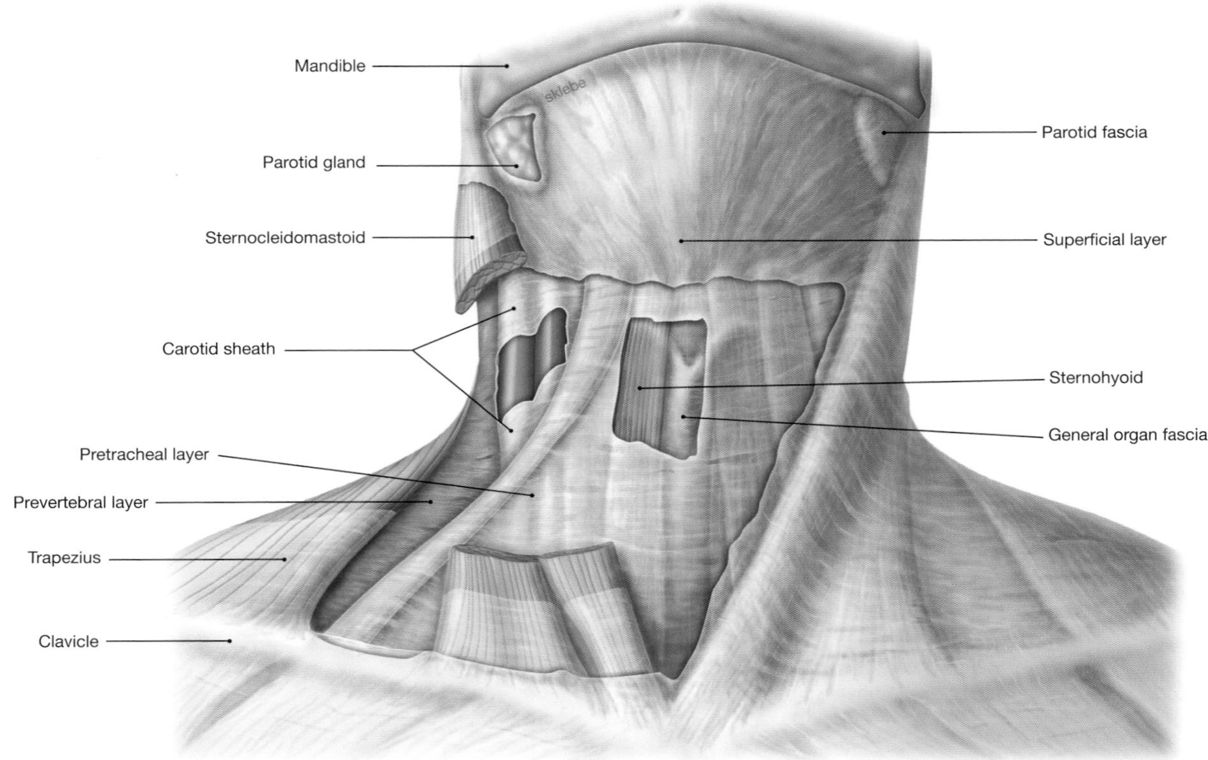
Mandible
Parotid gland
Sternocleidomastoid
Carotid sheath
Pretracheal layer
Prevertebral layer
Trapezius
Clavicle
Parotid fascia
Superficial layer
Sternohyoid
General organ fascia

**Fig. 11.9 Muscle fascia of the neck;** ventral view.
The platysma was removed on both sides. On the right side, the superficial layer of the cervical fascia is intact and ensheathes the sternocleidomastoid. On the left side, most of the muscles and the superficial layer of the cervical fascia were resected. Above the larynx, a small part of the middle cervical fascia was removed to demonstrate the sternohyoid, a muscle normally ensheathed by the middle cervical fascia, and the general organ fascia located below. The fenestrated carotid sheath and the deep cervical fascia are visible at the posterior margin of the omohyoid.

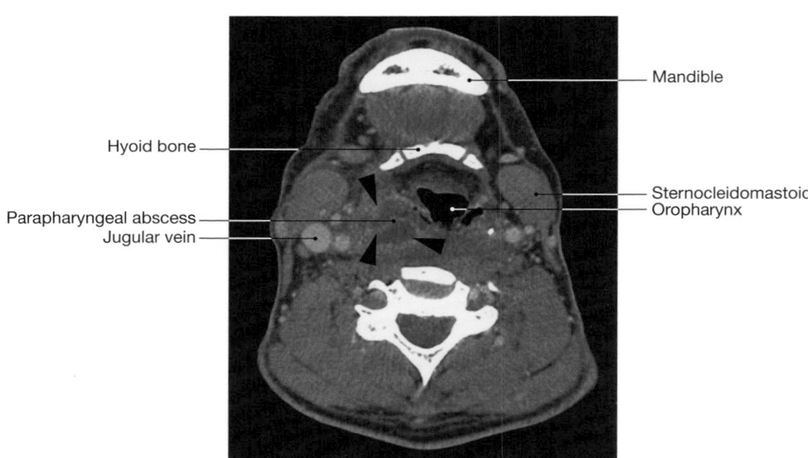
Mandible
Hyoid bone
Sternocleidomastoid
Oropharynx
Parapharyngeal abscess
Jugular vein

**Fig. 11.10 Parapharyngeal abscess, left side;** ventral view. [13]
The abscess extends along the anatomically defined space (lateropharyngeal space) in the cervical region (black arrow tips).

### Clinical Remarks

During surgical procedures in the cervical region (e.g. neck dissection), the fascial laminae of the neck and the spaces of connective tissue delineated by them serve as reference structures for the surgeon. Bleedings and abscesses can distribute in between the fascial laminae and descend caudally into the mediastinum. The weakness of the walls of the pharynx can result in an invasion of microorganisms into the parapharyngeal and retropharyngeal spaces (**parapharyngeal** [peripharyngeal], → Fig. 11.10, or **retropharyngeal abscess**).

## Fasciae of the neck

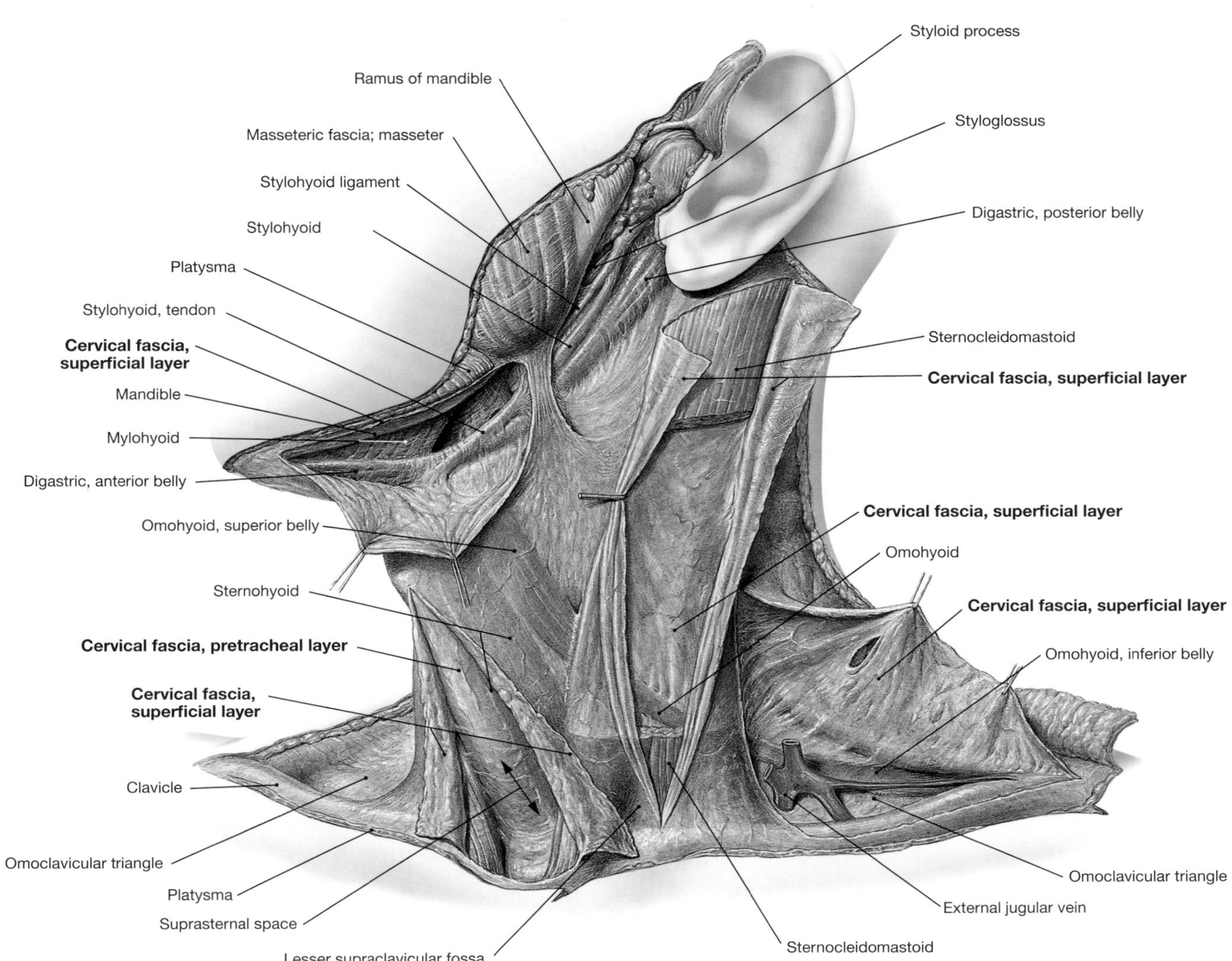
Styloid process
Ramus of mandible
Styloglossus
Masseteric fascia; masseter
Stylohyoid ligament
Digastric, posterior belly
Stylohyoid
Platysma
Stylohyoid, tendon
Sternocleidomastoid
Cervical fascia, superficial layer
Cervical fascia, superficial layer
Mandible
Mylohyoid
Digastric, anterior belly
Cervical fascia, superficial layer
Omohyoid, superior belly
Omohyoid
Sternohyoid
Cervical fascia, superficial layer
Cervical fascia, pretracheal layer
Omohyoid, inferior belly
Cervical fascia, superficial layer
Clavicle
Omoclavicular triangle
Omoclavicular triangle
Platysma
External jugular vein
Suprasternal space
Sternocleidomastoid
Lesser supraclavicular fossa

**Fig. 11.11 Cervical fascia, left side;** ventrolateral view.
The superficial layer of the cervical fascia has been opened and detached in various places. The superficial layer of the cervical fascia that ensheathes the sternocleidomastoid has been opened also and the middle portion of the sternocleidomastoid has been resected. Thus, the fascial sheath and the deep part of the superficial fascia become visible. From the jugular notch of the sternum to the level of the larynx, the superficial layer of the cervical fascia has been slit open and folded sideways to open up the suprasternal space. Upon removal of the adipose tissue (frequently the jugular venous arch can be found here, → Fig. 11.17), the pretracheal (middle) layer of the cervical fascia becomes visible, which forms the posterior wall of the suprasternal space. In addition, the superficial layer of the cervical fascia has been resected at the mandible and was folded downwards to demonstrate the tendon of the stylohyoid, the mylohyoid, and the anterior belly of the digastric. In the posterior triangle of the neck, the superficial cervical fascia has been removed from the clavicle and folded upwards. Beneath, the external jugular vein and the inferior belly of the omohyoid, ensheathed by the middle cervical fascia, are visible.

## Pharyngeal muscles

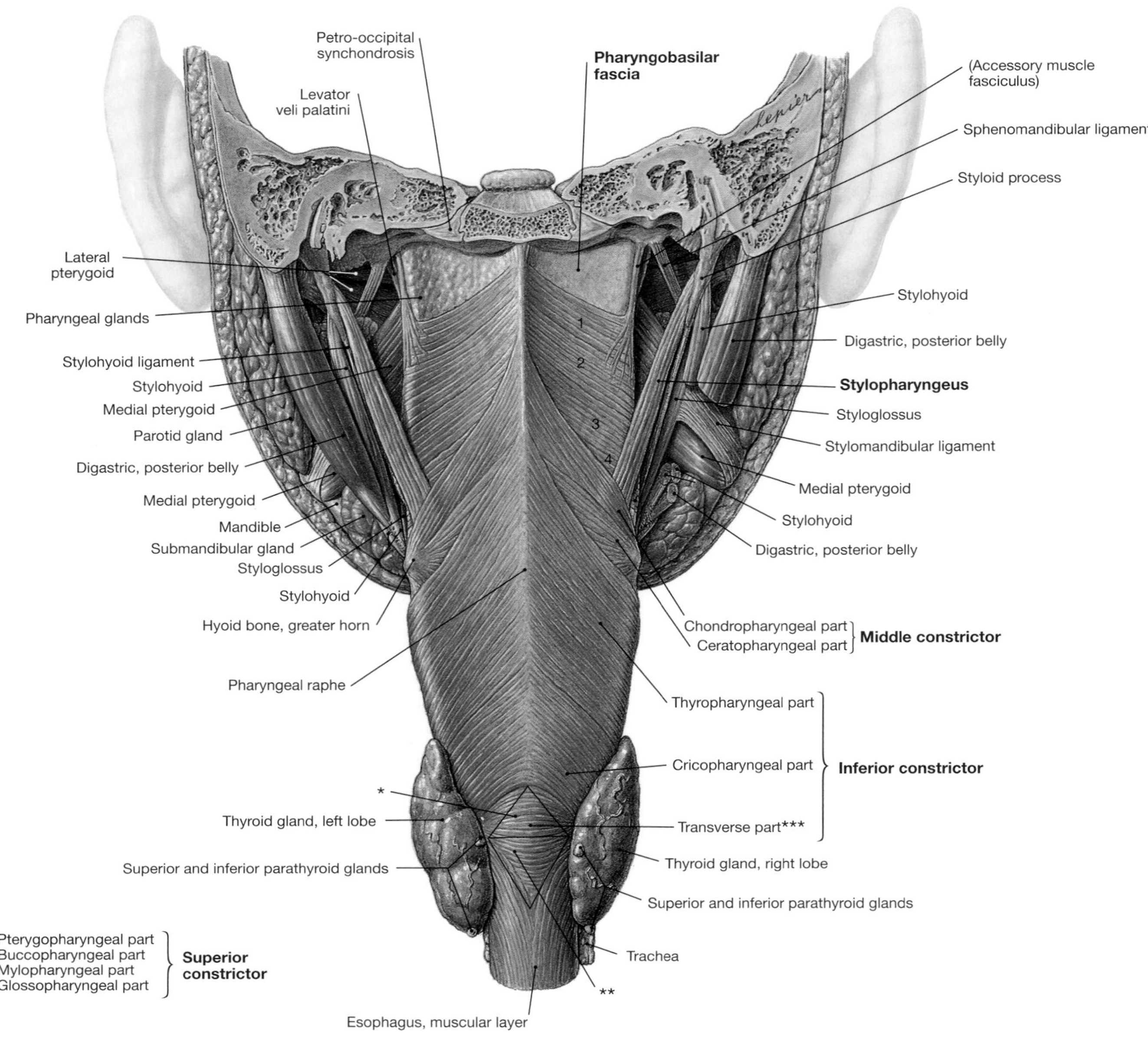
Petro-occipital synchondrosis
Levator veli palatini
Pharyngobasilar fascia
(Accessory muscle fasciculus)
Sphenomandibular ligament
Styloid process
Lateral pterygoid
Pharyngeal glands
Stylohyoid ligament
Stylohyoid
Medial pterygoid
Parotid gland
Digastric, posterior belly
Medial pterygoid
Mandible
Submandibular gland
Styloglossus
Stylohyoid
Hyoid bone, greater horn
Pharyngeal raphe
Stylohyoid
Digastric, posterior belly
Stylopharyngeus
Styloglossus
Stylomandibular ligament
Medial pterygoid
Stylohyoid
Digastric, posterior belly
Chondropharyngeal part
Ceratopharyngeal part
Middle constrictor
Thyropharyngeal part
Cricopharyngeal part
Inferior constrictor
Transverse part***
Thyroid gland, right lobe
Superior and inferior parathyroid glands
Trachea
**
*
Thyroid gland, left lobe
Superior and inferior parathyroid glands
1 Pterygopharyngeal part
2 Buccopharyngeal part
3 Mylopharyngeal part
4 Glossopharyngeal part
Superior constrictor
Esophagus, muscular layer

**Fig. 11.12 Pharyngeal muscles;** dorsal view.
The muscle layer of pharynx consists of the **constrictor muscles** and three paired **levator muscles** elevating the pharynx. Submucosa and adventitia combine to form the pharyngobasilar fascia in a muscle-free upper part of the pharyngeal wall. Constricting and elevating pharyngeal muscles mainly act during swallowing, choking, and during speaking and singing.
The superior, middle, and inferior **constrictors muscles** consist of different parts. The muscles enclose the pharyngeal lumen like a horseshoe and overlap, with the lower muscle slightly covering the lower margin of the muscle above. The cricopharyngeal part of the inferior constrictor is composed of two muscle parts which together form a triangle weak in muscle fibers (KILLIAN's dehiscence, also called KILLIAN's triangle). On the dorsal side, at the transition from the fundiform part of the inferior constrictor to the esophagus, muscle fibers projecting upwards from the esophagus form a muscular triangle (LAIMER's triangle). The tip of the LAIMER's triangle points in the opposite direction to the tip of the KILLIAN's triangle. The fundiform part of the cricopharyngeal part of the inferior constrictor is the base of both triangles.
The muscles elevating the pharynx are the **palatopharyngeus, salpingopharyngeus,** and **stylopharyngeus.**

* KILLIAN's triangle or dehiscence
** LAIMER's triangle
*** Pars fundiformis of the Pars cricopharyngea (KILLIAN's muscle)

→T 5

## Clinical Remarks

The KILLIAN's triangle or dehiscence marks a weak spot in the pharyngeal muscles and often creates a problem in aged men. The increased intraluminal pressure causes the pharyngeal wall to bulge out through the muscular weak spot and creates a **pharyngo-esophageal diverticulum** (ZENKER's diverticulum) into the retropharyngeal space. This can cause regurgitation of ingested food back into the mouth.

## Facial and pharyngeal muscles

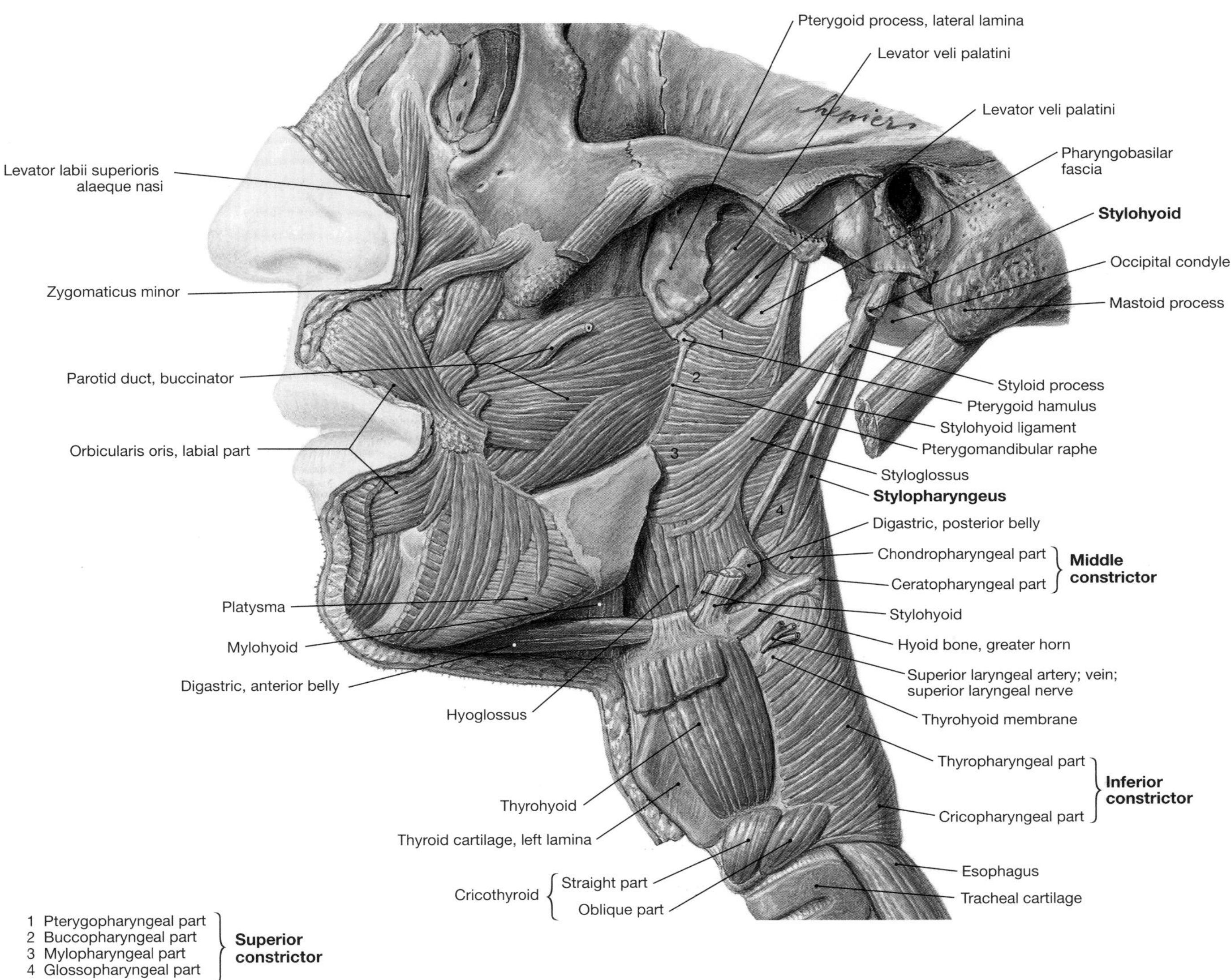
Pterygoid process, lateral lamina
Levator veli palatini
Levator veli palatini
Pharyngobasilar fascia
Stylohyoid
Occipital condyle
Mastoid process
Styloid process
Pterygoid hamulus
Stylohyoid ligament
Pterygomandibular raphe
Styloglossus
Stylopharyngeus
Digastric, posterior belly
Chondropharyngeal part
Ceratopharyngeal part
Middle constrictor
Stylohyoid
Hyoid bone, greater horn
Superior laryngeal artery; vein; superior laryngeal nerve
Thyrohyoid membrane
Thyropharyngeal part
Cricopharyngeal part
Inferior constrictor
Esophagus
Tracheal cartilage
Levator labii superioris alaeque nasi
Zygomaticus minor
Parotid duct, buccinator
Orbicularis oris, labial part
Platysma
Mylohyoid
Digastric, anterior belly
Hyoglossus
Thyrohyoid
Thyroid cartilage, left lamina
Cricothyroid
Straight part
Oblique part
1 Pterygopharyngeal part
2 Buccopharyngeal part
3 Mylopharyngeal part
4 Glossopharyngeal part
Superior constrictor

**Fig. 11.13 Pharyngeal muscles and facial muscles, left side;** lateral view.
The pharyngeal muscles divide into constrictor muscles (superior, middle, and inferior constrictor) and levator muscles (stylopharyngeus, salpingopharyngeus, and palatopharyngeus). This lateral view displays the different parts of the constrictor muscles and the stylopharyngeus.

→T 1e, 5

## Clinics

Straight variant of the internal carotid artery

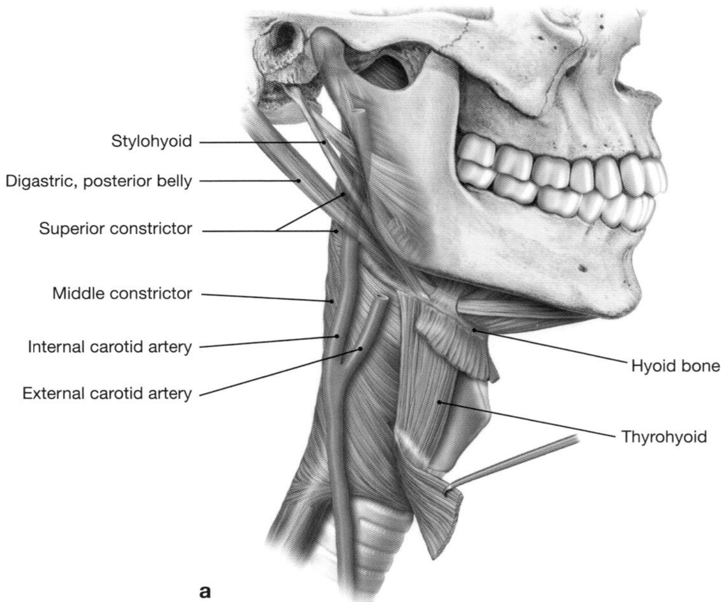
Stylohyoid
Digastric, posterior belly
Superior constrictor
Middle constrictor
Internal carotid artery
External carotid artery
Hyoid bone
Thyrohyoid
a

Curved variant of the internal carotid artery

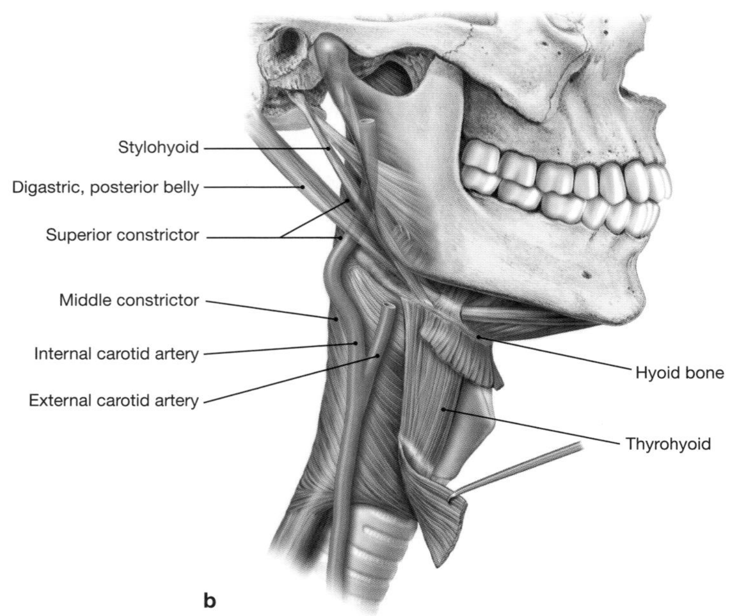
Stylohyoid
Digastric, posterior belly
Superior constrictor
Middle constrictor
Internal carotid artery
External carotid artery
Hyoid bone
Thyrohyoid
b

S-shaped course of the internal carotid artery (kinking)

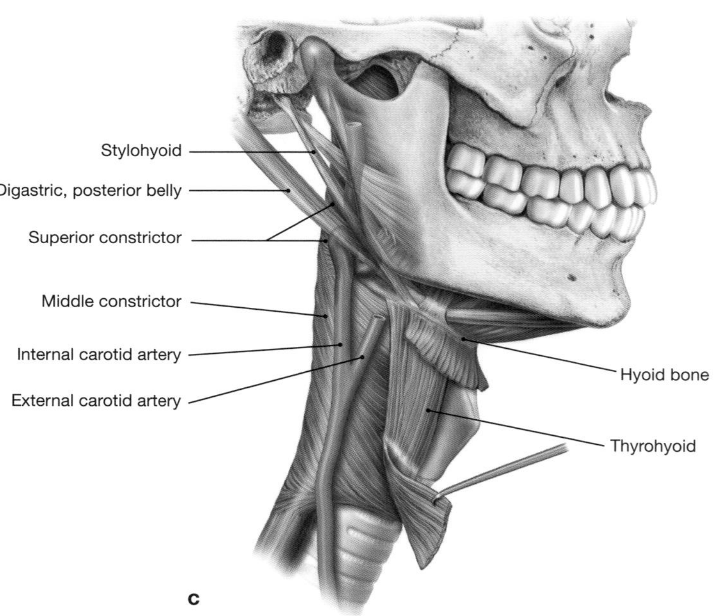
Stylohyoid
Digastric, posterior belly
Superior constrictor
Middle constrictor
Internal carotid artery
External carotid artery
Hyoid bone
Thyrohyoid
c

Loop formation of the internal carotid artery (coiling)

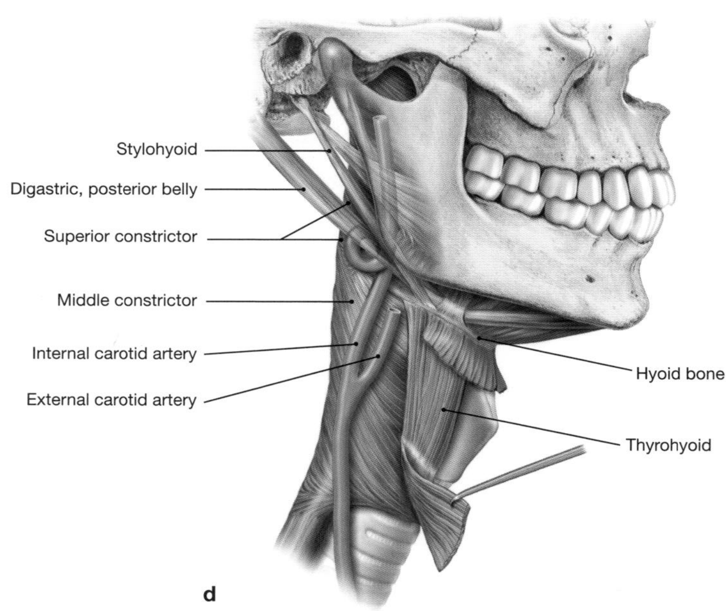
Stylohyoid
Digastric, posterior belly
Superior constrictor
Middle constrictor
Internal carotid artery
External carotid artery
Hyoid bone
Thyrohyoid
d

**Figs. 11.14a to d Variations in the course of the cervical part of the internal carotid artery in relation to the pharyngeal wall.**

- **a** Straight variant (frequency 66%)
- **b** Curved variant (frequency 26.2%)
- **c** S-shaped course (frequency 6%, 2.8% thereof in close association with the pharyngeal wall)
- **d** Loop formation (frequency 1.8%, 2.8% thereof in close association with the pharyngeal wall)

The S-shaped course and the loop formation are classified as **dangerous carotid loops** (**c** and **d**).

## Clinical Remarks

The close topographic relationship between the internal carotid artery and the tonsils (location of the palatine tonsil at the posterior margin of the isthmus of fauces [oropharyngeal isthmus]) and the presence of a **dangerous carotid loop** can result in injuries to the carotid artery with accidental fatal bleeding during tonsillectomy or opening of a peritonsillar abscess.

Clinics

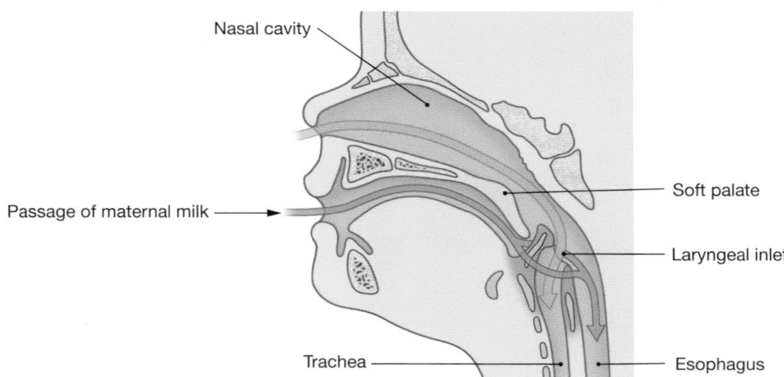
Nasal cavity
Passage of maternal milk
Soft palate
Laryngeal inlet
Trachea
Esophagus

**Fig. 11.15 Head of an infant;** midsagittal section at the level of the nose and larynx. [9]
Contrary to adults and children, an infant can drink and breathe simultaneously. Since the larynx locates relatively high in the neck, the epiglottis reaches the nasopharynx. Fluids (e.g. the breast milk from the mother) pass through the piriform recess of the larynx into the esophagus without entering the lower airways.

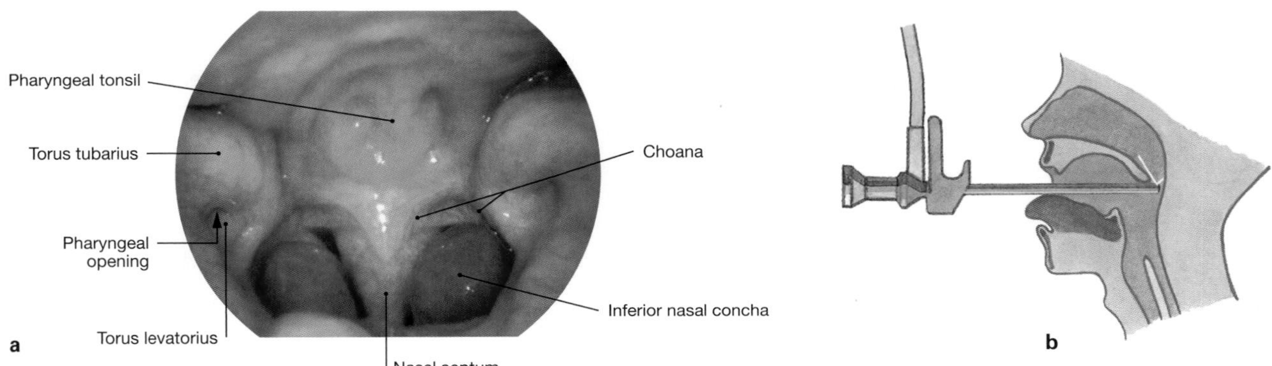
Pharyngeal tonsil
Torus tubarius
Pharyngeal opening
Torus levatorius
Choana
Inferior nasal concha
Nasal septum
a
b

**Figs. 11.16a and b Nasopharynx;** endoscopy of the nasopharynx; posterior view at the choanae, the opening of the auditory tube and the pharyngeal tonsil.
The endoscopic view from posterior into the nasopharyngeal space shows the posterior tips of the inferior nasal conchae on both sides and the pharyngeal opening of the auditory tube (pharyngeal opening of the auditory tube). The inconspicuous pharyngeal tonsil locates at the roof of the pharynx.

## Clinical Remarks

Hyperplasia of the pharyngeal tonsil **(adenoids)** occurs frequently in children. It can lead to the occlusion of the opening of the auditory tube, and cause recurring middle ear infections. In young children, this condition can result in hearing impairment and subsequently causes a delay in development. In these cases a surgical removal of the pharyngeal tonsil **(adenectomy)** is indicated. Pharyngeal pituitary tissue **(pharyngeal hypophysis)** represents remnant tissue derived from the stalk of the embryonic RATHKE's pouch and can be found in the connective tissue located anterior to the pharyngeal tonsil underneath the sphenoidal bone. The pharyngeal hypophysis can be the source of a **craniopharyngeoma** in young people.

## Inner relief of the pharynx

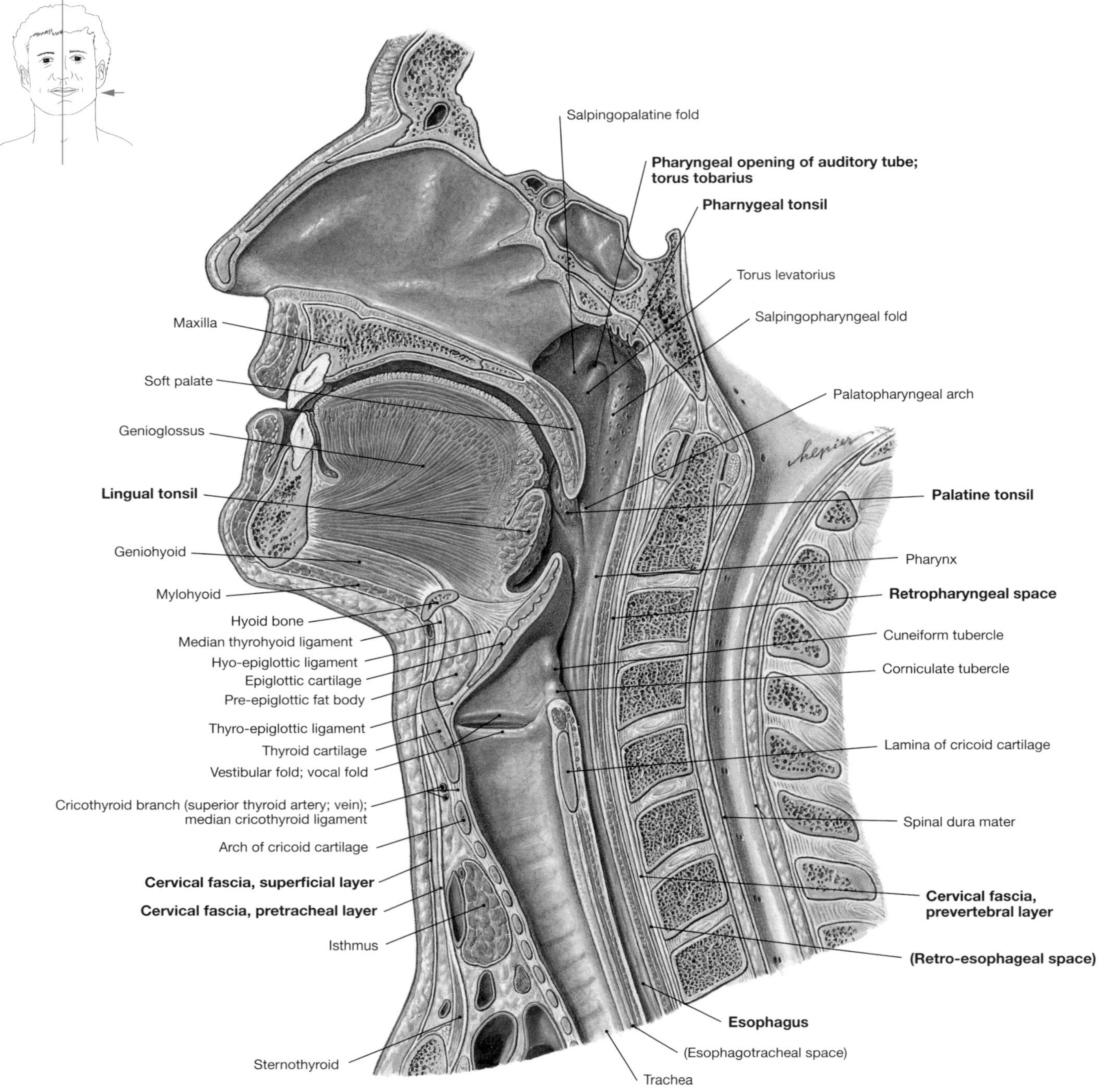
Salpingopalatine fold
Pharyngeal opening of auditory tube; torus tobarius
Pharnygeal tonsil
Torus levatorius
Salpingopharyngeal fold
Palatopharyngeal arch
Maxilla
Soft palate
Genioglossus
Lingual tonsil
Palatine tonsil
Geniohyoid
Pharynx
Mylohyoid
Retropharyngeal space
Hyoid bone
Median thyrohyoid ligament
Hyo-epiglottic ligament
Epiglottic cartilage
Pre-epiglottic fat body
Cuneiform tubercle
Corniculate tubercle
Thyro-epiglottic ligament
Thyroid cartilage
Vestibular fold; vocal fold
Lamina of cricoid cartilage
Cricothyroid branch (superior thyroid artery; vein); median cricothyroid ligament
Spinal dura mater
Arch of cricoid cartilage
Cervical fascia, superficial layer
Cervical fascia, pretracheal layer
Cervical fascia, prevertebral layer
Isthmus
(Retro-esophageal space)
Esophagus
(Esophagotracheal space)
Sternothyroid
Trachea

**Fig. 11.17 Oral cavity, pharynx, and larynx;** midsagittal section.
Relationships of the different levels of the pharynx to neighbouring structures:

- The **nasopharynx** connects with the nasal cavity and the middle ear through the choanae and the auditory tube, respectively.
- The **oropharynx** represents the junction between the superior and inferior pharyngeal levels and connects with the oral cavity through the isthmus of fauces.
- The **laryngopharynx** has an anterior connection with the larynx through the laryngeal inlet and transitions caudally into the esophagus. Airways and alimentary passage cross within the pharynx.

The WALDEYER's ring consists of lympho-epithelial tissue, and is part of the immune defence of the body. Situated in the transitional space between the nasal and oral cavity, the WALDEYER's ring is composed of the pharyngeal, tubal (not shown), palatine and lingual tonsils as well as lateral strands of lymphoid tissue located on the salpingopharyngeal folds.

## Clinical Remarks

**Ingested foreign bodies** frequently reach the epiglottic vallecula at the base of the tongue and, by exerting pressure on the epiglottis, can occlude the airways. Death can occur from a **bolus** aspiration, if an oversized bite (bolus) becomes irreversibly stuck in the laryngopharynx and cannot be expelled by coughing. This can cause reflexive cardiovascular arrest due to vagal stimulation of the highly sensitive network of nerves in the pharynx and larynx which responds to the acute stimulation by the ingested bolus. Smaller pointed foreign bodies, like fish bones or pieces of chicken bones, most often get stuck in the palatine tonsil.

## Levels and innervation of the pharynx

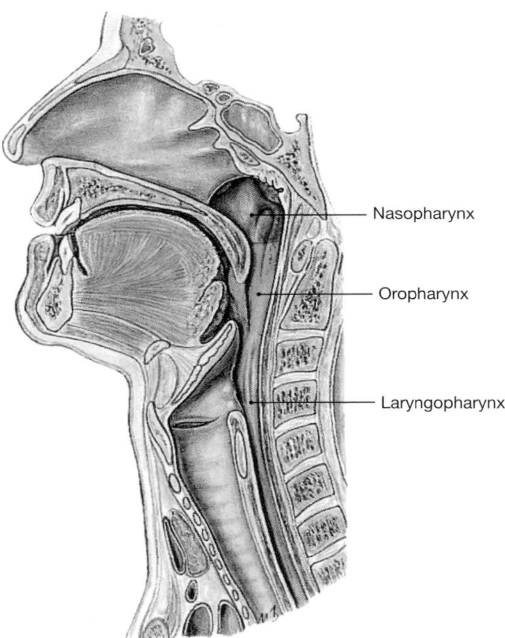
Nasopharynx
Oropharynx
Laryngopharynx

**Fig. 11.18 Levels of the pharynx;** midsagittal section.
According to its openings, the pharynx can be devided into three levels:

- upper level: epipharynx, nasopharynx
- middle level: mesopharynx, oropharynx
- lower level: hypopharynx, laryngopharynx

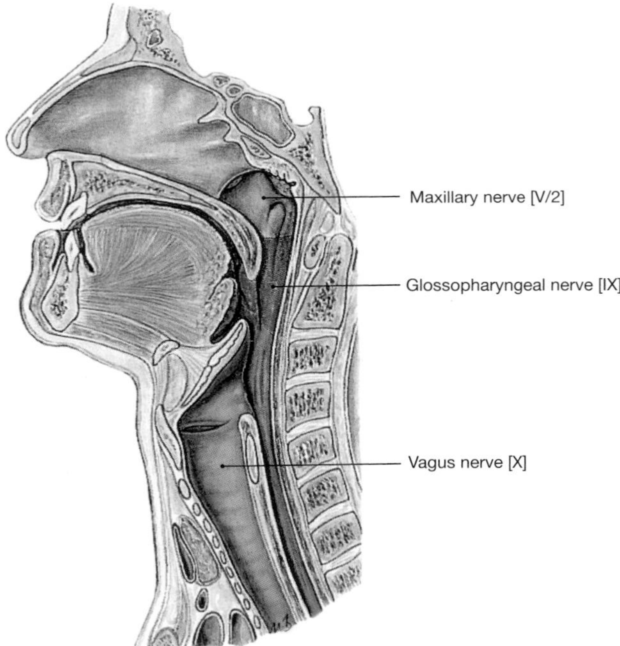
Maxillary nerve [V/2]
Glossopharyngeal nerve [IX]
Vagus nerve [X]

**Fig. 11.19 Sensory innervation of the pharynx;** midsagittal section. Sensory fibers of the second trigeminal branch (pharyngeal branch, a branch of the ganglionary branches [pterygopalatine nerves] of the maxillary nerve [V/2]) contribute to the innervation of the nasopharynx. Branches of the glossopharyngeal nerve [IX] and the vagus nerve [X] (superior laryngeal nerve) innervate the rest of the pharynx. Together with autonomic nerve fibers of the sympathetic trunk, these fibers form a neuronal network at the outer surface of the pharynx **(pharyngeal plexus).** Afferent and efferent fibers of this pharyngeal plexus are part of the vital swallowing and choking reflexes which remain active during sleep. The coordination of these complex reflexes takes place in the medulla oblongata.

## Vessels and nerves of the parapharyngeal space

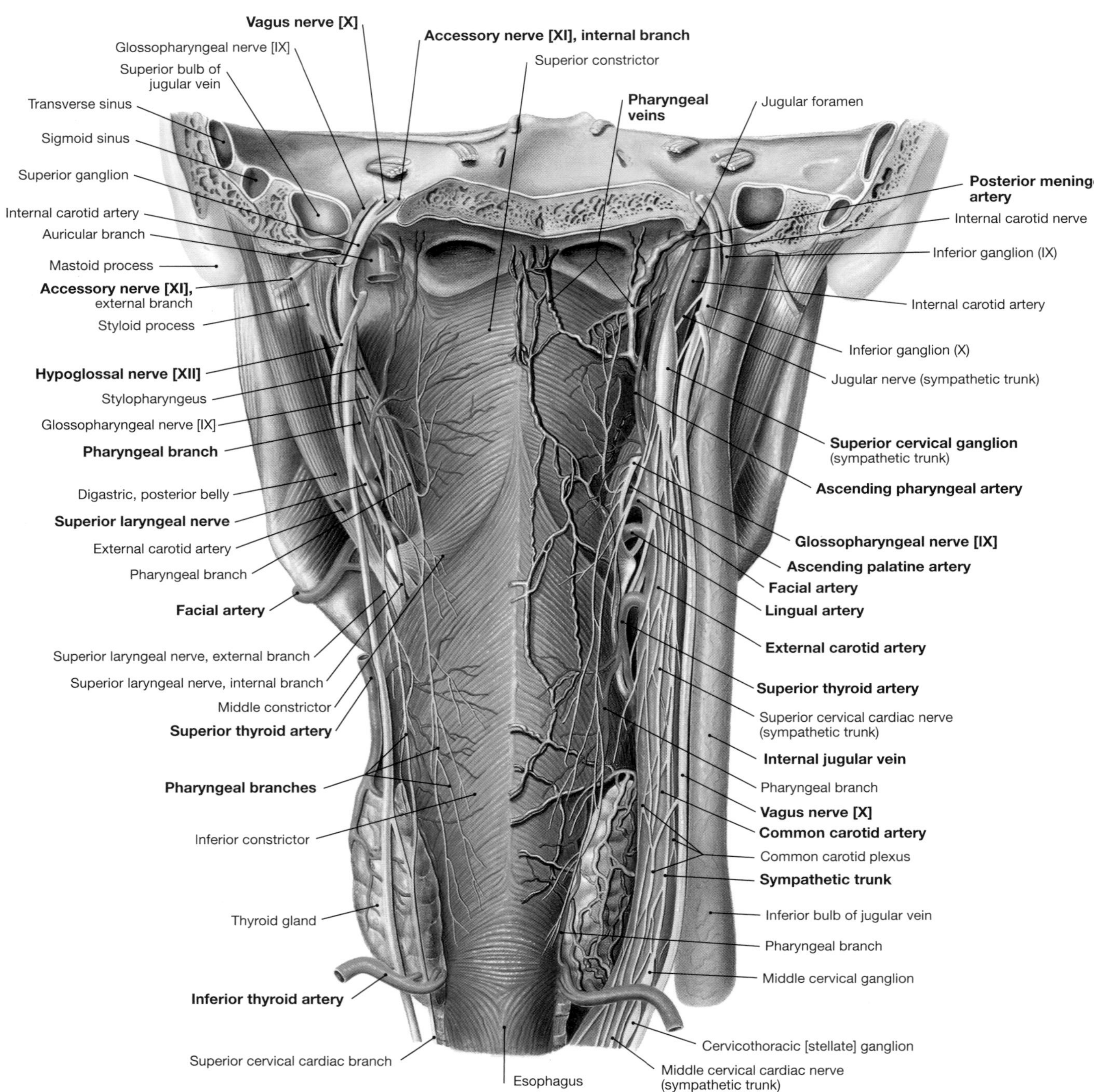
Vagus nerve [X]
Glossopharyngeal nerve [IX]
Superior bulb of jugular vein
Accessory nerve [XI], internal branch
Superior constrictor
Pharyngeal veins
Jugular foramen
Transverse sinus
Sigmoid sinus
Superior ganglion
Internal carotid artery
Auricular branch
Mastoid process
Accessory nerve [XI], external branch
Styloid process
Hypoglossal nerve [XII]
Stylopharyngeus
Glossopharyngeal nerve [IX]
Pharyngeal branch
Digastric, posterior belly
Superior laryngeal nerve
External carotid artery
Pharyngeal branch
Facial artery
Superior laryngeal nerve, external branch
Superior laryngeal nerve, internal branch
Middle constrictor
Superior thyroid artery
Pharyngeal branches
Inferior constrictor
Thyroid gland
Inferior thyroid artery
Superior cervical cardiac branch
Esophagus
Posterior meningeal artery
Internal carotid nerve
Inferior ganglion (IX)
Internal carotid artery
Inferior ganglion (X)
Jugular nerve (sympathetic trunk)
Superior cervical ganglion (sympathetic trunk)
Ascending pharyngeal artery
Glossopharyngeal nerve [IX]
Ascending palatine artery
Facial artery
Lingual artery
External carotid artery
Superior thyroid artery
Superior cervical cardiac nerve (sympathetic trunk)
Internal jugular vein
Pharyngeal branch
Vagus nerve [X]
Common carotid artery
Common carotid plexus
Sympathetic trunk
Inferior bulb of jugular vein
Pharyngeal branch
Middle cervical ganglion
Cervicothoracic [stellate] ganglion
Middle cervical cardiac nerve (sympathetic trunk)

**Fig. 11.20 Vessels and nerves of the pharynx and the parapharyngeal space;** dorsal view.

The main source of blood supply is the ascending pharyngeal artery. This artery ascends to the base of the skull in the parapharyngeal space medial of the neurovascular bundle of the neck. Its terminal branch, the posterior meningeal artery, enters the posterior cranial fossa through the jugular foramen. Additional blood supply comes from the ascending palatine artery in the region of the pharyngeal opening of the auditory tube (pharyngeal opening of the auditory tube) and from the inferior thyroid artery in the hypopharynx.

The entire submucosa of the pharynx contains a venous plexus (pharyngeal plexus). The **venous drainage** is performed by the pharyngeal veins into the internal jugular vein and into the meningeal veins in the nasopharyngeal region.

The **lymphatic drainage** of the pharyngeal tonsil and the pharyngeal wall reaches the retropharyngeal lymph nodes and the deep cervical lymph nodes (not shown).

**Innervation:** In addition to the pharyngeal plexus and the pharyngeal nerve coming off the maxillary nerve [V/2] (see sensory innervation of the pharynx → Figs. 11.19 and 12.144), the glossopharyngeal nerve [IX] provides motor innervation for the superior and upper part of the middle constrictor and for the levator pharyngeal muscles; the vagus nerve [X] innervates the lower part of the middle constrictor and the inferior constrictor.

## Vessels and nerves of the parapharyngeal space

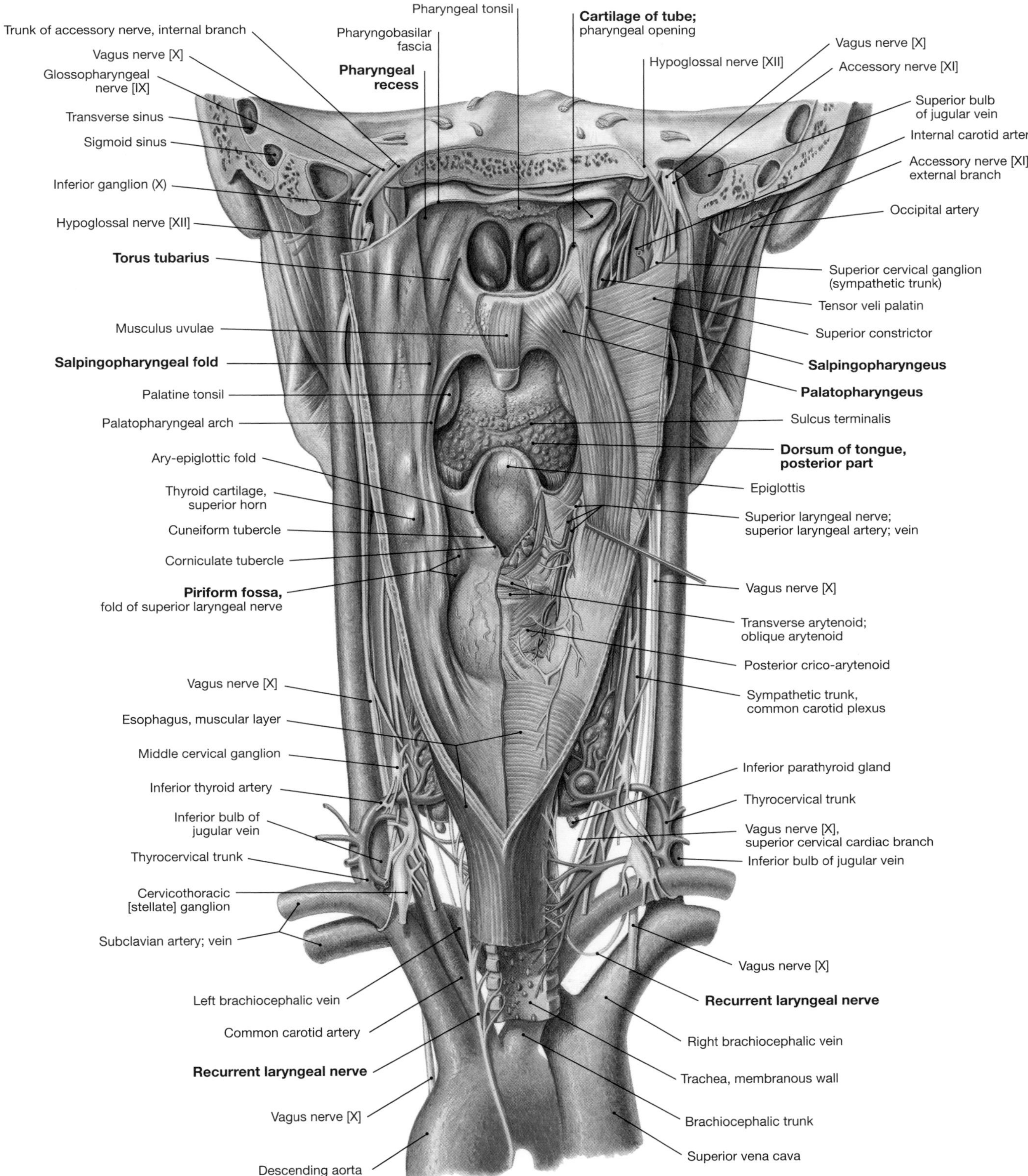
Trunk of accessory nerve, internal branch
Vagus nerve [X]
Glossopharyngeal nerve [IX]
Transverse sinus
Sigmoid sinus
Inferior ganglion (X)
Hypoglossal nerve [XII]
Torus tubarius
Musculus uvulae
Salpingopharyngeal fold
Palatine tonsil
Palatopharyngeal arch
Ary-epiglottic fold
Thyroid cartilage, superior horn
Cuneiform tubercle
Corniculate tubercle
Piriform fossa, fold of superior laryngeal nerve
Vagus nerve [X]
Esophagus, muscular layer
Middle cervical ganglion
Inferior thyroid artery
Inferior bulb of jugular vein
Thyrocervical trunk
Cervicothoracic [stellate] ganglion
Subclavian artery; vein
Left brachiocephalic vein
Common carotid artery
Recurrent laryngeal nerve
Vagus nerve [X]
Descending aorta
Pharyngeal tonsil
Pharyngobasilar fascia
Pharyngeal recess
Cartilage of tube; pharyngeal opening
Hypoglossal nerve [XII]
Vagus nerve [X]
Accessory nerve [XI]
Superior bulb of jugular vein
Internal carotid artery
Accessory nerve [XI], external branch
Occipital artery
Superior cervical ganglion (sympathetic trunk)
Tensor veli palatin
Superior constrictor
Salpingopharyngeus
Palatopharyngeus
Sulcus terminalis
Dorsum of tongue, posterior part
Epiglottis
Superior laryngeal nerve; superior laryngeal artery; vein
Vagus nerve [X]
Transverse arytenoid; oblique arytenoid
Posterior crico-arytenoid
Sympathetic trunk, common carotid plexus
Inferior parathyroid gland
Thyrocervical trunk
Vagus nerve [X], superior cervical cardiac branch
Inferior bulb of jugular vein
Vagus nerve [X]
Recurrent laryngeal nerve
Right brachiocephalic vein
Trachea, membranous wall
Brachiocephalic trunk
Superior vena cava

**Fig. 11.21 Vessels and nerves of the pharynx and the parapharyngeal space;** dorsal view. Pharynx opened from the dorsal side.
The pharyngeal opening of the auditory tube lies roughly at the level of the inferior nasal meatus. At its posterior and superior side, this opening displays an elevation, the **torus tubarius.** Caudally, the torus tubarius extends into a longitudinal mucosal fold (salpingopharyngeal fold) which is created by the salpingopharyngeus. The inferior part of the pharyngeal opening of the auditory tube displays another elevation, the **torus levatorius,** which is formed by the levator veli palatini. This orifice is the entrance to the auditory tube (EUSTACHIAN tube) and connects the nasal part of the pharynx with the tympanic cavity. Immediately behind the torus tubarius there is a fossa (pharyngeal recess, fossa of ROSENMÜLLER) extending upwards to the roof of the pharynx. The palatopharyngeus creates the lateral margin of the isthmus of fauces. The dorsal view also shows the dorsum of the tongue, the dorsal side of the laryngeal wall, and the entrance to the esophagus. On either side of the posterior laryngeal wall lies the piriform recess. Note the side difference in the course of the recurrent laryngeal nerve; on the left side the nerve winds around the aortic arch and on the right side around the subclavian artery.

## Skeleton of the larynx

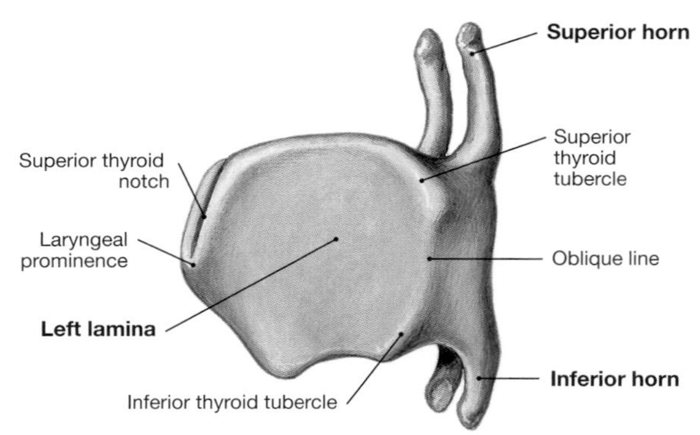
Superior horn
Superior thyroid notch
Superior thyroid tubercle
Laryngeal prominence
Oblique line
Left lamina
Inferior horn
Inferior thyroid tubercle

**Fig. 11.22 Thyroid cartilage;** view from the left side.
The thyroid cartilage is composed of two laminae (right and left lamina) with a superior and an inferior horn.

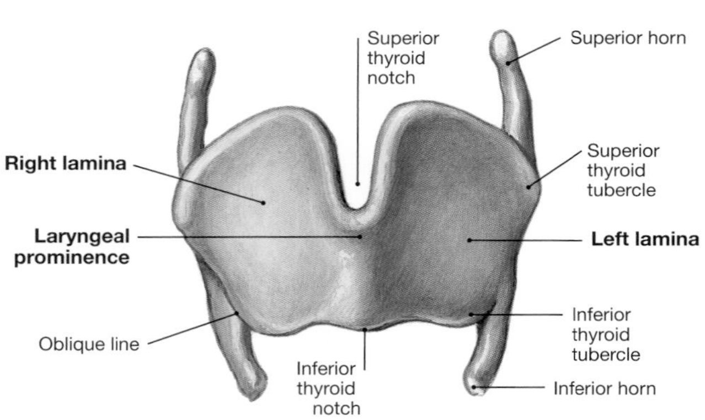
Superior thyroid notch
Superior horn
Right lamina
Superior thyroid tubercle
Laryngeal prominence
Left lamina
Inferior thyroid tubercle
Oblique line
Inferior thyroid notch
Inferior horn

**Fig. 11.23 Thyroid cartilage;** ventral view.
Both lamina of the thyroid cartilage join at an angle of 90° and 120° in men and women, respectively.

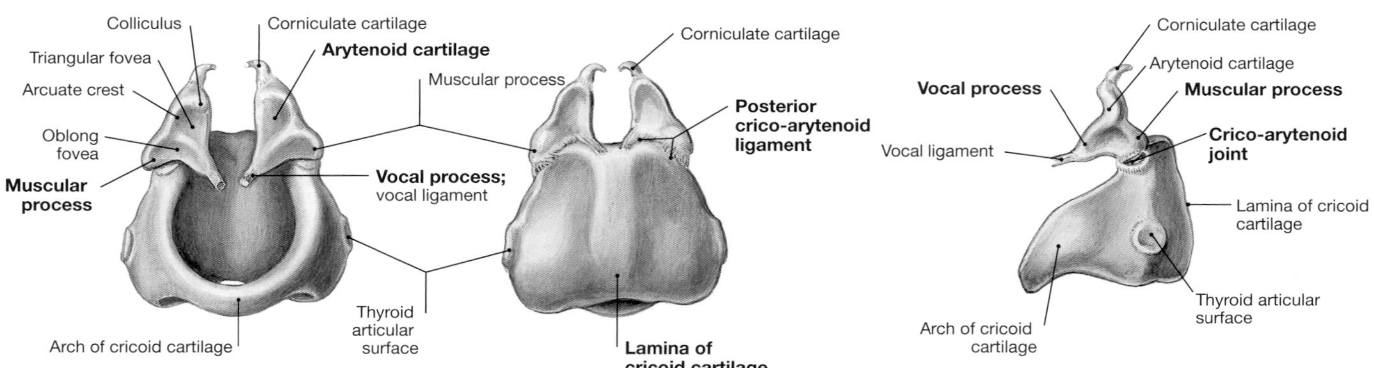
Colliculus
Corniculate cartilage
Triangular fovea
Arytenoid cartilage
Corniculate cartilage
Arcuate crest
Muscular process
Posterior crico-arytenoid ligament
Oblong fovea
Muscular process
Vocal process; vocal ligament
Thyroid articular surface
Arch of cricoid cartilage
Lamina of cricoid cartilage
Corniculate cartilage
Arytenoid cartilage
Vocal process
Muscular process
Crico-arytenoid joint
Vocal ligament
Lamina of cricoid cartilage
Thyroid articular surface
Arch of cricoid cartilage

**Fig. 11.24 Cricoid cartilage and arytenoid cartilages;** ventral and dorsal views.
The posterior crico-arytenoid ligament extends between the cricoid and arytenoid cartilages.

**Fig. 11.25 Cricoid cartilage and arytenoid cartilages;** view from the left side.
The crico-arytenoid joint, a diarthrotic joint, connects the cricoid and arytenoid cartilages.

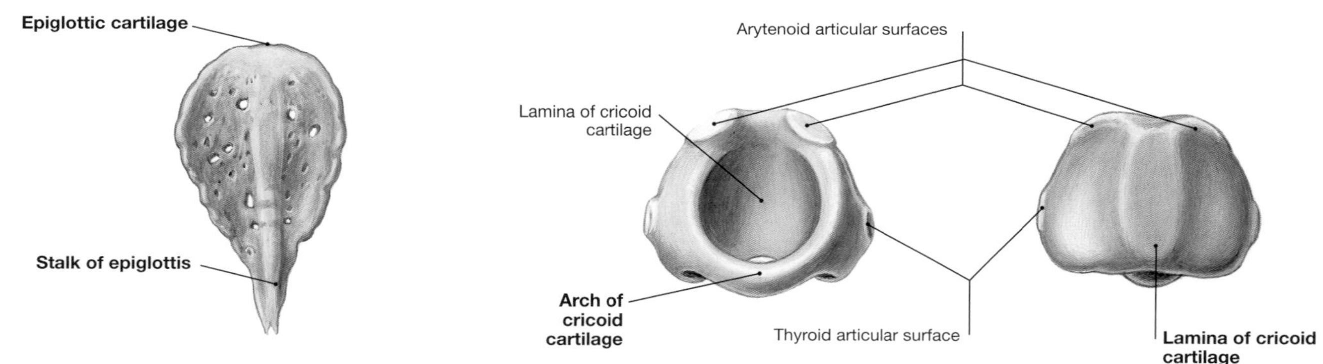
Epiglottic cartilage
Stalk of epiglottis
Arytenoid articular surfaces
Lamina of cricoid cartilage
Arch of cricoid cartilage
Thyroid articular surface
Lamina of cricoid cartilage

**Fig. 11.26 Epiglottic cartilage;** dorsal view.
In contrast to the other major hyaline laryngeal cartilages, the epiglottis is made of elastic cartilage.

**Fig. 11.27 Cricoid cartilage;** ventral and dorsal views.
The cricoid cartilage has the shape of a signet ring.

### Clinical Remarks

At about 30 years of age, the ossification of the hyaline laryngeal cartilage (thyroid, cricoid, and arytenoid cartilages) begins and progresses with age, with men displaying stronger ossification than women. **Fractures of the laryngeal skeleton** (e.g. car accidents) can result in severe obstruction of the airways with difficulties in phonation and breathing.

After surgical excision of the thyroid cartilage, for example during the **hemilaryngectomy** of a laryngeal carcinoma, the remaining laminae of the thyroid cartilage can be adjusted and connected with material used for osteosynthesis.
In rare cases, a congenital softening of the laryngeal cartilage **(laryngomalacia)** can cause difficulties in breathing (dyspnoea).

## Hyoid bone and skeleton of the larynx

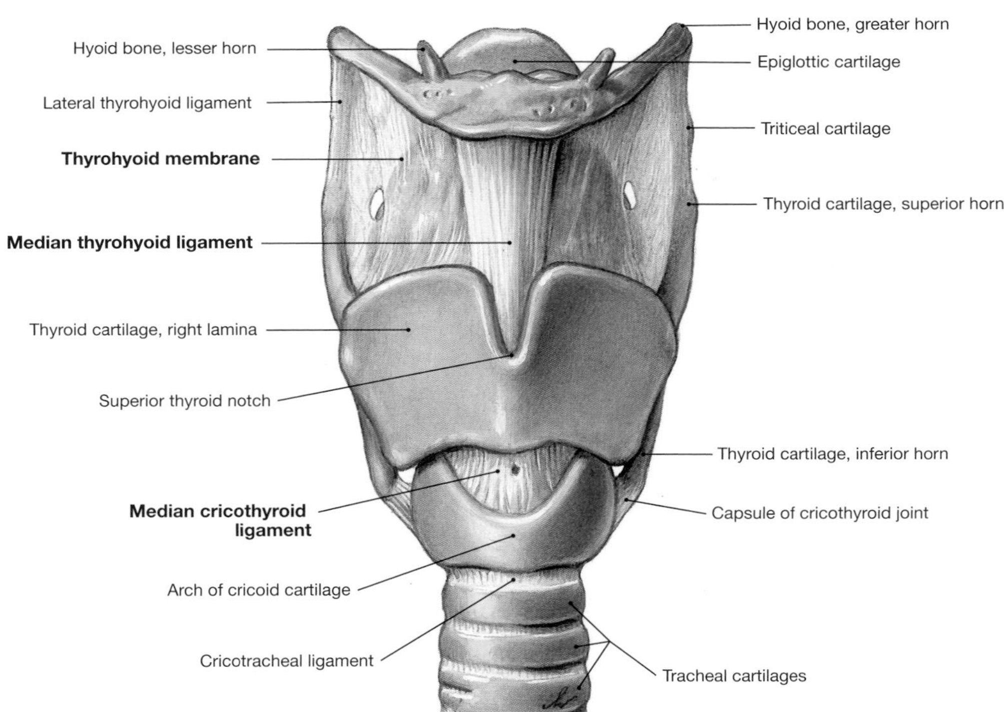
Hyoid bone, lesser horn
Lateral thyrohyoid ligament
Thyrohyoid membrane
Median thyrohyoid ligament
Thyroid cartilage, right lamina
Superior thyroid notch
Median cricothyroid ligament
Arch of cricoid cartilage
Cricotracheal ligament
Hyoid bone, greater horn
Epiglottic cartilage
Triticeal cartilage
Thyroid cartilage, superior horn
Thyroid cartilage, inferior horn
Capsule of cricothyroid joint
Tracheal cartilages

**Fig. 11.28 Larynx and hyoid bone;** ventral view.
Developmentally and functionally, the hyoid bone has a close relationship with the laryngeal skeleton. The individual parts of the laryngeal skeleton connect by **syndesmoses** and true joints **(diarthroses).**

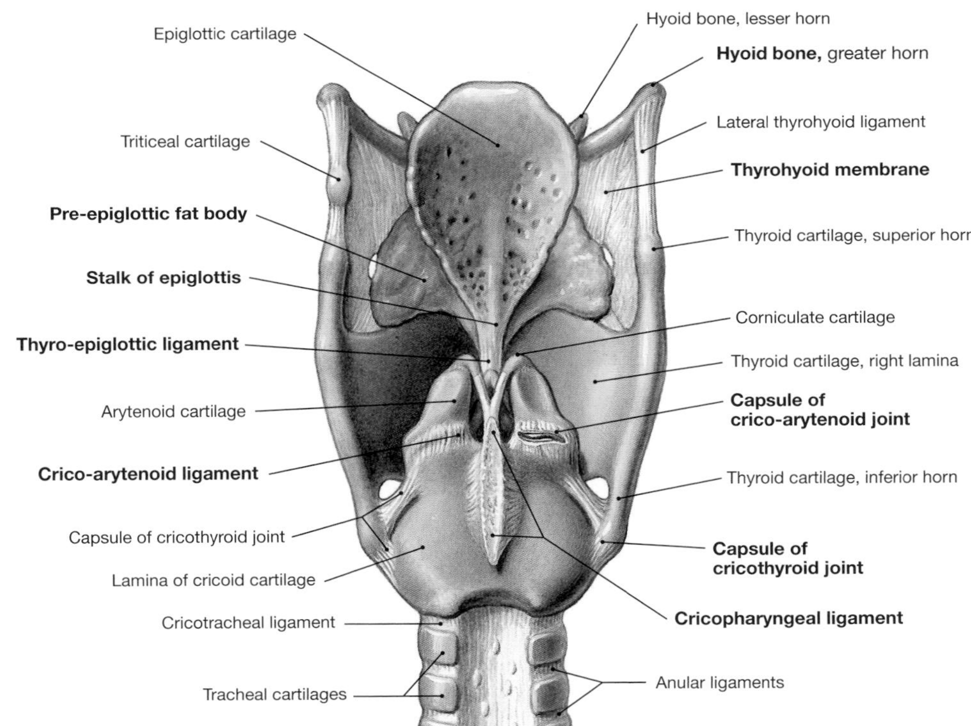
Epiglottic cartilage
Triticeal cartilage
Pre-epiglottic fat body
Stalk of epiglottis
Thyro-epiglottic ligament
Arytenoid cartilage
Crico-arytenoid ligament
Capsule of cricothyroid joint
Lamina of cricoid cartilage
Cricotracheal ligament
Tracheal cartilages
Hyoid bone, lesser horn
Hyoid bone, greater horn
Lateral thyrohyoid ligament
Thyrohyoid membrane
Thyroid cartilage, superior horn
Corniculate cartilage
Thyroid cartilage, right lamina
Capsule of crico-arytenoid joint
Thyroid cartilage, inferior horn
Capsule of cricothyroid joint
Cricopharyngeal ligament
Anular ligaments

**Fig. 11.29 Laryngeal cartilages and hyoid bone;** dorsal view.
Beneath the thyrohyoid membrane an adipose body (pre-epiglottic fat body) extends in a cranial direction to the hyo-epiglottic ligament and in a dorsocaudal direction to the frontal side of the epiglottis. The thyro-epiglottic ligament attaches the stalk of the epiglottis to the inside of the thyroid cartilage.

True joints of the larynx are the **cricothyroid joint,** the paired joint between the cricoid cartilage and the inferior horns of the thyroid cartilage as well as the **crico-arytenoid joint** between the cricoid and arytenoid cartilages. The crico-arytenoid ligament and the cricopharyngeal ligament act as dorsal reins for the arytenoid cartilage.

## Hyoid bone and skeleton of the larynx

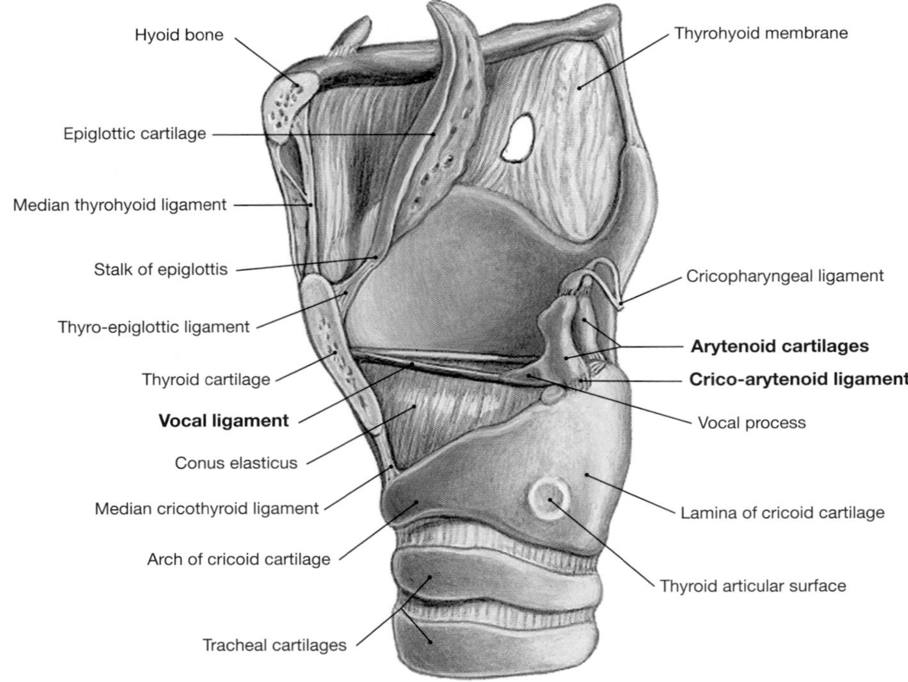
Hyoid bone
Thyrohyoid membrane
Epiglottic cartilage
Median thyrohyoid ligament
Stalk of epiglottis
Cricopharyngeal ligament
Thyro-epiglottic ligament
Arytenoid cartilages
Thyroid cartilage
Crico-arytenoid ligament
Vocal ligament
Vocal process
Conus elasticus
Median cricothyroid ligament
Lamina of cricoid cartilage
Arch of cricoid cartilage
Thyroid articular surface
Tracheal cartilages

**Fig. 11.30 Larynx and hyoid bone;** view onto the vocal ligament and the arytenoid cartilage from the left side; the left lamina of thyroid cartilage has been removed.
The cricoid and arytenoid cartilages articulate in the crico-arytenoid joint. The articular surfaces of the cricoid cartilage are convex and oval in size (cylinder-shaped, → Fig. 11.27); the articular surface of the arytenoid cartilage is concave and more round. This shape of the articular cartilaginous components and the crico-arytenoid ligament (posterior) provide stability to the joint. Functionally, this ligament guides the arytenoid cartilage and counteracts the forces of the vocal ligament.

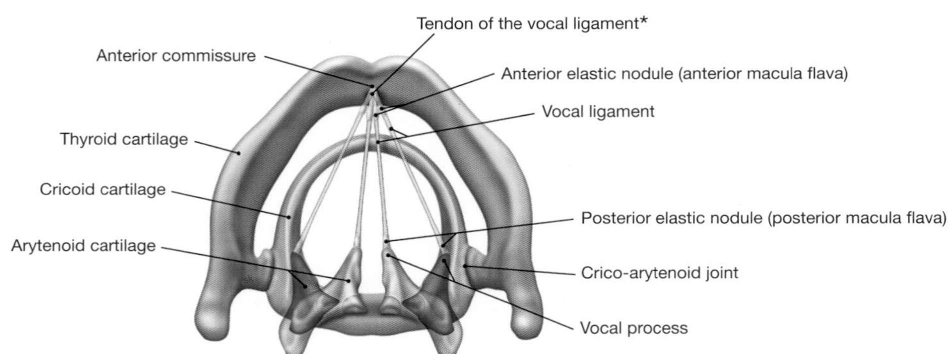
Tendon of the vocal ligament*
Anterior commissure
Anterior elastic nodule (anterior macula flava)
Vocal ligament
Thyroid cartilage
Cricoid cartilage
Posterior elastic nodule (posterior macula flava)
Arytenoid cartilage
Crico-arytenoid joint
Vocal process

**Fig. 11.31 Larynx and hyoid bone;** superior view.
The crico-arytenoid joint permits hinge and sliding motions parallel to the cylindrical axis; this joint primarily supports the opening and closure of the space between the vocal ligaments (glottis, rima glottidis) and also keeps tension on the vocal ligament. A hinge-like outward rotation results in elevation and abduction of the vocal process and, consecutively, an **opening of the glottis.** Inward rotation through the hinge as well as depression and adduction of the vocal process cause the **occlusion of the glottis.** These hinge-like movements can combine with gliding motions, whereby ventral or dorsal movement occurs during abduction and adduction of the arytenoid cartilage, respectively. The vocal ligament and the vestibular ligament connect the arytenoid and thyroid cartilages.

* BROYLE's tendon

### Clinical Remarks

Dislocation of the arytenoid cartilage in a dorsolateral or medioventral direction, called **aryluxation,** is a potential complication during endotracheal intubation or extubation, laryngoscopy, and bronchoscopy. The patient has a hoarse voice since the vocal ligament on the affected side is immobile. Displacement of the arytenoid cartilage can be caused by bleeding into the articular cavity or inflammatory swelling upon injury of synovial membrane folds. The displaced arytenoid cartilage is kept in place by muscle contractions. This condition can result in adhesions of articular surfaces and subsequently ankylosis can occur. An aryluxation must be distinguished from a nerve lesion.

# Skeleton of the larynx

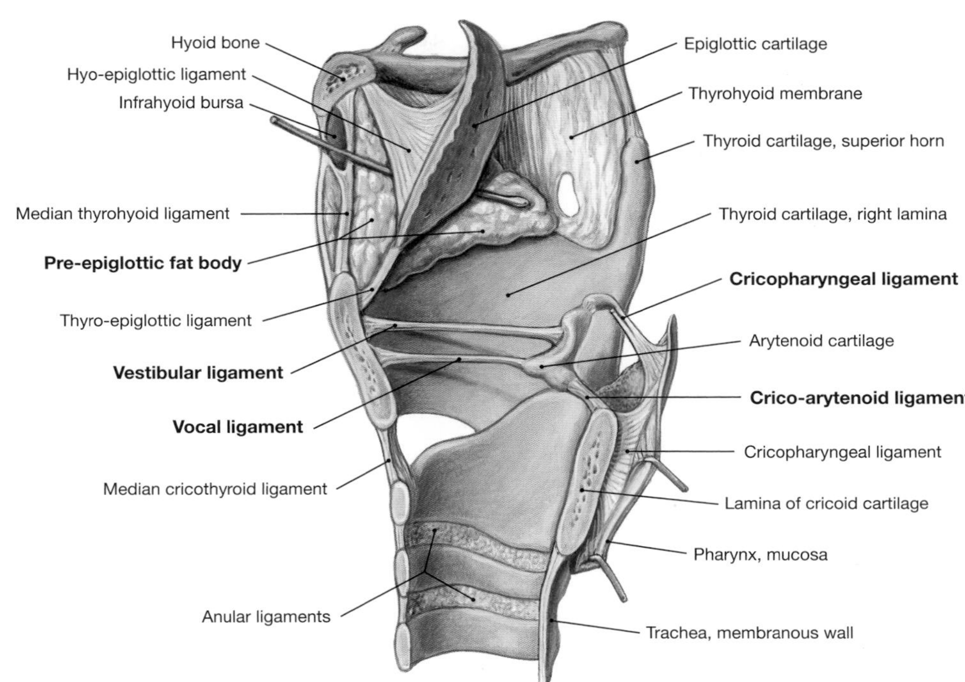
Hyoid bone
Hyo-epiglottic ligament
Infrahyoid bursa
Median thyrohyoid ligament
Pre-epiglottic fat body
Thyro-epiglottic ligament
Vestibular ligament
Vocal ligament
Median cricothyroid ligament
Anular ligaments
Epiglottic cartilage
Thyrohyoid membrane
Thyroid cartilage, superior horn
Thyroid cartilage, right lamina
Cricopharyngeal ligament
Arytenoid cartilage
Crico-arytenoid ligament
Cricopharyngeal ligament
Lamina of cricoid cartilage
Pharynx, mucosa
Trachea, membranous wall

**Fig. 11.32 Larynx and hyoid bone;** median section, medial view.
The cricothyroid joints connect thyroid and cricoid cartilages. The cricoid and arytenoid cartilages articulate in the crico-arytenoid joint. The arytenoid and thyroid cartilages are connected by the vocal ligament and the vestibular ligament. The crico-arytenoid ligament and cricopharyngeal ligament act as a dorsal rein of the arytenoid cartilage. Lateral and in front of the epiglottis the pre-epiglottic fat body is visible.

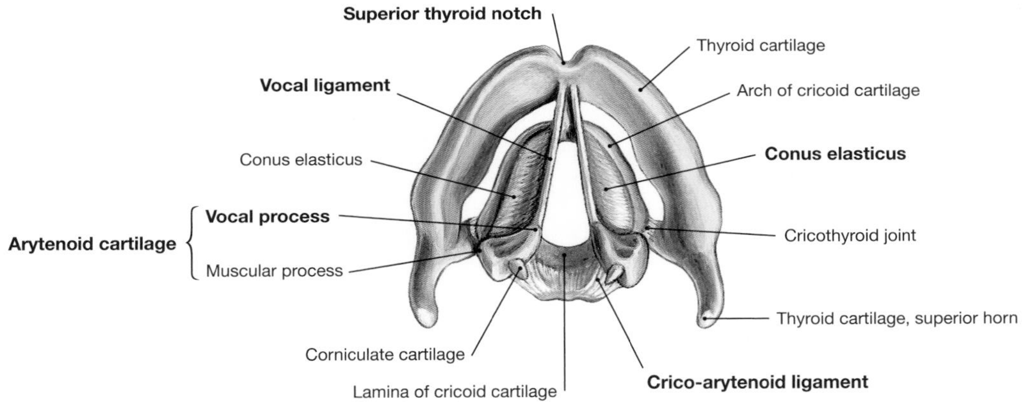
Superior thyroid notch
Vocal ligament
Conus elasticus
Arytenoid cartilage
Vocal process
Muscular process
Corniculate cartilage
Lamina of cricoid cartilage
Thyroid cartilage
Arch of cricoid cartilage
Conus elasticus
Cricothyroid joint
Thyroid cartilage, superior horn
Crico-arytenoid ligament

**Fig. 11.33 Laryngeal cartilages and vocal ligament;** cranioventral view.
The paired vocal ligament stretches between the vocal process of the arytenoid cartilage and the inside of the thyroid cartilage shortly below the superior thyroid notch. The conus elasticus (cricovocal membrane) is an elastic membrane and extends between the vocal ligament and the upper rim of the cricoid cartilage. The conus elasticus directs the airflow from the lungs in the direction of the vocal ligaments. The strong crico-arytenoid ligament is visible on the dorsal aspect of the arytenoid cartilage.

## Clinical Remarks

The crico-arytenoid joint not only contains the same extracellular matrix as joints of the extremities, but can also be afflicted by the same joint diseases as the larger joints of the limbs. Degenerative alterations of the cartilage (**arthrosis** or **degenerative arthritis**) are common in older persons and affect phonation and quality of voice due to improper occlusion of the glottis by the vocal ligaments. In addition, the crico-arytenoid joint can develop **infectious arthritis** and **rheumatoid arthritis.**

## Laryngeal muscles

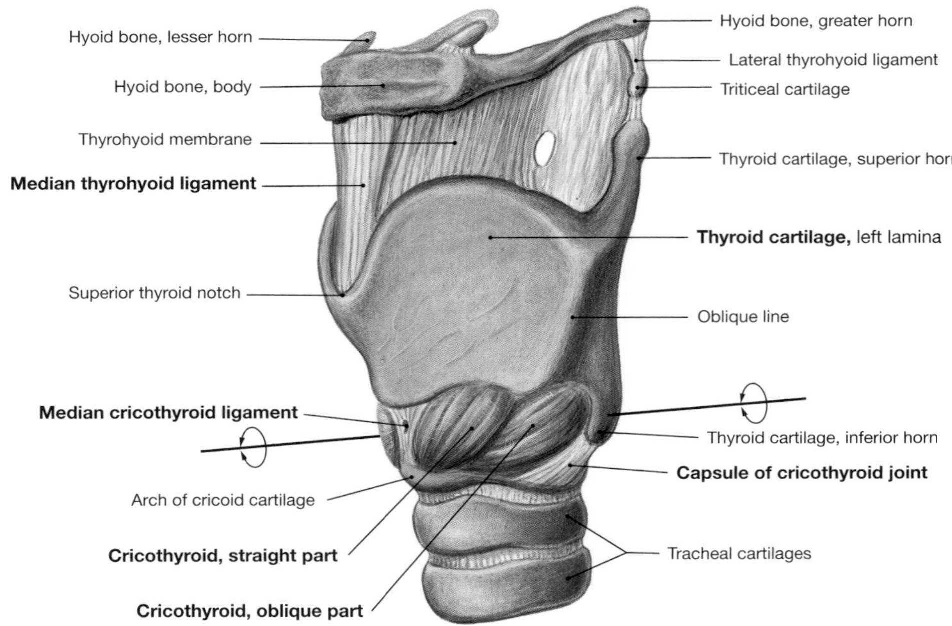
Hyoid bone, lesser horn
Hyoid bone, body
Thyrohyoid membrane
Median thyrohyoid ligament
Superior thyroid notch
Median cricothyroid ligament
Arch of cricoid cartilage
Cricothyroid, straight part
Cricothyroid, oblique part
Hyoid bone, greater horn
Lateral thyrohyoid ligament
Triticeal cartilage
Thyroid cartilage, superior horn
Thyroid cartilage, left lamina
Oblique line
Thyroid cartilage, inferior horn
Capsule of cricothyroid joint
Tracheal cartilages

**Fig. 11.34 Cricothyroid muscle;** ventral view from the left side.
The cricoid cartilage and the thyroid cartilage articulate in the left and right cricothyroid joint. These are spheroidal joints with a firm joint capsule. This joint allows hinge-like motions in the transverse axis and small gliding (translatory) movements in the sagittal plane. Contraction of the cricothyroid increases the tension of the vocal folds (→ Fig. 11.35).

→T 6

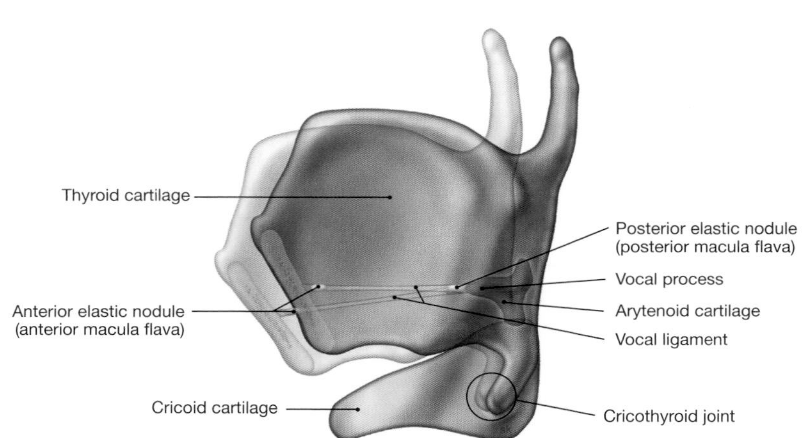
Thyroid cartilage
Anterior elastic nodule
(anterior macula flava)
Cricoid cartilage
Posterior elastic nodule
(posterior macula flava)
Vocal process
Arytenoid cartilage
Vocal ligament
Cricothyroid joint

**Fig. 11.35 Cricothyroid muscle;** lateral view.
Contraction of the cricothyroid causes the anterior part of the thyroid cartilage to rock towards the arch of the cricoid cartilage. This results in the elongation of the vocal ligament which is now under increased tension. During this rocking movement, the arytenoid cartilages are stabilized by the actions of the posterior crico-arytenoid and the crico-arytenoid ligament.

**Biomechanics of the vocal folds:** The structures at the insertion site of the vocal ligaments (**anterior** and **posterior elastic nodules,** BROYLE's tendon of the vocal ligament, → Fig. 11.48) have biomechanical functions during the vibration of the vocal folds by equalizing the different elastic modules of the vocal ligament, cartilage, and bone. This prevents the vocal ligaments from rupturing at their insertion points during vibration.

→T 6

### Clinical Remarks

Benign or malignant **alterations in the region of the vocal folds** result in incomplete occlusion of the glottis, hoarseness, and in dyspnoea breathing at advanced stages of the disease. The median cricothyroid ligament (ligamentum conicum) extends between the thyroid and cricoid cartilages and can be easily palpated here. In an emergency case, if breathing functions are compromised, the ligament can be split to insert a breathing tube (→ Fig. 11.4).

## Laryngeal muscles

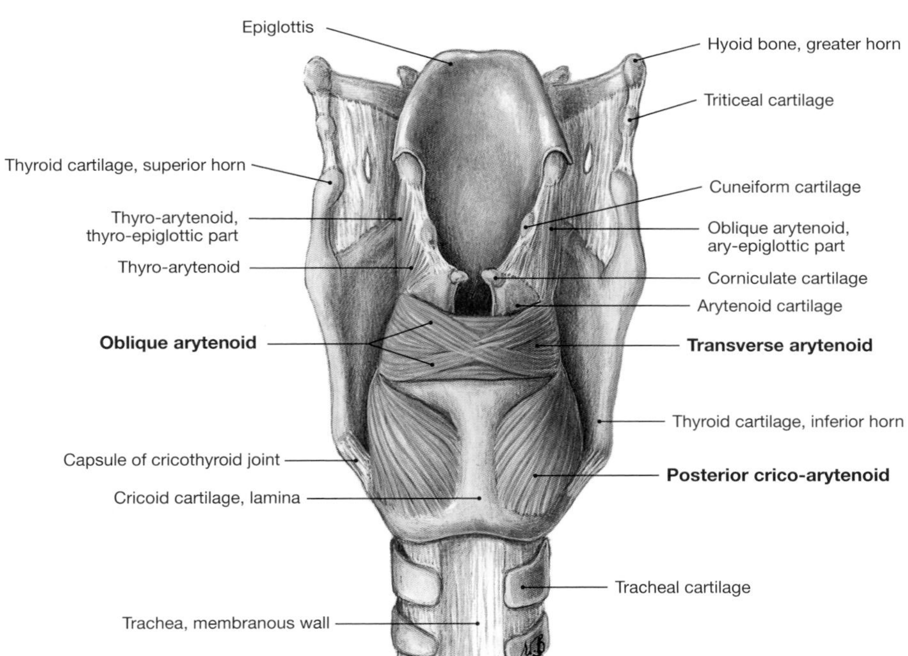
Epiglottis
Hyoid bone, greater horn
Triticeal cartilage
Thyroid cartilage, superior horn
Cuneiform cartilage
Thyro-arytenoid, thyro-epiglottic part
Oblique arytenoid, ary-epiglottic part
Thyro-arytenoid
Corniculate cartilage
Arytenoid cartilage
Oblique arytenoid
Transverse arytenoid
Thyroid cartilage, inferior horn
Capsule of cricothyroid joint
Posterior crico-arytenoid
Cricoid cartilage, lamina
Tracheal cartilage
Trachea, membranous wall

**Fig. 11.36 Laryngeal muscles;** dorsal view.
The actions of the laryngeal muscles determine the shape of the rima glottidis and the tension of the vocal ligament. The **posterior crico-arytenoid ("posticus")** is mainly responsible for the abduction and elevation of the vocal process of the arytenoid cartilage resulting in the widening of the glottis as part of the inspiration. All other muscles that act on the space between the vocal folds cause the narrowing of the glottis and include the **transverse arytenoid** and **oblique arytenoid** as well as the **lateral crico-arytenoid** (→ Fig. 11.37). Whispering is made possible by the isolated contraction of the lateral crico-arytenoideus, which results in the so-called **"whispering triangle"**, the formation of a small triangular opening in the posterior part of the rima glottidis (→ Fig. 11.43).

→T 6

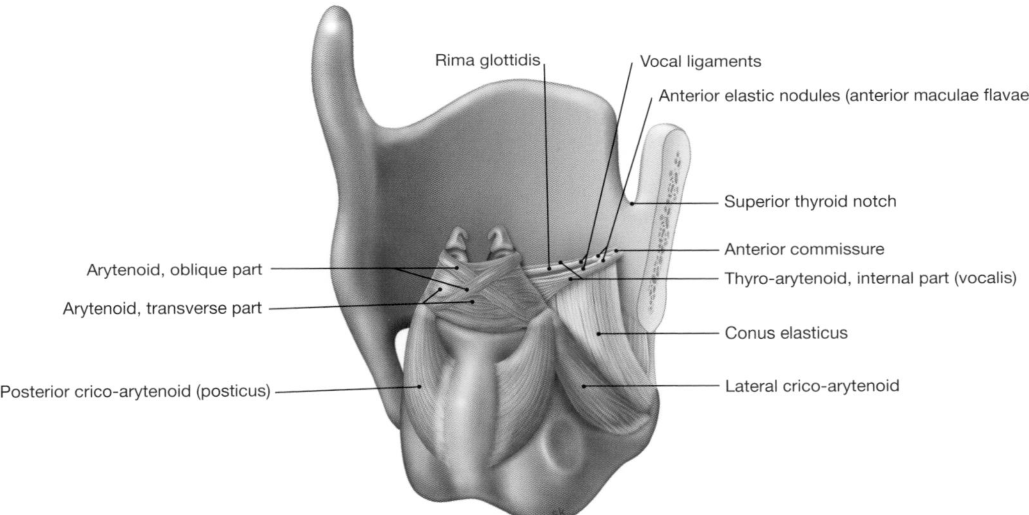
Rima glottidis
Vocal ligaments
Anterior elastic nodules (anterior maculae flavae)
Superior thyroid notch
Anterior commissure
Arytenoid, oblique part
Thyro-arytenoid, internal part (vocalis)
Arytenoid, transverse part
Conus elasticus
Posterior crico-arytenoid (posticus)
Lateral crico-arytenoid

**Fig. 11.37 Laryngeal muscles;** dorsal view from an oblique angle.
In this particular view, the lateral crico-arytenoid and the internal part of the thyro-arytenoid (vocalis muscle) are visible. The lateral crico-arytenoid closes the rima glottidis. **"Fine-tuning" of the vocal folds** is performed by the **vocalis** (internal part of the thyro-arytenoid). Its muscle fibers run parallel to the vocal ligament and to the vocal fold. The muscle creates a cushion which acts like the mouthpiece of a pipe. The tension of this mouthpiece is regulated by isometric muscle contractions and its length is shortened by isotonic muscle contractions. Thus, the actions of the vocalis have an important impact on sound quality and vocalization.

→T 6

### Clinical Remarks

The paramedian positioning of the vocal fold is caused by the isolated unilateral **paralysis of the posterior crico-arytenoid;** its bilateral paralysis results in a narrowing of the glottis with difficulties in breathing and potential death by choking.

**Dysphonia** refers to all signs of a phonation disorder. This includes hoarseness of the voice in patients with unilateral paralysis of the posterior crico-arytenoid. **Aphonia** is the inability to speak.

## Levels and inner relief of the larynx

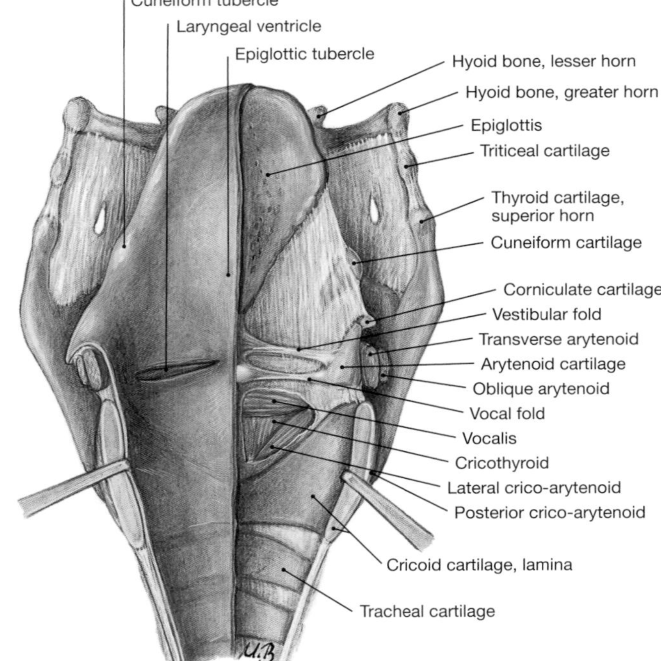
Cuneiform tubercle
Laryngeal ventricle
Epiglottic tubercle
Hyoid bone, lesser horn
Hyoid bone, greater horn
Epiglottis
Triticeal cartilage
Thyroid cartilage, superior horn
Cuneiform cartilage
Corniculate cartilage
Vestibular fold
Transverse arytenoid
Arytenoid cartilage
Oblique arytenoid
Vocal fold
Vocalis
Cricothyroid
Lateral crico-arytenoid
Posterior crico-arytenoid
Cricoid cartilage, lamina
Tracheal cartilage

**Fig. 11.38 Larynx;** dorsal view; the larynx was sectioned from dorsal in the median plane and separated with hooks.
On the left side, the mucosal lining is shown; on the right side, the laryngeal muscles (vocalis [= internal part of the thyro-arytenoid], cricothyroid and lateral crico-arytenoid), the cartilages (epiglottis, arytenoid, cricoid, and thyroid cartilages as well as the small laryngeal cartilages), and the mucosal folds (vestibular and vocal fold) are depicted.

→T 6

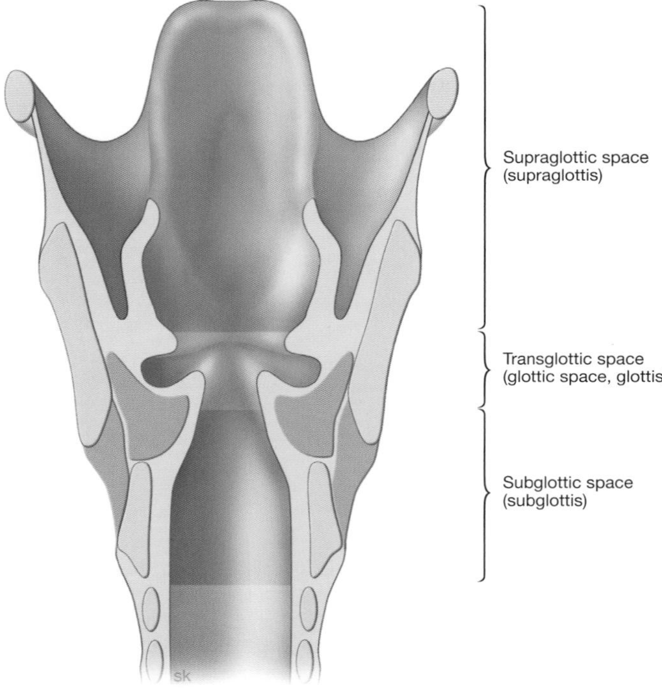
Supraglottic space (supraglottis)
Transglottic space (glottic space, glottis)
Subglottic space (subglottis)

**Fig. 11.39 Compartments of the larynx.**
Clinicians divide the larynx into the following spaces:
**Supraglottic space (supraglottis):** This space extends from the laryngeal inlet to the level of the vestibular folds and is divided into:
- epilarynx: laryngeal area of the epiglottis and ary-epiglottic folds
- laryngeal vestibule: stalk of epiglottis, vestibular folds = ventricular, laryngeal ventricle = MORGAGNI's ventricle

**Glottic space (glottis):** The area extends from the free rim of the vocal folds as opposed to the "transglottic space" which encompasses the space between glottis, vestibular folds, and laryngeal ventricle. The anterior part of the glottis, including the anterior commissure, is known as intermembranous part; the dorsal part of the glottis between the arytenoid cartilages is the intercartilaginous part (→ Fig. 11.43) and constitutes two-thirds of the rima glottidis. In their dorsal part, the vocal folds end at the transition of the intercartilaginous part into the interarytenoid fold (→ Fig. 11.43).
**Subglottic space (subglottis):** The subglottis is the space that extends below the vocal folds to the lower rim of the cricoid cartilage. It is a conical space between the free margin of the vocal fold, the area below the vocal fold, and the lower margin of the cricoid cartilage. The cranial border of the subglottis is the macroscopically visible inferior arcuate line (→ Fig. 11.49) of the vocal fold. The caudal border is at the level of the lower rim of the cricoid cartilage. Craniolaterally, it is confined by the conus elasticus, and further caudally by the cricoid cartilage. The caudal part of the subglottis assumes a cylindrical shape, and tapers off at its cranial end due to the shape of the conus elasticus. The ventral border is the median cricothyroid ligament (ligamentum conicum), and the cricoid cartilage is the dorsal demarcation.

### Clinical Remarks

The above mentioned compartmentalization of the larynx is important in diagnostic imaging techniques for the staging of the **extent of local tumor growth.** The spiral computed tomography (spiral CT) with thin slicing mode is the recommended diagnostic procedure for larynx imaging. Although magnetic resonance imaging (MRI) has the highest sensitivity of all imaging techniques for tumor staging, this method is prone to imaging artifacts by patient movements.

## Laryngoscopy

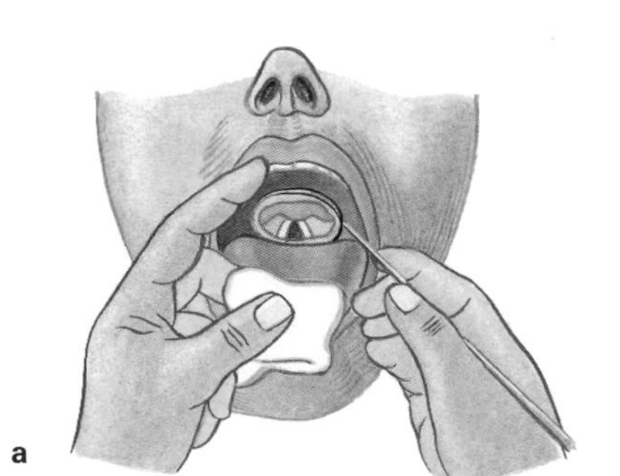
a

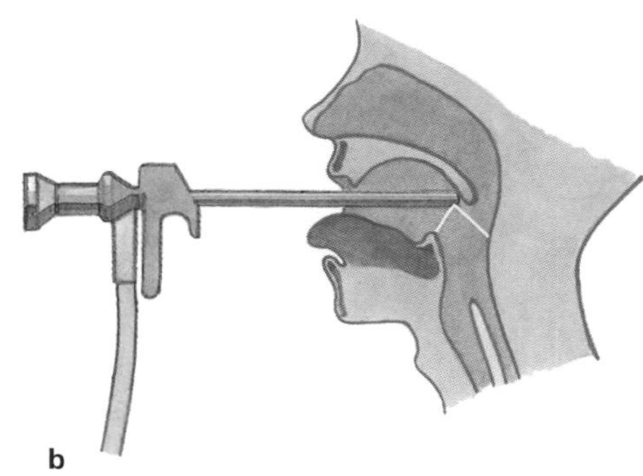
b

**Figs. 11.40a and b Laryngoscopy.**
**a** Indirect laryngoscopy
**b** Direct, endoscopic laryngoscopy

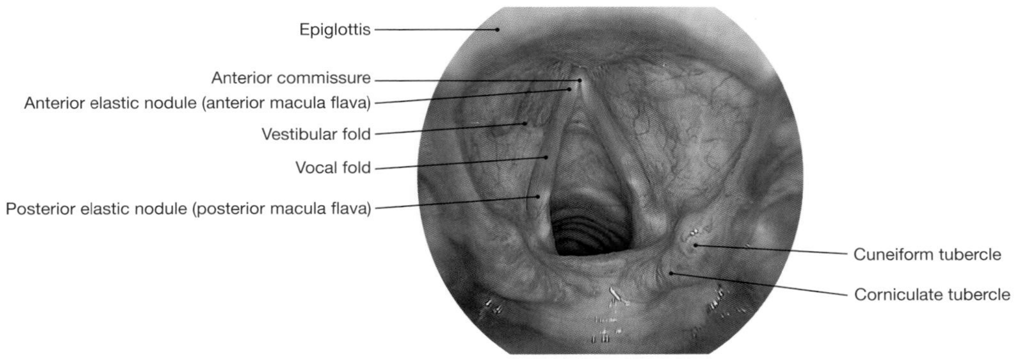
Epiglottis
Anterior commissure
Anterior elastic nodule (anterior macula flava)
Vestibular fold
Vocal fold
Posterior elastic nodule (posterior macula flava)
Cuneiform tubercle
Corniculate tubercle

**Fig. 11.41 Direct laryngoscopy;** respiratory position.

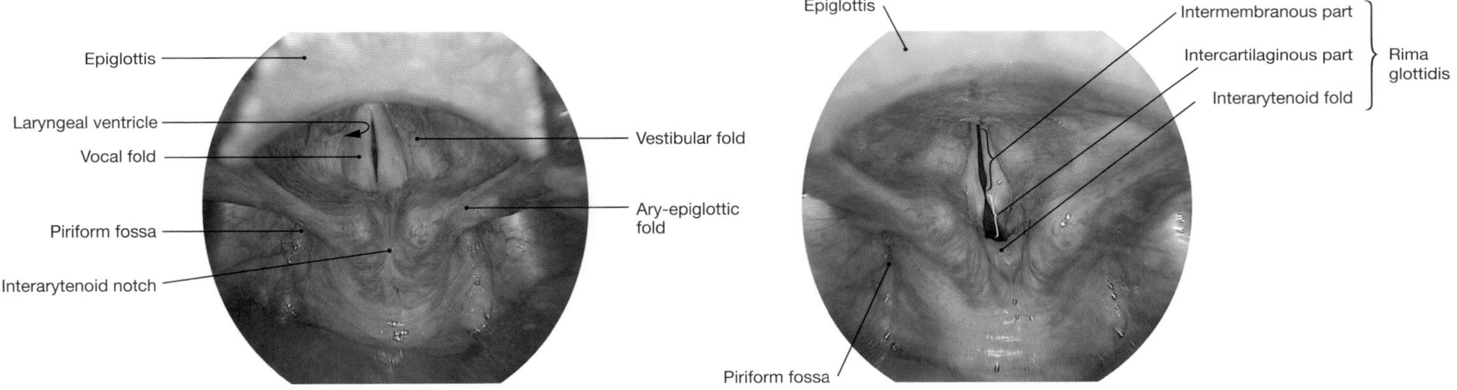
Epiglottis
Laryngeal ventricle
Vocal fold
Piriform fossa
Interarytenoid notch
Vestibular fold
Ary-epiglottic fold
Epiglottis
Intermembranous part
Intercartilaginous part
Interarytenoid fold
Rima glottidis
Piriform fossa

**Fig. 11.42 Direct laryngoscopy;** phonation position.

**Fig. 11.43 Direct laryngoscopy;** whispering position.

### Clinical Remarks

Persons who stress their voice in a strenuous or abusive manner are at risk of developing **vocal cord or singer's nodules** located at the free margin of the vocal ligament. Weakness of the arytenoid muscle may result in an incomplete occlusion of the intercartilaginous part of the glottis (open whisper triangle), resulting in a weak and breathy voice.

The most frequently observed benign tumors of the vocal fold are **polyps; squamous cell carcinomas** are the most frequent malignant tumors. Prolonged intubation can lead the formation of an **intubation granuloma** in the intercartilaginous part.

## Inner relief of the larynx

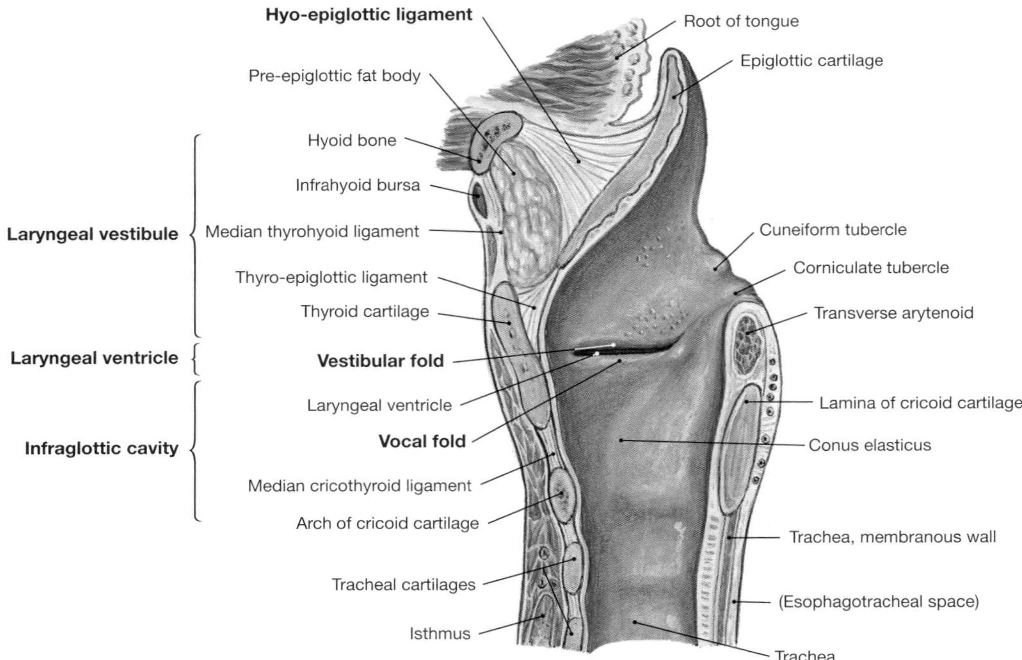
Hyo-epiglottic ligament
Root of tongue
Pre-epiglottic fat body
Epiglottic cartilage
Hyoid bone
Infrahyoid bursa
Laryngeal vestibule
Median thyrohyoid ligament
Cuneiform tubercle
Corniculate tubercle
Thyro-epiglottic ligament
Thyroid cartilage
Transverse arytenoid
Laryngeal ventricle
Vestibular fold
Laryngeal ventricle
Lamina of cricoid cartilage
Infraglottic cavity
Vocal fold
Conus elasticus
Median cricothyroid ligament
Arch of cricoid cartilage
Trachea, membranous wall
Tracheal cartilages
(Esophagotracheal space)
Isthmus
Trachea

**Fig. 11.44 Larynx;** midsagittal section.
The paired vocal fold locates below the paired vestibular fold in the middle laryngeal compartment. The largest part of the laryngeal cavity is lined by **respiratory epithelium. Non-keratinized stratified squamous epithelium** is commonly present in some areas of the larynx, while in other areas this type of surface epithelium is only observed occasionally with large interindividual variations. Non-keratinized stratified squamous epithelium is commonly localized to the vocal folds covering the vocal ligament. This epithelium spreads along the mucosal lining of the arytenoid cartilages and seamlessly transitions into the stratified squamous epithelium of the hypopharynx. Squamous epithelium covers the lingual area of the epiglottis. The distribution of respiratory and squamous epithelium on the vestibular folds and in the entire laryngeal cavity is subject to significant variations specific to each individual. With increasing age, laryngeal areas covered with squamous epithelium increase.

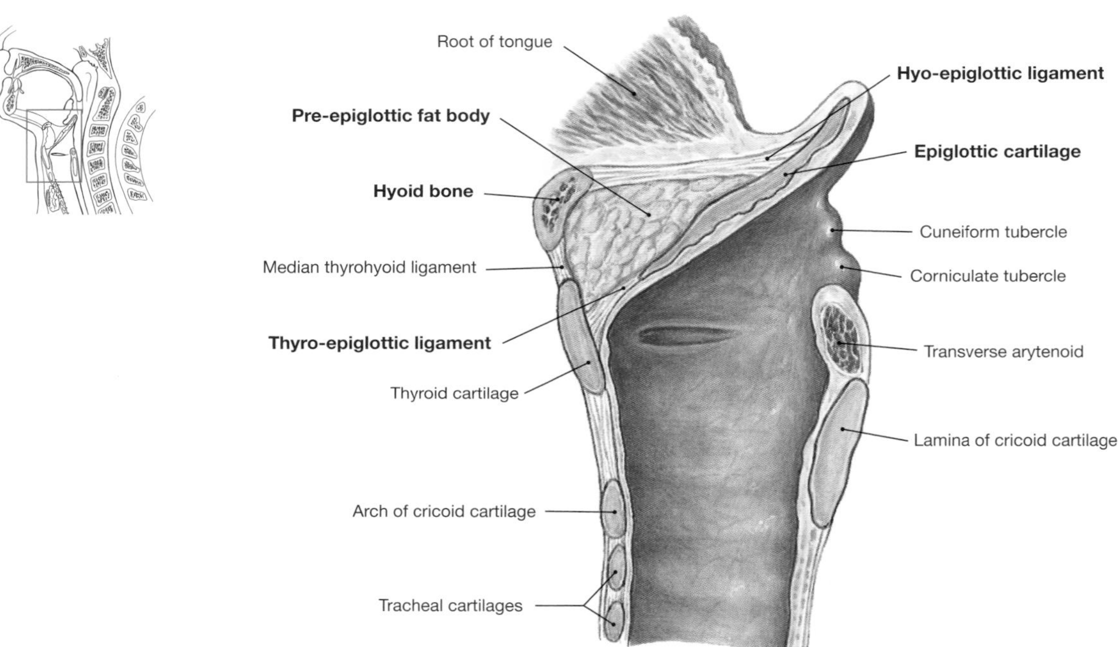
Root of tongue
Hyo-epiglottic ligament
Pre-epiglottic fat body
Epiglottic cartilage
Hyoid bone
Cuneiform tubercle
Median thyrohyoid ligament
Corniculate tubercle
Thyro-epiglottic ligament
Transverse arytenoid
Thyroid cartilage
Lamina of cricoid cartilage
Arch of cricoid cartilage
Tracheal cartilages

**Fig. 11.45 Larynx, position of the epiglottis during swallowing;** midsagittal section.

Swallowing involves a change in the position of the structures of the laryngeal orifice. The epiglottis is pushed downward. The pre-epiglottic fat body moves dorsally, the laryngeal inlet becomes narrow.

### Clinical Remarks

The clinical term "vocal cord" is anatomically incorrect; this term should be reserved for the vocal ligament.

In the larynx, the amount of squamous epithelium increases with age and can be the source of malignant laryngeal **squamous cell carcinoma.**

## Arteries and nerves of the larynx

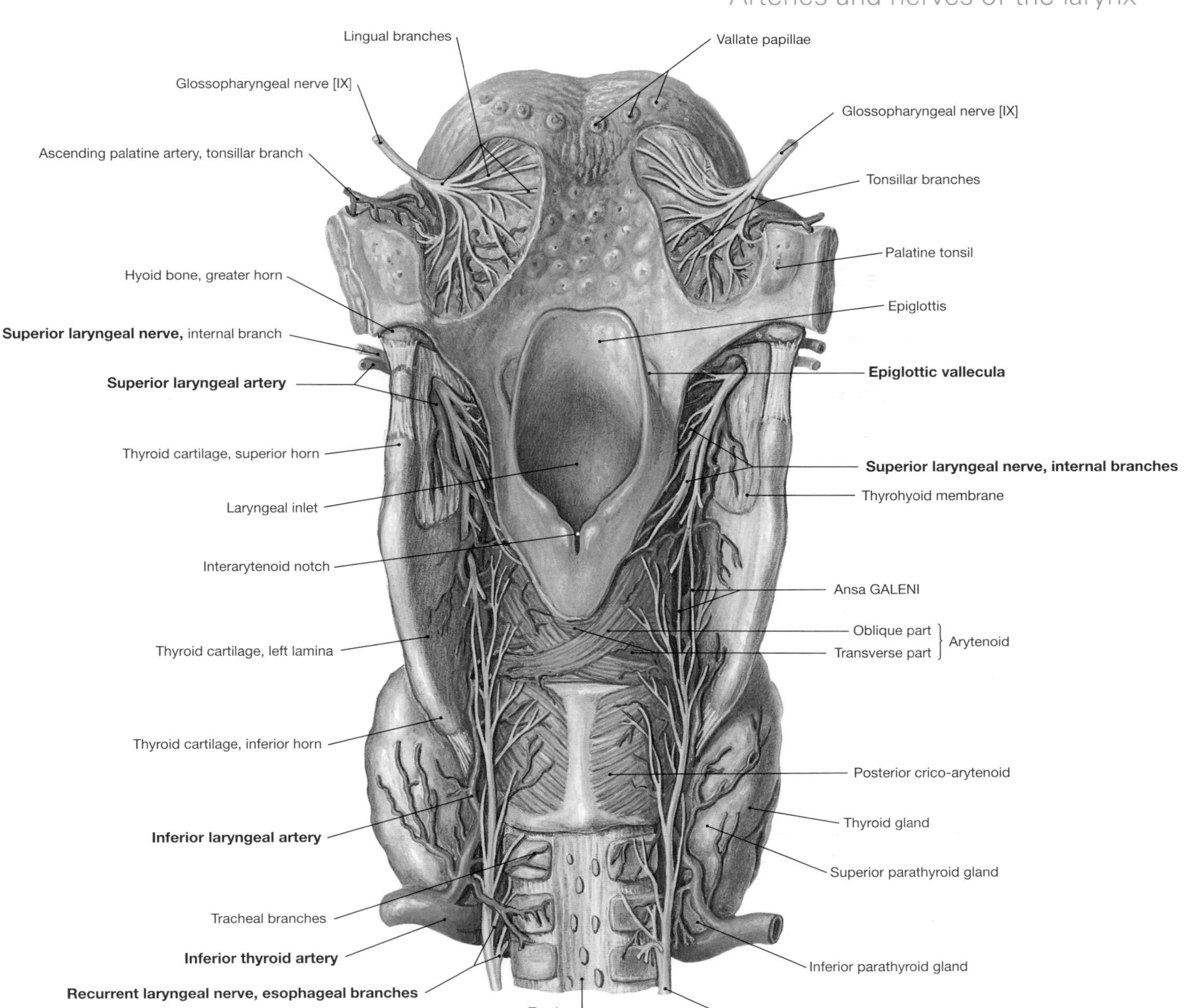

Lingual branches
Vallate papillae
Glossopharyngeal nerve [IX]
Glossopharyngeal nerve [IX]
Ascending palatine artery, tonsillar branch
Tonsillar branches
Palatine tonsil
Hyoid bone, greater horn
Epiglottis
Superior laryngeal nerve, internal branch
Superior laryngeal artery
Epiglottic vallecula
Thyroid cartilage, superior horn
Superior laryngeal nerve, internal branches
Thyrohyoid membrane
Laryngeal inlet
Interarytenoid notch
Ansa GALENI
Oblique part
Transverse part
Arytenoid
Thyroid cartilage, left lamina
Thyroid cartilage, inferior horn
Posterior crico-arytenoid
Thyroid gland
Inferior laryngeal artery
Superior parathyroid gland
Tracheal branches
Inferior thyroid artery
Inferior parathyroid gland
Recurrent laryngeal nerve, esophageal branches
Trachea
Recurrent laryngeal nerve


**Fig. 11.46 Arteries and nerves of the larynx and root of the tongue;** dorsal view.
The superior laryngeal artery branches off the superior thyroid artery, perforates the thyrohyoid membrane below the superior horn of the hyoid bone, and divides into smaller branches within the mucosa of the piriform recess. Here, the superior laryngeal artery has multiple anastomoses and collaterals with the inferior laryngeal artery.
The larynx receives bilateral innervation through **two branches of the vagus nerve [X]:**

- The **superior laryngeal nerve** divides into an internal branch and an external branch (→ Fig. 11.81). The internal branch projects into the wall of the pharynx from lateral and, jointly with the superior laryngeal artery, passes through the thyrohyoid membrane into the larynx where it provides sensory innervation for the supraglottic mucosa, the mucosa of the epiglottic valleculae, and the epiglottis. Sensory innervation of the laryngeal mucosa is very dense (cough reflex). Apart from its motor and sensory fibers, the superior laryngeal nerve also contains many parasympathetic fibers for the innervation of glands.
- The **recurrent laryngeal nerve** (inferior) provides motor innervation for the inner laryngeal muscles. The innervation of the paired posterior crico-arytenoid and arytenoid on the posterior side of the larynx is shown. The connection between the superior laryngeal nerve and the inferior laryngeal nerve is called GALEN's anastomosis. For demonstration of the course of the recurrent laryngeal nerves → Figs. 11.21 and 11.56.

## Clinical Remarks

**Lesions of the superior laryngeal nerve** cause a reduction in sensory abilities (frequent choking), and paralysis of the cricothyroid. Insufficient tension on the vocal folds will result in the incomplete occlusion of the glottis and phonation disorders.

**Acute edema at the entrance of the larynx** (e.g. due to allergic reactions) can develop quickly in the loose connective tissue and cause severe difficulties in breathing.
**Acute bacterial infections of the epiglottis** occur most frequently in children and can cause acute and life-threatening obstructions of the airways.

## Larynx, transverse sections

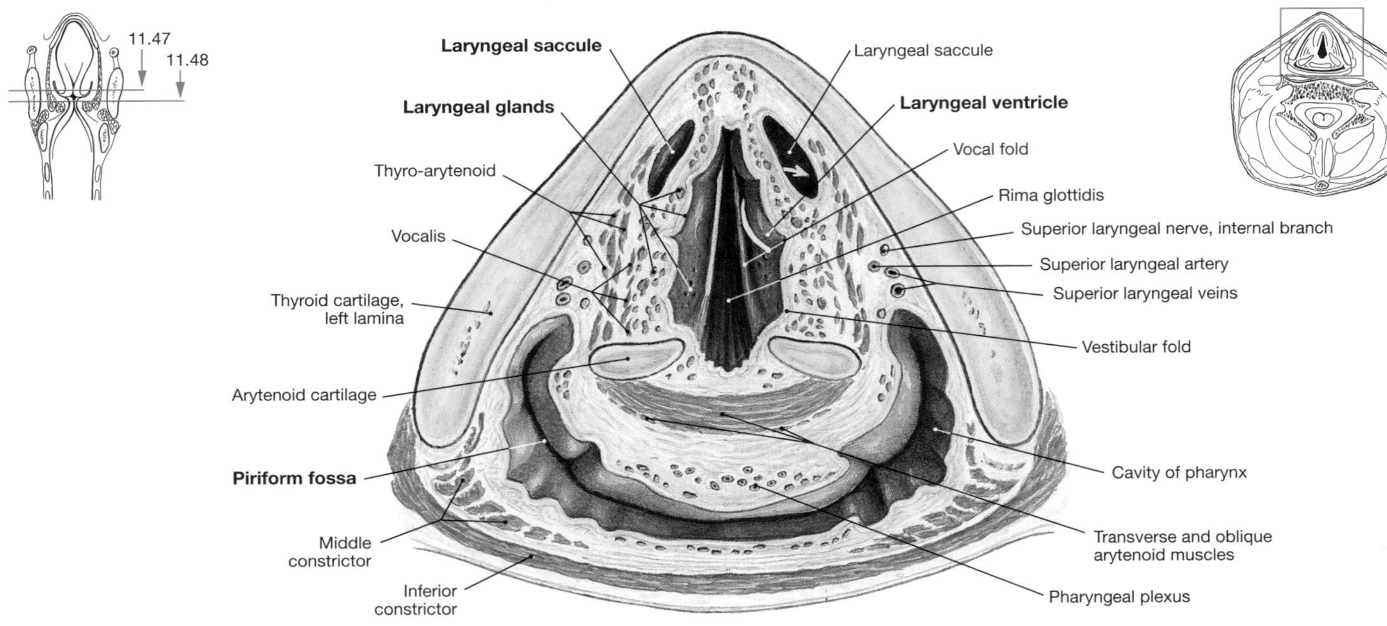
11.47
11.48
Laryngeal saccule
Laryngeal glands
Thyro-arytenoid
Vocalis
Thyroid cartilage, left lamina
Arytenoid cartilage
Piriform fossa
Middle constrictor
Inferior constrictor
Laryngeal saccule
Laryngeal ventricle
Vocal fold
Rima glottidis
Superior laryngeal nerve, internal branch
Superior laryngeal artery
Superior laryngeal veins
Vestibular fold
Cavity of pharynx
Transverse and oblique arytenoid muscles
Pharyngeal plexus

**Fig. 11.47 Larynx;** transverse section at the level of the vestibular folds.
The vestibular folds contain multiple seromucous glands (laryngeal glands) which serve to moisten the vocal folds. The white arrow indicates the connection between the laryngeal ventricle and the laryngeal saccule. Posterior to the larynx, the laryngopharynx with the piriform recess is visible.

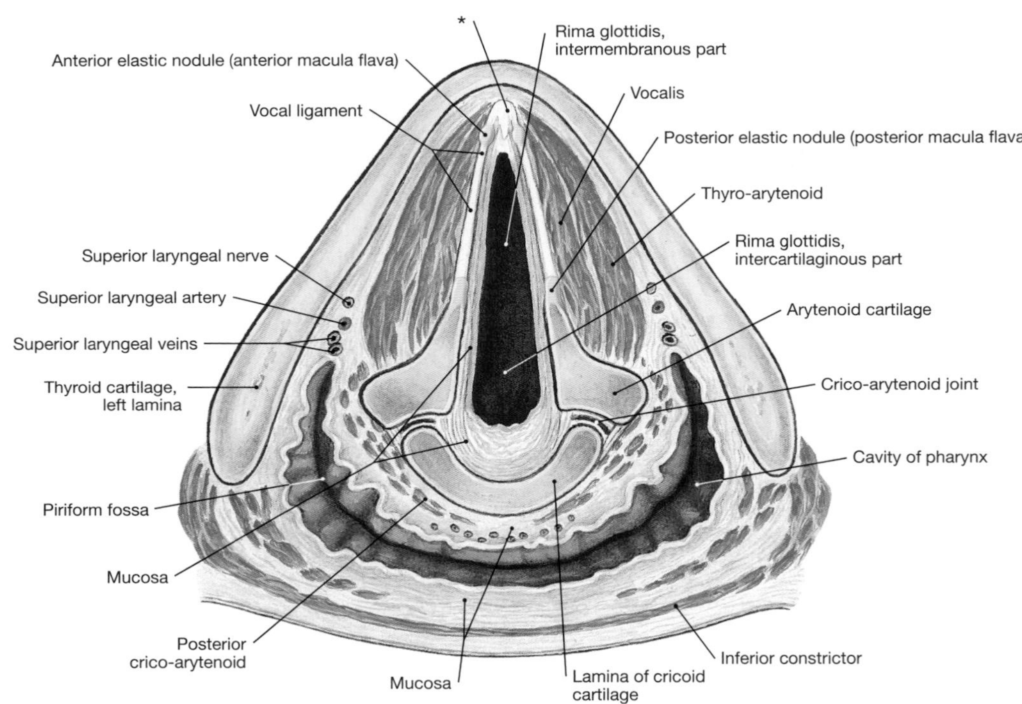
*
Anterior elastic nodule (anterior macula flava)
Vocal ligament
Superior laryngeal nerve
Superior laryngeal artery
Superior laryngeal veins
Thyroid cartilage, left lamina
Piriform fossa
Mucosa
Posterior crico-arytenoid
Mucosa
Rima glottidis, intermembranous part
Vocalis
Posterior elastic nodule (posterior macula flava)
Thyro-arytenoid
Rima glottidis, intercartilaginous part
Arytenoid cartilage
Crico-arytenoid joint
Cavity of pharynx
Inferior constrictor
Lamina of cricoid cartilage

**Fig. 11.48 Larynx;** transverse section at the level of the vocal folds.
The section at the level of the true opening of the vocal ligaments (glottis, rima glottidis) displays the mucosa of the vocal ligaments. The following structures are arranged from the inside to the outside of the glottis: the vocal ligament, the vocalis (internal part of the thyro-arytenoid), and the external part of the thyro-arytenoid. The cartilage-free part of the vocal fold is the intermembranous part, the part between the two arytenoid cartilages is the intercartilaginous part (→ Fig. 11.43). In the front, the vocal folds converge on the thyroid cartilage. The insertion site is described as the anterior commissure. Here, the vocal folds insert via anterior elastic nodules and the tendon of the vocal ligament (BROYLE's tendon*) at the thyroid cartilage. Dorsally, the vocal ligament attaches at the vocal process of the arytenoid cartilage via the posterior elastic nodule.

## Larynx, frontal section

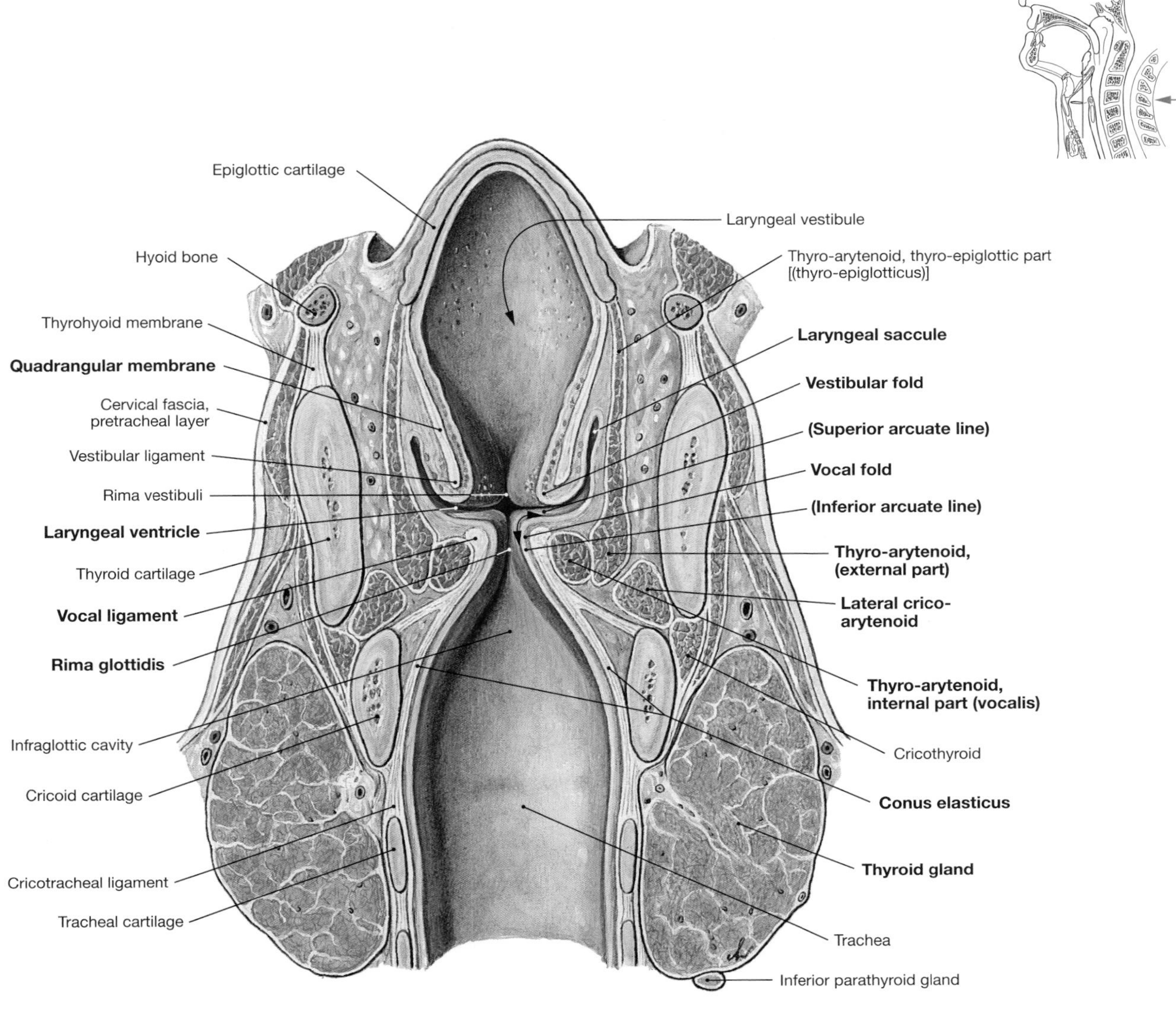
Epiglottic cartilage
Hyoid bone
Thyrohyoid membrane
Quadrangular membrane
Cervical fascia, pretracheal layer
Vestibular ligament
Rima vestibuli
Laryngeal ventricle
Thyroid cartilage
Vocal ligament
Rima glottidis
Infraglottic cavity
Cricoid cartilage
Cricotracheal ligament
Tracheal cartilage
Laryngeal vestibule
Thyro-arytenoid, thyro-epiglottic part [(thyro-epiglotticus)]
Laryngeal saccule
Vestibular fold
(Superior arcuate line)
Vocal fold
(Inferior arcuate line)
Thyro-arytenoid, (external part)
Lateral crico-arytenoid
Thyro-arytenoid, internal part (vocalis)
Cricothyroid
Conus elasticus
Thyroid gland
Trachea
Inferior parathyroid gland

**Fig. 11.49 Larynx and thyroid gland;** frontal section.
Normally, the vocal folds extend beyond the vestibular folds and protrude more into the lumen of the Larynx, which makes them accessible for inspection by laryngoscopy. The vocal folds are composed of an outer mucosa, the vocal ligament, followed caudally by the conus elasticus, and the vocalis (internal part of the thyro-arytenoid), and the external part of the thyro-arytenoid. Located at both sides is the lateral crico-arytenoid. Both vocal folds demarcate the opening of the vocal ligaments (glottis, rima glottidis) which represents the part of the larynx responsible for phonation.

The vocal ligament is lined by a loose subepithelial connective tissue layer between the superior arcuate line and the inferior arcuate line which provides a flexible potential space (REINKE's space, arrow). The laryngeal ventricle extends in between the vocal and vestibular folds. The elastic quadrangular membrane forms the connective tissue framework for the laryngeal ventricle. The thyroid gland with its two lobes is located between the cricoid cartilage and the upper tracheal semicircular cartilages.

### Clinical Remarks

An accumulation of fluid in the REINKE's space creates a swelling of the vocal folds, which extends into the glottis and results in hoarseness and dyspnoea **(REINKE's edema).** The REINKE's edema has to be distinguished from a **glottic edema.** In the latter, fluid collects in the mucosa in the supraglottic space (e.g. due to allergic reactions) and, thus, the edema is located above the glottis. The edema restricts the airflow through the glottis. Its symptoms can range from stridor (pitched wheezing sound) to hoarseness, dyspnoea and potentially asphyxia.

## Thyroid gland

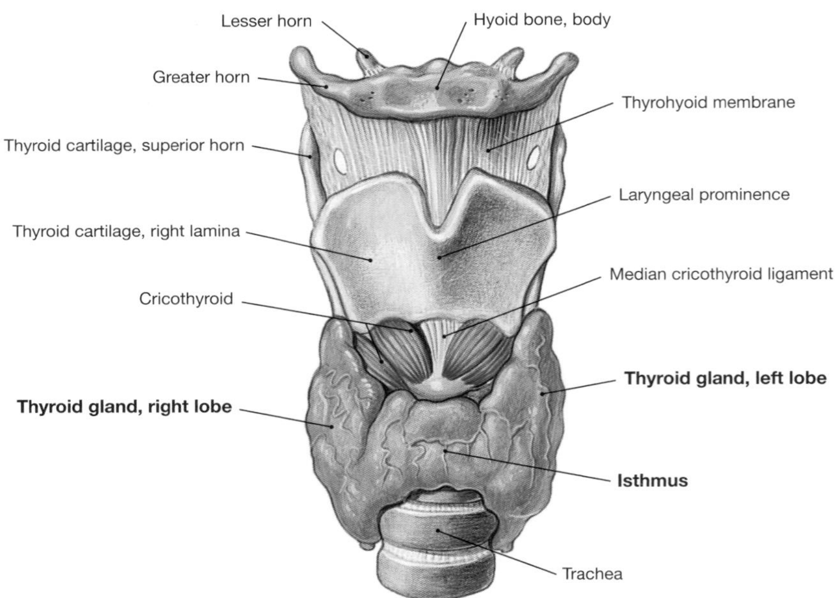
Lesser horn
Hyoid bone, body
Greater horn
Thyrohyoid membrane
Thyroid cartilage, superior horn
Laryngeal prominence
Thyroid cartilage, right lamina
Median cricothyroid ligament
Cricothyroid
Thyroid gland, left lobe
Thyroid gland, right lobe
Isthmus
Trachea

**Fig. 11.50 Position of the thyroid gland;** ventral view.
The thyroid gland (weight in an adult 20–25 g) is located below the larynx. The thyroid gland surrounds the upper part of the trachea with bilateral lobes (right and left lobe) and an anterior isthmus.

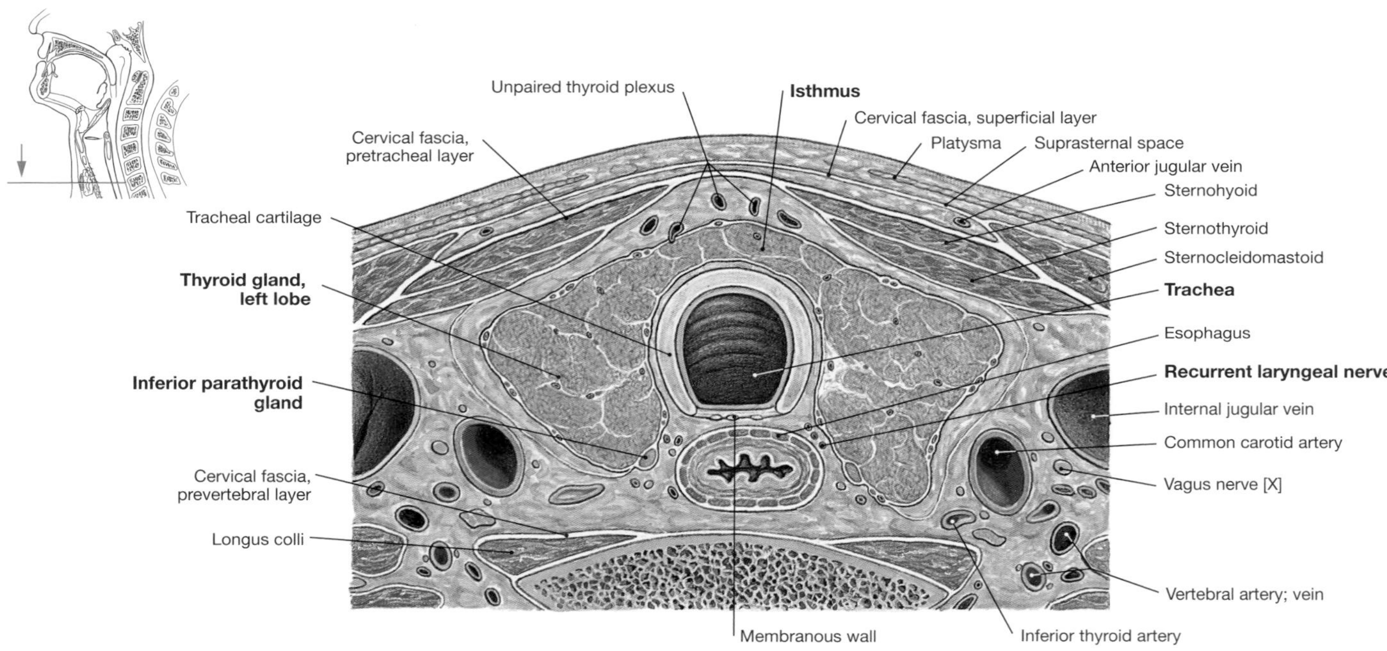
Unpaired thyroid plexus
Isthmus
Cervical fascia, superficial layer
Cervical fascia, pretracheal layer
Platysma
Suprasternal space
Anterior jugular vein
Sternohyoid
Tracheal cartilage
Sternothyroid
Sternocleidomastoid
Thyroid gland, left lobe
Trachea
Esophagus
Inferior parathyroid gland
Recurrent laryngeal nerve
Internal jugular vein
Common carotid artery
Cervical fascia, prevertebral layer
Vagus nerve [X]
Longus colli
Vertebral artery; vein
Membranous wall
Inferior thyroid artery

**Fig. 11.51 Thyroid gland;** horizontal section.
The thyroid gland covers the upper tracheal part from lateral and ventral. It is the largest endocrine gland in the body and secretes the hormones thyroxine (tetraiodothyronine, $T_4$), triiodothyronine ($T_3$), and calcitonin. The gland is ensheathed in its own capsule and, together with the larynx, trachea, esophagus, and pharynx, is surrounded by the general organ fascia.

Placed at the posterior side of each glandular lobe there are two grain-sized epithelial bodies **(parathyroid glands)** weighing 12–50 mg, which produce the parathyroid hormone (PTH).
On both sides, the **recurrent laryngeal nerve** courses between the trachea and the esophagus. The nerve is located outside of the special organ fasciae but inside the general organ fascia.

### Clinical Remarks

**Thyroid gland surgery** requires the ventral opening of the pretracheal fascia and the joint special and general organ fascia at the anterior side of the thyroid gland. Surgeons refer to it as outer (pretracheal fascia) and inner (organ fascia) capsule of the thyroid gland. Hyperplasia, adenoma, or carcinoma of the parathyroid glands can result in a hyperfunction with the development of a primary **hyperparathyroidism.** The increased secretion of parathyroid hormone (PTH) causes an increase of the serum calcium levels and is associated with complications affecting the bones, kidneys, and gastrointestinal tract.

## Development of the thyroid gland

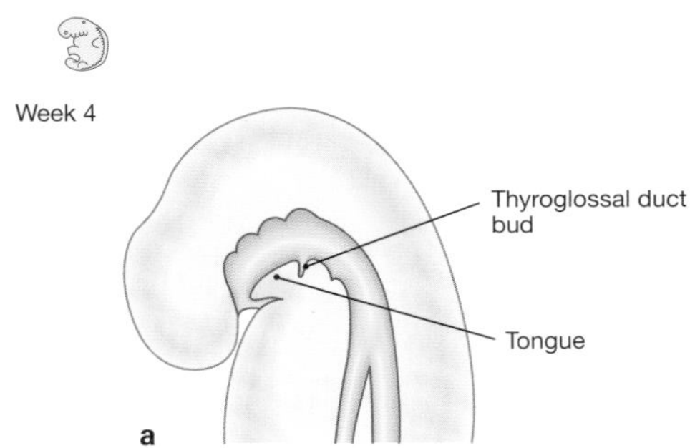
Week 4
Thyroglossal duct bud
Tongue
a

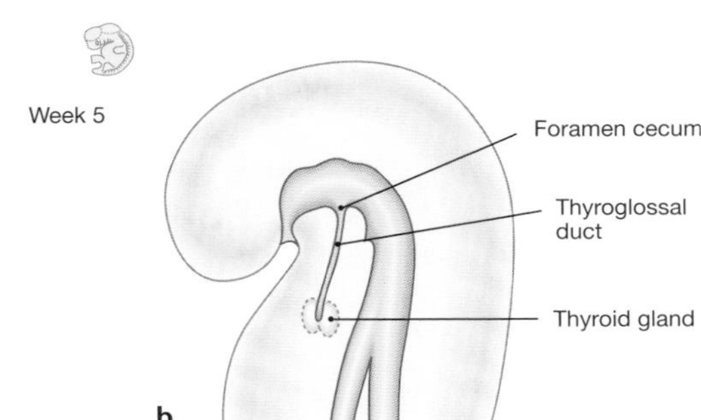
Week 5
Foramen cecum
Thyroglossal duct
Thyroid gland
b

**Figs. 11.52a and b Development of the thyroid gland.** [21]
From day 24 after fertilization onwards, epithelium from the ektodermal stomodaeum grows caudally past the hyoid bone and the larynx to form the **thyroglossal duct** (**a**). When the thyroglossal duct has reached its final location at the thyroid cartilage of the larynx at week 7, it forms the isthmus and the two lobes of the thyroid gland (**b**). The cranial part of the thyroglossal duct regresses. The proximal opening of the thyroglossal duct persists as **foramen cecum** behind the terminal sulcus and frequently a **pyramidal lobe** (thyroid gland tissue) is found along the passageway of the primitive thyroglossal duct (→ Fig. 8.162). Protruding from the fifth pharyngeal pouch, the ultimobranchial body gives rise to C-cells (produce calcitonin) which migrate into the thyroid gland. The epithelial bodies (produce parathyroid hormone) derive from the third and fourth pharyngeal pouches.

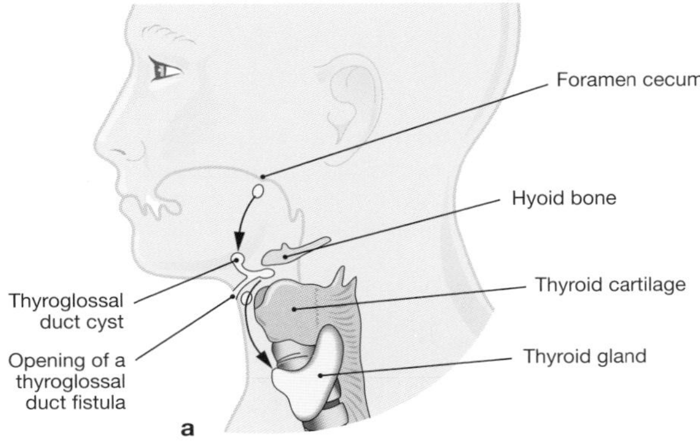
Foramen cecum
Hyoid bone
Thyroid cartilage
Thyroglossal duct cyst
Opening of a thyroglossal duct fistula
Thyroid gland
a

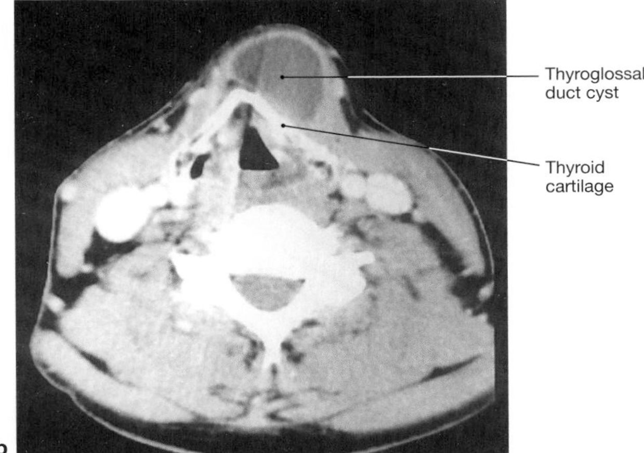
Thyroglossal duct cyst
Thyroid cartilage
b

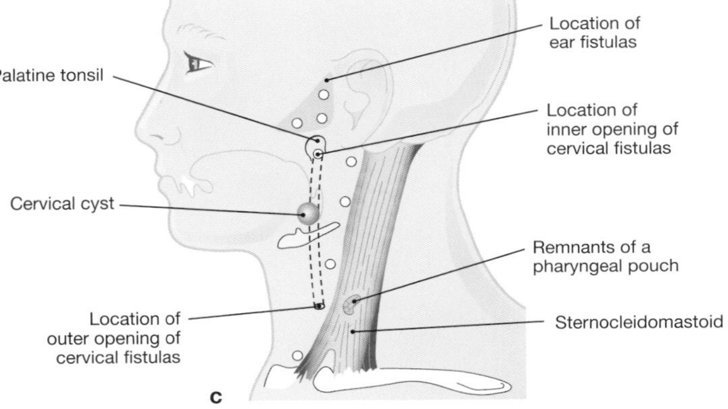
Location of ear fistulas
Palatine tonsil
Location of inner opening of cervical fistulas
Cervical cyst
Remnants of a pharyngeal pouch
Location of outer opening of cervical fistulas
Sternocleidomastoid
c

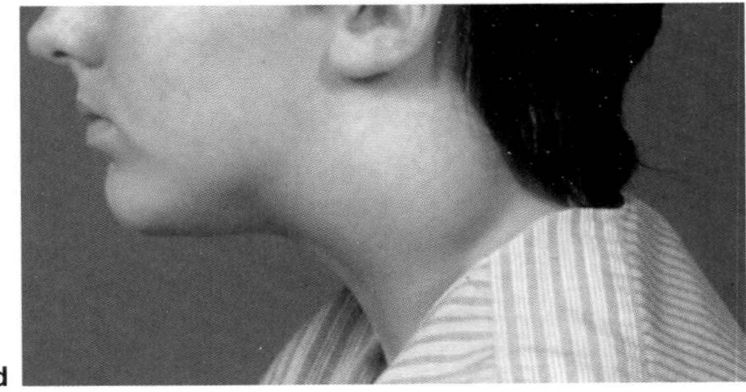
d

**Figs. 11.53a to d Cervical cysts and cervical fistulas.** [20]

- **a** Possible locations of cysts derived from the thyroglossal duct (arrows show the location of the thyroglossal duct during the descent of the thyroid gland from the foramen cecum to the final position in the anterior cervical region)
- **b** Computed tomography of a thyroglossal duct cyst in front of the thyroid cartilage
- **c** Possible locations of cervical cysts and cervical fistulas
- **d** Lateral cervical cyst; notice the swelling on the lateral side of the neck.

### Clinical Remarks

Persistence of parts of the thyroglossal duct can lead to a **median cervical cyst** or a **median cervical fistula** (→ Figs. 11.53a and b). Clinically, both only become a concern when infected.
A lateral cervical fistula or cyst is caused by the imperfect obliteration of the lateral aspects of the branchial clefts or the cervical sinus. **Lateral cervical fistulas** usually open at the anterior margin of the sternocleidomastoid (→ Fig. 11.53c); the accumulation of fluid within the **lateral cervical cysts** results in a swelling at the side of the neck (→ Fig. 11.53d).

## Vessels and nerves of the thyroid gland

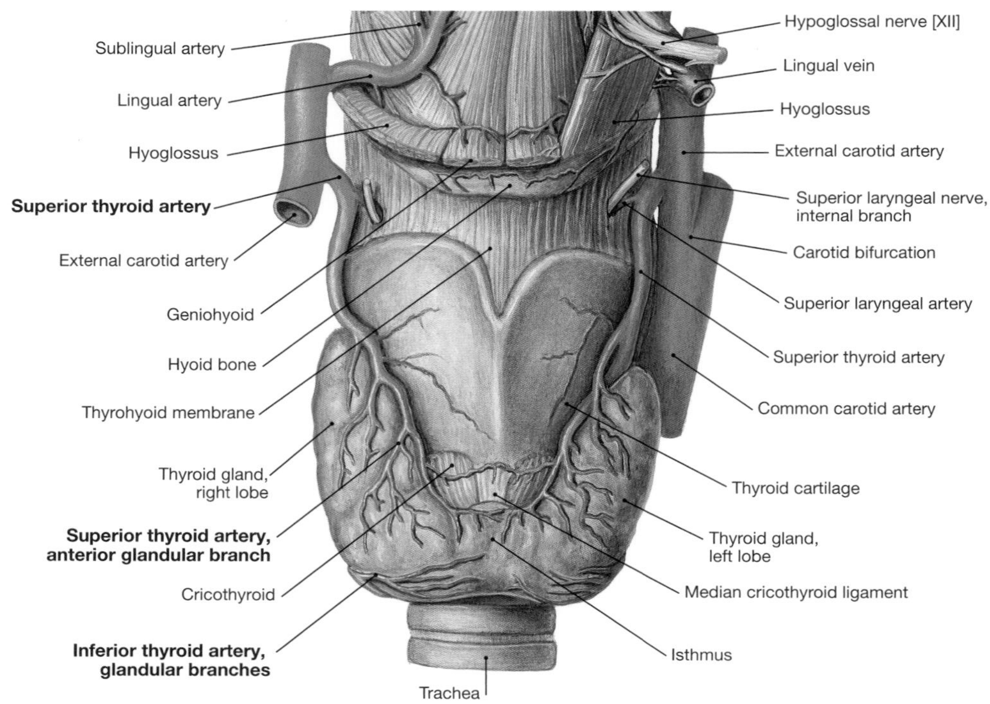
Sublingual artery
Lingual artery
Hyoglossus
Superior thyroid artery
External carotid artery
Geniohyoid
Hyoid bone
Thyrohyoid membrane
Thyroid gland, right lobe
Superior thyroid artery, anterior glandular branch
Cricothyroid
Inferior thyroid artery, glandular branches
Trachea
Hypoglossal nerve [XII]
Lingual vein
Hyoglossus
External carotid artery
Superior laryngeal nerve, internal branch
Carotid bifurcation
Superior laryngeal artery
Superior thyroid artery
Common carotid artery
Thyroid cartilage
Thyroid gland, left lobe
Median cricothyroid ligament
Isthmus

**Fig. 11.54 Arteries of the thyroid gland;** ventral view.
Being an endocrine organ, the thyroid gland has an exquisite blood supply through the **superior thyroid artery** (with anterior and posterior glandular branches) from the **external carotid artery** as well as through the **inferior thyroid artery** from the thyrocervical trunk. Sometimes, a small thyroid ima artery from the brachiocephalic trunk or the aortic arch also contributes to the blood supply (not shown). The blood vessels also supply blood to the epithelial bodies (→ Fig. 11.56).

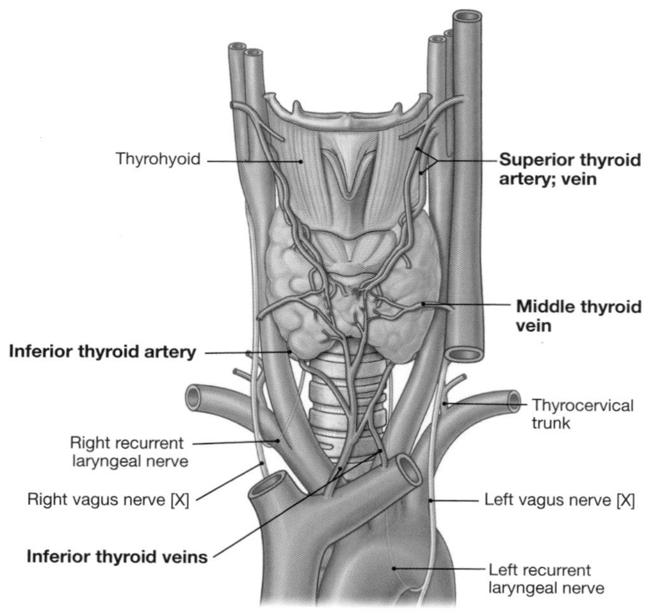
Thyrohyoid
Superior thyroid artery; vein
Middle thyroid vein
Inferior thyroid artery
Thyrocervical trunk
Right recurrent laryngeal nerve
Right vagus nerve [X]
Left vagus nerve [X]
Inferior thyroid veins
Left recurrent laryngeal nerve

**Fig. 11.55 Veins of the thyroid gland;** ventral view. [8]
Three paired veins collect the blood of the thyroid gland. The **superior and medial thyroid veins** drain into the internal jugular vein, whereas the **inferior thyroid vein** leads the blood into the left brachiocephalic vein.

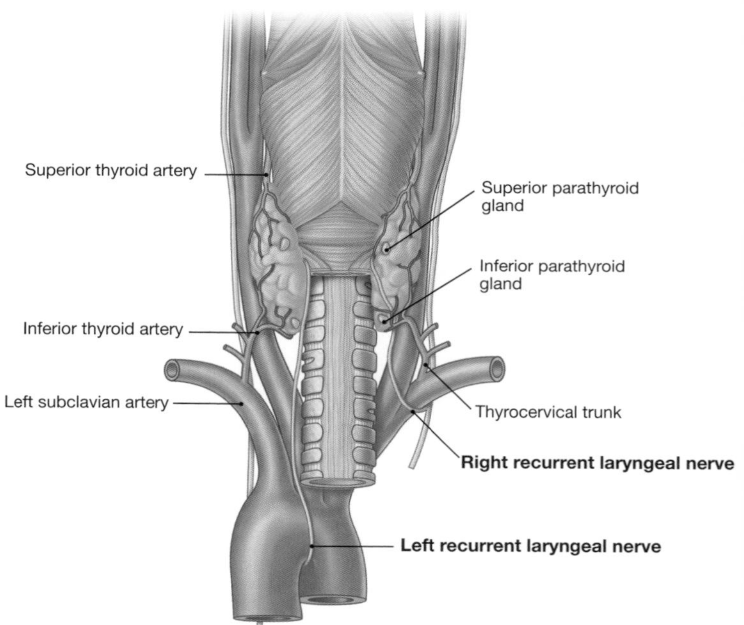
Superior thyroid artery
Superior parathyroid gland
Inferior parathyroid gland
Inferior thyroid artery
Left subclavian artery
Thyrocervical trunk
Right recurrent laryngeal nerve
Left recurrent laryngeal nerve

**Fig. 11.56 Superior and inferior thyroid arteries as well as left and right recurrent laryngeal nerve;** dorsal view. [8]
The thyroid gland has a close topographic relationship with the recurrent laryngeal nerves (inferior laryngeal nerves). Located within the groove between the trachea and the esophagus, these nerves course cranially to the larynx (→ Fig. 11.46).

## Clinical Remarks

Resection of a goitre (thyroidectomy; mostly performed as subtotal strumectomy) is the most frequent cause of **paralysis of the laryngeal muscles.** The enlargement of the thyroid gland disrupts the normal topography of the recurrent laryngeal nerve. Even in the case of a goitre the nerve maintains close relationships with the thyroid gland and the inferior thyroid artery, but is more difficult to localize and can be injured easily. An enlarged thyroid gland can compress the trachea. In advanced stages this can result in dyspnoea and often requires surgical intervention.

## Imaging and clinics

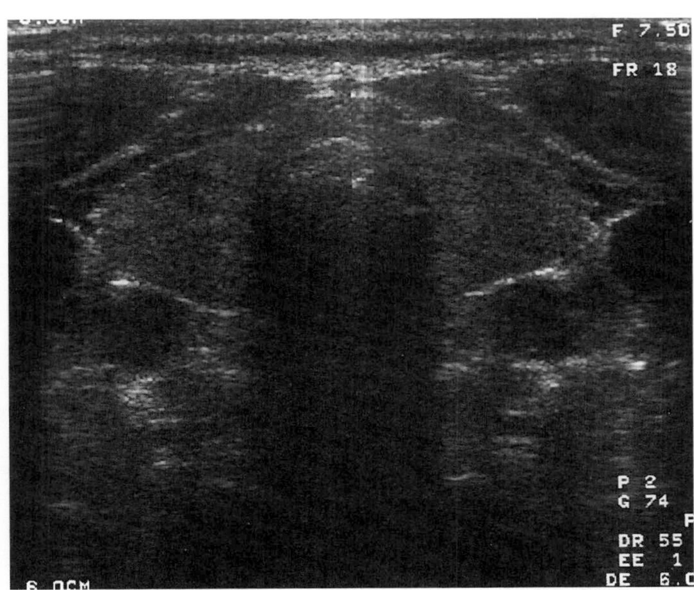
F 7.50
FR 18
P 2
G 74
DR 55
EE 1

**Fig. 11.57 Thyroid gland;** ultrasound image, normal thyroid, transverse section at the level of the isthmus of the thyroid gland. [27]

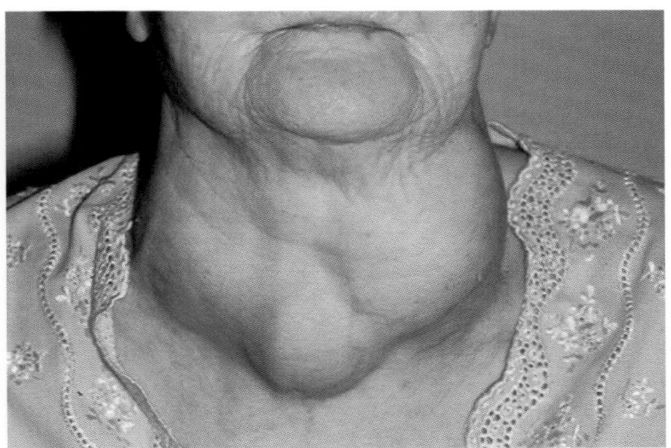

**Fig. 11.58 Enlargement of the thyroid gland (struma multinodosa).**
Three large nodes are visible (multinodular goitre).

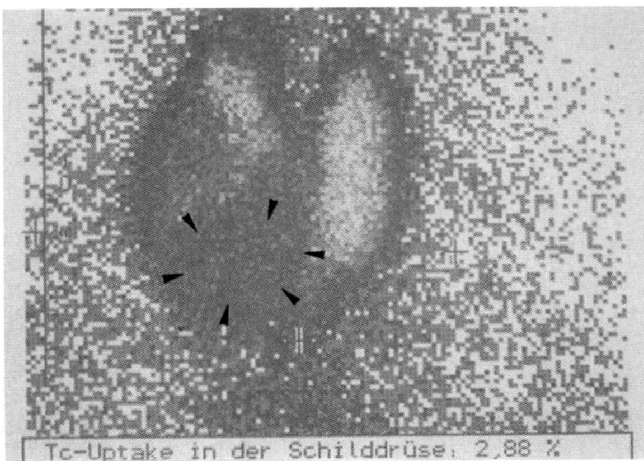
Tc-Uptake in der Schilddrüse: 2,88 %

**Fig. 11.59 Thyroid gland;** scintigraphic scan, ventral view. [6]
Scintigraphy is a diagnostic procedure which provides topographic and functional information of the thyroid gland. This image was taken 20 minutes after intravenous injection of technetium-99m-pertechnetate and shows a "cold nodule" (arrowheads) in the right thyroid lobe extending into the isthmus. The left thyroid lobe displays a homogeneous distribution of nuclides. The "cold node" represents functionally inactive thyroid tissue.

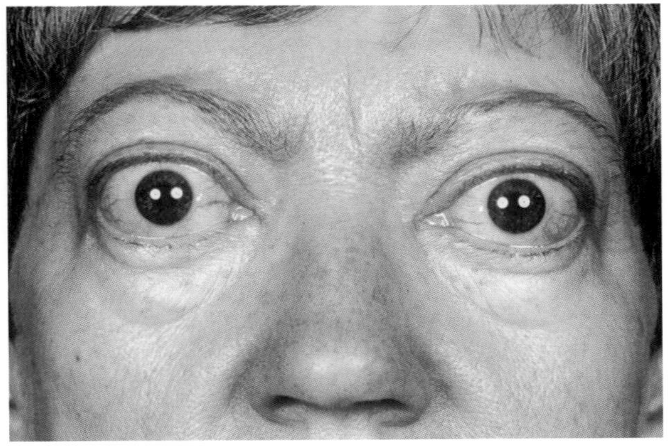

**Fig. 11.60 Patient with endocrine ophthalmopathy:** exophthalmus and retraction of the upper eyelid due to hyperthyroidism. [5]

## Clinical Remarks

The pathology of the thyroid gland is complex. **Diffuse** (→ Fig. 11.58) and **focal** (→ Fig. 11.59) **alterations in the thyroid gland** can be distinguished. Both types may have multiple causes. In addition, a deficient **(hypothyroidism)** or excessive production **(hyperthyroidism)** of the hormones thyroxine and triiodothyronine can occur. One example is the hyperthyroidism associated with diffuse goitre **(GRAVES' disease)** caused by immunological (autoimmune) processes. It is frequently associated with orbitopathy. This is likely the result of circulating antibodies against an antigen derived from the external ocular muscles. These antibodies cross-react with the microsomal fraction of the thyroid follicular epithelial cells. An **exophthalmus** can result from a retro-orbital edema, deposition of glycosaminoglycans, lymphocytic infiltrates and progressive fibrosis (→ Fig. 11.60).

## Vessels and nerves of the neck

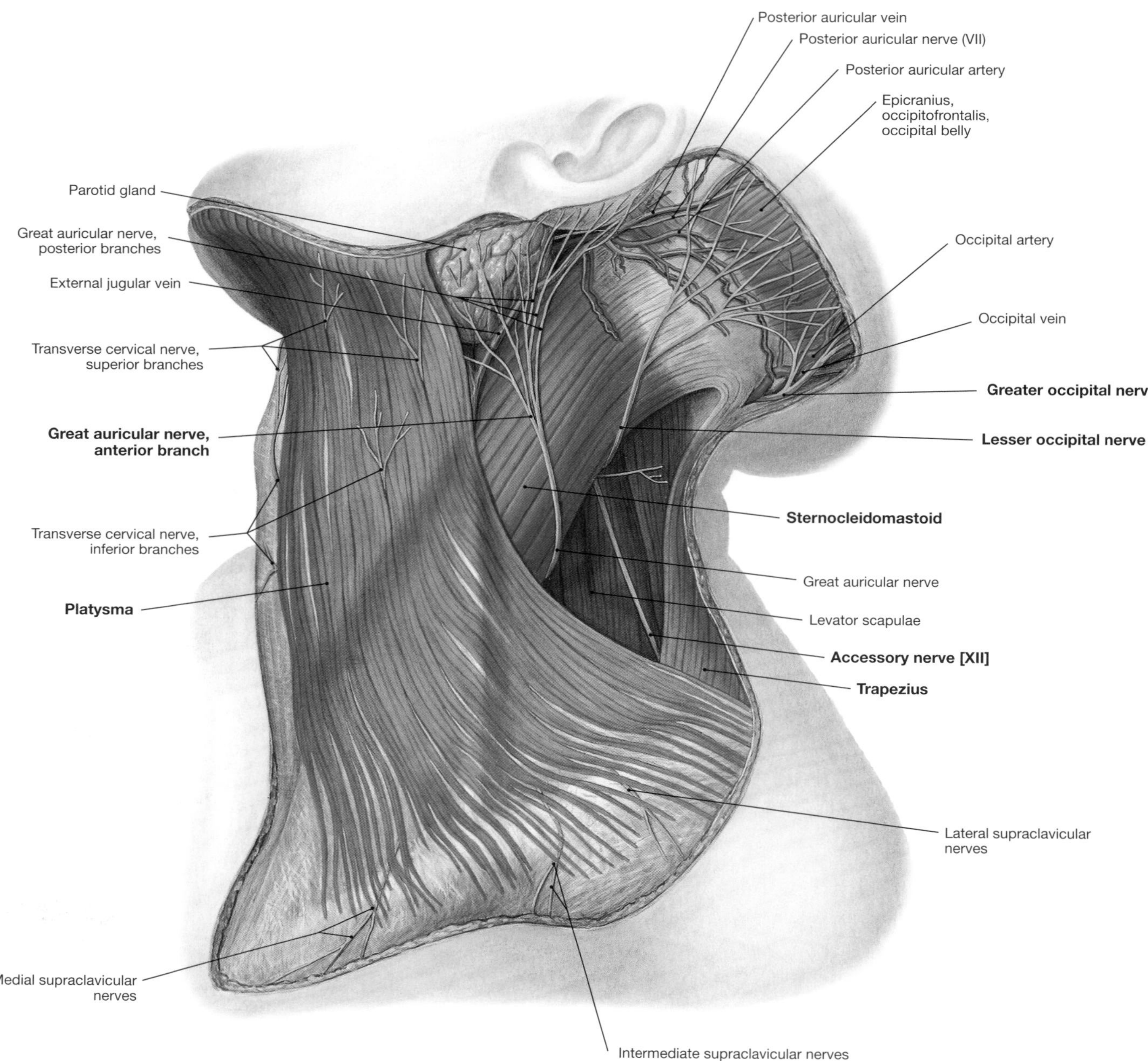
Posterior auricular vein
Posterior auricular nerve (VII)
Posterior auricular artery
Epicranius, occipitofrontalis, occipital belly
Parotid gland
Great auricular nerve, posterior branches
External jugular vein
Occipital artery
Occipital vein
Transverse cervical nerve, superior branches
Greater occipital nerve
Great auricular nerve, anterior branch
Lesser occipital nerve
Sternocleidomastoid
Transverse cervical nerve, inferior branches
Great auricular nerve
Platysma
Levator scapulae
Accessory nerve [XII]
Trapezius
Lateral supraclavicular nerves
Medial supraclavicular nerves
Intermediate supraclavicular nerves

**Fig. 11.61 Vessels and nerves of the anterior and lateral cervical region;** lateral view.

The superficial fascia of the neck has been removed dorsally of the platysma. The **great auricular nerve** and the **lesser occipital nerve** come from behind the sternocleidomastoid and curve around this muscle in an anterior and superior direction. Both are sensory nerves derived from the cervical plexus (C1–C4) and innervate the skin in front of and below the auricle to the occiput region. The **greater occipital nerve** passes through the tendinous origin of the trapezius at the superior nuchal line and provides the sensory cutaneous innervation to the occipital region. It is the dorsal branch of the spinal nerve C2. The **accessory nerve [XI]** lies on top of the levator scapulae and courses through the lateral triangle of the neck from the sternocleidomastoid to the trapezius, the two muscles innervated by this nerve. The accessory nerve [XI] has its origin in the brain stem and the upper cervical spinal cord (→ Fig. 12.160).

## Clinical Remarks

The **accessory nerve [XI]** is at risk of being injured during surgical interventions in the lateral cervical region (e.g. during removal of lymph nodes or neck dissection). Nerve lesions in this cervical region most frequently affect the function of the trapezius (paresis). As a result, the patient is unable to elevate the arm above the horizontal plane.

## Vessels and nerves of the neck

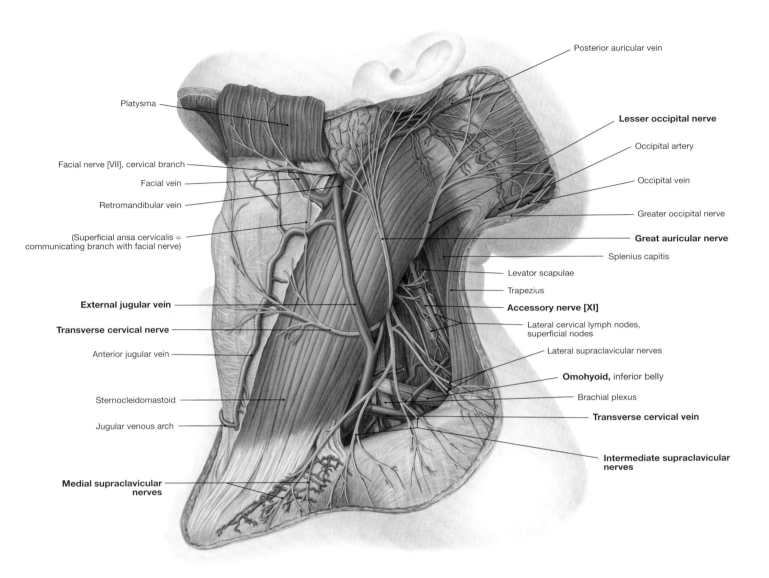

Posterior auricular vein
Platysma
**Lesser occipital nerve**
Occipital artery
Facial nerve [VII], cervical branch
Facial vein
Occipital vein
Retromandibular vein
Greater occipital nerve
(Superficial ansa cervicalis = communicating branch with facial nerve)
**Great auricular nerve**
Splenius capitis
Levator scapulae
Trapezius
**External jugular vein**
**Accessory nerve [XI]**
**Transverse cervical nerve**
Lateral cervical lymph nodes, superficial nodes
Anterior jugular vein
Lateral supraclavicular nerves
**Omohyoid,** inferior belly
Sternocleidomastoid
Brachial plexus
**Transverse cervical vein**
Jugular venous arch
**Intermediate supraclavicular nerves**
**Medial supraclavicular nerves**

**Fig. 11.62 Blood vessels and nerves of the lateral cervical region, left side;** lateral view. Parts of the platysma were deflected upwards, and the superficial layer of the cervical fascia was largely removed.
The sensory nerves of the cervical plexus emerge at the posterior margin of the sternocleidomastoid and penetrate the superficial fascia of the neck. The supraclavicular nerves, transverse cervical nerve, and the greater auricular nerve all emerge in a confined area, called **punctum nervosum** (ERB's point), midway of the sternocleidomastoid. ERB's point also includes the lesser occipital nerve although it exits far more cranially. The accessory nerve [XI], the omohyoid, and the transverse cervical vein are visible in the posterior triangle of the neck. The transverse cervical vein drains into the external jugular vein, which has a variable course across the sternocleidomastoid.

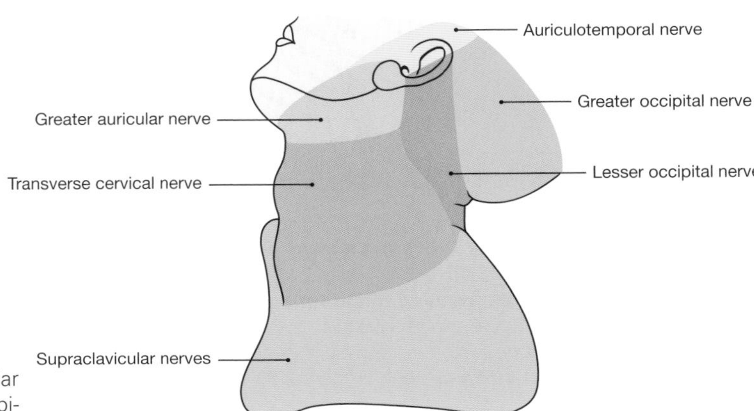
Auriculotemporal nerve
Greater occipital nerve
Greater auricular nerve
Lesser occipital nerve
Transverse cervical nerve
Supraclavicular nerves

**Fig. 11.63 Sensory innervation of the skin in the cervical region (cutaneous nerves).**
The sensory innervation of the skin is provided by the supraclavicular nerves, transverse cervical nerve, greater auricular nerve, lesser occipital nerve, greater occipital nerve and third occipital nerve (not shown).

## Vessels and nerves of the neck

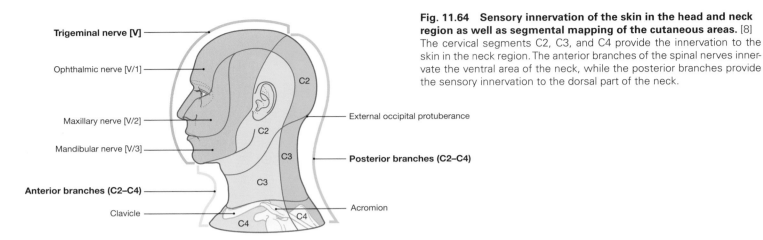

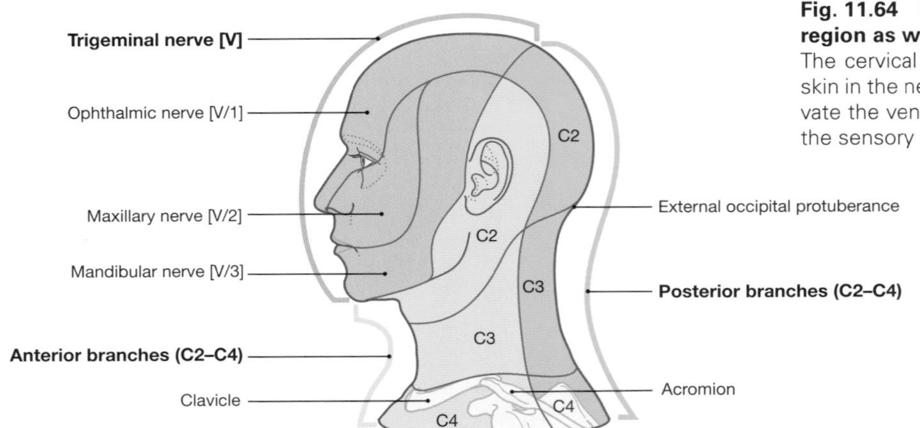
Trigeminal nerve [V]
Ophthalmic nerve [V/1]
Maxillary nerve [V/2]
Mandibular nerve [V/3]
Anterior branches (C2–C4)
Clavicle
C2
C2
C3
C3
C4
C4
External occipital protuberance
Posterior branches (C2–C4)
Acromion

**Fig. 11.64 Sensory innervation of the skin in the head and neck region as well as segmental mapping of the cutaneous areas.** [8]
The cervical segments C2, C3, and C4 provide the innervation to the skin in the neck region. The anterior branches of the spinal nerves innervate the ventral area of the neck, while the posterior branches provide the sensory innervation to the dorsal part of the neck.

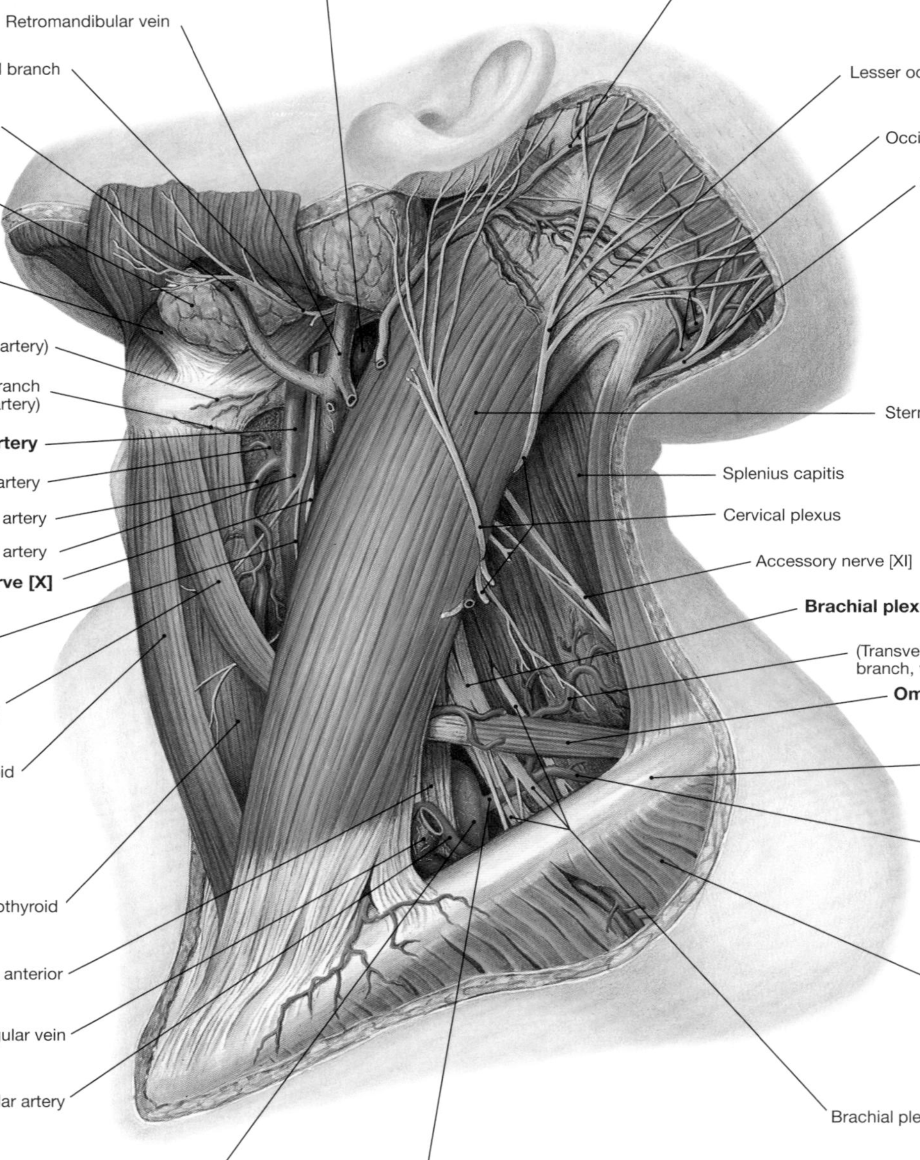

Internal jugular vein
Retromandibular vein
Facial nerve [VII], cervical branch
Facial vein
Submandibular gland
Digastric, anterior belly
Suprahyoid branch (lingual artery)
Infrahyoid branch (superior thyroid artery)
External carotid artery
Superior laryngeal artery
Superior thyroid artery
Common carotid artery
Vagus nerve [X]
(Deep ansa cervicalis), superior root (cervical plexus)
Omohyoid, superior belly
Sternohyoid
Sternothyroid
Scalenus anterior
External jugular vein
Suprascapular artery
Subclavian artery
Transverse cervical artery
Posterior auricular vein
Lesser occipital nerve
Occipital artery; vein
Greater occipital nerve
Sternocleidomastoid
Splenius capitis
Cervical plexus
Accessory nerve [XI]
Brachial plexus, superior trunk
(Transverse cervical artery, superficial branch, var.)
Omohyoid, inferior belly
Clavicle
(Transverse cervical artery, deep branch, var.)
Deltoid
Brachial plexus, supraclavicular part

**Fig. 11.65 Vessels and nerves of the anterior and lateral cervical region, left side;** lateral view; after removal of the superficial and middle fascia of the neck.
The anterior triangle of the neck depicts structures normally covered by the carotid sheath (external carotid artery, vagus nerve [X], internal jugular vein); displayed in the posterior triangle of the neck are the brachial plexus and the subclavian artery in the scalene hiatus, which are crossed by the inferior belly of the omohyoid.

## Vessels and nerves of the neck

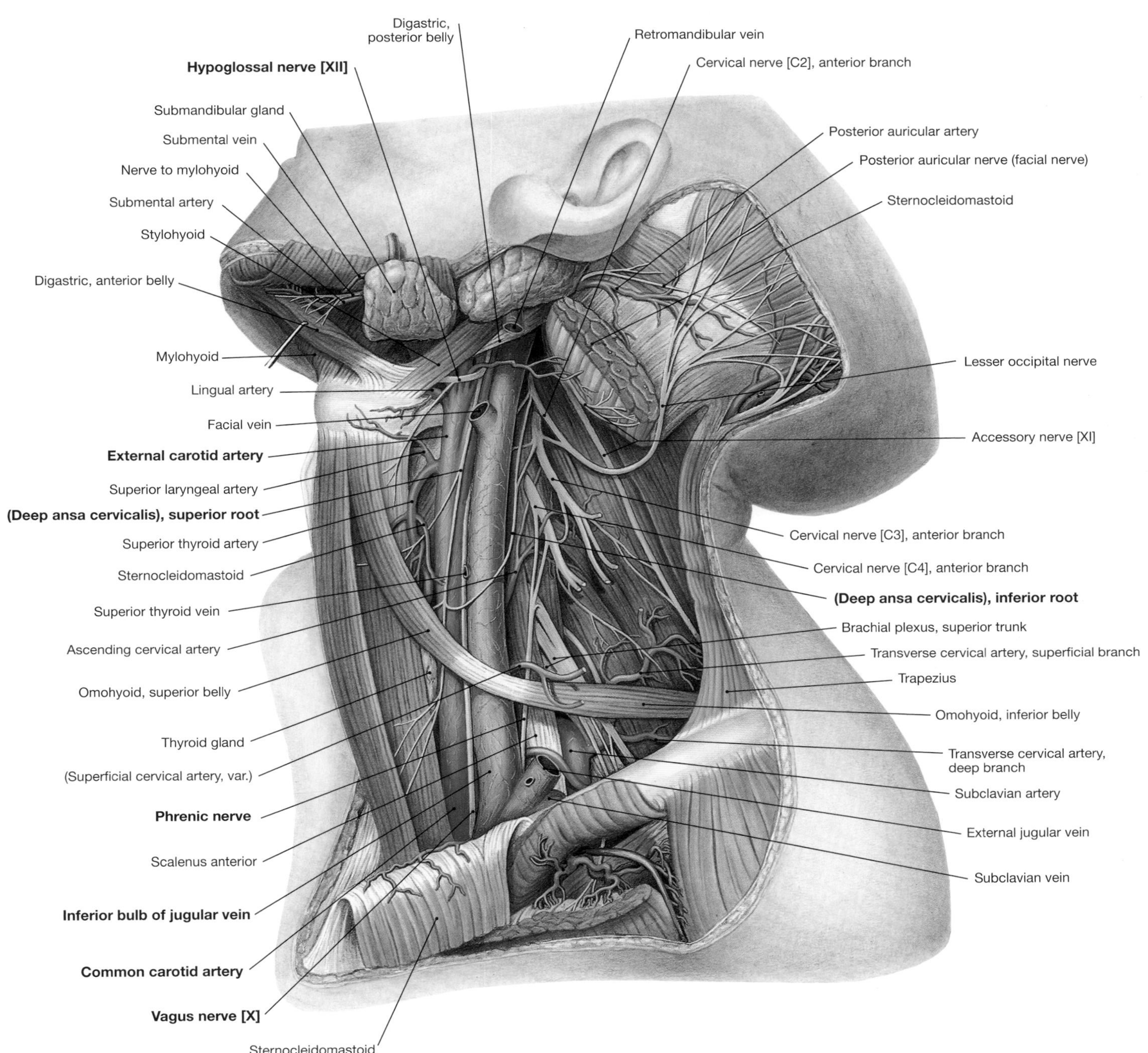
Digastric, posterior belly
Retromandibular vein
Cervical nerve [C2], anterior branch
Hypoglossal nerve [XII]
Submandibular gland
Submental vein
Nerve to mylohyoid
Submental artery
Stylohyoid
Digastric, anterior belly
Posterior auricular artery
Posterior auricular nerve (facial nerve)
Sternocleidomastoid
Mylohyoid
Lingual artery
Facial vein
External carotid artery
Superior laryngeal artery
(Deep ansa cervicalis), superior root
Superior thyroid artery
Sternocleidomastoid
Superior thyroid vein
Ascending cervical artery
Omohyoid, superior belly
Thyroid gland
(Superficial cervical artery, var.)
Phrenic nerve
Scalenus anterior
Inferior bulb of jugular vein
Common carotid artery
Vagus nerve [X]
Sternocleidomastoid
Lesser occipital nerve
Accessory nerve [XI]
Cervical nerve [C3], anterior branch
Cervical nerve [C4], anterior branch
(Deep ansa cervicalis), inferior root
Brachial plexus, superior trunk
Transverse cervical artery, superficial branch
Trapezius
Omohyoid, inferior belly
Transverse cervical artery, deep branch
Subclavian artery
External jugular vein
Subclavian vein

**Fig. 11.66 Vessels and nerves of the lateral cervical region, left side;** lateral view; after almost complete removal of the sternocleidomastoid.

The removal of the sternocleidomastoid permits an unobstructed view of the **common carotid artery** in the lower neck region, the **external carotid artery** in the upper cervical region as well as the **vagus nerve [X]** and the **internal jugular vein.** In the upper cervical region, the **(deep) ansa cervicalis** with its superior and inferior roots encloses the internal jugular vein. The superior and inferior roots provide branches to the infrahyoid muscles. Lateral to the internal jugular vein, the **phrenic nerve** branches off the cervical plexus and crosses the scalenus anterior in the lower cervical region to reach the upper thoracic aperture. In the upper cervical region, the **hypoglossal nerve** [XII] projects forward and crosses the external carotid artery close to the branching points of the lingual artery and the facial artery to disappear below the stylohyoid.

## Vessels and nerves of the neck

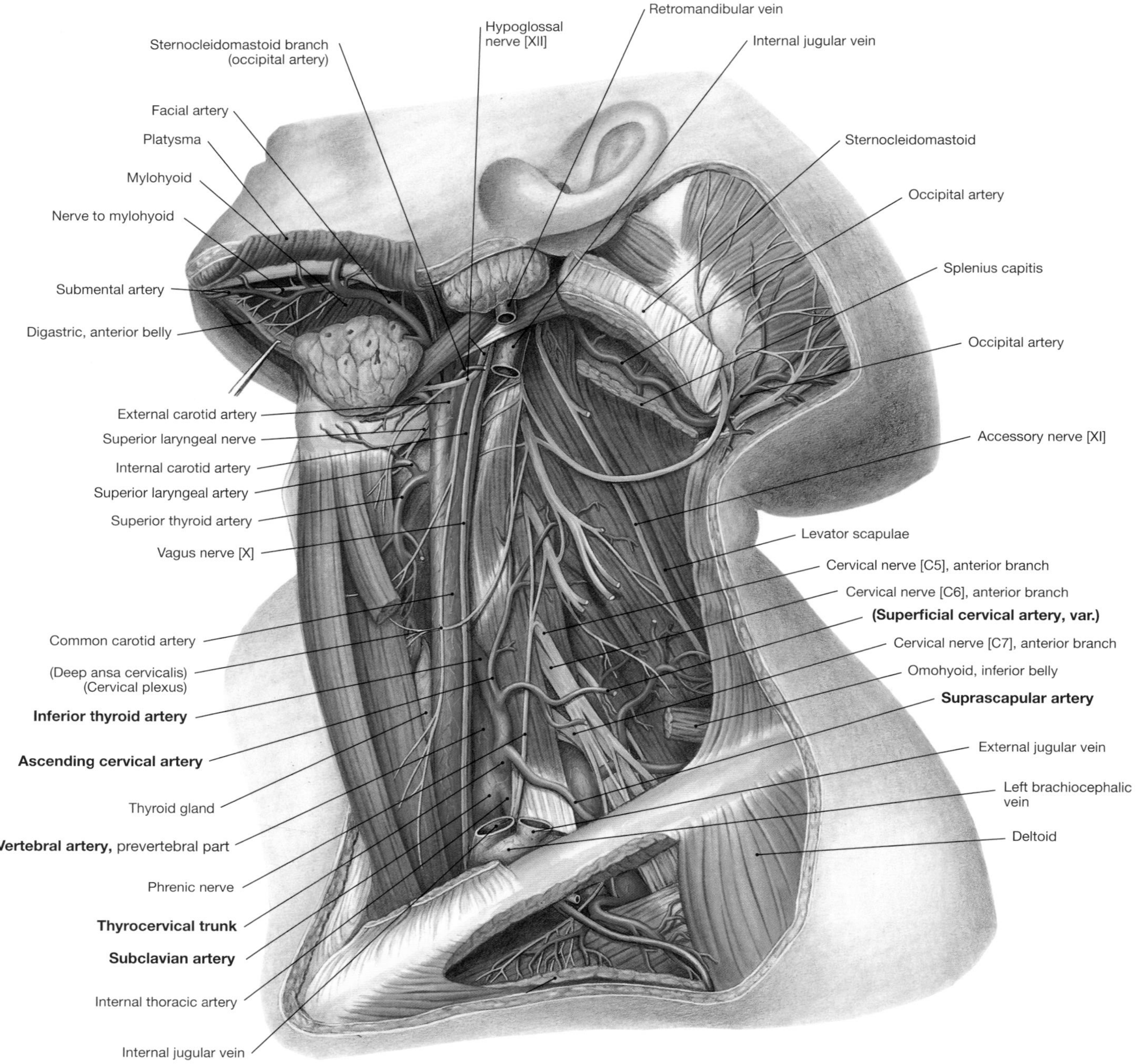
Sternocleidomastoid branch (occipital artery)
Hypoglossal nerve [XII]
Retromandibular vein
Internal jugular vein
Facial artery
Platysma
Mylohyoid
Nerve to mylohyoid
Submental artery
Digastric, anterior belly
Sternocleidomastoid
Occipital artery
Splenius capitis
Occipital artery
External carotid artery
Superior laryngeal nerve
Internal carotid artery
Superior laryngeal artery
Superior thyroid artery
Vagus nerve [X]
Accessory nerve [XI]
Levator scapulae
Cervical nerve [C5], anterior branch
Cervical nerve [C6], anterior branch
(Superficial cervical artery, var.)
Common carotid artery
Cervical nerve [C7], anterior branch
(Deep ansa cervicalis) (Cervical plexus)
Omohyoid, inferior belly
Inferior thyroid artery
Suprascapular artery
Ascending cervical artery
External jugular vein
Thyroid gland
Left brachiocephalic vein
Vertebral artery, prevertebral part
Deltoid
Phrenic nerve
Thyrocervical trunk
Subclavian artery
Internal thoracic artery
Internal jugular vein

**Fig. 11.67 Vessels and nerves of the lateral cervical region, deep layer, left side;** lateral view.
Upon removal of the internal jugular vein, the medially located **subclavian artery,** the **vertebral artery** and the **thyrocervical trunk** branching off the subclavian artery are visible. The subclavian artery courses dorsal to the scalenus anterior and, together with the brachial plexus, passes through the scalene hiatus.

| Branches of the Thyrocervical Trunk | |
|---|---|
| • Inferior thyroid artery<br>– Inferior laryngeal artery<br>– Glandular branches<br>– Pharyngeal branches<br>– Esophageal branches<br>– Tracheal branches | • Suprascapular artery<br>– Acromial branch<br><br>• Transverse cervical artery<br>– Superficial branch<br>– Deep branch |
| • Ascending cervical artery<br>– Spinal branches | • (Dorsal scapular artery) |

### Clinical Remarks

A proximal high-grade stenosis (narrowing) of the left subclavian artery, less frequently of the right subclavian artery, can result in a retrograde (reversed) flow into the vertebral artery of the affected side during intense physical activity of the arm **(subclavian steal syndrome; SSS).** The resulting reduction in the blood perfusion of the brain can cause dizziness and headaches.

## Vessels and nerves of neck and axilla

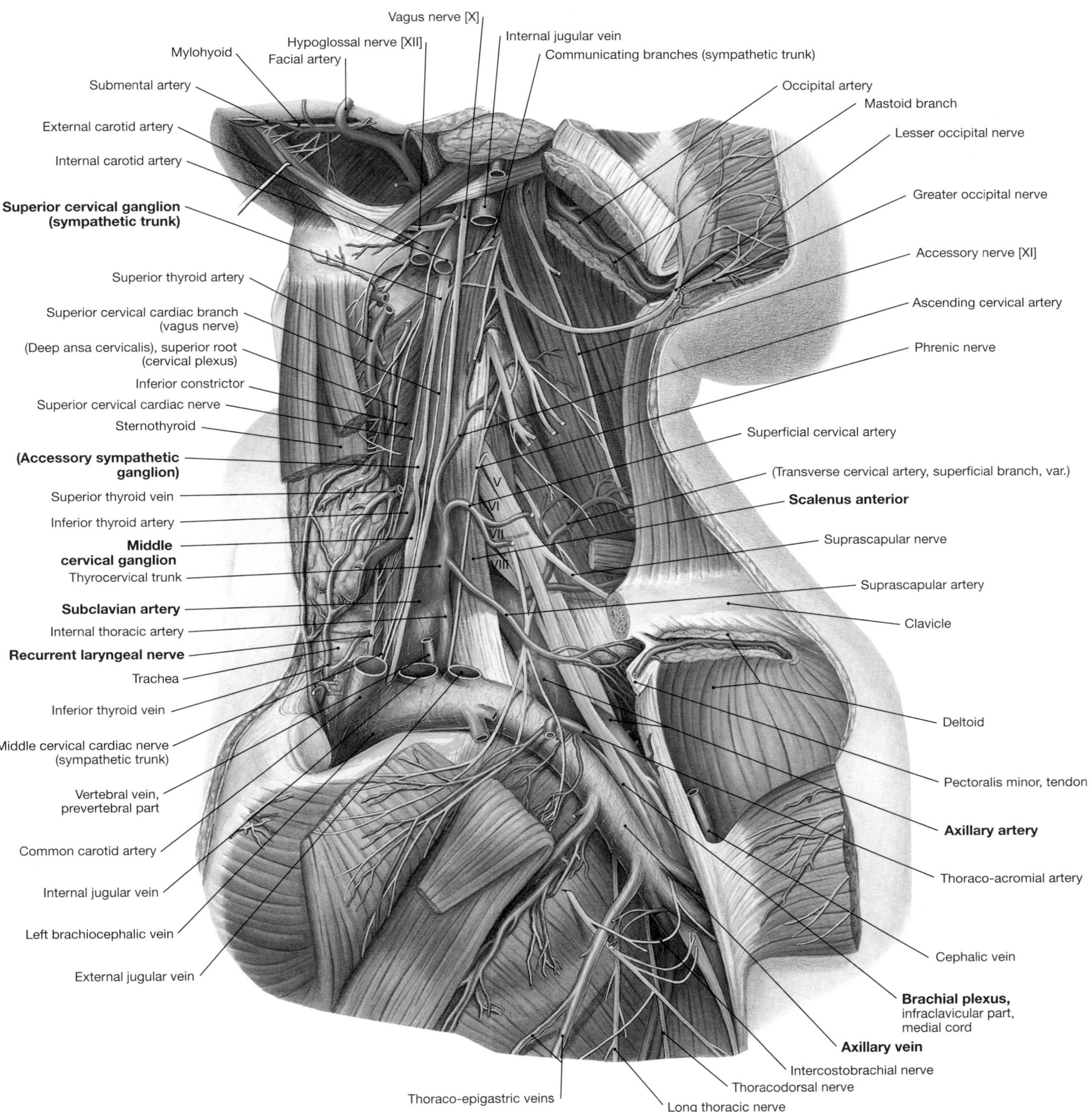

Vagus nerve [X]
Internal jugular vein
Hypoglossal nerve [XII]
Mylohyoid
Facial artery
Communicating branches (sympathetic trunk)
Submental artery
Occipital artery
Mastoid branch
External carotid artery
Lesser occipital nerve
Internal carotid artery
Superior cervical ganglion (sympathetic trunk)
Greater occipital nerve
Accessory nerve [XI]
Superior thyroid artery
Ascending cervical artery
Superior cervical cardiac branch (vagus nerve)
Phrenic nerve
(Deep ansa cervicalis), superior root (cervical plexus)
Inferior constrictor
Superior cervical cardiac nerve
Sternothyroid
Superficial cervical artery
(Accessory sympathetic ganglion)
(Transverse cervical artery, superficial branch, var.)
Superior thyroid vein
Scalenus anterior
Inferior thyroid artery
Middle cervical ganglion
Suprascapular nerve
Thyrocervical trunk
Suprascapular artery
Subclavian artery
Internal thoracic artery
Clavicle
Recurrent laryngeal nerve
Trachea
Inferior thyroid vein
Deltoid
Middle cervical cardiac nerve (sympathetic trunk)
Pectoralis minor, tendon
Vertebral vein, prevertebral part
Axillary artery
Common carotid artery
Thoraco-acromial artery
Internal jugular vein
Left brachiocephalic vein
Cephalic vein
External jugular vein
Brachial plexus, infraclavicular part, medial cord
Axillary vein
Intercostobrachial nerve
Thoracodorsal nerve
Thoraco-epigastric veins
Long thoracic nerve
V
VI
VII
VIII


**Fig. 11.68 Vessels and nerves of the lateral cervical region and the axillary region.**
The numbers V to VIII mark the ventral branches of the corresponding cervical nerves.
After the removal of the anterior two-thirds of the clavicle, the **brachial plexus** and the **subclavian artery** passing through the scalene hiatus (between scalenus anterior and scalenus medius), and the course of the subclavian vein (in front of the scalenus anterior) across rib I into the upper extremity are visible. In some cases, the upper part of the brachial plexus can penetrate the scalenus medius. In the cervical region, the brachial plexus provides a number of smaller branches and, after multiple exchanges of fibers, forms fascicles which are located shortly below the clavicle lateral of the subclavian artery. Only in the middle of the axilla they reach the topographic position depicted in their name.
On top of the deep cervical muscles lies the **sympathetic trunk** with the superius and middle cervical ganglion (in the upper cervical region the sympathetic trunk runs within the general organ fascia, in the lower cervical region between the prevertebral fascia and the general organ fascia, not shown). The recurrent laryngeal nerve is visible below the thyroid gland between the trachea and the esophagus.

## Cervical plexus

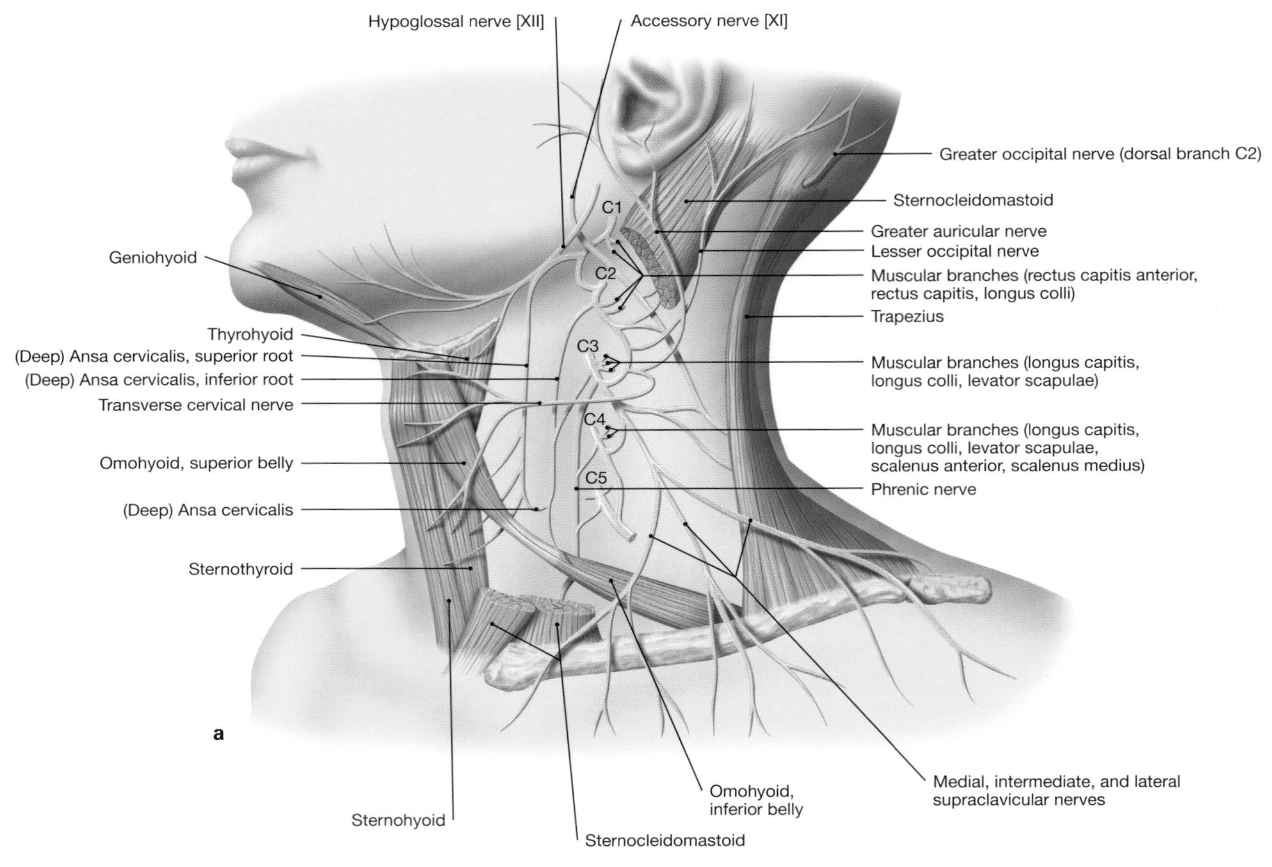
Hypoglossal nerve [XII]
Accessory nerve [XI]
Greater occipital nerve (dorsal branch C2)
Sternocleidomastoid
Greater auricular nerve
Lesser occipital nerve
Muscular branches (rectus capitis anterior, rectus capitis, longus colli)
Trapezius
Muscular branches (longus capitis, longus colli, levator scapulae)
Muscular branches (longus capitis, longus colli, levator scapulae, scalenus anterior, scalenus medius)
Phrenic nerve
Medial, intermediate, and lateral supraclavicular nerves
Geniohyoid
Thyrohyoid
(Deep) Ansa cervicalis, superior root
(Deep) Ansa cervicalis, inferior root
Transverse cervical nerve
Omohyoid, superior belly
(Deep) Ansa cervicalis
Sternothyroid
C1
C2
C3
C4
C5
a
Sternohyoid
Sternocleidomastoid
Omohyoid, inferior belly

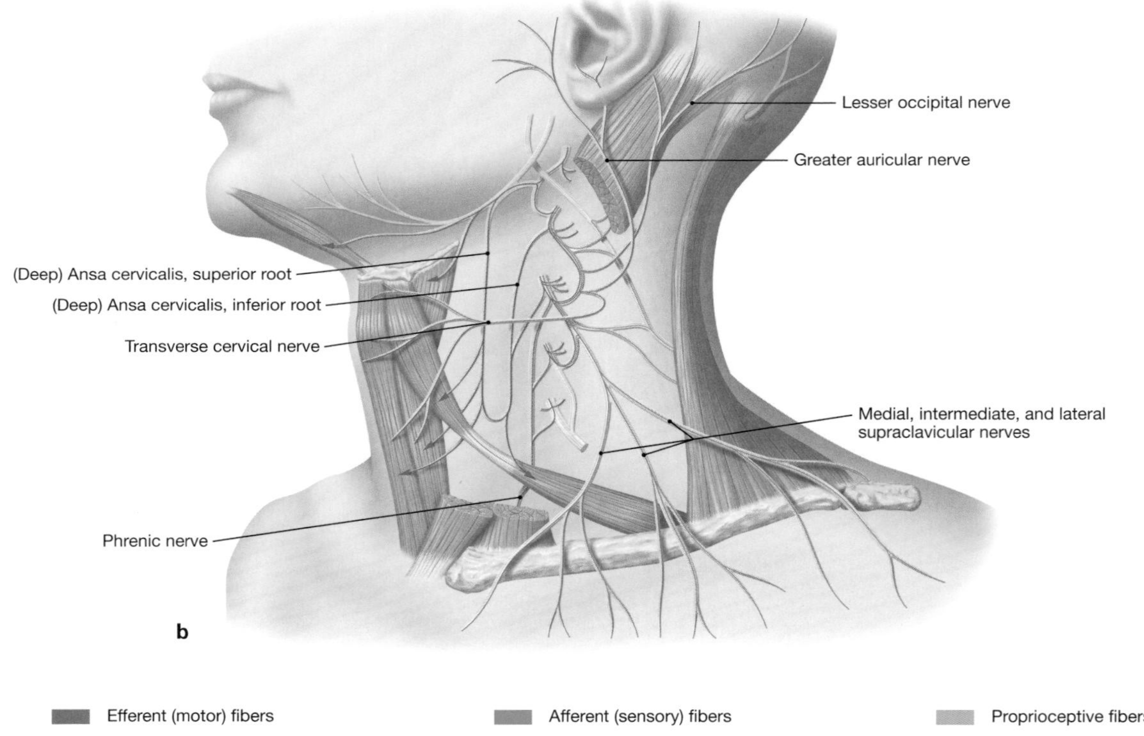
Lesser occipital nerve
Greater auricular nerve
(Deep) Ansa cervicalis, superior root
(Deep) Ansa cervicalis, inferior root
Transverse cervical nerve
Medial, intermediate, and lateral supraclavicular nerves
Phrenic nerve
b

Efferent (motor) fibers | Afferent (sensory) fibers | Proprioceptive fibers

**Figs. 11.69a and b Cervical plexus, sensory and motor branches.** The **deep ansa cervicalis** and the phrenic nerve constitute the motor branches of the brachial plexus. The deep ansa cervicalis consisting of a superior root (limb) from segment C1 and an inferior root (limb) from segments C2 and C3 serves to innervate the infrahyoid muscles (thyrohyoid, sternohyoid, sternothyroid, and omohyoid). Additional motor branches innervate the suprahyoid located geniohyoid muscle, the prevertebral muscles, the rectus capitis anterior, the scaleni anterior and medius as well as parts of the levator scapulae. The **phrenic nerve** derives from the segments C3 to C5, runs caudally, and enters the thoracic cavity through the upper thoracic aperture.

→ T 7

## Vertebral artery and costocervical trunk

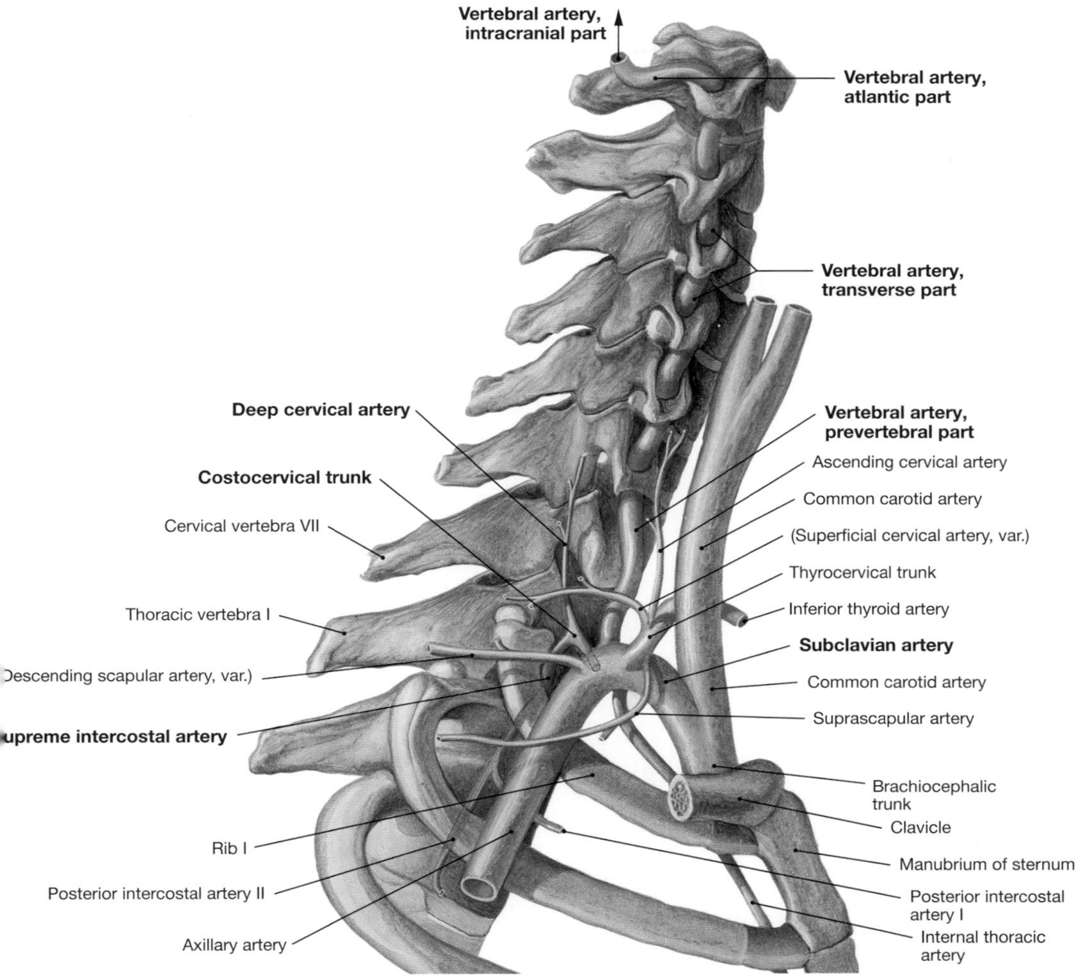

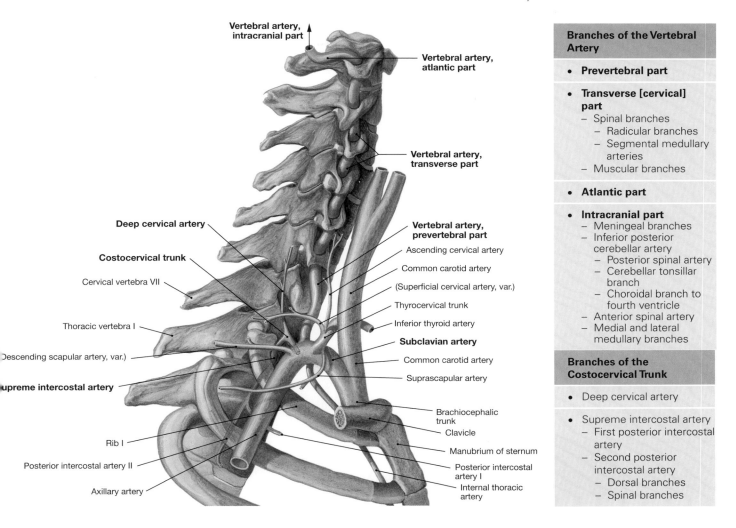

Vertebral artery, intracranial part
Vertebral artery, atlantic part
Vertebral artery, transverse part
Deep cervical artery
Vertebral artery, prevertebral part
Costocervical trunk
Ascending cervical artery
Common carotid artery
Cervical vertebra VII
(Superficial cervical artery, var.)
Thyrocervical trunk
Thoracic vertebra I
Inferior thyroid artery
Subclavian artery
(Descending scapular artery, var.)
Common carotid artery
Supreme intercostal artery
Suprascapular artery
Brachiocephalic trunk
Clavicle
Rib I
Manubrium of sternum
Posterior intercostal artery II
Posterior intercostal artery I
Axillary artery
Internal thoracic artery

**Fig. 11.70 Branches of the subclavian artery, the vertebral artery, and the costocervical trunk;** lateral view.

| Branches of the Vertebral Artery |
|---|
| • **Prevertebral part** |
| • **Transverse [cervical] part**<br>– Spinal branches<br>  – Radicular branches<br>  – Segmental medullary arteries<br>– Muscular branches |
| • **Atlantic part** |
| • **Intracranial part**<br>– Meningeal branches<br>– Inferior posterior cerebellar artery<br>  – Posterior spinal artery<br>  – Cerebellar tonsillar branch<br>  – Choroidal branch to fourth ventricle<br>– Anterior spinal artery<br>– Medial and lateral medullary branches |

| Branches of the Costocervical Trunk |
|---|
| • Deep cervical artery |
| • Supreme intercostal artery<br>– First posterior intercostal artery<br>– Second posterior intercostal artery<br>  – Dorsal branches<br>  – Spinal branches |

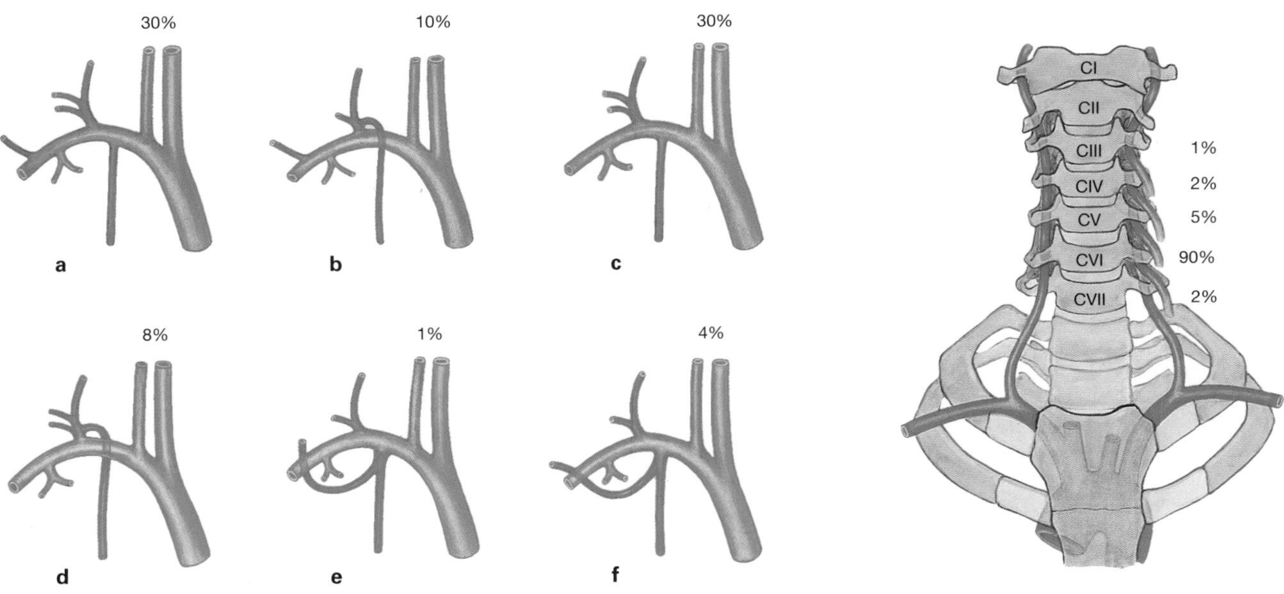
30%
10%
30%
a
b
c
8%
1%
4%
d
e
f
CI
CII
CIII
CIV
CV
CVI
CVII
1%
2%
5%
90%
2%

**Figs. 11.71a to f Variations in branching types of the subclavian artery and the costocervical trunk.**

**Fig. 11.72 Variations in the level of entry of the vertebral artery into the foramina transversaria.**

## Veins of the neck

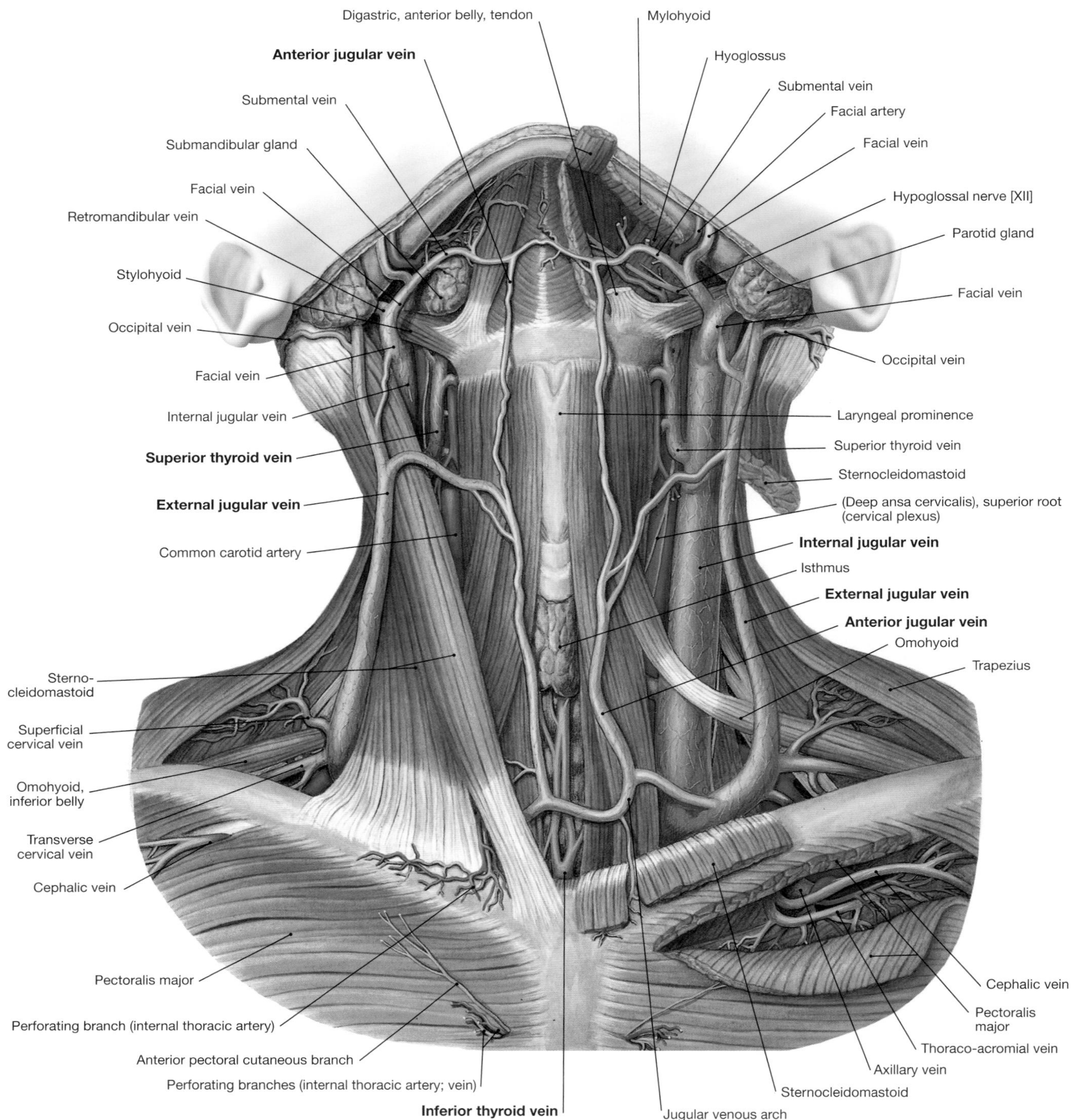
Digastric, anterior belly, tendon
Mylohyoid
Anterior jugular vein
Hyoglossus
Submental vein
Submental vein
Facial artery
Submandibular gland
Facial vein
Facial vein
Hypoglossal nerve [XII]
Retromandibular vein
Parotid gland
Stylohyoid
Facial vein
Occipital vein
Occipital vein
Facial vein
Internal jugular vein
Laryngeal prominence
Superior thyroid vein
Superior thyroid vein
Sternocleidomastoid
External jugular vein
(Deep ansa cervicalis), superior root (cervical plexus)
Common carotid artery
Internal jugular vein
Isthmus
External jugular vein
Anterior jugular vein
Omohyoid
Trapezius
Sterno-cleidomastoid
Superficial cervical vein
Omohyoid, inferior belly
Transverse cervical vein
Cephalic vein
Pectoralis major
Cephalic vein
Pectoralis major
Perforating branch (internal thoracic artery)
Thoraco-acromial vein
Axillary vein
Anterior pectoral cutaneous branch
Perforating branches (internal thoracic artery; vein)
Sternocleidomastoid
Inferior thyroid vein
Jugular venous arch

**Fig. 11.73 Veins of the neck;** ventral view. The sternocleidomastoid was largely removed on the left side. All fasciae of the neck have also been removed.
**Superficial** veins of the neck are the anterior jugular vein and the external jugular vein which drain venous blood into the internal jugular vein, subclavian vein, and brachiocephalic vein.
**Deep** veins of the neck are the internal jugular vein, the superior thyroid veins, the inferior thyroid vein and the unpaired thyroid plexus (not shown). The course of the superficial veins is very variable.

### Clinical Remarks

**Intravenous (IV) therapy** is one of the most frequently employed invasive procedures in the emergency case prior to reaching a hospital. The external jugular vein provides a good accessibility for IV treatment, even if the other superficial veins are in a poor condition. The guidelines for cardiovascular resuscitation recommend this IV access route as the first choice.

## Vessels and nerves of the neck and upper thoracic aperture

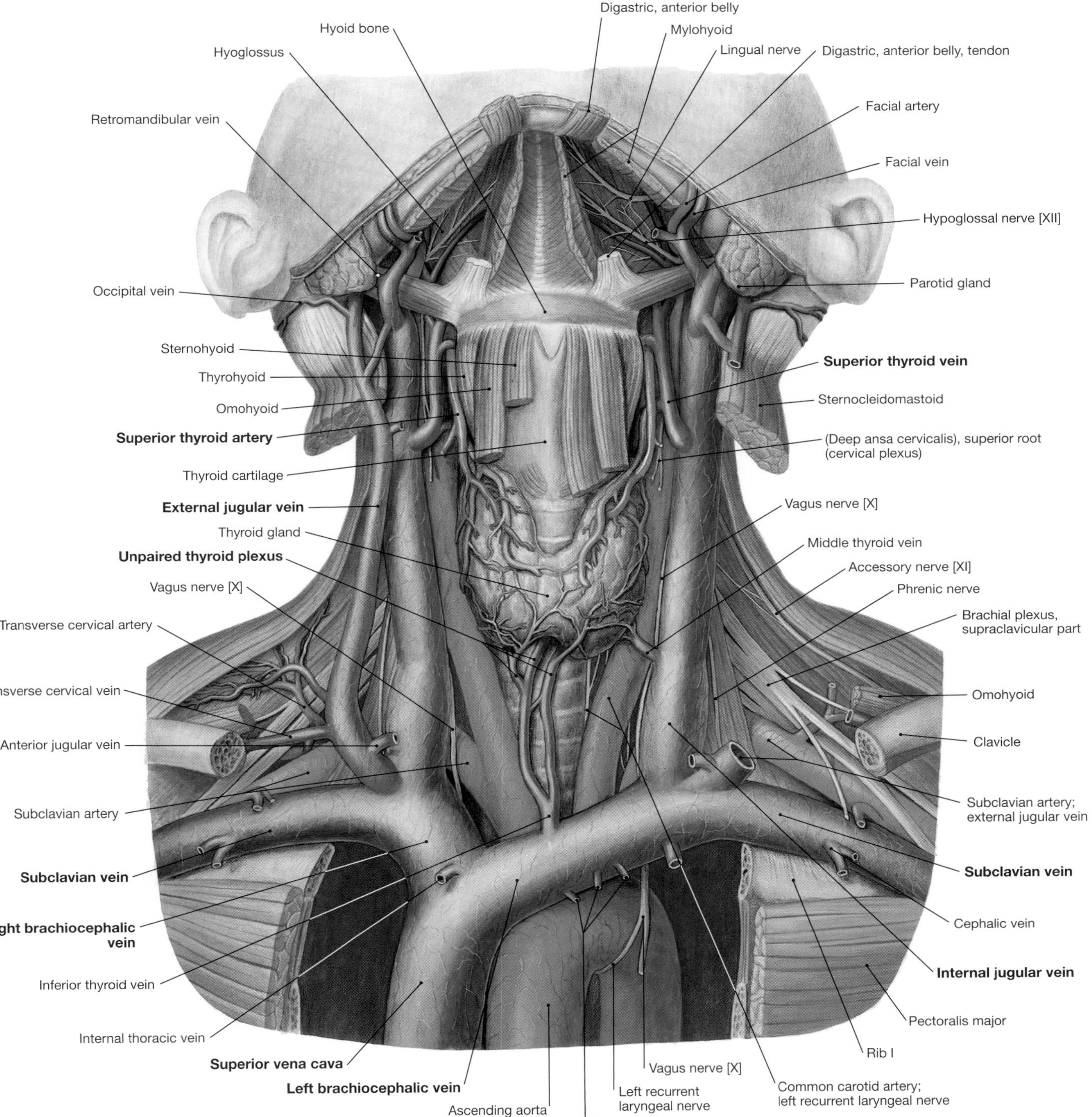
Digastric, anterior belly
Hyoid bone
Mylohyoid
Hyoglossus
Lingual nerve
Digastric, anterior belly, tendon
Retromandibular vein
Facial artery
Facial vein
Hypoglossal nerve [XII]
Occipital vein
Parotid gland
Sternohyoid
Superior thyroid vein
Thyrohyoid
Omohyoid
Sternocleidomastoid
Superior thyroid artery
(Deep ansa cervicalis), superior root (cervical plexus)
Thyroid cartilage
External jugular vein
Vagus nerve [X]
Thyroid gland
Middle thyroid vein
Unpaired thyroid plexus
Accessory nerve [XI]
Vagus nerve [X]
Phrenic nerve
Transverse cervical artery
Brachial plexus, supraclavicular part
Transverse cervical vein
Omohyoid
Anterior jugular vein
Clavicle
Subclavian artery
Subclavian artery; external jugular vein
Subclavian vein
Subclavian vein
Right brachiocephalic vein
Cephalic vein
Inferior thyroid vein
Internal jugular vein
Pectoralis major
Internal thoracic vein
Rib I
Superior vena cava
Vagus nerve [X]
Left brachiocephalic vein
Left recurrent laryngeal nerve
Common carotid artery; left recurrent laryngeal nerve
Ascending aorta
Thymic veins

**Fig. 11.74 Vessels and nerves of the neck and the upper thoracic aperture;** ventral view. The sternum, parts of the clavicle, sternocleidomastoid, and parts of the infrahyoid muscles were removed. Presentation of the venous tributary of the **superior vena cava** (brachiocephalic, internal jugular, external jugular, and subclavian veins) with particular emphasis on the venous drainage of the thyroid gland (→ Fig. 11.55). Also visible are the brachial plexus as well as the subclavian artery and vein running between the clavicle and rib I, the course of the phrenic nerve across the scalenus anterior, and the left recurrent laryngeal nerve curving around the aortic arch.

### Clinical Remarks

The term **PANCOAST's tumor** (apical sulcus tumor) describes a rapidly growing peripheral bronchial carcinoma at the apex of lung (→ Fig. 11.79) which quickly expands onto the ribs, soft tissues of the neck, brachial plexus, and vertebrae. Other structures affected may involve the phrenic nerve, the recurrent laryngeal nerve, the subclavian artery and vein, and the stellate ganglion (with HORNER's syndrome: enophthalmus, miosis, ptosis [drooping of upper eyelid]).

## Lymph vessels and lymph nodes of the neck

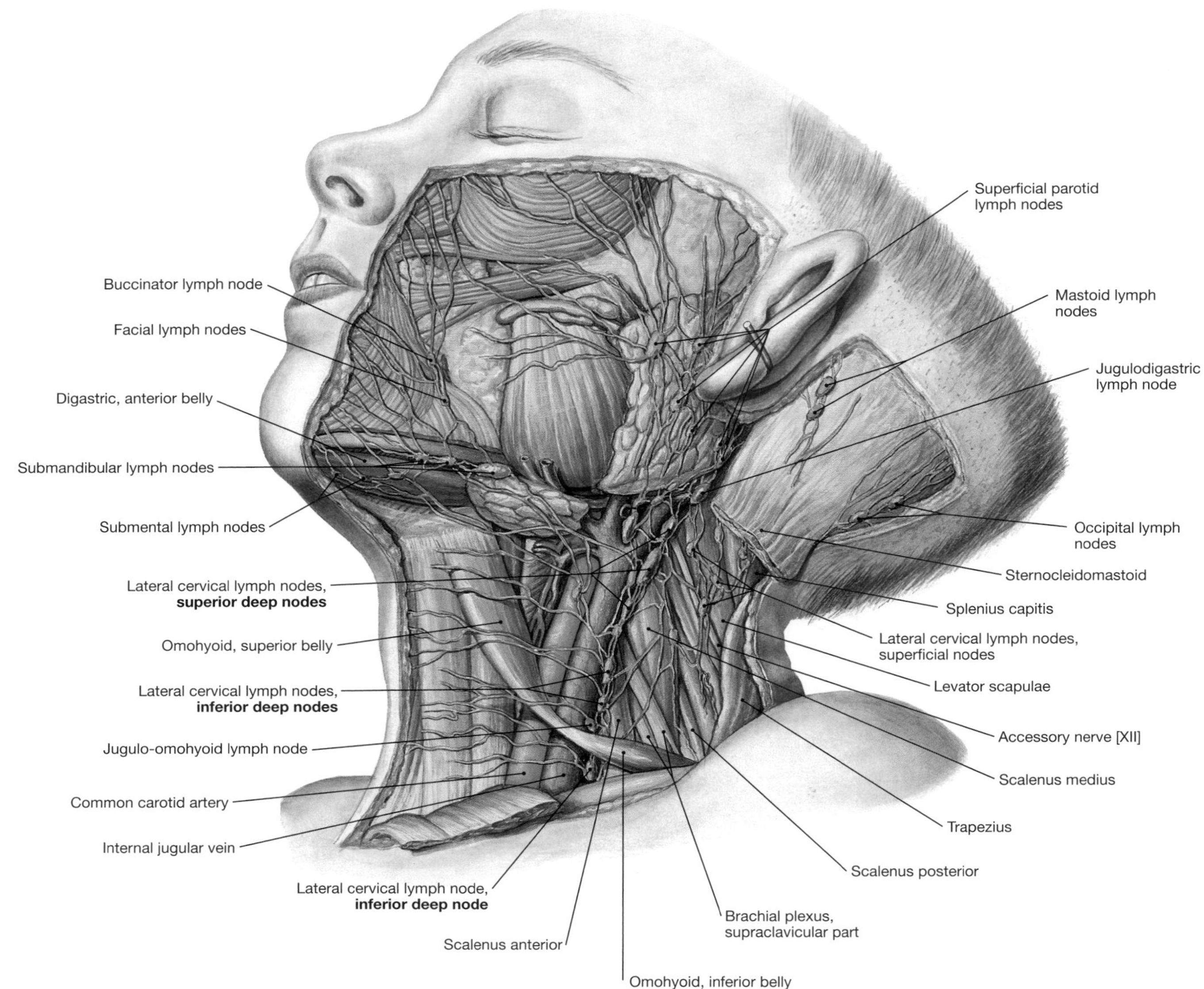
Superficial parotid lymph nodes
Buccinator lymph node
Mastoid lymph nodes
Facial lymph nodes
Jugulodigastric lymph node
Digastric, anterior belly
Submandibular lymph nodes
Submental lymph nodes
Occipital lymph nodes
Sternocleidomastoid
Lateral cervical lymph nodes, **superior deep nodes**
Splenius capitis
Lateral cervical lymph nodes, superficial nodes
Omohyoid, superior belly
Levator scapulae
Lateral cervical lymph nodes, **inferior deep nodes**
Accessory nerve [XII]
Jugulo-omohyoid lymph node
Scalenus medius
Common carotid artery
Trapezius
Internal jugular vein
Scalenus posterior
Lateral cervical lymph node, **inferior deep node**
Brachial plexus, supraclavicular part
Scalenus anterior
Omohyoid, inferior belly

**Fig. 11.75 Superficial lymph vessels and lymph nodes of the head and neck of a child.**
The neck region contains 200 to 300 lymph nodes. The majority thereof assemble in groups along the neurovascular bundle (→ table, → Fig. 8.85).

Lymphatic fluid of the right side of the head and neck drains into the **right lymphatic duct** (→ Fig. 8.86), whereas the left side of the head and neck drains into the **thoracic duct.** For entry of the thoracic duct into the left venous angle → Fig. 11.81.

| Lymph Nodes of the Neck | |
|---|---|
| **Anterior cervical lymph nodes** | **Lateral cervical lymph nodes** |
| • Superficial lymph nodes | • Superficial lymph nodes |
| • Deep lymph nodes<br>– Infrahyoid lymph nodes<br>– Prelaryngeal lymph nodes<br>– Thyroid lymph nodes<br>– Pretracheal lymph nodes<br>– Paratracheal lymph nodes<br>– Retropharyngeal lymph nodes | • Superior deep lymph nodes<br>– Jugulodigastric lymph nodes<br>– Lateral lymph nodes<br>– Anterior lymph nodes |
| | • Inferior deep lymph nodes<br>– Jugulo-omohyoid lymph nodes<br>– Lateral lymph nodes<br>– Anterior lymph nodes |
| | • Supraclavicular lymph nodes |
| | • Accessory lymph nodes<br>– Retropharyngeal lymph nodes |

## Lymph vessels and lymph nodes of the neck

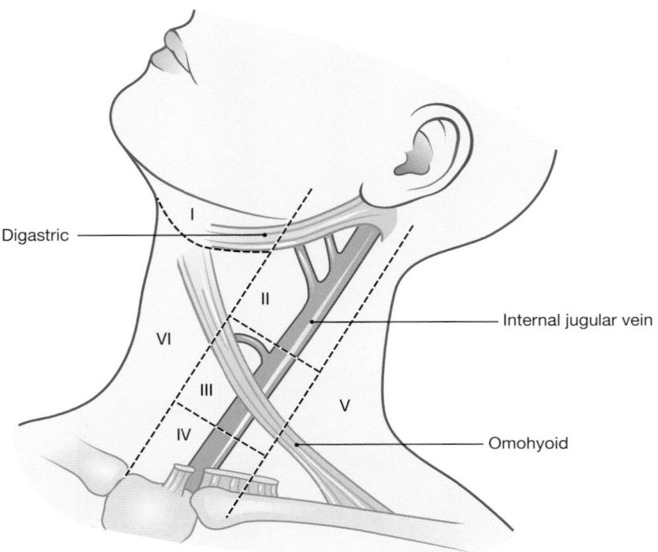
Digastric
I
II
VI
III
IV
V
Internal jugular vein
Omohyoid

**Fig. 11.76 Classification of drainage regions of the head and neck into compartments;** according to the classification of the American Joint Committee of Cancer (AJCC).

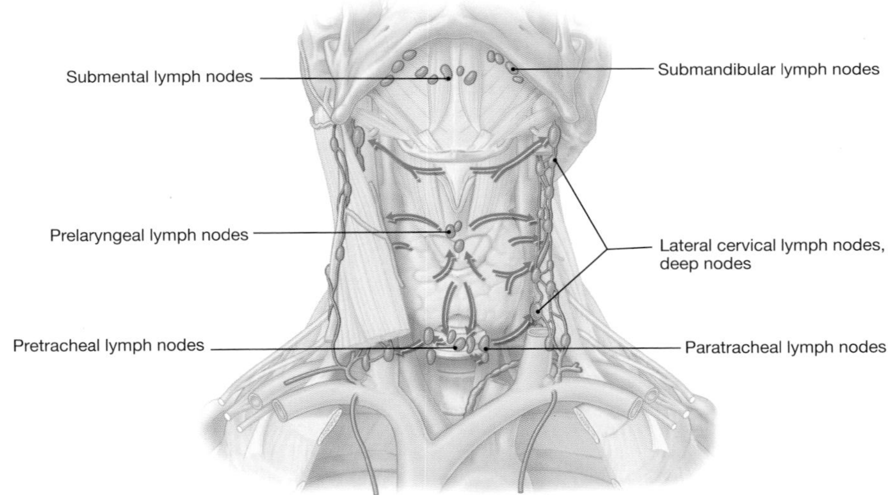
Submental lymph nodes
Submandibular lymph nodes
Prelaryngeal lymph nodes
Lateral cervical lymph nodes, deep nodes
Pretracheal lymph nodes
Paratracheal lymph nodes

**Fig. 11.77 Lymph vessels and lymph nodes of the larynx, thyroid gland, and trachea;** ventral view. [10]
All three organs drain into the deep lymph nodes of the neck.

### Clinical Remarks

According to the classification of the American Joint Committee of Cancer (AJCC), **lymph node metastases** of the neck are divided into six zones (**compartments I–VI;** → Fig. 11.76). These compartments serve as reference zones for the elective surgical removal of metastases in lymph nodes due to the lymphogenic spread of malignant tumors of the head and neck region (neck dissection). Injuries to the thoracic duct during surgical interventions in the neck region can lead to the development of a **chylous fistula.**

## Vessels and nerves of the submandibular triangle

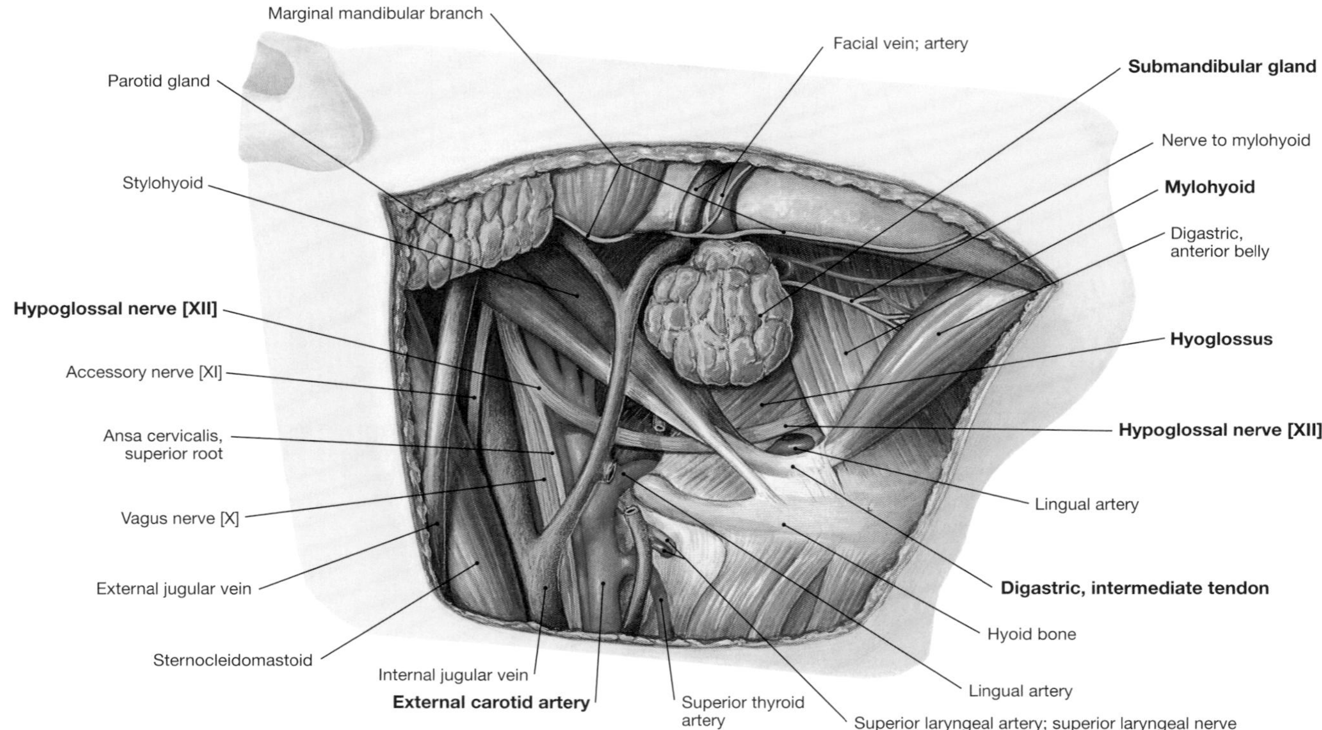
Marginal mandibular branch
Facial vein; artery
Submandibular gland
Parotid gland
Nerve to mylohyoid
Stylohyoid
Mylohyoid
Digastric, anterior belly
Hypoglossal nerve [XII]
Hyoglossus
Accessory nerve [XI]
Ansa cervicalis, superior root
Hypoglossal nerve [XII]
Lingual artery
Vagus nerve [X]
External jugular vein
Digastric, intermediate tendon
Hyoid bone
Sternocleidomastoid
Internal jugular vein
External carotid artery
Superior thyroid artery
Lingual artery
Superior laryngeal artery; superior laryngeal nerve

**Fig. 11.78 Vessels and nerves of the submandibular triangle;** inferolateral view.
Upon dissection of the submandibular gland and the neurovascular bundle as well as after the removal of the fascial layers, the **hypoglossal nerve** [XII] becomes visible. This cranial nerve separates from the neurovascular bundle in the parapharyngeal space, crosses the external carotid artery and passes between the hyoglossus and the intermediate tendon of the digastric until it disappears beneath the mylohyoid.

## Clinical Remarks

Inflammations in the region of the lower premolars and molars can lead to an **abscess formation in the fascial compartment of the submandibular gland** and the sublingual compartment. Abscesses from the wisdom teeth can even reach the fascial compartment of the retromandibular fossa and descend from here along the fascia of the neck into the mediastinum to cause a life-threatening infection.

**Injury to the hypoglossal nerve [XII],** e.g. as a result of a tumor infiltration into a cervical lymph node (metastasis), is easily diagnosed: when stretched out, the tongue deviates to the side with impaired nerve function, since the muscle force generated on the healthy side of the tongue exceeds that of the affected side.

## Vessels and nerves of the neck and upper thoracic aperture

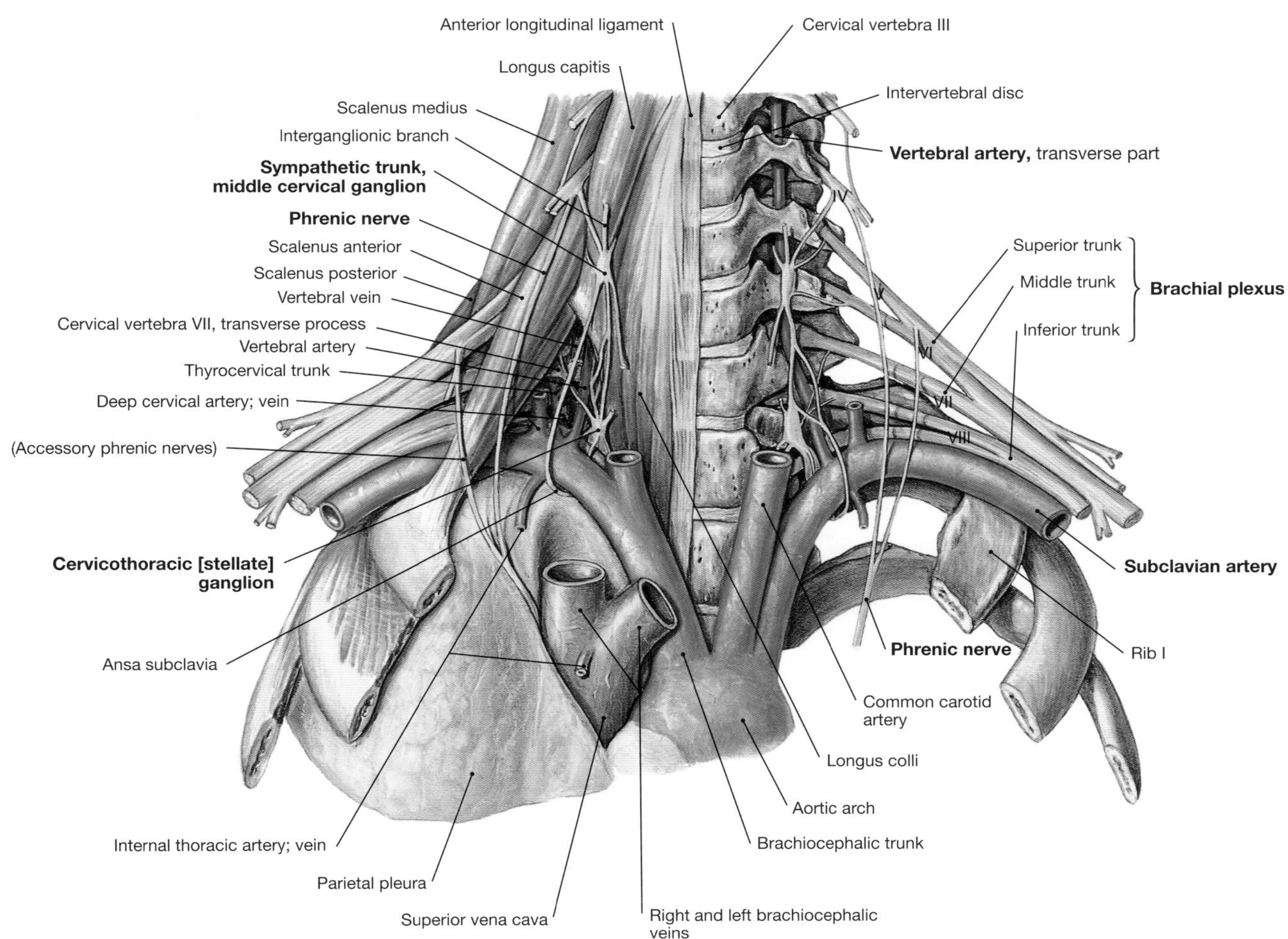
Anterior longitudinal ligament
Cervical vertebra III
Longus capitis
Intervertebral disc
Scalenus medius
Interganglionic branch
Vertebral artery, transverse part
Sympathetic trunk, middle cervical ganglion
Phrenic nerve
Superior trunk
Scalenus anterior
Middle trunk
Brachial plexus
Scalenus posterior
Vertebral vein
Cervical vertebra VII, transverse process
Inferior trunk
Vertebral artery
Thyrocervical trunk
Deep cervical artery; vein
(Accessory phrenic nerves)
Subclavian artery
Cervicothoracic [stellate] ganglion
Ansa subclavia
Phrenic nerve
Rib I
Common carotid artery
Longus colli
Aortic arch
Internal thoracic artery; vein
Brachiocephalic trunk
Parietal pleura
Superior vena cava
Right and left brachiocephalic veins

**Fig. 11.79 Vessels and nerves in the transition zone from the neck to the thorax and to the upper extremity.**
Visible are the pleural cupula, the scalene hiatus, the middle cervical ganglion (on top of the longus colli) and the inferior cervical ganglion (cervicothoracic/stellate; on top of the head of rib I) of the sympathetic trunk, the course of the phrenic nerve, the course of the vertebral artery, trunks of the brachial plexus and the subclavian artery.

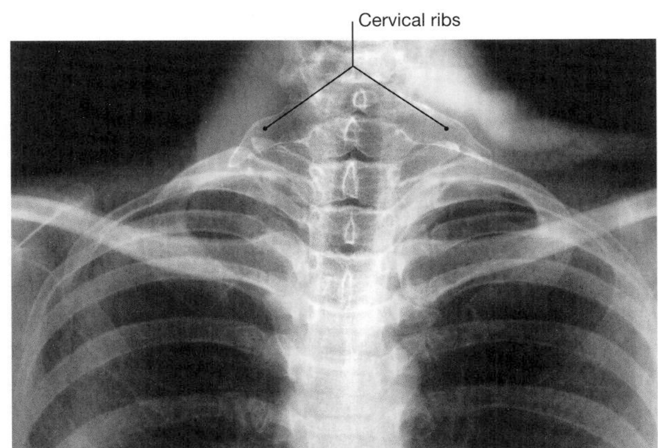
Cervical ribs

**Fig. 11.80 Neck;** radiograph in anteroposterior (AP) beam projection. [8]
Bilateral cervical ribs are visible.

## Clinical Remarks

Anatomic variations in the region of the scalene hiatus (cervical rib [cervical rib syndrome], narrow scalene hiatus, accessory scalenus minimus, or aberrant muscular fibers [collectively called scalenus anticus syndrome], or narrowing of the space between rib I and clavicle [costoclavicular syndrome]) are the cause for the **thoracic outlet syndrome (TOS).** TOS can result in the compression of the brachial plexus and the subclavian artery.
The scalene hiatus is also the site for the administration of an **interscalene brachial plexus block.**

## Pleural cupula and entry of the thoracic duct

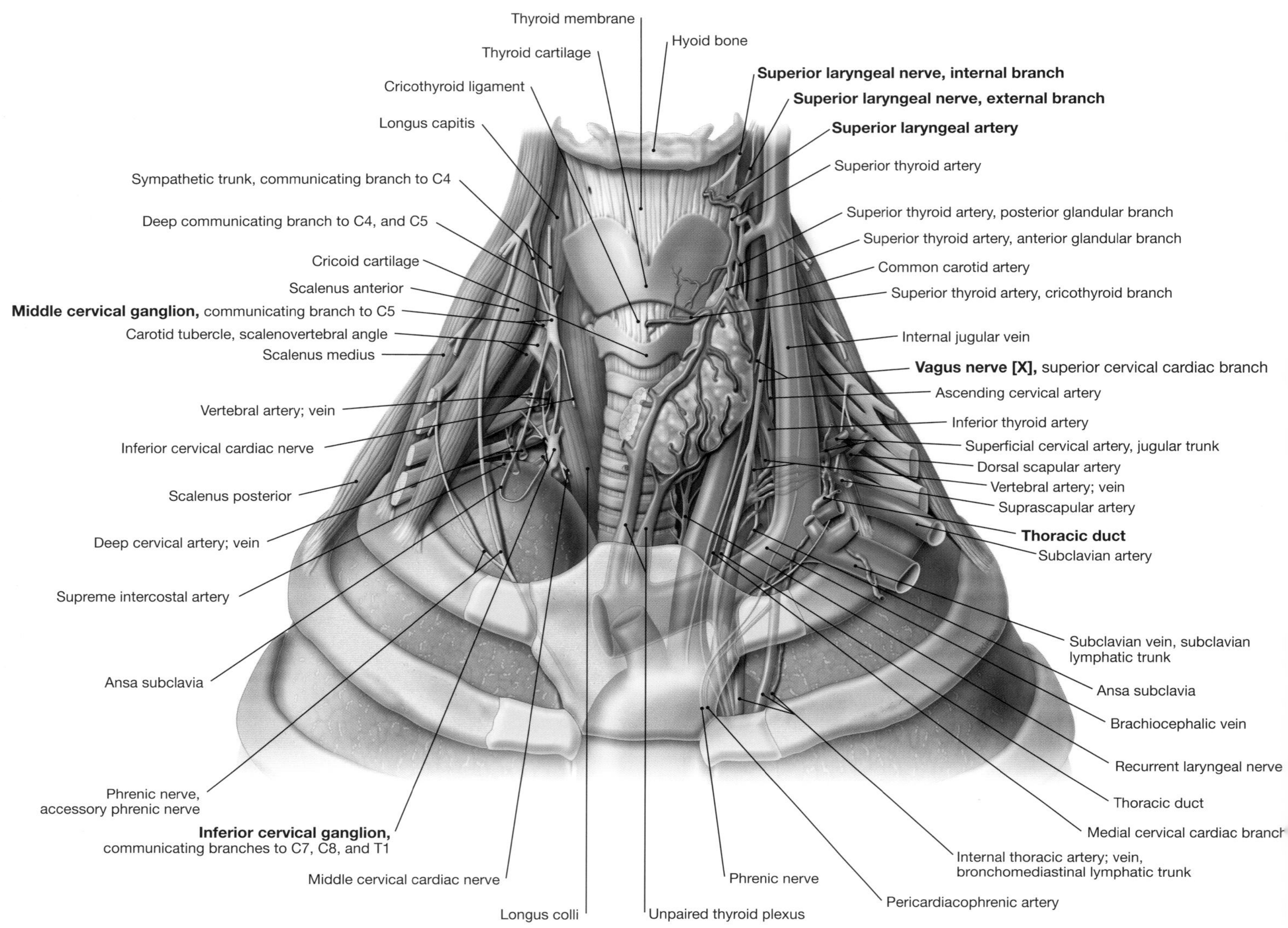
Thyroid membrane
Thyroid cartilage
Hyoid bone
Cricothyroid ligament
Superior laryngeal nerve, internal branch
Superior laryngeal nerve, external branch
Longus capitis
Superior laryngeal artery
Superior thyroid artery
Sympathetic trunk, communicating branch to C4
Deep communicating branch to C4, and C5
Superior thyroid artery, posterior glandular branch
Superior thyroid artery, anterior glandular branch
Cricoid cartilage
Common carotid artery
Scalenus anterior
Superior thyroid artery, cricothyroid branch
Middle cervical ganglion, communicating branch to C5
Carotid tubercle, scalenovertebral angle
Internal jugular vein
Scalenus medius
Vagus nerve [X], superior cervical cardiac branch
Ascending cervical artery
Vertebral artery; vein
Inferior thyroid artery
Inferior cervical cardiac nerve
Superficial cervical artery, jugular trunk
Dorsal scapular artery
Scalenus posterior
Vertebral artery; vein
Suprascapular artery
Deep cervical artery; vein
Thoracic duct
Subclavian artery
Supreme intercostal artery
Subclavian vein, subclavian lymphatic trunk
Ansa subclavia
Ansa subclavia
Brachiocephalic vein
Recurrent laryngeal nerve
Phrenic nerve, accessory phrenic nerve
Thoracic duct
Inferior cervical ganglion, communicating branches to C7, C8, and T1
Medial cervical cardiac branch
Internal thoracic artery; vein, bronchomediastinal lymphatic trunk
Middle cervical cardiac nerve
Phrenic nerve
Pericardiacophrenic artery
Longus colli
Unpaired thyroid plexus

**Fig. 11.81 Prevertebral and paravertebral structures of the neck and the upper thoracic aperture;** ventral view.
On the right side of the body, the great blood vessels were removed to permit an unobstructed view onto the pleural cupula and the sympathetic trunk. The **inferior cervical ganglion** (cervicothoracic [stellate] ganglion) rests on the head of rib I and the **middle cervical ganglion** lies on top of the longus colli. The pleural cupula extends beyond the upper thoracic aperture. On the left side, the great blood vessels and the left thyroid lobe were left in place. Visible are the blood supply to the thyroid gland, the internal branch of the superior laryngeal nerve and the superior laryngeal vessels, the entry of the thoracic duct into the left venous angle as well as the course of the vagus nerve [X] between the common carotid artery and the internal jugular vein.

# Brain and Spinal Cord



12

# The Central Nervous System – Pressing Constriction and Open Expanse

Commonly the term "central" refers to those parts of the nervous system, the brain (encephalon) and spinal cord, which are located within the cranial cavity and in the vertebral canal, respectively. The locations where cranial and spinal nerves (12 cranial nerves, 31 spinal nerves) enter and exit the central nervous system (CNS) mark the border between the CNS and the peripheral nervous system (PNS). Distal to this border in the PNS, nerve fibers are coated with an insulating sheath formed by SCHWANN's cells; in the CNS this insulating layer is provided by oligodendrocytes.

## The Maters

Three membranes, known as meninges, completely surround the brain and spinal cord. Directly beneath the outer, tough, parchment-like membrane, the dura mater ("tough mother"), lies a softer membrane, the arachnoid mater ("spider-like mother"), from which fine and cobwebbed fibers emerge to the surface of the CNS. The narrow space between the arachnoid mater and pia mater – the subarachnoid space – is filled with cerebrospinal fluid (CSF), in which the CNS floats. Directly on the surface of the CNS lies the very delicate pia mater ("tender mother"), which serves as an attachment site for the fibers of the arachnoid mater.

## Brain ...

The skull is a space of pressing constriction: the brain fills the cranial cavity almost completely, only in a few areas (especially in the area of the occipital foramen, foramen magnum), the subarachnoid space extends beyond a few millimetres. The brain of an adult weighs on average 1300 grams. In the dissection laboratory – that is in its fixed state – the brain has a rubber-like consistency. In the natural unfixed state, its consistency is more that of a soft pudding. This consistency is due to its high moisture content: The brain consists of 85% water, whereas the rest of the body only contains about 65% water.

The embryonic brain comprises five parts and consists of five successively arranged hollow cysts. In the adult brain, only three parts are still recognizable. The brain is hollow inside. The inner cavities are called ventricles and contain cerebrospinal fluid. The largest of the three brain parts is the **cerebrum,** which takes up almost the entire interior of the skull with the exception of the area above the foramen magnum. The cerebrum consists of a right and a left hemisphere. The surface of these hemispheres is enlarged by coarse gyri and is called the cerebral cortex. Likewise, the **cerebellum** consists of two hemispheres and lies in the "postero-inferior" region of the skull, above of and bilateral to the foramen magnum. Its surfaces also contain folds which are much finer and more regular. These leaf-resembling folds are called folia of cerebellum, encompassing the cerebellar cortex, the cerebellum's own cortex. The unpaired **brainstem** is about as thick as a thumb, located at the cranial base and extends through the foramen magnum into the spinal cord. Extensive peduncles connect the brainstem to the cerebrum and cerebellum. Ten out of twelve cranial nerves emerge from the brainstem. In contrast to the cerebrum and cerebellum, its surface appears white, because it is mainly composed of nerve fibers (white matter), whereas the gray cortices mainly consist of cell bodies (gray matter).

## ... and Spinal Cord

The spinal cord has a white surface and resides in a spacious spinal canal. The spinal cord is about as thick as a pencil; however, the inner diameter of the vertebral canal almost reaches the width of a thumb. More caudally towards the sacral bone the vertebral canal becomes narrower; in this lower region, it does not contain any spinal cord, but rather roots of lumbar and sacral spinal nerves, each exiting the spinal canal "much lower" through their respective intervertebral foramina. The subarachnoid space is relatively wide, and a space filled with abundant adipose tissue and veins remains in between the dura mater and the bony wall of the vertebral canal. Encompassing the spinal cord, the dural sac extends downwards to the coccyx. However, the caudal tip of the spinal cord concludes at the level of the second lumbar vertebra.

The **diameter of the spinal cord** varies. Compared to the segments that innervate the less muscular trunk, the cervical spinal cord is thicker at the site of the motor neurons responsible for the innervation of the arm muscles. The caudal part of the spinal cord providing innervation to the lower extremities again shows an increased diameter. These two enlarged regions are termed cervical enlargement and lumbosacral enlargement.

The **radicular filaments** of the dorsal sensory roots of the spinal nerves enter the spinal cord bilaterally along two longitudinal lines at its dorsal surface. On its ventral surface, the radicular filaments of the ventral motor roots exit in a similar manner. Five to ten radicular filaments bundle to form the dorsal (posterior) and ventral (anterior) roots; in the intervertebral foramen, anterior and posterior roots merge to form the spinal nerve, which passes through the intervertebral foramen and exits both the vertebral column and the dural sac.

## Caveat!

"Beware!" applies to the CNS and especially to the brain. The above summary is about the surface of the organ and – deliberately – superficial in a contextual sense. Internally, no other organ is as complex as the brain: If one has seen and understood a small part of the liver, one comprehends the entire liver. However, if one has seen a part of the brain, one cannot draw conclusions about the other parts, as no two cells are identical (although they can be classified). Only a synoptic approach, involving the anatomy, physiology, and psychology/psychiatry, lets one appreciate the brain's complexity.
It should be noted also that the relationship of the brain to its products, the thoughts, is still a mystery. This mystery and the complexity of the brain are often exploited as an excuse to indulge in superlatives, to speak of "the miracles" of the brain, to unite human and brain, and to emphasize uniqueness by saying: "Look, this and only this is YOU!"
Sometimes, establishing an essentially sarcastic distance to this "miraculous organ" as well as to one's own thoughts is helpful. For example, with the (slightly altered) words of the physiologist Carl Vogt (1817–1895), a notorious scoffer: "The brain treats the thought as the liver the bile and the kidney the urine: it discharges its products".

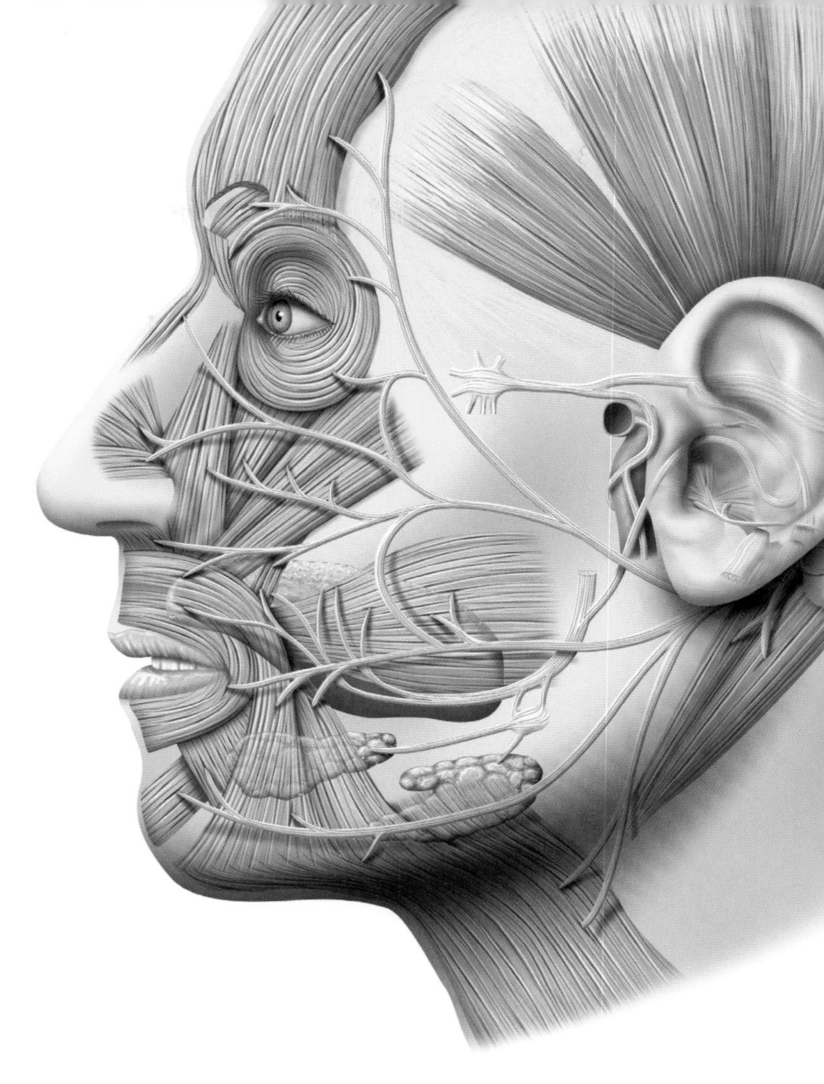

## Clinical Remarks

Comprising about 15% of all fatalities, **stroke** is the third most frequent cause of death in Western industrialized countries, only surpassed by myocardial infarction (MI) and malignant tumors as the first and second most frequent causes of death. Ischemic strokes form the largest group (85%). Strokes are the most frequent cause of acquired disability in adults resulting in need of care. There are 182 stroke cases per 100,000 in the population. Annually, 150,000 new cases of stroke and 15,000 recurrences occur. The major neurological diseases of the elderly are ALZHEIMER's disease (progressive impairment of cognitive functions), PARKINSON's disease, and cerebral microangiopathy (BINSWANGER's disease).

**ALZHEIMER's disease** is a neurodegenerative disease. In its most frequent form, it affects elderly people over 65 years of age and comprises approximately 60% of the about 24 million cognitively impaired (dementia) patients worldwide.

**PARKINSON's disease** is a degenerative disease affecting the extrapyramidal motor system. Typical symptoms include slowness of movement (bradykinesia), increased muscle tonus (rigidity), resting tremor, as well as various sensory, autonomic, psychological, and cognitive impairments. Currently, some 10 million people are estimated to suffer from PARKINSON's disease worldwide.

**BINSWANGER's disease** is the most frequent cause of vascular dementia. This is the result of a subcortical arteriosclerotic encephalopathy with arterial hypertension and subsequent microangiopathy. An incidence of more than 3% in the advanced age group can be estimated.

These three age-related diseases commonly share many symptoms. Patients with PARKINSON's disease often suffer from dementia, and many patients with BINSWANGER's disease display the same impairment in movement as patients with PARKINSON's disease. Patients with stroke are predisposed to develop ALZHEIMER's disease; PARKINSON's disease increases the risk of stroke. No causal treatment is available for these three neurodegenerative diseases and the damage to the brain is irreparable.

***→ Dissection Link***

Upon removal of the brain from the skull, the blood vessels and cranial nerves in the region of the cranial base and at the base of the brain as well as the removed brain itself are inspected. For visualization of the superficial cerebral veins, the arachnoid mater is removed from the brain. The cerebral arterial circle with adjacent vessels is dissected next. The cerebral arterial circle is detached at the branching points of the blood vessels, glued to a sheet of paper and labelled. For the dissection of the ventricles, remnants of the leptomeninx (arachnoid mater and pia mater) are removed, and the remaining blood vessels are traced, studied and removed. With the brain knife, a horizontal cut above the corpus callosum is now being conducted and the lateral ventricles are opened from cranial. Severing the two crura of fornix and deflecting of the fornix opens the third ventricle. In the following step, the dissection of the inferior (temporal) horn of the lateral ventricle, located in the temporal lobe, exposes the hippocampus formation. Thereafter, the cerebellum is inspected externally, dissected, the cerebellar nuclei are examined and the cerebellar peduncles are removed from the brainstem, exposing the fourth ventricle. The brainstem is severed; the midbrain (mesencephalon), pons, and spinal cord are sectioned in planes for examination. Frontal and horizontal sections through each of the brain hemispheres serve to study the basal ganglia. Finally, medial and lateral tracts (including the visualization of the insula, internal capsule, and optic tract) as well as the pyramidal tract, and the middle and upper cerebellar peduncles are examined. The spinal cord is best visualized on the preserved prosected demonstration specimen, where the spinal cord, the enlargements, the cauda equina surrounded by meninges and the outgoing spinal nerve pairs are visible in the opened vertebral canal.

## EXAM CHECK LIST

• Structure of the nervous system • superficial arterial and venous systems of the skull • meninges: subarachnoid space, types of bleeding injuries (epidural, subdural, subarachnoid bleedings), dura mater, course of the internal carotid artery, cavernous sinus, dural venous sinuses and arachnoid mater • development and structure of the CNS • telencephalon: cerebral cortex, hemispheres, gyri, sulci, cerebral cortical areas, fornix, hippocampus, basal ganglia, limbic system, clinical relevance • diencephalon: epithalamus (pineal gland, habenulae), thalamus and hypothalamus (pituitary gland) • cerebral trunk: mesencephalon, tectum, tectal (quadrigeminal) plate, tegmentum, reticular formation, red nucleus, substantia nigra, cerebral crura, ascending and descending pathways • pons: pontine nuclei, medulla oblongata, raphe nuclei and olivary nuclei • cerebellum: structure, cerebellar nuclei, cerebellar tracts and ataxia • tracts: association, commissural, projecting tracts, pyramidal tract with internal capsule and blood supply • ventricular system: ventricles and subarachnoid space, lateral ventricles, third ventricle, fourth ventricle, choroid plexus and hydrocephalus • circumventricular organs • blood supply: arterial circle, brain arteries and venous drainage • cranial nerves: olfactory bulb and olfactory nerve [I], projections, visual tract, nuclei of the brainstem, exit from the brainstem, cerebellopontine angle, course, fiber qualities and cranial nerve lesions • spinal cord: structure, enlargements, roots, cauda equina, spinal meninges, blood supply, segments, gray substance, white substance (anterior, lateral, and posterior funiculus), position of the tracts in cross-sections of the spinal cord, spinal cord injuries (hemisection and quadriplegia or paraplegia)

## Nervous system, overview

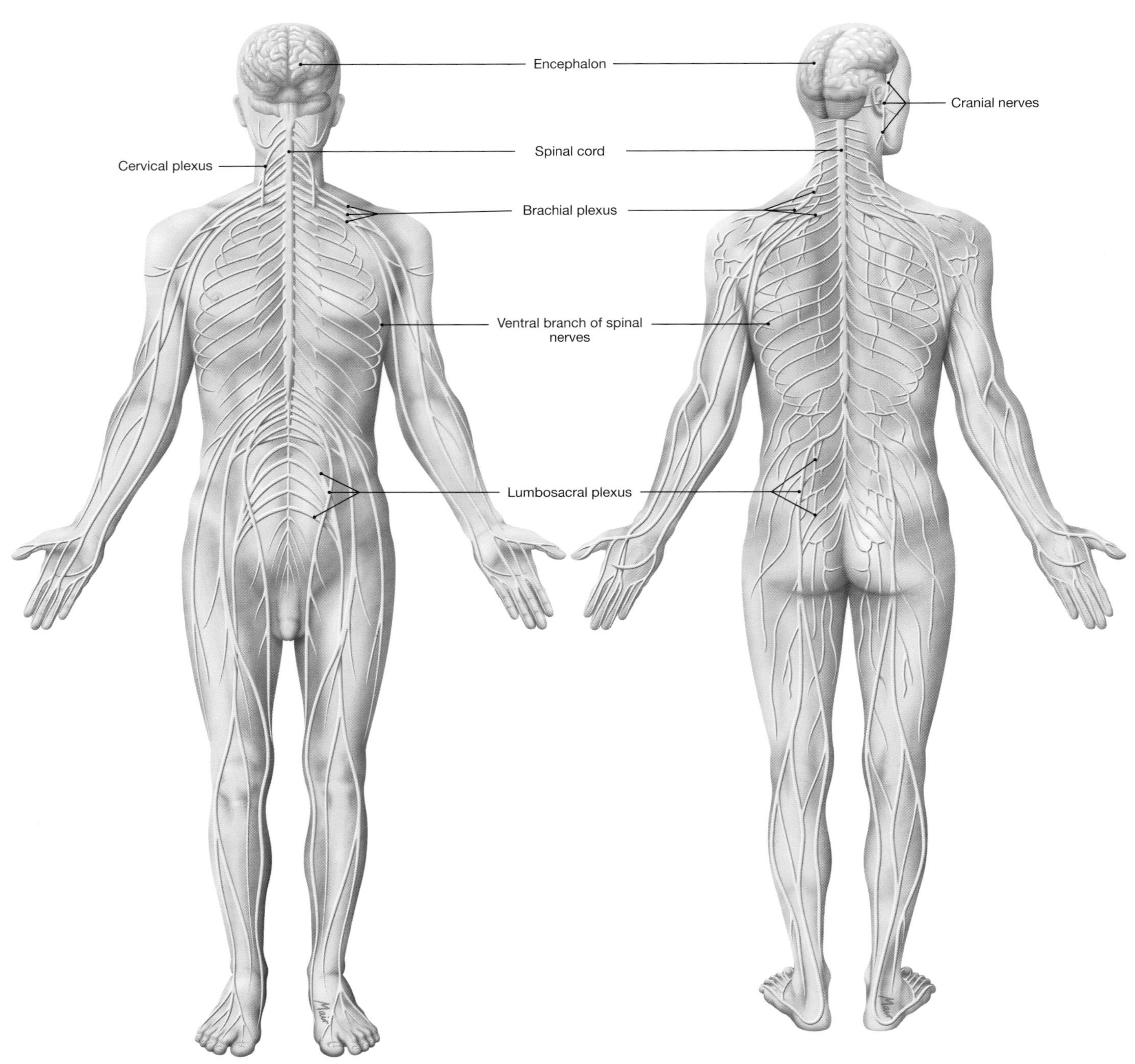
Encephalon
Cranial nerves
Spinal cord
Cervical plexus
Brachial plexus
Ventral branch of spinal nerves
Lumbosacral plexus

**Fig. 12.1 Structure of the nervous system;** ventral and dorsal views.

The nervous system is divided into a central (CNS) and a peripheral nervous system (PNS).

The brain and spinal cord constitute the **CNS** which regulates complex functions, including the storage of experiences (memory), the creation of imaginations (thoughts) and emotions. The CNS assists the whole body in adapting quickly to changes occurring in the environment and within the body. The **PNS** is mainly composed of spinal nerves (with connections to the spinal cord) and cranial nerves (with connections to the brain). Its function is to enable communication between the organs and the CNS, to control the activity of muscles and viscera, and to provide an essential link between the surrounding environment and the body interior.

Functionally, the nervous system is divided into an **autonomic** (vegetative visceral, control of visceral activity, mostly involuntary) and a **somatic** (animalic, innervation of skeletal muscles, voluntary perception of sensory input, communication with the surrounding environment) nervous system. Both systems are closely interlaced and interact with each other.

Besides the nervous system, the endocrine system also participates in the regulation of body functions.

## Directional and positional informations

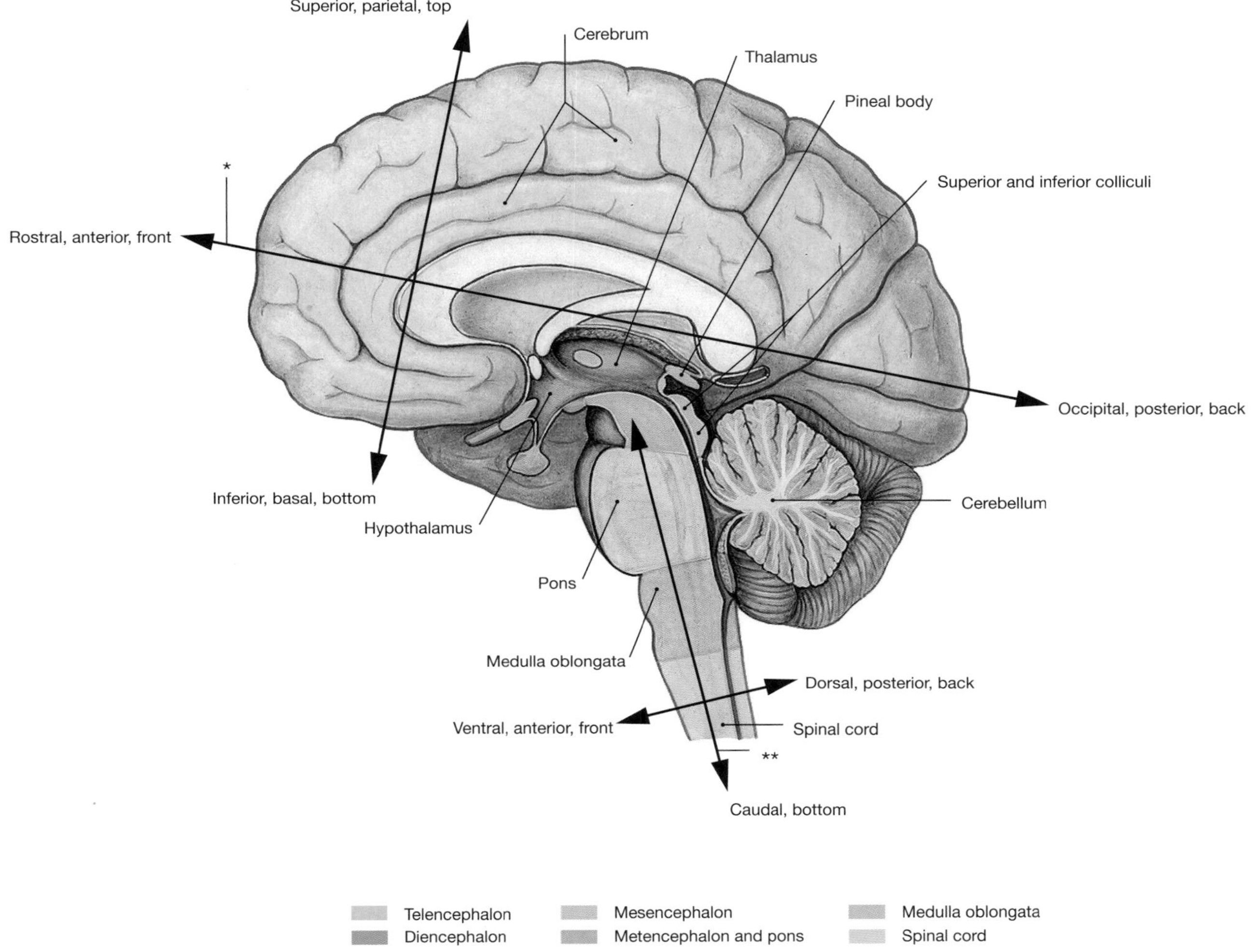
Superior, parietal, top
Cerebrum
Thalamus
Pineal body
Superior and inferior colliculi
*
Rostral, anterior, front
Occipital, posterior, back
Inferior, basal, bottom
Hypothalamus
Cerebellum
Pons
Medulla oblongata
Dorsal, posterior, back
Ventral, anterior, front
Spinal cord
**
Caudal, bottom
Telencephalon
Diencephalon
Mesencephalon
Metencephalon and pons
Medulla oblongata
Spinal cord

**Fig. 12.2 Directional and positional informations concerning the central nervous system (CNS and spinal cord);** median section.
During brain development, the neural tube bends and, thus, the longitudinal axis of the forebrain (prosencephalon = diencephalon and telencephalon) tilts forward. Consequently, a unique nomenclature was generated as is shown in the figure. For example, parts formerly positioned dorsally, e.g. the metencephalon, relocated to a parietal site, yet, their position is still referred to as dorsal.
The **FOREL's axis** (*) refers to the topographic axis between the telencephalon and diencephalon, while the axis projecting through the center of the brainstem is called **MEYNERT's axis** (**).

## Arteries of the head

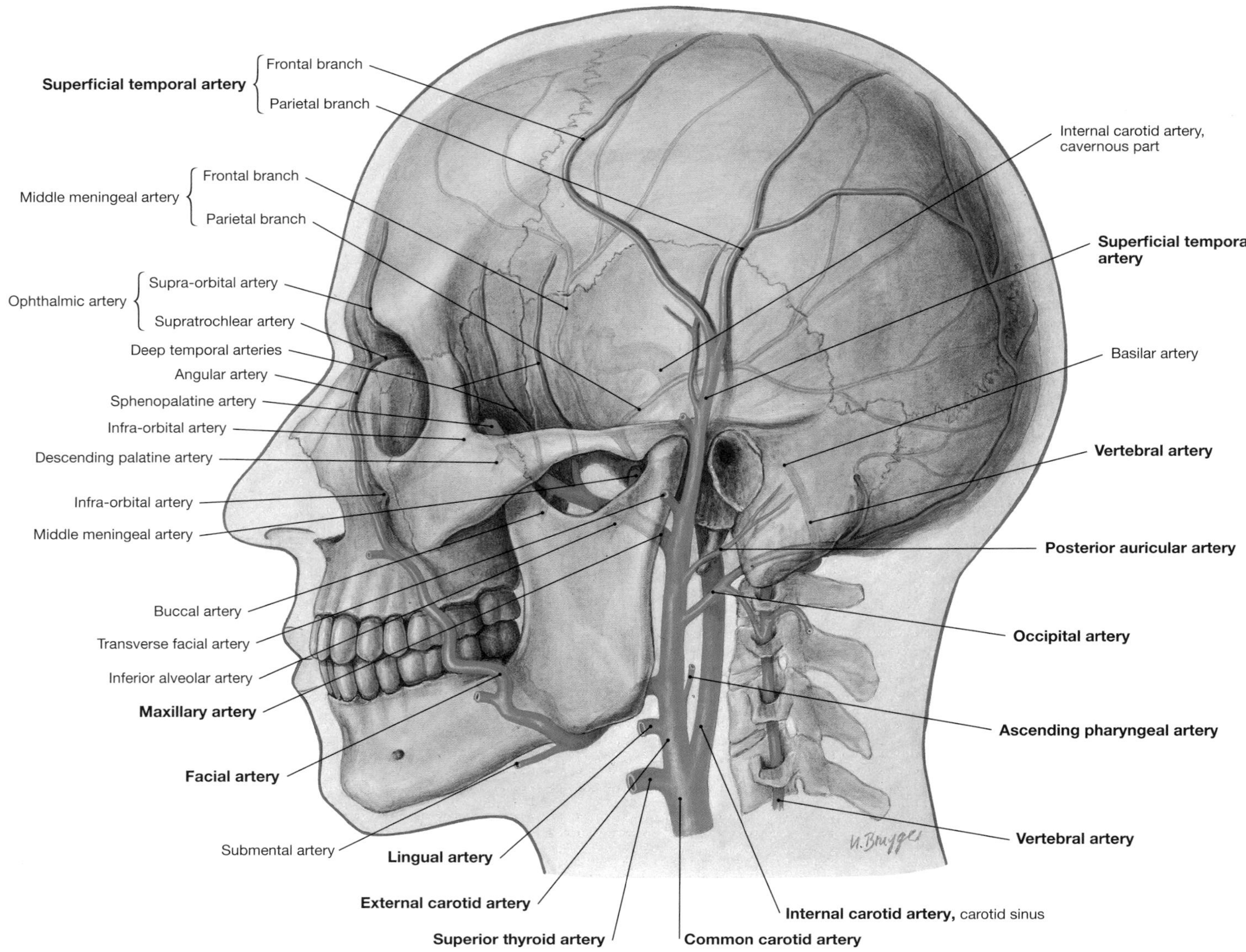
Superficial temporal artery
Frontal branch
Parietal branch
Middle meningeal artery
Frontal branch
Parietal branch
Ophthalmic artery
Supra-orbital artery
Supratrochlear artery
Deep temporal arteries
Angular artery
Sphenopalatine artery
Infra-orbital artery
Descending palatine artery
Infra-orbital artery
Middle meningeal artery
Buccal artery
Transverse facial artery
Inferior alveolar artery
Maxillary artery
Facial artery
Submental artery
Lingual artery
External carotid artery
Superior thyroid artery
Common carotid artery
Internal carotid artery, carotid sinus
Vertebral artery
Ascending pharyngeal artery
Occipital artery
Posterior auricular artery
Vertebral artery
Basilar artery
Superficial temporal artery
Internal carotid artery, cavernous part

**Fig. 12.3 External arteries of the head.**
The common carotid artery bifurcates into the external carotid artery and the internal carotid artery at the level of the fourth cervical vertebra. The **external carotid artery** provides the following arterial branches: superior thyroid, lingual, facial, ascending pharyngeal, occipital, posterior auricular, maxillary, and superficial temporal artery; the **internal carotid artery** ascends cranially without giving off any branches in its cervical part (→ Fig. 12.15), passes through the skull base into the cranial cavity, and primarily supplies blood to the brain.

## Clinical Remarks

Frequently, the carotid bifurcation is the site of **pathological alterations in vasculature** (extracranial arteriosclerosis: plaques, stenosis, and occlusion). Located within the carotid bifurcation is the carotid body (not shown in the figure, → Fig. 12.155). As a paraganglion, it contains chemoreceptors wich respond to changes of the pH, $O_2$, and $CO_2$ content of the blood.

The **carotid sinus syndrome** constitutes a hypersensitivity of the pressoreceptors located in the carotid sinus. Frequently, rotational movements of the head can trigger a reflex causing a sudden decrease in heart beat (vasovagal reflex). This can result in major circulatory complications and cardiac arrest.

## Arteries of the head

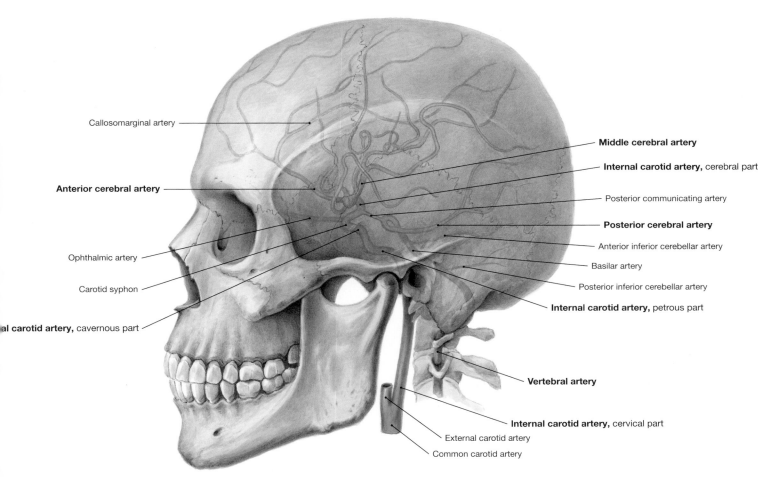


Callosomarginal artery
**Anterior cerebral artery**
Ophthalmic artery
Carotid syphon
**al carotid artery,** cavernous part
**Middle cerebral artery**
**Internal carotid artery,** cerebral part
Posterior communicating artery
**Posterior cerebral artery**
Anterior inferior cerebellar artery
Basilar artery
Posterior inferior cerebellar artery
**Internal carotid artery,** petrous part
**Vertebral artery**
**Internal carotid artery,** cervical part
External carotid artery
Common carotid artery


**Fig. 12.4 Internal arteries of the head.**
Four large arteries supply blood to the brain: the paired internal carotid arteries and the paired vertebral arteries. These four blood vessels feed into the **cerebral arterial circle** (**circle of WILLIS** → Fig. 12.95) located at the base of the brain, which creates an anastomosis between the internal carotid arteries and the vertebral arteries and releases paired branches of the anterior, middle, and posterior cerebral arteries.

The anastomosing blood vessels within the cerebral arterial circle (circle of WILLIS) often are so narrow that they will not permit a sufficient exchange of blood.
At normal intracranial pressure, the ipsilateral **internal carotid artery** and the **posterior cerebral artery** usually supply blood to each cerebral hemisphere. In about 10% of cases, both anterior cerebral arteries branch off the same internal carotid artery on one side. Also, in 10% of cases the posterior cerebral artery derives from the posterior communicating artery, which, in turn, branches off the internal carotid artery.

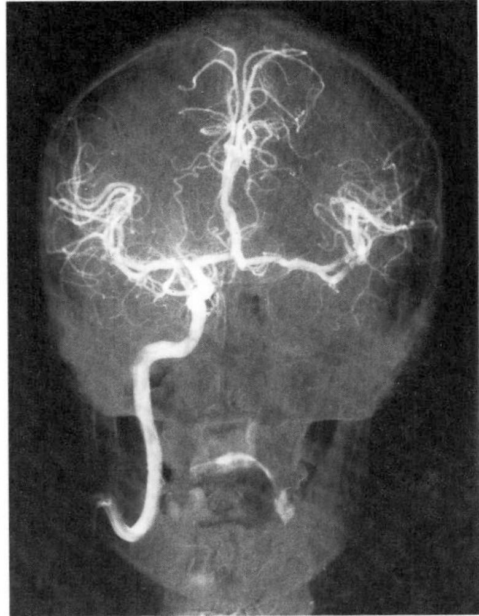
a

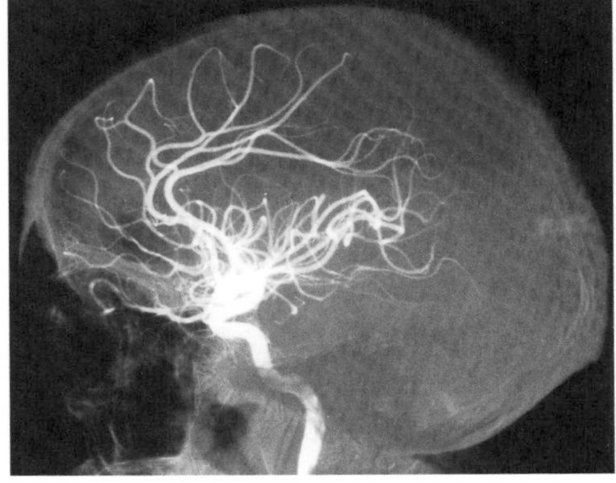
b

**Figs. 12.5a and b Internal carotid artery;** radiographs after unilateral injection of contrast medium (angiograms).
The contrast medium distributes to the vessels of the contralateral side via the cerebral arterial circle (circle of WILLIS).

**a** AP radiograph, digital subtraction angiography (DSA)
**b** Lateral radiograph, digital subtraction angiography (DSA)

## Veins of the head

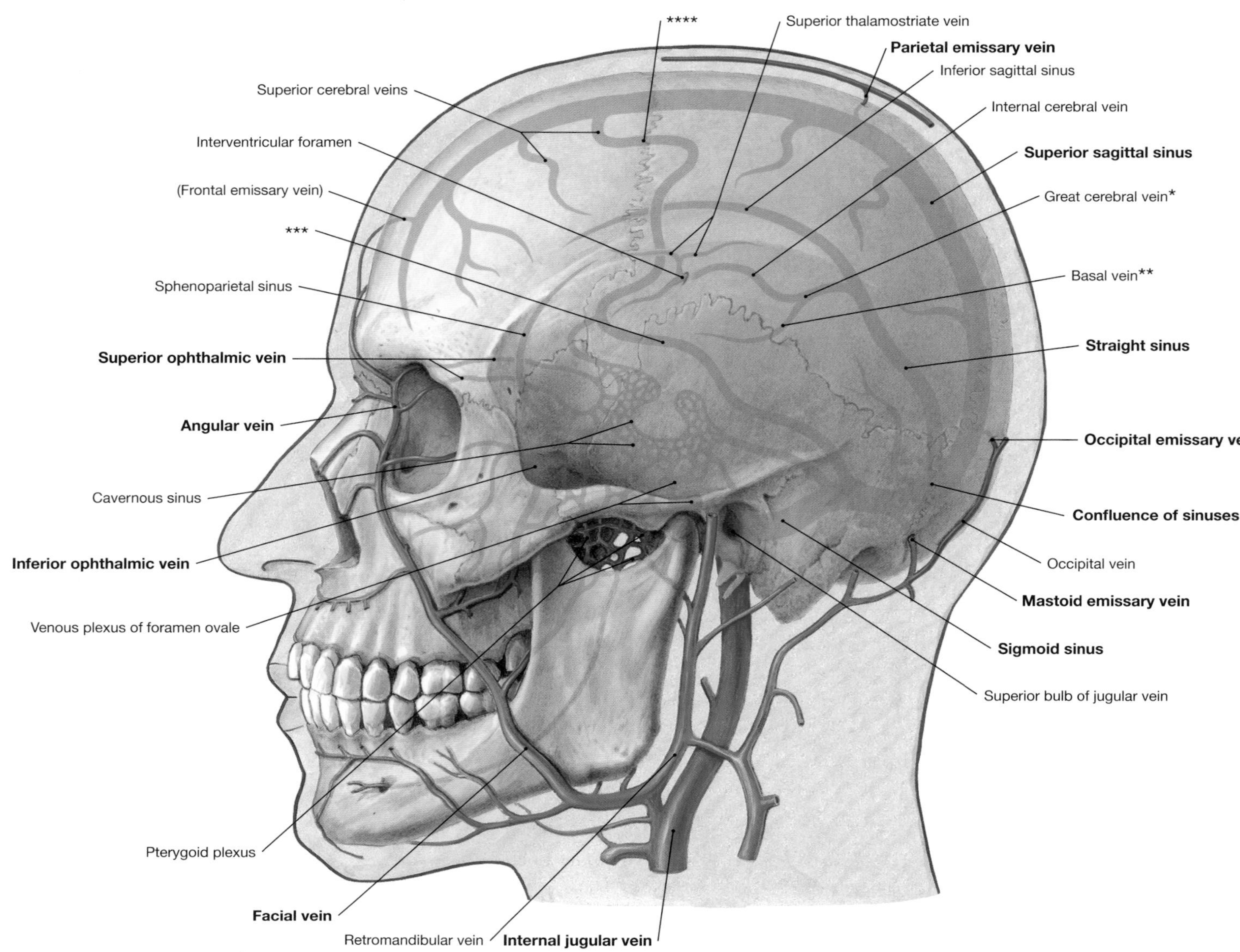
****
Superior thalamostriate vein
Parietal emissary vein
Inferior sagittal sinus
Superior cerebral veins
Internal cerebral vein
Interventricular foramen
Superior sagittal sinus
(Frontal emissary vein)
Great cerebral vein*
***
Sphenoparietal sinus
Basal vein**
Straight sinus
Superior ophthalmic vein
Angular vein
Occipital emissary ve
Cavernous sinus
Confluence of sinuses
Inferior ophthalmic vein
Occipital vein
Mastoid emissary vein
Venous plexus of foramen ovale
Sigmoid sinus
Superior bulb of jugular vein
Pterygoid plexus
Facial vein
Retromandibular vein
Internal jugular vein

**Fig. 12.6 Internal and external veins of the head.**
The internal and external veins of the head communicate via by numerous anastomoses. This includes the emissary veins, ophthalmic veins, and the venous plexus.

* vein of GALEN
** ROSENTHAL's vein
*** vein of LABBÉ
**** TROLARD's vein

## Clinical Remarks

Injuries to the scalp can result in the **spread of germs via the emissary veins** and the diploic veins of the diploë (→ Fig. 12.8) into the dural venous sinuses and the intracranial space.

**Emissary Veins – Passage Through the Skull**

| Emissary vein | Site of Passage |
|---|---|
| Parietal emissary vein | Parietal foramen |
| Mastoid emissary vein | Mastoid foramen |
| Occipital emissary vein | Passage in the region of the external occipital protuberence |
| Condylar emissary vein | Condylar canal |
| Venous plexus of hypoglossal canal | Hypoglossal canal |
| Venous plexus of foramen ovale | Foramen ovale |
| Internal carotid venous plexus | Carotid canal |

## Veins of the head

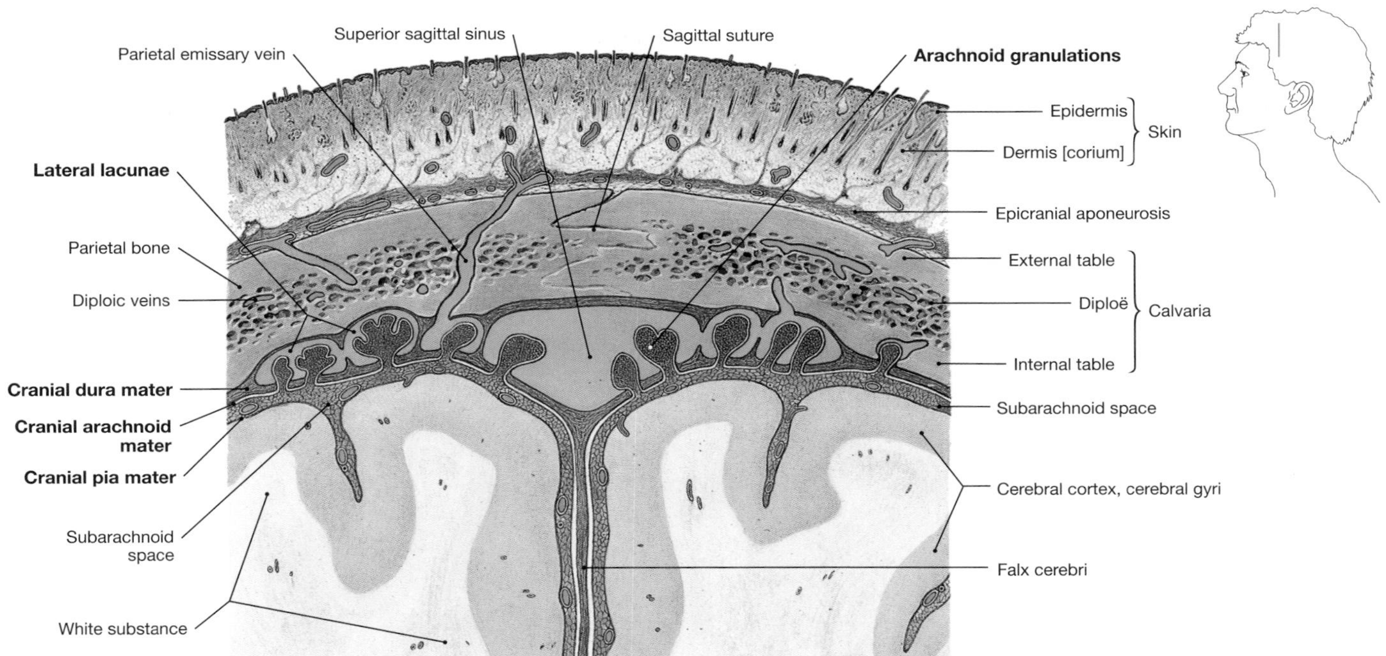

Superior sagittal sinus
Sagittal suture
Parietal emissary vein
Arachnoid granulations
Lateral lacunae
Epidermis
Dermis [corium]
Skin
Epicranial aponeurosis
Parietal bone
External table
Diploic veins
Diploë
Calvaria
Internal table
Cranial dura mater
Subarachnoid space
Cranial arachnoid mater
Cranial pia mater
Cerebral cortex, cerebral gyri
Subarachnoid space
Falx cerebri
White substance


**Fig. 12.7 Calvaria, meninges, and dural venous sinuses;** frontal section.

In the adult, the cerebrospinal fluid is mainly reabsorbed into the venous system through the **PACCHIONIAN granulations** (arachnoid granulations, arachnoid protrusions into the superior sagittal sinus or the lateral lacunae) along the superior sagittal sinus. Additionally, reabsorption occurs through the lymphatic sheaths of small vessels of the cranial pia mater and through the perineural sheaths of the cranial and the spinal nerves (not shown).

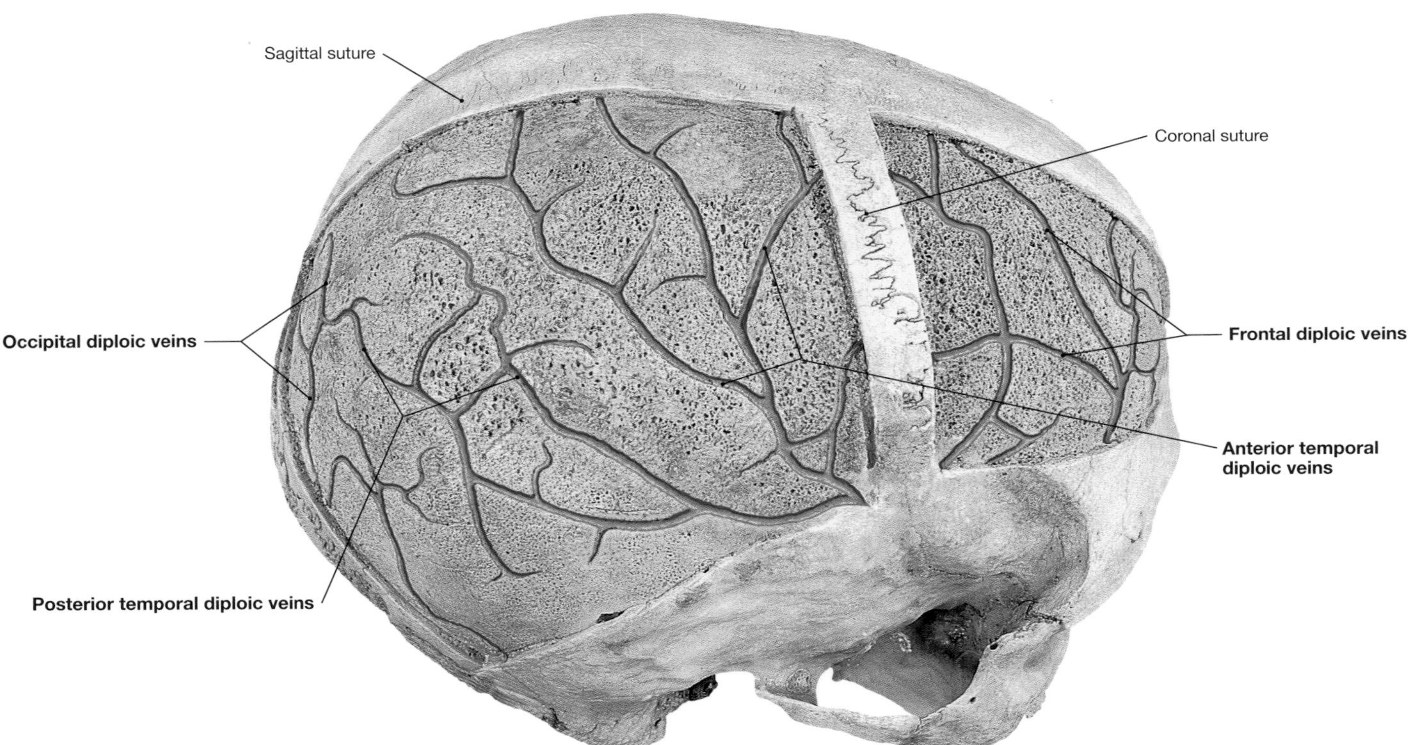

Sagittal suture
Coronal suture
Occipital diploic veins
Frontal diploic veins
Anterior temporal diploic veins
Posterior temporal diploic veins


**Fig. 12.8 Diploic canals and diploic veins of the calvaria, right side;** superior oblique view; after the external layer of the compact bone has been removed from the calvaria.

Passing through the diploic space are diploic canals, which harbor the diploic veins. They communicate with the emissary veins and the dural venous sinus.

## Blood supply of the dura mater

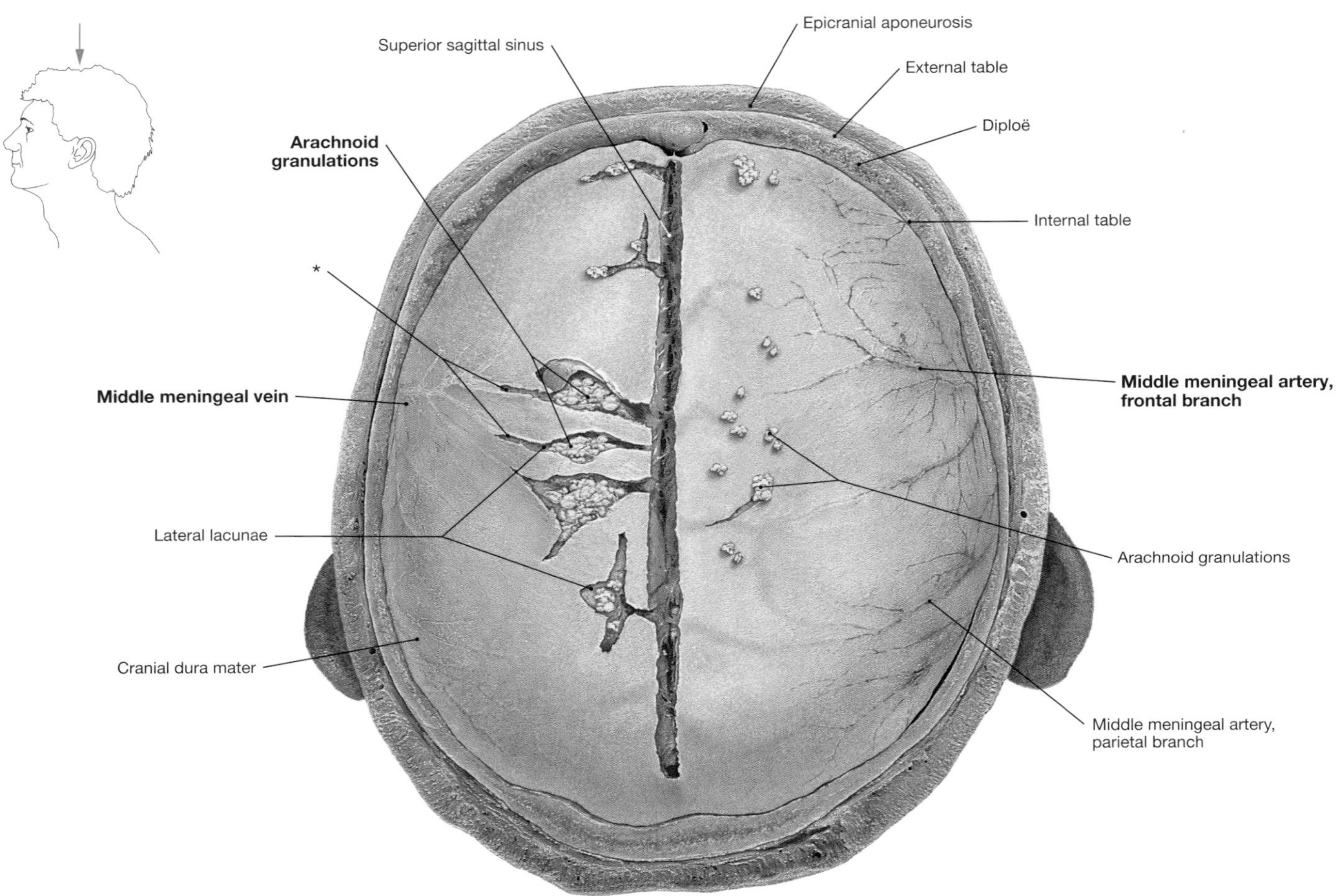
Superior sagittal sinus
Epicranial aponeurosis
External table
Diploë
Arachnoid granulations
Internal table
*
Middle meningeal vein
Middle meningeal artery, frontal branch
Lateral lacunae
Arachnoid granulations
Cranial dura mater
Middle meningeal artery, parietal branch

**Fig. 12.9 Cranial dura mater and superior sagittal sinus with some lateral lacunae;** superior view.
The calvaria has been removed. On the left side of the body, the cranial dura mater has been opened along the **lateral lacunae** and the confluence of the **medial meningeal veins** into the lacunae is shown. The PACCHIONIAN granulations (arachnoid granulations) reside within the lacunae. On the right side of the body, the arachnoid granulations are visible as they rise above the level of the dura. The latter extend into the calvarian bone. Here they generate characteristic impressions and communicate with the diploic veins.

* confluence of the medial meningeal veins into the lateral lacunae

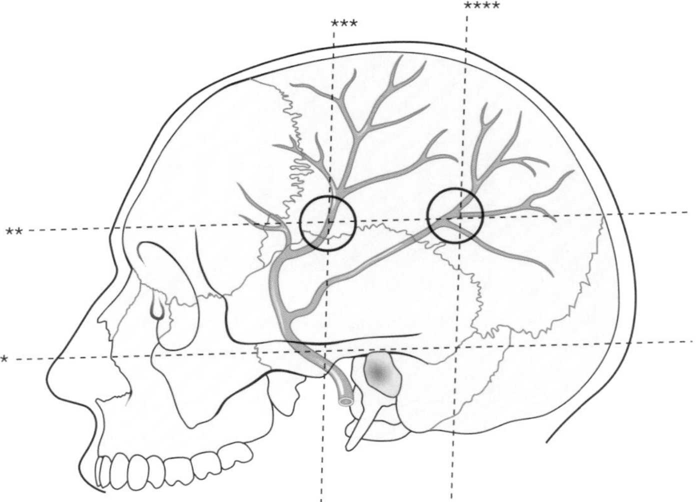
***
****
**
*

**Fig. 12.10 Projection of the frontal and parietal branches of the medial meningeal artery onto the side of the skull.** Circles mark the projections of the main branches of the medial meningeal artery. The main branches of the medial meningeal artery are located where the upper horizontal line crosses the vertical line passing through the middle of the zygomatic arch and the vertical line passing through the posterior part of the mastoid process.

- * clinical term: auriculo-orbital horizontal line (FRANKFORT horizontal line)
- ** clinical term: supra-orbital horizontal line
- *** vertical line through the middle of the zygomatic arch
- **** vertical line through the posterior part of the mastoid process

### Clinical Remarks

**Meningioma** are the most frequent benign intracranial tumors. Often, they develop in the region of the PACCHIONIAN granulations (arachnoid granulations), alongside the falx cerebri, in the region of the sphenoidal wings, and in the olfactory pit. A blunt impact trauma against the side of the head can result in a **fracture of the skull.** The most likely location for a fracture is where the upper horizontal line (positioned above the orbit) crosses the two vertical lines passing midway through the zygomatic arch or through the posterior part of the mastoid process. An **epidural hematoma** results in the event of a rupture of either the frontal branch or the parietal branch of the medial meningeal artery (→ Fig. 12.11).

## Intracranial bleeding

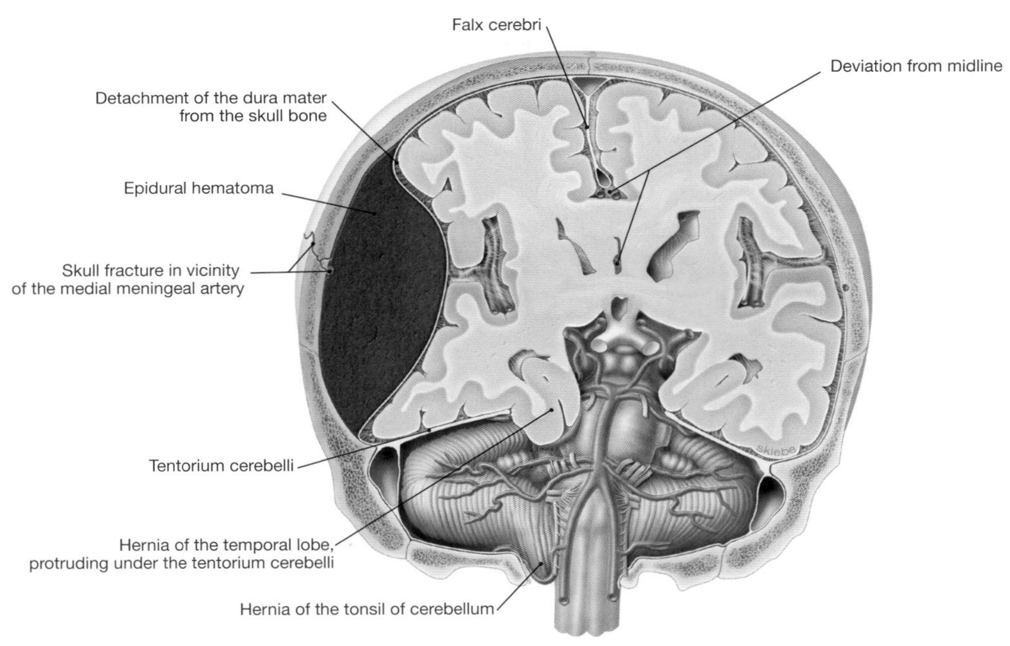
Falx cerebri
Deviation from midline
Detachment of the dura mater from the skull bone
Epidural hematoma
Skull fracture in vicinity of the medial meningeal artery
Tentorium cerebelli
Hernia of the temporal lobe, protruding under the tentorium cerebelli
Hernia of the tonsil of cerebellum

**Fig. 12.11 Epidural hematoma;** frontal section; frontal view.
An injury to the medial meningeal artery on the right side of the body has resulted in an arterial bleeding between the calvarian bone and dura mater. The pressure of the hematoma causes the midline to deviate sideways and results in parts of the temporal lobe being squeezed underneath the tentorium cerebelli through the tentorial notch.

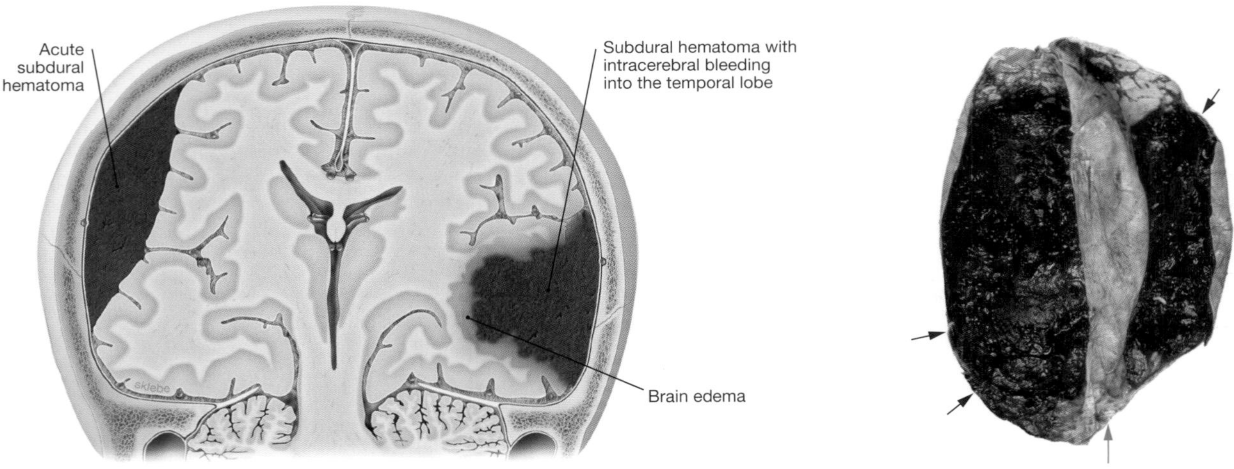
Acute subdural hematoma
Subdural hematoma with intracerebral bleeding into the temporal lobe
Brain edema

**Fig. 12.12 Subdural hematoma and intracerebral bleeding;** frontal section; frontal view.
Ruptures of bridging veins resulted in an acute subdural hematoma on the right side and a subdural hematoma with intracerebral bleeding into the temporal lobe on the left side.

**Fig. 12.13 Subdural hematoma;** superior view at the brain. [5]
Large fresh bilateral traumatic subdural hematoma (arrows) on the inner aspect of the dura mater (red arrow = falx cerebri). The dura above the hematoma has been deflected.

## Clinical Remarks

Head trauma, e.g. caused by car accidents, can result in injuries to the medial meningeal artery, which supplies blood to the dura mater. Often, the patient seems to have no apparent injuries and remains without symptoms during the first 30 minutes. The onset of an arterial bleeding causes the dura mater to detach from the inside of the skull and an **epidural hematoma** develops. This results in the displacement of parts of the brain and increasing pressure on the brain, brainstem, and cranial nerves with serious neurological deficits and pathological reflexes. Elderly people often have more fragile veins and even small injuries can lead to the rupture of bridging veins (connecting veins between cranial veins and dural venous sinuses), causing the formation of a **subdural hematoma.** Thereby, acutely or in a more subtle way (sometimes over weeks), venous blood collects between the dura mater and the arachnoid mater. Patients show general and uncharacteristic symptoms like dizziness, headache, fatigue, listlessness, or confusion. Subdural hematoma can also coincide with intracerebral bleeding and corresponding acute neurological deficits (→ pp. 240, 256, 267, and 270).

## Dural venous sinuses and parts of the internal carotid artery

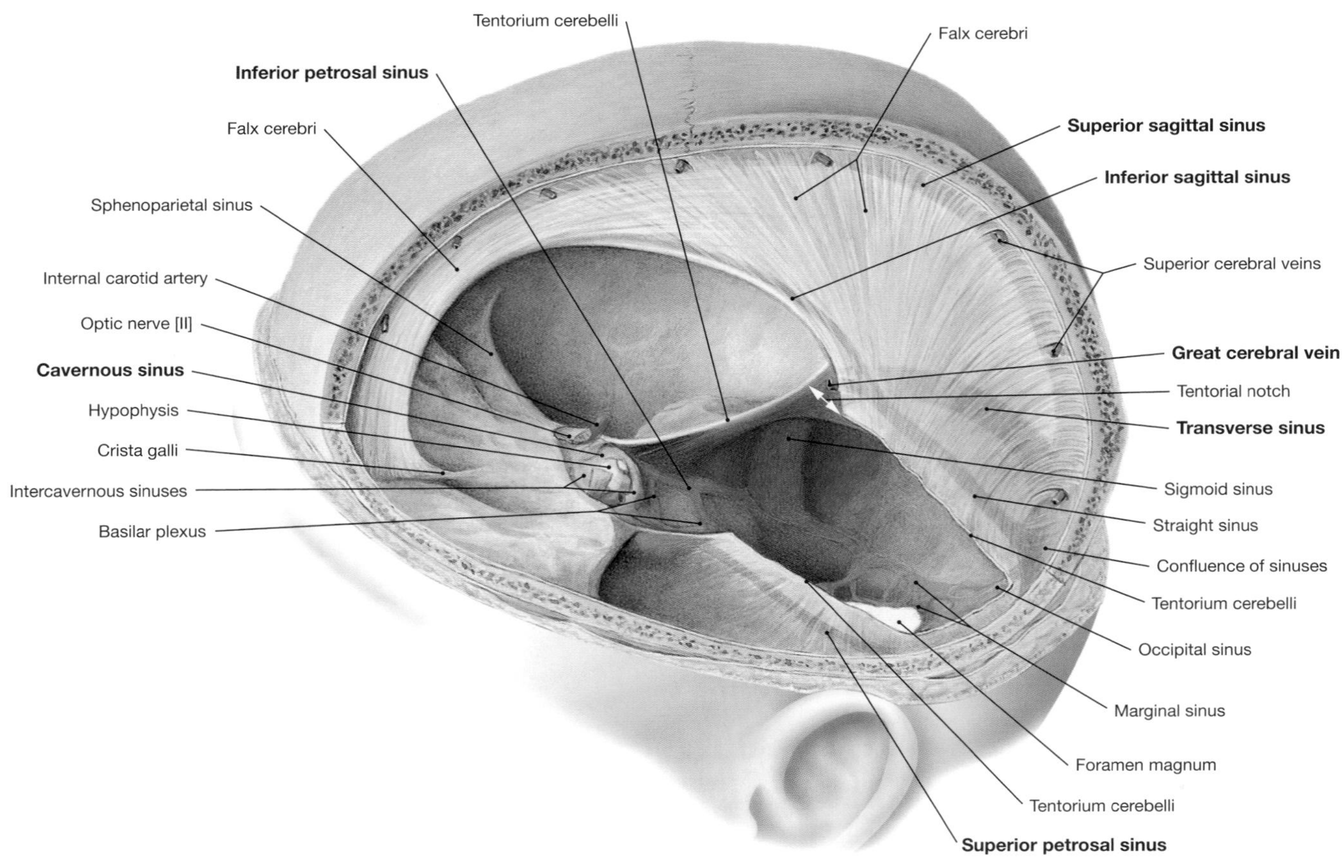
Tentorium cerebelli
Falx cerebri
Inferior petrosal sinus
Falx cerebri
Superior sagittal sinus
Inferior sagittal sinus
Sphenoparietal sinus
Superior cerebral veins
Internal carotid artery
Optic nerve [II]
Great cerebral vein
Cavernous sinus
Tentorial notch
Hypophysis
Transverse sinus
Crista galli
Sigmoid sinus
Intercavernous sinuses
Straight sinus
Basilar plexus
Confluence of sinuses
Tentorium cerebelli
Occipital sinus
Marginal sinus
Foramen magnum
Tentorium cerebelli
Superior petrosal sinus

**Fig. 12.14 Cranial dura mater and dural venous sinuses;** superior oblique view; tentorium cerebelli partially removed.
The cranial dura mater lines the cranial cavity completely and tightly adheres to the skull bones. The dural venous sinuses course within the dura. The **falx cerebri** protrudes in the sagittal plane in a sickle-like shape and stretches from the crista galli to the ridge of the **tentorium cerebelli.** This, in turn, spans the posterior cranial fossa and is attached along the transverse sinus and the pyramidal edge. The margins of the tentorial notch envelope the midbrain (mesencephalon) and taper off into the petroclinoid folds which project to the anterior and posterior clinoid process. The falx cerebri and the tentorium cerebelli divide the cranial cavity into three spaces that are incompletely separated from one another, containing the two cerebral hemispheres and the cerebellum.

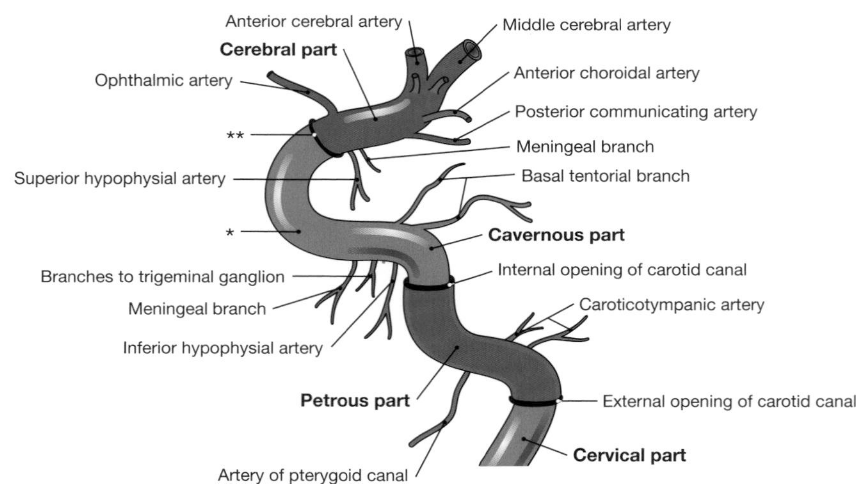
Anterior cerebral artery
Middle cerebral artery
Cerebral part
Ophthalmic artery
Anterior choroidal artery
Posterior communicating artery
**
Meningeal branch
Superior hypophysial artery
Basal tentorial branch
*
Cavernous part
Branches to trigeminal ganglion
Internal opening of carotid canal
Meningeal branch
Caroticotympanic artery
Inferior hypophysial artery
Petrous part
External opening of carotid canal
Cervical part
Artery of pterygoid canal

**Fig. 12.15 Parts of the internal carotid artery.** [8]
The internal carotid artery divides into four parts: cervical part, petrous part, cavernous part, and cerebral part. Along its course through the base of the skull, the internal carotid artery passes through the external opening of carotid canal, the internal opening of carotid canal, and through the dura mater. Small vessels branch off in the cervical part.

* carotid artery siphon
** passage through the cranial dura mater in the region of the sellar diaphragm

## Cavernous sinus

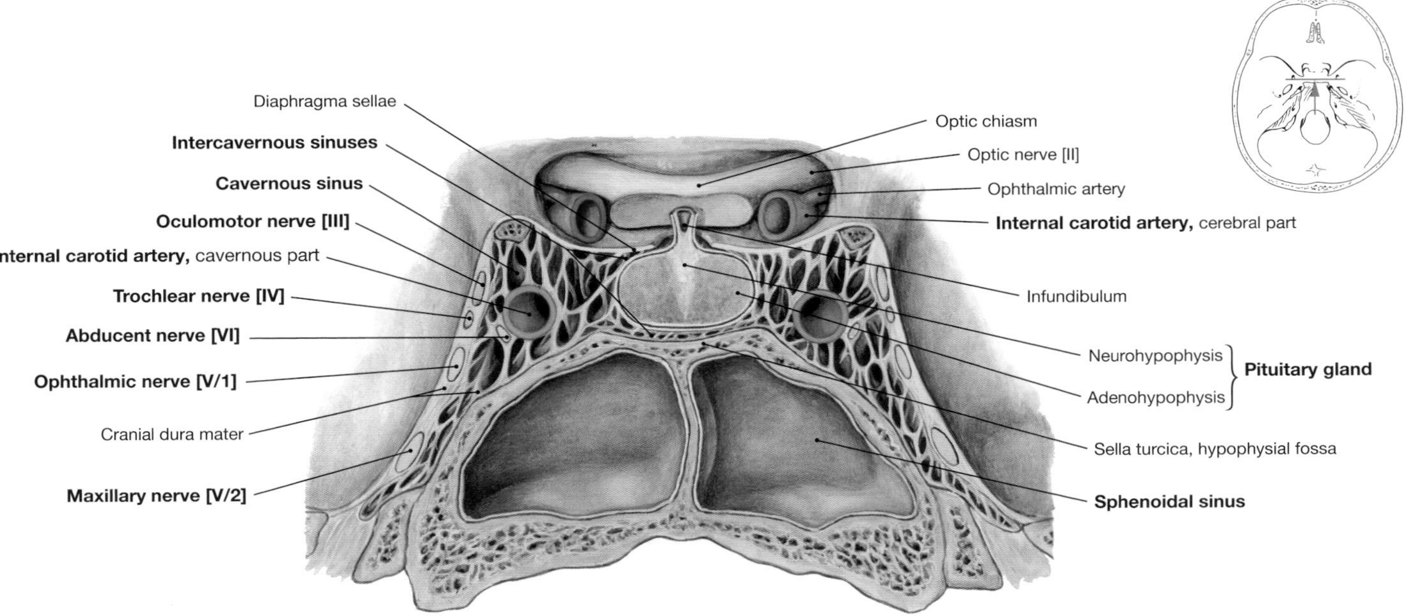
Diaphragma sellae
Intercavernous sinuses
Cavernous sinus
Oculomotor nerve [III]
Internal carotid artery, cavernous part
Trochlear nerve [IV]
Abducent nerve [VI]
Ophthalmic nerve [V/1]
Cranial dura mater
Maxillary nerve [V/2]
Optic chiasm
Optic nerve [II]
Ophthalmic artery
Internal carotid artery, cerebral part
Infundibulum
Neurohypophysis
Adenohypophysis
Pituitary gland
Sella turcica, hypophysial fossa
Sphenoidal sinus

**Fig. 12.16 Pituitary gland and cavernous sinus;** frontal section; posterior view.
The pituitary gland is surrounded by the right and left cavernous sinus, which communicate via the intercavernous sinuses. The internal carotid artery and lateral thereof the abducent nerve [VI] run through the center of the the cavernous sinus; the oculomotor [III], trochlear [IV], ophthalmic [V/1], and maxillary nerve [V/2] are located in the wall of the cavernous sinus. The sphenoidal sinus is located beneath the sella turcica which harbors the pituitary gland.

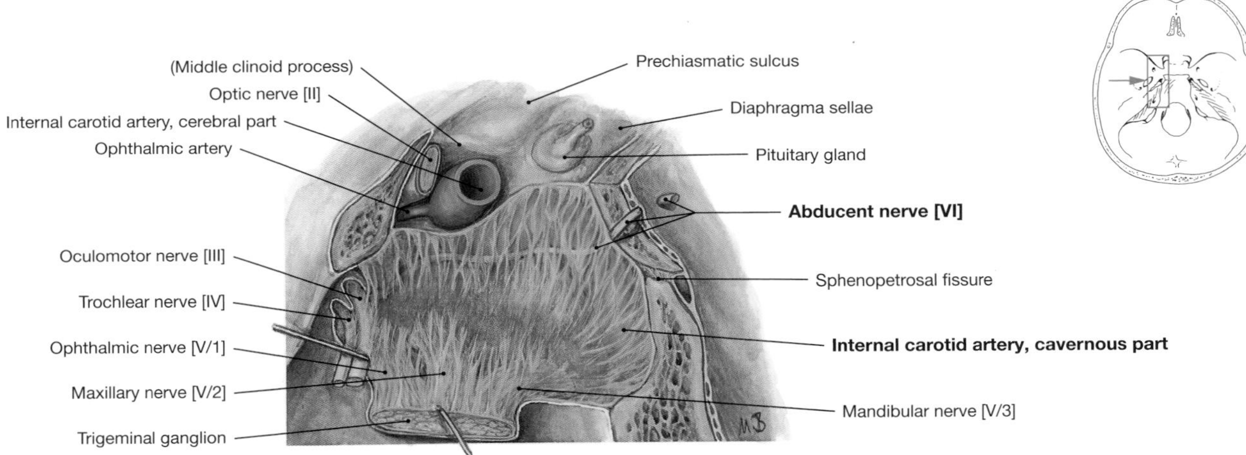
(Middle clinoid process)
Optic nerve [II]
Internal carotid artery, cerebral part
Ophthalmic artery
Oculomotor nerve [III]
Trochlear nerve [IV]
Ophthalmic nerve [V/1]
Maxillary nerve [V/2]
Trigeminal ganglion
Prechiasmatic sulcus
Diaphragma sellae
Pituitary gland
Abducent nerve [VI]
Sphenopetrosal fissure
Internal carotid artery, cavernous part
Mandibular nerve [V/3]

**Fig. 12.17 Cavernous sinus, left side;** lateral view; the lateral part of the dura mater contributing to the formation of the sinus wall has been removed; the trigeminal ganglion was deflected laterally.
The course of the cavernous part of the internal carotid artery and the passage of the abducent nerve [VI] through the cavernous sinus is shown.

## Clinical Remarks

A disease of the cavernous sinus (**cavernous sinus syndrome;** cavernous sinus thrombosis, tumor, metastasis, aneurysm of the internal carotid artery, inflammatory infiltration) coincides with unilateral palsy of the abducent and oculomotor nerves in combination with sensory deficits of the first trigeminal branch (ophthalmic nerve [V/1]). Acute onset of these symptoms in combination with signs of impaired venous drainage, like venous stasis of the content of the orbit with a swelling of eyelids and conjunctiva as well as a protrusion of the eyeball (proptosis, exophthalmus) suggest a venous thrombosis and/or a fistula between the internal carotid artery and the cavernous sinus.
**Arteriosclerotic alterations in the vascular wall** are relatively frequent at the site where the internal carotid artery branches off the common carotid artery as well as in the cavernous part of the internal carotid artery.

## Dural venous sinuses

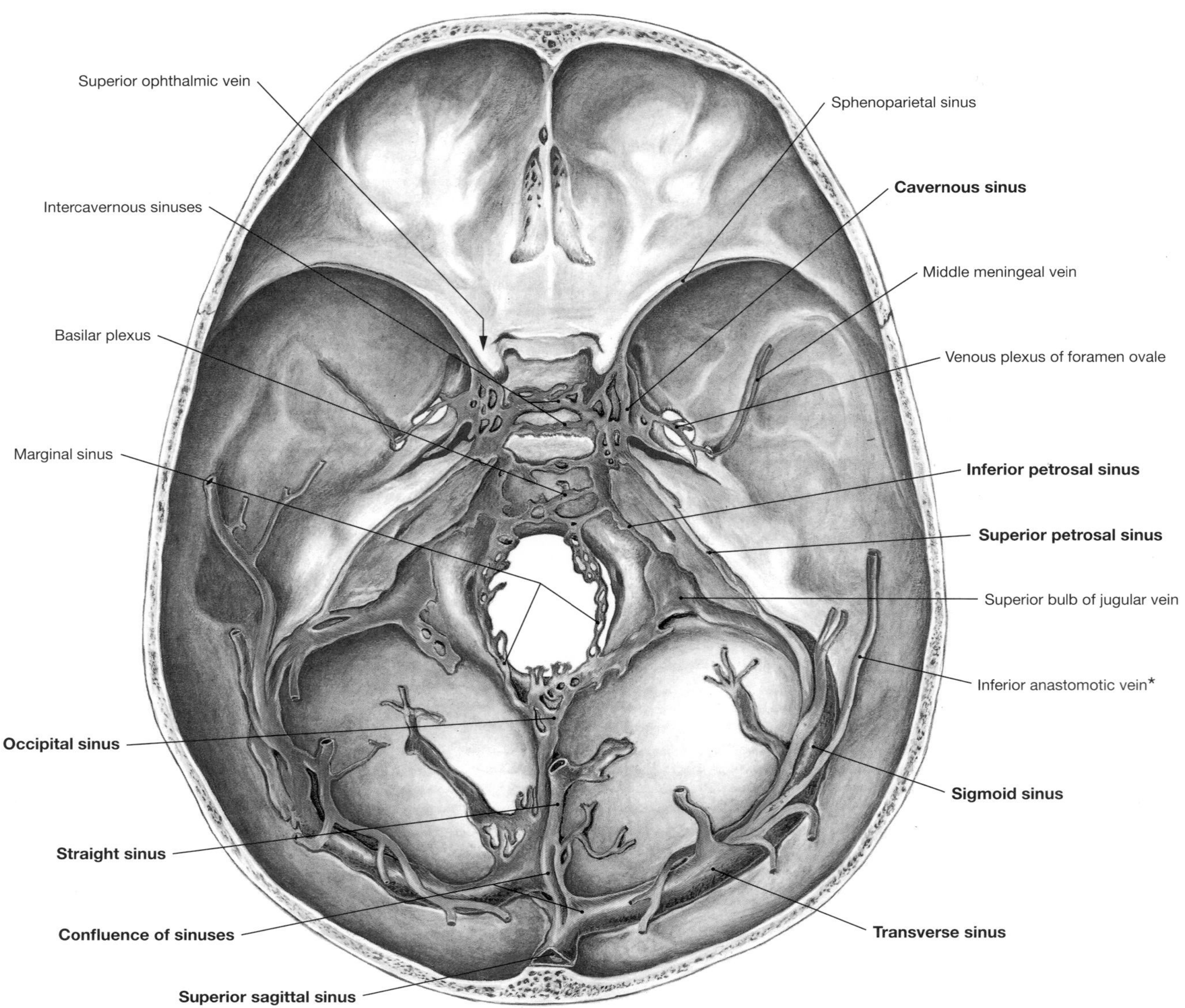
Superior ophthalmic vein
Sphenoparietal sinus
Intercavernous sinuses
Cavernous sinus
Middle meningeal vein
Basilar plexus
Venous plexus of foramen ovale
Marginal sinus
Inferior petrosal sinus
Superior petrosal sinus
Superior bulb of jugular vein
Inferior anastomotic vein*
Occipital sinus
Sigmoid sinus
Straight sinus
Confluence of sinuses
Transverse sinus
Superior sagittal sinus

**Fig. 12.18 Dural venous sinuses;** corrosion cast; superior view.
The dural venous sinuses are rigid venous canals devoid of valves that drain the venous blood from the brain via so-called bridging veins. The main drainage from within the skull occurs via the paired **sigmoid sinuses** into the internal jugular veins (initially forming the superior bulb of jugular vein). Additionally, the superior ophthalmic veins (in the orbit, not visible but indicated by the arrow, communication via the superior orbital fissure) and the highly variable emissary veins (→ Fig. 12.6) form a series of smaller, likewise valveless, venous connections between the intra- and extracranial regions.
The two **cavernous sinuses** assume a central position by being situated in the middle cranial fossa to both sides of the sella turcica. They communicate with each other through the intercavernous sinuses and either directly or indirectly with most other sinuses and with the veins of the orbit and the infratemporal fossa.

* vein of LABBÉ to the superficial middle cerebral veins

## Clinical Remarks

**Thrombosis in the dural venous sinuses,** e.g. caused by cerebral contusion or inflammations like middle ear infections, can lead to a partial or complete blockage with resulting brain edema and hemorrhagic infarction due to a stasis-induced diapedetic bleeding. Symptoms include headaches, nausea, vomiting, and epileptic seizures.

## Superficial vessels of the brain

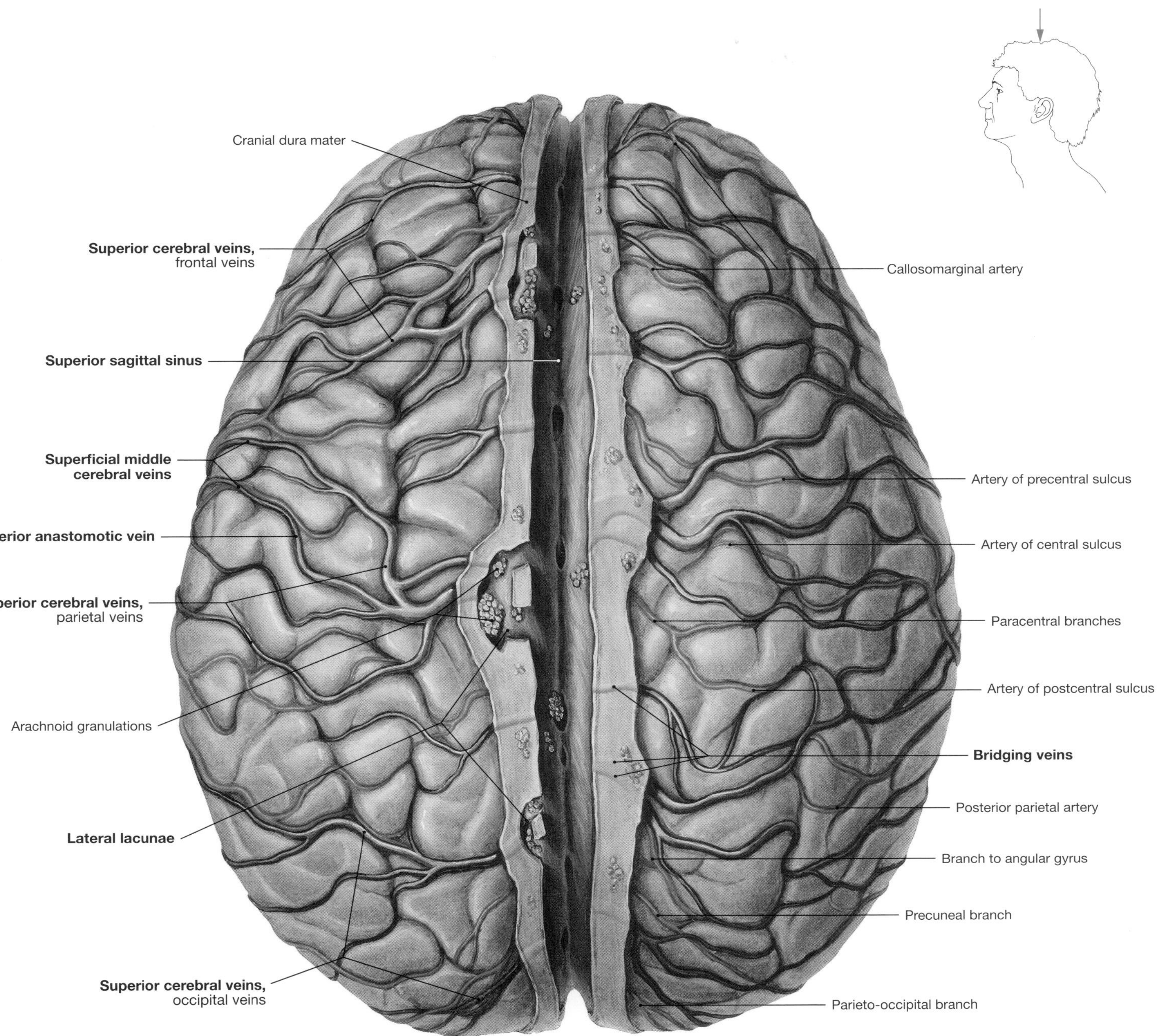
Cranial dura mater
Superior cerebral veins, frontal veins
Superior sagittal sinus
Superficial middle cerebral veins
uperior anastomotic vein
Superior cerebral veins, parietal veins
Arachnoid granulations
Lateral lacunae
Superior cerebral veins, occipital veins
Callosomarginal artery
Artery of precentral sulcus
Artery of central sulcus
Paracentral branches
Artery of postcentral sulcus
Bridging veins
Posterior parietal artery
Branch to angular gyrus
Precuneal branch
Parieto-occipital branch

**Fig. 12.19 Superficial arteries and veins of the brain;** superior view; after removal of the cranial dura mater and sectioning of the superior sagittal sinus; cranial arachnoid mater removed.
The superficial arteries and veins supply the cerebral cortex and the subjacent basal ganglia. Superficial veins are the superior cerebral veins, the superficial middle cerebral vein, and the inferior cerebral veins (not shown). Anastomoses usually connect the larger veins (superior anastomotic vein [TROLARD's vein, → Fig. 12.6] and inferior anastomotic vein [vein of LABBÉ, → Figs. 12.6 and 12.18]). The superior cerebral veins drain into the superior sagittal sinus directly or, via small bridging veins piercing the dura mater, connect with the lateral lacunae which then drain into the superior sagittal sinus.

## Clinical Remarks

**Injuries to the bridging veins** result in the accumulation of blood between the dura and the arachnoid mater and can cause a subdural hematoma (→ Fig. 12.12). Particularly those elderly patients with age-related atrophy of the brain and fragile bridging veins have a greater tendency to develop a **chronic subdural hematoma.** This type of hematoma is overlooked easily due to the subtle nature of the venous bleeding and the inability of the patient to recall the initiating small trauma.

## Leptomeninx

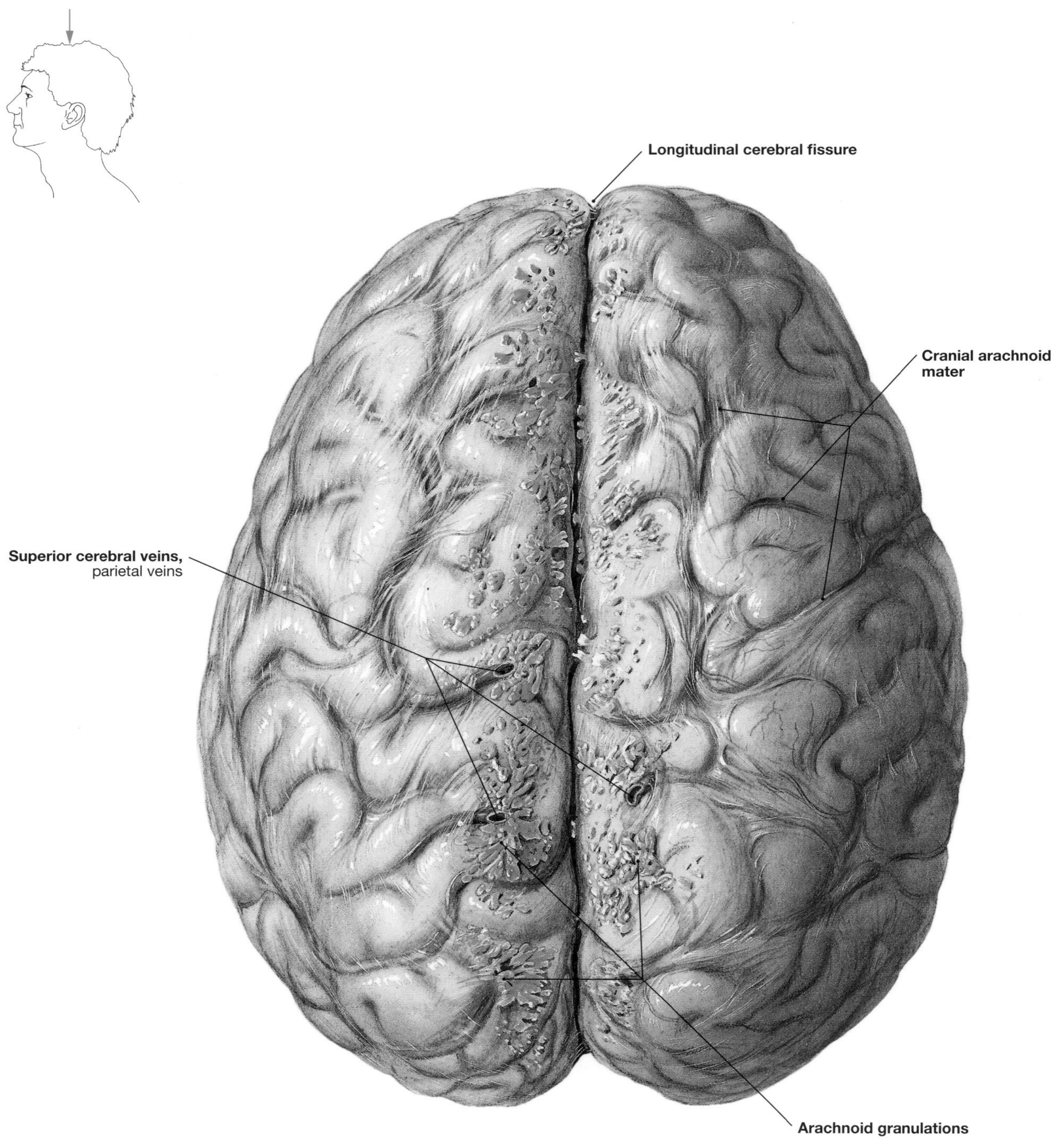
Longitudinal cerebral fissure
Cranial arachnoid mater
Superior cerebral veins, parietal veins
Arachnoid granulations

**Fig. 12.20 Brain with cranial arachnoid mater;** superior view.
The cranial arachnoid mater covers the brain. The falx cerebri (a duplication of the cranial dura mater), normally residing within the **longitudinal cerebral fissure,** divides the two cerebral hemispheres into a right and a left half and extends down to the callosal commissure (corpus callosum, not visible). To both sides of the longitudinal cerebral fissure, multiple PACCHIONIAN granulations (arachnoid granulations) are visible. These extend above the level of the arachnoid mater and assist in the reabsorption of cerebrospinal fluid. In addition, a number of cerebral veins (superior cerebral veins, parietal veins) are visible, which were severed from the bridging veins (small veins piercing the cranial dura mater on their way to the superior sagittal sinus) during the removal of the brain from the skull.

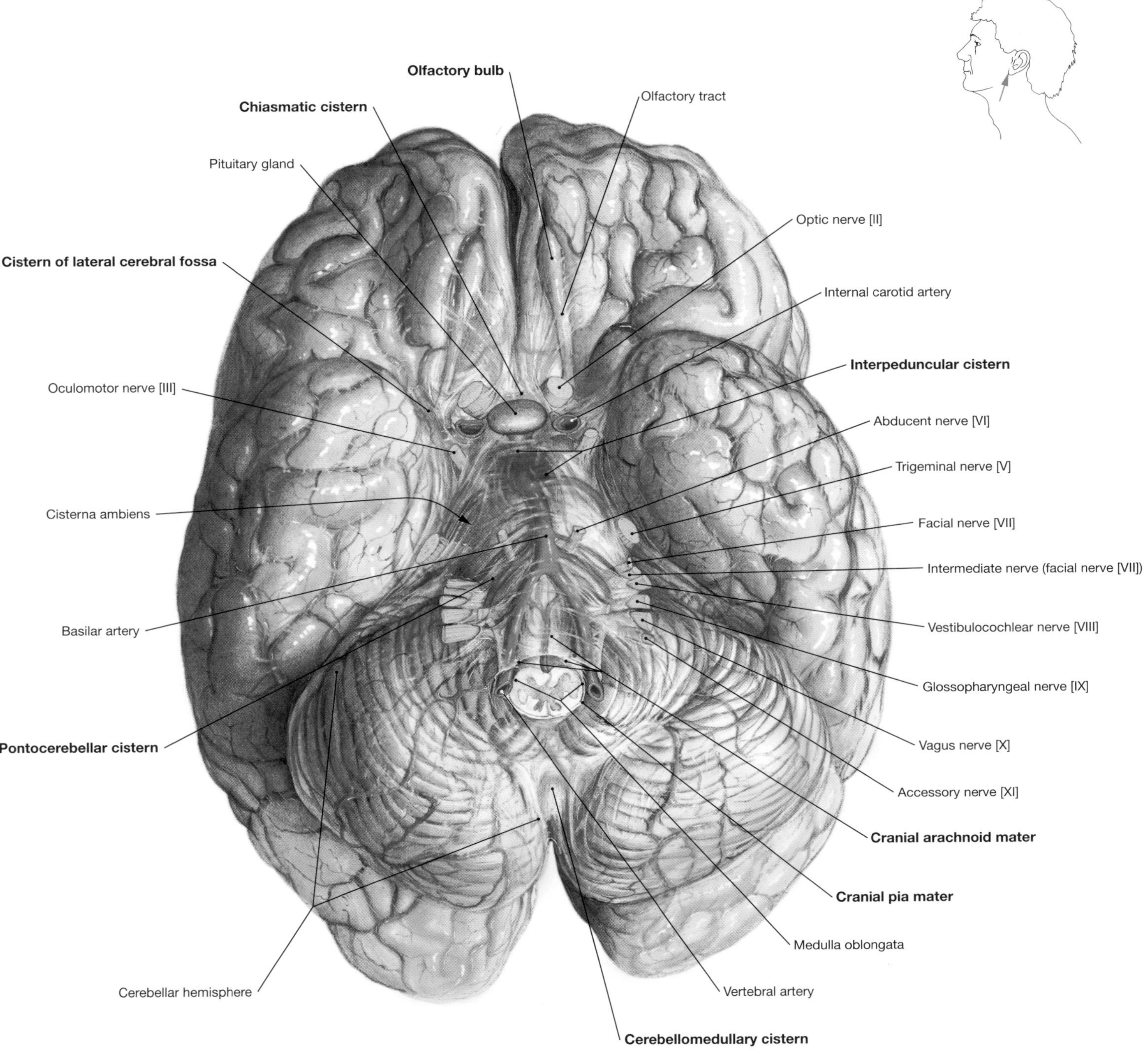
Olfactory bulb
Chiasmatic cistern
Olfactory tract
Pituitary gland
Optic nerve [II]
Cistern of lateral cerebral fossa
Internal carotid artery
Interpeduncular cistern
Oculomotor nerve [III]
Abducent nerve [VI]
Trigeminal nerve [V]
Cisterna ambiens
Facial nerve [VII]
Intermediate nerve (facial nerve [VII])
Basilar artery
Vestibulocochlear nerve [VIII]
Glossopharyngeal nerve [IX]
Pontocerebellar cistern
Vagus nerve [X]
Accessory nerve [XI]
Cranial arachnoid mater
Cranial pia mater
Medulla oblongata
Cerebellar hemisphere
Vertebral artery
Cerebellomedullary cistern

**Fig. 12.21 Brain with cranial arachnoid mater;** inferior view.
Removal of the brain from the skull was accomplished by cutting the brainstem at the level of the medulla oblongata and severing the vertebral arteries, the carotid arteries, and the twelve pairs of cranial nerves (the olfactory nerves of the first cranial nerve are teared off at the olfactory bulb). The cranial arachnoid mater covers the brain. Nerves and vessels run in the subarachnoid space. The caudal part of the frontal, temporal, and occipital lobes and the cerebellum are shown. The cerebral arterial circle (circle of WILLIS) is preserved but only partially visible. Further, the location of the cerebral cisterns is demonstrated.

## Development of the brain

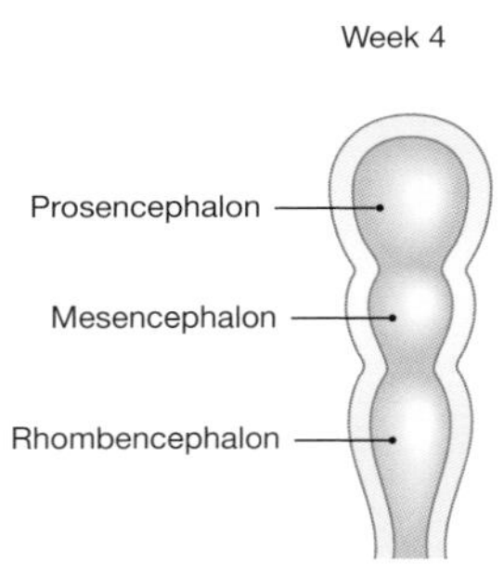
Week 4
Prosencephalon
Mesencephalon
Rhombencephalon
Primary brain vesicles

**Fig. 12.22 Development of the brain: primary brain vesicles;** schematic frontal section. [21]
The neural tube openings are closed in **week 4.** The rostral end begins to enlarge and forms the three successive **primary brain vesicles:** forebrain (prosencephalon), midbrain (mesencephalon), and hindbrain (rhombencephalon).

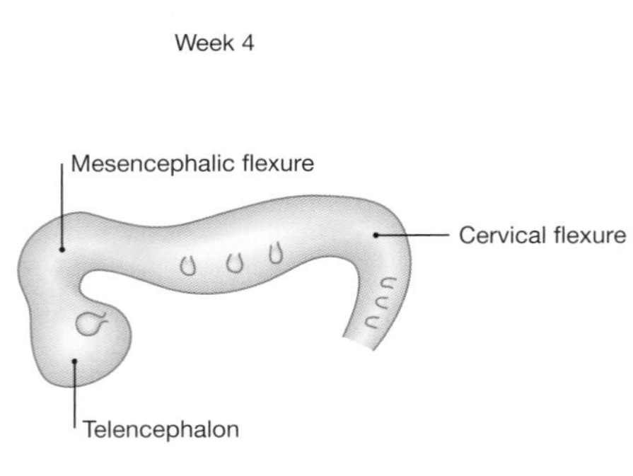
Week 4
Mesencephalic flexure
Cervical flexure
Telencephalon
Primary brain vesicles

**Fig. 12.23 Development of the brain: primary brain vesicles;** schematic lateral view. [21]
During **week 4,** the **midbrain flexure** (mesencephalic flexure) forms between the forebrain (prosencephalon) and the midbrain (mesencephalon). The **cervical flexure** develops between the hindbrain (rhombencephalon) and the spinal cord.

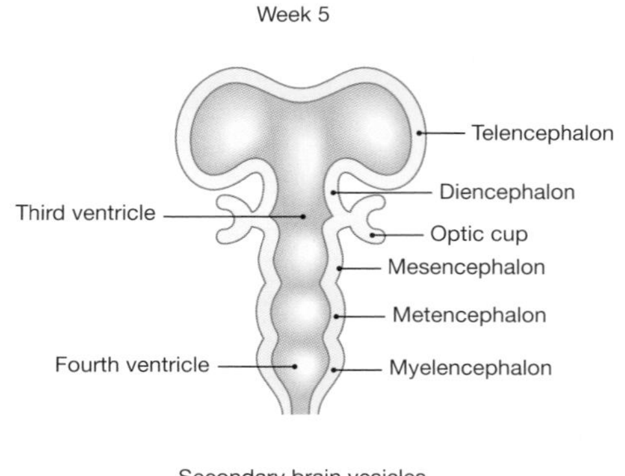
Week 5
Telencephalon
Diencephalon
Third ventricle
Optic cup
Mesencephalon
Metencephalon
Fourth ventricle
Myelencephalon
Secondary brain vesicles

**Fig. 12.24 Development of the brain: secondary brain vesicles;** schematic frontal section. [21]
In **week 5,** parts of the prosencephalon located on the right and left side of the midline enlarge to form the **telencephalon** which generates the cerebral hemispheres. In addition, the diencephalon derives from the prosencephalon. The third ventricle evolves between the diencephalon and mesencephalon. Forming beneath the **mesencephalon** is the metencephalon with its two main components, the pons and the cerebellum. The **myelencephalon** follows caudally; it includes the fourth ventricle and the medulla oblongata and transitions into the spinal cord.
The three primary brain vesicles gave rise to six **secondary brain vesicles** (the paired vesicles of the telencephalon and the di-, mes-, met-, and myelencephalon).

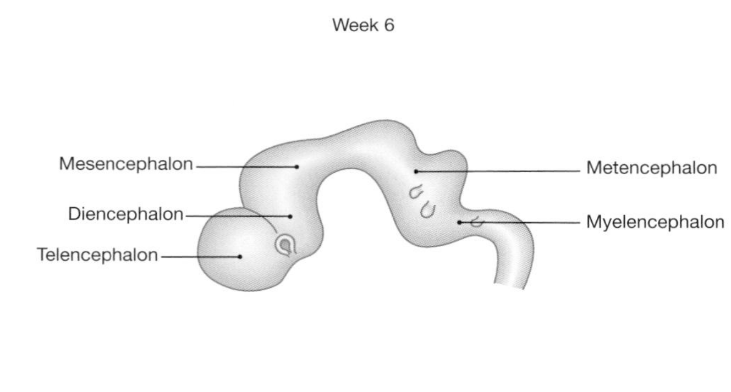
Week 6
Mesencephalon
Metencephalon
Diencephalon
Myelencephalon
Telencephalon
Secondary brain vesicles

**Fig. 12.25 Development of the brain: secondary brain vesicles;** schematic lateral view. [21]
In **week 6,** the telencephalon, diencephalon, mesencephalon, metencephalon, and myelencephalon are clearly delineated. The optic cups become visible between the telencephalon and the diencephalon. The development of the cerebellum starts as a lateral extension of the rhombencephalon. The developing cerebellum is visible at the dorsal aspect of the metencephalon.

### Clinical Remarks

Failure of the neural tube to close in its rostral section (open rostral neuropore) prevents the proper development of the three brain vesicles. Misguided induction processes merely cause the formation of diffuse, underdeveloped neuronal tissue. This lack of proper brain development entails improper skull formation. A facial skull (viscerocranium) is formed but brain and brain case (neurocranium) are not present **(anencephaly).** This malformation is fatal.

## Development of the brain

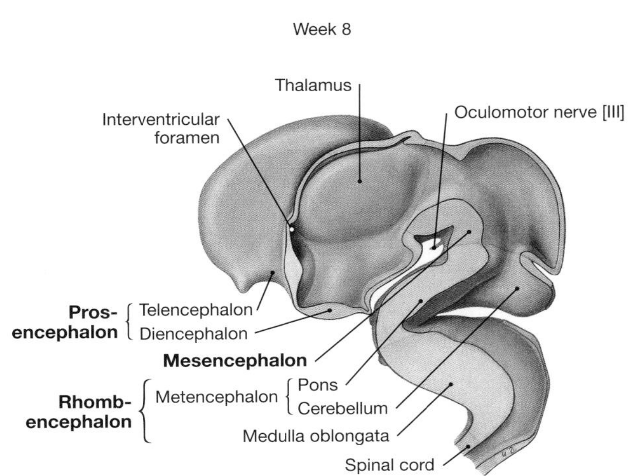
Week 8
Thalamus
Interventricular foramen
Oculomotor nerve [III]
Pros-encephalon
Telencephalon
Diencephalon
Mesencephalon
Rhomb-encephalon
Metencephalon
Pons
Cerebellum
Medulla oblongata
Spinal cord

**Fig. 12.26 Development of the brain;** median section.
In **week 8** the individual brain structures are clearly distinguishable. Telencephalon and diencephalon derived from the prosencephalon. The thalamus in the diencephalon and the oculomotor nerve [III] exiting the mesencephalon become visible. The rhombencephalon has differentiated into the metencephalon and the medulla oblongata (myeloencephalon). Pons and cerebellum derive from the metencephalon. The medulla oblongata is followed by the spinal cord.

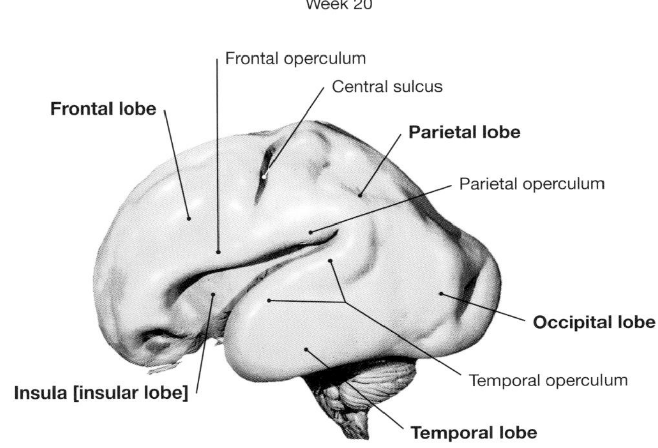
Week 20
Frontal operculum
Central sulcus
Frontal lobe
Parietal lobe
Parietal operculum
Occipital lobe
Temporal operculum
Insula [insular lobe]
Temporal lobe

**Fig. 12.27 Development of the brain;** view from the left side.
At **week 20** (with a foetal crown-rump length of 20 cm), the growth of the telencephalon has progressed significantly. It is already composed of the frontal, parietal, occipital and temporal lobes. However, the insular lobe is not yet fully covered by the frontal, parietal, and temporal lobes. Of all the structures of the brainstem, only parts of the pons, the cerebellum, and the medulla oblongata are still visible.

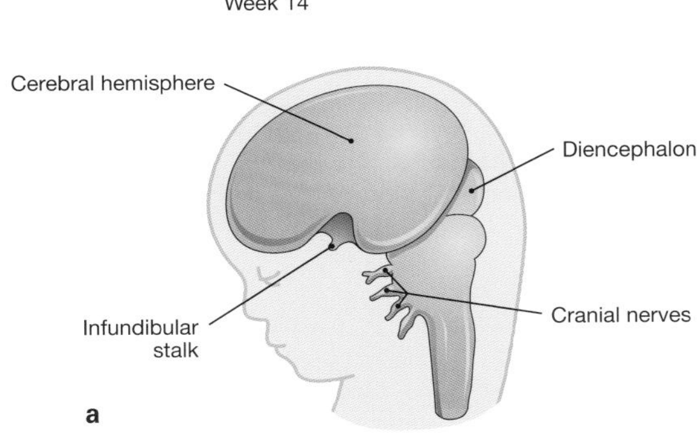
Week 14
Cerebral hemisphere
Diencephalon
Infundibular stalk
Cranial nerves
a

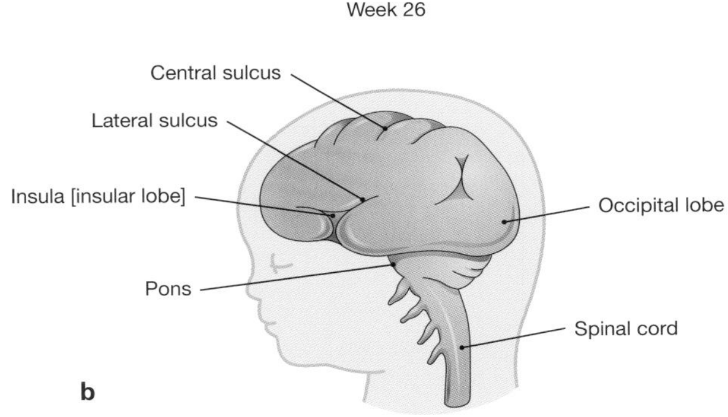
Week 26
Central sulcus
Lateral sulcus
Insula [insular lobe]
Occipital lobe
Pons
Spinal cord
b

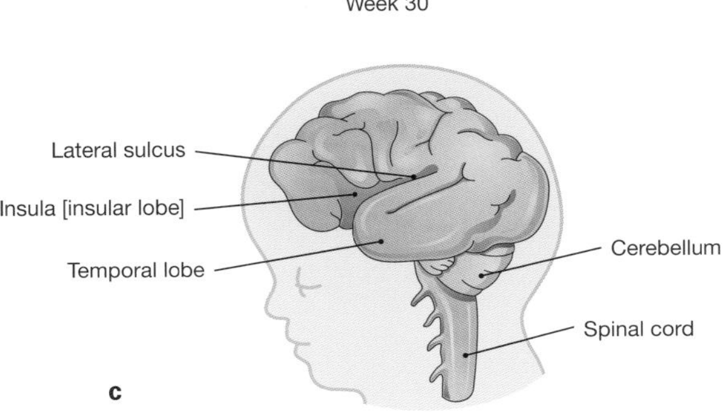
Week 30
Lateral sulcus
Insula [insular lobe]
Temporal lobe
Cerebellum
Spinal cord
c

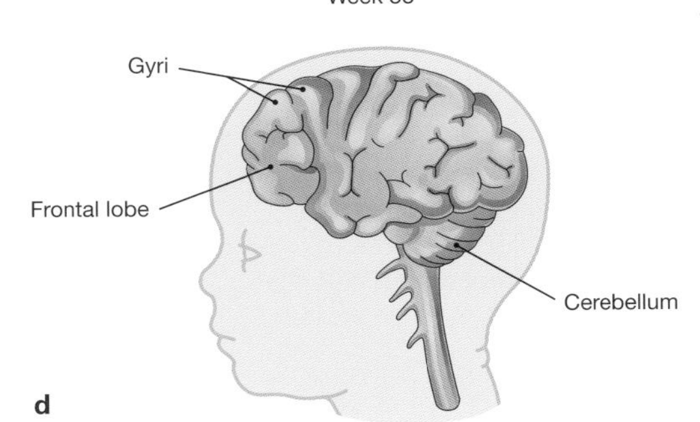
Week 38
Gyri
Frontal lobe
Cerebellum
d

**Figs. 12.28a to d Development of the left cerebral hemisphere, diencephalon and brainstem;** schematic drawings; lateral view. [20]
At week 14, the surface of the telencephalon is still smooth. Thereafter, the cerebral cortex undergoes successive stages in the **development of grooves (sulci) and convolutions (gyri).** In addition, the formation of the insula becomes overlapped by the frontal, parietal, and temporal lobes.

## Development of the brain

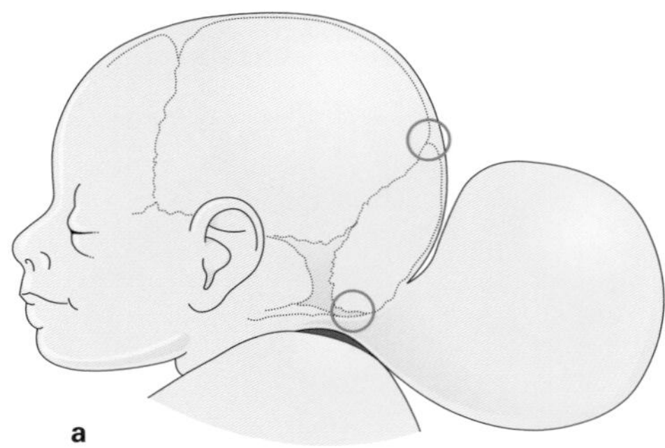
a

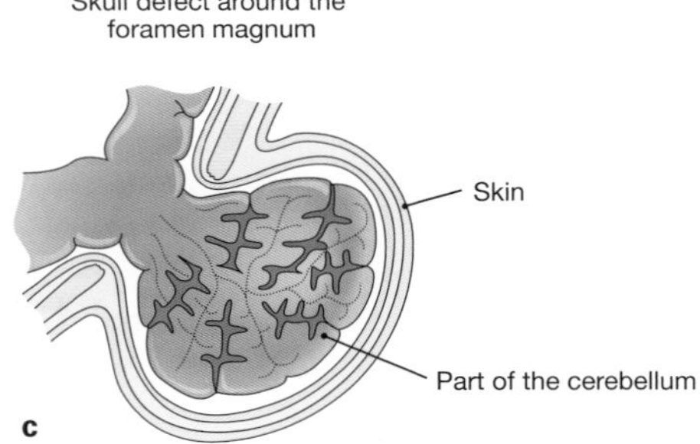
Skull defect around the foramen magnum
Skin
Part of the cerebellum
c

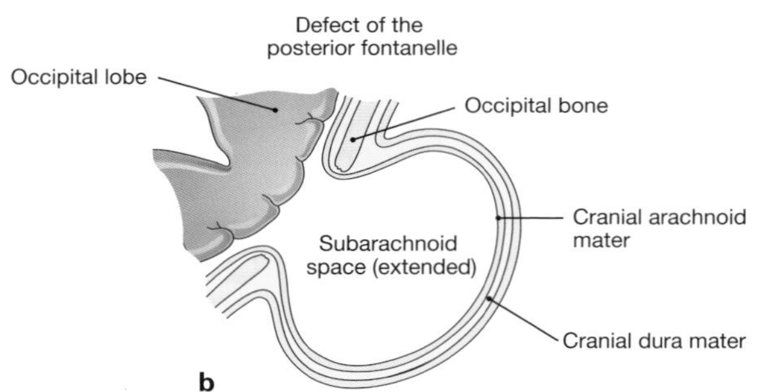
Defect of the posterior fontanelle
Occipital lobe
Occipital bone
Cranial arachnoid mater
Subarachnoid space (extended)
Cranial dura mater
b

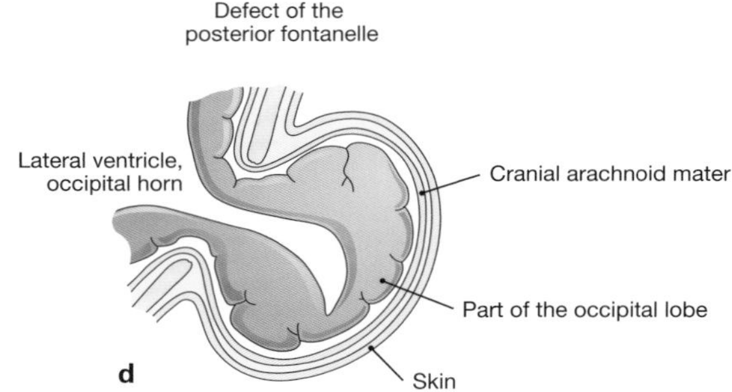
Defect of the posterior fontanelle
Lateral ventricle, occipital horn
Cranial arachnoid mater
Part of the occipital lobe
Skin
d

**Figs. 12.29a to d Cranium bifidum formation and various types of herniation of the brain and/or meninges,** schematic presentation. [20]

- **a** Head of a newborn with an extensive herniation in the occipital region. The upper red circle marks the defect of the small fontanelle, the lower red circle indicates the defect in the area of the foramen magnum.
- **b Meningocele:** the herinal sac is formed by skin and meninges and is filled with cerebrospinal fluid.
- **c Meningoencephalocele:** the herinal sac comprises prolapsed parts of the cerebellum and is covered by meninges and skin.
- **d Meningohydroencephalocele:** the herinal sac consists of prolapsed parts of the occipital lobe and of the posterior horn of the lateral ventricle.

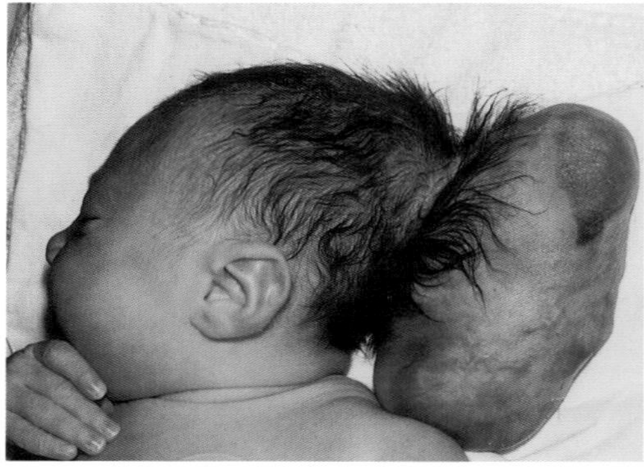

**Fig. 12.30 Meningoencephalocele.** [20]

### Clinical Remarks

An **encephalocele** (cerebral hernia, outer brain prolapse, cranium bifidum) is a defect caused by incomplete closure of the neural tube during foetal development with a median gap in the skull (at the root of the nose, forehead, cranial base, or occiput). Parts of the meninges **(meningocele)** or brain **(meningoencephalocele)** without participation of brain ventricles **(cenencephalocele),** or including ventricular parts **(encephalocystocele, meningohydroencephalocele)** can protrude into the gap.

## Organization of the brain

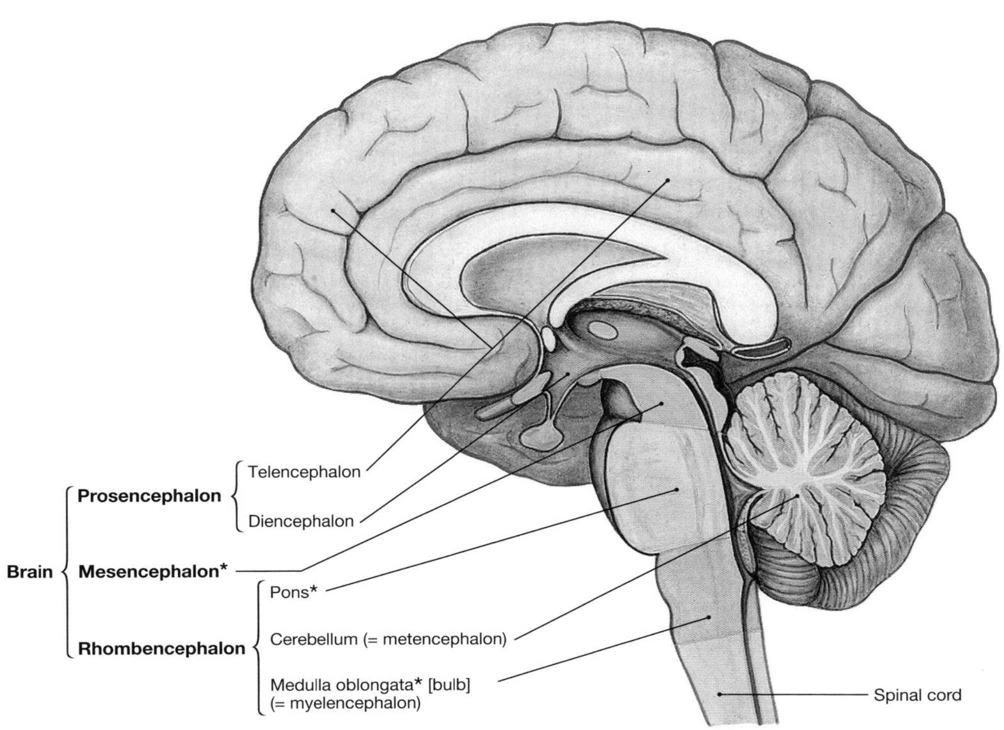
Brain
Prosencephalon
Telencephalon
Diencephalon
Mesencephalon*
Rhombencephalon
Pons*
Cerebellum (= metencephalon)
Medulla oblongata* [bulb]
(= myelencephalon)
Spinal cord

**Fig. 12.31 Organization of the central nervous system;** median section; schematic drawing. The parts of the brain that constitute the brainstem are marked by a star (*).
Based on the development of the brain from three primary brain vesicles (forebrain [prosencephalon], midbrain [mesencephalon], and hindbrain [rhombencephalon]) the brain divides into telencephalon, diencephalon, mesencephalon, pons, cerebellum (metencephalon), and medulla oblongata.

## Clinical Remarks

The **average brain volume** is between 1000 and 1400 $cm^3$. Often but not always, smaller brain volumes coincide with mental impairment. However, no correlation exists between the size of a brain and intelligence. On the other hand, not all cases of mental impairment coincide with a small brain size.

## Telencephalon, cortex

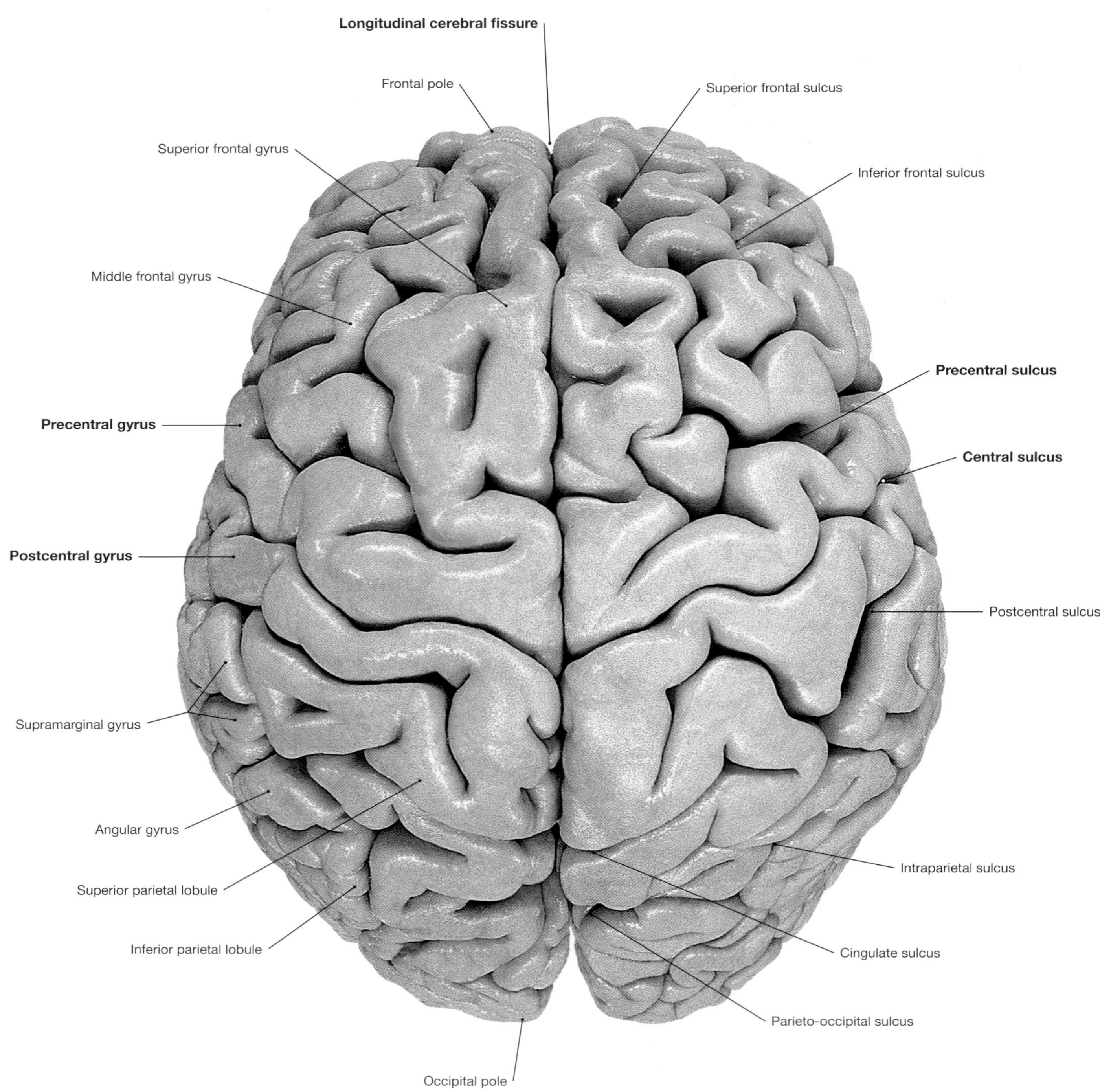
Longitudinal cerebral fissure
Frontal pole
Superior frontal sulcus
Superior frontal gyrus
Inferior frontal sulcus
Middle frontal gyrus
Precentral sulcus
Precentral gyrus
Central sulcus
Postcentral gyrus
Postcentral sulcus
Supramarginal gyrus
Angular gyrus
Intraparietal sulcus
Superior parietal lobule
Inferior parietal lobule
Cingulate sulcus
Parieto-occipital sulcus
Occipital pole

**Fig. 12.32 Cerebrum;** superior view, after removal of the leptomeninx.

The cerebrum constitutes the major part of the brain. It is composed of **two hemispheres** which are separated by the **longitudinal cerebral fissure.** During early stages of development, the surface of the cerebrum is smooth. Strong growth results in the formation of quite variable grooves **(sulci)** and convolutions **(gyri).** This folding dramatically increases the cerebral surface area and, as a result, two-thirds of the cerebral surface area are invisible to the eye.

### Clinical Remarks

**Atrophy of the brain** occurs with advanced age. This coincides with enlarged sulci and narrowed gyri. The progressive difficulty to memorize with advancing age is not a direct result of atrophy of the brain but is caused foremost by the shorter duration of slow-wave sleep (deep sleep) phases. The deep sleep phases diminish significantly with advancing age. While deep sleep makes up to 19% of the sleep in individuals up to 26 years of age, this proportion decreases to 3% in the age groups of 36 to 50 years. Studies demonstrated that this correlates with decreased memory functions.

## Telencephalon, organization of the lobes

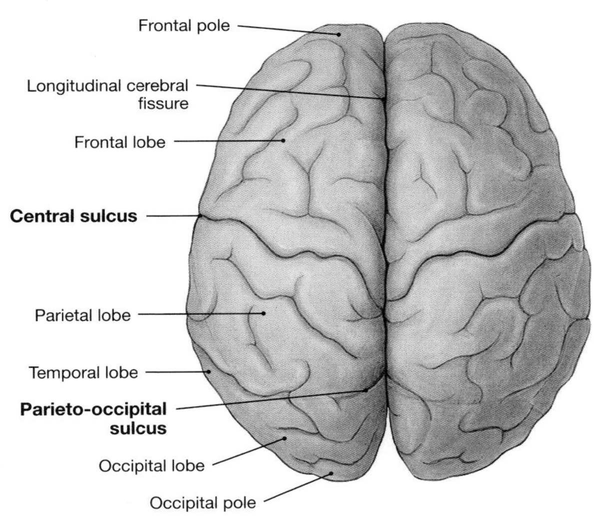
Frontal pole
Longitudinal cerebral fissure
Frontal lobe
Central sulcus
Parietal lobe
Temporal lobe
Parieto-occipital sulcus
Occipital lobe
Occipital pole

**Fig. 12.33 Cerebral lobes;** superior view.
Towards the end of the 8th month of foetal development, the primary grooves become visible (→ Table). These are regularly present in all humans. The view from the top shows the central sulcus and the parieto-occipital sulcus.

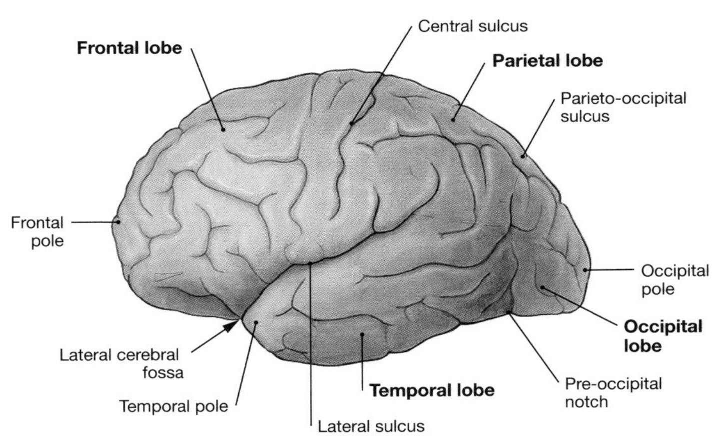
Frontal lobe
Central sulcus
Parietal lobe
Parieto-occipital sulcus
Frontal pole
Occipital pole
Occipital lobe
Lateral cerebral fossa
Temporal pole
Temporal lobe
Pre-occipital notch
Lateral sulcus

**Fig. 12.34 Cerebral lobes;** view from the left side. Each cerebral hemisphere divides into four lobes:

- frontal lobe
- parietal lobe
- temporal lobe
- occipital lobe

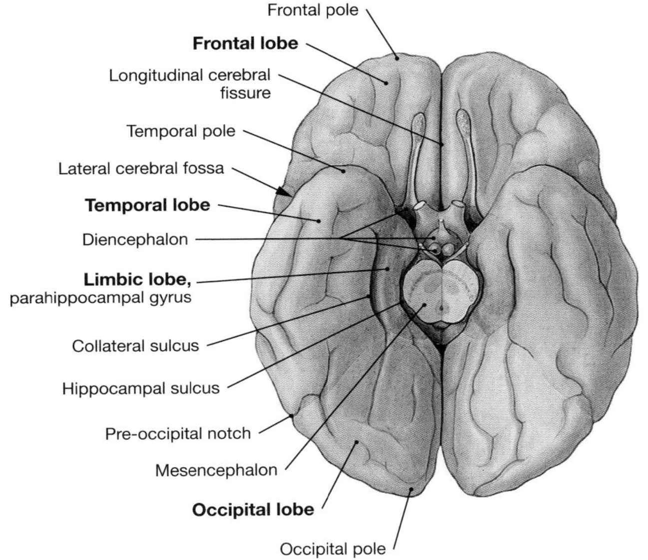
Frontal pole
Frontal lobe
Longitudinal cerebral fissure
Temporal pole
Lateral cerebral fossa
Temporal lobe
Diencephalon
Limbic lobe, parahippocampal gyrus
Collateral sulcus
Hippocampal sulcus
Pre-occipital notch
Mesencephalon
Occipital lobe
Occipital pole

**Fig. 12.35 Cerebral lobes;** inferior view.
In addition to the four cerebral lobes listed in the legend to → Fig. 12.34, the **limbic lobe** (composed mainly of the cingulate gyrus and the parahippocampal gyrus with the uncus) and the insular lobe (insula, not visible, since covered by the opercula of the frontal, parietal, and temporal lobes) can be distinguished.

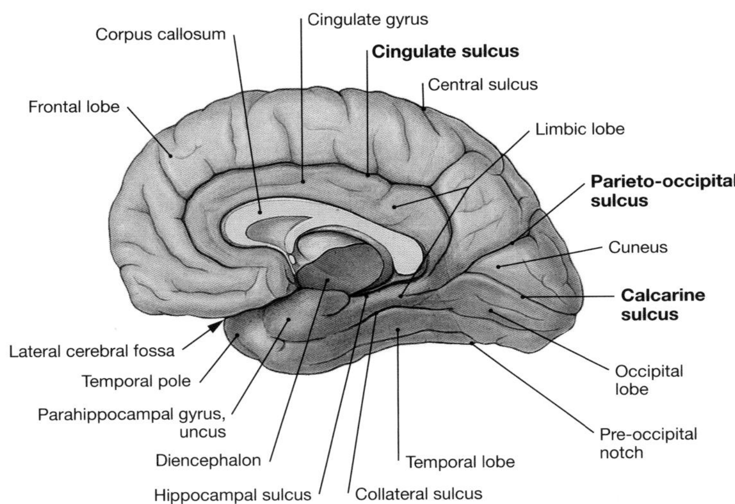
Corpus callosum
Cingulate gyrus
Cingulate sulcus
Central sulcus
Frontal lobe
Limbic lobe
Parieto-occipital sulcus
Cuneus
Calcarine sulcus
Lateral cerebral fossa
Temporal pole
Parahippocampal gyrus, uncus
Diencephalon
Hippocampal sulcus
Collateral sulcus
Temporal lobe
Occipital lobe
Pre-occipital notch

**Fig. 12.36 Cerebral lobes;** medial view.
Secondary and tertiary grooves in the telencephalon show individual variability. In many places, the margins drawn between the individual lobes are arbitrary (e.g. pre-occipital notch).

**Primary Grooves of the Cerebral Cortex**

| Sulcus | Location/Projection |
|---|---|
| Central sulcus | Extends between the frontal and parietal lobes; separates the (motor) precentral gyrus from the (sensory) postcentral gyrus |
| Lateral sulcus | Separates the frontal, parietal, and temporal lobes; deep within lie the lateral fossa and the insula |
| Parieto-occipital sulcus | Extends from the upper rim at the medial surface of the hemisphere to the calcarine sulcus; separates the parietal and occipital lobes |
| Calcarine sulcus | Like the parieto-occipital sulcus it extends at the medial surface of the hemisphere and both enclose the cuneus |
| Cingulate sulcus | Separates the cingulate gyrus (limbic lobe) from the frontal and parietal lobes |

## Telencephalon, cortex

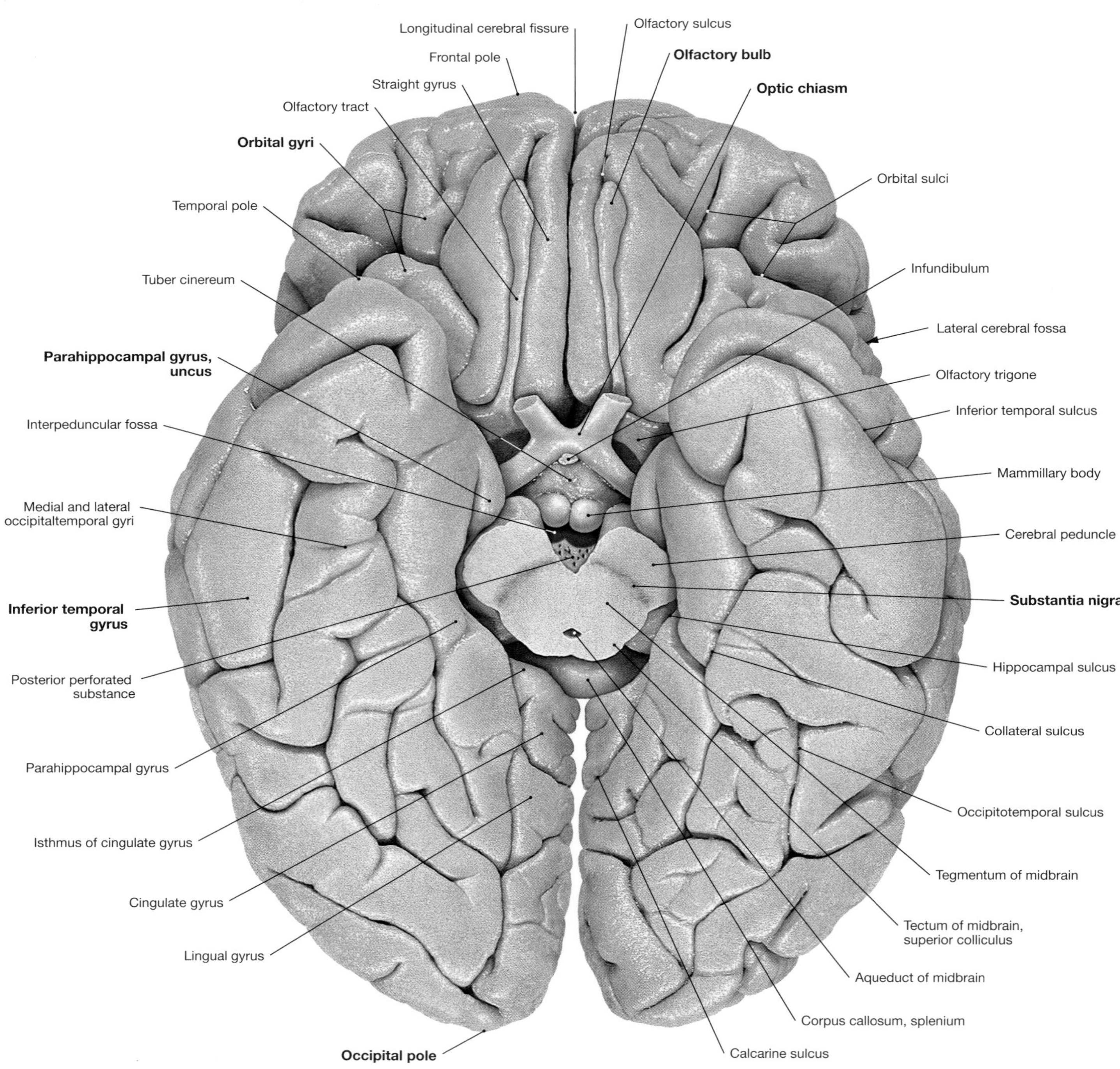
Longitudinal cerebral fissure
Olfactory sulcus
Frontal pole
Olfactory bulb
Straight gyrus
Optic chiasm
Olfactory tract
Orbital gyri
Orbital sulci
Temporal pole
Infundibulum
Tuber cinereum
Lateral cerebral fossa
Parahippocampal gyrus, uncus
Olfactory trigone
Inferior temporal sulcus
Interpeduncular fossa
Mammillary body
Medial and lateral occipitaltemporal gyri
Cerebral peduncle
Inferior temporal gyrus
Substantia nigra
Hippocampal sulcus
Posterior perforated substance
Collateral sulcus
Parahippocampal gyrus
Occipitotemporal sulcus
Isthmus of cingulate gyrus
Tegmentum of midbrain
Cingulate gyrus
Tectum of midbrain, superior colliculus
Lingual gyrus
Aqueduct of midbrain
Corpus callosum, splenium
Occipital pole
Calcarine sulcus

**Fig. 12.37 Gyri and grooves of the cerebral hemispheres;** inferior view; the midbrain has been sectioned.
The telencephalon occupies the majority of the cerebral base. Here, the olfactory bulb and olfactory tract overlying the orbital gyri are located. In addition, the optic chiasm, the parahippocampal gyrus in the temporal lobe with its characteristic anterior bend, the uncus, the temporal gyri, and the occipital pole are also visible. The dark colored substantia nigra is clearly visible in the mesencephalon.

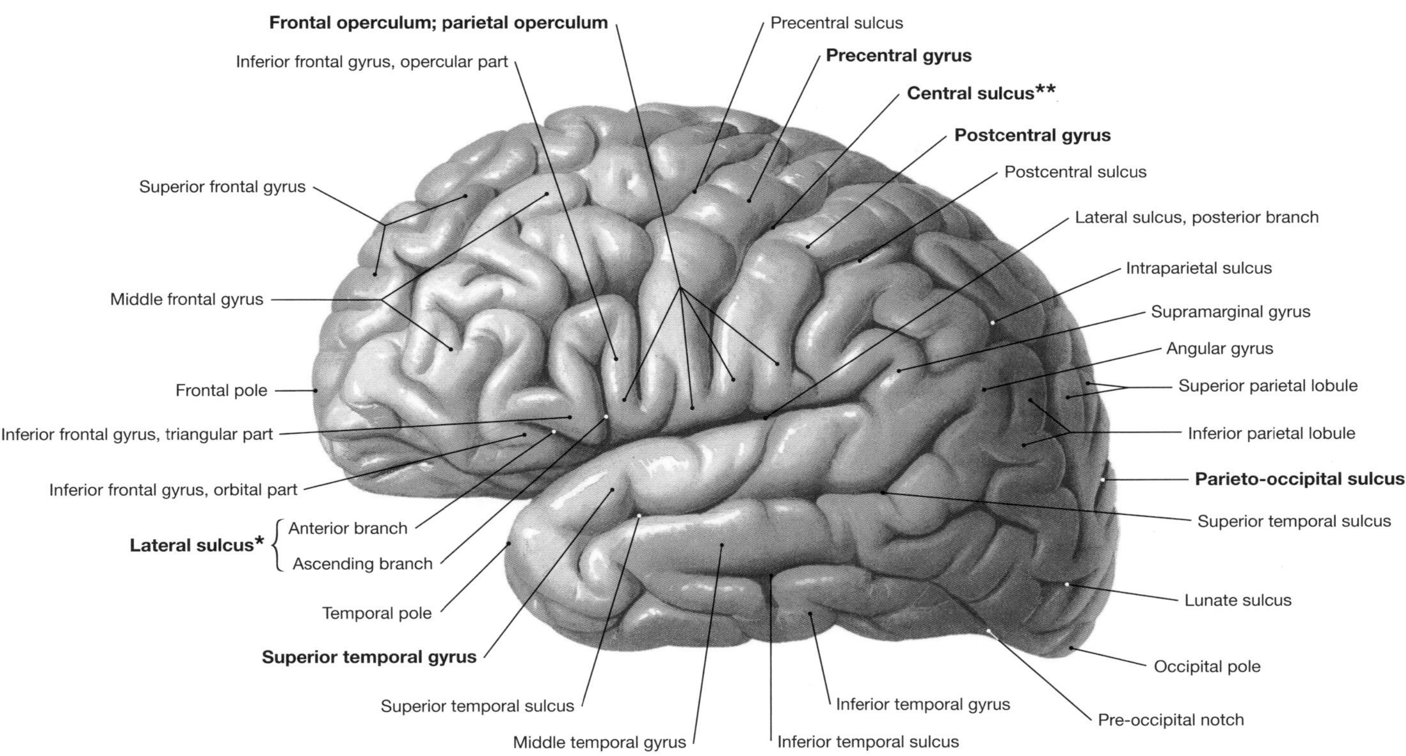
Frontal operculum; parietal operculum
Inferior frontal gyrus, opercular part
Precentral sulcus
Precentral gyrus
Central sulcus**
Postcentral gyrus
Postcentral sulcus
Lateral sulcus, posterior branch
Intraparietal sulcus
Supramarginal gyrus
Angular gyrus
Superior parietal lobule
Inferior parietal lobule
Parieto-occipital sulcus
Superior temporal sulcus
Lunate sulcus
Occipital pole
Pre-occipital notch
Superior frontal gyrus
Middle frontal gyrus
Frontal pole
Inferior frontal gyrus, triangular part
Inferior frontal gyrus, orbital part
Lateral sulcus*
Anterior branch
Ascending branch
Temporal pole
Superior temporal gyrus
Superior temporal sulcus
Middle temporal gyrus
Inferior temporal gyrus
Inferior temporal sulcus

**Fig. 12.38 Gyri and grooves of the cerebral hemispheres;** view from the left side.
Although the indicated gyri and sulci are present in each human brain (e.g. central sulcus, lateral sulcus, or superior temporal gyrus), no two brains or even two hemispheres of the same brain display an identical pattern of gyri and sulci. Similar to a fingerprint, the cerebral cortex is unique.

* SYLVIAN fissure
** fissure of ROLANDO or central fissure

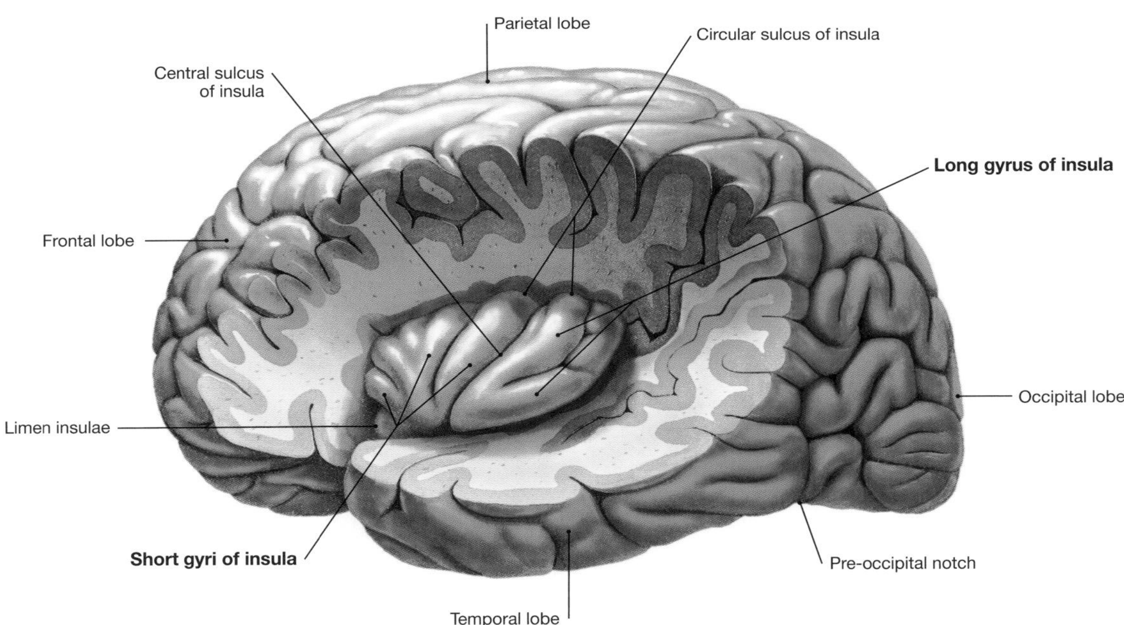
Parietal lobe
Circular sulcus of insula
Central sulcus of insula
Long gyrus of insula
Frontal lobe
Occipital lobe
Limen insulae
Short gyri of insula
Pre-occipital notch
Temporal lobe

**Fig. 12.39 Gyri and grooves of the cerebral hemispheres;** view from the left side; after removal of the parts of the frontal, parietal, and temporal lobes covering the insula.
The cortical regions of the frontal, parietal and temporal lobes that surround the lateral sulcus are called the opercula and have been removed to demonstrate the insula (→ Fig. 12.38). In the insula olfactory, gustatory, and visceral information is processed. In general the insula is considered a lobe of its own.

## Telencephalon, cortex

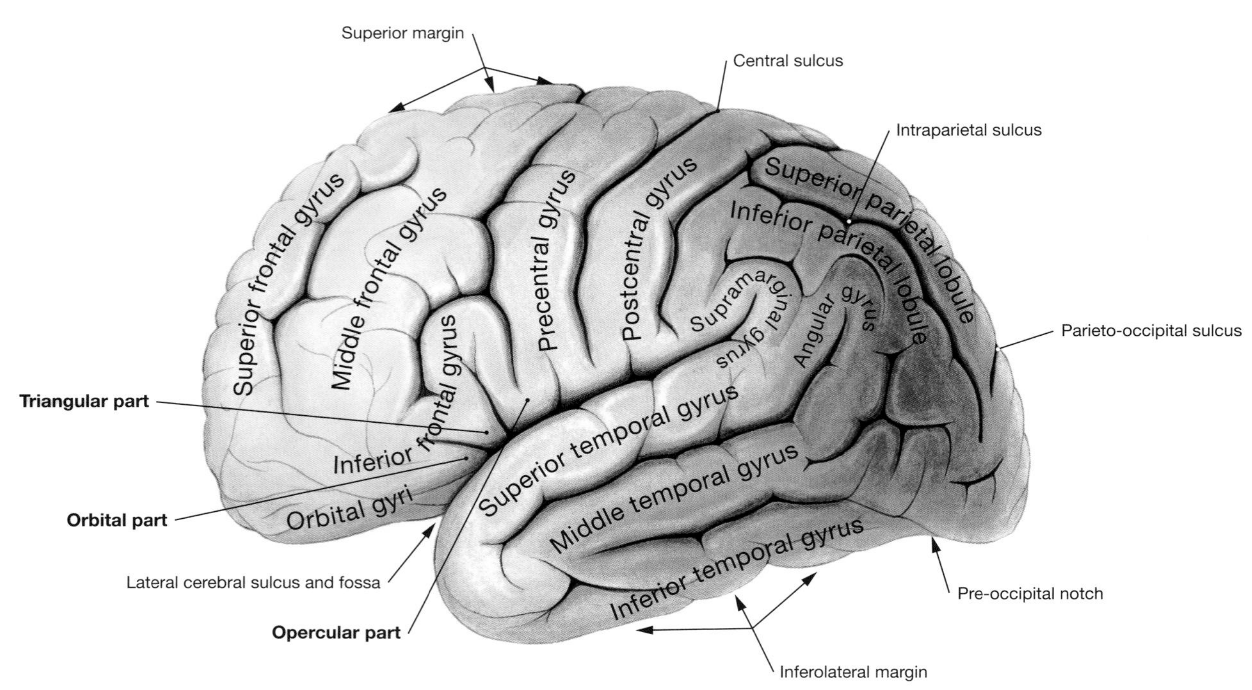
Superior margin
Central sulcus
Intraparietal sulcus
Superior parietal lobule
Inferior parietal lobule
Superior frontal gyrus
Middle frontal gyrus
Precentral gyrus
Postcentral gyrus
Supramarginal gyrus
Angular gyrus
Parieto-occipital sulcus
Triangular part
Inferior frontal gyrus
Superior temporal gyrus
Middle temporal gyrus
Orbital part
Orbital gyri
Lateral cerebral sulcus and fossa
Inferior temporal gyrus
Pre-occipital notch
Opercular part
Inferolateral margin

**Fig. 12.40 Gyri of the cerebral hemispheres;** view from the left side.

The frontal gyrus divides into an orbital part, a triangular part, and an opercular part.

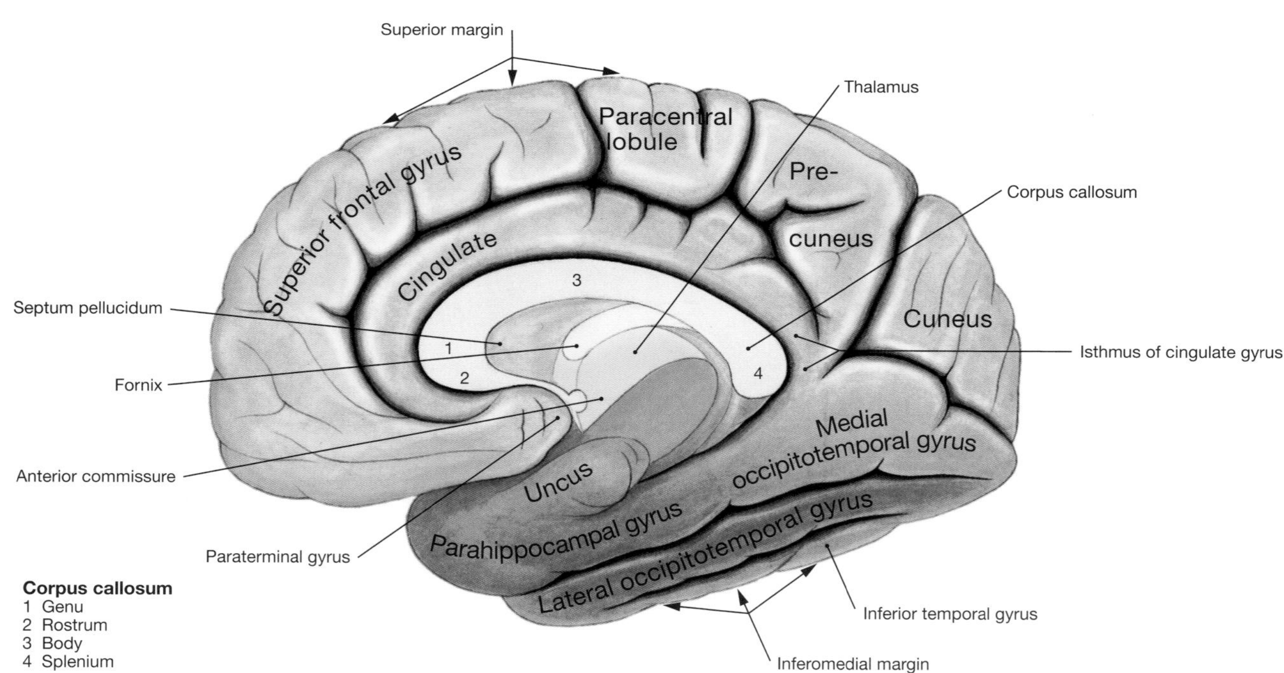
Superior margin
Thalamus
Paracentral lobule
Pre-cuneus
Superior frontal gyrus
Corpus callosum
Cingulate
3
Septum pellucidum
1
Cuneus
Isthmus of cingulate gyrus
Fornix
2
4
Medial occipitotemporal gyrus
Anterior commissure
Uncus
Parahippocampal gyrus
Paraterminal gyrus
Lateral occipitotemporal gyrus
Inferior temporal gyrus
Inferomedial margin
Corpus callosum
1 Genu
2 Rostrum
3 Body
4 Splenium

**Fig. 12.41 Gyri of the cerebral hemispheres;** medial view. The corpus callosum is composed of the rostrum, genu, trunk (body), and splenium. In addition, the fornix, the anterior commissure, the thalamus, and the septum pellucidum are visible.

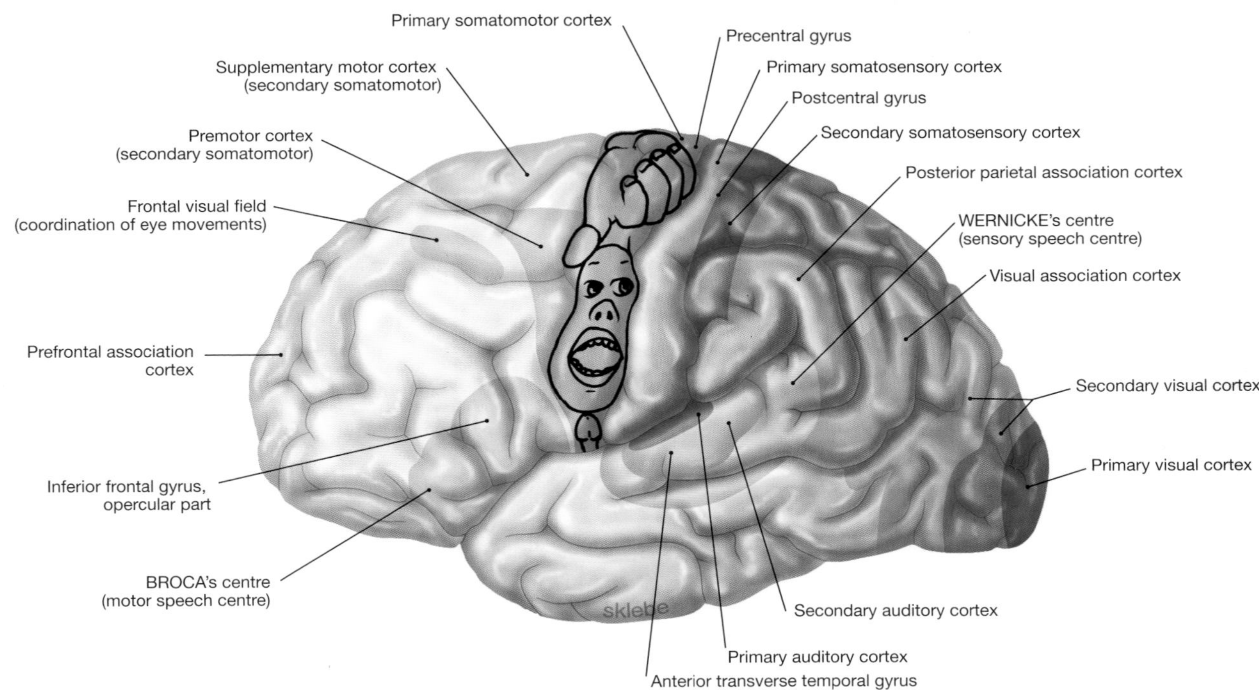
Primary somatomotor cortex
Precentral gyrus
Supplementary motor cortex (secondary somatomotor)
Primary somatosensory cortex
Postcentral gyrus
Premotor cortex (secondary somatomotor)
Secondary somatosensory cortex
Posterior parietal association cortex
Frontal visual field (coordination of eye movements)
WERNICKE's centre (sensory speech centre)
Visual association cortex
Prefrontal association cortex
Secondary visual cortex
Primary visual cortex
Inferior frontal gyrus, opercular part
BROCA's centre (motor speech centre)
Secondary auditory cortex
Primary auditory cortex
Anterior transverse temporal gyrus
sklebe

**Fig. 12.42 Functional cortical areas of the cerebral hemispheres;** view from the left side.
Higher cortical functions, like speech, require the cooperation of multiple different cortical areas. One can distinguish primary cortical areas (e.g. precentral gyrus, primary somatomotor cortex) from secondary and association areas of the cortex (e.g. premotor cortex, supplementary motor cortex). **Primary** and **secondary cortical areas** process specific sensory informations (e.g. perception and interpretation of visual impulses by the visual cortex in the occipital lobe). **Cortical association areas** (e.g. prefrontal association cortex) occupy most of the cortex and serve to integrate different and complex information patterns.
The outline of the human-like character (homunculus) reflects the somatotopic structure in the primary somatomotor cortex. Primary and secondary auditory cortices and the WERNICKE's center extend along the upper rim and inner surface of the temporal lobe.

→T 59

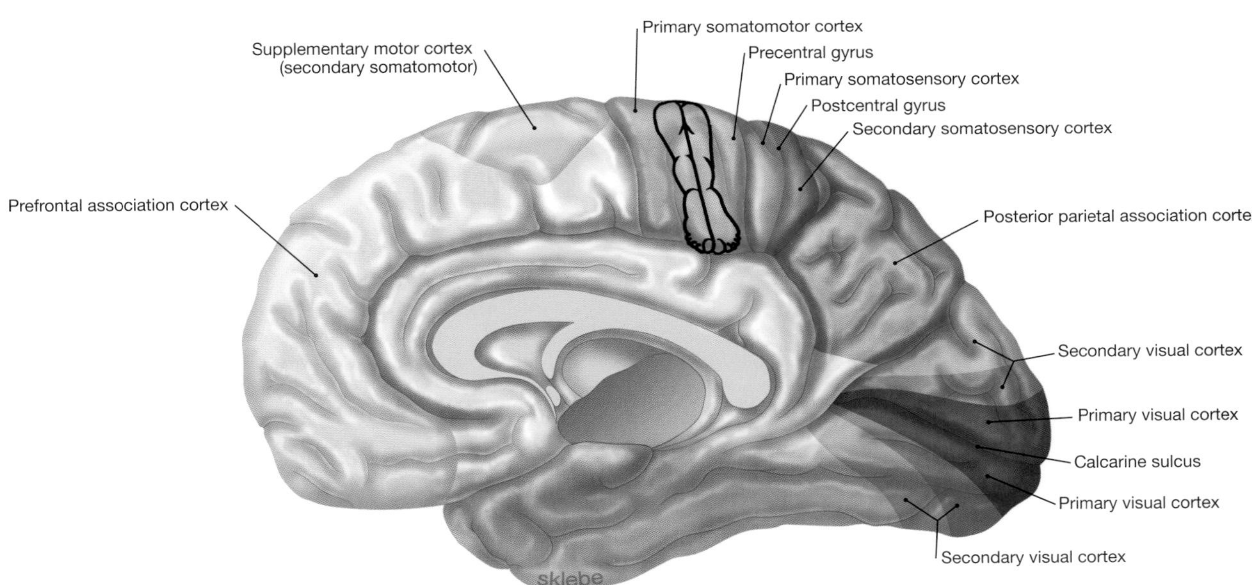
Primary somatomotor cortex
Supplementary motor cortex (secondary somatomotor)
Precentral gyrus
Primary somatosensory cortex
Postcentral gyrus
Secondary somatosensory cortex
Prefrontal association cortex
Posterior parietal association cortex
Secondary visual cortex
Primary visual cortex
Calcarine sulcus
Primary visual cortex
Secondary visual cortex
sklebe

**Fig. 12.43 Functional cortical areas of the cerebral hemispheres;** medial view.

The schematic outline of the homunculus illustrated in this figure and in → Fig. 12.42 roughly reflects the somatotopic organization.

→T 59

## Telencephalon, fornix

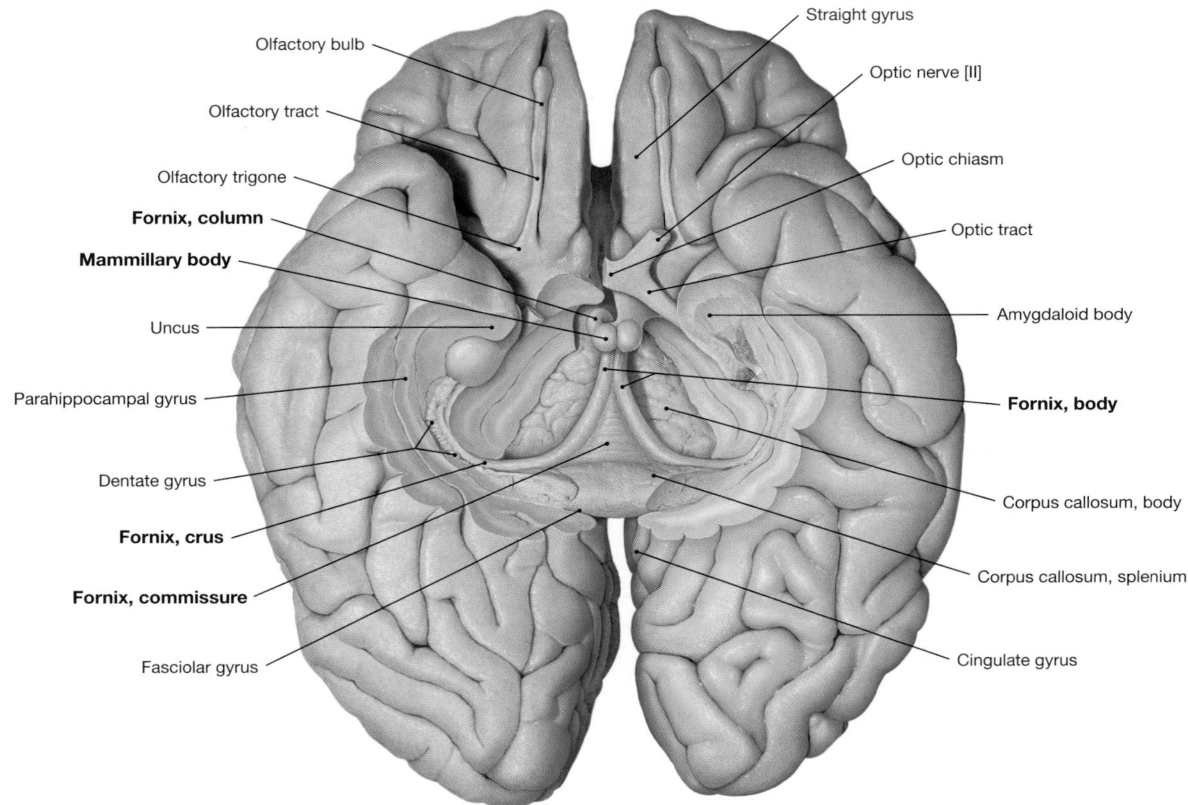
Olfactory bulb
Olfactory tract
Olfactory trigone
Fornix, column
Mammillary body
Uncus
Parahippocampal gyrus
Dentate gyrus
Fornix, crus
Fornix, commissure
Fasciolar gyrus
Straight gyrus
Optic nerve [II]
Optic chiasm
Optic tract
Amygdaloid body
Fornix, body
Corpus callosum, body
Corpus callosum, splenium
Cingulate gyrus

**Fig. 12.44 Fornix;** inferior view; after removal of the basal parts of the brain.
The fornix is a paired structure composed of the crus, commissure, body and column. It originates from the hippocampus and the subiculum in the temporal lobe and arches above the third ventricle towards the mamillary body. The fornices from both sides merge (commissure) before they reach the mamillary bodies. At the commissure, an **exchange of fibers** occurs.

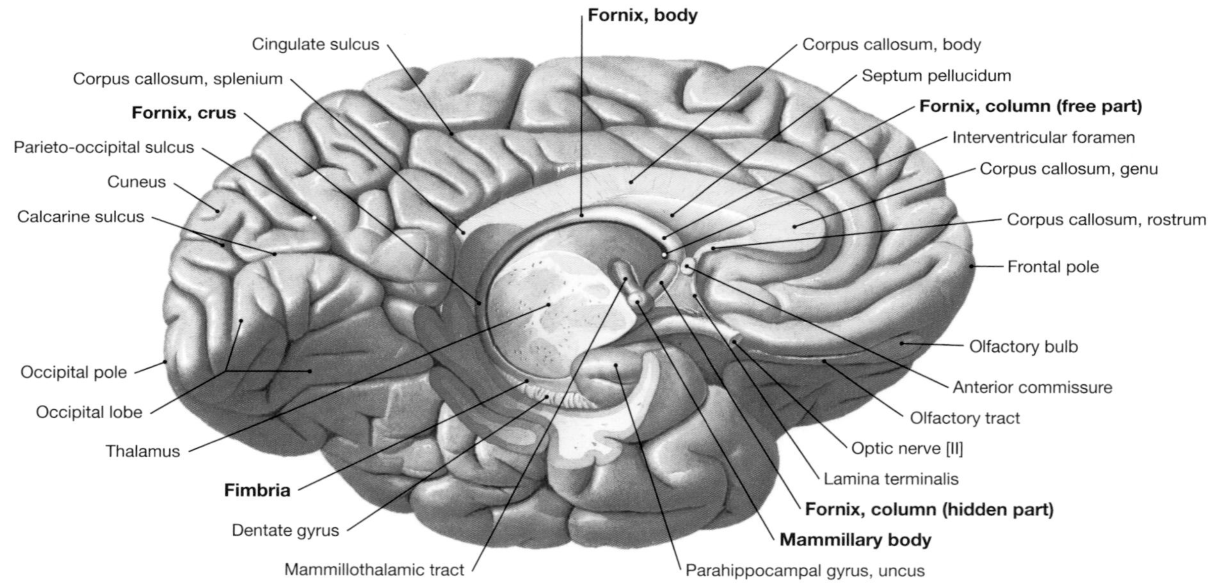
Fornix, body
Cingulate sulcus
Corpus callosum, splenium
Fornix, crus
Parieto-occipital sulcus
Cuneus
Calcarine sulcus
Occipital pole
Occipital lobe
Thalamus
Fimbria
Dentate gyrus
Mammillothalamic tract
Corpus callosum, body
Septum pellucidum
Fornix, column (free part)
Interventricular foramen
Corpus callosum, genu
Corpus callosum, rostrum
Frontal pole
Olfactory bulb
Anterior commissure
Olfactory tract
Optic nerve [II]
Lamina terminalis
Fornix, column (hidden part)
Mammillary body
Parahippocampal gyrus, uncus

**Fig. 12.45 Fornix;** inferior medial view.
The fornix is an important tract of the limbic system. **Fiber connections** exist to the anterior hypothalamic nuclei, the thalamus, and the habenulae. The figure shows the topographic relationships of the fornix.

### Clinical Remarks

Like the fornix and the hippocampus, the mamillary bodies are part of the limbic system. Although their exact role is unknown, the mamillary bodies are likely involved in memory processes. Chronic alcoholism can result in the destruction of the mamillary bodies with memory loss, disorientation, and confabulation (creation of false memory and beliefs) **(KORSAKOFF's syndrome).** The patient tries to create false "stories" to conceal his memory gaps.

## Telencephalon, fornix and anterior commissure

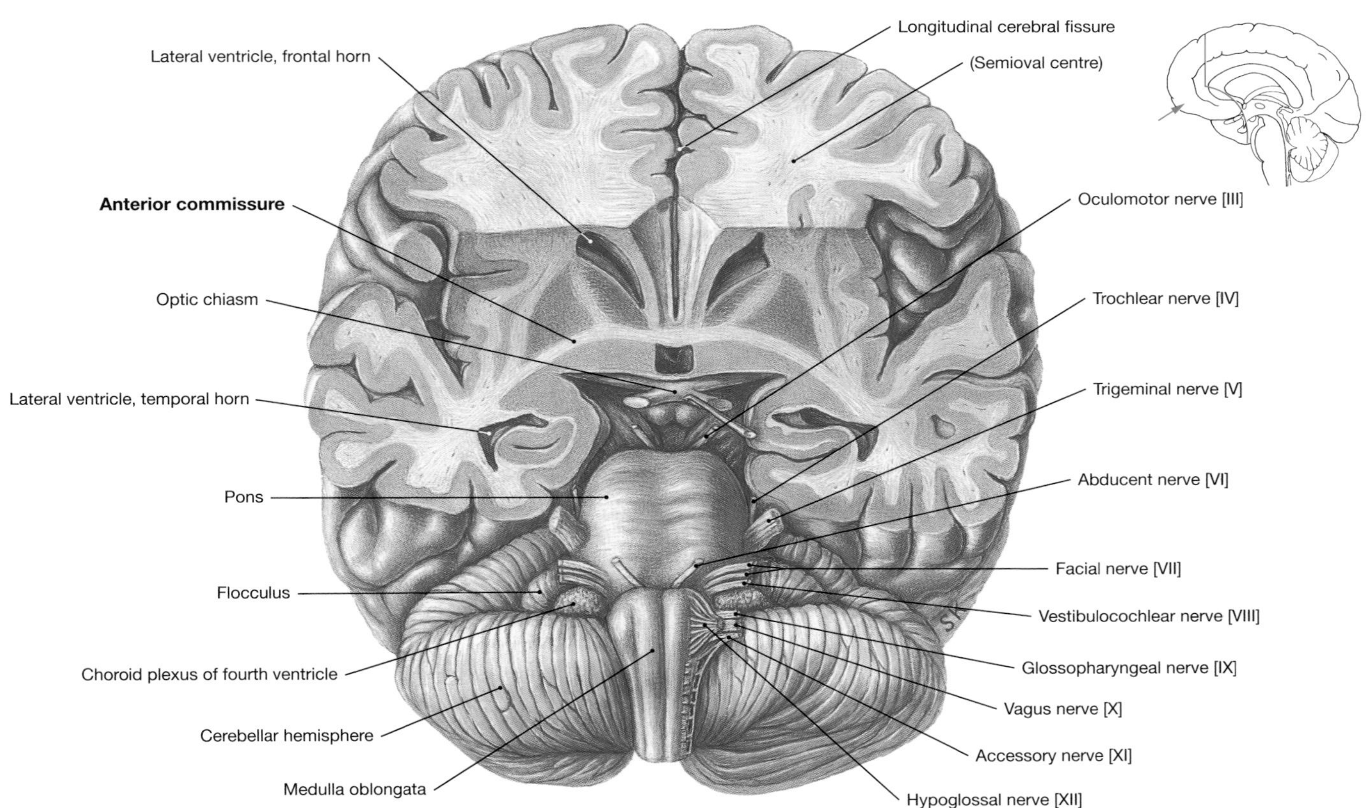
Lateral ventricle, frontal horn
Anterior commissure
Optic chiasm
Lateral ventricle, temporal horn
Pons
Flocculus
Choroid plexus of fourth ventricle
Cerebellar hemisphere
Medulla oblongata
Longitudinal cerebral fissure
(Semioval centre)
Oculomotor nerve [III]
Trochlear nerve [IV]
Trigeminal nerve [V]
Abducent nerve [VI]
Facial nerve [VII]
Vestibulocochlear nerve [VIII]
Glossopharyngeal nerve [IX]
Vagus nerve [X]
Accessory nerve [XI]
Hypoglossal nerve [XII]

**Fig. 12.46 Anterior commissure and brainstem;** inferior view; after partial removal of the basal parts of the cerebrum.
The anterior commissure is composed of commissural fibers. Located in the anterior wall of the third ventricle, it represents the commissural system of the paleocortex. The rostral part of the anterior commissure is small and connects the two olfactory tracts with the olfactory cortex of both hemispheres. The much more developed dorsal part facilitates the exchange of fibers between the rostral parts of the temporal lobes (particularly the cortex and amygdaloid body).

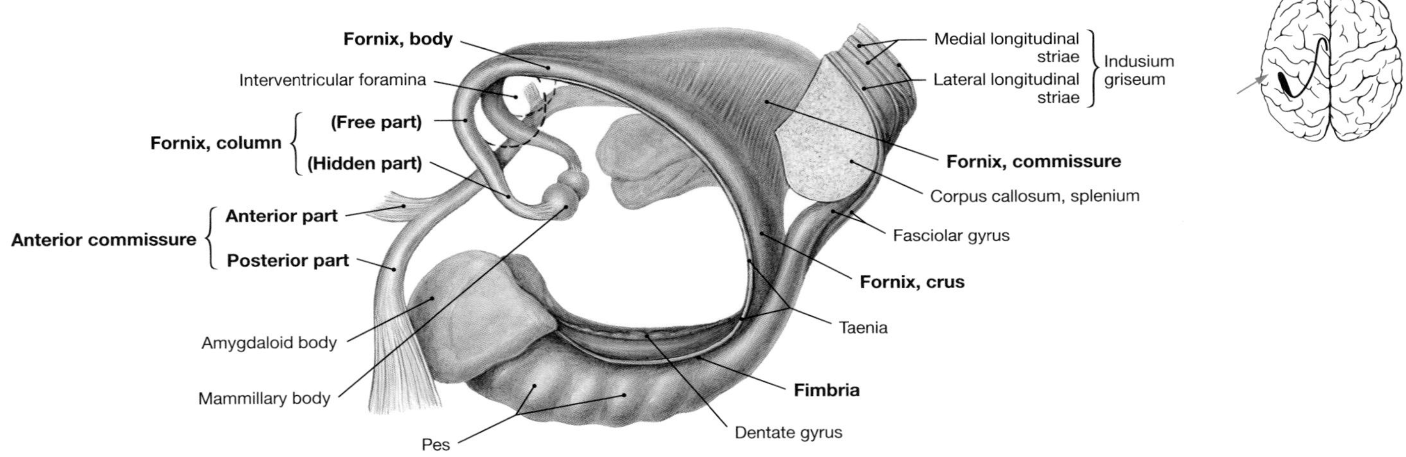
Fornix, body
Interventricular foramina
Fornix, column
(Free part)
(Hidden part)
Anterior commissure
Anterior part
Posterior part
Amygdaloid body
Mammillary body
Pes
Medial longitudinal striae
Lateral longitudinal striae
Indusium griseum
Fornix, commissure
Corpus callosum, splenium
Fasciolar gyrus
Fornix, crus
Taenia
Fimbria
Dentate gyrus

**Fig. 12.47 Anterior commissure, fornix and hippocampus formation, indusium griseum;** view from the left side.
All structures shown here are part of the **limbic system,** a functional concept with input from the telencephalon, diencephalon, and mesencephalon. Relevant structures are the hippocampi, the amygdaloid bodies, the cingulate gyri, and the septal nuclei. The limbic system regulates numerous functions, such as impulse, learning, memory, emotions, but also the regulation of food intake, digestion, and reproduction by the autonomic nervous system.
The **anterior commissure** is a fiber system (commissural fibers) composed of an anterior and posterior part. The anterior part connects the olfactory tracts and the olfactory cortices of both sides. The posterior part connects the rostral parts of the temporal lobes (particularly cortex and amygdaloid bodies). The amygdaloid body connects with the hippocampus.
The **hippocampus** displays the hippocampal digitations of the pes and the fimbria which transition into the crus of fornix. An exchange of fibers occurs in the region of the column. In its rostral part, the columns of the fornix continue as free and tectal parts and the tectal part connects to the mamillary bodies.

## Telencephalon, basal ganglia

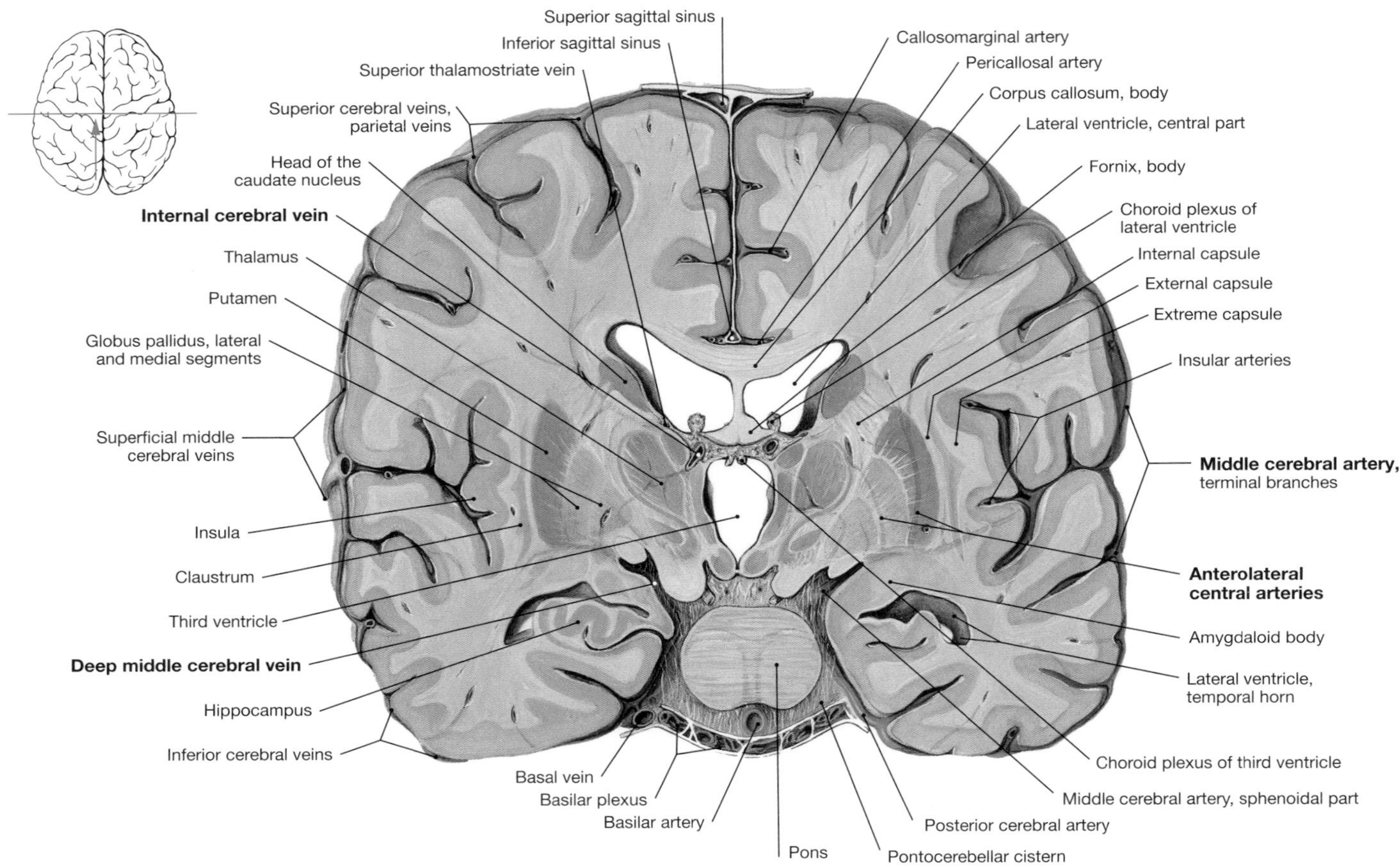
Superior sagittal sinus
Inferior sagittal sinus
Superior thalamostriate vein
Superior cerebral veins, parietal veins
Head of the caudate nucleus
Internal cerebral vein
Thalamus
Putamen
Globus pallidus, lateral and medial segments
Superficial middle cerebral veins
Insula
Claustrum
Third ventricle
Deep middle cerebral vein
Hippocampus
Inferior cerebral veins
Basal vein
Basilar plexus
Basilar artery
Pons
Pontocerebellar cistern
Posterior cerebral artery
Middle cerebral artery, sphenoidal part
Choroid plexus of third ventricle
Lateral ventricle, temporal horn
Amygdaloid body
Anterolateral central arteries
Middle cerebral artery, terminal branches
Insular arteries
Extreme capsule
External capsule
Internal capsule
Choroid plexus of lateral ventricle
Fornix, body
Lateral ventricle, central part
Corpus callosum, body
Pericallosal artery
Callosomarginal artery

**Fig. 12.48 Blood supply of the basal ganglia;** frontal section; posterior view; the arteries are shown on the right side and the veins on the left side.

The basal ganglia are supplied by the branches of the middle cerebral artery. On its way to the lateral fossa, the middle cerebral artery provides the anterolateral central arteries (anterolateral thalamostriate arteries, lenticulostriate arteries) for the basal ganglia and the internal capsule. The venous blood is drained by the deep middle cerebral vein and the internal cerebral vein.

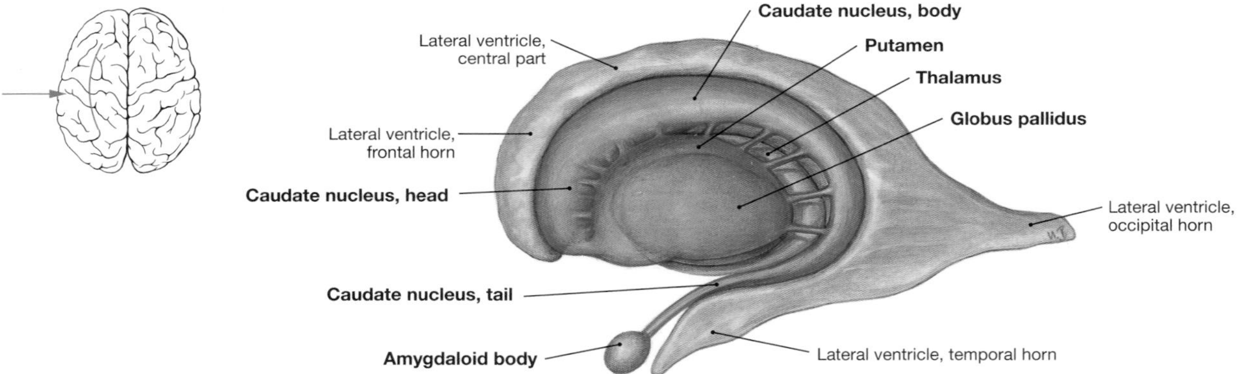
Lateral ventricle, central part
Caudate nucleus, body
Putamen
Thalamus
Globus pallidus
Lateral ventricle, frontal horn
Caudate nucleus, head
Lateral ventricle, occipital horn
Caudate nucleus, tail
Amygdaloid body
Lateral ventricle, temporal horn

**Fig. 12.49 Basal ganglia and thalamus;** view from the left side.

This figure depicts the topographic relationships between the lateral ventricle, caudate nucleus, amygdaloid body, putamen, globus pallidus, and thalamus. Many of these nuclei are collectively named basal ganglia. This includes the illustrated striatum (caudate nucleus and putamen) and the globus pallidus as well as the subthalamic nucleus and the substantia nigra in the mesencephalon (both not visible).

The basal ganglia are an integral part of different cortical feedback loops (cortex – basal ganglia – thalamus – cortex) and participate in the **motor cortical output.** Their main function is to modulate the motor activity (strength, direction, range of movement). Impulses reaching the basal ganglia are modulated either to directly enhance onto indirectly inhibit motor activity.

### Clinical Remarks

The **anterolateral central arteries** branch off the middle cerebral artery in an almost right angle and this can easily lead to turbulences in blood flow and a secondary formation of arteriosclerotic plaques at these sites. Individuals with high blood pressure (arterial hypertension) frequently develop **occlusions** at these critical branching points.

Occlusions as well as **bleedings** from these blood vessels cause a necrosis in the region of the basal ganglia and the internal capsule with resulting contralateral hemiplegia. Depending on the location of the **damage to the basal ganglia,** a severe hyperkinetic or hypokinetic movement disorder can result (dystonia).

## Diencephalon

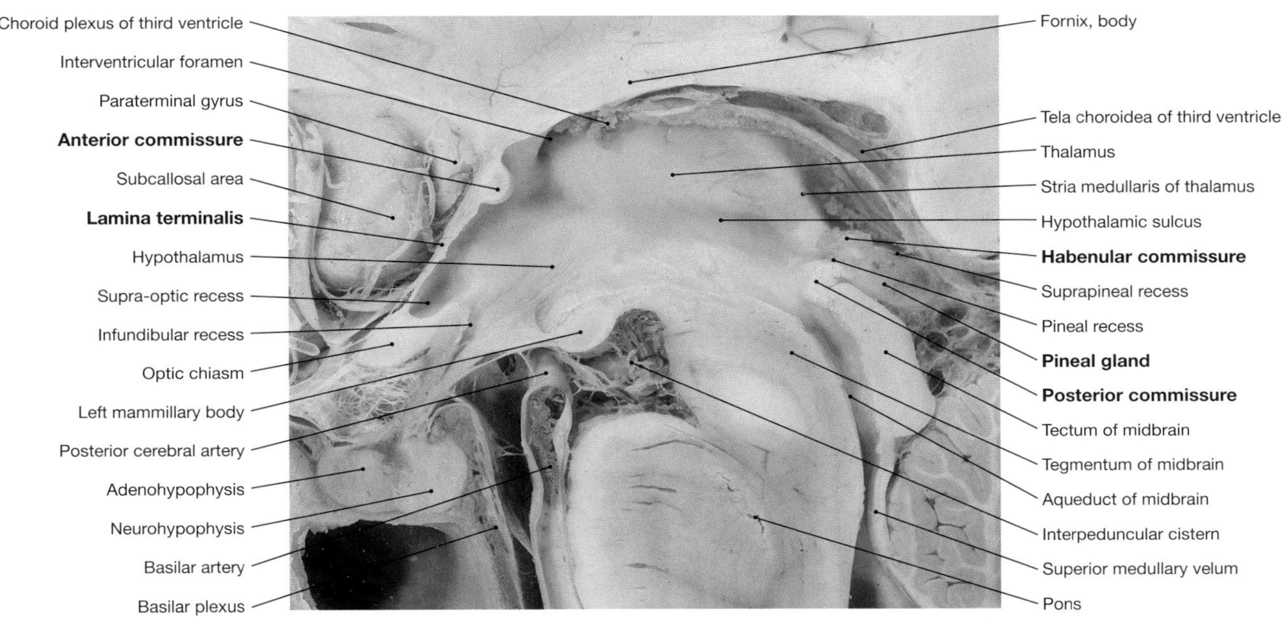
Choroid plexus of third ventricle
Interventricular foramen
Paraterminal gyrus
Anterior commissure
Subcallosal area
Lamina terminalis
Hypothalamus
Supra-optic recess
Infundibular recess
Optic chiasm
Left mammillary body
Posterior cerebral artery
Adenohypophysis
Neurohypophysis
Basilar artery
Basilar plexus
Fornix, body
Tela choroidea of third ventricle
Thalamus
Stria medullaris of thalamus
Hypothalamic sulcus
Habenular commissure
Suprapineal recess
Pineal recess
Pineal gland
Posterior commissure
Tectum of midbrain
Tegmentum of midbrain
Aqueduct of midbrain
Interpeduncular cistern
Superior medullary velum
Pons

**Fig. 12.50 Third ventricle and diencephalon;** median section.
Phylogenetically, the diencephalon derives from the prosencephalon and is located between the telencephalon and the mesencephalon. The diencephalon surrounds the third ventricle and divides into the epithalamus, thalamus (dorsal), hypothalamus, and the subthalamus (ventral).

The anterior commissure and the lamina terminalis represent the rostral margin of the diencephalon (anterior commissure to the optic chiasm). The posterior commissure, the habenular commissure, and the pineal gland constitute the inferior margin of the diencephalon.

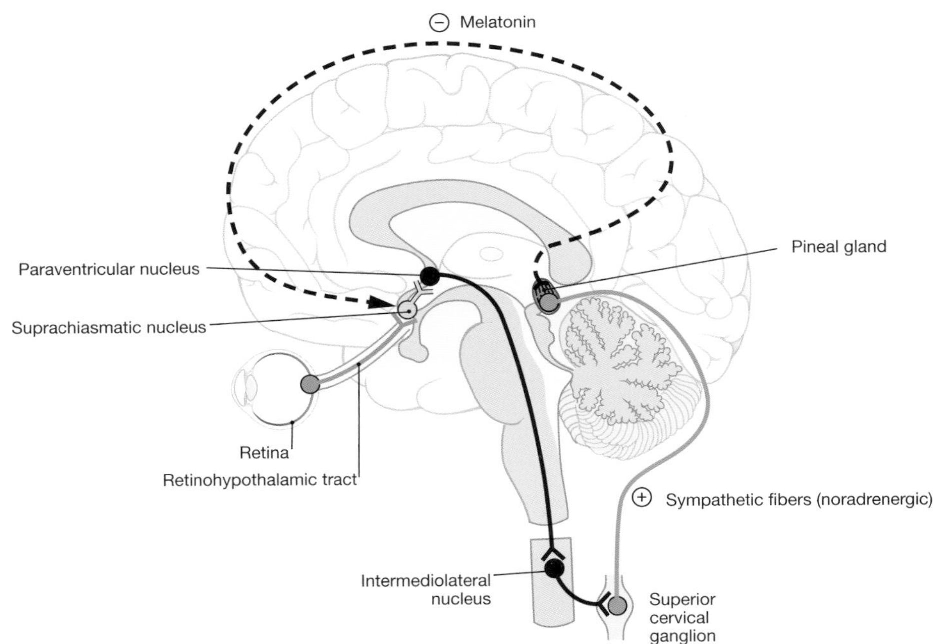
⊖ Melatonin
Paraventricular nucleus
Suprachiasmatic nucleus
Retina
Retinohypothalamic tract
Pineal gland
⊕ Sympathetic fibers (noradrenergic)
Intermediolateral nucleus
Superior cervical ganglion

**Fig. 12.51 Neural circuitry involved in the regulation of the pineal gland;** schematic median section. (according to [2])
The epithalamus is composed of the striae medullares of thalamus, the habenulae, the habenular nuclei, the habenular commissure, the posterior (epithalamic) commissure, the pretectal area, and the pineal gland. The production of **melatonin** in pinealocytes of the pineal gland is light dependent. Melatonin is an important regulator of circadian rhythms and does so by affecting the function of other endocrine organs. In addition, melatonin acts on the suprachiasmatic nucleus and via a feedback loop modulates its role in synchronizing endogenous with environmental rhythms.
The **circuitry** initiates at the photoreceptors of the retina which send signals to the suprachiasmatic nucleus in the hypothalamus (retinohypothalamic tract). This information is conveyed to the hypothalamic paraventricular nucleus, from here projects to the superior cervical ganglion of the sympathetic system, and then reaches the pinealocytes of the pineal gland. The production of melatonin increases in the dark.

## Diencephalon, thalamus

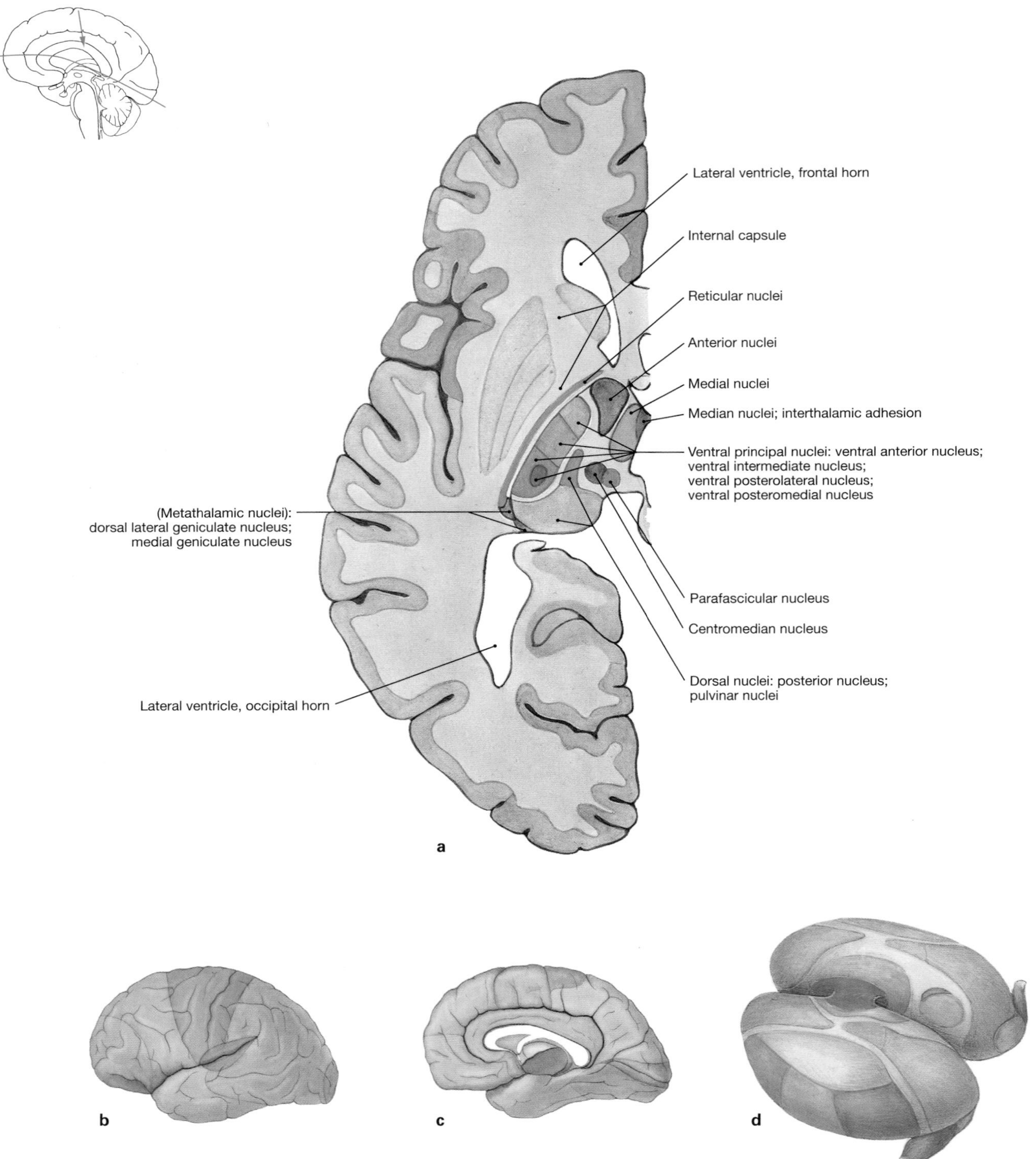
Lateral ventricle, frontal horn
Internal capsule
Reticular nuclei
Anterior nuclei
Medial nuclei
Median nuclei; interthalamic adhesion
Ventral principal nuclei: ventral anterior nucleus; ventral intermediate nucleus; ventral posterolateral nucleus; ventral posteromedial nucleus
(Metathalamic nuclei): dorsal lateral geniculate nucleus; medial geniculate nucleus
Parafascicular nucleus
Centromedian nucleus
Dorsal nuclei: posterior nucleus; pulvinar nuclei
Lateral ventricle, occipital horn
a
b
c
d

**Figs. 12.52a to d Nuclei and cortical projections of the thalamus.** Corresponding nuclei and cortical projections are indicated by the same color.

**a** Horizontal section through the left cerebral hemisphere
**b** Left cerebral hemisphere from the left (lateral) side
**c** Right cerebral hemisphere from the medial side
**d** View onto both thalami from a superior oblique angle

The thalamus is regarded as the **"gateway to consciousness".** All sensory input to the body is synapsed and integrated in the thalamus (with the exception of olfactory sensations) prior to this information reaching the cortex. In addition, the thalamus participates in the modulation of autonomic and motor activities. The thalamus is composed of specific and nonspecific groups of nuclei (more than 100 nuclear regions, including the lateral and medial geniculate bodies [see visual and auditory pathways; → Fig. 12.59]). **Specific thalamic nuclei** (palliothalamus) connect with defined cortical regions (primary cortical projection and association fields); **nonspecific thalamic nuclei** (truncothalamus) project broadly into the brainstem and diffusely into some cortical areas.

→ T 60

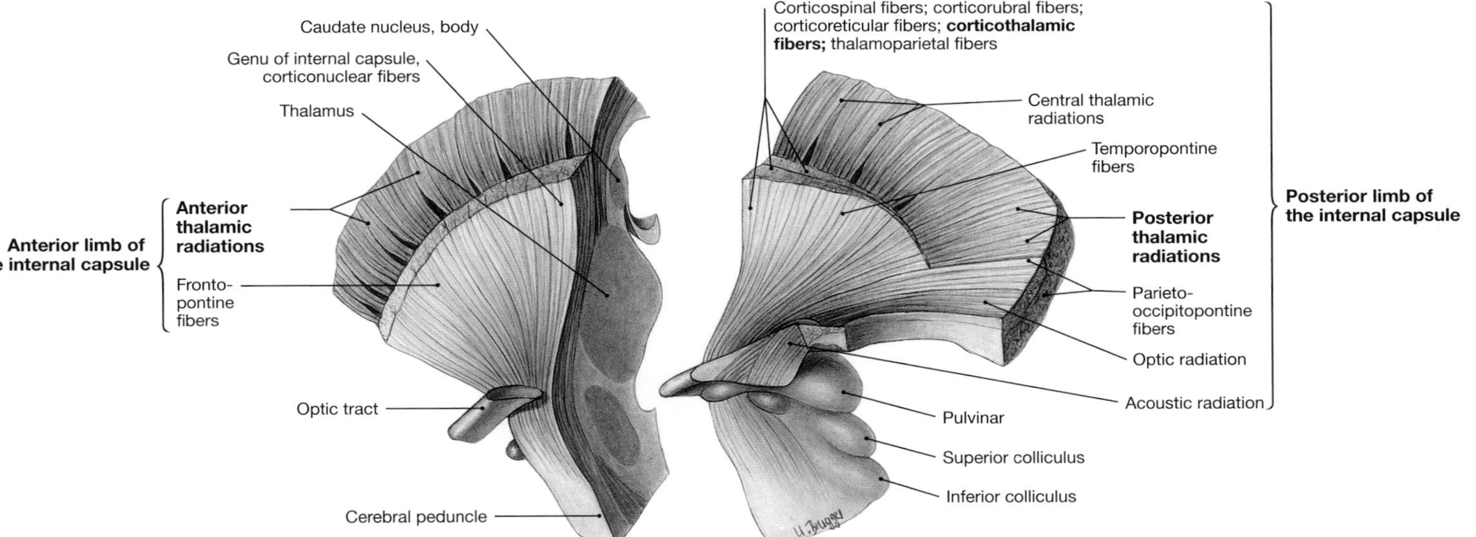
Caudate nucleus, body
Genu of internal capsule, corticonuclear fibers
Thalamus
Anterior thalamic radiations
Anterior limb of the internal capsule
Fronto-pontine fibers
Optic tract
Cerebral peduncle
Corticospinal fibers; corticorubral fibers; corticoreticular fibers; corticothalamic fibers; thalamoparietal fibers
Central thalamic radiations
Temporopontine fibers
Posterior thalamic radiations
Parieto-occipitopontine fibers
Optic radiation
Acoustic radiation
Posterior limb of the internal capsule
Pulvinar
Superior colliculus
Inferior colliculus

**Fig. 12.53 Thalamic radiation and internal capsule;** view from the left side; divided into two parts by a frontal section.
Thalamic nuclei mainly project into the cortex. Their projections contribute to the formation of the anterior limb and the posteror limb of the internal capsule. The anterior and posterior thalamic radiations are part of these projections as are the corticothalamic fibers and the thalamoparietal fibers.

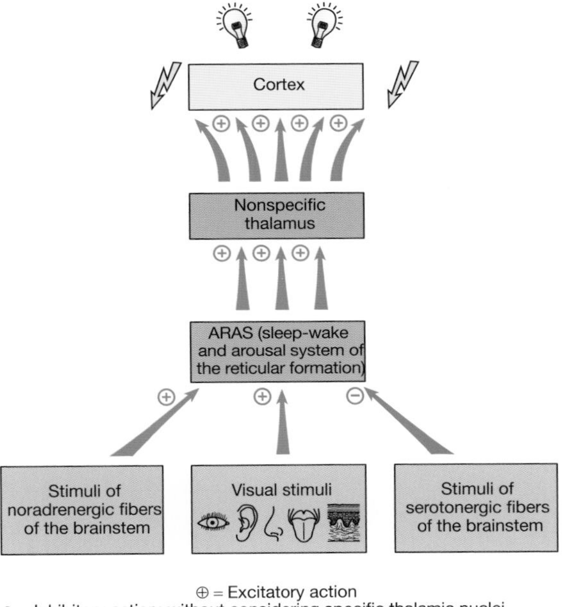
Cortex
Nonspecific thalamus
ARAS (sleep-wake and arousal system of the reticular formation)
Stimuli of noradrenergic fibers of the brainstem
Visual stimuli
Stimuli of serotonergic fibers of the brainstem
⊕ = Excitatory action
⊖ = Inhibitory action; without considering specific thalamic nuclei

**Fig. 12.54 Ascending reticular activation system (ARAS);** specific thalamic nuclei have been excluded. [23]
The **median nuclei of thalamus** and the **intralaminar group of nuclei,** of which the centromedian nucleus is the largest nucleus, belong to the group of nonspecific thalamic nuclei. Corresponding to the broad and diffuse connections with the cortex, the intralaminar group of nuclei is involved in the nonspecific and general excitation of the cortex. This puts the body in a state of alertness and readiness. This state of arousal is controlled by signals from the ARAS of the reticular formation reaching the intralaminar thalamic nuclei which then activate the entire cortex via the nonspecific connections.

## Clinical Remarks

**Lesions of the nonspecific thalamic nuclei,** e.g. due to disturbances in blood circulation, result in an impaired consciousness with reduced awareness.
Depending on the location, damage to the **specific thalamic nuclei** may cause sensory impairment (ventral posterolateral nucleus), hemianopsia, pain (thalamic pain), motor disorders like paralysis, ataxia (anterior ventrolateral nucleus) as well as personality changes.

## Diencephalon, hypothalamus and pituitary gland

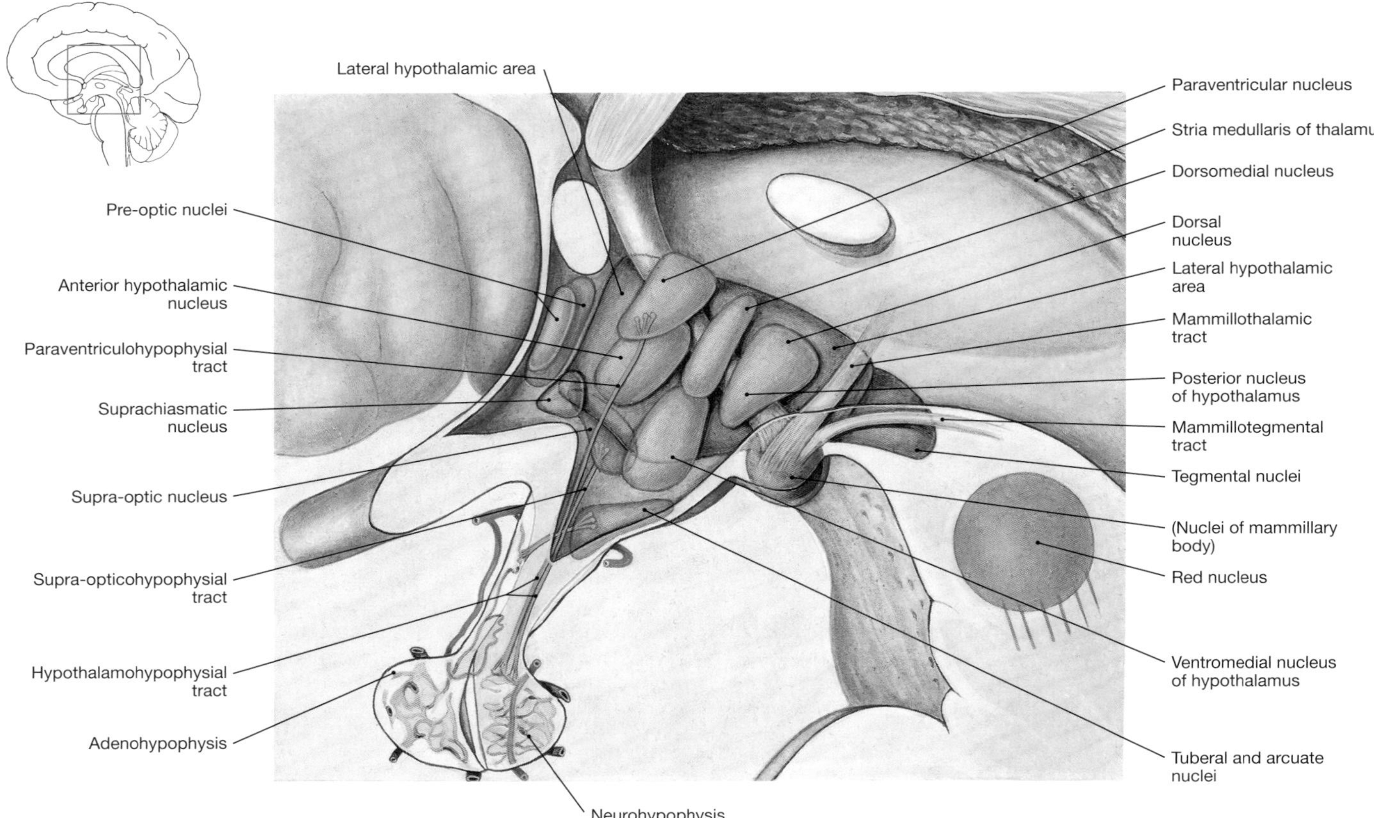
Lateral hypothalamic area
Paraventricular nucleus
Stria medullaris of thalamus
Dorsomedial nucleus
Pre-optic nuclei
Dorsal nucleus
Lateral hypothalamic area
Anterior hypothalamic nucleus
Mammillothalamic tract
Paraventriculohypophysial tract
Posterior nucleus of hypothalamus
Suprachiasmatic nucleus
Mammillotegmental tract
Tegmental nuclei
Supra-optic nucleus
(Nuclei of mammillary body)
Supra-opticohypophysial tract
Red nucleus
Hypothalamohypophysial tract
Ventromedial nucleus of hypothalamus
Adenohypophysis
Tuberal and arcuate nuclei
Neurohypophysis

**Fig. 12.55 Hypothalamus;** medial view; overview, nuclei illustrated translucently.
Forming the floor of the diencephalon, the hypothalamus is the supervisory regulatory center of the autonomic nervous system.
The hypothalamus is composed of multiple groups of nuclei, which, according to their location, divide into the anterior, middle, and posterior groups of hypothalamic nuclei:

- The **anterior group** of hypothalamic nuclei comprises the suprachiasmatic nucleus (central pacemaker of the circadian rhythm, sleep-wake cycle, body temperature, blood pressure), the paraventricular and supra-optic nuclei (production of antidiuretic hormone [ADH] and oxytocin and axonal transport [hypothalamohypophysial tract] to the neurohypophysis), and the preoptic nuclei (participation in the regulation of blood pressure, body temperature, sexual behaviour, menstrual cycle, gonadotropin).
- The **middle group** of hypothalamic nuclei comprises the tuberal, dorsomedial, ventromedial, and arcuate [infundibular = semilunar] nuclei (production and secretion of releasing and release-inhibiting hormones, participation in the regulation of water and food intake).
- The **posterior group** of hypothalamic nuclei comprises the nuclei of mammilary body in the mammilary bodies which are integrated into the limbic system by receiving afferent fibers from the fornix and projecting efferent fibers to the thalamus (mamillothalamic fasciculus). They modulate sexual functions and play an important role in activities related to memory and emotions. These nuclei connect to the tegmentum of midbrain via the mamillotegmental fasciculus.

In the caudal aspect of the hypothalamus, the infundibulum (pituitary stalk) connects the pituitary gland to the rest of the hypothalamus. The pituitary gland divides into the anterior (adenohypophysis) and posterior (neurohypophysis) lobes.

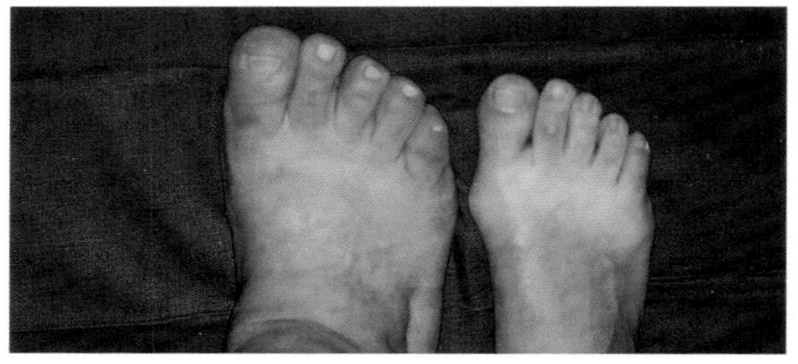

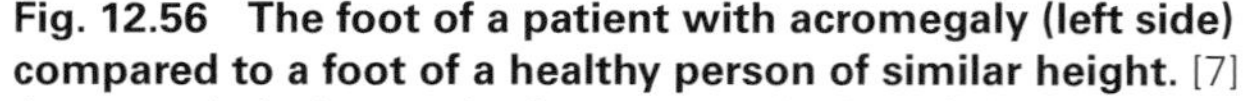

**Fig. 12.56 The foot of a patient with acromegaly (left side) compared to a foot of a healthy person of similar height.** [7]
Acromegaly is the result of an overproduction of the growth hormone somatotropin (STH) in the adenohypophysis caused by a benign tumor in the anterior lobe of the pituitary gland, a part of the diencephalon.

### Clinical Remarks

Damage to the paraventricular nucleus and particularly to the supra-optic nucleus causes a deficiency in **ADH.** Consequently, the inability to reabsorb water in the renal collecting tubules results in **diabetes insipidus.** Patients urinate excessively and excrete up to 20 liters of urine daily.
**Acromegaly** describes the distinct enlargement of the limbs and protruding body parts (acra) like hands, feet (→ Fig. 12.56), chin, mandible, ears, nose, eyebrows, or genitals. This is caused by an overproduction of the growth hormone **STH** in the anterior lobe of the pituitary gland, mainly resulting from a benign and more rarely from a malignant tumor. **Gigantism** with excessive growth and height results from an STH-producing tumor in the anterior lobe of the pituitary gland that has formed prior to the completion of the growth phase. Once the epiphyseal plates (growth plates) are closed, enlargement is restricted to the acra.

## Mesencephalon

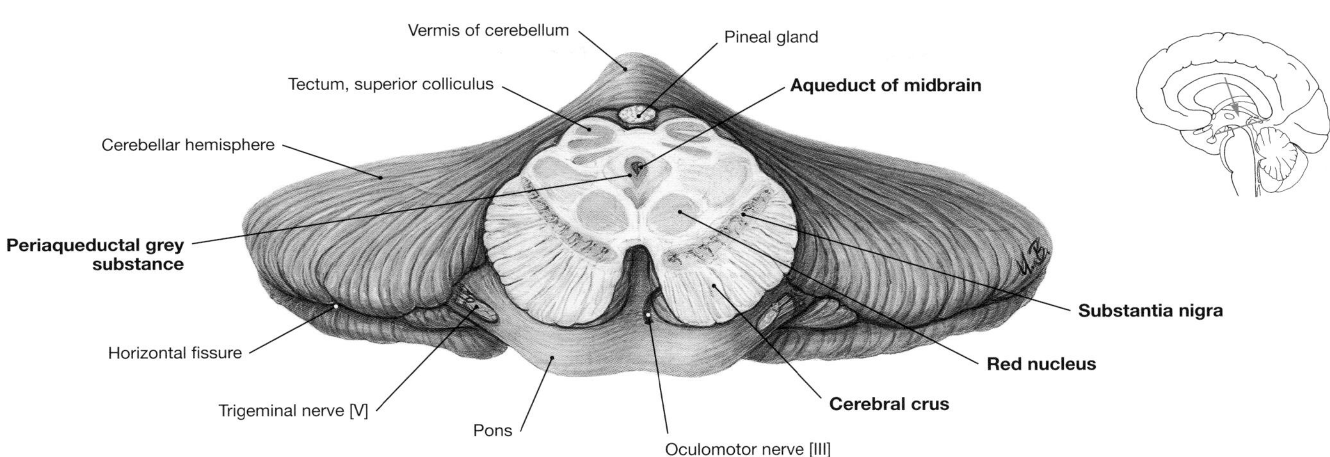
Vermis of cerebellum
Pineal gland
Tectum, superior colliculus
Aqueduct of midbrain
Cerebellar hemisphere
Periaqueductal grey substance
Substantia nigra
Horizontal fissure
Red nucleus
Trigeminal nerve [V]
Cerebral crus
Pons
Oculomotor nerve [III]

**Fig. 12.57 Mesencephalon, midbrain;** cross-section at the level of the superior colliculi; anterior view.

The mesencephalon is composed of the base, the tegmentum, and the tectum. Both, tegmentum and base of midbrain are collectively named cerebral peduncles.

The **base of midbrain** comprises the cerebral crura which contain different fiber tracts (e.g. corticonuclear fibers).

The **tegmentum of midbrain** comprises the central (periaqueductal) gray substance surrounding the aqueduct of midbrain (participates in the central suppression of pain, facilitates fear and flight reflexes, regulates autonomic nervous processes) and the substantia nigra as part of the basal ganglia. Additional structures of the tegmentum of midbrain include the red nucleus, an important relay station of the motor system, the mesencephalic parts of the reticular formation, the nuclei of the cranial nerves II and IV, as well as ascending and descending tracts.

The **tectum of midbrain** (tectal plate [quadrigeminal plate]) includes the paired superior and inferior colliculi. These are important relay stations for visual reflexes (superior colliculi) and the central auditory pathway (inferior colliculi).

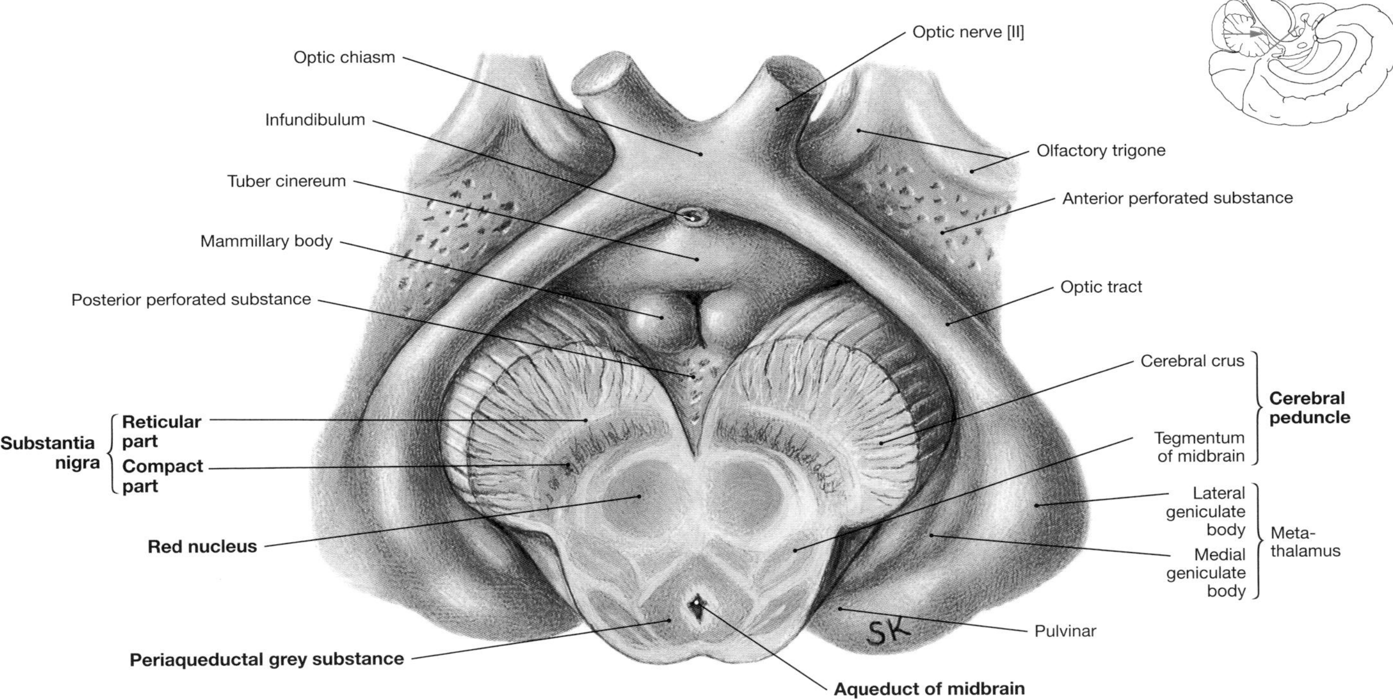
Optic nerve [II]
Optic chiasm
Infundibulum
Olfactory trigone
Tuber cinereum
Anterior perforated substance
Mammillary body
Optic tract
Posterior perforated substance
Cerebral crus
Tegmentum of midbrain
Cerebral peduncle
Substantia nigra
Reticular part
Compact part
Lateral geniculate body
Medial geniculate body
Metathalamus
Red nucleus
Pulvinar
Periaqueductal grey substance
Aqueduct of midbrain

**Fig. 12.58 Mesencephalon, midbrain, and diencephalon;** inferior view; after oblique section of the midbrain.

The illustration demonstrates the division of the mesencephalon into basis, tegmentum, and tectum of midbrain. Structures distinctly separate of the midbrain are the substantia nigra, the red nucleus, and the aqueduct of midbrain with the surrounding central (periaqueductal) gray substance. The substantia nigra subdivides into the reticular part and the compact part.

## Clinical Remarks

The primary cause of **PARKINSON's disease** is the greatly reduced dopamine synthesis, particularly in the substantia nigra. The decrease in dopamine results in a syndrome (paralysis agitans, shaking palsy) characterized by hypokinesis, rigor, and resting tremor. In addition, these patients suffer from increased secretion of saliva, tears, sweat, and sebum. Also, these patients display cognitive and mood disturbances. PARKINSON's disease affects approximately 1% of individuals over 60 years of age. A PARKINSON-like disease can develop after encephalitis, intoxications, long-term psychotropic drug medication, etc.

**Lesions of the red nucleus** cause symptoms similar to cerebellar lesions, including cerebellar (intention) tremor and reduced muscular tonus, due to the inclusion of this nucleus in the important neuronal circuitry between "cerebellum – red nucleus – cerebellum – inferior olivary nucleus – cerebellum".

## Mesencephalon and brainstem

**Fig. 12.59 Brainstem;** lateral view; oblique view on the floor of the fourth ventricle after sectioning of the cerebellar peduncles.
The brainstem consists of the mesencephalon (midbrain), pons, and medulla oblongata. The **mesencephalon** extends from the diencephalon to the upper margin of the pons. The cerebral peduncle is located at its anterior side. The superior and inferior colliculi of the tectum of midbrain form the dorsal side and create the particular shape of the quadrigeminal plate (tectal plate). The pineal gland and the fourth ventricle are positioned superior and inferior to the quadrigeminal plate, respectively.
The **cerebellum** has been sectioned at the cerebellar peduncles. Visible are the cranial nerves IV, V, and VII to XII exiting the brainstem. Their nuclei are located in the brainstem. The nuclei of the cranial nerves III and VI are also located in the brainstem but these nerves exit at the anterior side and, thus, are not visible in this figure.

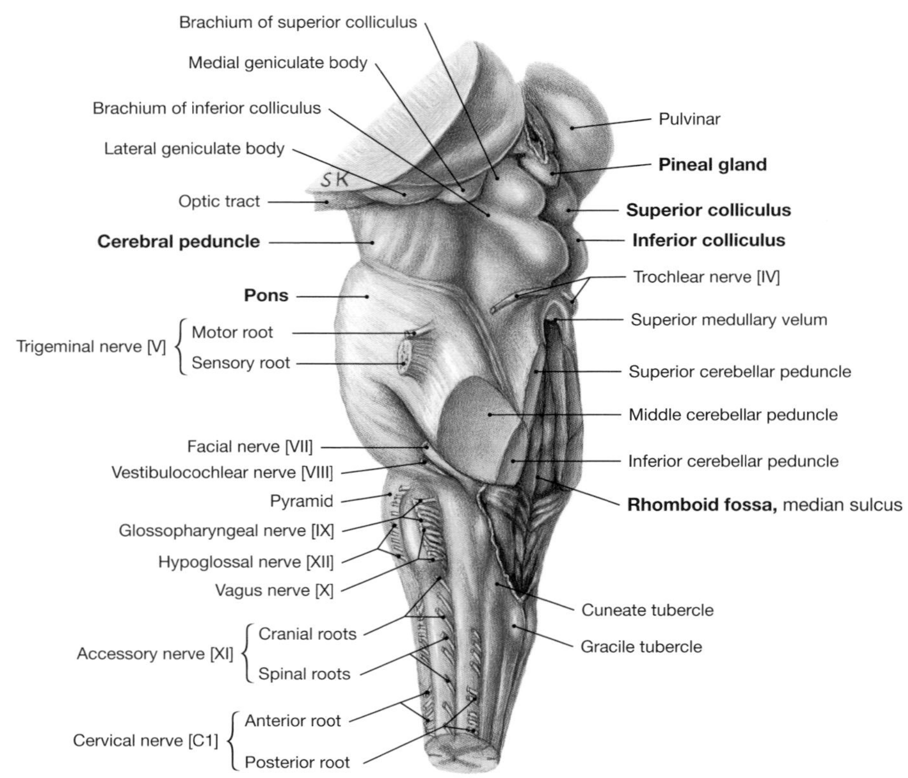
Brachium of superior colliculus
Medial geniculate body
Brachium of inferior colliculus
Lateral geniculate body
Optic tract
Cerebral peduncle
Pons
Trigeminal nerve [V]
Motor root
Sensory root
Facial nerve [VII]
Vestibulocochlear nerve [VIII]
Pyramid
Glossopharyngeal nerve [IX]
Hypoglossal nerve [XII]
Vagus nerve [X]
Accessory nerve [XI]
Cranial roots
Spinal roots
Cervical nerve [C1]
Anterior root
Posterior root
Pulvinar
Pineal gland
Superior colliculus
Inferior colliculus
Trochlear nerve [IV]
Superior medullary velum
Superior cerebellar peduncle
Middle cerebellar peduncle
Inferior cerebellar peduncle
Rhomboid fossa, median sulcus
Cuneate tubercle
Gracile tubercle

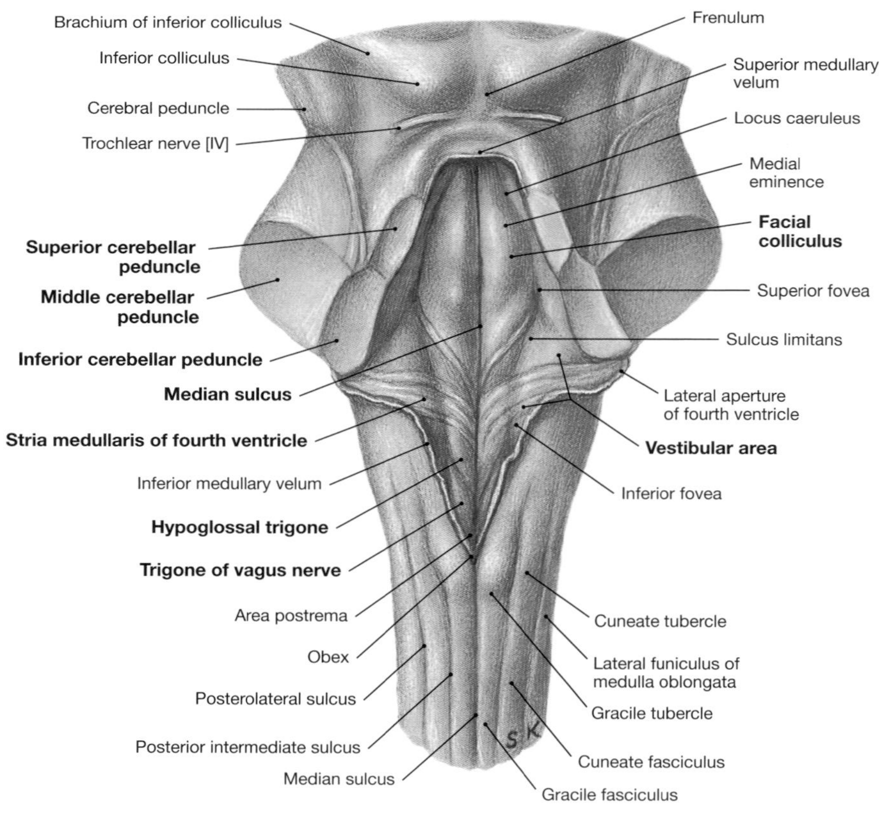
Brachium of inferior colliculus
Inferior colliculus
Cerebral peduncle
Trochlear nerve [IV]
Superior cerebellar peduncle
Middle cerebellar peduncle
Inferior cerebellar peduncle
Median sulcus
Stria medullaris of fourth ventricle
Inferior medullary velum
Hypoglossal trigone
Trigone of vagus nerve
Area postrema
Obex
Posterolateral sulcus
Posterior intermediate sulcus
Median sulcus
Frenulum
Superior medullary velum
Locus caeruleus
Medial eminence
Facial colliculus
Superior fovea
Sulcus limitans
Lateral aperture of fourth ventricle
Vestibular area
Inferior fovea
Cuneate tubercle
Lateral funiculus of medulla oblongata
Gracile tubercle
Cuneate fasciculus
Gracile fasciculus

**Fig. 12.60 Rhomboid fossa;** posterior view; view onto the floor of the fourth ventricle after dissection of the cerebellar peduncles.
The rhomboid fossa forms the floor of the fourth ventricle. The cerebellar peduncles, pons, and medulla oblongata provide the margins of the rhomboid fossa. As part of the area of the rhomboid fossa, important nuclei responsible for the **regulation of the systemic circulation** and the **nuclei of the cranial nerves** V to X, and partially cranial nerves XI and XII, are located in the pons and medulla oblongata. In the rhomboid fossa one can distinguish the median sulcus, the facial colliculus (fibers of the facial nerve [VII]), the medullary stria of fourth ventricle as part of the central auditory pathway, the vestibular area (vestibular nuclei), the hypoglossal trigone (trigone of hypoglossal nerve – nucleus of the hypoglossal nerve [XII]), the vagal trigone (trigone of vagal nerve – nuclei of the vagus nerve [X] and glossopharyngeal nerve [IX]), and the area postrema (vomiting center, see circumventricular organs, → Fig. 12.91).

## Mesencephalon and brainstem

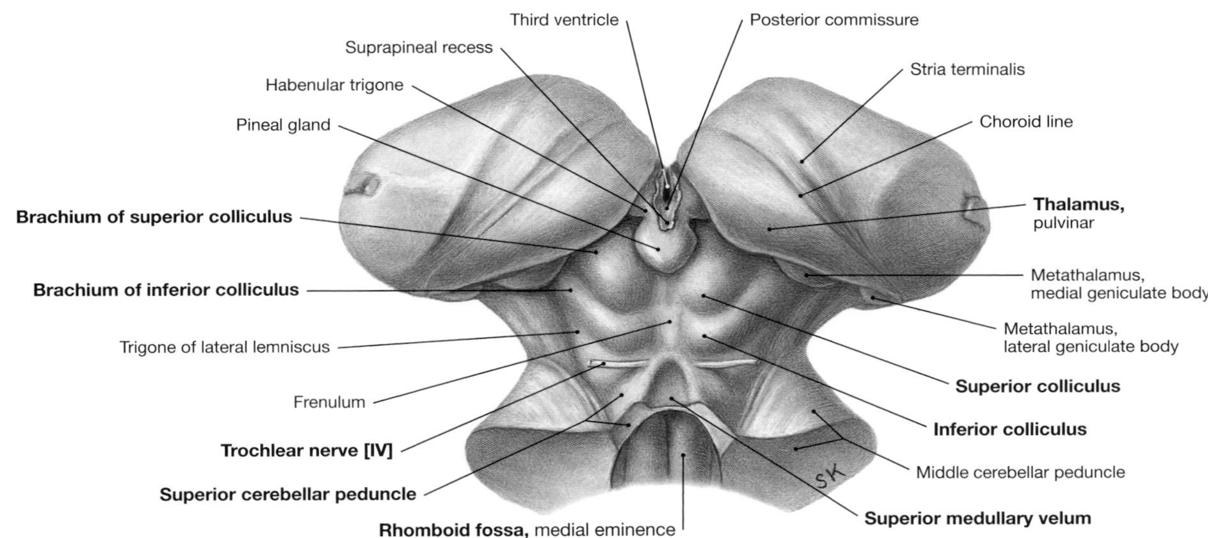
Third ventricle
Posterior commissure
Suprapineal recess
Stria terminalis
Habenular trigone
Choroid line
Pineal gland
Brachium of superior colliculus
Thalamus, pulvinar
Brachium of inferior colliculus
Metathalamus, medial geniculate body
Trigone of lateral lemniscus
Metathalamus, lateral geniculate body
Superior colliculus
Frenulum
Inferior colliculus
Trochlear nerve [IV]
Middle cerebellar peduncle
Superior cerebellar peduncle
Superior medullary velum
Rhomboid fossa, medial eminence

**Fig. 12.61 Mesencephalon, midbrain, and pineal gland;** posterior superior view.
At the dorsal side of the brainstem, the midbrain extends from the diencephalon to the cerebellar peduncles, the superior medullary velum, and the rhomboid fossa (floor of fourth ventricle). The quadrigeminal plate (tectal plate) is the characteristic feature of the dorsal side. It is composed of the superior colliculi and the inferior colliculi and forms the tectum of midbrain. To each side, the corresponding colliculi connect with the diencephalon (medial and lateral geniculate bodies) through fiber bundles (brachium of superior and inferior colliculus). Below the inferior colliculi, the trochlear nerve [VI] is the only cranial nerve to exit the brainstem at its dorsal side.

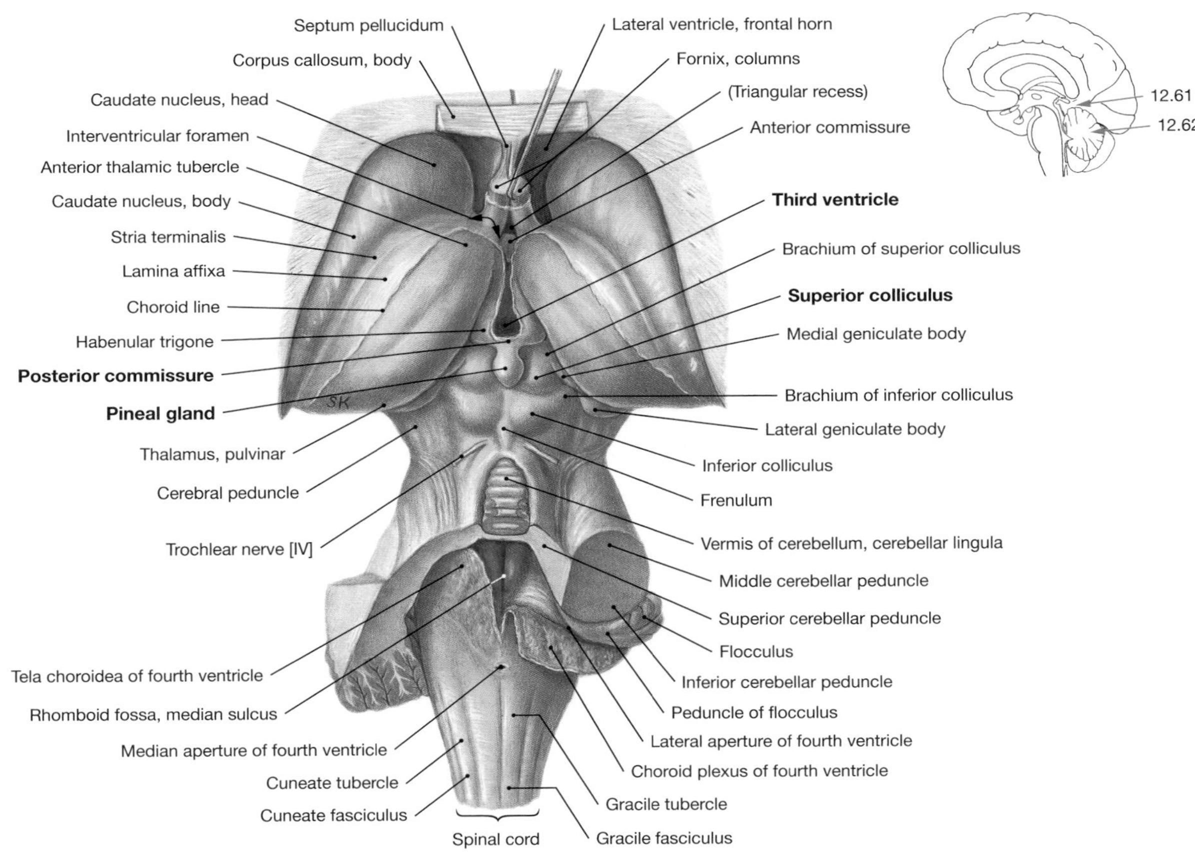
Septum pellucidum
Lateral ventricle, frontal horn
Corpus callosum, body
Fornix, columns
Caudate nucleus, head
(Triangular recess)
Interventricular foramen
Anterior commissure
Anterior thalamic tubercle
Caudate nucleus, body
Third ventricle
Stria terminalis
Brachium of superior colliculus
Lamina affixa
Superior colliculus
Choroid line
Medial geniculate body
Habenular trigone
Posterior commissure
Brachium of inferior colliculus
Pineal gland
Lateral geniculate body
Thalamus, pulvinar
Inferior colliculus
Cerebral peduncle
Frenulum
Trochlear nerve [IV]
Vermis of cerebellum, cerebellar lingula
Middle cerebellar peduncle
Superior cerebellar peduncle
Flocculus
Tela choroidea of fourth ventricle
Inferior cerebellar peduncle
Rhomboid fossa, median sulcus
Peduncle of flocculus
Lateral aperture of fourth ventricle
Median aperture of fourth ventricle
Choroid plexus of fourth ventricle
Cuneate tubercle
Gracile tubercle
Cuneate fasciculus
Spinal cord
Gracile fasciculus
12.61
12.62

**Fig. 12.62 Brainstem;** posterior superior view; the pons and major parts of the cerebellum have been removed, the choroid membrane of the fourth ventricle has been sectioned in the median plane and reflected to the right side.
The pineal gland attaches to the posterior commissure and is located between the two superior colliculi. The third ventricle lies above. The brainstem contains important centers (red, pontine, inferior olivary, and vestibular nuclei as well as the reticular formation) which coordinate critical life-saving functions, including circulation, breathing, and consciousness (ARAS → Fig. 12.54).

## Brainstem and cerebellum

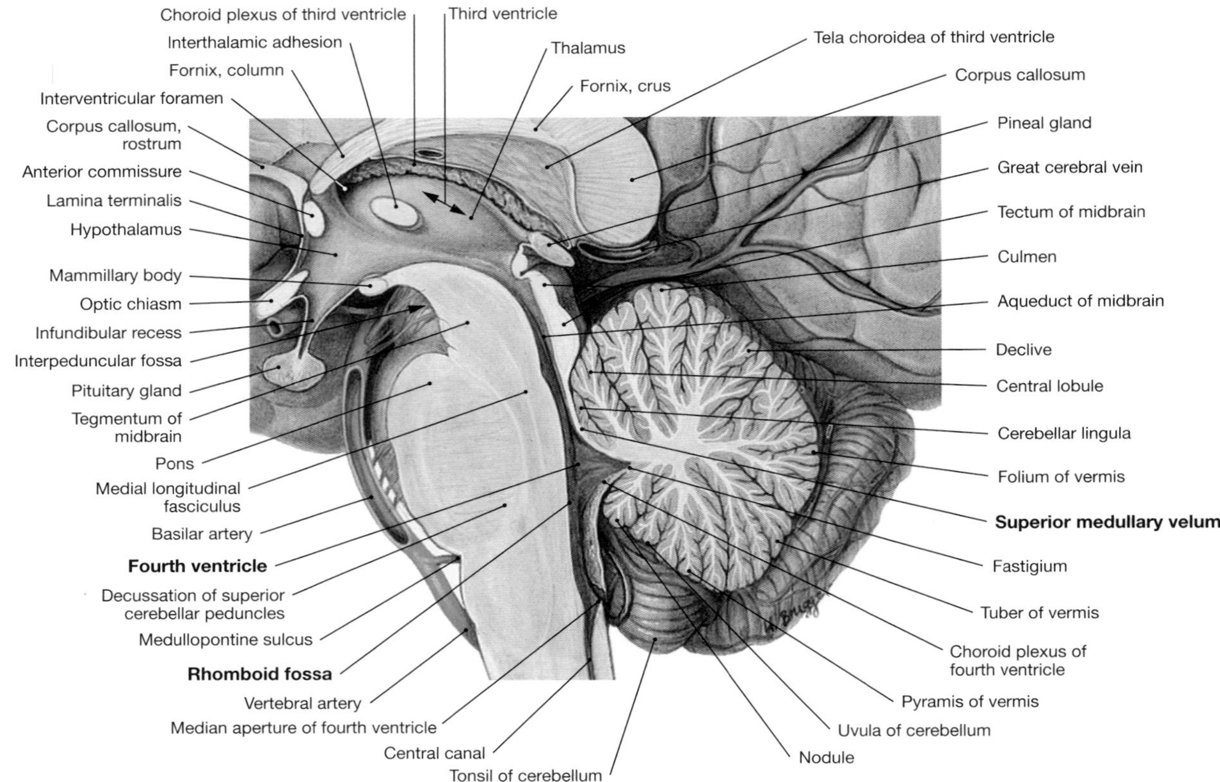
Choroid plexus of third ventricle
Third ventricle
Interthalamic adhesion
Thalamus
Tela choroidea of third ventricle
Fornix, column
Fornix, crus
Corpus callosum
Interventricular foramen
Corpus callosum, rostrum
Pineal gland
Anterior commissure
Great cerebral vein
Lamina terminalis
Tectum of midbrain
Hypothalamus
Culmen
Mammillary body
Aqueduct of midbrain
Optic chiasm
Infundibular recess
Declive
Interpeduncular fossa
Central lobule
Pituitary gland
Tegmentum of midbrain
Cerebellar lingula
Pons
Folium of vermis
Medial longitudinal fasciculus
Superior medullary velum
Basilar artery
Fastigium
Fourth ventricle
Decussation of superior cerebellar peduncles
Tuber of vermis
Medullopontine sulcus
Choroid plexus of fourth ventricle
Rhomboid fossa
Pyramis of vermis
Vertebral artery
Median aperture of fourth ventricle
Uvula of cerebellum
Central canal
Nodule
Tonsil of cerebellum

**Fig.12.63 Brainstem with fourth ventricle and cerebellum;** median section.
The median section reveals the characteristic structure of the so-called tree of life **(Arbor vitae)** of the cerebellum created by the distinct grooves (surface enlargement) of the cerebellar cortex.
The rhomboid fossa lies anterior to the cerebellum and forms the floor of the fourth ventricle. The brainstem with mesencephalon, pons, and medulla oblongata are positioned anterior to the fourth ventricle and even further anterior the basilar artery runs alongside the brainstem. In the median section, the superior medullary velum constitutes the rostral wall of the fourth ventricle and stretches from the cerebellum to the quadrigeminal plate (tectal plate). The pineal gland and the corpus callosum are located on top.

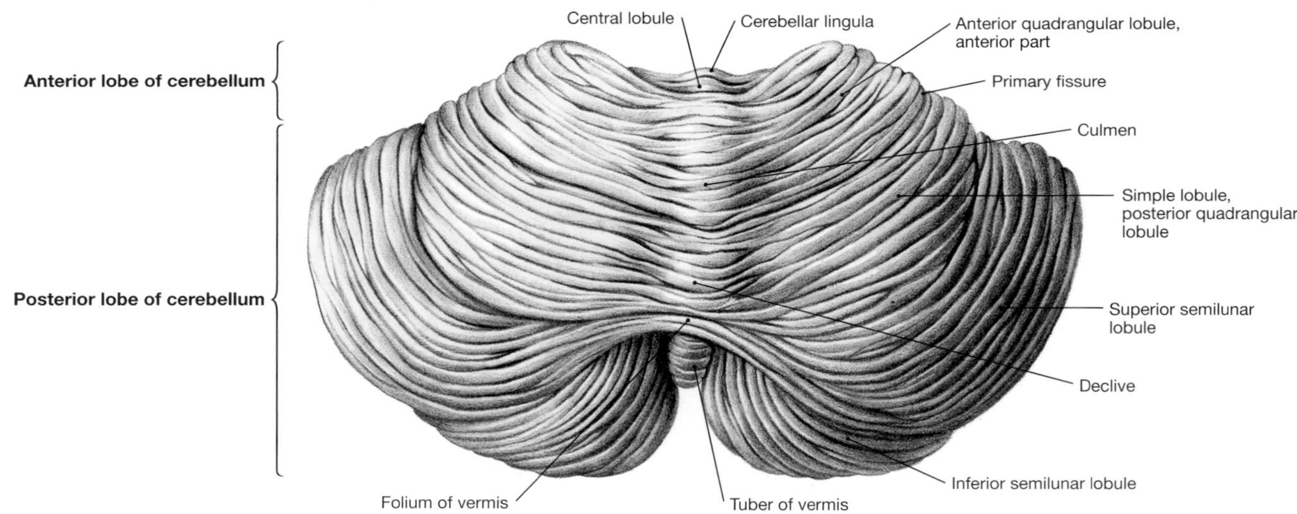
Central lobule
Cerebellar lingula
Anterior quadrangular lobule, anterior part
Anterior lobe of cerebellum
Primary fissure
Culmen
Simple lobule, posterior quadrangular lobule
Posterior lobe of cerebellum
Superior semilunar lobule
Declive
Inferior semilunar lobule
Folium of vermis
Tuber of vermis

**Fig. 12.64 Cerebellum;** posterior superior view.
The cerebellum divides into the **vermis** of cerebellum and two **hemispheres** of cerebellum. The tuber of vermis, folium, declive, culmen, as well as the central lobule and the lingula are shown. The cerebellar hemispheres divide into **three lobes** (→ Fig. 12.71):

- anterior lobe of cerebellum
- posterior lobe of cerebellum
- flocculonodular lobe (nodule + flocculus → Figs. 12.65 and 12.66)

The lobes subdivide further into **lobuli,** such as anterior quadrangular lobule, posterior quadrangular lobule (simple lobule), and the superior and inferior semilunar lobules (ansiform lobules).

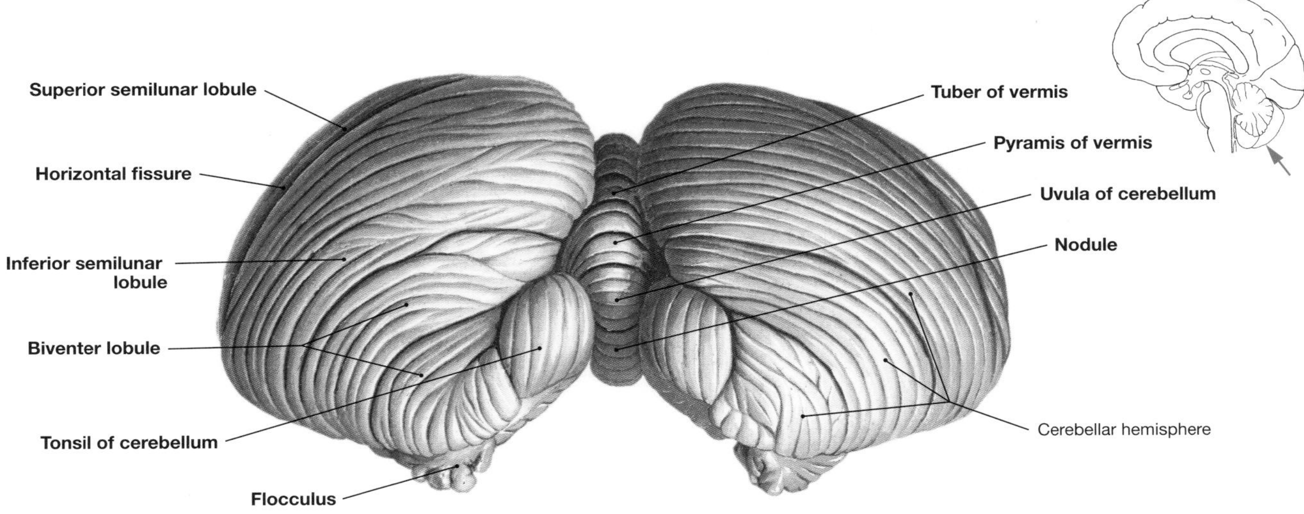
Superior semilunar lobule
Horizontal fissure
Inferior semilunar lobule
Biventer lobule
Tonsil of cerebellum
Flocculus
Tuber of vermis
Pyramis of vermis
Uvula of cerebellum
Nodule
Cerebellar hemisphere

**Fig. 12.65 Cerebellum;** posterior inferior view.
The tuber of vermis, pyramis, uvula, and nodule become visible from this angle. Visible are also the paired tonsils of the cerebellum as well as the superior and inferior semilunar lobules, separated by the horizontal fissure. The biventral lobule is located below the inferior semilunar lobule and above the flocculus.

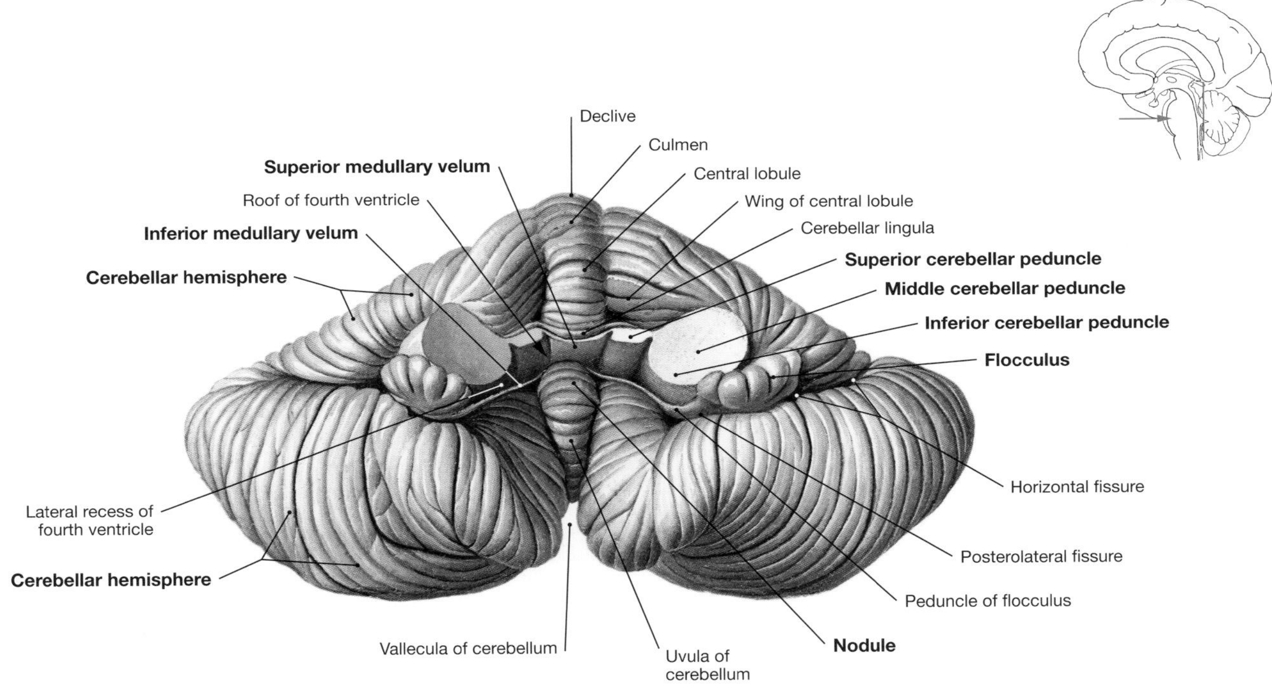
Declive
Culmen
Superior medullary velum
Central lobule
Roof of fourth ventricle
Wing of central lobule
Inferior medullary velum
Cerebellar lingula
Cerebellar hemisphere
Superior cerebellar peduncle
Middle cerebellar peduncle
Inferior cerebellar peduncle
Flocculus
Horizontal fissure
Lateral recess of fourth ventricle
Posterolateral fissure
Cerebellar hemisphere
Peduncle of flocculus
Vallecula of cerebellum
Nodule
Uvula of cerebellum

**Fig. 12.66 Cerebellum;** anterior view; after dissection of the cerebellar peduncles.
The anterior surface depicts the cerebellar peduncles which connect the cerebellum to the brainstem: superior, middle, and inferior cerebellar peduncles. The superior medullary velum divides the vermis of cerebellum and connects both cerebellar peduncles. The paired inferior medullary velum located on the left and right side of the nodule continues bilaterally towards the flocculus. The cerebellar hemispheres constitute the outer parts.

## Clinical Remarks

In the event of increased intracranial pressure (e.g. due to a tumor or bleeding), the most caudal structure of the cerebellum, the area of the cerebellar tonsils, is at risk of being squeezed between bone and medulla oblongata in the region of the foramen magnum. The resulting pressure exerted on the medulla oblongata can cause a loss of vital functions, e.g. respiration, and cause death. This tonsillar herniation, also named downward cerebellar herniation, resembles an **infratentorial herniation** type, which must be distinguished from a **supratentorial herniation,** like the central herniation, also named transtentorial herniation. Here, squeezing of the parts of the diencephalon and mesencephalon in the tentorial notch can result in a loss of function of the reticular formation and corticobulbar and rubrospinal tracts. The supratentorial herniation can precede an infratentorial herniation.

## Nuclei of the cerebellum

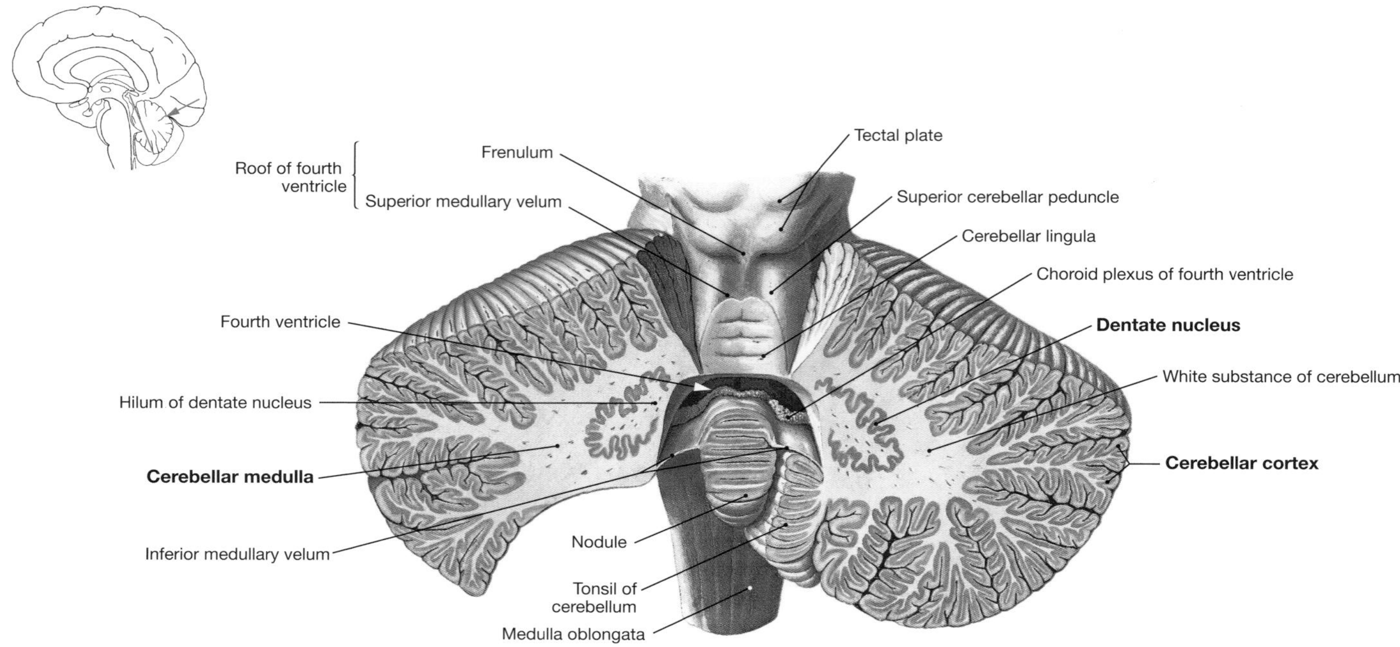
Roof of fourth ventricle
Frenulum
Superior medullary velum
Tectal plate
Superior cerebellar peduncle
Cerebellar lingula
Choroid plexus of fourth ventricle
Fourth ventricle
Dentate nucleus
White substance of cerebellum
Hilum of dentate nucleus
Cerebellar medulla
Cerebellar cortex
Inferior medullary velum
Nodule
Tonsil of cerebellum
Medulla oblongata

**Fig. 12.67 Cerebellum;** oblique section; posterior view.
An oblique section through the cerebellum reveals the structure of the gray substance which consists of the cerebellar cortex and medulla. Visible in the cerebellar medulla is the biggest of the four cerebellar nuclei, the **dentate nucleus,** with its gray substance showing a jagged and gyral configuration. This nucleus is not only located in both cerebellar hemispheres (pontocerebellum) but also has multiple close functional connections with the cerebellar cortex.

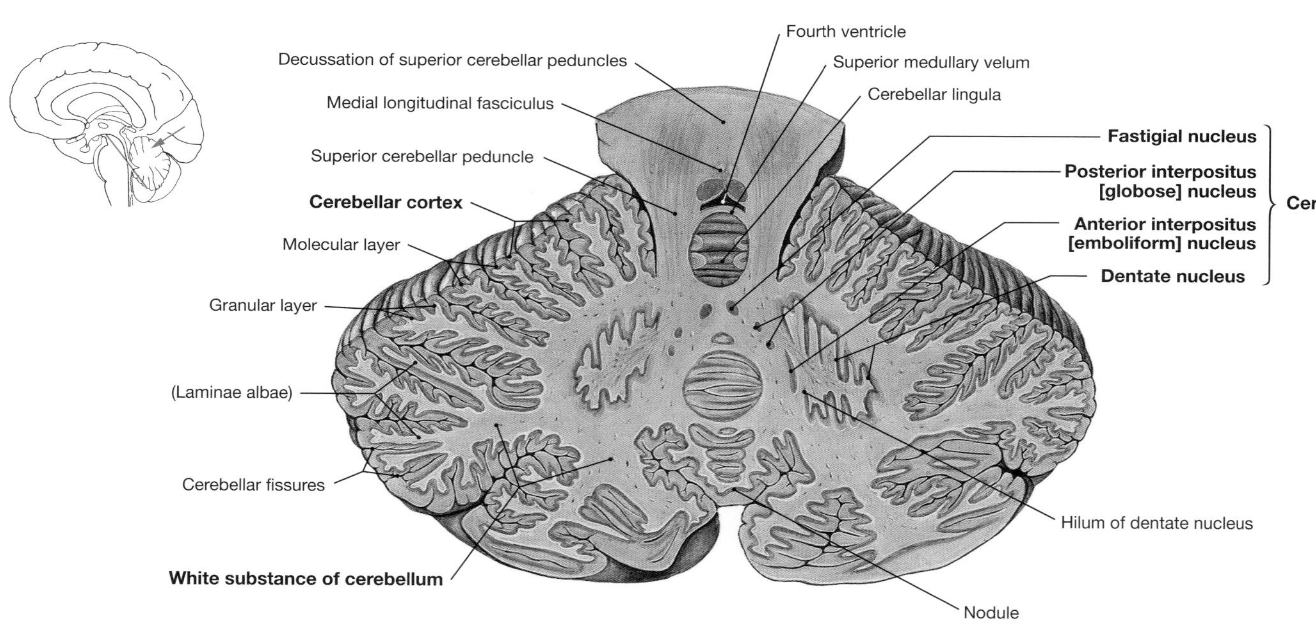
Fourth ventricle
Decussation of superior cerebellar peduncles
Superior medullary velum
Cerebellar lingula
Medial longitudinal fasciculus
Superior cerebellar peduncle
Fastigial nucleus
Posterior interpositus [globose] nucleus
Cerebellar nuclei
Cerebellar cortex
Anterior interpositus [emboliform] nucleus
Molecular layer
Dentate nucleus
Granular layer
(Laminae albae)
Cerebellar fissures
Hilum of dentate nucleus
White substance of cerebellum
Nodule

**Fig. 12.68 Cerebellum with cerebellar nuclei;** oblique section through the upper cerebellar peduncles; posterior view.
The cerebellum is composed of the white substance of cerebellum **(medullary center)** with embedded cerebellar nuclei and the surrounding **cerebellar cortex.** The oblique section reveals all four cerebellar nuclei in both hemispheres (pontocerebellum). The dentate nucleus is U-shaped and jagged. Medial to the dentate nucleus lies the anterior interpositus nucleus (emboliform nucleus) and even further medial the posterior interpositus nucleus (globose nucleus), both collectively named **interpositus nucleus.** Both nuclei share functional similarities and connect with the paravermal and vermal zone of the cerebellum (spinocerebellum). Located in the medulla of the vermis are the right and left fastigial nucleus (fastigial nucleus or nucleus medialis cerebelli) which have close functional connections with the cortex of the flocculonodular lobe (vestibulocerebellum) (→ Figs. 12.65 and 12.66).

## Cerebellar connections

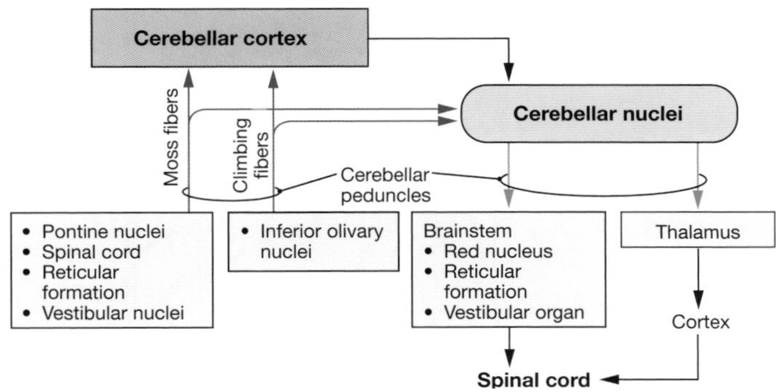
Cerebellar cortex
Moss fibers
Climbing fibers
Cerebellar nuclei
Cerebellar peduncles
• Pontine nuclei
• Spinal cord
• Reticular formation
• Vestibular nuclei
• Inferior olivary nuclei
Brainstem
• Red nucleus
• Reticular formation
• Vestibular organ
Thalamus
Cortex
Spinal cord

**Fig. 12.69 Schematic structure of the basic flow of information from and to the cerebellum.** [14]
Blue arrows indicate the systems providing input for the cerebellum, red arrows demonstrate the parts of the CNS receiving output information from the cerebellum.

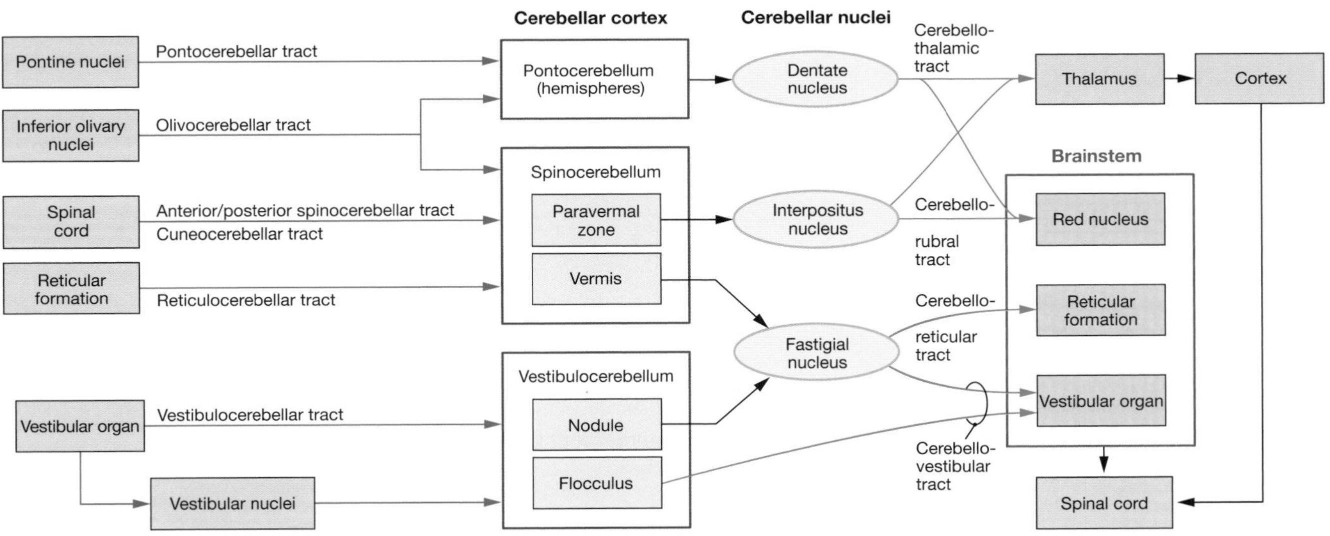
Cerebellar cortex
Cerebellar nuclei
Pontine nuclei
Pontocerebellar tract
Pontocerebellum (hemispheres)
Dentate nucleus
Cerebello-thalamic tract
Thalamus
Cortex
Inferior olivary nuclei
Olivocerebellar tract
Spinocerebellum
Brainstem
Spinal cord
Anterior/posterior spinocerebellar tract
Cuneocerebellar tract
Paravermal zone
Interpositus nucleus
Cerebello-rubral tract
Red nucleus
Reticular formation
Reticulocerebellar tract
Vermis
Cerebello-reticular tract
Reticular formation
Fastigial nucleus
Vestibulocerebellum
Vestibular organ
Vestibulocerebellar tract
Nodule
Vestibular organ
Cerebello-vestibular tract
Vestibular nuclei
Flocculus
Spinal cord

**Fig. 12.70 Schematic presentation of the cerebellar compartments with corresponding afferent and efferent connections.** [14]

## Cerebellum, organization

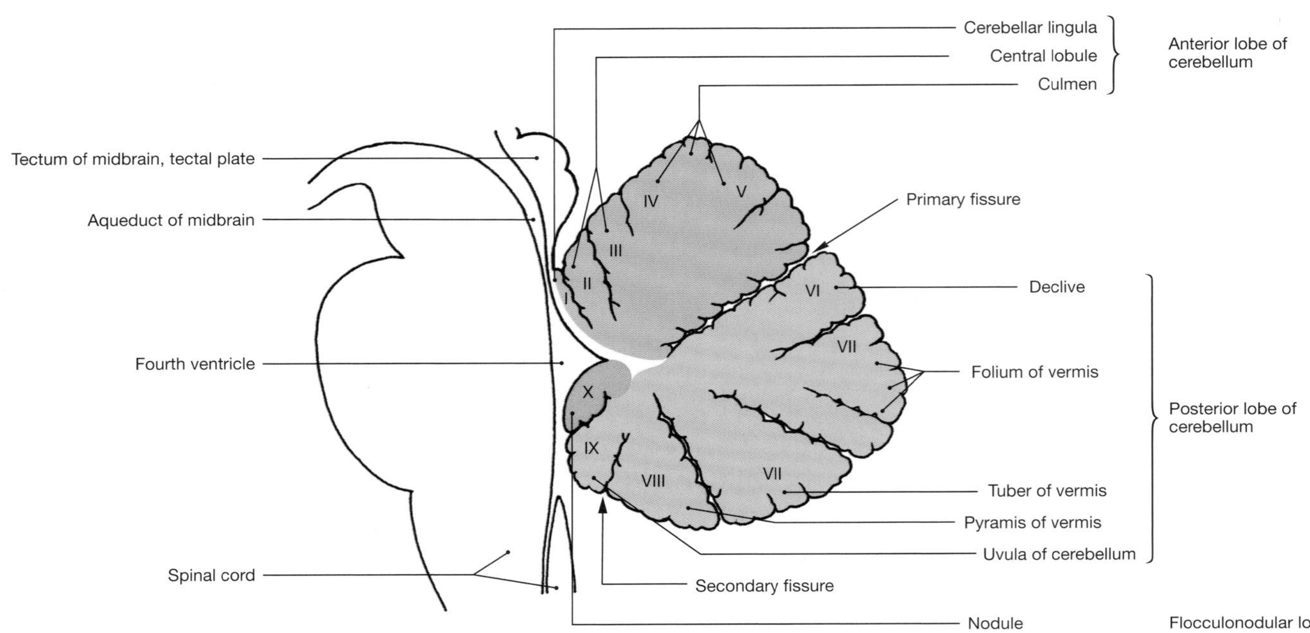
Cerebellar lingula
Central lobule
Culmen
Anterior lobe of cerebellum
Tectum of midbrain, tectal plate
Aqueduct of midbrain
Primary fissure
Declive
Fourth ventricle
Folium of vermis
Posterior lobe of cerebellum
Tuber of vermis
Pyramis of vermis
Uvula of cerebellum
Spinal cord
Secondary fissure
Nodule
Flocculonodular lobe
I
II
III
IV
V
VI
VII
VIII
IX
X

**Fig. 12.71 Parts of the cerebellar vermis, I to X;** median section; overview.
The **spinocerebellum** consists of the vermis, the bilateral paravermal zone and the major part of the anterior lobe of cerebellum with the exception of the nodule. Functionally, it controls the muscular tonus and regulates body and limb movements. The spinocerebellum receives the majority of its afferent proprioception input from the spinal cord (anterior and posterior spinocerebellar tracts, cuneocerebellar tract). Additional afferent fibers come from the reticular formation and the inferior olivary nuclei. The nodule is part of the **vestibulocerebellum.**

| **Structure of the Cerebellar Vermis** (Roman numbers according to the classification by LARSELL) | |
|---|---|
| I | Lingula |
| II, III | Central lobe |
| IV, V | Culmen |
| **Primary (preclival) fissure** | |
| VI | Declive |
| VII A | Folium of vermis |
| **Horizontal (intercrural) fissure** | |
| VII B | Tuber |
| VIII | Pyramis |
| **Secondary (post-pyramidal) fissure** | |
| IX | Uvula |
| **Posterolateral fissure** | |
| X | Nodule |

## Clinical Remarks

**Lesions of the spinocerebellum** result in largely irreparable deficits in the coordination movement sequences. Loss or severely impaired coordination between muscle agonists and antagonists results in postural maladjustment with wide-based stance, gait ataxia and lack of coordination of movements (dysmetria).
Intention tremor is a typical symptom of **lesions of the pontocerebellum.** This tremor becomes more intense in the extremities during voluntary movements and is particularly severe towards the end of the movement. The disturbed muscular coordination involves asynergies as demonstrated by dysmetria (incoordinated movements of the hand, arm, leg, or eye undershooting or overshooting an intended position) and dysdiadochokinesis (inability to execute rapid changes of antagonistic movements)

## Cerebellum, organization

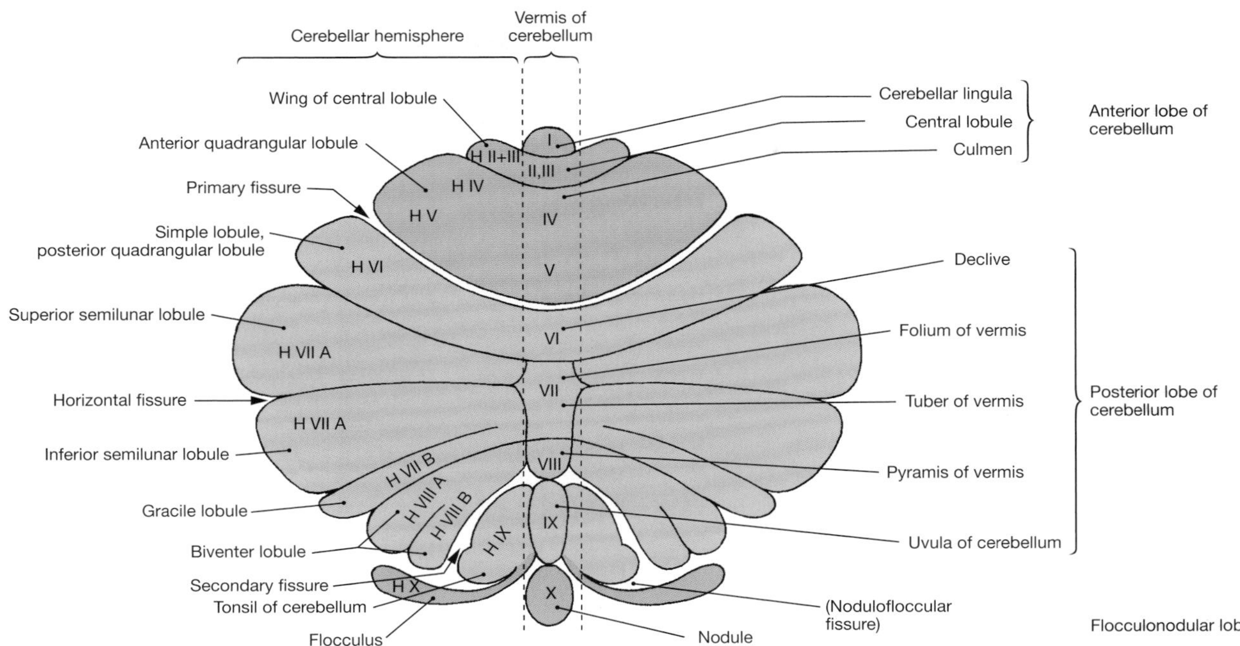
Cerebellar hemisphere
Vermis of cerebellum
Wing of central lobule
Anterior quadrangular lobule
Primary fissure
Simple lobule, posterior quadrangular lobule
Superior semilunar lobule
Horizontal fissure
Inferior semilunar lobule
Gracile lobule
Biventer lobule
Secondary fissure
Tonsil of cerebellum
Flocculus
H II+III
H IV
H V
H VI
H VII A
H VII B
H VIII A
H VIII B
H IX
H X
I
II,III
IV
V
VI
VII
VIII
IX
X
Cerebellar lingula
Central lobule
Culmen
Anterior lobe of cerebellum
Declive
Folium of vermis
Tuber of vermis
Pyramis of vermis
Uvula of cerebellum
Posterior lobe of cerebellum
(Nodulofloccular fissure)
Nodule
Flocculonodular lobe

**Fig. 12.72 Cerebellar cortex and cerebellar vermis;** diagram of the cerebellar cortex outstretched; overview.

With the exception of the anterior lobe of cerebellum, the hemispheres are separated by the vermis and include the areas H II to H IX of LARSELL's classification. They constitute the **pontocerebellum** (cerebrocerebellum). The pontocerebellum receives its afferent fibers primarily from the pontine nuclei. This part of the cerebellum has close connections with the cerebral cortex via the pons and participates in the planning of voluntary movements. Collectively named the **flocculonodular lobe,** the nodule and flocculus (X and H X) are the essential components of the **vestibulocerebellum.** The extensive connections with the vestibular system of the inner ear provide the majority of afferent fibers to the vestibulocerebellum. The main function of the vestibulocerebellum is to regulate balance.

| **Structure of the Cerebellar Hemispheres** (Roman numbers according to the classification by LARSELL) | |
|---|---|
| H II, III | Wing of central lobe |
| H IV, V | Anterior quadrangular lobule |
| **Primary (preclival) fissure** | |
| HVI | Posterior quadrangular lobule (simple lobule) |
| HVII A | Superior semilunar lobule (first crus of ansiform lobule) |
| **Horizontal (intercrural) fissure** | |
| HVII A | Inferior semilunar lobule (second crus of ansiform lobule) |
| HVII B | Gracile lobule (paramedian lobule) |
| HVIII A und B | Biventral lobule |
| **Secondary (post-pyramidal) fissure** | |
| H IX | Tonsil of cerebellum (ventral paraflocculus) |
| **Posterolateral fissure** | |
| H X | Flocculus |

## Clinical Remarks

**Lesions of the vestibulocerebellum** mainly result in an impaired balance and control of eye movements. This includes the inability to translate vestibular input during head turns into coordinated eye movements and causes difficulties in controlling the postural muscles during standing, walking, or sitting (ataxia affecting the torso, stance, and gait; incoordination of movement). The incoordination of eye movements results in spontaneous nystagmus and involuntary saccadic eye movements.

## Association and commissural tracts

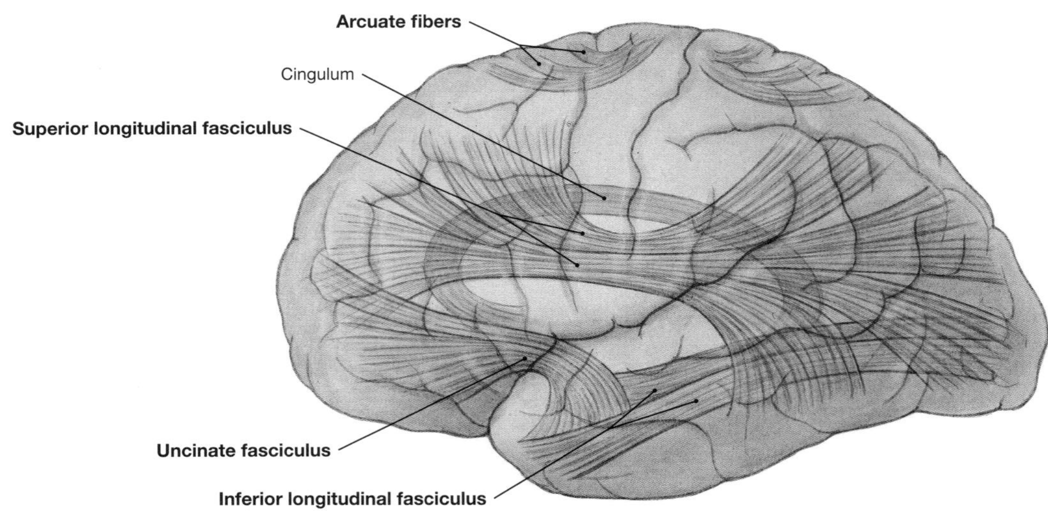
Arcuate fibers
Cingulum
Superior longitudinal fasciculus
Uncinate fasciculus
Inferior longitudinal fasciculus

**Fig. 12.73 Association tracts and arcuate fibers;** overview; view from the left side.
The majority of fibers in the white matter are association fibers. They connect different regions within one hemisphere and facilitate association and integrative functions by linking functionally distinct areas.
**Short association fibers,** known as cerebral arcuate fibers, are located near the cortex and their U-shaped structure is ideally suited in connecting neighboring gyri. **Long association fibers** located deeper in the medulla interconnect the lobes.
Functionally important association tracts are the superior longitudinal fasciculus, the inferior longitudinal fasciculus, the uncinate fasciculus as well as the arcuate fibers and the cingulum.

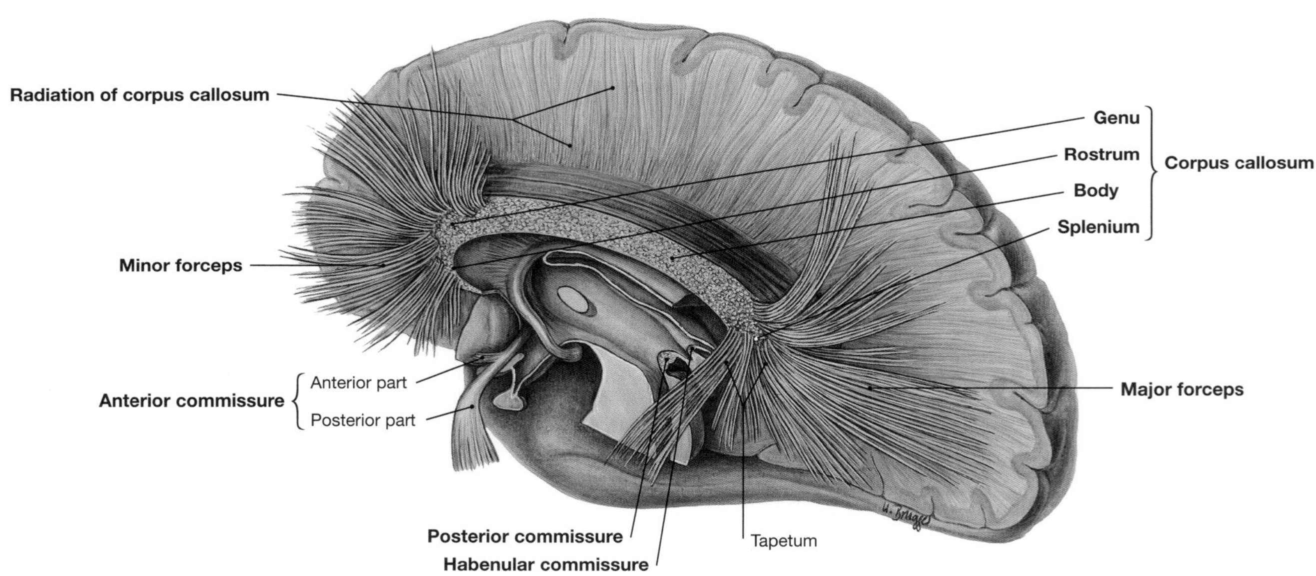
Radiation of corpus callosum
Genu
Rostrum
Body
Splenium
Corpus callosum
Minor forceps
Anterior commissure
Anterior part
Posterior part
Major forceps
Posterior commissure
Habenular commissure
Tapetum

**Fig. 12.74 Commissural tracts;** topographic overview; view from the left side; after extensive removal of the corpus callosum in the paramedian plane, single fibers of the corpus callosum are shown.
Commissural (transverse) fibers facilitate the information exchange between the two cerebral hemispheres, e.g. to generate a complete visual image composed of the visual input to each cerebral hemisphere. **Homotopic** commissural fibers connect corresponding cerebral areas, **heterotopic** commissural fibers facilitate the exchange between non-corresponding cerebral areas.
Each phylogenetic cerebral part has its own commissure: for the paleocortex, this is the anterior commissure, for the archicortex, it is the commissure of fornix, and the corpus callosum serves this function in the neocortex. The latter consists of the rostrum, genu, trunk, and splenium. The corpus callosum is shorter than the cerebral hemispheres and, thus, the rostral and occipital fibers create fan-shaped projections into the corresponding lobes (**radiation of corpus callosum;** projections of the corpus callosum with minor (frontal) forceps and major (occipital) forceps). However, some homotopic cerebral areas do not connect via commissural fibers. These include the primary visual cortex, the primary auditory cortex, and the somatosensory areas for hand and foot.

# Projection tracts

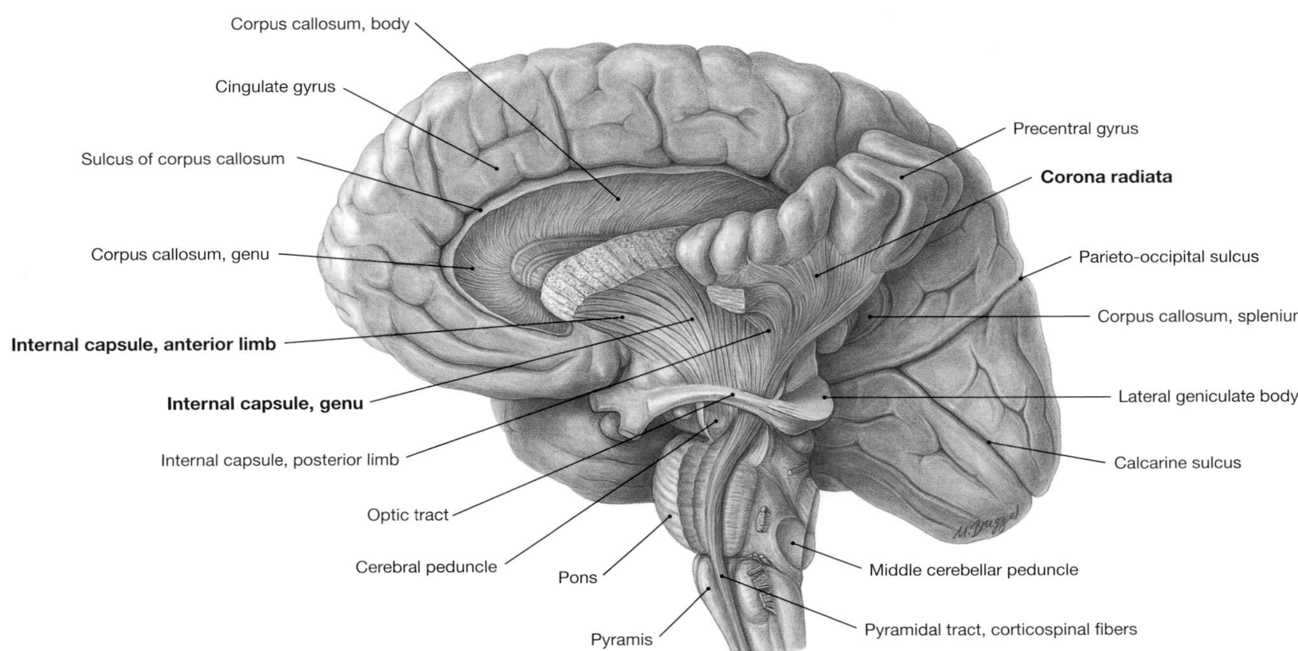

Corpus callosum, body
Cingulate gyrus
Sulcus of corpus callosum
Corpus callosum, genu
Internal capsule, anterior limb
Internal capsule, genu
Internal capsule, posterior limb
Optic tract
Cerebral peduncle
Pons
Pyramis
Precentral gyrus
Corona radiata
Parieto-occipital sulcus
Corpus callosum, splenium
Lateral geniculate body
Calcarine sulcus
Middle cerebellar peduncle
Pyramidal tract, corticospinal fibers


**Fig. 12.75 Projection tracts;** view from the left side; the internal capsule and the pyramidal tract have been exposed.
Projection tracts consist of projection fibers which connect the cortex with subjacent structures of the CNS (e.g. thalamus, brainstem). In the area of the striatum and pallidum, these fibers have to pass through narrow spaces where all fibers converge. These bottleneck areas are the internal capsule and the external capsule between the lentiform nucleus and claustrum as well as the extreme capsule between the insular cortex and the claustrum. The **internal capsule** is the main passageway for projection fibers. The **external capsule** and the **extreme capsule** mainly contain long association fibers. The **corona radiata** describes the radial arrangement of projection fibers between the cerebral cortex and the internal capsule.

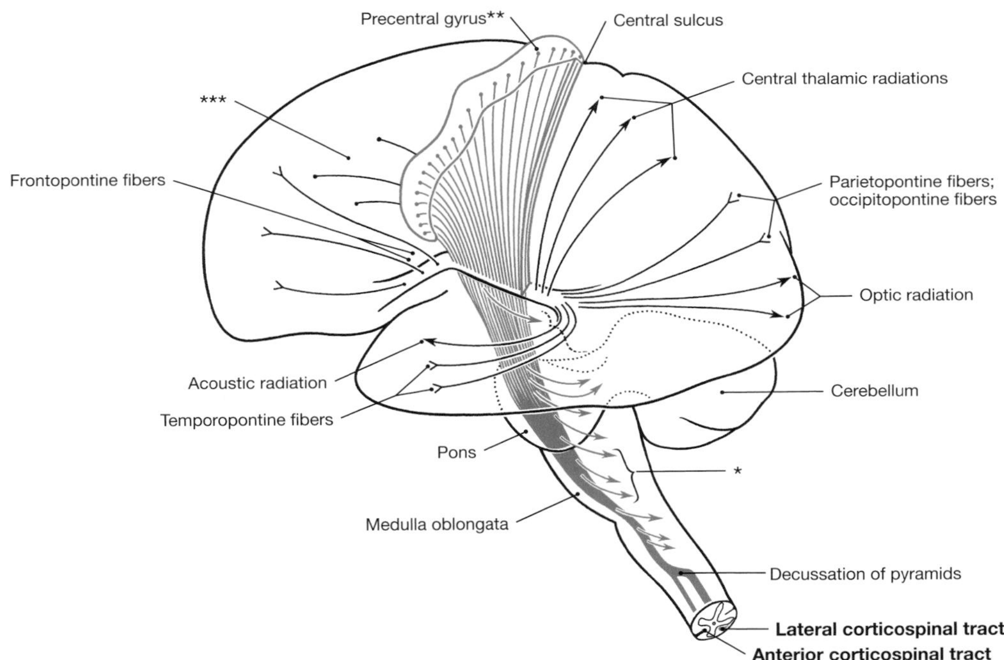

Precentral gyrus**
Central sulcus
***
Central thalamic radiations
Frontopontine fibers
Parietopontine fibers; occipitopontine fibers
Optic radiation
Acoustic radiation
Temporopontine fibers
Cerebellum
Pons
*
Medulla oblongata
Decussation of pyramids
Lateral corticospinal tract
Anterior corticospinal tract


**Fig. 12.76 Internal capsule and pyramidal tract;** functional overview; view from the left side.
At the internal capsule, almost all cortical projection tracts converge in a narrow space. This is examplified with the **pyramidal tract** derived from the precentral gyrus shown in red, which continues as lateral and anterior corticospinal tracts into the spinal cord.

* fibers to the quadrigeminal plate and to the nuclei of the rhombencephalon
** perikarya of the pyramidal tract
*** perikarya of area 6 and 8 (premotor cortical field)

## Internal capsule

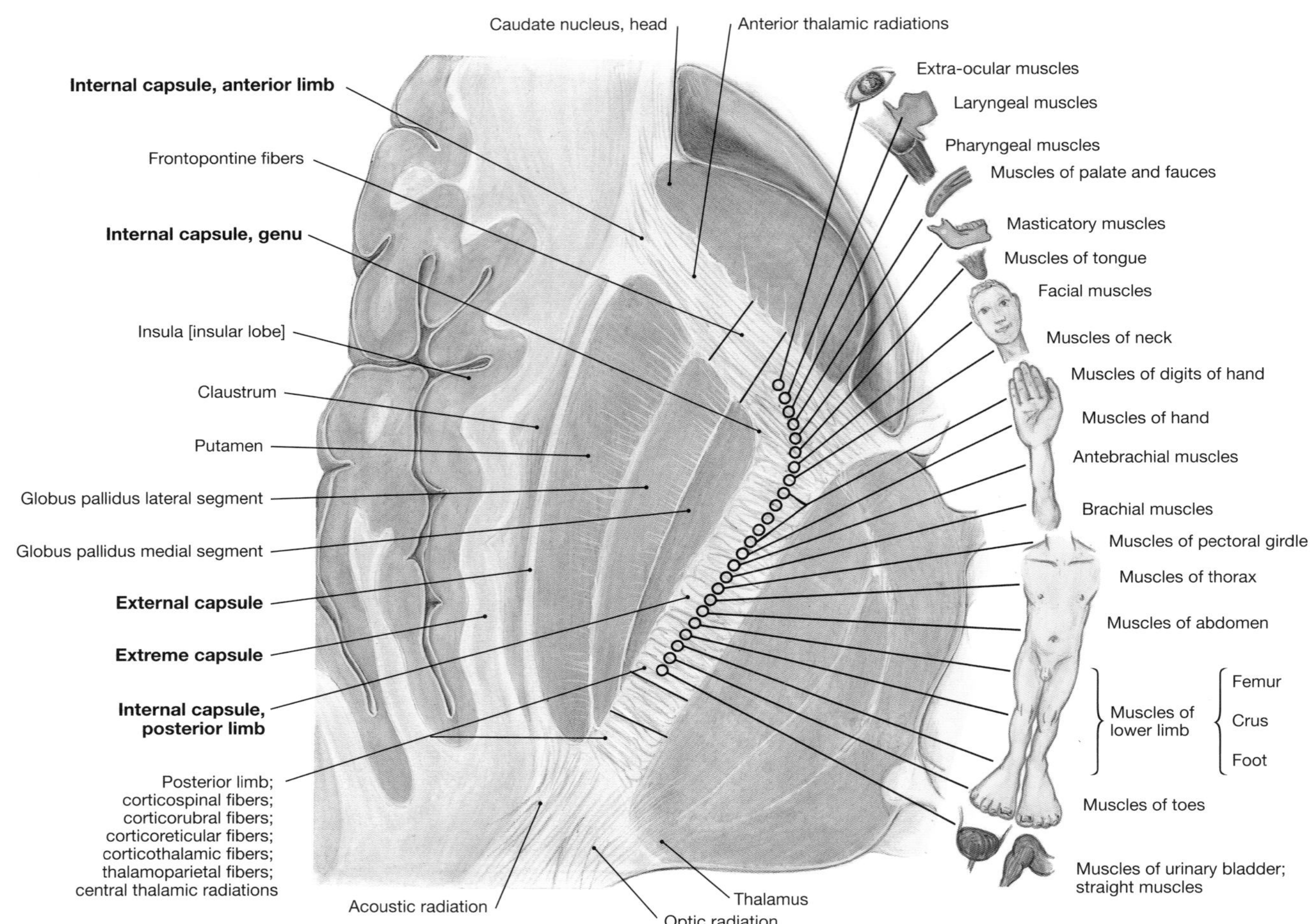
Caudate nucleus, head
Anterior thalamic radiations
Internal capsule, anterior limb
Frontopontine fibers
Internal capsule, genu
Insula [insular lobe]
Claustrum
Putamen
Globus pallidus lateral segment
Globus pallidus medial segment
External capsule
Extreme capsule
Internal capsule, posterior limb
Posterior limb; corticospinal fibers; corticorubral fibers; corticoreticular fibers; corticothalamic fibers; thalamoparietal fibers; central thalamic radiations
Acoustic radiation
Optic radiation
Thalamus
Extra-ocular muscles
Laryngeal muscles
Pharyngeal muscles
Muscles of palate and fauces
Masticatory muscles
Muscles of tongue
Facial muscles
Muscles of neck
Muscles of digits of hand
Muscles of hand
Antebrachial muscles
Brachial muscles
Muscles of pectoral girdle
Muscles of thorax
Muscles of abdomen
Muscles of lower limb
Femur
Crus
Foot
Muscles of toes
Muscles of urinary bladder; straight muscles

**Fig. 12.77 Internal capsule;** functional structure.
The internal capsule is clinically highly relevant because it contains almost all **cortical projection tracts** concentrated in a small space. The margins of the internal capsule are formed by the caudate nucleus in the anterior medial part, the thalamus in the posterior medial section, and the globus pallidus and putamen laterally. In the horizontal section, the internal capsule has a bend shape. An anterior limb, a genu of internal capsule, and a posterior limb are distinguishable. The descending tracts within the internal capsule have a **somatotopic** arrangement. The corticonuclear fibers run in the genu, while the corticospinal fibers for the upper extremity, torso, and lower extremity are somatotopically arranged in an anterior to posterior direction in the posterior limb.

**Tracts and Arterial Blood Supply of the Internal Capsule** [14]

| **Locations** | **Tracts** (due to clinical practice the terms fibers and tracts are used interchangeably here) | **Blood Supply** |
|---|---|---|
| Anterior limb | • Frontopontine fibers (from frontal lobe to pons)<br>• Anterior thalamic radiation (from thalamus to frontal cortex) | Anteromedial central arteries (from anterior cerebral artery) |
| Genu of internal capsule | • Corticonuclear fibers (part of the pyramidal tract) | Anterolateral central arteries (from middle cerebral artery) = lenticulostriate arteries |
| Posterior limb | • Corticospinal fibers<br>• Corticorubral fibers and corticoreticular fibers<br>• Central thalamic radiation (from rostral thalamic nuclei to motor cortex)<br>• Posterior thalamic radiation (from lateral geniculate body and additional thalamic nuclei to the parietal and occipital lobes)<br>• Parietotemporopontine fibers and occipitopontine fibers (from temporal or occipital lobe to pons)<br>• Optic radiation (geniculocalcarine fibers; from laterale geniculate body to occipital lobe)<br>• Acoustic radiation (auditory radiation; from medial geniculate body to temporal lobe) | Branches to internal capsule (from anterior choroid artery) |

## Clinical Remarks

The blood vessels to the internal capsule are terminal arteries. Not infrequently, **vascular occlusion** or **mass bleeding** into the internal capsule caused by rupture of blood vessels (particularly the anterolateral central arteries) occurs. Destruction of the fiber tracts and stroke are the consequences. The extent of the **stroke** depends on its location within the internal capsule and can involve a contralateral paralysis (hemiplegia), sensory deficits, and blindness on the contralateral visual field (hemianopsia).

## Pyramidal tract

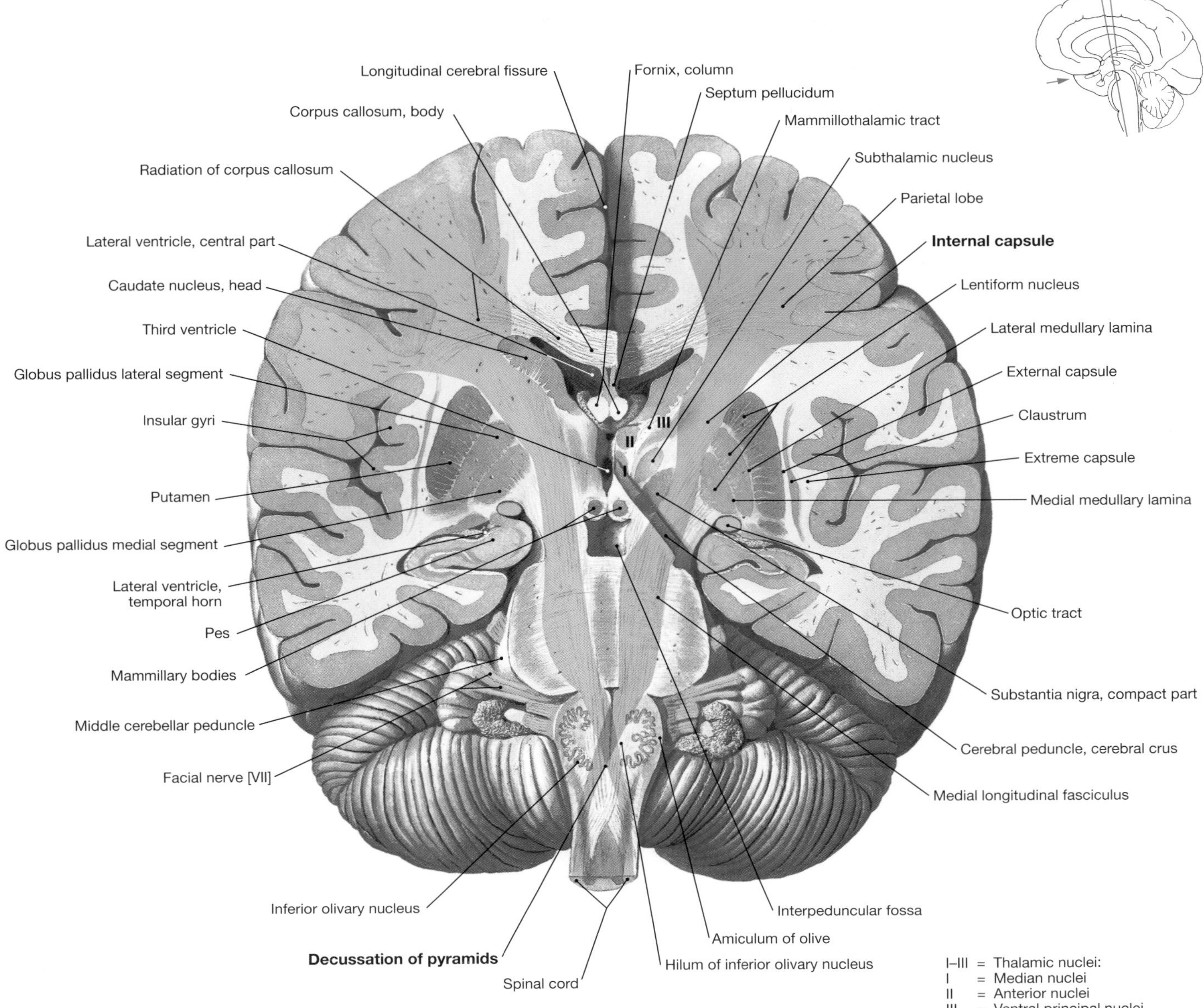
Longitudinal cerebral fissure
Fornix, column
Septum pellucidum
Mammillothalamic tract
Corpus callosum, body
Radiation of corpus callosum
Subthalamic nucleus
Parietal lobe
Internal capsule
Lateral ventricle, central part
Caudate nucleus, head
Lentiform nucleus
Third ventricle
Lateral medullary lamina
Globus pallidus lateral segment
External capsule
Insular gyri
Claustrum
Extreme capsule
Putamen
Medial medullary lamina
Globus pallidus medial segment
Lateral ventricle, temporal horn
Optic tract
Pes
Mammillary bodies
Substantia nigra, compact part
Middle cerebellar peduncle
Cerebral peduncle, cerebral crus
Facial nerve [VII]
Medial longitudinal fasciculus
Inferior olivary nucleus
Interpeduncular fossa
Amiculum of olive
Decussation of pyramids
Hilum of inferior olivary nucleus
Spinal cord
I
II
III
I–III = Thalamic nuclei:
I = Median nuclei
II = Anterior nuclei
III = Ventral principal nuclei

**Fig. 12.78 Pyramidal tract and basal ganglia;** oblique staggered section through the posterior limb of the internal capsule, the cerebral peduncles, and the medulla oblongata; anterior view; pyramidal tracts shown in color, right: pink, left: green.

The pyramidal tract transmits motor impulses from the motor cortex to the motor efferent nuclei of the cranial nerves (corticonuclear fibers) and the motor neurons in the anterior horn of the spinal cord (corticospinal fibers). The fibers **originate** in the precentral gyrus, in secondary motor fields, and in somatosensory cortical areas. The **converging** fibers create the corona radiata. Somatotopically arranged, the fibers pass through the genu and posterior limb of the internal capsule (→ Fig. 12.77). In the mesencephalon, the fibers enter the **cerebral crura.** Along the way through the brainstem, the corticonuclear fibers exit the pyramidal tract at different levels. At the **decussation of pyramids,** the major part of the remaining fibers (corticospinal fibers) cross to the opposite side, a smaller fraction courses on the ipsilateral side downwards and crosses to the opposite side only within the spinal cord.

## Clinical Remarks

**Lesions of the pyramidal tract** first result in a flaccid paralysis of the muscles on the contralateral side, despite the fact that propagation of action potentials remains intact in the peripheral nervous system and in the muscles. Particularly, fine motor skills of the hands and feet are impaired, while gross movement patterns in the proximal extremities and the torso are usually unaffected. Pyramidal lesions evoke primitive reflexes previously blocked by the corticospinal motor system, like the **BABINSKI's reflex.** Up to 2 years of age, the nerve fibers of the pyramidal tract are not fully myelinated and, thus, primitive reflexes, such as the BABINSKI's reflex (scratching of the lateral side of the foot sole causes a dorsal extension of the big toe) are considered as a normal and thereafter as a pathological reflex response.

With time, patients with a lesion of the pyramidal tract develop an increased muscular tonus and extensor reflexes, but weakened flexor reflexes. However, this syndrome of spastic paralysis reflects an additional damage to reticulospinal (extrapyramidal) tracts.

## Ventricles of the brain

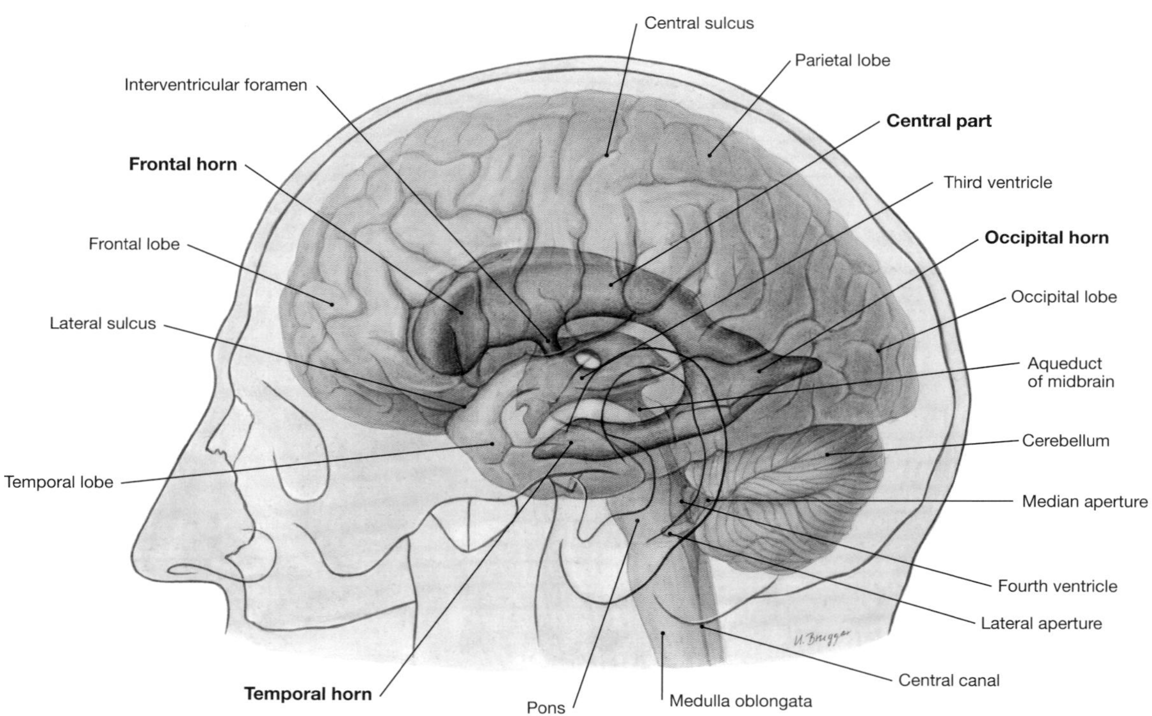
Central sulcus
Parietal lobe
Interventricular foramen
Central part
Frontal horn
Third ventricle
Frontal lobe
Occipital horn
Occipital lobe
Lateral sulcus
Aqueduct of midbrain
Cerebellum
Temporal lobe
Median aperture
Fourth ventricle
Lateral aperture
Central canal
Temporal horn
Pons
Medulla oblongata

**Fig. 12.79 Ventricles of the brain;** view from the left side.
The inner subarachnoid space consists of the ventricular system and the central canal of the spinal cord. The ventricular system is composed of the **paired lateral ventricles** with frontal (anterior) horn, central part, occipital (posterior) horn, and temporal (inferior) horn, the **third ventricle,** the aqueduct of midbrain (cerebral aqueduct), and the **fourth ventricle.**

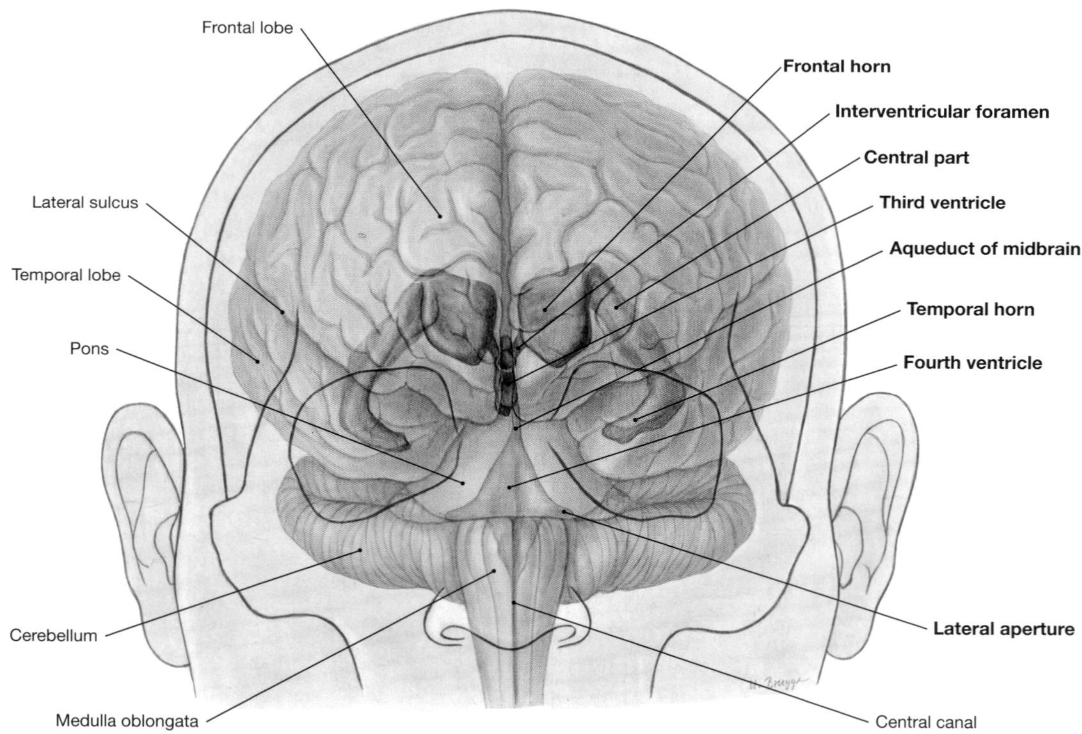
Frontal lobe
Frontal horn
Interventricular foramen
Central part
Lateral sulcus
Third ventricle
Aqueduct of midbrain
Temporal lobe
Temporal horn
Pons
Fourth ventricle
Lateral aperture
Cerebellum
Medulla oblongata
Central canal

**Fig. 12.80 Ventricles of the brain;** anterior view.
In this anterior view, the paired lateral ventricles and the medially located third and fourth ventricles have been projected onto the brain.

## Inner and outer subarachnoid spaces

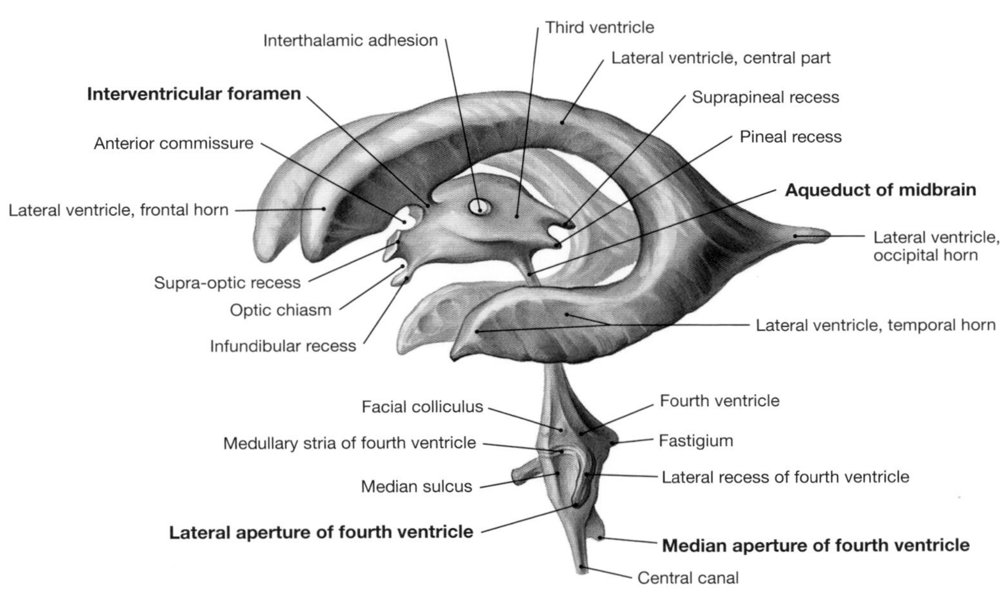
Interthalamic adhesion
Third ventricle
Lateral ventricle, central part
Interventricular foramen
Suprapineal recess
Anterior commissure
Pineal recess
Aqueduct of midbrain
Lateral ventricle, frontal horn
Lateral ventricle, occipital horn
Supra-optic recess
Optic chiasm
Infundibular recess
Lateral ventricle, temporal horn
Facial colliculus
Fourth ventricle
Medullary stria of fourth ventricle
Fastigium
Median sulcus
Lateral recess of fourth ventricle
Lateral aperture of fourth ventricle
Median aperture of fourth ventricle
Central canal

**Fig. 12.81 Inner subarachnoid spaces; corrosion cast specimen;** oblique view from the left side.
Each of the lateral ventricles connects with the third ventricle by a separate interventricular foramen **(foramen of MONRO).** The third ventricle communicates with the fourth ventricle through the **aqueduct of midbrain.** The fourth ventricle contains three openings to the outer subarachnoid space: the median aperture (foramen of MAGENDIE) and the paired lateral apertures (foramina of LUSCHKA).

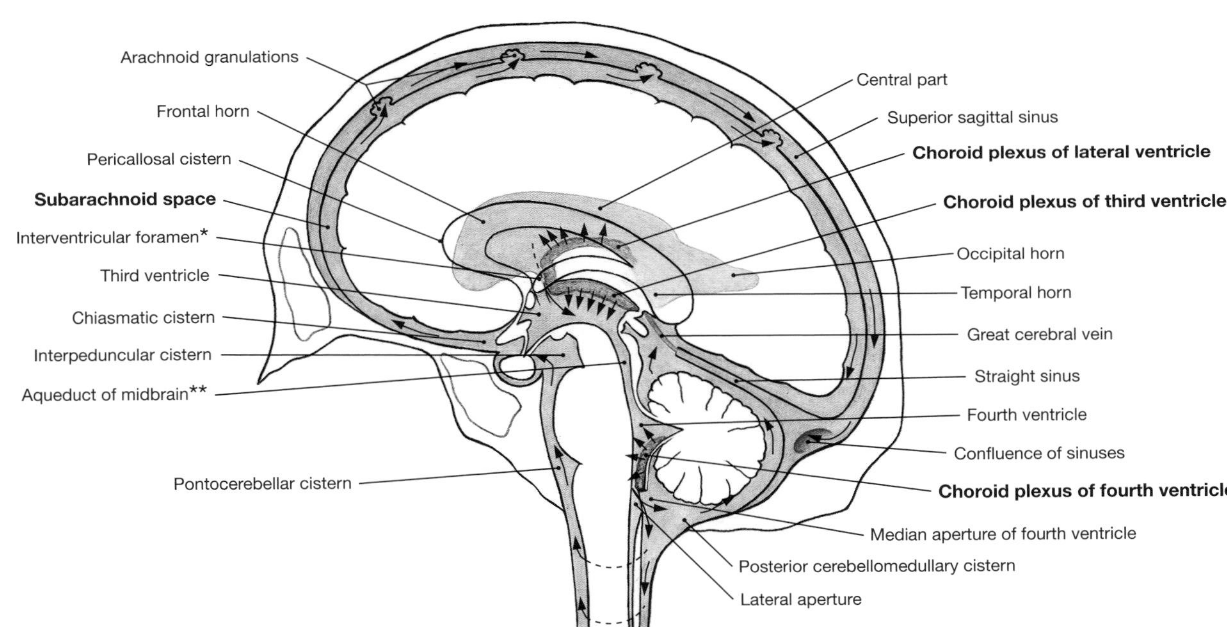
Arachnoid granulations
Frontal horn
Pericallosal cistern
Subarachnoid space
Interventricular foramen*
Third ventricle
Chiasmatic cistern
Interpeduncular cistern
Aqueduct of midbrain**
Pontocerebellar cistern
Central part
Superior sagittal sinus
Choroid plexus of lateral ventricle
Choroid plexus of third ventricle
Occipital horn
Temporal horn
Great cerebral vein
Straight sinus
Fourth ventricle
Confluence of sinuses
Choroid plexus of fourth ventricle
Median aperture of fourth ventricle
Posterior cerebellomedullary cistern
Lateral aperture

**Fig. 12.82 Ventricles of the brain and subarachnoid space;** schematic drawing of the circulation (arrows) of the cerebrospinal fluid from the inner to the outer subarachnoid space.
The space in between the arachnoid and pia mater constitutes the outer subarachnoid space. It surrounds the brain as well as the spinal cord. The choroid plexus in the ventricles produce the major part of the cerebrospinal fluid (CSF).
The circulating fluid volume (150 ml) is exchanged permanently (daily production volume approx. 500 ml).

The cerebrospinal fluid has multiple **functions.** It serves as a cushion to protect the CNS from mechanical forces, reduces the weight of the CNS (the CSF creates buoyancy which causes a 97% weight reduction from 1400 g to 45 g), supports the metabolism of the CNS, removes toxic substances, and transports hormones (e.g. leptin).

* clinical term: foramen of MONRO
** clinical term: aqueduct of SYLVIUS

## Ventricles

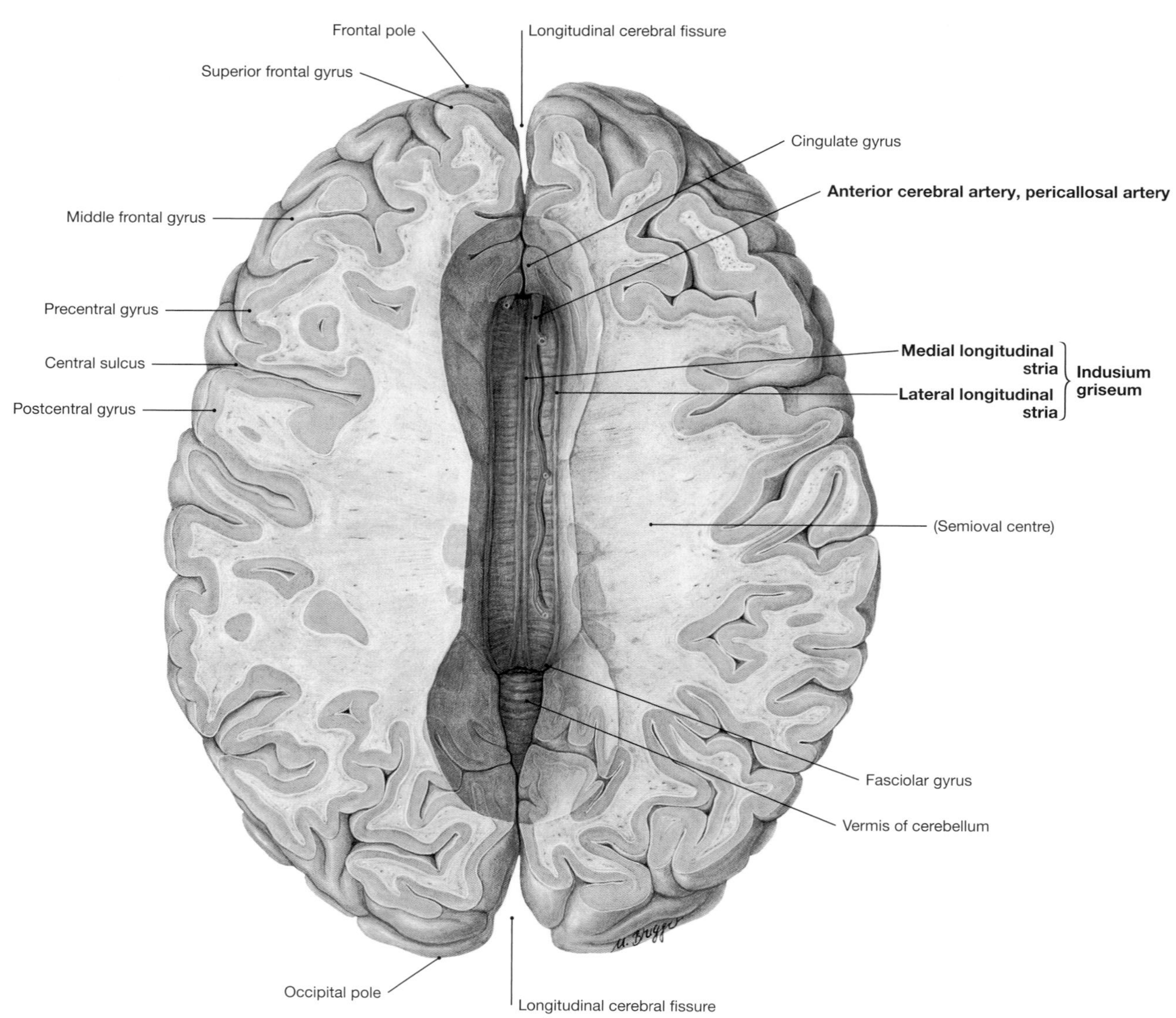
Frontal pole
Longitudinal cerebral fissure
Superior frontal gyrus
Cingulate gyrus
Anterior cerebral artery, pericallosal artery
Middle frontal gyrus
Precentral gyrus
Central sulcus
Postcentral gyrus
Medial longitudinal stria
Lateral longitudinal stria
Indusium griseum
(Semioval centre)
Fasciolar gyrus
Vermis of cerebellum
Occipital pole
Longitudinal cerebral fissure

**Fig. 12.83 Corpus callosum;** superior view; after removal of the upper parts of the cerebral hemispheres.

A superior view onto the corpus callosum reveals the rostral to occipital orientation of the medial and lateral longitudinal stria of the indusium griseum (considered a cortical part of the limbic system) as well as the pericallosal artery (from the anterior cerebral artery). The corpus callosum consists of the rostrum, genu, trunk, and a thickened posterior end (splenium; → Fig. 12.127). It creates the roof of the lateral ventricles and is composed of commissural fibers connecting one hemisphere with the other. It contains approximately 200 million axones.

The **function** of the corpus callosum involves the information exchange and coordination between the two hemispheres, with each hemisphere having partially different tasks in the processing of information.

## Clinical Remarks

The surgical sectioning of the corpus callosum has been used for the treatment of some severe forms of epilepsy (almost always the splenium was kept intact). The rationale for this drastic therapy was to prevent the propagation of the irregular brain excitations onto the unaffected cerebral hemisphere. A significant reduction in the frequency and severity of epileptic seizures occurs. However, this operation, also known as **split-brain operation** or **callosotomia,** results in patients suffering from severe cognitive impairment and a split-brain syndrome. Therefore, this surgery has been largely abandonded. A vivid description of a patient with **split-brain syndrome** is presented in the book by Oliver Sacks, a neurologist and author of the 1985 novel "The Man Who Mistook His Wife for a Hat".

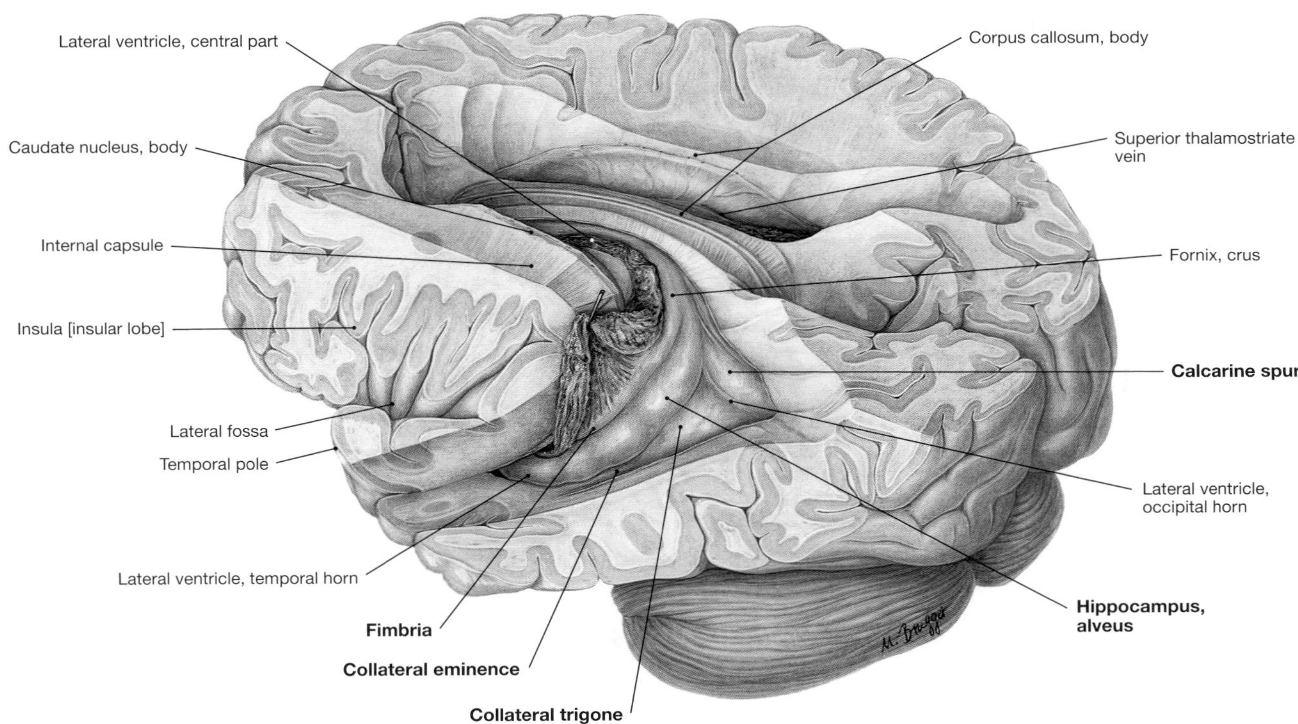
Lateral ventricle, central part
Caudate nucleus, body
Internal capsule
Insula [insular lobe]
Lateral fossa
Temporal pole
Lateral ventricle, temporal horn
Fimbria
Collateral eminence
Collateral trigone
Corpus callosum, body
Superior thalamostriate vein
Fornix, crus
Calcarine spur
Lateral ventricle, occipital horn
Hippocampus, alveus

**Fig. 12.84 Lateral ventricles;** posterior superior view from the left side; after removal of the upper parts of the cerebral hemispheres. View into both lateral ventricles. The course of the **choroid plexus** is visible in the left lateral ventricle. The choroid plexus has been lifted up with a probe at the transition from the central part to the temporal part of the lateral ventricle. The choroid plexus **produces cerebrospinal fluid.**
The roof and the lateral wall of the occipital horn are formed by the tapetum (radiation of corpus callosum, optic radiation) (not visible). The calcar avis forms the medial wall, and the collateral trigone and the collateral eminence create the floor. The roof and lateral wall of the temporal horn are part of the tail of caudate nucleus and the tapetum (not visible), the hippocampal fimbria, and the choroid plexus form the medial wall, and the floor consists of the collateral eminence and the alveus of hippocampus (→ Figs. 12.87, 12.123 to 12.126).

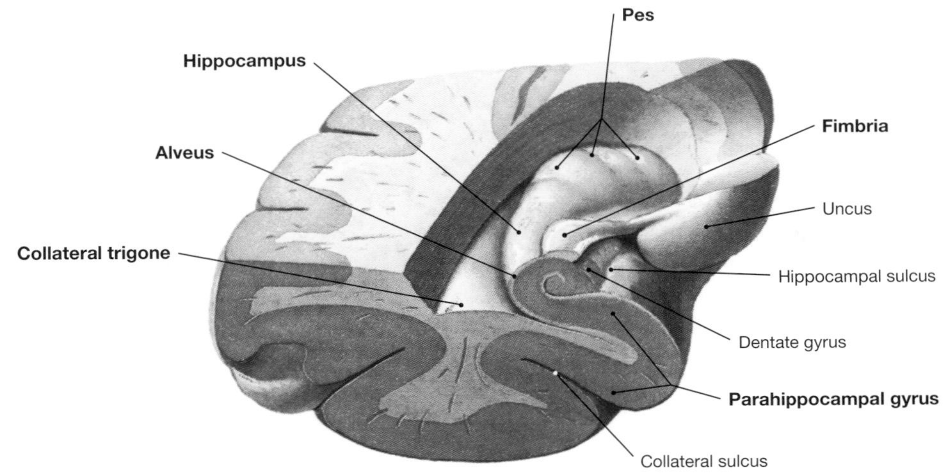
Pes
Hippocampus
Alveus
Collateral trigone
Fimbria
Uncus
Hippocampal sulcus
Dentate gyrus
Parahippocampal gyrus
Collateral sulcus

**Fig. 12.85 Left temporal horn of the lateral ventricle;** frontal section after removal of the temporal wall; posterior superior view.
The alveus, fimbria, and pes of the hippocampus form parts of the floor of the temporal horn of the lateral ventricle. The collateral trigone is also visible. The hippocampus formation with the parahippocampal gyrus is visible in the frontal section. The **hippocampus** is a central element of the limbic system (→ Fig. 12.47) and is involved in processes of learning, memory, and emotions.

## Ventricles

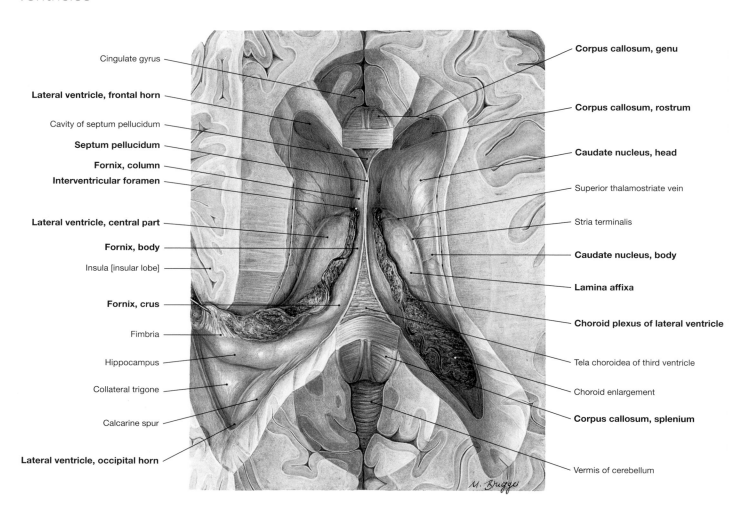

Cingulate gyrus
**Lateral ventricle, frontal horn**
Cavity of septum pellucidum
**Septum pellucidum**
**Fornix, column**
**Interventricular foramen**
**Lateral ventricle, central part**
**Fornix, body**
Insula [insular lobe]
**Fornix, crus**
Fimbria
Hippocampus
Collateral trigone
Calcarine spur
**Lateral ventricle, occipital horn**
**Corpus callosum, genu**
**Corpus callosum, rostrum**
**Caudate nucleus, head**
Superior thalamostriate vein
Stria terminalis
**Caudate nucleus, body**
**Lamina affixa**
**Choroid plexus of lateral ventricle**
Tela choroidea of third ventricle
Choroid enlargement
**Corpus callosum, splenium**
Vermis of cerebellum
M. Brugger

**Fig. 12.86 Lateral ventricles;** superior view; after removal of the upper part of the cerebral hemispheres and the central part of the corpus callosum.
This view shows the frontal horn, the central part, and the occipital horn as well as the transition of both lateral ventricles to the temporal horn. The margins of the **frontal horn** are the genu of the corpus callosum (anterior wall), the trunk of the corpus callosum (roof, not visible, because the corpus callosum was detached at the genu and the splenium), the septum pellucidum (medial wall), the head of the caudate nucleus (lateral wall), as well as the rostrum of the corpus callosum (floor). The interventricular foramina **(foramina of MONRO)** in the frontal horn are also visible. Like the frontal part, the roof of the central part is formed by the trunk of the corpus callosum (removed). The crus of the fornix and the septum pellucidum create the medial wall, the body of the caudate nucleus forms the lateral wall, and the floor consists of the lamina affixa of the choroid plexus and the crus of the fornix.

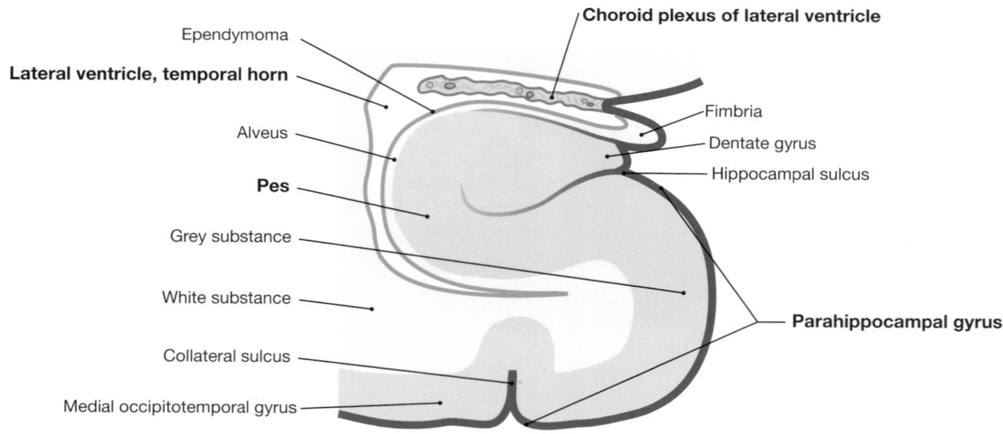
Ependymoma
Lateral ventricle, temporal horn
Alveus
Pes
Grey substance
White substance
Collateral sulcus
Medial occipitotemporal gyrus
Choroid plexus of lateral ventricle
Fimbria
Dentate gyrus
Hippocampal sulcus
Parahippocampal gyrus

**Fig. 12.87 Temporal horn of the lateral ventricle;** schematic frontal section.
The scheme demonstrates the topographic relationship of the lateral ventricle and the hippocampus formation. The choroid plexus protrudes into the lateral ventricle. The walls of the ventricle are colored in bright green, while the cerebrospinal fluid and the internal ventricular space are shown in white.

## Ventricles

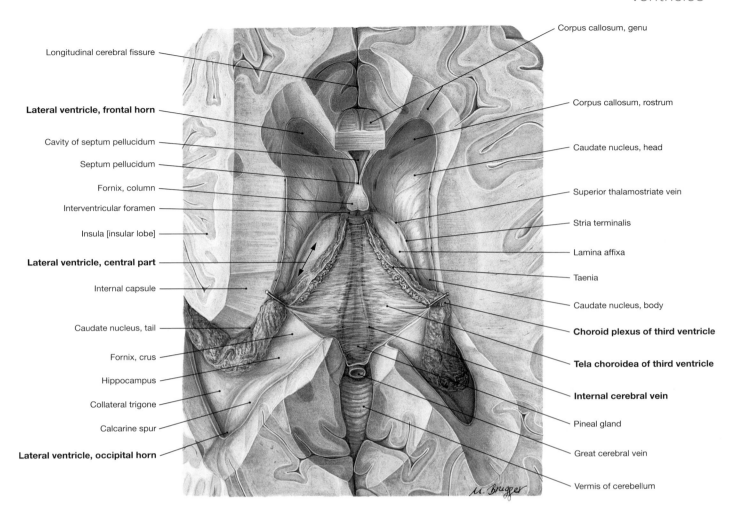

Longitudinal cerebral fissure
**Lateral ventricle, frontal horn**
Cavity of septum pellucidum
Septum pellucidum
Fornix, column
Interventricular foramen
Insula [insular lobe]
**Lateral ventricle, central part**
Internal capsule
Caudate nucleus, tail
Fornix, crus
Hippocampus
Collateral trigone
Calcarine spur
**Lateral ventricle, occipital horn**
Corpus callosum, genu
Corpus callosum, rostrum
Caudate nucleus, head
Superior thalamostriate vein
Stria terminalis
Lamina affixa
Taenia
Caudate nucleus, body
**Choroid plexus of third ventricle**
**Tela choroidea of third ventricle**
**Internal cerebral vein**
Pineal gland
Great cerebral vein
Vermis of cerebellum

**Fig. 12.88 Lateral ventricles;** superior view; after removal of the central part of the corpus callosum and the columns of the fornix. Shown is the choroid membrane overarching the third ventricle. The internal cerebral veins gleam through and drain into the great cerebral vein. The frontal horn, central part, and occipital horn of the lateral ventricles are visible. Laterally, the **choroid plexus** continues alongside the hippocampus into the temporal horn.

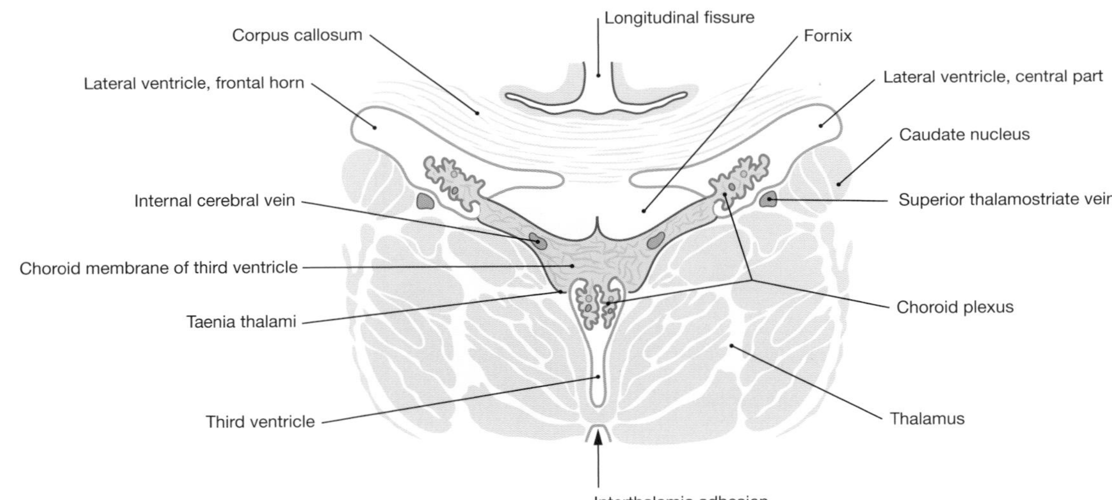
Corpus callosum
Longitudinal fissure
Fornix
Lateral ventricle, frontal horn
Lateral ventricle, central part
Caudate nucleus
Internal cerebral vein
Superior thalamostriate vein
Choroid membrane of third ventricle
Taenia thalami
Choroid plexus
Third ventricle
Thalamus
Interthalamic adhesion

**Fig. 12.89 Choroid plexus in the lateral ventricles and third ventricle;** schematic frontal section. (according to [2])
The **choroid plexus** produces cerebrospinal fluid (CSF) and is present in the paired lateral ventricles (left first and right second lateral ventricle) as well as in the third and the fourth ventricles (not shown). In the choroid plexus, capillary blood and CSF space are separated by a **blood-CSF barrier.**

## Ventricles

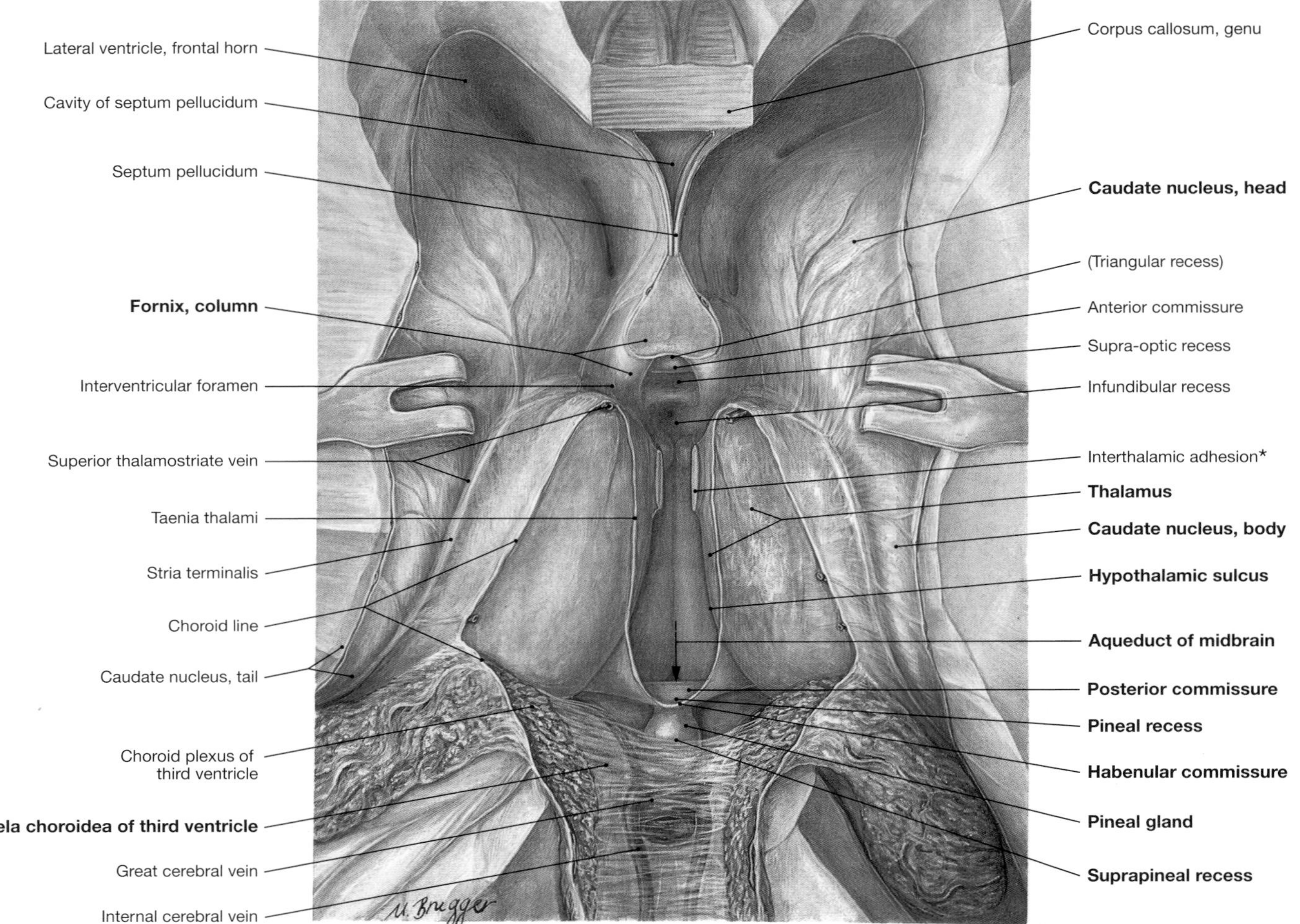
Lateral ventricle, frontal horn
Cavity of septum pellucidum
Septum pellucidum
Fornix, column
Interventricular foramen
Superior thalamostriate vein
Taenia thalami
Stria terminalis
Choroid line
Caudate nucleus, tail
Choroid plexus of third ventricle
Tela choroidea of third ventricle
Great cerebral vein
Internal cerebral vein
Corpus callosum, genu
Caudate nucleus, head
(Triangular recess)
Anterior commissure
Supra-optic recess
Infundibular recess
Interthalamic adhesion*
Thalamus
Caudate nucleus, body
Hypothalamic sulcus
Aqueduct of midbrain
Posterior commissure
Pineal recess
Habenular commissure
Pineal gland
Suprapineal recess

**Fig. 12.90 Lateral ventricles and third ventricle;** superior view; parts of the cerebral hemispheres, the central part of the corpus callosum as well as the fornix and the choroid plexus have been removed, the choroid membrane of the third ventricle has been reflected.

**The margins of the third ventricle are:**

- roof: choroid membrane and choroid plexus
- anterior wall: columna of fornix, anterior commissure, lamina terminalis, triangular recess, and supra-optic recess
- lateral wall: thalamus, stria medullaris of thalamus, hypothalamic sulcus, and hypothalamus (wall)
- posterior wall: habenular commissure, posterior commissure, suprapineal recess, and pineal recess
- floor: infundibular recess

* interthalamic adhesion (massa intermedia) cut in the median plane

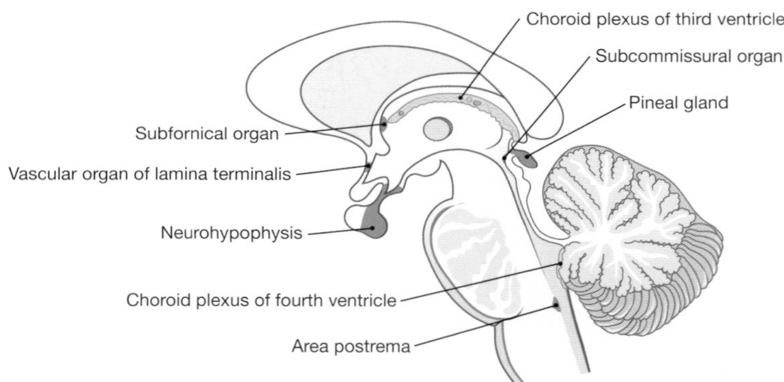
Choroid plexus of third ventricle
Subcommissural organ
Pineal gland
Subfornical organ
Vascular organ of lamina terminalis
Neurohypophysis
Choroid plexus of fourth ventricle
Area postrema

**Fig. 12.91 Circumventricular organs,** median sagittal section. Characteristic features of the circumventricular organs are strong vascularization, a modified ependyme (tanycytes with tight junctions), and the formation of a blood-CSF barrier instead of a blood-brain barrier. Circumventricular organs include the neurohypophysis, the median eminence, the pineal gland as well as the vascular organ of lamina terminalis and the subfornical organ (both: regulation of blood volume and blood pressure, secretion of hormones like angiotensin, somatostatin, inducing fever), the subcommissural organ (present only in the foetus and newborn, secretion of a glycoprotein-rich product), and the area postrema (triggers vomiting).

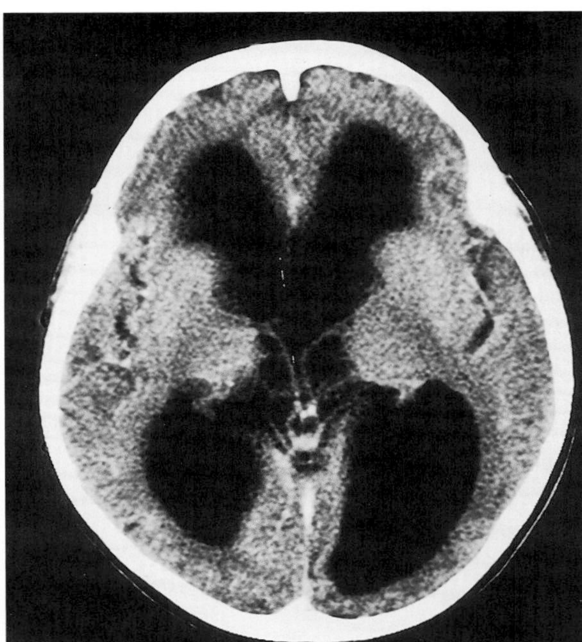
a

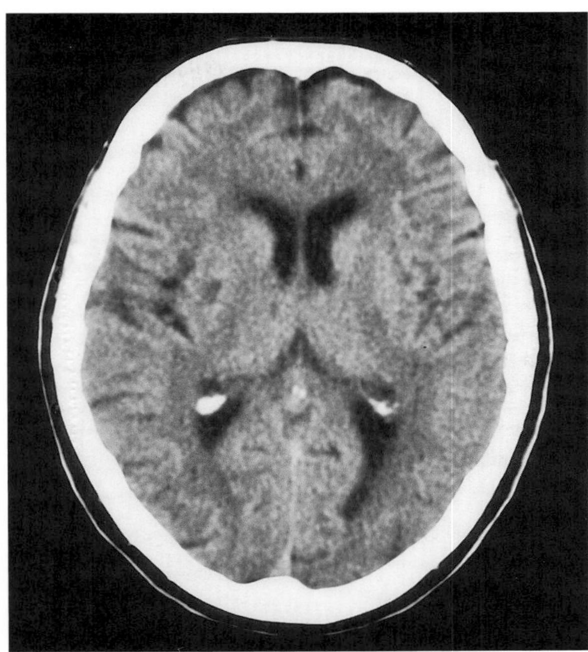
b

**Figs. 12.92a and b Computed tomographic (CT) cross-sections of the head.** [23]
**a** CT scan of a patient with a cerebrospinal fluid block caused by obstruction in the cerebral aqueduct (aqueduct of midbrain). The cerebral ventricles are greatly enlarged (hydrocephalus) at the expense of the cerebral parenchyma. The patient showed massive mental disabilities and significantly impaired gait.
**b** CT scan of a healthy person

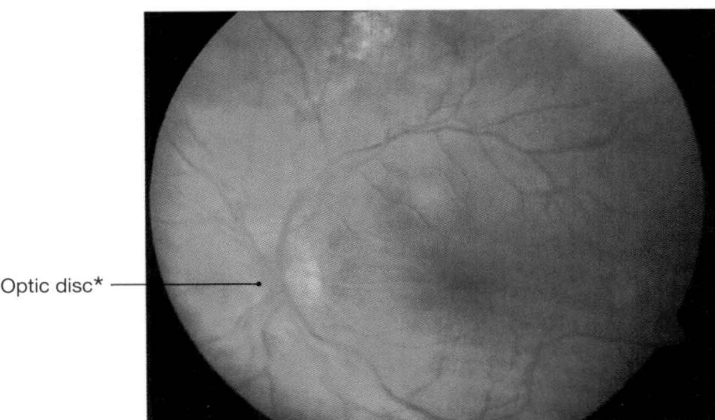
Optic disc*

**Fig. 12.93 Ocular fundus; left side;** anterior view; ophthalmoscopic image of the central area with papilledema caused by increased intracranial pressure.
The examination of the ocular fundus reveals a swelling of the optic disc resulting from an intraventricular neurocytoma WHO grade II. As the optic nerve [II] is surrounded by meninges and cerebrospinal fluid, the optic disc bulges out into the eyeball.

* clinical term: blind spot

## Clinical Remarks

The circumventricular organs (→ Fig. 12.91) lack the **blood-brain barrier** and, thus, are capable of monitoring the plasma-blood milieu. This is not only of pharmacological interest. The area postrema contains numerous dopamine and serotonin receptors. Dopamine and serotonin antagonists are effective anti-emetic drugs. In addition, the activation of chemoreceptors in the area of the area postrema presents a protective mechanism for the body as exemplified by the centrally induced vomiting as a response to the ingestion of spoiled food. This will remove the major part of potentially harmful substances from the body.

The **impaired drainage of cerebrospinal fluid** (CSF) can be the result of tumors, deformities, bleedings, or other causes and, due to the increased intracranial pressure, coincide with headaches, nausea, and optic papilla protrusion (papilloedema) (→ Fig. 12.93). An **internal hydrocephalus** (→ Fig. 12.92) is caused by the blockage of the inner (intracerebral) subarachnoid space with accumulation of CSF in the ventricles, whereas accumulation of CSF in the outer subarachnoid space is a characteristic feature of an **external hydrocephalus.** A **hydrocephalus ex vacuo** results from an increase in ventricular size due to a rarefication of brain matter, as it occurs in ALZHEIMER's disease.

## Arteries at the cranial base

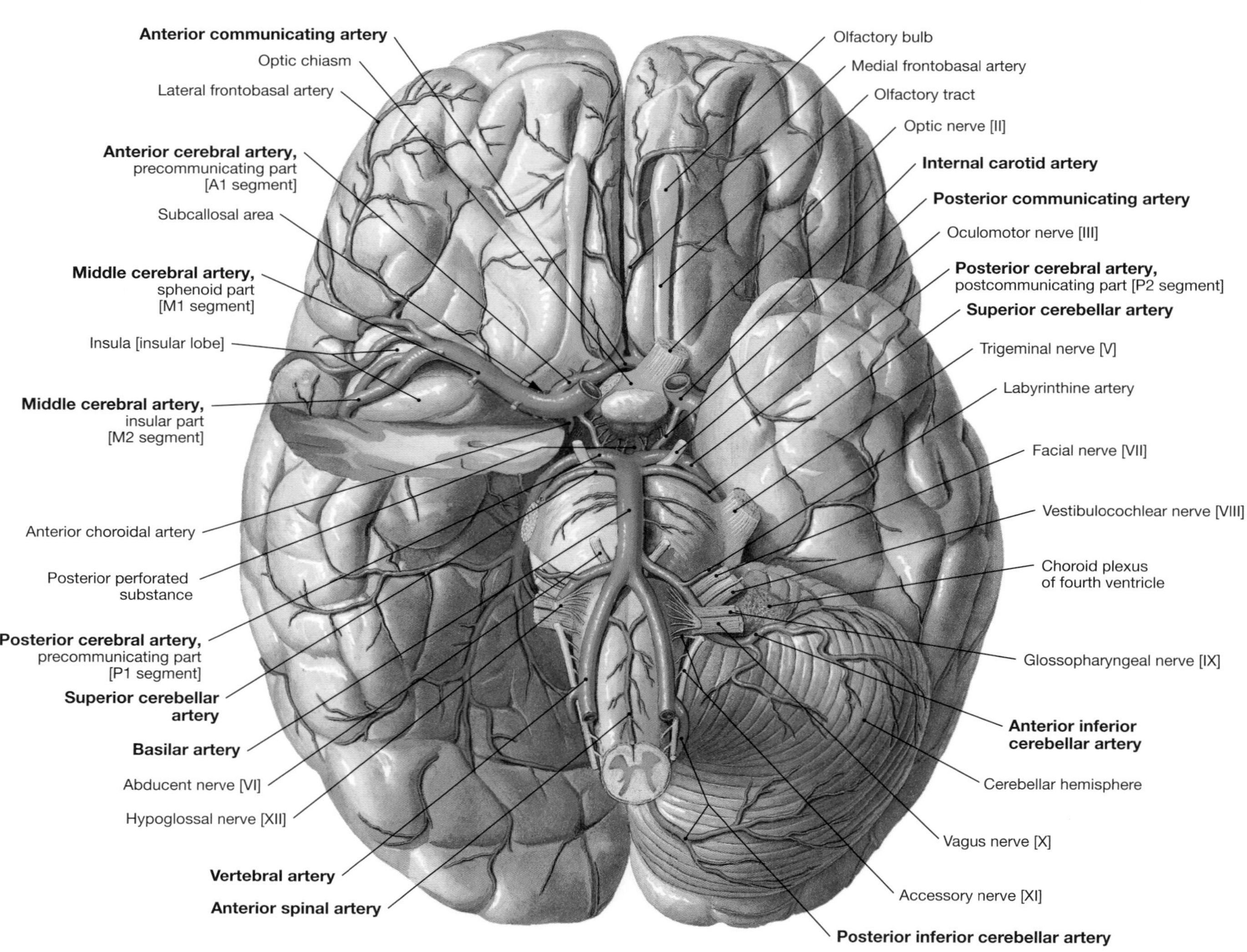
Anterior communicating artery
Optic chiasm
Lateral frontobasal artery
Anterior cerebral artery, precommunicating part [A1 segment]
Subcallosal area
Middle cerebral artery, sphenoid part [M1 segment]
Insula [insular lobe]
Middle cerebral artery, insular part [M2 segment]
Anterior choroidal artery
Posterior perforated substance
Posterior cerebral artery, precommunicating part [P1 segment]
Superior cerebellar artery
Basilar artery
Abducent nerve [VI]
Hypoglossal nerve [XII]
Vertebral artery
Anterior spinal artery
Olfactory bulb
Medial frontobasal artery
Olfactory tract
Optic nerve [II]
Internal carotid artery
Posterior communicating artery
Oculomotor nerve [III]
Posterior cerebral artery, postcommunicating part [P2 segment]
Superior cerebellar artery
Trigeminal nerve [V]
Labyrinthine artery
Facial nerve [VII]
Vestibulocochlear nerve [VIII]
Choroid plexus of fourth ventricle
Glossopharyngeal nerve [IX]
Anterior inferior cerebellar artery
Cerebellar hemisphere
Vagus nerve [X]
Accessory nerve [XI]
Posterior inferior cerebellar artery

**Fig. 12.94 Arteries of the brain;** inferior view.
The figure demonstrates the location of the arteries at the cranial base. The vertebral arteries converge to form the basilar artery which releases the posterior cerebral arteries and branches for the brainstem, the cerebellum, and the inner ear (so-called **vertebralis tributary**). Small connecting arteries (posterior communicanting arteries) provide the link between the posterior cerebral arteries and the two internal carotid arteries. Each of the latter contributes one middle cerebral artery and one anterior cerebral artery which collectively provide the major part of the blood for the hemispheres (so-called **carotis tributary**). The anterior communicating artery connects both anterior cerebral arteries.
Clinically, the anterior, middle, and posterior cerebral artery are divided into segments. The A1 segment (precommunicating part) corresponds to the part of the anterior cerebral artery proximal to the anterior communicating artery and the part distal of the anterior communicating artery is the A2 segment (infracallosal or postcommunicating part). The A3 segment (precallosal part) describes the part of the anterior cerebral artery located in front of the corpus callosum and the part located on top of the corpus callosum constitutes the A4 segment (supracallosal part). Clinicians call the part of the anterior cerebral artery distal to the anterior communicating artery the pericallosal artery. The middle cerebral artery is composed of the segments M1 (sphenoidal or horizontal part), M2 (insular part), M3 (opercular part), and M4 (terminal part). The posterior cerebral artery divides into four segments: P1 (precommunicating part; proximal to the posterior communicating artery), P2 (postcommunicating part; up to the posterior rim of the brainstem), P3 (quadrigeminal part; up to the point where the posterior cerebral artery enters the calcarine fissure), and P4 (no specific name; division into two arterial branches). Some segments are visible in the figure.

### Clinical Remarks

One of the most frequent forms of cerebral ischemia in the vertebralis tributary is called **WALLENBERG's syndrome** (dorsolateral medulla oblongata syndrome). Caused by an occluded or largely blocked posterior inferior cerebellar artery, the symptoms include nystagmus, difficulties in equilibrium and swallowing (dysphagia), uncontrollable singultus, dysphonia, and dizziness.

## Arteries at the cranial base, arterial circle of the brain

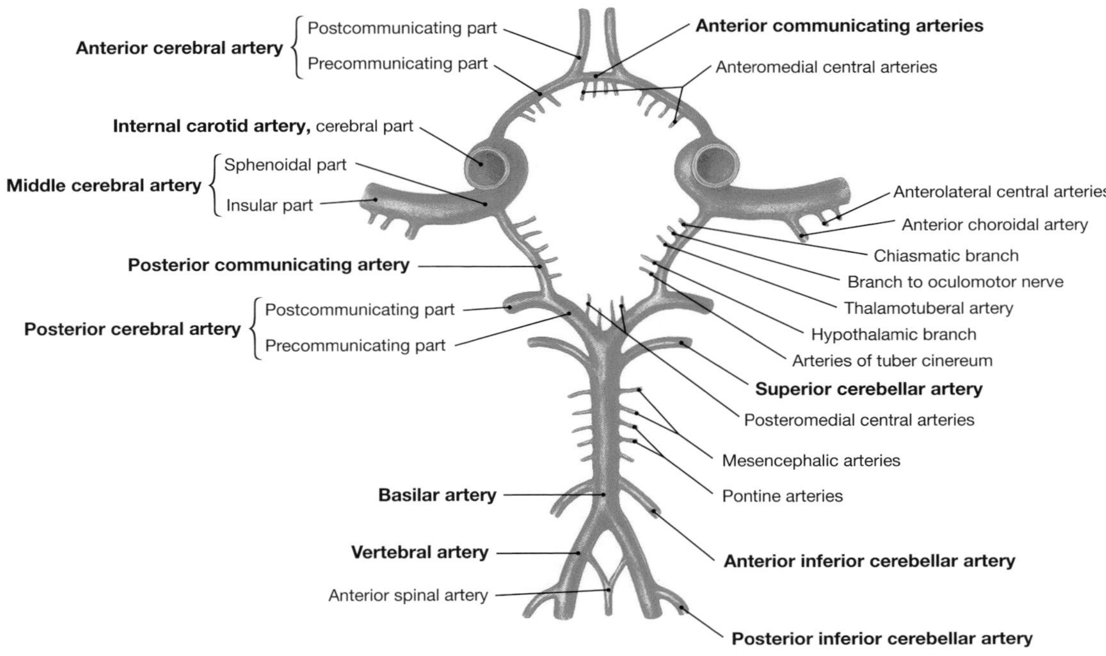
Anterior cerebral artery
Postcommunicating part
Precommunicating part
Anterior communicating arteries
Anteromedial central arteries
Internal carotid artery, cerebral part
Middle cerebral artery
Sphenoidal part
Insular part
Anterolateral central arteries
Anterior choroidal artery
Posterior communicating artery
Chiasmatic branch
Branch to oculomotor nerve
Posterior cerebral artery
Postcommunicating part
Precommunicating part
Thalamotuberal artery
Hypothalamic branch
Arteries of tuber cinereum
Superior cerebellar artery
Posteromedial central arteries
Mesencephalic arteries
Basilar artery
Pontine arteries
Vertebral artery
Anterior inferior cerebellar artery
Anterior spinal artery
Posterior inferior cerebellar artery

**Fig. 12.95 Arterial circle of the brain (circle of WILLIS);** superior view.
The posterior communicating artery connects the posterior cerebral artery with the cerebral parts of the internal carotid artery on both sides. In front, the anterior communicating artery connects the two anterior cerebral arteries. This generates a closed arterial circle which provides an anastomosis between the two internal carotid arteries and the vertebralis tributary.

## Clinical Remarks

Of all **cerebral aneurysms,** more than 90% occur at the cerebral vessels that make up the cerebral arterial circle (circle of WILLIS). The anterior communicating artery followed by the internal carotid artery are the most frequently affected cerebral vessels. Most cerebral aneurysms are the result of congenital defects in the tunica media of the vascular wall close to branching points. Often, aneurysms are associated with other diseases, such as polycystic kidneys or fibromuscular dysplasia. Most of the aneurysms are asymptomatic. However, the aneurysmal sac may cause a compression of neighboring cranial nerves.
Cerebral aneurysms have a tendency to **rupture** and are the most frequent cause of subarachnoid bleedings. Upon rupture, immediate and strong headaches combined with vomiting and changes in consciousness occur.

## Vessels and nerves at the cranial base

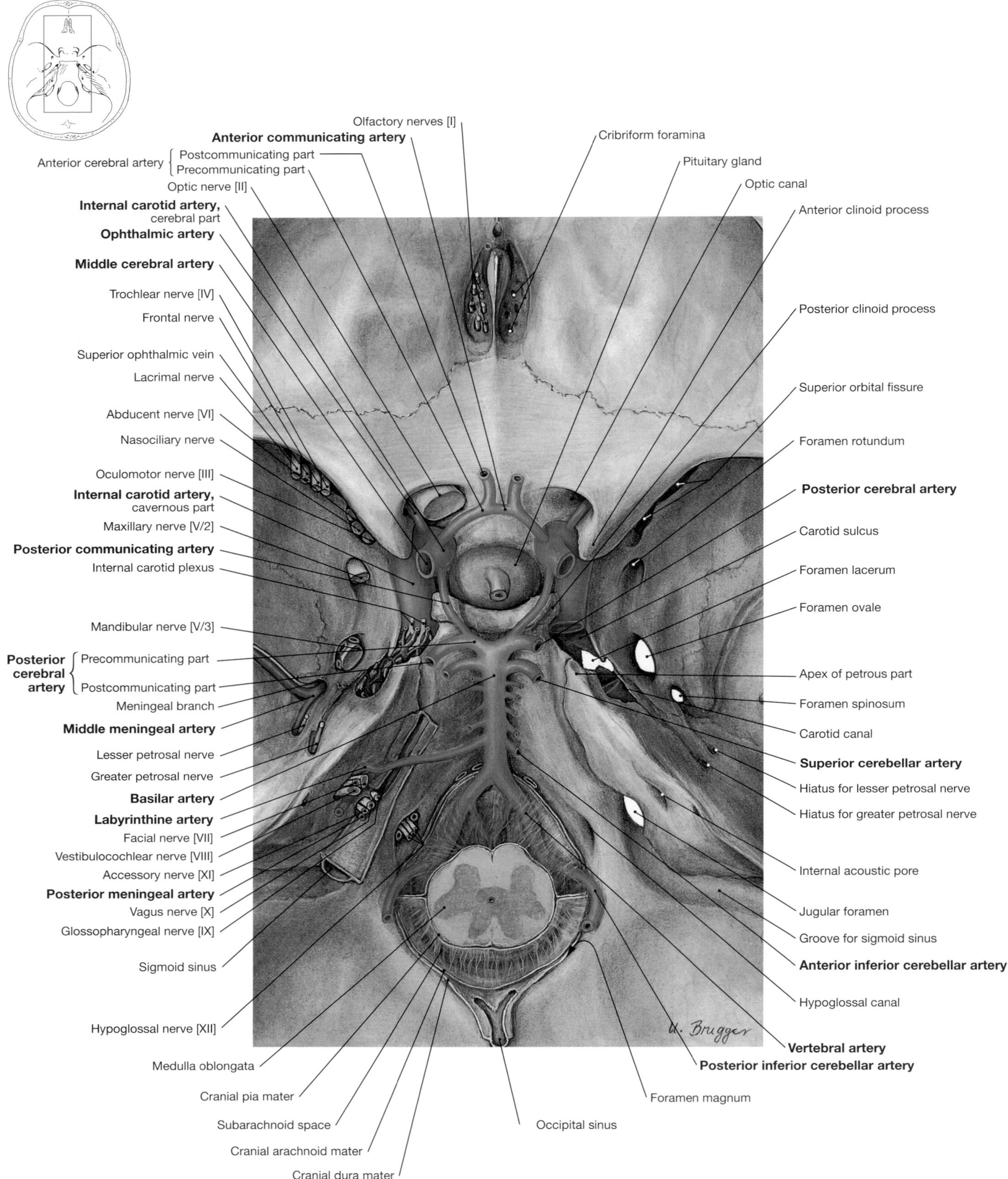
Olfactory nerves [I]
Anterior communicating artery
Anterior cerebral artery
Postcommunicating part
Precommunicating part
Optic nerve [II]
Internal carotid artery, cerebral part
Ophthalmic artery
Middle cerebral artery
Trochlear nerve [IV]
Frontal nerve
Superior ophthalmic vein
Lacrimal nerve
Abducent nerve [VI]
Nasociliary nerve
Oculomotor nerve [III]
Internal carotid artery, cavernous part
Maxillary nerve [V/2]
Posterior communicating artery
Internal carotid plexus
Mandibular nerve [V/3]
Posterior cerebral artery
Precommunicating part
Postcommunicating part
Meningeal branch
Middle meningeal artery
Lesser petrosal nerve
Greater petrosal nerve
Basilar artery
Labyrinthine artery
Facial nerve [VII]
Vestibulocochlear nerve [VIII]
Accessory nerve [XI]
Posterior meningeal artery
Vagus nerve [X]
Glossopharyngeal nerve [IX]
Sigmoid sinus
Hypoglossal nerve [XII]
Medulla oblongata
Cranial pia mater
Subarachnoid space
Cranial arachnoid mater
Cranial dura mater
Occipital sinus
Foramen magnum
Cribriform foramina
Pituitary gland
Optic canal
Anterior clinoid process
Posterior clinoid process
Superior orbital fissure
Foramen rotundum
Posterior cerebral artery
Carotid sulcus
Foramen lacerum
Foramen ovale
Apex of petrous part
Foramen spinosum
Carotid canal
Superior cerebellar artery
Hiatus for lesser petrosal nerve
Hiatus for greater petrosal nerve
Internal acoustic pore
Jugular foramen
Groove for sigmoid sinus
Anterior inferior cerebellar artery
Hypoglossal canal
Vertebral artery
Posterior inferior cerebellar artery
U. Brugger

**Fig. 12.96 Passageways of vessels and nerves through the internal surface of the cranial base and the cerebral arterial circle (circle of WILLIS);** superior view.

From a superior view, the cerebral arterial circle projects onto the hypophysial fossa. The ophthalmic artery branches off the **internal carotid artery** at the optic canal and, together with the optic nerve [II], enters the orbit through this bony canal. The **basilar artery** runs on top of the clivus. The **anterior inferior cerebellar artery** derives from the basilar artery and releases the **labyrinthine artery** while passing the internal acoustic pore or entering it in an S-shaped detour.

For an overview of the passageways through the internal surface of the cranial base → Figs. 8.16 and 8.17.

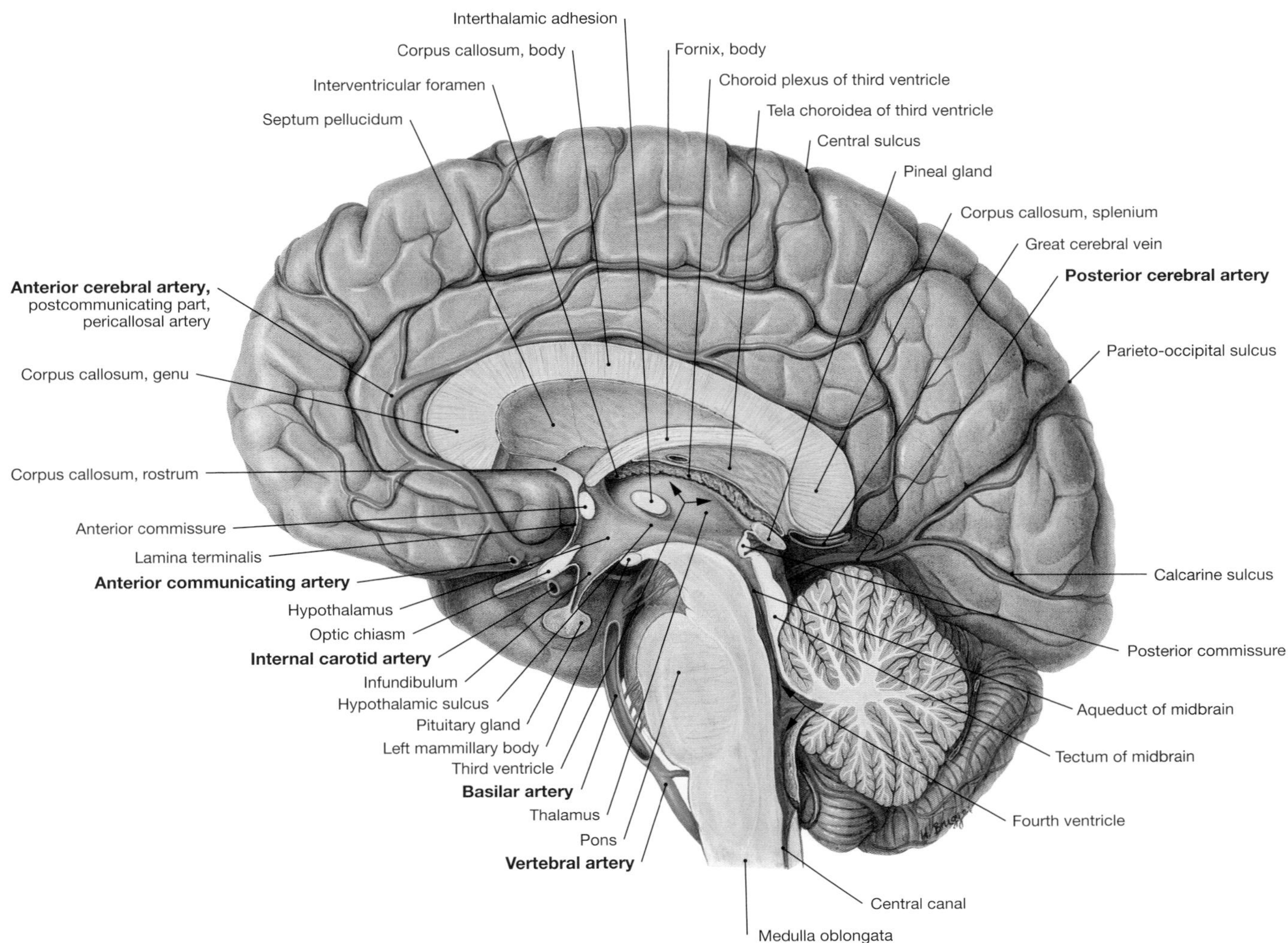
Interthalamic adhesion
Corpus callosum, body
Fornix, body
Interventricular foramen
Choroid plexus of third ventricle
Tela choroidea of third ventricle
Septum pellucidum
Central sulcus
Pineal gland
Corpus callosum, splenium
Great cerebral vein
Posterior cerebral artery
Anterior cerebral artery, postcommunicating part, pericallosal artery
Parieto-occipital sulcus
Corpus callosum, genu
Corpus callosum, rostrum
Anterior commissure
Lamina terminalis
Anterior communicating artery
Calcarine sulcus
Hypothalamus
Optic chiasm
Internal carotid artery
Posterior commissure
Infundibulum
Hypothalamic sulcus
Aqueduct of midbrain
Pituitary gland
Left mammillary body
Tectum of midbrain
Third ventricle
Basilar artery
Thalamus
Fourth ventricle
Pons
Vertebral artery
Central canal
Medulla oblongata

**Fig. 12.97 Medial surface of the brain, diencephalon, and brainstem;** staggered median section; view from the left side.
Once the anterior communicating artery has branched off the **anterior cerebral artery,** the postcommunicating part (pericallosal artery) of the latter passes around the rostrum and genu of the corpus callosum and runs alongside the upper surface of the corpus callosum. Its extensions reach the parietooccipital sulcus. The anterior cerebral artery supplies blood to the medial area of the frontal and parietal lobes as well as the hemispherical rim and a small area alongside thereof at the cerebral convexity (→ p. 271).
The **posterior cerebral artery** courses to the occipital lobe, basal part of the temporal lobe, lower part of the striatum (not visible), and thalamus.

## Arteries of the brain

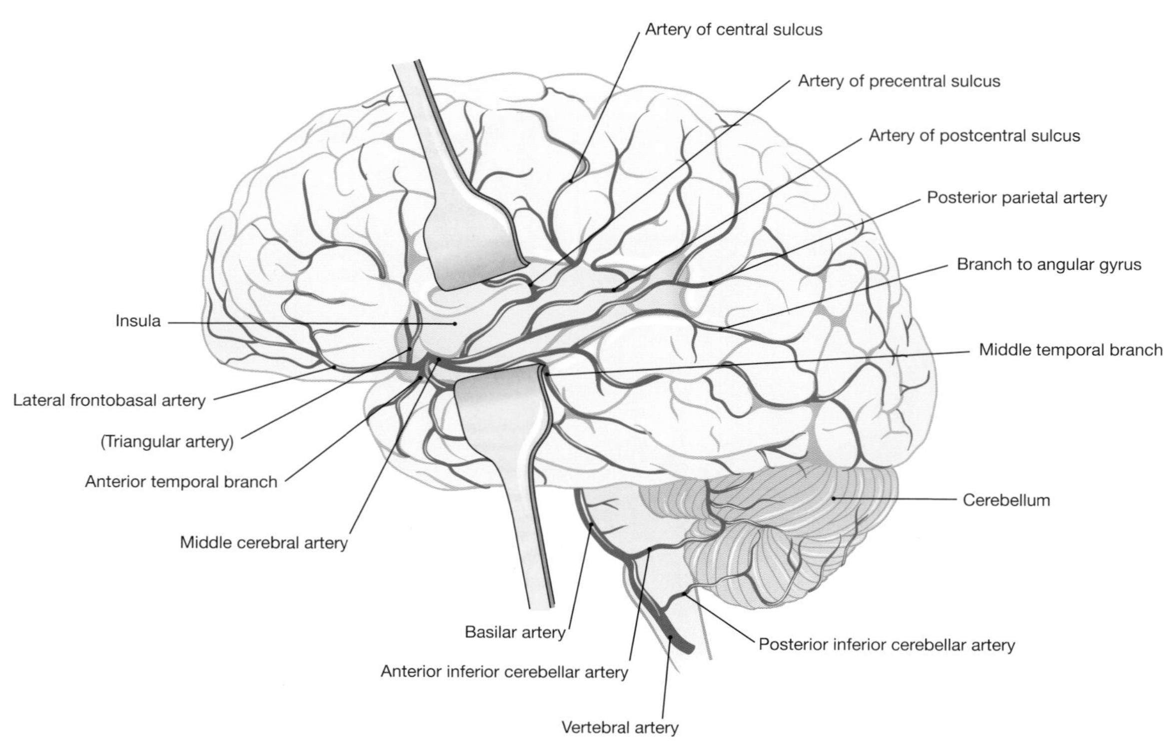
Artery of central sulcus
Artery of precentral sulcus
Artery of postcentral sulcus
Posterior parietal artery
Branch to angular gyrus
Middle temporal branch
Insula
Lateral frontobasal artery
(Triangular artery)
Anterior temporal branch
Middle cerebral artery
Cerebellum
Basilar artery
Anterior inferior cerebellar artery
Posterior inferior cerebellar artery
Vertebral artery

**Fig. 12.98 Branches of the middle cerebral artery in the insular region and at the outer cerebral cortex;** view from the left side. (according to [2])

The **middle cerebral artery** enters the lateral fossa from the lateral side and divides into four parts (→ Fig. 12.94):

- sphenoidal part (not visible; M1)
- insular part with short branches for the insular cortex (M2)
- opercular part for the cortex of the temporal lobe (lateralis frontobasal artery and temporal arteries; M3)
- inferior and superior terminal branches (terminal part; M4) for the cortex in the area of the central sulcus and the parietal lobe

## Clinical Remarks

Occlusion of the middle cerebral artery shortly after branching from the internal carotid artery due to arteriosclerosis or embolus results in **cerebral infarction** (ischemic stroke) with severe symptoms. These include a contralateral, predominantly brachiofacial hemiplegia with weakness and loss of sensation (hypesthesia, local or general decrease in touch and pressure sensation of the skin). If the dominant hemisphere is affected, additional symptoms occur. These include aphasia (speech impairment), agraphia (inability to write words or text, despite existing motor and intellectual capabilities), and alexia (inability to read). In patients with high blood pressure (hypertension), changes in the wall of cerebral vessels can cause a vascular rupture and bleeding into the cerebral parenchyma (up to the extent of a massive bleeding). The basal ganglia are particularly prone to this scenario.

# Arteries of the brain

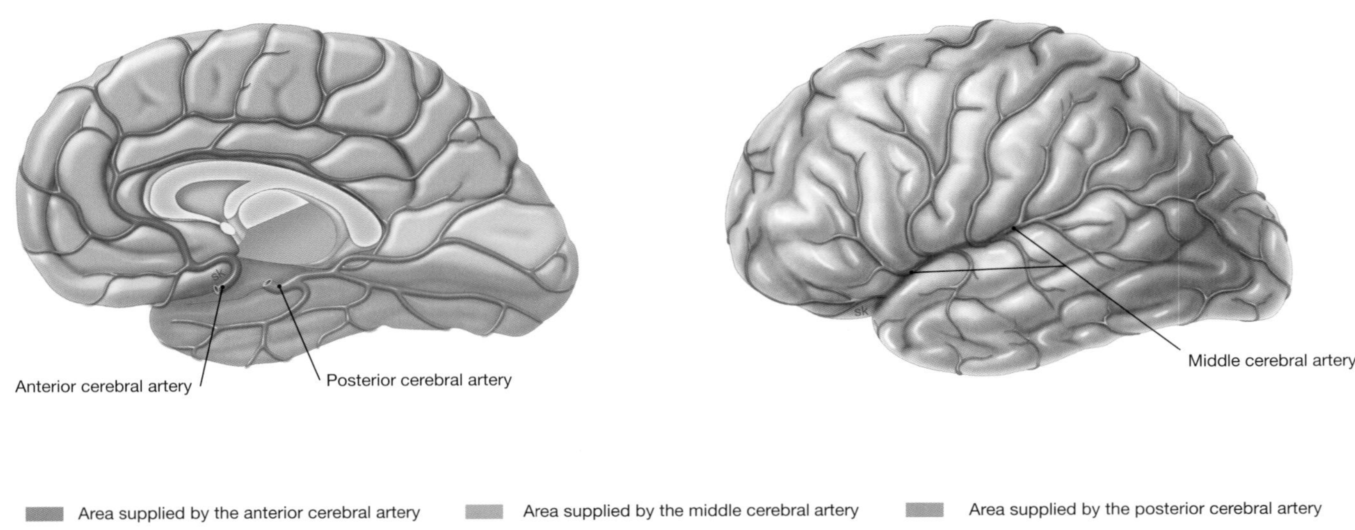
Anterior cerebral artery
Posterior cerebral artery
Middle cerebral artery
Area supplied by the anterior cerebral artery
Area supplied by the middle cerebral artery
Area supplied by the posterior cerebral artery

**Fig. 12.99 Arteries of the right hemisphere of the brain;** view from the left side.
The **anterior cerebral artery** supplies the medial side of the frontal and parietal lobes extending past the hemispheral rim and up to the parieto-occipital sulcus. The occipital lobe and the base of the temporal lobe receive their blood supply from the **posterior cerebral artery.**

**Fig. 12.100 Arteries of the left hemisphere of the brain; view from the left side.**
The **anterior cerebral artery** supplies blood to an area of the frontal and parietal cerebral cortex extending approximately 1 cm past the hemispheral rim onto the cortex convexity. The **posterior cerebral artery** supplies blood to the occipital pole and the inferior rim of the temporal lobe. The remaining outer cortical area receives blood from the **middle cerebral artery.** The areas of the precentral and postcentral gyri receive blood via both the anterior cerebral artery and the middle cerebral artery.

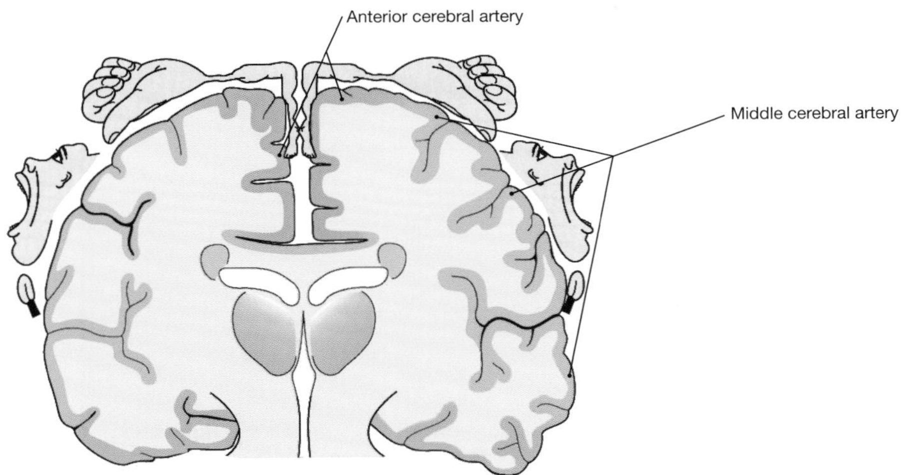
Anterior cerebral artery
Middle cerebral artery

**Fig. 12.101 Arteries in the region of the precentral gyrus and their tributaries in relation to the homunculus of the primary motor cortex.**
The **anterior cerebral artery** supplies blood to the cortex of the precentral gyrus up to approximately 1 cm past the hemispheral rim onto the cortical convexity. It supplies those precentral cortical areas representing the lower extremity, the pelvis, and the thorax as depicted by the homunculus. The **middle cerebral artery** supplies the representational cortex areas representing the upper extremity and the entire head.

## Clinical Remarks

Due to the blood supply of the particular cortical area in the the precentral gyrus, a blockage of the anterior cerebral artery results in **paralyses predominantly of the lower extremities;** an impaired perfusion by the middle cerebral artery causes **predominantly brachiofacial paralyses.** The symptoms of the patient (lower extremity or brachiofacial paralysis) can indicate the affected cerebral blood vessel.

## Arteries and veins of the brain

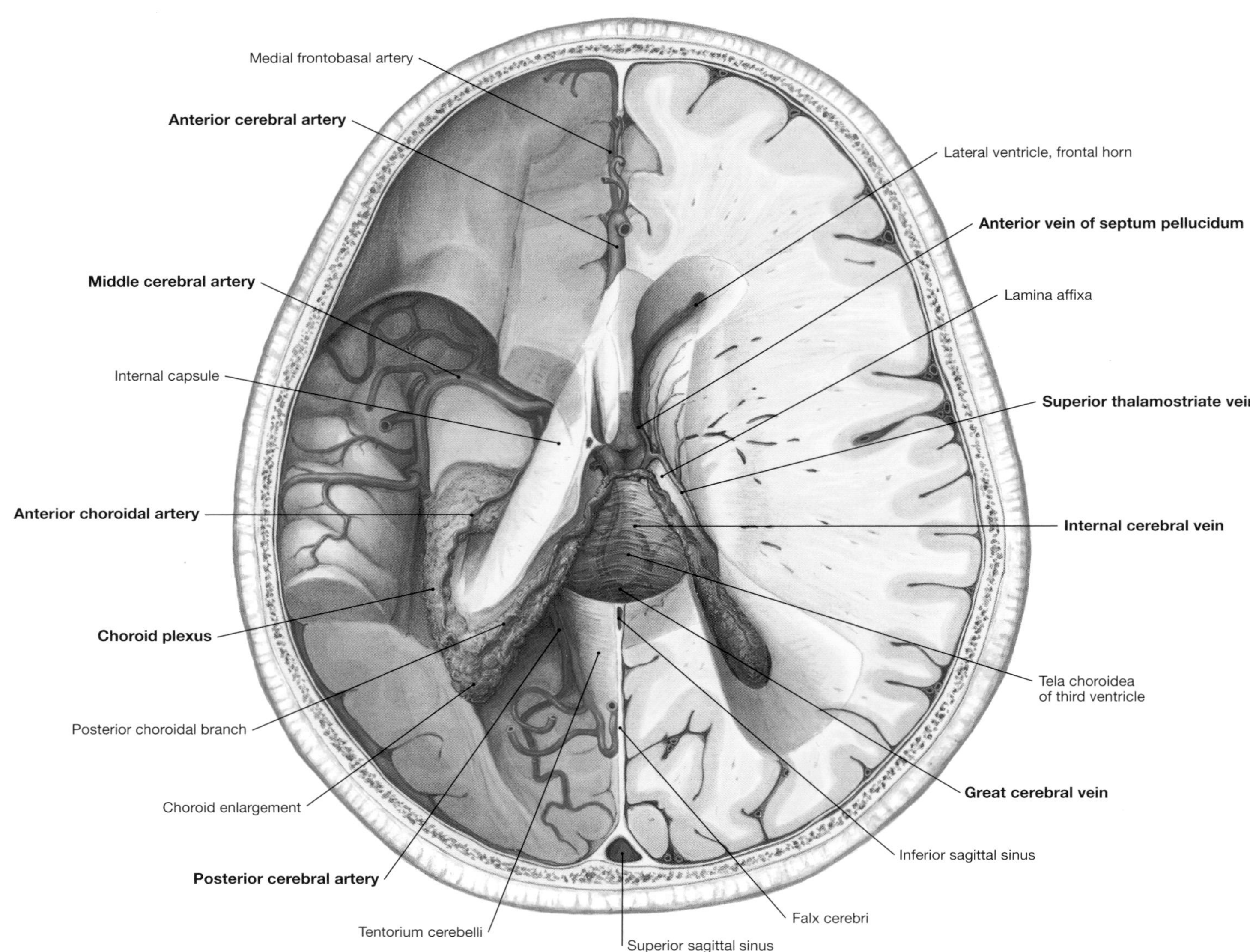
Medial frontobasal artery
Anterior cerebral artery
Middle cerebral artery
Internal capsule
Anterior choroidal artery
Choroid plexus
Posterior choroidal branch
Choroid enlargement
Posterior cerebral artery
Tentorium cerebelli
Superior sagittal sinus
Falx cerebri
Inferior sagittal sinus
Great cerebral vein
Tela choroidea of third ventricle
Internal cerebral vein
Superior thalamostriate vein
Lamina affixa
Anterior vein of septum pellucidum
Lateral ventricle, frontal horn

**Fig. 12.102 Arteries and veins of the brain;** superior view.
Upon removal of the parietal parts of the brain the otherwise hidden courses of the anterior, middle, and posterior cerebral arteries become visible on the **left side of the body.** The anterior choroid artery derives from the middle cerebral artery and supplies the choroid plexus of the lateral ventricle. The anterior choroid artery continues as a posterior choroid branch which extends into the tip of the choroid plexus of the frontal horn in the lateral ventricle.

On the **right side of the body** at the floor of the frontal horn of the lateral ventricle lies the anterior vein of septum pellucidum and further posterior the superior thalamostriate vein. Both drain blood into the internal cerebral vein which drains into the great cerebral vein (vein of GALEN). This group of veins drains the venous blood from the ventricular system, the basal ganglia, and the internal capsule.

## Veins of the brain

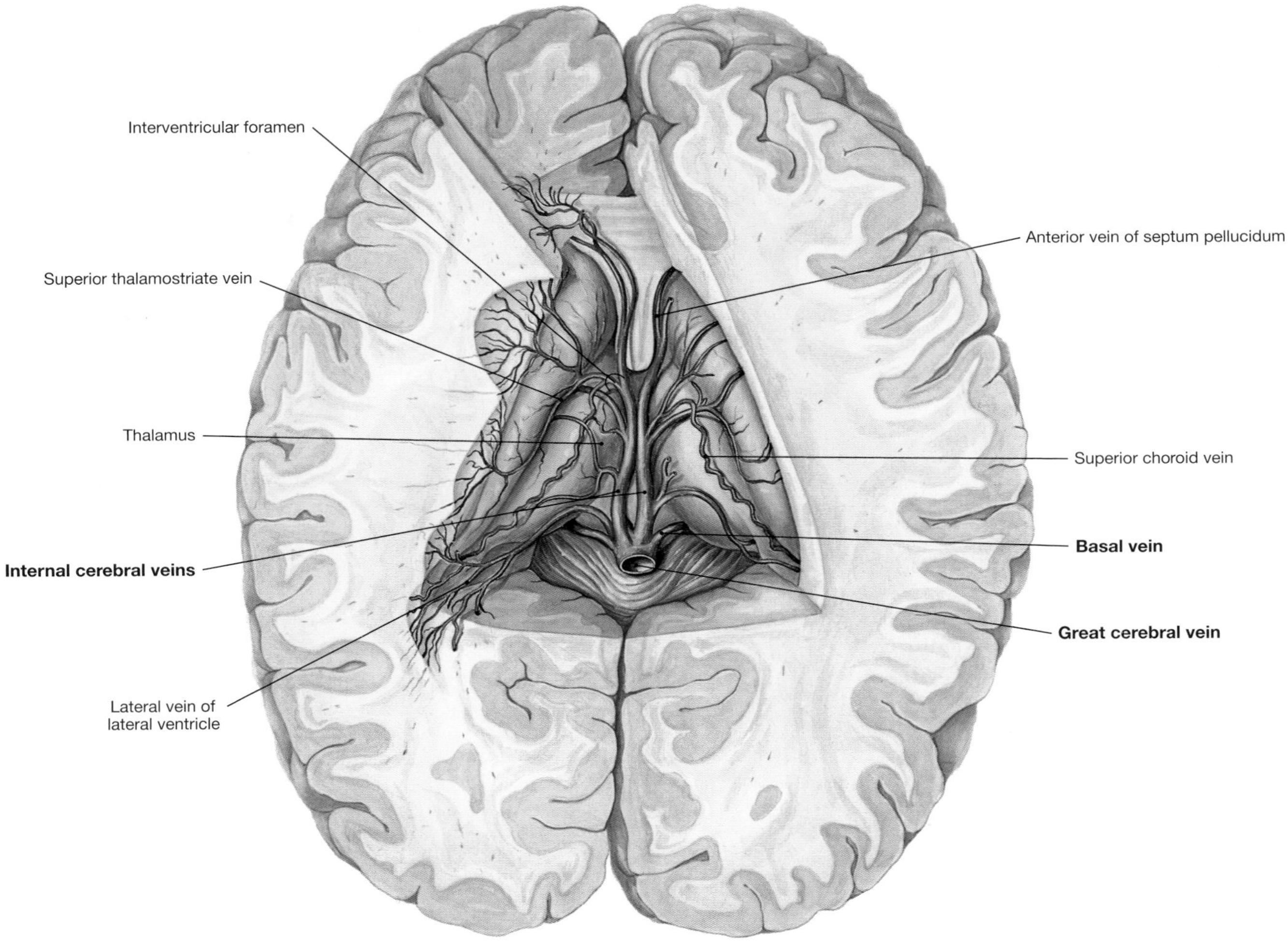

Interventricular foramen
Superior thalamostriate vein
Thalamus
**Internal cerebral veins**
Lateral vein of lateral ventricle
Anterior vein of septum pellucidum
Superior choroid vein
**Basal vein**
**Great cerebral vein**

**Fig. 12.103 Deep veins of the brain;** superior view.
The internal cerebral veins run in the choroid membrane of the third ventricle. The veins of the ventricular system, the basal ganglia, and the internal capsule belong to the deep veins of the brain. The blood from these structures is drained through the superior thalamostriate veins into the internal cerebral veins and from here into the great cerebral vein (vein of GALEN).

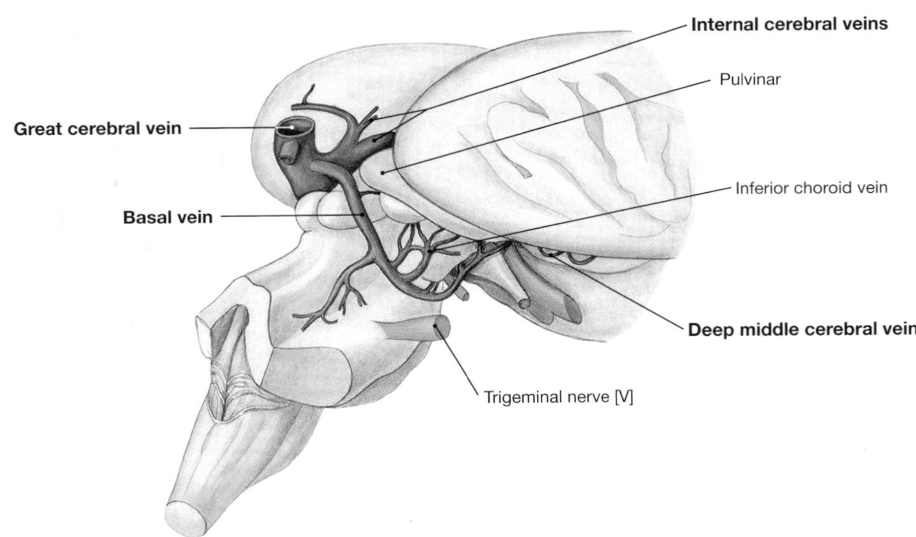
Internal cerebral veins
Pulvinar
Great cerebral vein
Inferior choroid vein
Basal vein
Deep middle cerebral vein
Trigeminal nerve [V]

**Fig. 12.104 Deep veins of the brain;** posterior view from the right side.
After removal of the cerebellum, the basal veins draining the rhombencephalon, mesencephalon, and insula become visible. Like the internal cerebral veins, the venous blood vessels of this region, the paired deep middle cerebral vein and the basal vein (ROSENTHAL's vein), drain into the great cerebral vein (vein of GALEN).

## Brain, MRI

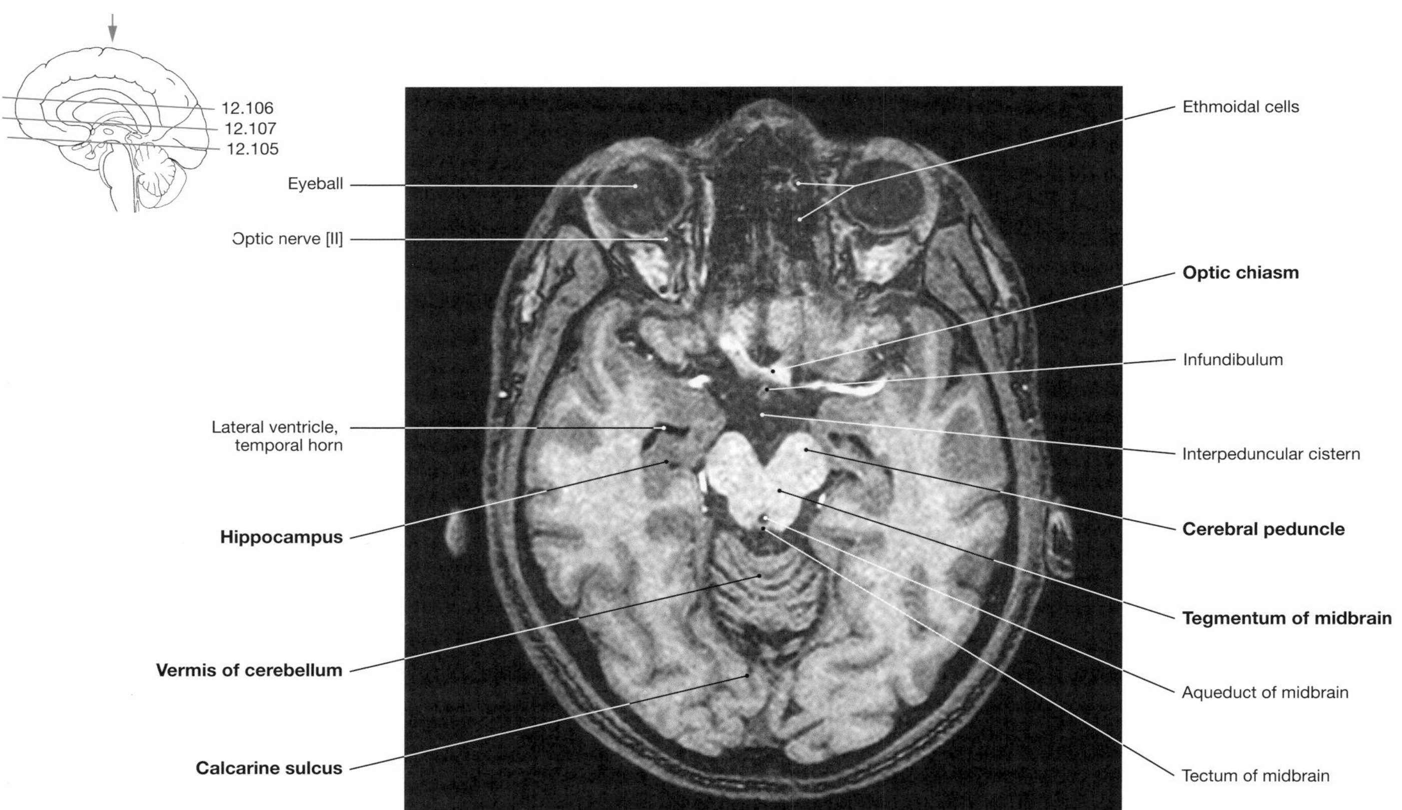
12.106
12.107
12.105
Eyeball
Optic nerve [II]
Lateral ventricle, temporal horn
Hippocampus
Vermis of cerebellum
Calcarine sulcus
Ethmoidal cells
Optic chiasm
Infundibulum
Interpeduncular cistern
Cerebral peduncle
Tegmentum of midbrain
Aqueduct of midbrain
Tectum of midbrain

**Fig. 12.105 Brain;** magnetic resonance tomographic image (MRI); horizontal section at the level of the mesencephalon and the temporal horns of the lateral ventricle; superior view.

The optic chiasm and the cerebral peduncles of the mesencephalon are visible. In addition, the cerebellar vermis appears in this sectional plane. The calcarine sulcus is discernible in the occipital lobe.

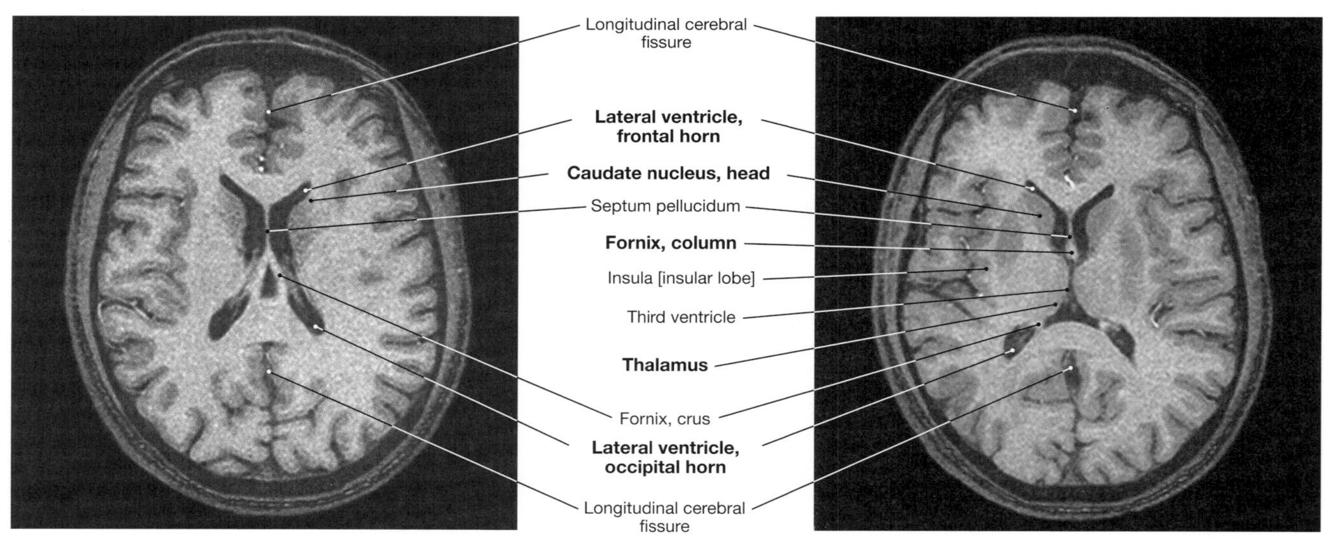
Longitudinal cerebral fissure
Lateral ventricle, frontal horn
Caudate nucleus, head
Septum pellucidum
Fornix, column
Insula [insular lobe]
Third ventricle
Thalamus
Fornix, crus
Lateral ventricle, occipital horn
Longitudinal cerebral fissure

**Fig. 12.106 Brain;** magnetic resonance tomographic image (MRI); horizontal section at the level of the central parts of the lateral ventricles; superior view.
Visible are the frontal and occipital horn, the septum pellucidum, and the crus of fornix. The left side of the image also shows the insular lobe.

**Fig. 12.107 Brain;** magnetic resonance tomographic image (MRI); horizontal section at the level of the third ventricle and the temporal horns of the lateral ventricles; superior view.
In addition to the insular lobes and the structures shown in → Fig. 12.106, the thalamus and the column of fornix are visible.

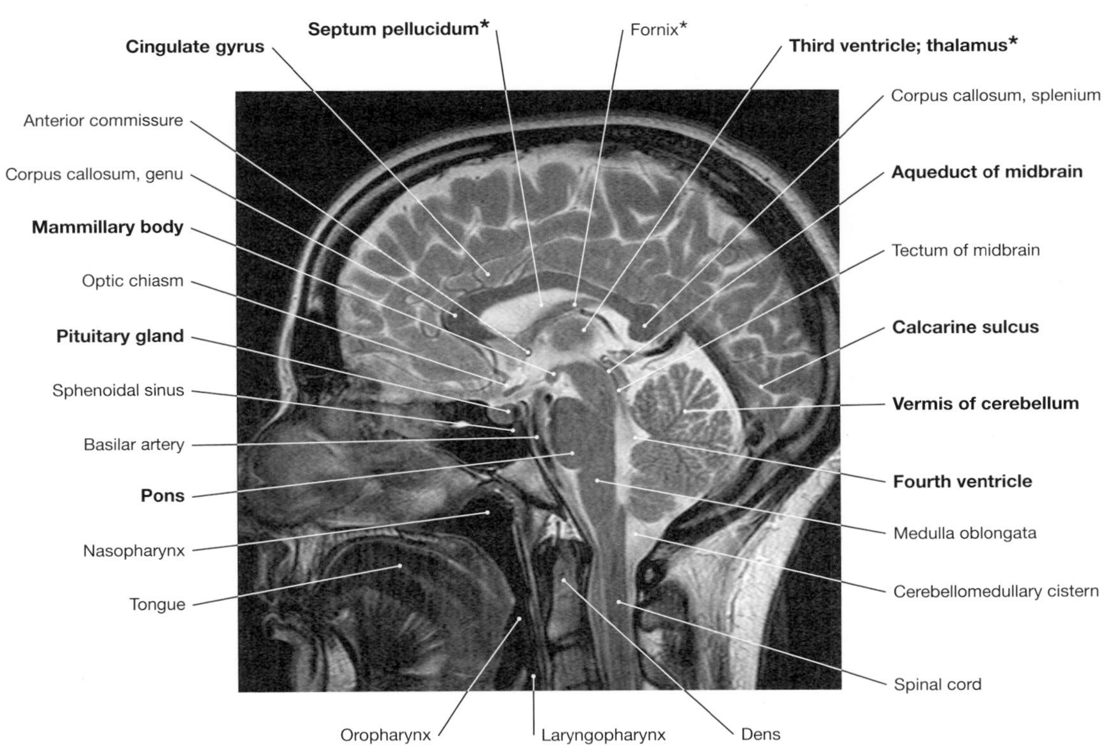
Cingulate gyrus
Septum pellucidum*
Fornix*
Third ventricle; thalamus*
Corpus callosum, splenium
Anterior commissure
Corpus callosum, genu
Aqueduct of midbrain
Mammillary body
Tectum of midbrain
Optic chiasm
Calcarine sulcus
Pituitary gland
Sphenoidal sinus
Vermis of cerebellum
Basilar artery
Pons
Fourth ventricle
Medulla oblongata
Nasopharynx
Cerebellomedullary cistern
Tongue
Spinal cord
Oropharynx
Laryngopharynx
Dens

**Fig. 12.108 Brain;** magnetic resonance tomographic image (MRI); median section.
This MRI scan clearly delineates all brain structures, for example the cingular gyrus, septum pellucidum, third ventricle, thalamus, aqueduct of midbrain, mamillary body, hypothalamus, pituitary gland, mesencephalon, pons, cerebellum, and medulla oblongata.
The structures marked with a star (*) appear partly falsified as a consequence of the "partial volume effect".

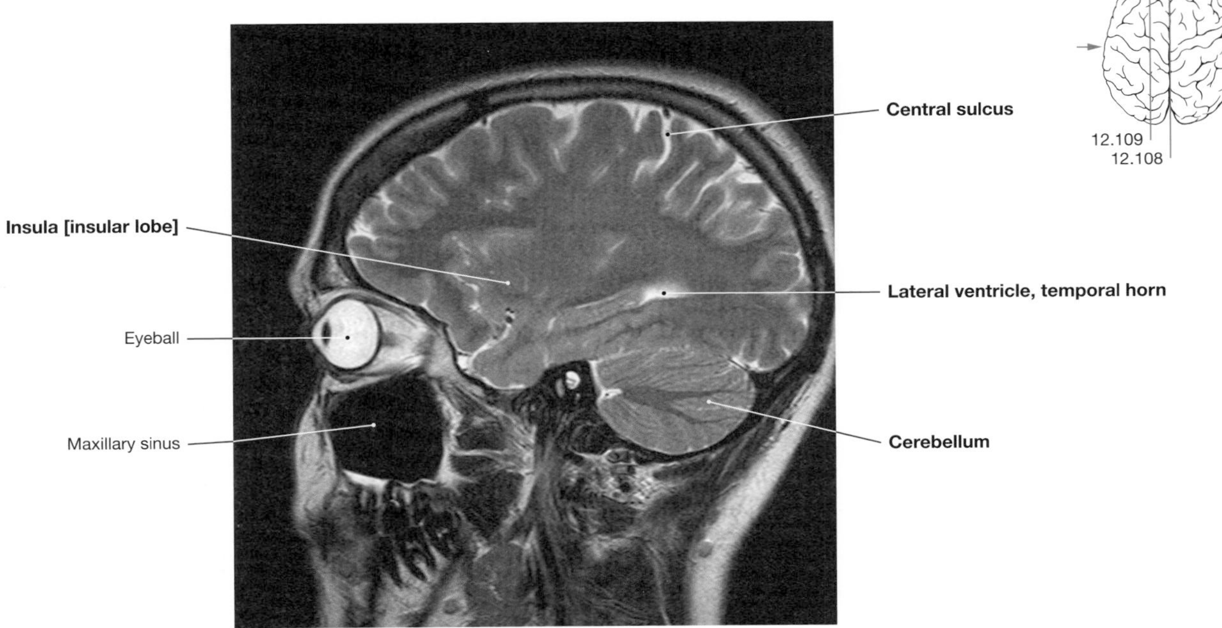
Central sulcus
12.109
12.108
Insula [insular lobe]
Lateral ventricle, temporal horn
Eyeball
Maxillary sinus
Cerebellum

**Fig. 12.109 Brain;** magnetic resonance tomographic image (MRI); sagittal section at the level of the mesencephalon and the temporal horns of the lateral ventricle; view from the left side.

The sagittal section includes the cerebellum and the central sulcus. A small part of the temporal horn of the lateral ventricle also lies within this sectional plane.

## Brain, MRI

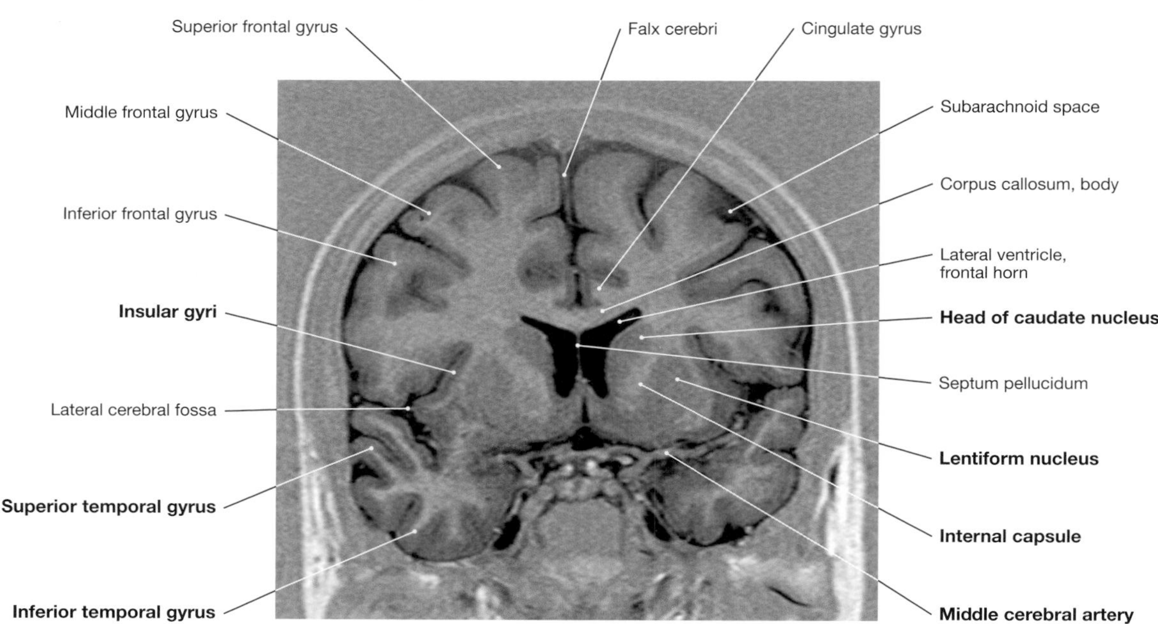
Superior frontal gyrus
Falx cerebri
Cingulate gyrus
Middle frontal gyrus
Subarachnoid space
Inferior frontal gyrus
Corpus callosum, body
Lateral ventricle, frontal horn
Insular gyri
Head of caudate nucleus
Septum pellucidum
Lateral cerebral fossa
Lentiform nucleus
Superior temporal gyrus
Internal capsule
Inferior temporal gyrus
Middle cerebral artery

**Fig. 12.110 Brain;** magnetic resonance tomographic image (MRI); frontal section at the level of the anterior part of the third ventricle; anterior view.
On the right side, the course of the middle cerebral artery projecting towards the lateral sulcus is visible. On both sides, the large gyri of the frontal lobe and the temporal lobe are shown. Among the basal ganglia, this imaging technique allows the caudate nucleus, the internal capsule, and the lentiform nucleus to be distinguished.

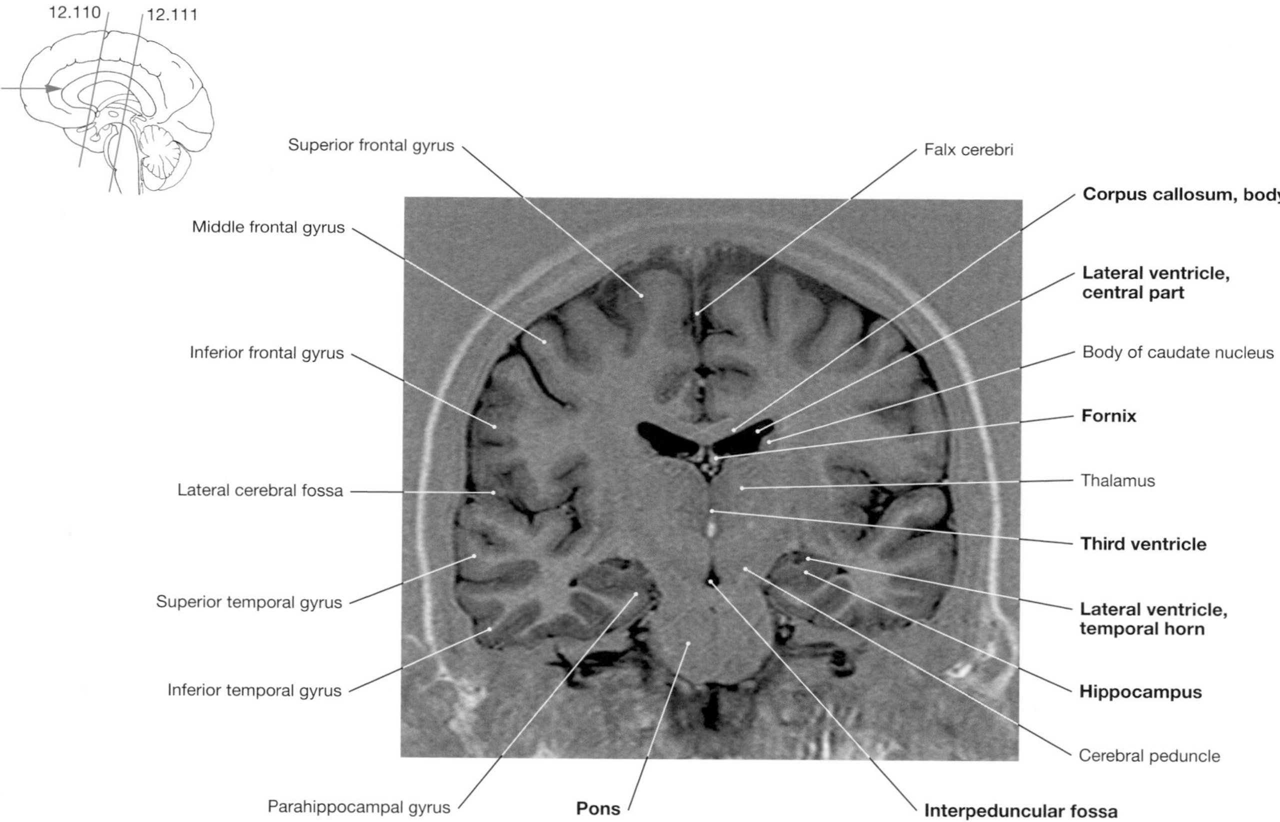
12.110
12.111
Superior frontal gyrus
Falx cerebri
Corpus callosum, body
Middle frontal gyrus
Lateral ventricle, central part
Inferior frontal gyrus
Body of caudate nucleus
Fornix
Thalamus
Lateral cerebral fossa
Third ventricle
Lateral ventricle, temporal horn
Superior temporal gyrus
Hippocampus
Inferior temporal gyrus
Cerebral peduncle
Parahippocampal gyrus
Pons
Interpeduncular fossa

**Fig. 12.111 Brain;** magnetic resonance tomographic image (MRI); frontal section at the level of the thalamus; anterior view.
This image shows the temporal horn of the lateral ventricles and the hippocampus. Further cranial, the central part of the lateral ventricle is imaged. In the midline from cranial to caudal, the trunk of the corpus callosum, the fornix, the third ventricle, the interpeduncular fossa of the brainstem, and the pons can be distinguished.

## Brain, frontal sections

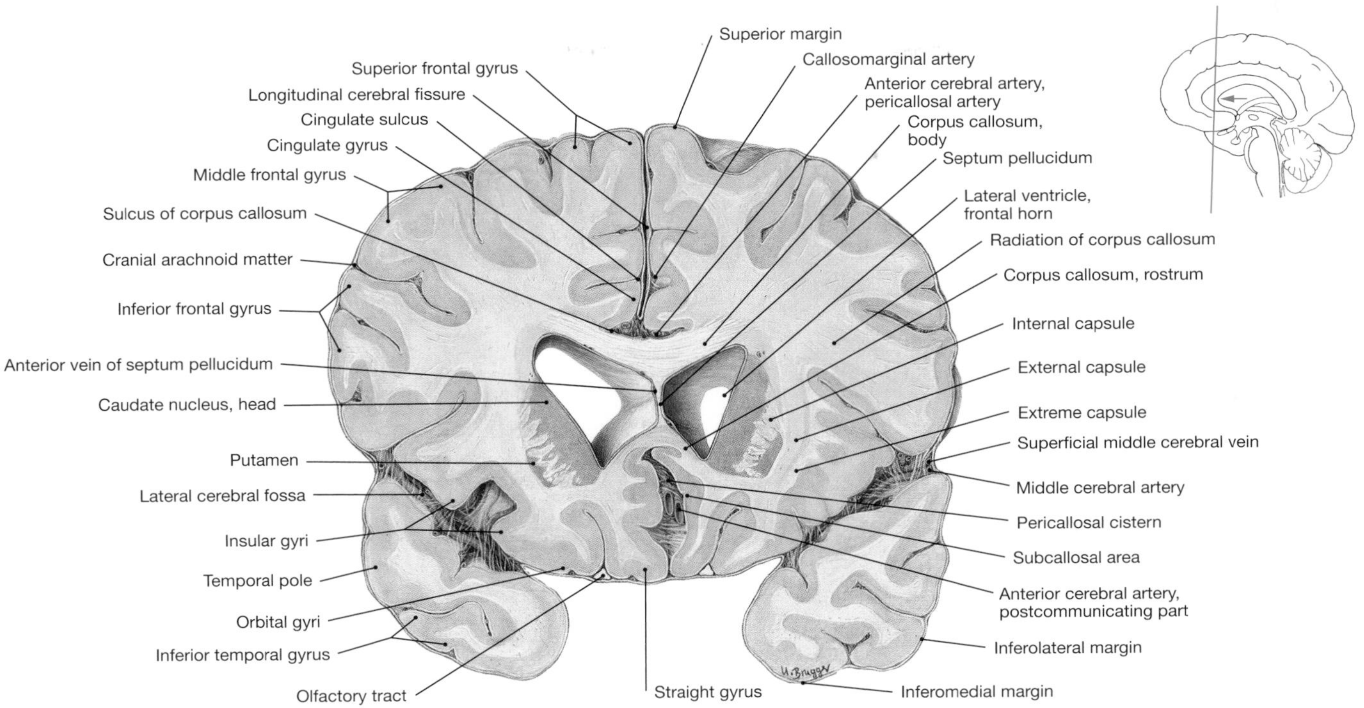
Superior margin
Callosomarginal artery
Anterior cerebral artery, pericallosal artery
Corpus callosum, body
Septum pellucidum
Lateral ventricle, frontal horn
Radiation of corpus callosum
Corpus callosum, rostrum
Internal capsule
External capsule
Extreme capsule
Superficial middle cerebral vein
Middle cerebral artery
Pericallosal cistern
Subcallosal area
Anterior cerebral artery, postcommunicating part
Inferolateral margin
Inferomedial margin
Straight gyrus
Olfactory tract
Inferior temporal gyrus
Orbital gyri
Temporal pole
Insular gyri
Lateral cerebral fossa
Putamen
Caudate nucleus, head
Anterior vein of septum pellucidum
Inferior frontal gyrus
Cranial arachnoid matter
Sulcus of corpus callosum
Middle frontal gyrus
Cingulate gyrus
Cingulate sulcus
Longitudinal cerebral fissure
Superior frontal gyrus

**Fig. 12.112 Brain;** frontal section at the level of the anterior parts of the frontal horns of the lateral ventricles; posterior view.
Visible are the two lateral ventricles, above them the corpus callosum, and lateral to them the caudate nucleus and the putamen.

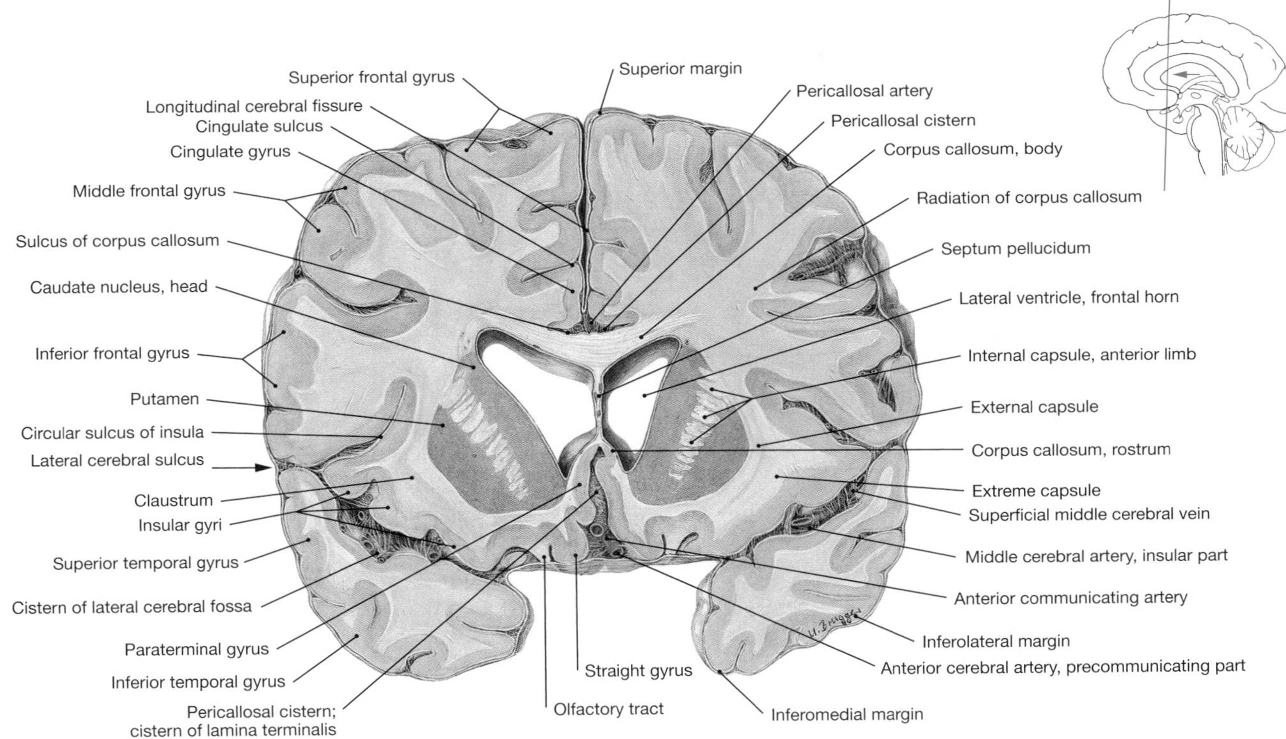
Superior margin
Pericallosal artery
Pericallosal cistern
Corpus callosum, body
Radiation of corpus callosum
Septum pellucidum
Lateral ventricle, frontal horn
Internal capsule, anterior limb
External capsule
Corpus callosum, rostrum
Extreme capsule
Superficial middle cerebral vein
Middle cerebral artery, insular part
Anterior communicating artery
Inferolateral margin
Anterior cerebral artery, precommunicating part
Inferomedial margin
Straight gyrus
Olfactory tract
Pericallosal cistern; cistern of lamina terminalis
Inferior temporal gyrus
Paraterminal gyrus
Cistern of lateral cerebral fossa
Superior temporal gyrus
Insular gyri
Claustrum
Lateral cerebral sulcus
Circular sulcus of insula
Putamen
Inferior frontal gyrus
Caudate nucleus, head
Sulcus of corpus callosum
Middle frontal gyrus
Cingulate gyrus
Cingulate sulcus
Longitudinal cerebral fissure
Superior frontal gyrus

**Fig. 12.113 Brain;** frontal section at the level of the posterior parts of the frontal horns of the lateral ventricles; posterior view.
Above the lateral ventricles, the trunk of the corpus callosum is discernible. Lateral to the lateral ventricles lie the head of the caudate nucleus and the putamen, and between them the anterior limb of the internal capsule is visible.

## Brain, frontal sections

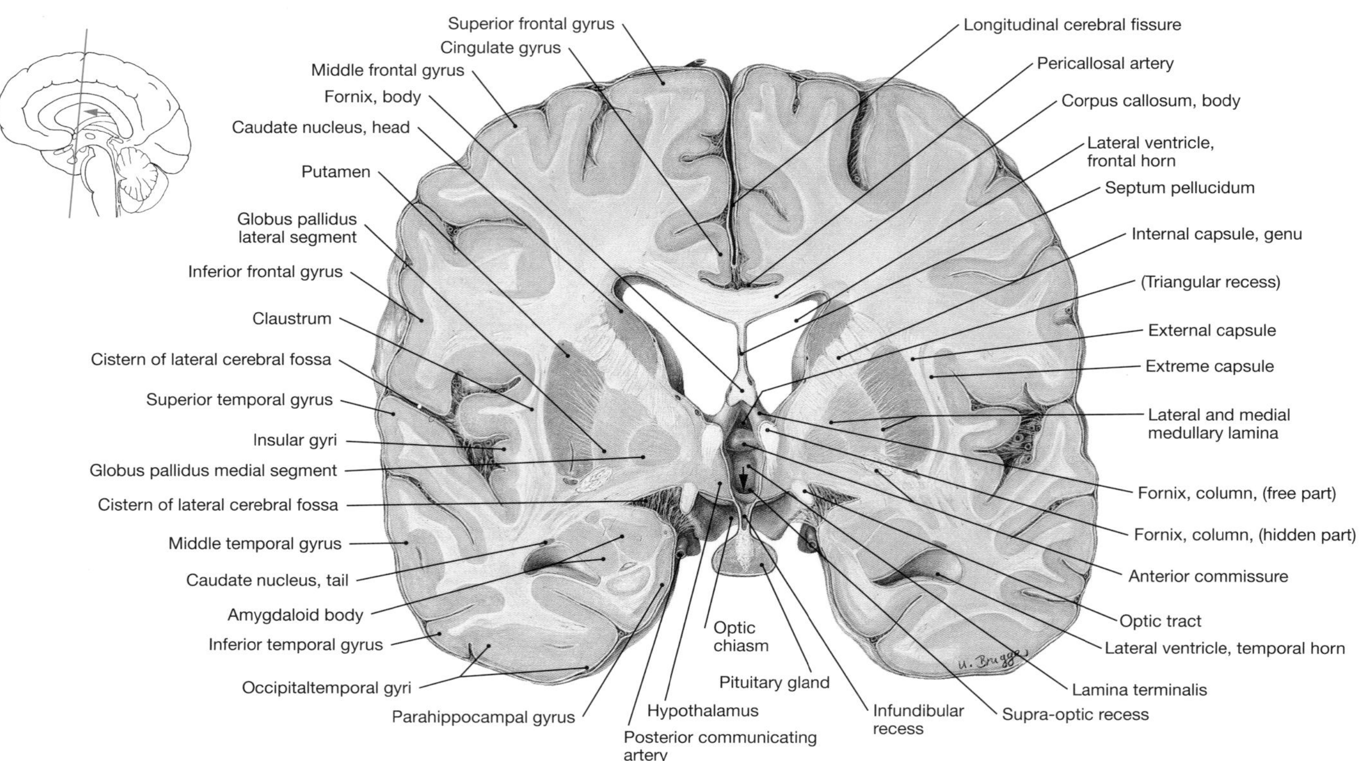
Superior frontal gyrus
Cingulate gyrus
Middle frontal gyrus
Fornix, body
Caudate nucleus, head
Putamen
Globus pallidus lateral segment
Inferior frontal gyrus
Claustrum
Cistern of lateral cerebral fossa
Superior temporal gyrus
Insular gyri
Globus pallidus medial segment
Cistern of lateral cerebral fossa
Middle temporal gyrus
Caudate nucleus, tail
Amygdaloid body
Inferior temporal gyrus
Occipitaltemporal gyri
Parahippocampal gyrus
Hypothalamus
Posterior communicating artery
Optic chiasm
Pituitary gland
Infundibular recess
Supra-optic recess
Lamina terminalis
Lateral ventricle, temporal horn
Optic tract
Anterior commissure
Fornix, column, (hidden part)
Fornix, column, (free part)
Lateral and medial medullary lamina
Extreme capsule
External capsule
(Triangular recess)
Internal capsule, genu
Septum pellucidum
Lateral ventricle, frontal horn
Corpus callosum, body
Pericallosal artery
Longitudinal cerebral fissure

**Fig. 12.114 Brain;** frontal section at the level of the interventricular foramina; posterior view.
The pituitary gland is sectioned in the center. Inferior to the lateral ventricles the head of the caudate nucleus, the internal capsule, the globus pallidus, the putamen, the claustrum, and some insular gyri are visible.

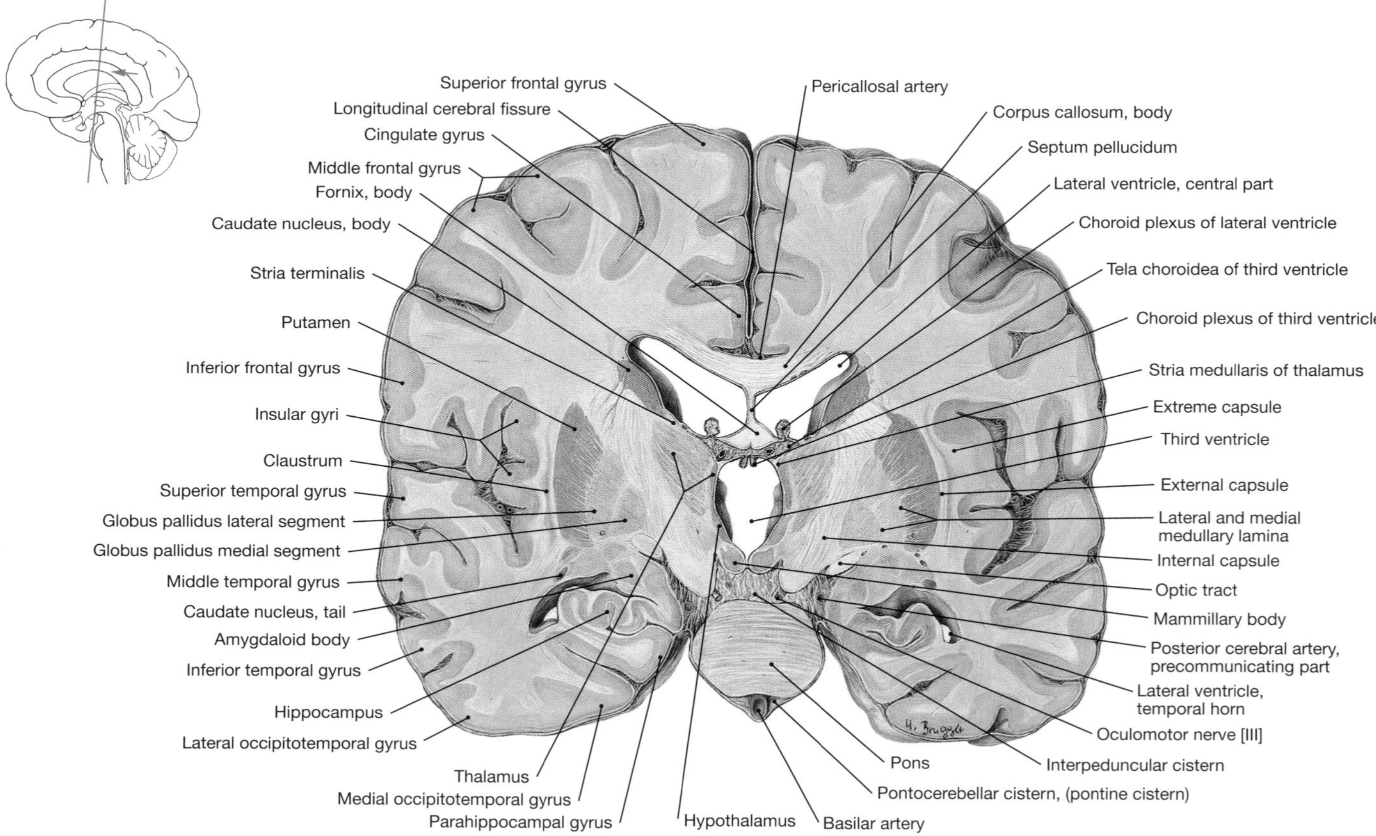
Superior frontal gyrus
Longitudinal cerebral fissure
Cingulate gyrus
Middle frontal gyrus
Fornix, body
Caudate nucleus, body
Stria terminalis
Putamen
Inferior frontal gyrus
Insular gyri
Claustrum
Superior temporal gyrus
Globus pallidus lateral segment
Globus pallidus medial segment
Middle temporal gyrus
Caudate nucleus, tail
Amygdaloid body
Inferior temporal gyrus
Hippocampus
Lateral occipitotemporal gyrus
Thalamus
Medial occipitotemporal gyrus
Parahippocampal gyrus
Hypothalamus
Basilar artery
Pontocerebellar cistern, (pontine cistern)
Pons
Interpeduncular cistern
Oculomotor nerve [III]
Lateral ventricle, temporal horn
Posterior cerebral artery, precommunicating part
Mammillary body
Optic tract
Internal capsule
Lateral and medial medullary lamina
External capsule
Third ventricle
Extreme capsule
Stria medullaris of thalamus
Choroid plexus of third ventricle
Tela choroidea of third ventricle
Choroid plexus of lateral ventricle
Lateral ventricle, central part
Septum pellucidum
Corpus callosum, body
Pericallosal artery

**Fig. 12.115 Brain;** frontal section at the level of the mamillary body; posterior view.
At the level of the mamillary bodies, the lumen of the third ventricle is located below the lateral ventricle. Lateral thereof from inside to outside lie the thalamus, internal capsule, globus pallidus, putamen, external capsule, claustrum, extreme capsule, and insular gyri.

## Brain, frontal sections

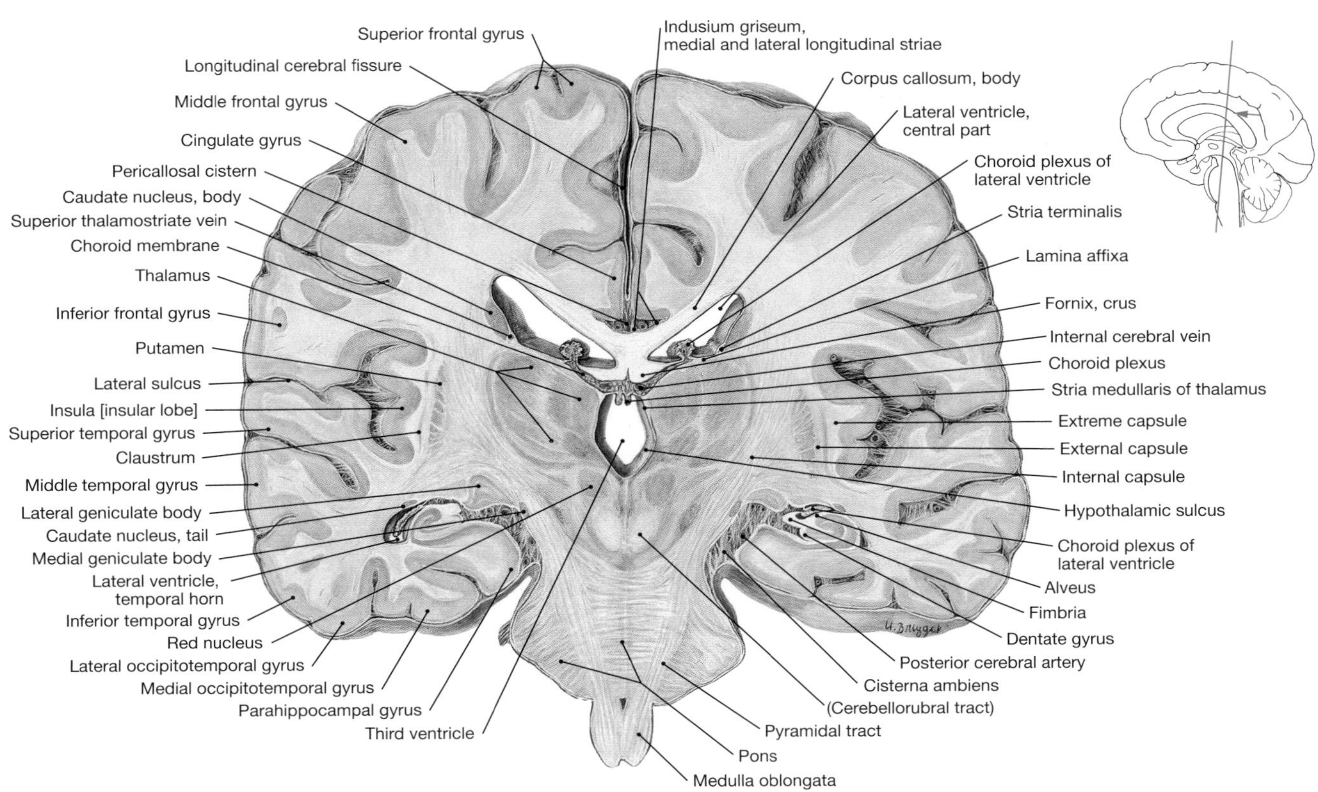
Superior frontal gyrus
Longitudinal cerebral fissure
Middle frontal gyrus
Cingulate gyrus
Pericallosal cistern
Caudate nucleus, body
Superior thalamostriate vein
Choroid membrane
Thalamus
Inferior frontal gyrus
Putamen
Lateral sulcus
Insula [insular lobe]
Superior temporal gyrus
Claustrum
Middle temporal gyrus
Lateral geniculate body
Caudate nucleus, tail
Medial geniculate body
Lateral ventricle, temporal horn
Inferior temporal gyrus
Red nucleus
Lateral occipitotemporal gyrus
Medial occipitotemporal gyrus
Parahippocampal gyrus
Third ventricle
Indusium griseum, medial and lateral longitudinal striae
Corpus callosum, body
Lateral ventricle, central part
Choroid plexus of lateral ventricle
Stria terminalis
Lamina affixa
Fornix, crus
Internal cerebral vein
Choroid plexus
Stria medullaris of thalamus
Extreme capsule
External capsule
Internal capsule
Hypothalamic sulcus
Choroid plexus of lateral ventricle
Alveus
Fimbria
Dentate gyrus
Posterior cerebral artery
Cisterna ambiens
(Cerebellorubral tract)
Pyramidal tract
Pons
Medulla oblongata

**Fig. 12.116 Brain;** frontal section at the level of the central part of the third ventricle; posterior view.
At this level, the right and left thalamus are often cross-connected by the interthalamic adhesion. Inferior to the thalamus the red nucleus is visible. The pons and the pyramidal tract present prominently in the brainstem.

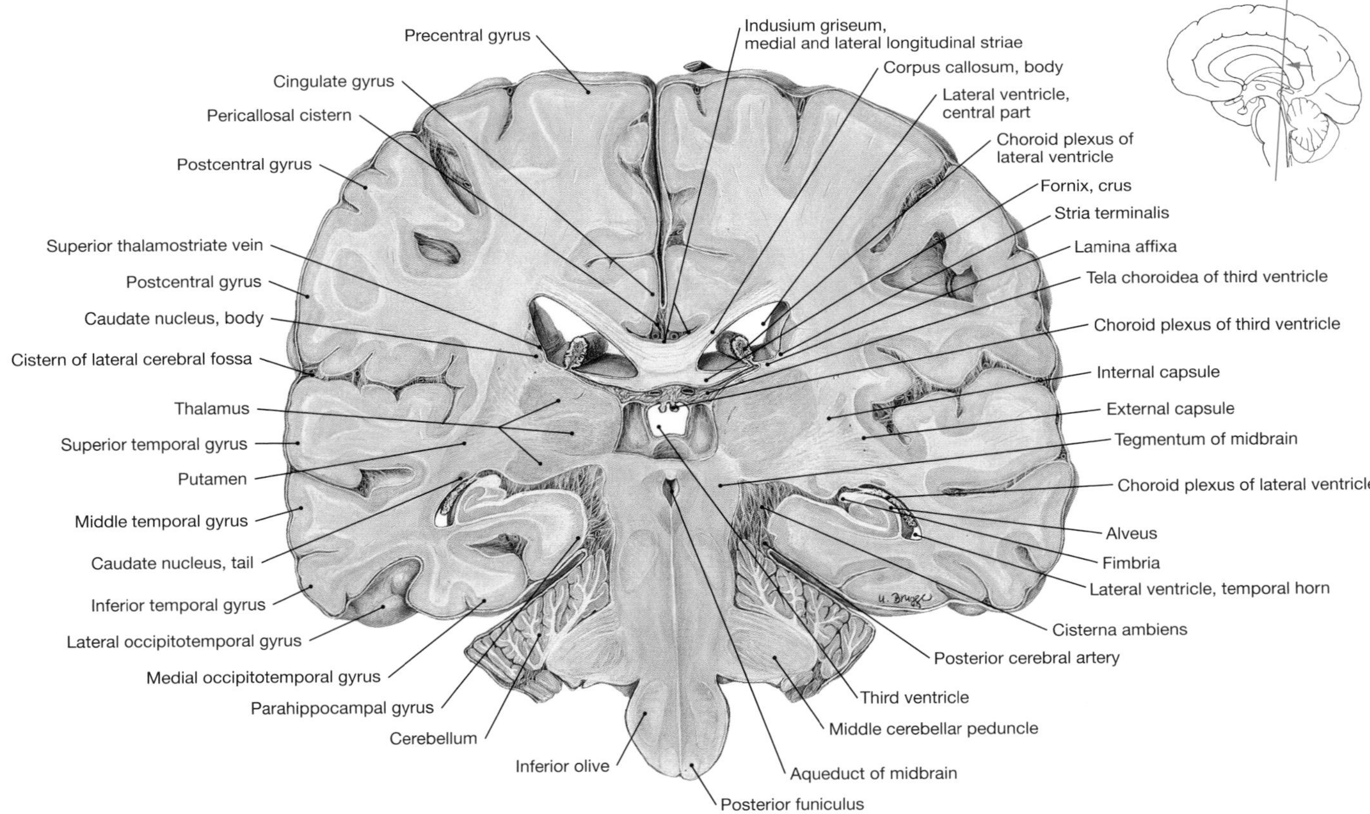
Precentral gyrus
Cingulate gyrus
Pericallosal cistern
Postcentral gyrus
Superior thalamostriate vein
Postcentral gyrus
Caudate nucleus, body
Cistern of lateral cerebral fossa
Thalamus
Superior temporal gyrus
Putamen
Middle temporal gyrus
Caudate nucleus, tail
Inferior temporal gyrus
Lateral occipitotemporal gyrus
Medial occipitotemporal gyrus
Parahippocampal gyrus
Cerebellum
Inferior olive
Indusium griseum, medial and lateral longitudinal striae
Corpus callosum, body
Lateral ventricle, central part
Choroid plexus of lateral ventricle
Fornix, crus
Stria terminalis
Lamina affixa
Tela choroidea of third ventricle
Choroid plexus of third ventricle
Internal capsule
External capsule
Tegmentum of midbrain
Choroid plexus of lateral ventricle
Alveus
Fimbria
Lateral ventricle, temporal horn
Cisterna ambiens
Posterior cerebral artery
Third ventricle
Middle cerebellar peduncle
Aqueduct of midbrain
Posterior funiculus

**Fig. 12.117 Brain;** frontal section at the level of the posterior wall of the third ventricle; posterior view.
Inferior to the lateral ventricles a number of thalamic nuclei are visible and further caudal the occipital part of the hippocampus is shown. The brainstem has been sectioned at the level of the aqueduct of midbrain.

## Brain, frontal sections

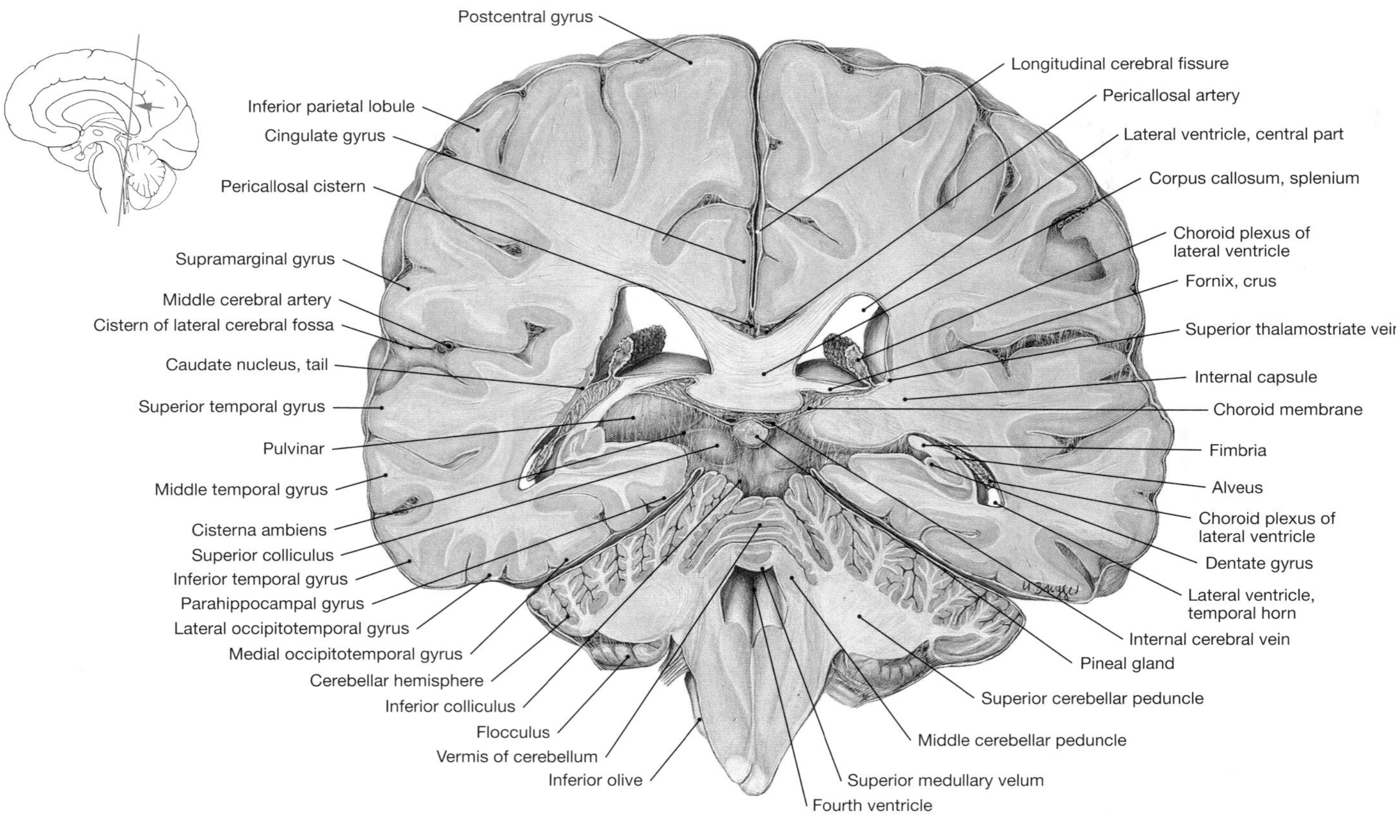
Postcentral gyrus
Inferior parietal lobule
Cingulate gyrus
Pericallosal cistern
Supramarginal gyrus
Middle cerebral artery
Cistern of lateral cerebral fossa
Caudate nucleus, tail
Superior temporal gyrus
Pulvinar
Middle temporal gyrus
Cisterna ambiens
Superior colliculus
Inferior temporal gyrus
Parahippocampal gyrus
Lateral occipitotemporal gyrus
Medial occipitotemporal gyrus
Cerebellar hemisphere
Inferior colliculus
Flocculus
Vermis of cerebellum
Inferior olive
Longitudinal cerebral fissure
Pericallosal artery
Lateral ventricle, central part
Corpus callosum, splenium
Choroid plexus of lateral ventricle
Fornix, crus
Superior thalamostriate vein
Internal capsule
Choroid membrane
Fimbria
Alveus
Choroid plexus of lateral ventricle
Dentate gyrus
Lateral ventricle, temporal horn
Internal cerebral vein
Pineal gland
Superior cerebellar peduncle
Middle cerebellar peduncle
Superior medullary velum
Fourth ventricle

**Fig. 12.118 Brain;** frontal section at the level of the pineal gland and the fourth ventricle; posterior view.
The splenium of the corpus callosum and the pineal gland are displayed in the center of the image. Lateral thereof the superior colliculi and the pulvinar are shown. The superior cerebellar peduncles are visible in the lateral brainstem slightly above the fourth ventricle.

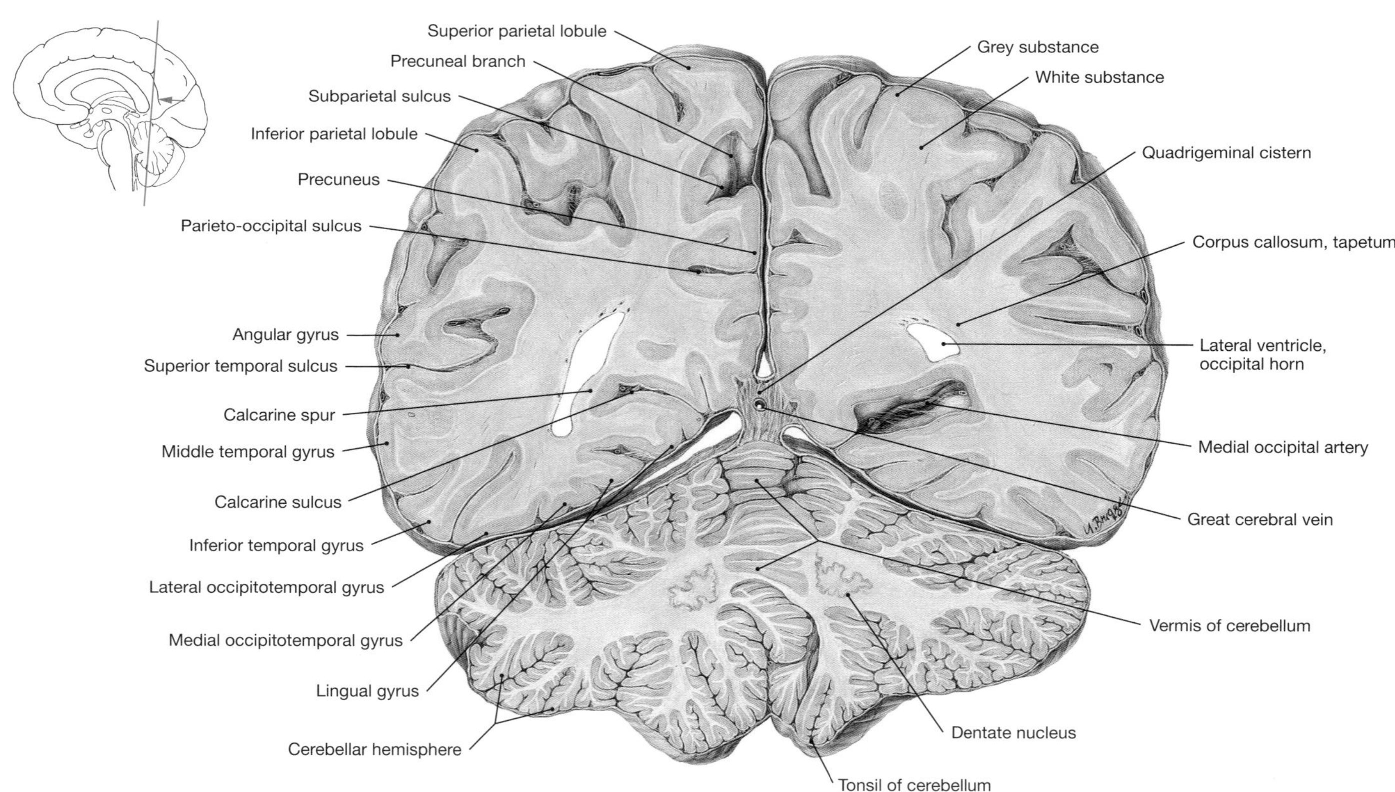
Superior parietal lobule
Precuneal branch
Subparietal sulcus
Inferior parietal lobule
Precuneus
Parieto-occipital sulcus
Angular gyrus
Superior temporal sulcus
Calcarine spur
Middle temporal gyrus
Calcarine sulcus
Inferior temporal gyrus
Lateral occipitotemporal gyrus
Medial occipitotemporal gyrus
Lingual gyrus
Cerebellar hemisphere
Grey substance
White substance
Quadrigeminal cistern
Corpus callosum, tapetum
Lateral ventricle, occipital horn
Medial occipital artery
Great cerebral vein
Vermis of cerebellum
Dentate nucleus
Tonsil of cerebellum

**Fig. 12.119 Brain;** frontal section at the level of the occipital horns of the lateral ventricles; posterior view.
The dentate nucleus and large parts of the vermis are discernible in the cerebellum.

## Brain, horizontal sections

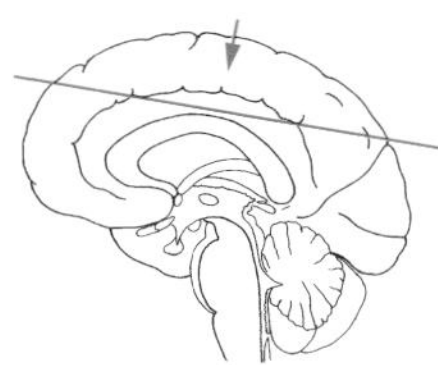

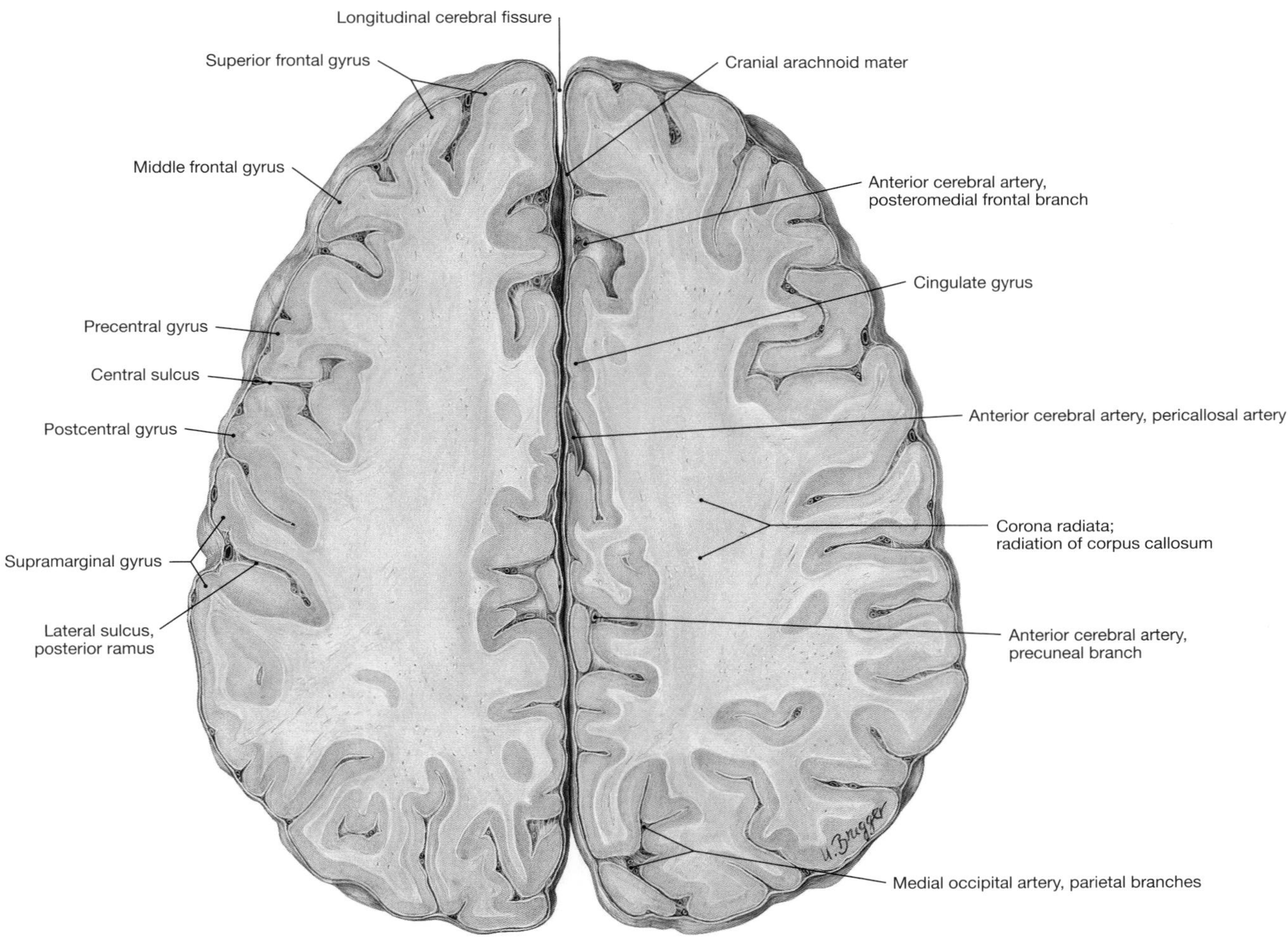
Longitudinal cerebral fissure
Superior frontal gyrus
Cranial arachnoid mater
Middle frontal gyrus
Anterior cerebral artery, posteromedial frontal branch
Cingulate gyrus
Precentral gyrus
Central sulcus
Anterior cerebral artery, pericallosal artery
Postcentral gyrus
Corona radiata; radiation of corpus callosum
Supramarginal gyrus
Lateral sulcus, posterior ramus
Anterior cerebral artery, precuneal branch
Medial occipital artery, parietal branches

**Fig. 12.120 Brain;** horizontal section just above the corpus callosum; superior view.
The brain has been sectioned immediately above the corpus callosum. At this level, there are still no nuclei visible. In the broad band of white matter, fibers projecting from the thalamus to the cortex (corona radiata) mix with commissural fibers of the corpus callosum connecting the two hemispheres (radiation of corpus callosum). In addition, fiber tracts converging on the internal capsule contribute to the white matter (→ Figs. 12.74 to 12.76). Age-related atrophy of the brain makes the subarachnoid space appear wider (→ Figs. 12.121 to 12.130).

## Brain, horizontal sections

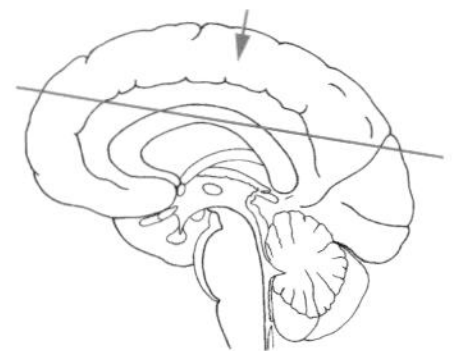

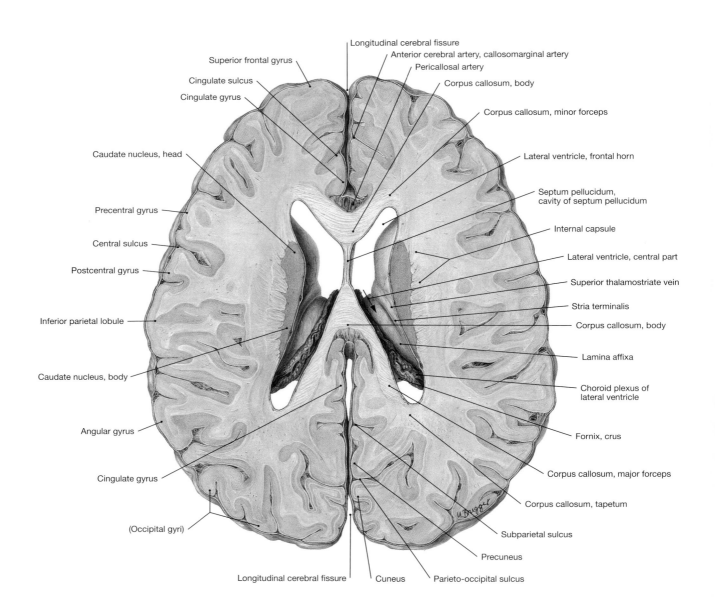

Longitudinal cerebral fissure
Anterior cerebral artery, callosomarginal artery
Pericallosal artery
Superior frontal gyrus
Cingulate sulcus
Corpus callosum, body
Cingulate gyrus
Corpus callosum, minor forceps
Caudate nucleus, head
Lateral ventricle, frontal horn
Septum pellucidum, cavity of septum pellucidum
Precentral gyrus
Internal capsule
Central sulcus
Lateral ventricle, central part
Postcentral gyrus
Superior thalamostriate vein
Stria terminalis
Inferior parietal lobule
Corpus callosum, body
Lamina affixa
Caudate nucleus, body
Choroid plexus of lateral ventricle
Angular gyrus
Fornix, crus
Cingulate gyrus
Corpus callosum, major forceps
Corpus callosum, tapetum
(Occipital gyri)
Subparietal sulcus
Precuneus
Longitudinal cerebral fissure
Cuneus
Parieto-occipital sulcus

**Fig. 12.121 Brain;** horizontal section at the level of the central part of the lateral ventricles; superior view.
The septum pellucidum extends between the body and fornix (not visible) of the corpus callosum and separates the lateral ventricles.

To both sides of the lateral ventricles, the head and body of the caudate nucleus are sectioned. The internal capsule is located lateral to the nucleus.

## Brain, horizontal sections

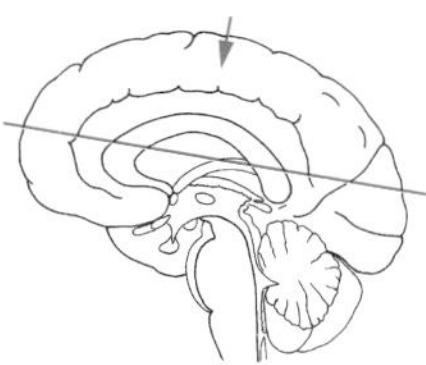

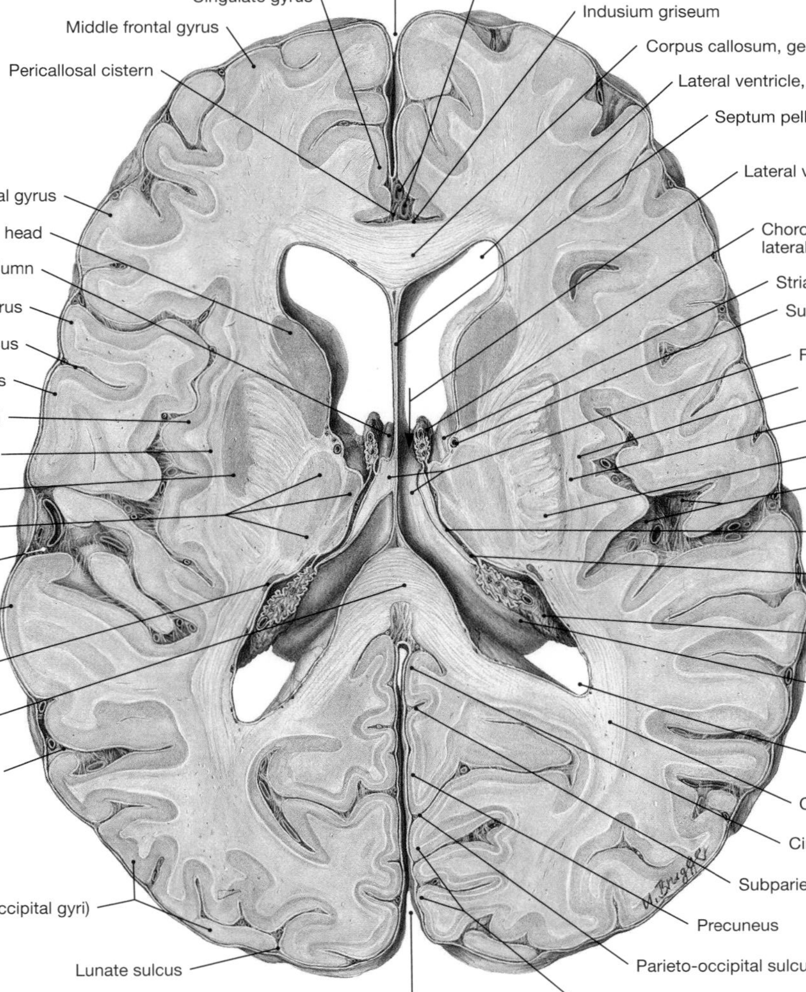

Longitudinal cerebral fissure
Cingulate gyrus
Middle frontal gyrus
Pericallosal cistern
Inferior frontal gyrus
Caudate nucleus, head
Fornix, column
Precentral gyrus
Central sulcus
Postcentral gyrus
Insula [insular lobe]
Claustrum
Putamen
Thalamus
Cistern of lateral cerebral fossa
Superior temporal gyrus
Caudate nucleus, tail
Corpus callosum, splenium
Superior temporal sulcus
(Occipital gyri)
Lunate sulcus
Longitudinal cerebral fissure
Anterior cerebral arteries, pericallosal arteries
Indusium griseum
Corpus callosum, genu
Lateral ventricle, frontal horn
Septum pellucidum
Lateral ventricle, central part
Choroid plexus of lateral ventricle
Stria terminalis
Superior thalamostriate vein
Fornix, body
Extreme capsule
External capsule
Internal capsule
Middle cerebral artery, terminal branches
Choroid membrane
Transverse cerebral fissure
Choroid plexus of lateral ventricle
Fornix, crus
Lateral ventricle, bulb of occipital horn
Corpus callosum, tapetum
Cingulate gyrus
Subparietal sulcus
Precuneus
Parieto-occipital sulcus
Cuneus

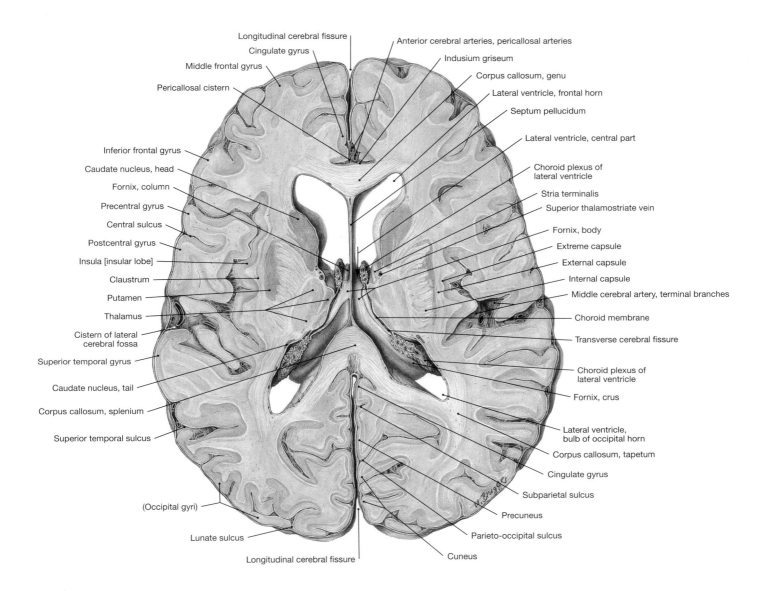

**Fig. 12.122 Brain;** horizontal section at the level of the floor of the central part of the lateral ventricles; superior view.
This central section shows parts of the thalamus lateral to the lateral ventricles. Anterior and posterior to the thalamus, the head and tail of the caudate nucleus are visible, respectively. Lateral to the thalamus, the internal capsule, putamen, external capsule, claustrum, extreme capsule, and insular gyri are arranged from medial to lateral. The genu of the corpus callosum locates to the anterior midline and its splenium is visible in the posterior midline.

## Brain, horizontal sections

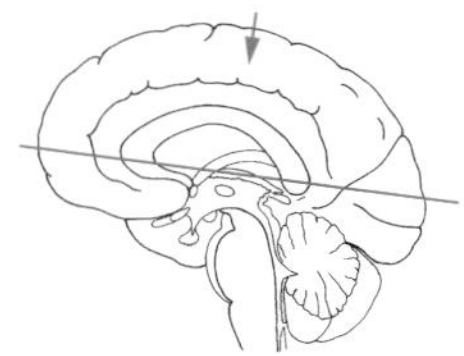

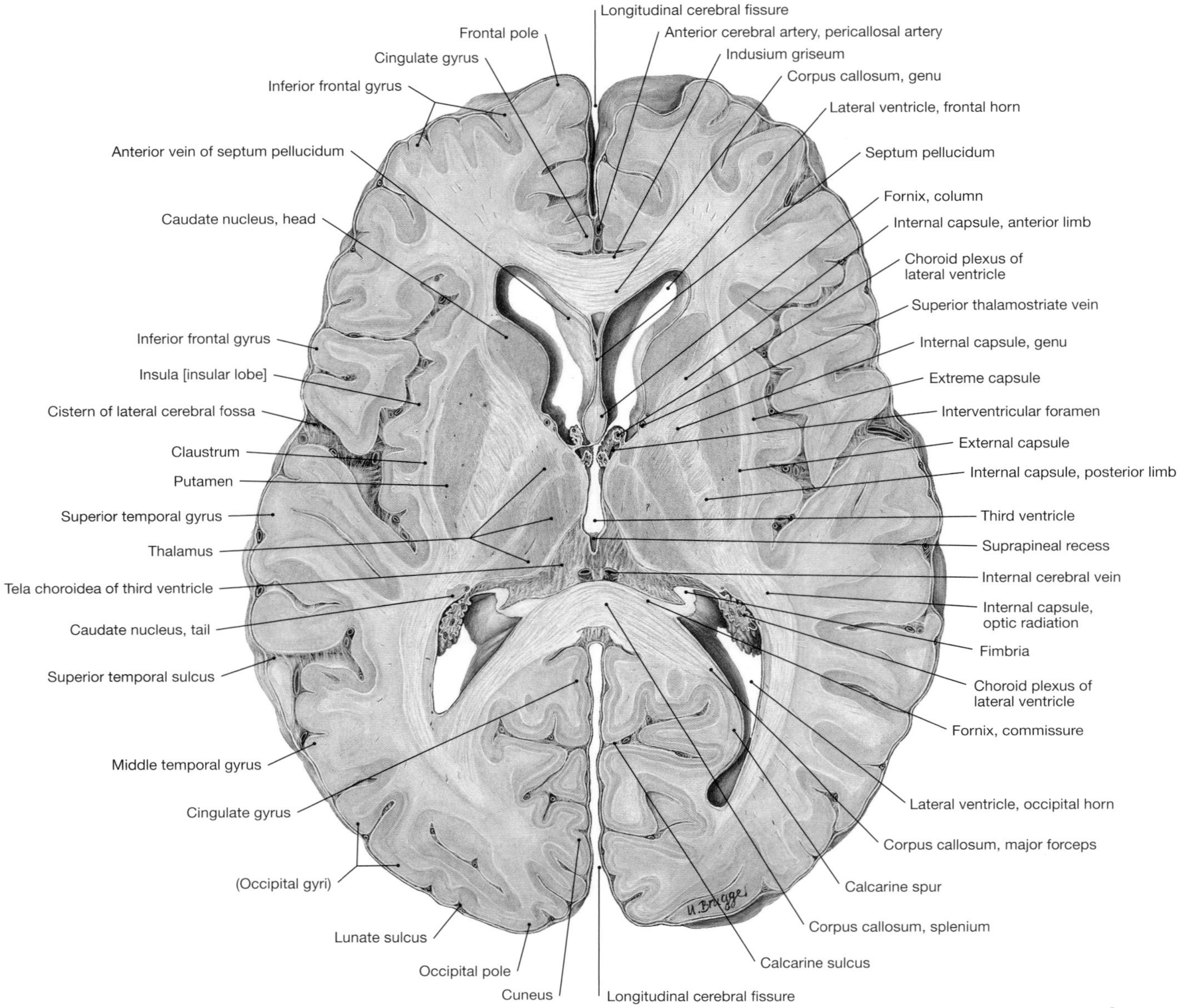

Longitudinal cerebral fissure
Frontal pole
Anterior cerebral artery, pericallosal artery
Cingulate gyrus
Indusium griseum
Corpus callosum, genu
Inferior frontal gyrus
Lateral ventricle, frontal horn
Anterior vein of septum pellucidum
Septum pellucidum
Fornix, column
Caudate nucleus, head
Internal capsule, anterior limb
Choroid plexus of lateral ventricle
Superior thalamostriate vein
Inferior frontal gyrus
Internal capsule, genu
Insula [insular lobe]
Extreme capsule
Cistern of lateral cerebral fossa
Interventricular foramen
External capsule
Claustrum
Internal capsule, posterior limb
Putamen
Third ventricle
Superior temporal gyrus
Suprapineal recess
Thalamus
Internal cerebral vein
Tela choroidea of third ventricle
Internal capsule, optic radiation
Caudate nucleus, tail
Fimbria
Superior temporal sulcus
Choroid plexus of lateral ventricle
Fornix, commissure
Middle temporal gyrus
Lateral ventricle, occipital horn
Cingulate gyrus
Corpus callosum, major forceps
(Occipital gyri)
Calcarine spur
Corpus callosum, splenium
Lunate sulcus
Calcarine sulcus
Occipital pole
Cuneus
Longitudinal cerebral fissure

**Fig. 12.123 Brain;** horizontal section at the level of the upper part of the third ventricle; superior view.
In the central part of the image, the third ventricle is shown, with parts of the lateral ventricles as well as the genu and splenium of the corpus callosum depicted anterior and posterior of the third ventricle. Head and tail of the caudate nucleus, thalamus, putamen, and claustrum constitute the cerebral **nuclei.** The internal capsule with its characteristic genu runs in between the large nuclei. In addition, the optic radiation of the internal capsule is visible.

# Brain, horizontal sections

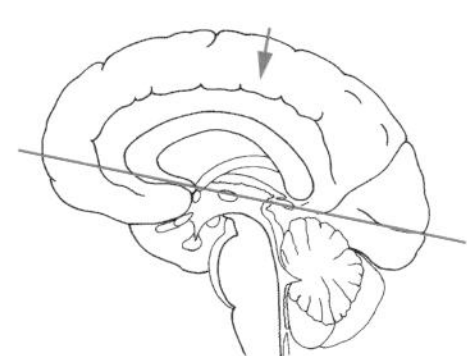

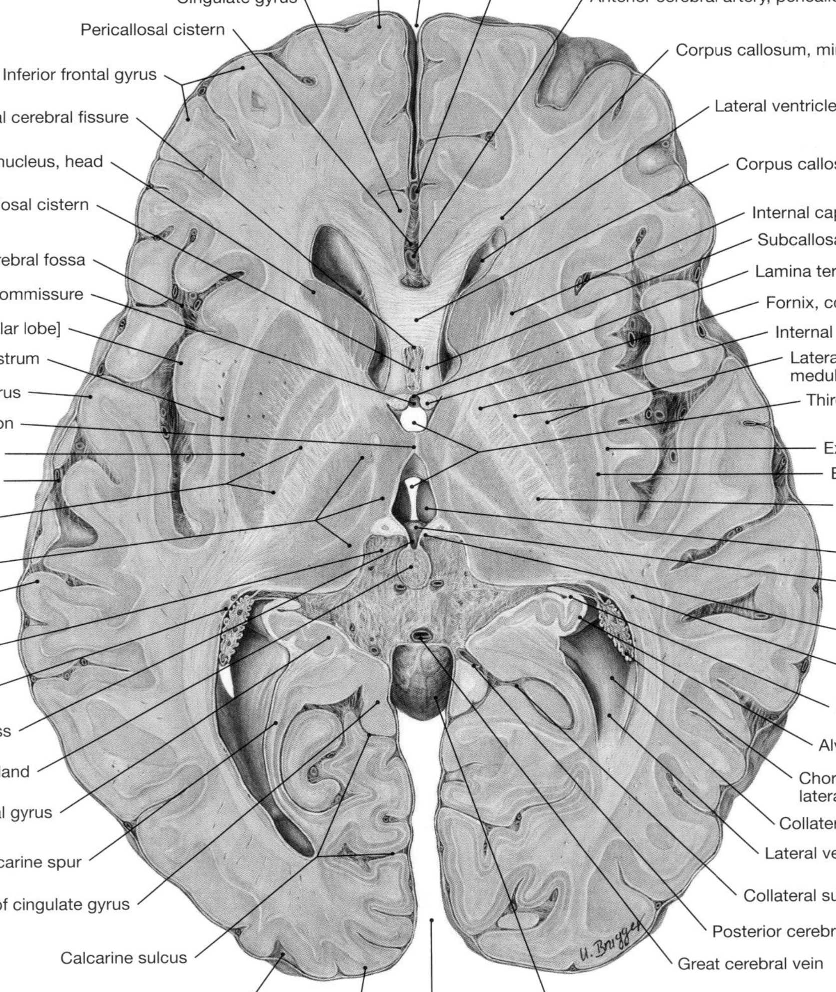

Longitudinal cerebral fissure
Frontal pole
Anterior cerebral artery, callosomarginal artery
Cingulate gyrus
Anterior cerebral artery, pericallosal artery
Pericallosal cistern
Corpus callosum, minor forceps
Inferior frontal gyrus
Lateral ventricle, frontal horn
Longitudinal cerebral fissure
Corpus callosum, rostrum
Caudate nucleus, head
Internal capsule, anterior limb
Pericallosal cistern
Subcallosal area
Cistern of lateral cerebral fossa
Lamina terminalis
Anterior commissure
Fornix, column
Insula [insular lobe]
Internal capsule, genu
Claustrum
Lateral and medial medullary laminae
Superior temporal gyrus
Third ventricle
Interthalamic adhesion
Putamen
Extreme capsule
Superior temporal sulcus
External capsule
Globus pallidus medial and lateral segments
Internal capsule, posterior limb
Thalamus
Hypothalamus
Middle temporal gyrus
Posterior commissure
Cisterna ambiens
Habenula
Caudate nucleus, tail
Internal capsule, optic radiation
Fimbria
Pineal recess
Alveus
Pineal gland
Choroid plexus of lateral ventricle
Parahippocampal gyrus
Collateral trigone
Calcarine spur
Lateral ventricle, occipital horn
Isthmus of cingulate gyrus
Collateral sulcus
Posterior cerebral artery
Calcarine sulcus
Great cerebral vein
Lunate sulcus
Vermis of cerebellum
Occipital pole
Longitudinal cerebral fissure

**Fig. 12.124 Brain;** horizontal section through the center of the third ventricle at the level of the interthalamic adhesion; superior view.
The section is centered through the pineal gland and the interthalamic adhesion. Lateral thereof, the thalamus, internal capsule, globus pallidus, putamen, external capsule, claustrum, extreme capsule, and the insular lobe are located. The hippocampal fimbria and alveus and the parahippocampal gyrus are also discernible.

## Brain, horizontal sections

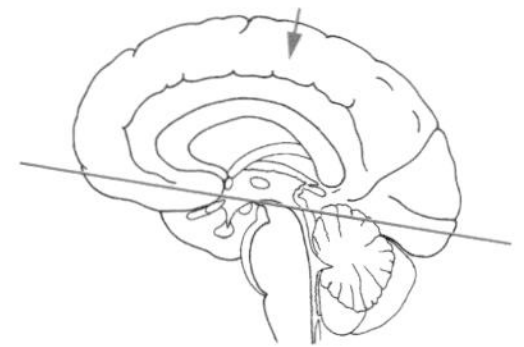

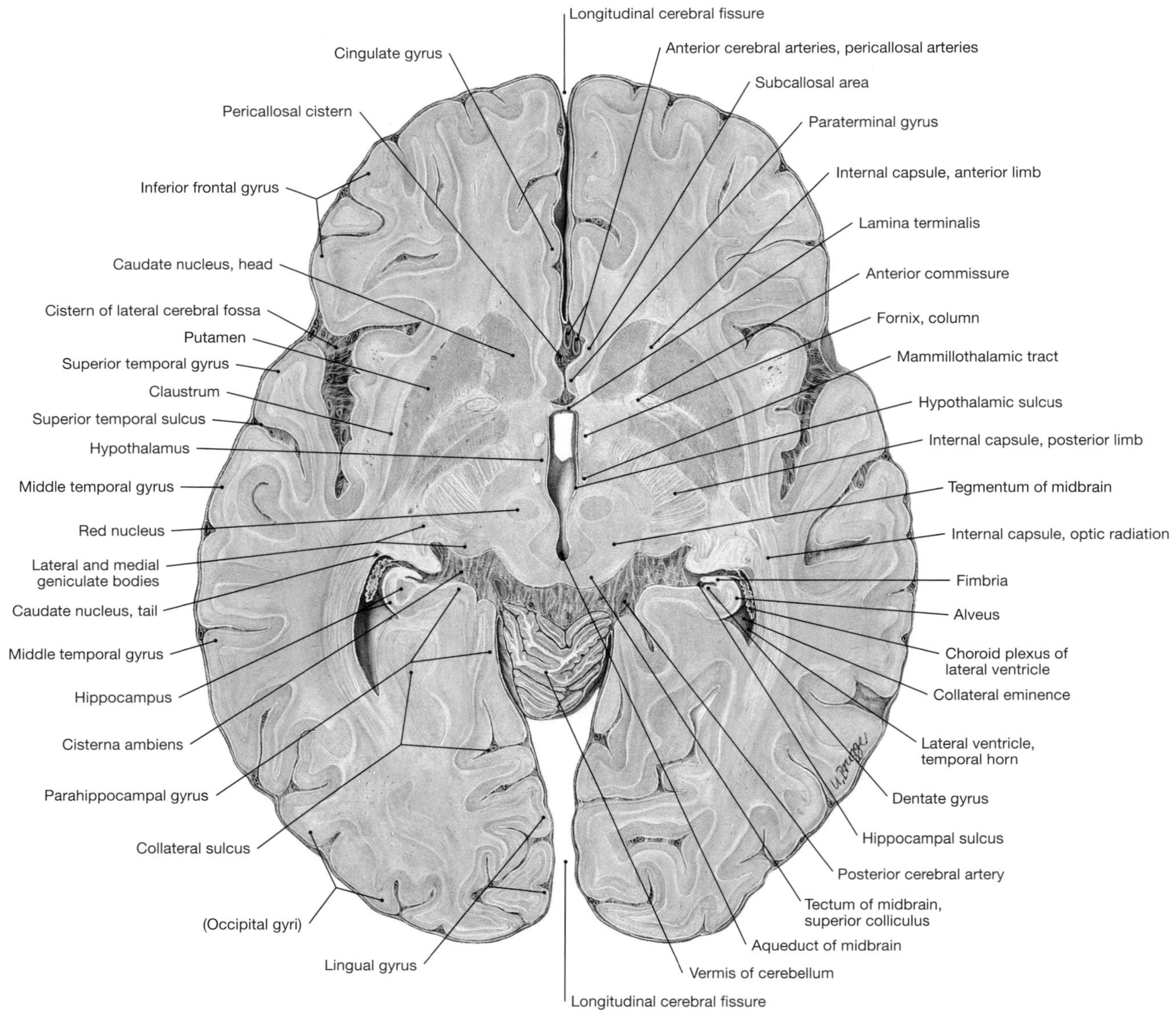

Longitudinal cerebral fissure
Cingulate gyrus
Pericallosal cistern
Inferior frontal gyrus
Caudate nucleus, head
Cistern of lateral cerebral fossa
Putamen
Superior temporal gyrus
Claustrum
Superior temporal sulcus
Hypothalamus
Middle temporal gyrus
Red nucleus
Lateral and medial geniculate bodies
Caudate nucleus, tail
Middle temporal gyrus
Hippocampus
Cisterna ambiens
Parahippocampal gyrus
Collateral sulcus
(Occipital gyri)
Lingual gyrus
Anterior cerebral arteries, pericallosal arteries
Subcallosal area
Paraterminal gyrus
Internal capsule, anterior limb
Lamina terminalis
Anterior commissure
Fornix, column
Mammillothalamic tract
Hypothalamic sulcus
Internal capsule, posterior limb
Tegmentum of midbrain
Internal capsule, optic radiation
Fimbria
Alveus
Choroid plexus of lateral ventricle
Collateral eminence
Lateral ventricle, temporal horn
Dentate gyrus
Hippocampal sulcus
Posterior cerebral artery
Tectum of midbrain, superior colliculus
Aqueduct of midbrain
Vermis of cerebellum
Longitudinal cerebral fissure

**Fig. 12.125 Brain;** horizontal section through the third ventricle at the level of the opening of the cerebral aqueduct (aqueduct of midbrain); superior view.
Due to its reddish coloration, the red nucleus prominently figures in this section plane. The close relationship between the caudate nucleus and the putamen also becomes obvious. The anterior limb of the internal capsule runs between both nuclear structures. The section is located at the transition from the third ventricle to the aqueduct of midbrain, with both structures being sectioned. The upper rim of the cerebellar vermis is sectioned as well.

## Brain, horizontal sections

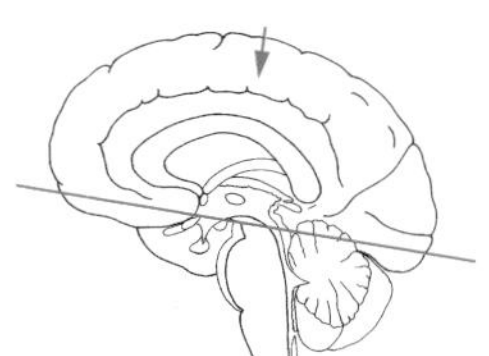

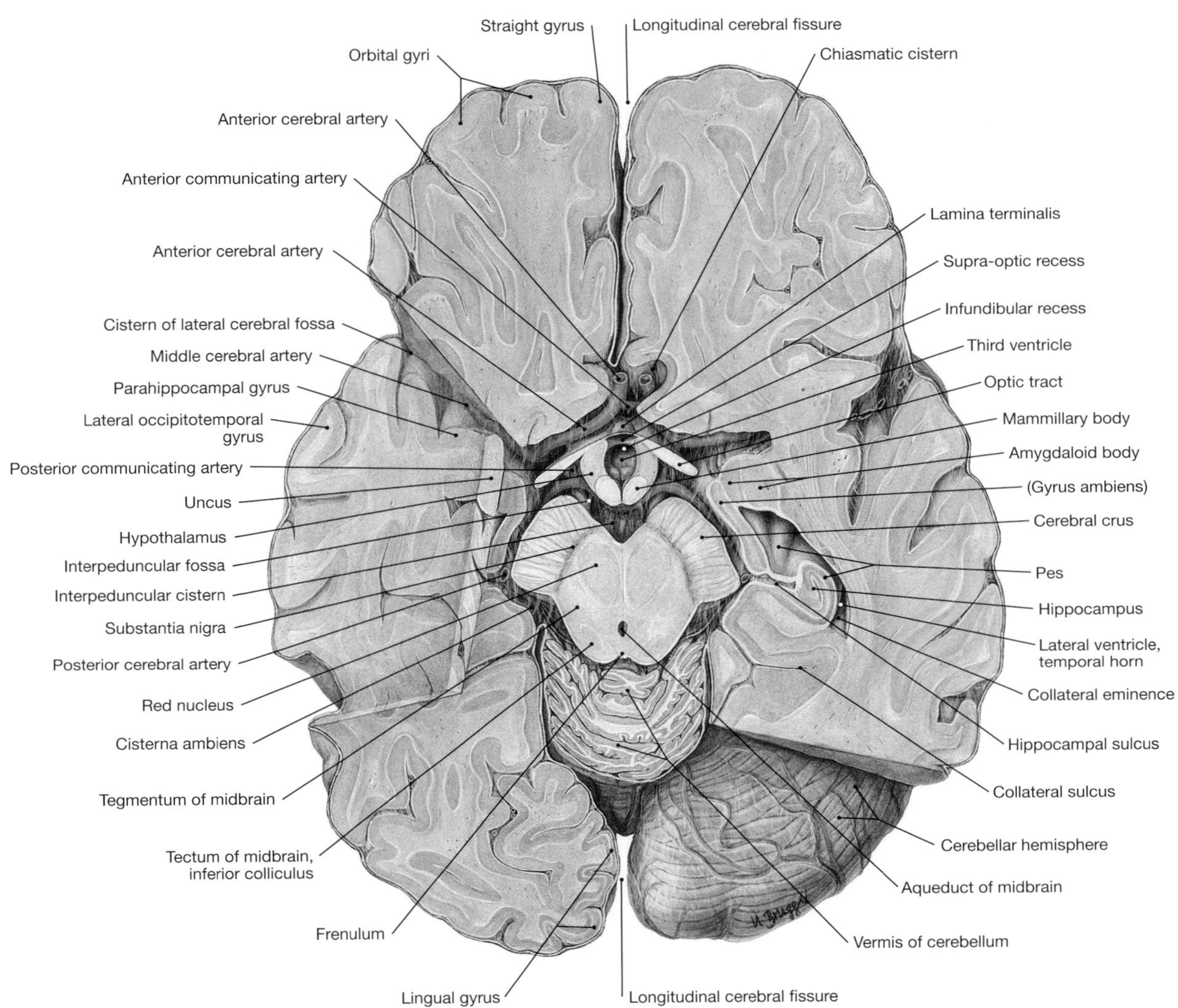
Straight gyrus
Longitudinal cerebral fissure
Orbital gyri
Chiasmatic cistern
Anterior cerebral artery
Anterior communicating artery
Lamina terminalis
Anterior cerebral artery
Supra-optic recess
Infundibular recess
Cistern of lateral cerebral fossa
Third ventricle
Middle cerebral artery
Optic tract
Parahippocampal gyrus
Mammillary body
Lateral occipitotemporal gyrus
Amygdaloid body
Posterior communicating artery
(Gyrus ambiens)
Uncus
Cerebral crus
Hypothalamus
Interpeduncular fossa
Pes
Interpeduncular cistern
Hippocampus
Substantia nigra
Lateral ventricle, temporal horn
Posterior cerebral artery
Collateral eminence
Red nucleus
Cisterna ambiens
Hippocampal sulcus
Collateral sulcus
Tegmentum of midbrain
Cerebellar hemisphere
Tectum of midbrain, inferior colliculus
Aqueduct of midbrain
Frenulum
Vermis of cerebellum
Lingual gyrus
Longitudinal cerebral fissure

**Fig. 12.126 Brain;** staggered horizontal section through the floor of the third ventricle at the level of the mamillary bodies; superior view. The optic tract, hypothalamus, mamillary bodies, cerebral crura, red nuclei, and inferior colliculi of the tectum of midbrain are sectioned. On the right side, the hippocampus is visible, on the left side the gray and white matter of the temporal and occipital lobes are shown. Removal of the occipital pole on the right side allows an unobstructed view on the cerebellar hemisphere.

## Brain, sagittal sections

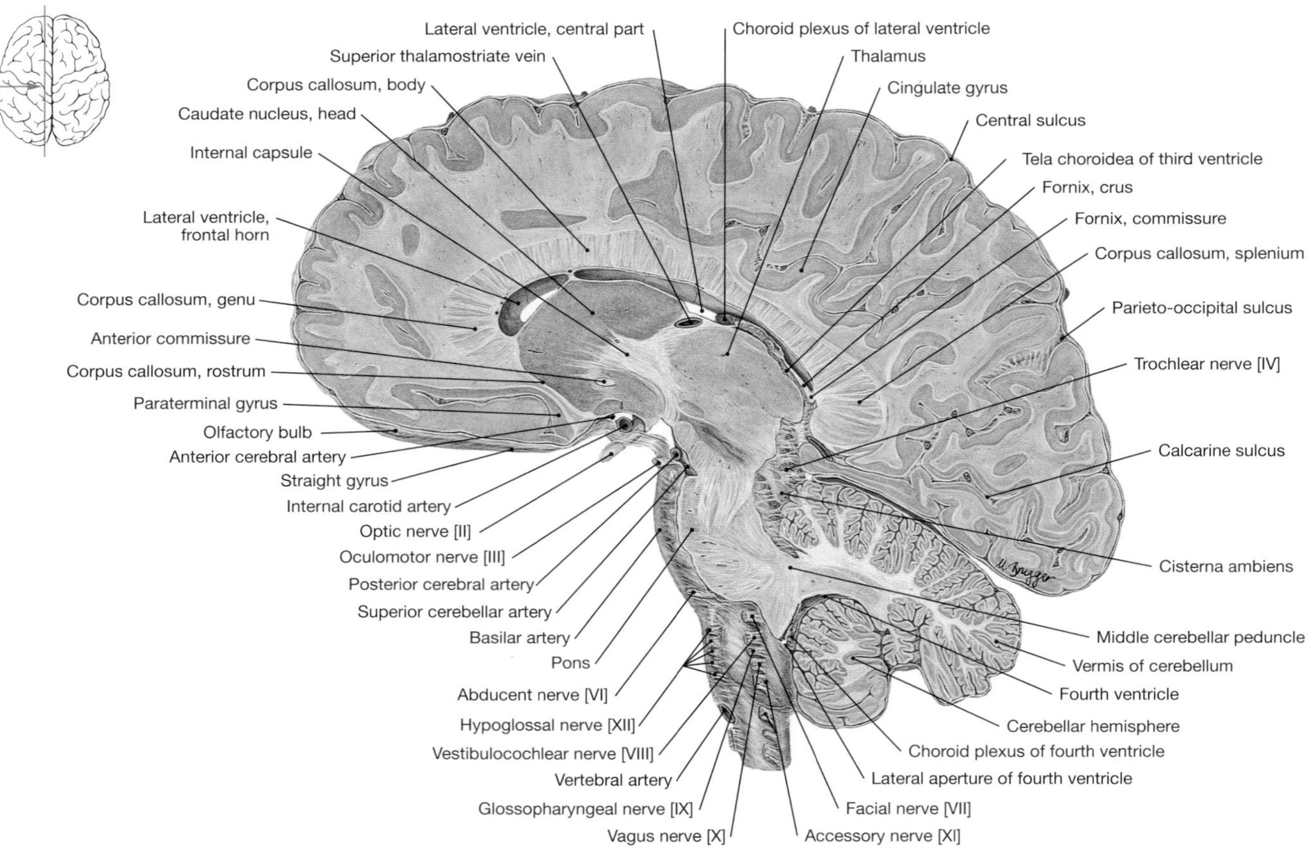
Lateral ventricle, central part
Choroid plexus of lateral ventricle
Superior thalamostriate vein
Thalamus
Corpus callosum, body
Cingulate gyrus
Caudate nucleus, head
Central sulcus
Internal capsule
Tela choroidea of third ventricle
Fornix, crus
Lateral ventricle, frontal horn
Fornix, commissure
Corpus callosum, splenium
Corpus callosum, genu
Parieto-occipital sulcus
Anterior commissure
Trochlear nerve [IV]
Corpus callosum, rostrum
Paraterminal gyrus
Olfactory bulb
Calcarine sulcus
Anterior cerebral artery
Straight gyrus
Internal carotid artery
Optic nerve [II]
Oculomotor nerve [III]
Cisterna ambiens
Posterior cerebral artery
Superior cerebellar artery
Middle cerebellar peduncle
Basilar artery
Vermis of cerebellum
Pons
Abducent nerve [VI]
Fourth ventricle
Hypoglossal nerve [XII]
Cerebellar hemisphere
Vestibulocochlear nerve [VIII]
Choroid plexus of fourth ventricle
Vertebral artery
Lateral aperture of fourth ventricle
Glossopharyngeal nerve [IX]
Facial nerve [VII]
Vagus nerve [X]
Accessory nerve [XI]

**Fig. 12.127 Brain;** sagittal section through the left hemisphere at the level of the head of the caudate nucleus; view from the left side.
A paramedian section shows the corpus callosum in its entire rostro-occipital dimension. The lateral ventricle positions below the corpus callosum and, further below, the caudate nucleus, thalamus, internal capsule, and optic nerve [II] are located. The basilar artery runs in front of the brainstem. The middle cerebellar peduncle marks the transition from the pons to the cerebellum.

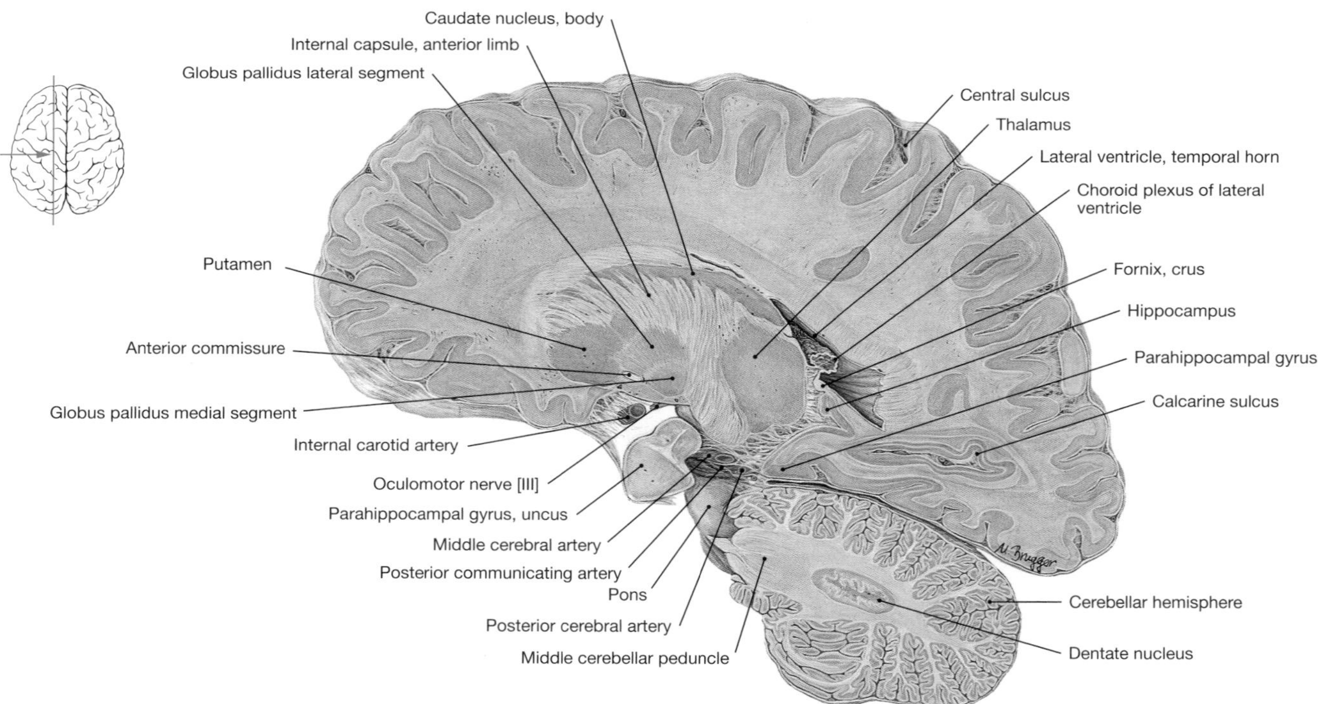
Caudate nucleus, body
Internal capsule, anterior limb
Globus pallidus lateral segment
Central sulcus
Thalamus
Lateral ventricle, temporal horn
Choroid plexus of lateral ventricle
Putamen
Fornix, crus
Hippocampus
Anterior commissure
Parahippocampal gyrus
Calcarine sulcus
Globus pallidus medial segment
Internal carotid artery
Oculomotor nerve [III]
Parahippocampal gyrus, uncus
Middle cerebral artery
Posterior communicating artery
Pons
Cerebellar hemisphere
Posterior cerebral artery
Middle cerebellar peduncle
Dentate nucleus

**Fig. 12.128 Brain;** sagittal section through the left hemisphere at the level of the body of the caudate nucleus; view from the left side.
Apart from the body of the caudate nucleus, the anterior limb of the internal capsule, the thalamus, the putamen, the globus pallidus, and the uncus of the parahippocampal gyrus have been sectioned. The dentate nucleus visualizes prominently in the section plane through the cerebellum.

## Brain, sagittal sections

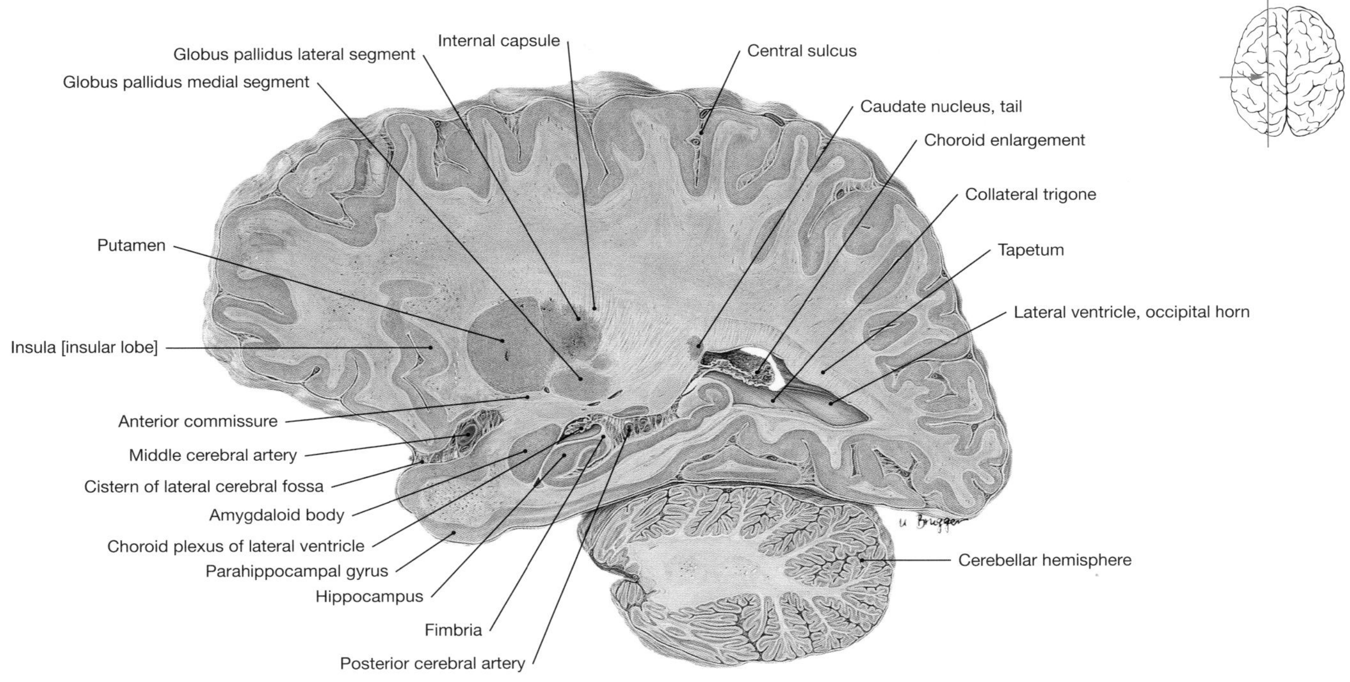
Globus pallidus lateral segment
Internal capsule
Central sulcus
Globus pallidus medial segment
Caudate nucleus, tail
Choroid enlargement
Collateral trigone
Putamen
Tapetum
Lateral ventricle, occipital horn
Insula [insular lobe]
Anterior commissure
Middle cerebral artery
Cistern of lateral cerebral fossa
Amygdaloid body
Choroid plexus of lateral ventricle
Parahippocampal gyrus
Hippocampus
Cerebellar hemisphere
Fimbria
Posterior cerebral artery

**Fig. 12.129 Brain;** sagittal section through the left hemisphere at the level of the amygdaloid body; view from the left side.
This section reveals the hippocampus, the hippocampal fimbria, and the tail of the caudate nucleus posterior to the amygdaloid body. In addition, the putamen, the globus pallidus, and the internal capsule are discernible. The inferior part of this section shows the cerebellar hemisphere.

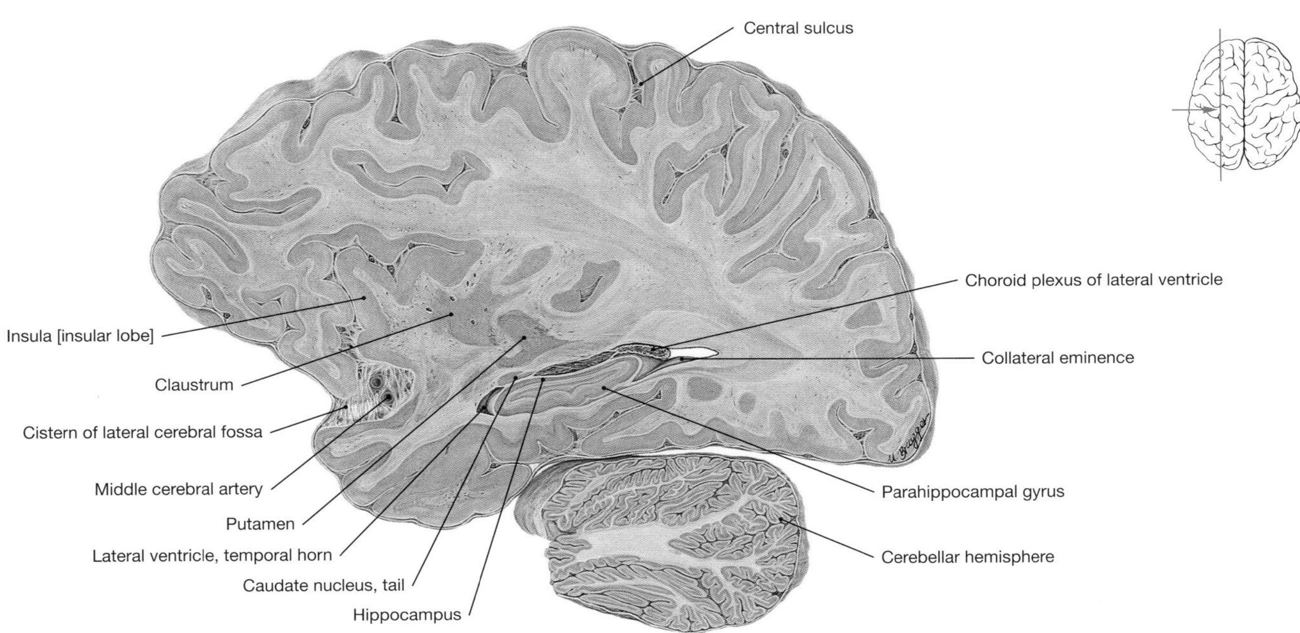
Central sulcus
Choroid plexus of lateral ventricle
Insula [insular lobe]
Collateral eminence
Claustrum
Cistern of lateral cerebral fossa
Middle cerebral artery
Parahippocampal gyrus
Putamen
Lateral ventricle, temporal horn
Cerebellar hemisphere
Caudate nucleus, tail
Hippocampus

**Fig. 12.130 Brain;** sagittal section through the left hemisphere at the level of the apex of the temporal horn of the lateral ventricle; view from the left side.
This lateral section shows the insular lobe and includes the hippocampus with the parahippocampal gyrus, the claustrum, and the putamen.

## Overview

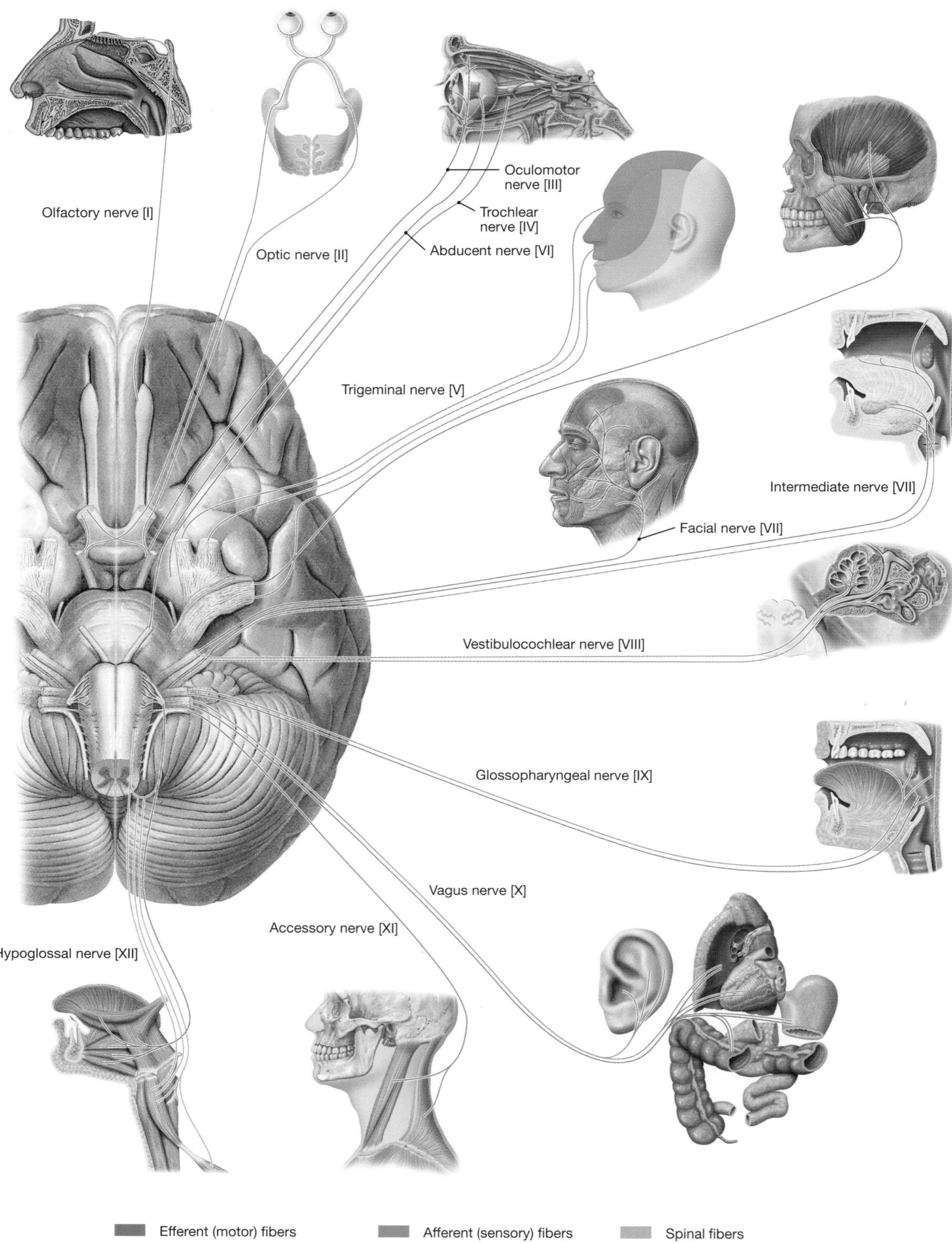
Olfactory nerve [I]
Optic nerve [II]
Oculomotor nerve [III]
Trochlear nerve [IV]
Abducent nerve [VI]
Trigeminal nerve [V]
Intermediate nerve [VII]
Facial nerve [VII]
Vestibulocochlear nerve [VIII]
Glossopharyngeal nerve [IX]
Vagus nerve [X]
Accessory nerve [XI]
Hypoglossal nerve [XII]
Efferent (motor) fibers
Afferent (sensory) fibers
Spinal fibers

**Fig. 12.131 Cranial nerves;** functional overview of the telencephalon, brainstem and cerebellum; inferior view.

Twelve pairs of cranial nerves exit the cranial base. They are numbered in Roman digits (I–XII) according to the order in which they exit the brainstem from anterior to posterior. The olfactory nerves constitute the first cranial nerve, collectively named **olfactory nerve [I].** Bipolar olfactory neurons in the mucosa (an unnamed sensory ganglion is located within the olfactory mucosa) project their axons into the olfactory bulb, a part of the telencephalon that was relocated cranially during development. Here, olfactory information from these axons is synapsed in layers of neuronal cells. The olfactory bulb represents the terminating nucleus for the olfactory nerve [I], with the exception that this nucleus does not reside in the brainstem but locates outside on the lamina cribrosa. The fact that the neurons of the first cranial nerve are very short and the terminating nucleus (olfactory bulb) resides outside of the brainstem are distinguishing features, separating the first from the other cranial nerves. The **optic nerve [II]** is exceptional as it includes the 3rd and possibly 4th neuron of the visual pathway. Contrary to all other cranial nerves, the optic nerve is a protrusion of the diencephalon and not actually a peripheral nerve.

→ T 56, 58

## Overview

**Overview of the Twelve Cranial Nerves and their Most Important Innervation Sites** [14]
A detailed presentation of the innervation sites for each cranial nerve is shown on pp. 296–323.
GSA: general somato-afferent; GSE: general somato-efferent; GVA: general viscero-afferent; GVE: general viscero-efferent; SSA: specific somato-afferent; SVA: specific viscero-afferent; SVE: specific viscero-efferent

| Cranial Nerve | Quality | Important Innervation Sites |
|---|---|---|
| Olfactory nerve [I] | SSA | Olfactory mucosa |
| Optic nerve [II] | SSA | Retina |
| Oculomotor nerve [III] | GSE, GVE | Intra-ocular and extra-ocular muscles |
| Trochlear nerve [IV] | GSE | Extra-ocular muscles |
| Trigeminal nerve [V] | SVE, GSA | Masticatory muscles, facial skin |
| Abducent nerve [VI] | GSE | Extra-ocular muscle |
| Facial nerve [VII] | GVE, SVE, SVA, GSA | Mimic muscles, gustatory organ, glands |
| Vestibulocochlear nerve [VIII] | SSA | Equilibrium and hearing |
| Glossopharyngeal nerve [IX] | GVE, SVE, GSA, GVA, SVA | Pharyngeal muscles, parotid gland |
| Vagus nerve [X] | GVE, SVE, GSA, GVA, SVA | Pharyngeal muscles, larynx, inner organs |
| Accessory nerve [XI] | SVE | Trapezius and sternocleidomastoid muscles |
| Hypoglossal nerve [XII] | GSE | Muscles of the tongue |

**Overview of Cranial Nerves with Two or More Nuclei in the Brainstem** [14]
The trochlear [IV], abducent [VI], accessory [XI], and hypoglossal nerve [XII] each possess only a single identically named nucleus and are therefore not mentioned here.

| Cranial Nerve | Corresponding Nuclei |
|---|---|
| Oculomotor nerve [III] | • Nucleus of oculomotor nerve<br>• Accessory nucleus of oculomotor nerve |
| Trigeminal nerve [V] | • Motor nucleus of trigeminal nerve<br>• Mesencephalic nucleus of trigeminal nerve<br>• Pontine (principal sensory) nucleus of trigeminal nerve<br>• Spinal nucleus of trigeminal nerve |
| Facial nerve [VII] | • Motor nucleus of facial nerve<br>• Superior salivatory nucleus<br>• Spinal nucleus of trigeminal nerve<br>• Nuclei of solitary tract |
| Vestibulocochlear nerve [VIII] | • Vestibular nuclei<br>• Cochlear nuclei |
| Glossopharyngeal nerve [IX] | • Inferior salivatory nucleus<br>• Nucleus ambiguus<br>• Spinal nucleus of trigeminal nerve<br>• Nuclei of solitary tract |
| Vagus nerve [X] | • Dorsal (posterior) nucleus of vagus nerve<br>• Nucleus ambiguus<br>• Spinal nucleus of trigeminal nerve<br>• Nuclei of solitary tract |

**Overview of Nuclei in the Brainstem with Divisions Allocated to Two or More Cranial Nerves** [14]
All other nuclei can be associated with a specific cranial nerve.

| Nucleus | Corresponding Cranial Nerve |
|---|---|
| Nucleus ambiguus | • Glossopharyngeal nerve [IX]<br>• Vagus nerve [X]<br>• Accessory nerve [XI] (cranial root) |
| Nuclei of solitary tract | • Facial nerve [VII]<br>• Glossopharyngeal nerve [IX]<br>• Vagus nerve [X] |
| Spinal nucleus of trigeminal nerve | • Trigeminal nerve [V]<br>• Facial nerve [VII]<br>• Glossopharyngeal nerve [IX]<br>• Vagus nerve [X] |

## Topography

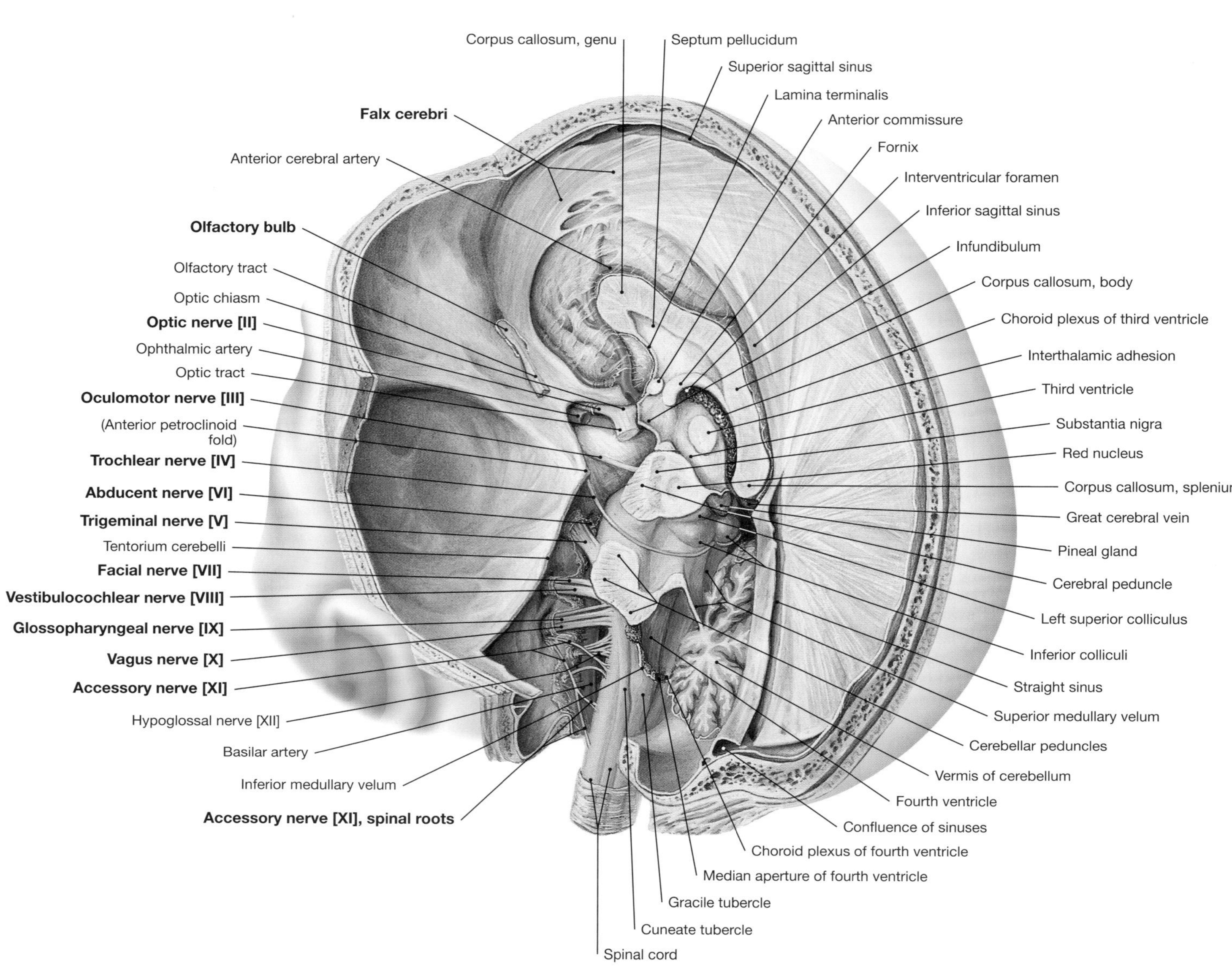
Corpus callosum, genu
Septum pellucidum
Superior sagittal sinus
Lamina terminalis
Falx cerebri
Anterior commissure
Fornix
Anterior cerebral artery
Interventricular foramen
Inferior sagittal sinus
Olfactory bulb
Infundibulum
Olfactory tract
Corpus callosum, body
Optic chiasm
Choroid plexus of third ventricle
Optic nerve [II]
Ophthalmic artery
Interthalamic adhesion
Optic tract
Third ventricle
Oculomotor nerve [III]
(Anterior petroclinoid fold)
Substantia nigra
Trochlear nerve [IV]
Red nucleus
Corpus callosum, splenium
Abducent nerve [VI]
Trigeminal nerve [V]
Great cerebral vein
Tentorium cerebelli
Pineal gland
Facial nerve [VII]
Cerebral peduncle
Vestibulocochlear nerve [VIII]
Glossopharyngeal nerve [IX]
Left superior colliculus
Vagus nerve [X]
Inferior colliculi
Accessory nerve [XI]
Straight sinus
Hypoglossal nerve [XII]
Superior medullary velum
Basilar artery
Cerebellar peduncles
Inferior medullary velum
Vermis of cerebellum
Accessory nerve [XI], spinal roots
Fourth ventricle
Confluence of sinuses
Choroid plexus of fourth ventricle
Median aperture of fourth ventricle
Gracile tubercle
Cuneate tubercle
Spinal cord

**Fig. 12.132 Course of the cranial nerves, in the subarachnoid space;** posterior superior view from the left side; the left hemisphere of the cerebrum and the cerebellum as well as the tentorium cerebelli have been removed.

The cranial nerves III–XII exit the brainstem in chronological order from cranial to caudal. Some exit as a loose bundle of nerve roots and form the actual cranial nerve (IX–XII) later. The trochlear nerve [IV] not only is the thinnest cranial nerve but also uniquely exits from the posterior side of the brainstem. The abducent nerve [VI] has the longest intradural course before exiting through its opening at the cranial base.

→ T 58

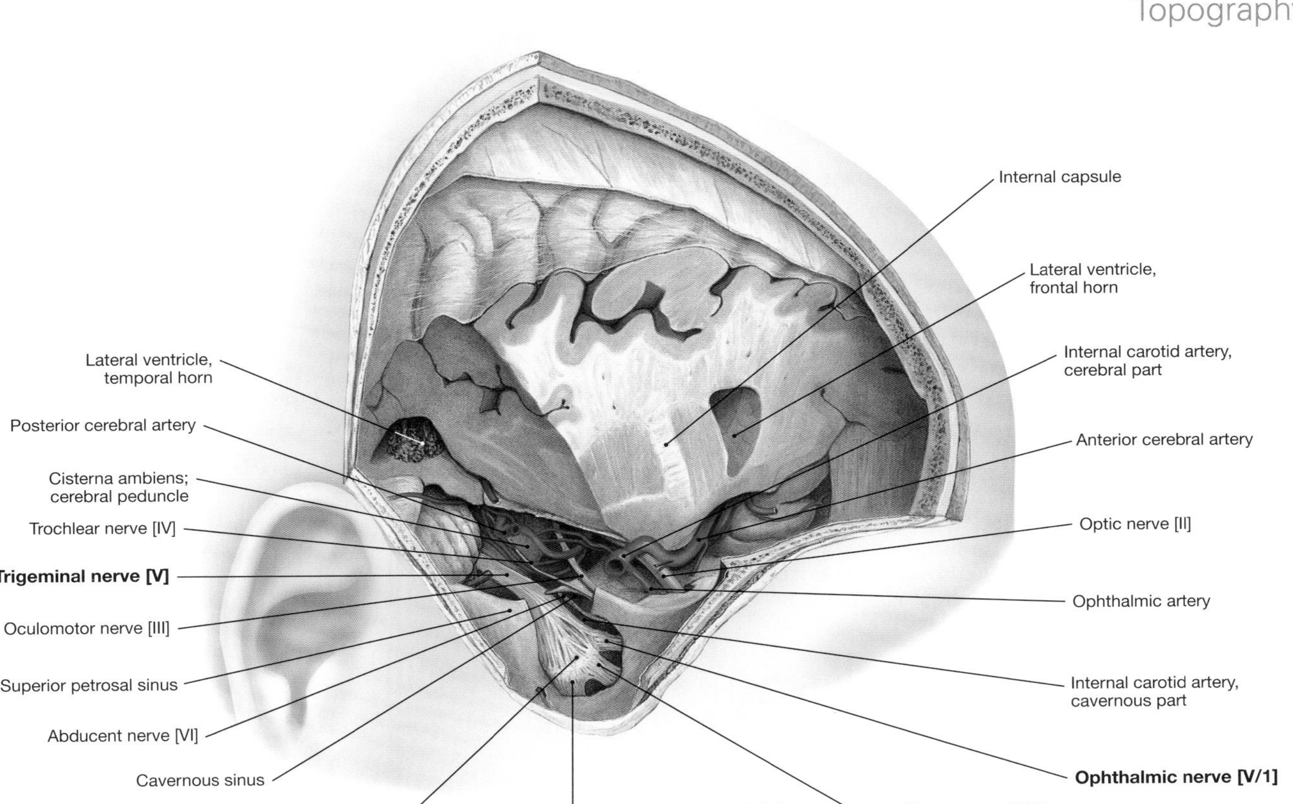
Internal capsule
Lateral ventricle, frontal horn
Internal carotid artery, cerebral part
Anterior cerebral artery
Optic nerve [II]
Ophthalmic artery
Internal carotid artery, cavernous part
Ophthalmic nerve [V/1]
Maxillary nerve [V/2]
Mandibular nerve [V/3]
Trigeminal ganglion
Cavernous sinus
Abducent nerve [VI]
Superior petrosal sinus
Oculomotor nerve [III]
Trigeminal nerve [V]
Trochlear nerve [IV]
Cisterna ambiens; cerebral peduncle
Posterior cerebral artery
Lateral ventricle, temporal horn

**Fig. 12.133 Course of the cranial nerves in the middle cranial fossa;** view from the right side.
Large parts of the frontal and temporal lobes were removed to allow an unobstructed view on the cranial base below. The trigeminal cavity (MECKEL's cave) has been opened. Located within is the **trigeminal ganglion** (V, semilunar ganglion, clinical term: GASSERIAN ganglion), with the three main branches of the trigeminal nerve (ophthalmic nerve [V/1], maxillary nerve [V/2], mandibular nerve [V/3]). In addition to the trigeminal nerve [V], parts of the optic nerve [II], oculomotor nerve [III] and trochlear nerve [IV] and arteries originating from the cerebral part of the internal carotid artery (ophthalmic artery, anterior cerebral artery) are visible.

→ T 58

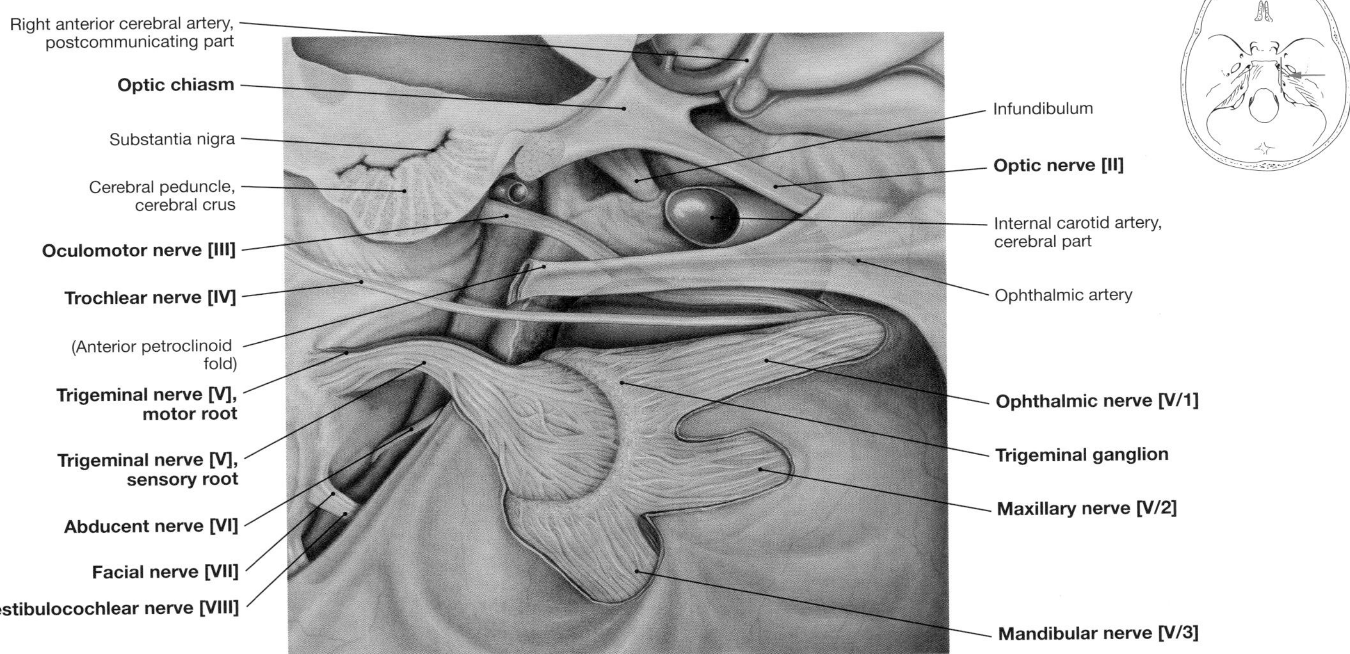
Right anterior cerebral artery, postcommunicating part
Optic chiasm
Substantia nigra
Cerebral peduncle, cerebral crus
Oculomotor nerve [III]
Trochlear nerve [IV]
(Anterior petroclinoid fold)
Trigeminal nerve [V], motor root
Trigeminal nerve [V], sensory root
Abducent nerve [VI]
Facial nerve [VII]
Vestibulocochlear nerve [VIII]
Infundibulum
Optic nerve [II]
Internal carotid artery, cerebral part
Ophthalmic artery
Ophthalmic nerve [V/1]
Trigeminal ganglion
Maxillary nerve [V/2]
Mandibular nerve [V/3]

**Fig. 12.134 Arteries and nerves in the region of the sella turcica and the cavernous sinus;** view from the right side.
The trigeminal cavity (MECKEL's cave) has been opened by removing the cranial dura mater and the arachnoid mater at this site. Visible is the **trigeminal ganglion** (V, semilunar ganglion, clinical term: GASSERIAN ganglion) with the three trigeminal nerve branches. In addition, the course of the cranial nerves III, IV, and VI to VIII from exiting the brainstem to entering the cranial base is shown. The cavernous part of the A internal carotid artery transitions into the cerebral part which lies close to the optic nerve [II]. The optic chiasm is located above the hypophyseal stalk (infundibulum).

→ T 58

## Nuclei of the cranial nerves

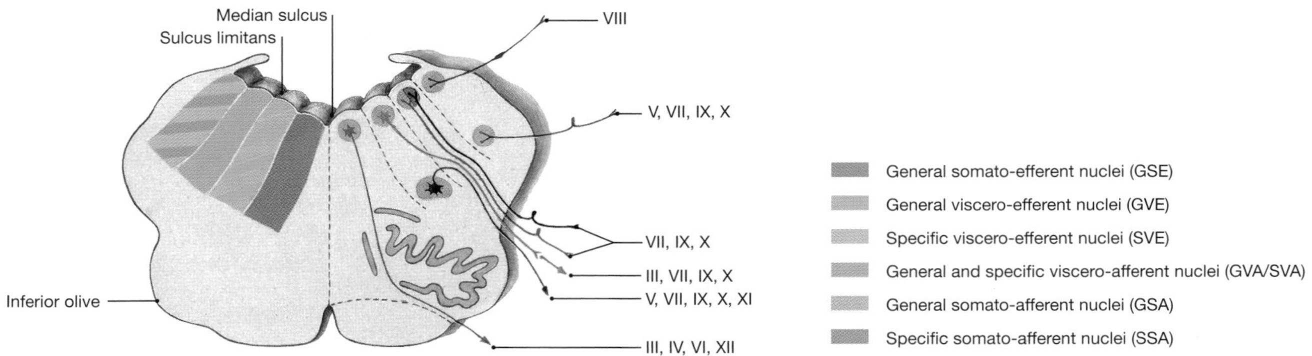
Median sulcus
Sulcus limitans
VIII
V, VII, IX, X
VII, IX, X
III, VII, IX, X
V, VII, IX, X, XI
III, IV, VI, XII
Inferior olive
General somato-efferent nuclei (GSE)
General viscero-efferent nuclei (GVE)
Specific viscero-efferent nuclei (SVE)
General and specific viscero-afferent nuclei (GVA/SVA)
General somato-afferent nuclei (GSA)
Specific somato-afferent nuclei (SSA)

**Fig. 12.135 Cranial nerves;** schematic cross-section through the rhomboid fossa demonstrating the nuclei.
In the brainstem, nuclei with similar functions are arranged in a column in a cranial to caudal direction. Due to spatial restrictions, the nuclei form four longitudinal **nuclear columns** and are arranged alongside each other. This includes in a medial to lateral direction a somato-efferent, a viscero-efferent, a viscero-afferent, and a somato-afferent column of nuclei. Within the viscero-efferent, the viscero-afferent, and the somato-afferent columns of nuclei, one can distinguish general and specific afferent nuclei.

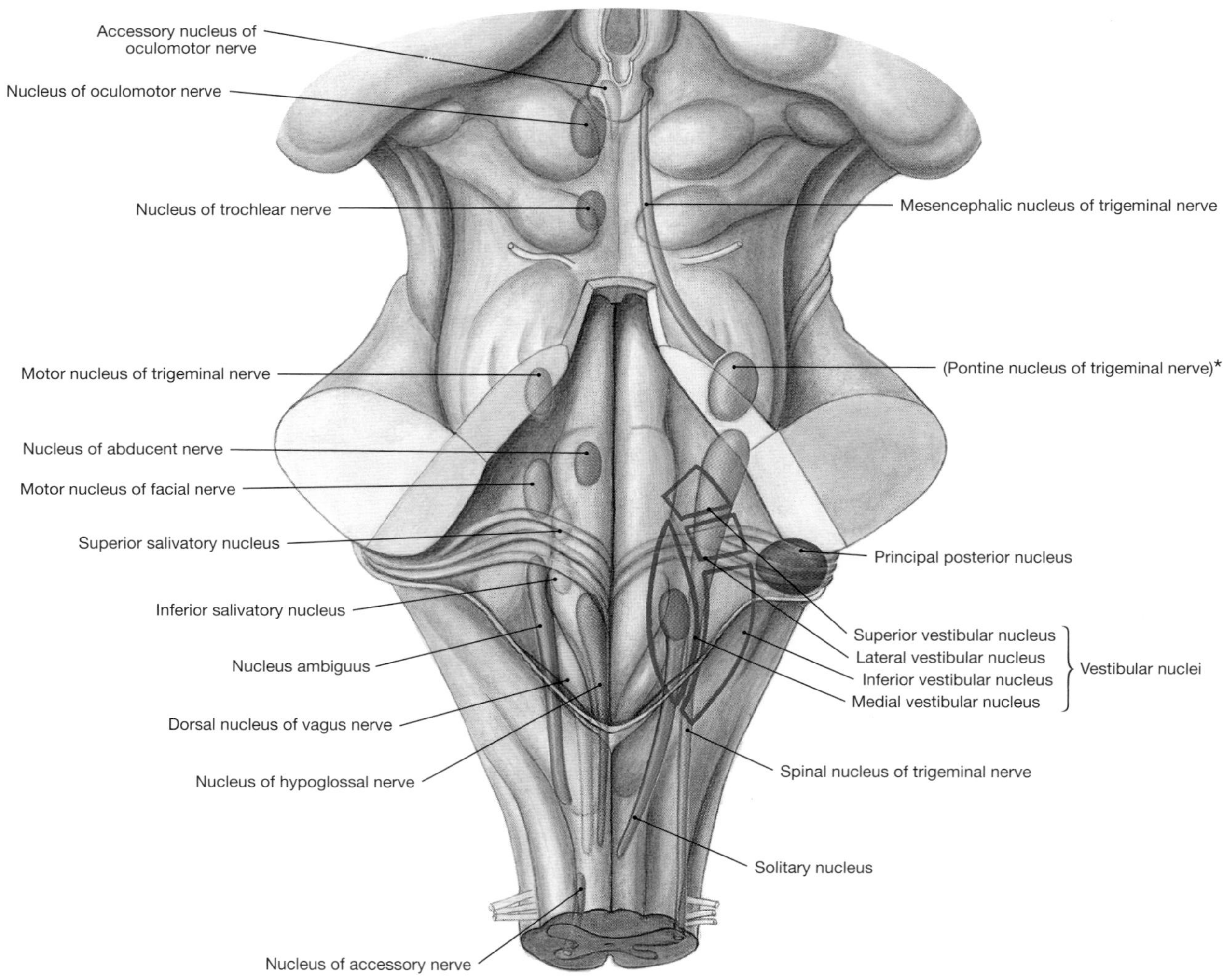
Accessory nucleus of oculomotor nerve
Nucleus of oculomotor nerve
Nucleus of trochlear nerve
Mesencephalic nucleus of trigeminal nerve
Motor nucleus of trigeminal nerve
(Pontine nucleus of trigeminal nerve)*
Nucleus of abducent nerve
Motor nucleus of facial nerve
Superior salivatory nucleus
Principal posterior nucleus
Inferior salivatory nucleus
Superior vestibular nucleus
Lateral vestibular nucleus
Inferior vestibular nucleus
Medial vestibular nucleus
Vestibular nuclei
Nucleus ambiguus
Dorsal nucleus of vagus nerve
Nucleus of hypoglossal nerve
Spinal nucleus of trigeminal nerve
Solitary nucleus
Nucleus of accessory nerve

**Fig. 12.136 Cranial nerves;** topographic overview of the nuclei; posterior view.
With the exception of the cranial nerves I and II, all cranial nerves (III–XII) have nuclei located in the brainstem. The mesencephalon contains the nuclei of the cranial nerves III and IV, the nuclei of the cranial nerves V to VII lie in the pons, and the medulla oblongata contains the nuclei of the cranial nerves VII to XII.
It is easy to understand the topographic arrangement of the nuclei of the cranial nerves if one keeps in mind the separation into functional nuclear columns (→ Fig. 12.135). On the left side are the nuclei of origin which contain the perikarya of the efferent neurons projecting into the periphery. In the terminal nuclei on the right side, the afferent fibers derived from the periphery synapse onto the 2nd neuron of the sensory tract.

* clinical term: principal sensory nucleus of trigeminal nerve

→T 57

## Nuclei of the cranial nerves

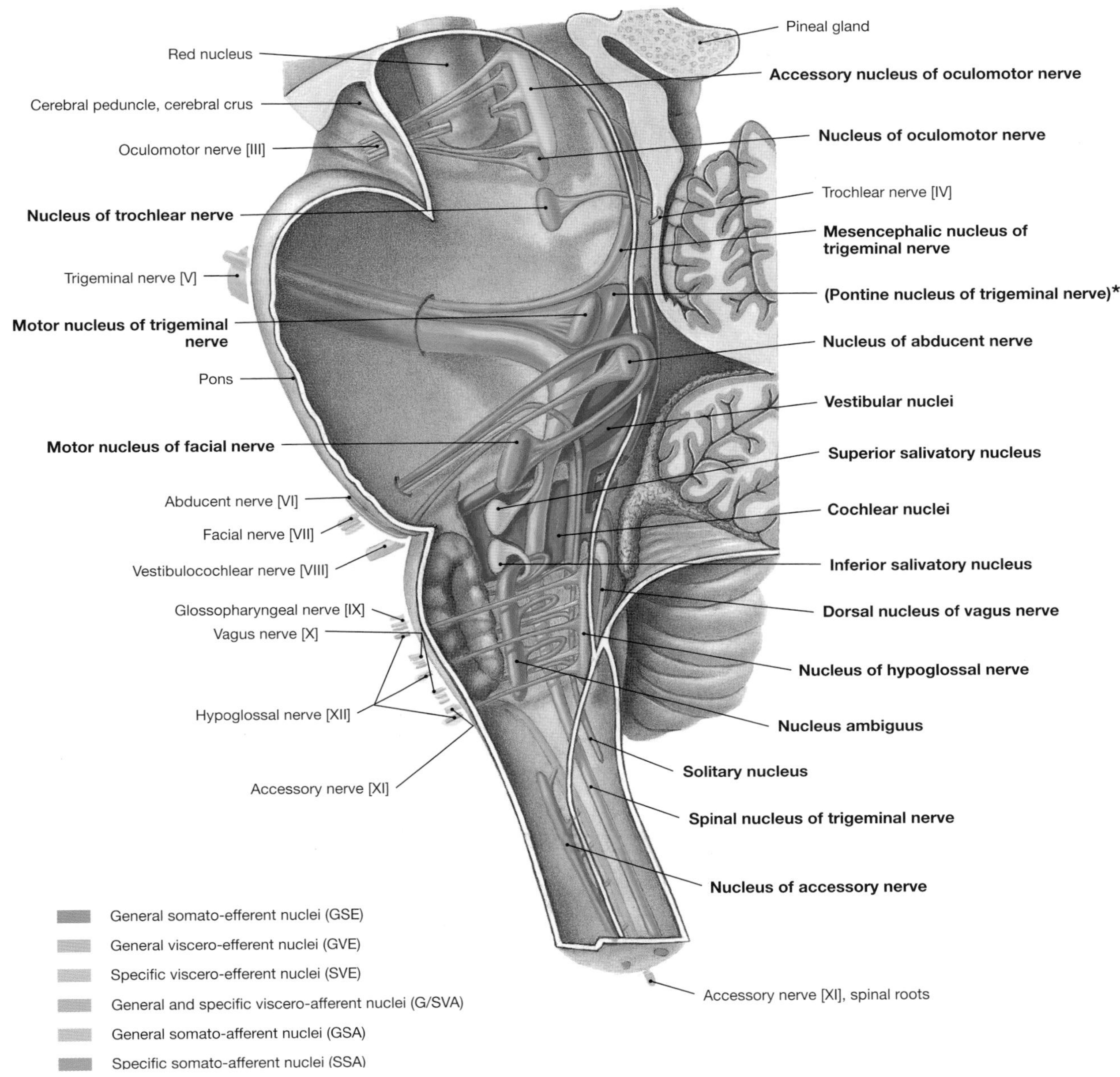

Red nucleus
Cerebral peduncle, cerebral crus
Oculomotor nerve [III]
Nucleus of trochlear nerve
Trigeminal nerve [V]
Motor nucleus of trigeminal nerve
Pons
Motor nucleus of facial nerve
Abducent nerve [VI]
Facial nerve [VII]
Vestibulocochlear nerve [VIII]
Glossopharyngeal nerve [IX]
Vagus nerve [X]
Hypoglossal nerve [XII]
Accessory nerve [XI]
Pineal gland
Accessory nucleus of oculomotor nerve
Nucleus of oculomotor nerve
Trochlear nerve [IV]
Mesencephalic nucleus of trigeminal nerve
(Pontine nucleus of trigeminal nerve)*
Nucleus of abducent nerve
Vestibular nuclei
Superior salivatory nucleus
Cochlear nuclei
Inferior salivatory nucleus
Dorsal nucleus of vagus nerve
Nucleus of hypoglossal nerve
Nucleus ambiguus
Solitary nucleus
Spinal nucleus of trigeminal nerve
Nucleus of accessory nerve
Accessory nerve [XI], spinal roots
General somato-efferent nuclei (GSE)
General viscero-efferent nuclei (GVE)
Specific viscero-efferent nuclei (SVE)
General and specific viscero-afferent nuclei (G/SVA)
General somato-afferent nuclei (GSA)
Specific somato-afferent nuclei (SSA)


**Fig. 12.137 Cranial nerves;** topographic overview of the nuclei of the cranial nerves III to XII in the median plane.

**Nuclei of origin** with perikarya of the efferent/motor fibers divide into:

- general somato-efferent nuclei (nuclei of oculomotor nerve [III, extra-ocular muscles], nucleus of trochlear nerve [IV, superior oblique], nucleus of abducent nerve [VI, lateral rectus], and nucleus of hypoglossal nerve [XII, muscles of the tongue])
- general viscero-efferent nuclei (accessory nuclei of oculomotor nerve [III, sphincter pupillae and ciliary muscle], superior salivatory nucleus [VII, submandibular, sublingual, lacrimal, nasal and palatine glands], inferior salivatory nucleus [IX, parotid gland], dorsal (posterior) nucleus of vagus nerve [X, visceral])
- special viscero-efferent nuclei (motor nucleus of trigeminal nerve [V, masticatory muscles, muscles of the floor of the mouth], motor nucleus of facial nerve [VII, mimic muscles], nucleus ambiguus [IX, X, cranial root of XI, pharyngeal and laryngeal muscles] and nucleus of accessory nerve [XI, spinal root, shoulder muscles])

**Terminal nuclei** are targeted by afferent/sensory fibers and divide into:

- general viscero-afferent nuclei (Nuclei of solitary tract, inferior part [IX, X, sensory innervation of smooth muscles (viscera)])
- special viscero-afferent nuclei (Nuclei of solitary tract, superior part [VII, IX, X], taste fibers)
- general somato-afferent nuclei (mesencephalic nucleus of trigeminal nerve [V, proprioception of masticatory muscles], pontine (principal sensory) nucleus of trigeminal nerve [V, touch, vibration, position of temporomandibular joint], spinalis nucleus of trigeminal nerve [V, pain and temperature sensation in the head region])
- special somato-afferent nuclei (superior, lateral, medial and inferior vestibular nuclei [VIII, vestibularis part, equilibrium] as well as anterior and posterior cochlear nuclei [VIII, cochlear part, hearing])

* clinical term: principal sensory nucleus of trigeminal nerve

→ T 57

## Olfactory nerve [I]

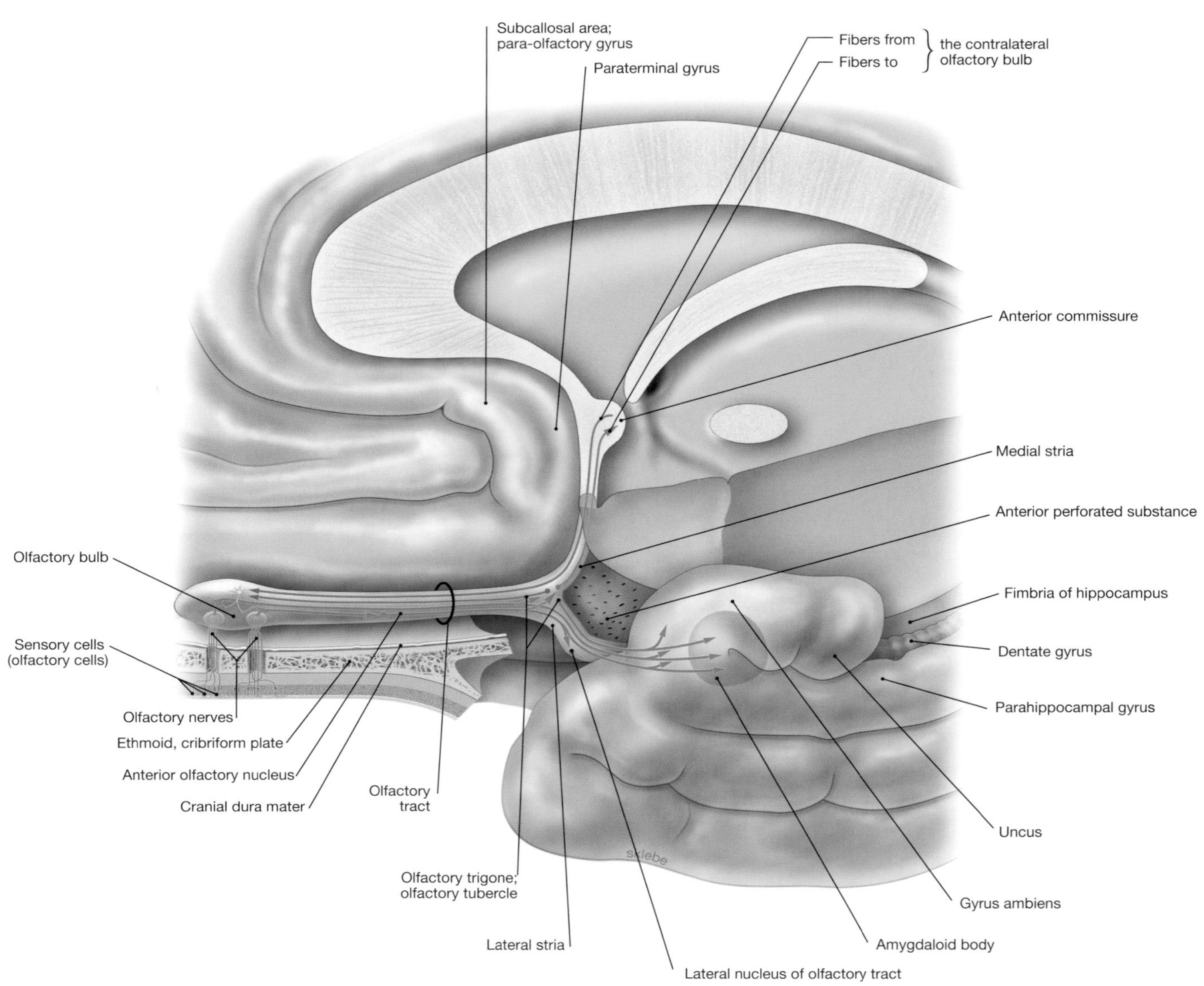
Subcallosal area;
para-olfactory gyrus
Paraterminal gyrus
Fibers from
Fibers to
the contralateral olfactory bulb
Anterior commissure
Medial stria
Anterior perforated substance
Olfactory bulb
Fimbria of hippocampus
Sensory cells (olfactory cells)
Dentate gyrus
Parahippocampal gyrus
Olfactory nerves
Ethmoid, cribriform plate
Anterior olfactory nucleus
Cranial dura mater
Olfactory tract
Uncus
Olfactory trigone; olfactory tubercle
Gyrus ambiens
Lateral stria
Amygdaloid body
Lateral nucleus of olfactory tract

**Fig. 12.138 Olfactory nerve [I] and olfactory tract;** view from the left side.

An area of 3 $cm^2$ of olfactory mucosa locates to both sides at the roof of the nasal cavity. It contains approximately 30 million receptor cells (olfactory sensory cells) which respond to chemical signals. These are bipolar neurons (olfactory neurons, 1st neuron, SSA). On the one side, they connect with the outer environment and on the other side their axons form the **olfactory nerves.** The olfactory neurons have a short life span of 30–60 days and are replaced by neuronal stem cells throughout life.

The olfactory nerves are collectively named olfactory nerve [I]. In each olfactory bulb, they converge onto approximately 1000 **glomeruli.** From here, the olfactory information reaches different areas at the cranial base and the temporal lobe (primary olfactory cortical area) and, through direct and indirect connections, projects to secondary olfactory cortical areas and other brain regions, including the hypothalamus. That way, the conscious realization of olfactory stimuli and the connection with other sensory perceptions is accomplished.

→ T 58a

## Olfactory nerve [I]

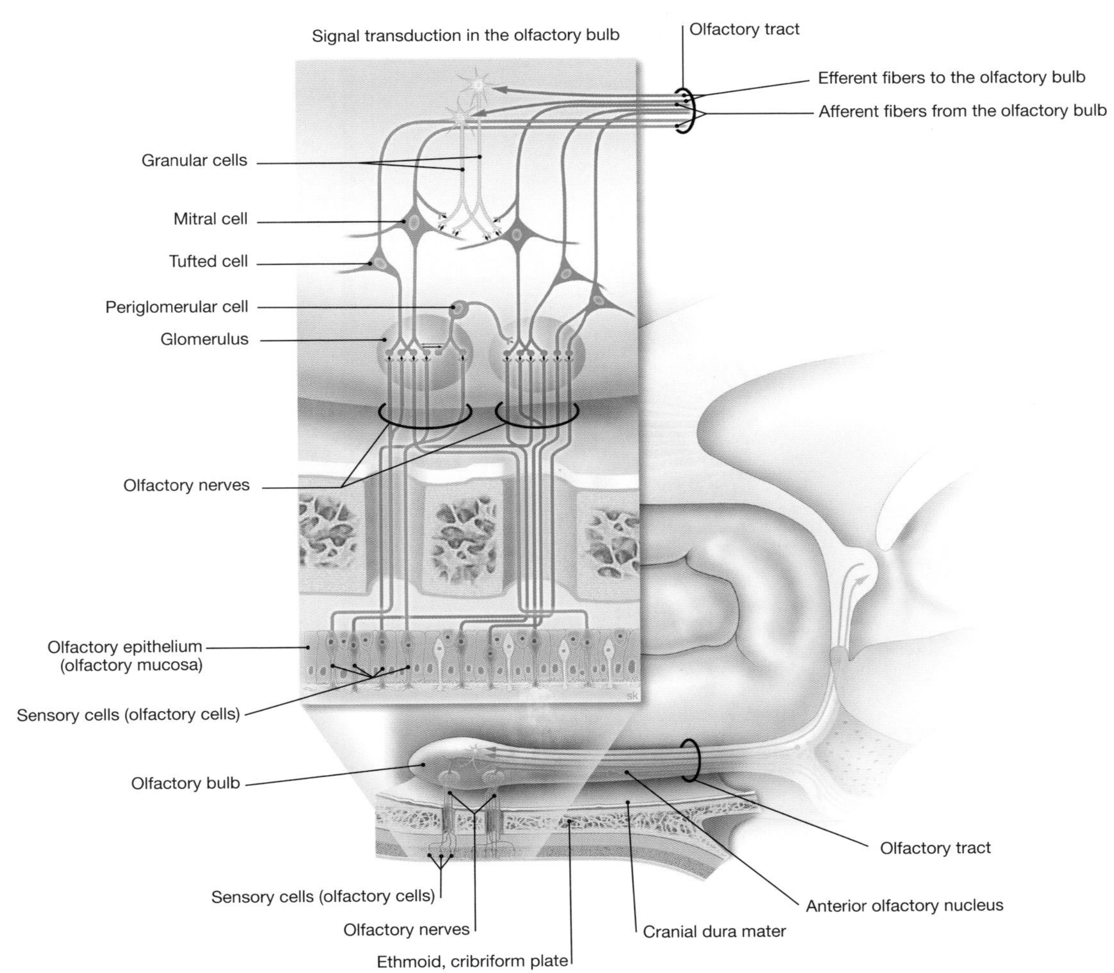
Signal transduction in the olfactory bulb
Olfactory tract
Efferent fibers to the olfactory bulb
Afferent fibers from the olfactory bulb
Granular cells
Mitral cell
Tufted cell
Periglomerular cell
Glomerulus
Olfactory nerves
Olfactory epithelium
(olfactory mucosa)
Sensory cells (olfactory cells)
Olfactory bulb
Olfactory tract
Anterior olfactory nucleus
Sensory cells (olfactory cells)
Olfactory nerves
Cranial dura mater
Ethmoid, cribriform plate

**Fig. 12.139 Scheme of the projections and synaptic connections of the olfactory nerves;** view from the left side.
In each olfactory bulb, all olfactory nerves converge onto approximately 1000 **glomeruli** (in the figure two glomeruli are demonstrated as an example) which collectively form the olfactory tract. Multiple synapses within the glomeruli finally converge on the **mitral cells** (2$^{nd}$ neuron). The axons of all neurons possessing the identical odorant receptor reach the glomerulus that is specific for each of the approximately 1000 different olfactory receptors. Mitral cells of the olfactory bulb project to different areas at the cranial base and the temporal lobe (→ Fig. 12.138). Feedback mechanisms increase the discrimination of odorant stimuli and involve granular cells that connect back with different mitral cells.

### Clinical Remarks

Viral infections, chronic sinusitis, obstruction of the nasal passage to the olfactory mucosa, e.g. due to allergy, side effects of medication, brain tumor or head trauma with injury to the olfactory nerves during their passage through the cribriform plate, can result in **hyposmia** (decreased ability to perceive odors) or **anosmia** (inability to perceive odors).

## Optic nerve [II]

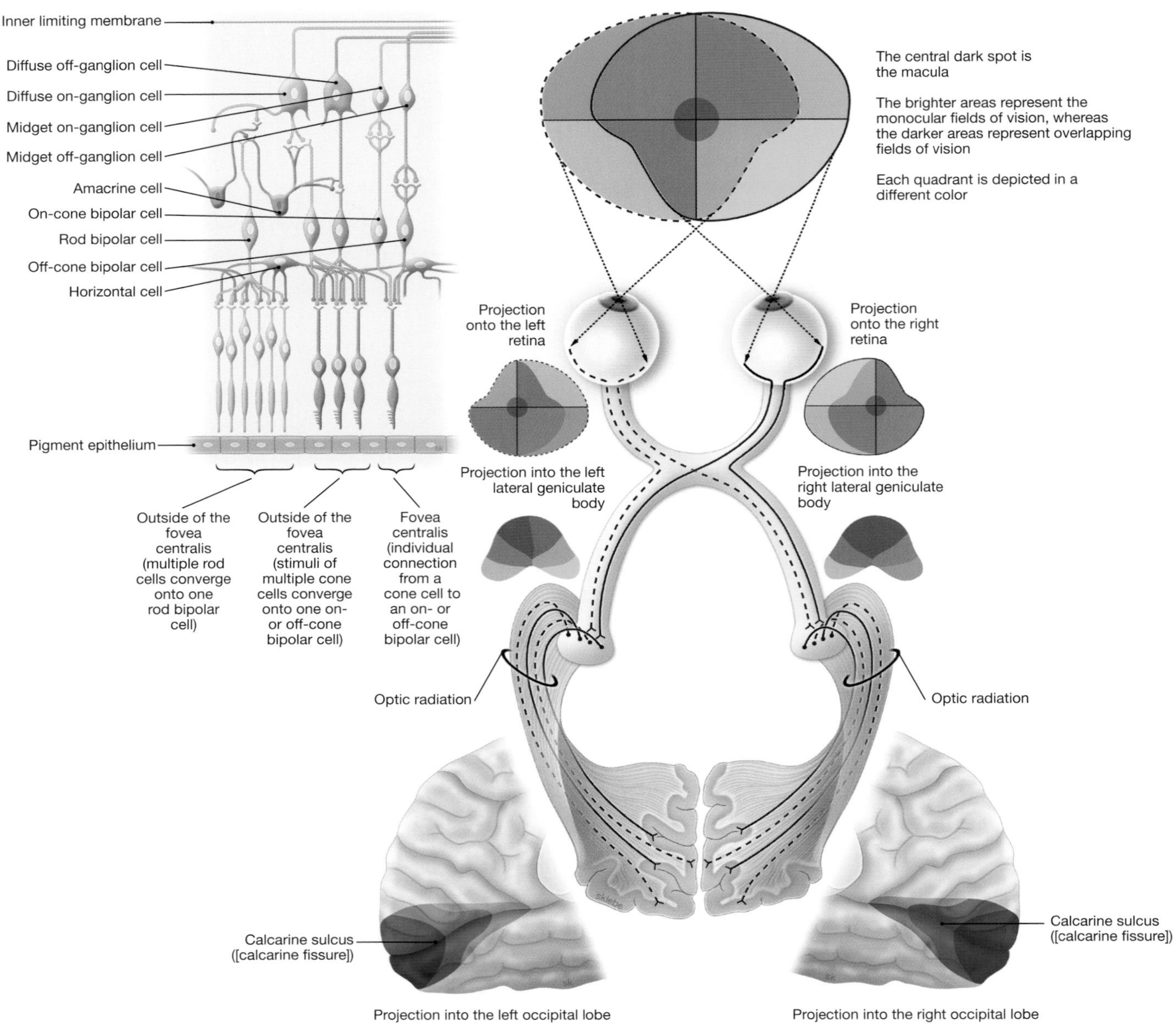

Inner limiting membrane
Diffuse off-ganglion cell
Diffuse on-ganglion cell
Midget on-ganglion cell
Midget off-ganglion cell
Amacrine cell
On-cone bipolar cell
Rod bipolar cell
Off-cone bipolar cell
Horizontal cell
Pigment epithelium
Outside of the fovea centralis (multiple rod cells converge onto one rod bipolar cell)
Outside of the fovea centralis (stimuli of multiple cone cells converge onto one on- or off-cone bipolar cell)
Fovea centralis (individual connection from a cone cell to an on- or off-cone bipolar cell)
The central dark spot is the macula
The brighter areas represent the monocular fields of vision, whereas the darker areas represent overlapping fields of vision
Each quadrant is depicted in a different color
Projection onto the left retina
Projection onto the right retina
Projection into the left lateral geniculate body
Projection into the right lateral geniculate body
Optic radiation
Optic radiation
Calcarine sulcus ([calcarine fissure])
Calcarine sulcus ([calcarine fissure])
Projection into the left occipital lobe
Projection into the right occipital lobe


**Fig. 12.140 Neuronal network in the retina and the central visual tract;** strongly simplified schematic representation.
**Cone cells** (1st neuron) direct the information to **cone bipolar cells** (2nd neuron) and **ganglion cells** (3rd neuron). Horizontal and amacrine cells modify the processing of information. The axons of the ganglion cells form the optic nerve [II]. The above-mentioned network of connections represented by an intraretinal chain of three neurons only applies to cone cells (for rod cells → Fig. 12.141 and textbooks of histology). For the central visual tract → pp. 131 and 132.

→ T 58b

## Optic nerve [II]

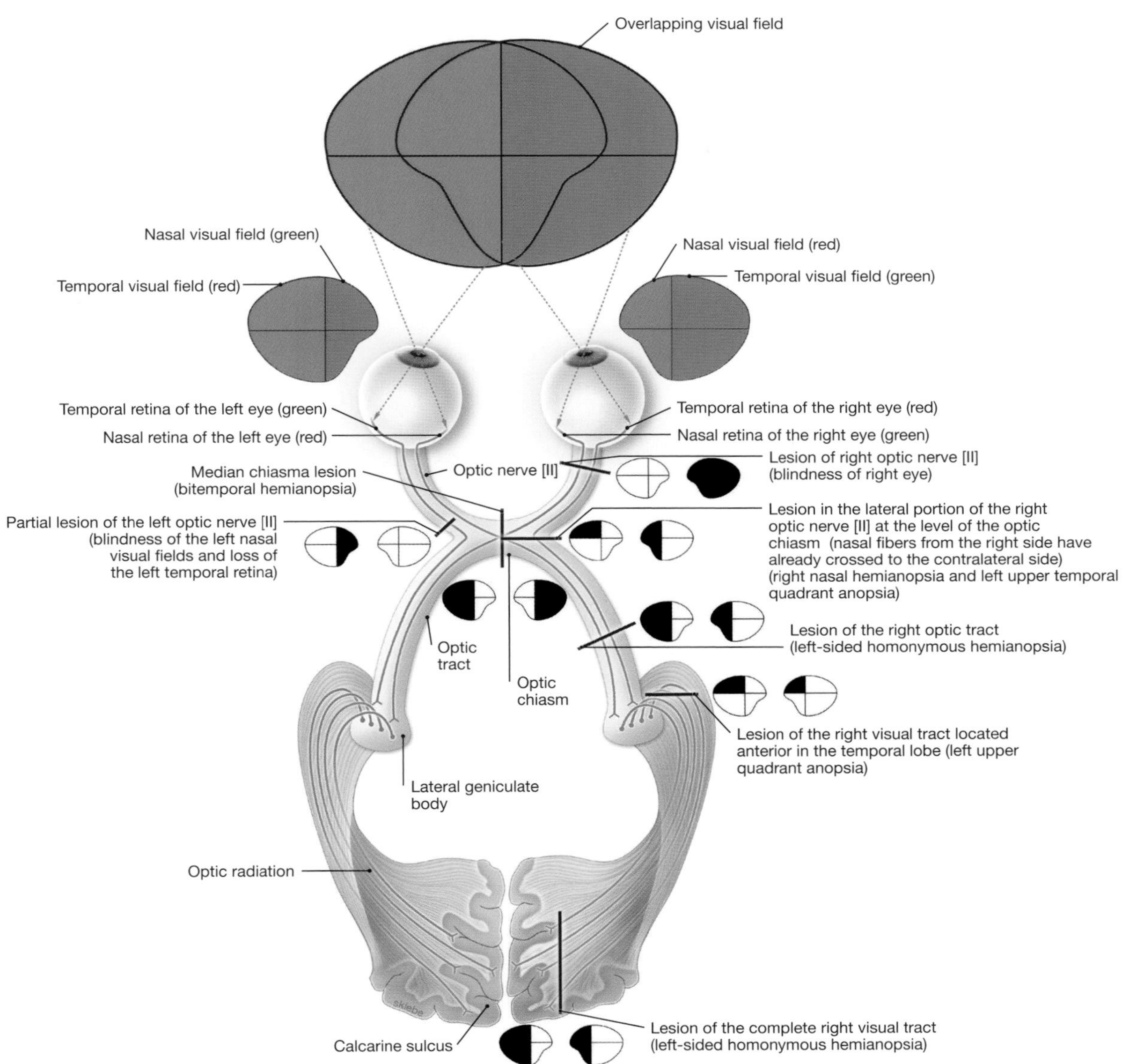
Overlapping visual field
Nasal visual field (green)
Temporal visual field (red)
Nasal visual field (red)
Temporal visual field (green)
Temporal retina of the left eye (green)
Nasal retina of the left eye (red)
Temporal retina of the right eye (red)
Nasal retina of the right eye (green)
Median chiasma lesion (bitemporal hemianopsia)
Optic nerve [II]
Lesion of right optic nerve [II] (blindness of right eye)
Partial lesion of the left optic nerve [II] (blindness of the left nasal visual fields and loss of the left temporal retina)
Lesion in the lateral portion of the right optic nerve [II] at the level of the optic chiasm (nasal fibers from the right side have already crossed to the contralateral side) (right nasal hemianopsia and left upper temporal quadrant anopsia)
Optic tract
Lesion of the right optic tract (left-sided homonymous hemianopsia)
Optic chiasm
Lesion of the right visual tract located anterior in the temporal lobe (left upper quadrant anopsia)
Lateral geniculate body
Optic radiation
Calcarine sulcus
Lesion of the complete right visual tract (left-sided homonymous hemianopsia)

**Fig. 12.141 Optic nerve [II] and visual tract.** [23]
The visual tract starts at the retina which contains the first three projection neurons and interneurons (horizontal cells, amacrine cells) (→ Fig. 12.140).
Up to 40 **rod cells** transmit their signals to a single **rod bipolar cell.** From here, the information is transmitted indirectly through amacrine cells (depending on the literature, today there are 20 to 50 different types described) to **ganglion cells.** Thus, an intraretinal chain of four neurons exists for the rod cells. The axons of the ganglion cells run in the optic nerve [II] to the **optic chiasm,** where the fibers of the nasal part of the retina cross to the opposite side (red). The fibers of the temporal part do not cross (green).
Directly following the optic chiasm is the optic tract which contains the fibers with visual information of the contralateral visual field. The major part of these fibers (lateral root) synapse in the lateral geniculate body (CGL). Some fibers (medial root) divert before reaching the CGL and project into the pretectal area, the superior colliculus, and into the hypothalamus. The **GRATIOLET's optic radiation** originates from the lateral geniculate body and projects into the region around the calcarine sulcus to the areas 17 and 18 of the cerebral cortex (striate area).

## Clinical Remarks

- Lesions of the optic nerve [II] anterior to the optic chiasm, e.g. caused by traumatic head and/or brain injury, result in blindness of the affected eye (→ Fig. 12.141).
- Lateral lesions of the optic nerve [II] at the level of the optic chiasm (right nasal fibers have already crossed to the contralateral side), e.g. caused by a tumor, result in a right nasal **hemianopsia** and **quadrant anopsia** of the left upper temporal quadrant (→ Fig. 12.141).
- Median lesions to the optic chiasm, mostly caused by pituitary tumors, result in a bitemporal hemianopsia (→ Fig. 12.141).
- Lesions to the optic tract on the right side (as exemplified in the figure), e.g. caused by a bleeding, result in left-sided homonymous hemianopsia (→ Fig. 12.141).
- Lesions of the anterior portion of the optic radiation located in the temporal lobe on the right side (as exemplified in the figure), e.g. due to ischemia, cause anopsia of the left-sided upper quadrants (→ Fig. 12.141).
- Lesions to the entire right optic radiation (as exemplified in the figure), e.g. caused by a mass bleeding, result in left-sided homonymous hemianopsia (→ Fig. 12.141).

## Oculomotor nerve [III], trochlear nerve [IV], abducent nerve [VI]

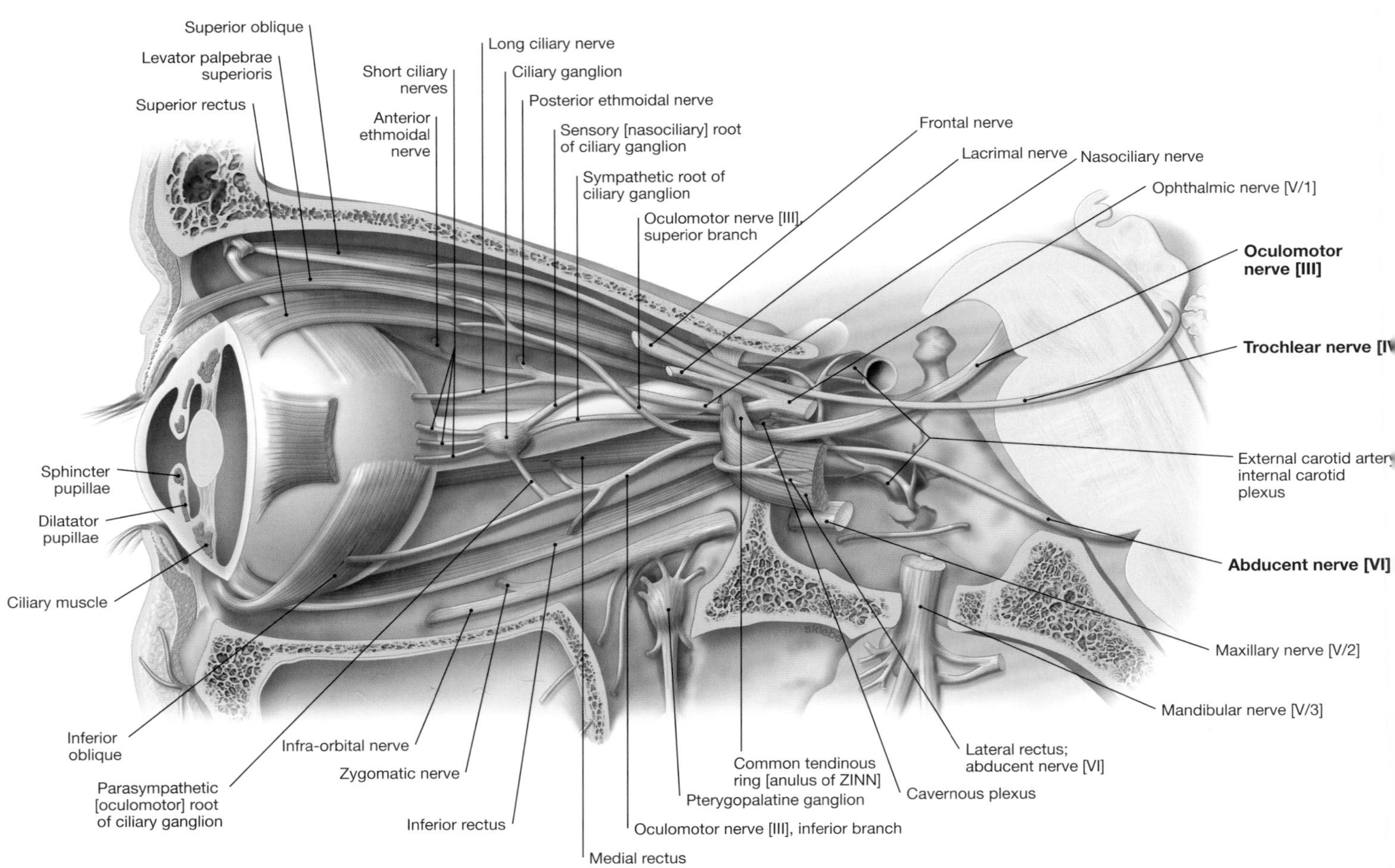
Superior oblique
Levator palpebrae superioris
Superior rectus
Short ciliary nerves
Anterior ethmoidal nerve
Long ciliary nerve
Ciliary ganglion
Posterior ethmoidal nerve
Sensory [nasociliary] root of ciliary ganglion
Sympathetic root of ciliary ganglion
Oculomotor nerve [III], superior branch
Frontal nerve
Lacrimal nerve
Nasociliary nerve
Ophthalmic nerve [V/1]
Oculomotor nerve [III]
Trochlear nerve [IV]
External carotid artery; internal carotid plexus
Abducent nerve [VI]
Maxillary nerve [V/2]
Mandibular nerve [V/3]
Sphincter pupillae
Dilatator pupillae
Ciliary muscle
Inferior oblique
Parasympathetic [oculomotor] root of ciliary ganglion
Infra-orbital nerve
Zygomatic nerve
Inferior rectus
Medial rectus
Oculomotor nerve [III], inferior branch
Pterygopalatine ganglion
Common tendinous ring [anulus of ZINN]
Cavernous plexus
Lateral rectus; abducent nerve [VI]

**Fig. 12.142 Oculomotor nerve [III], trochlear nerve [IV] and abducent nerve [VI], left side;** lateral view; orbit opened, orbital fat body removed, the lateral rectus was sectioned close to its insertion and deflected.
The oculomotor nerve [III] innervates the extra-ocular muscles with the exception of the superior oblique (trochlear nerve [IV]) and the lateral rectus (abducent nerve [VI]). The parasympathetic part of the cranial nerve III innervates the sphincter pupillae and the ciliary muscle (two intra-ocular muscles).

→ T 58c, d, f

# Oculomotor nerve [III], trochlear nerve [IV], abducent nerve [VI]

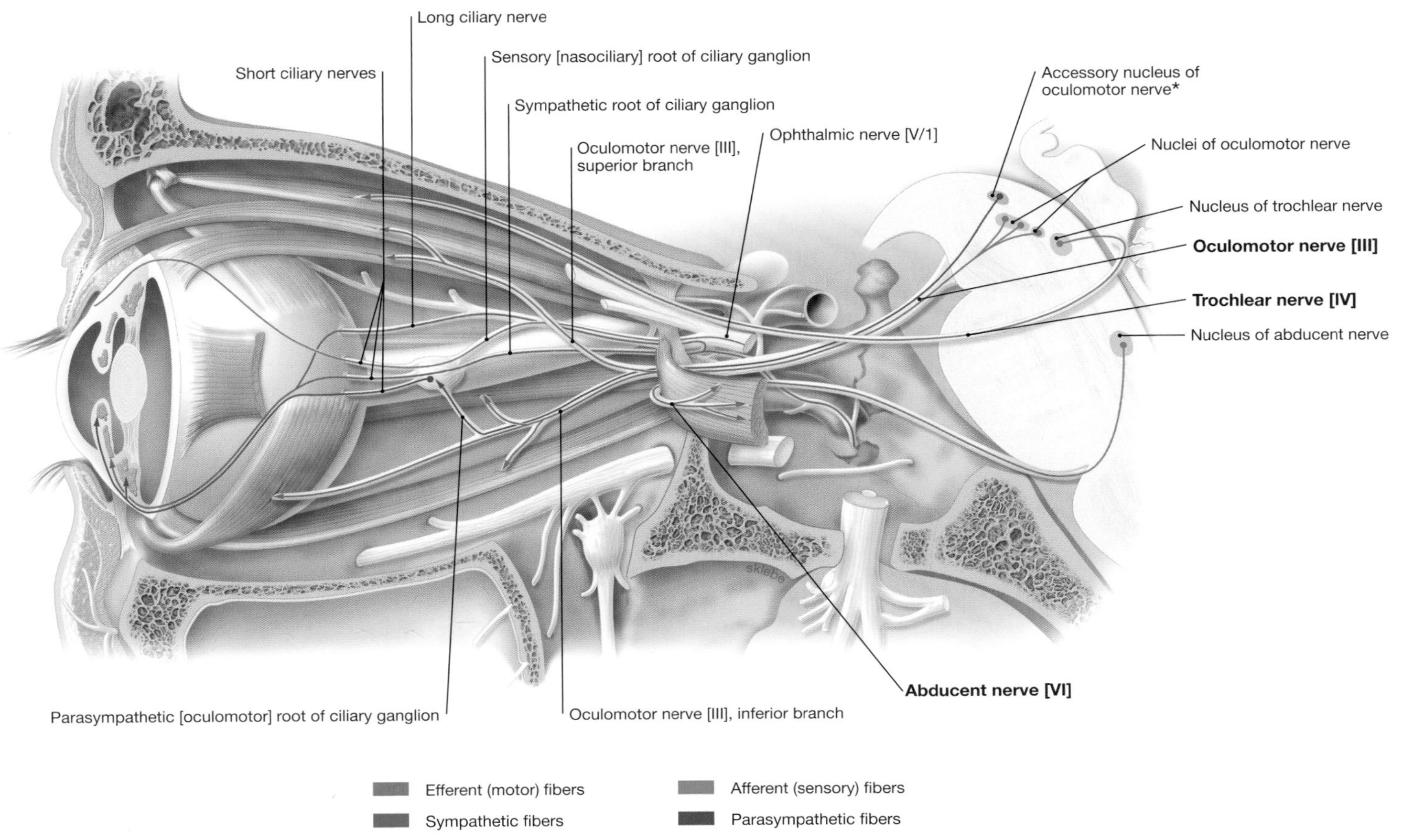
Long ciliary nerve
Sensory [nasociliary] root of ciliary ganglion
Short ciliary nerves
Sympathetic root of ciliary ganglion
Oculomotor nerve [III], superior branch
Ophthalmic nerve [V/1]
Accessory nucleus of oculomotor nerve*
Nuclei of oculomotor nerve
Nucleus of trochlear nerve
Oculomotor nerve [III]
Trochlear nerve [IV]
Nucleus of abducent nerve
Abducent nerve [VI]
Parasympathetic [oculomotor] root of ciliary ganglion
Oculomotor nerve [III], inferior branch
Efferent (motor) fibers
Sympathetic fibers
Afferent (sensory) fibers
Parasympathetic fibers

**Fig. 12.143 Fiber qualities of the oculomotor nerve [III], trochlear nerve [IV] and abducent nerve [VI], left side;** lateral view.
The **oculomotor nerve [III]** contains motor fibers (GSE) derived from the nucleus of oculomotor nerve for the major part of extra-ocular muscles. In the orbit, the nerve divides into a superior branch to innervate the superior rectus and levator palpebrae superioris and an inferior branch for the innervation of the medial rectus, inferior rectus, and inferior oblique. The accessory nucleus of oculomotor nerve (EDINGER-WESTPHAL nucleus) contributes parasympathetic fibers (GVE) which reach the ciliary ganglion through the inferior root as well as a parasympathic root (oculomotoria). In the ciliary ganglion, preganglionic parasympathetic fibers synapse onto postganglionic neurons. The postganglionic fibers project alongside the short ciliary nerves to the eyeball, traverse its wall, and reach the intra-ocular sphincter pupillae and ciliary muscle.
The **trochlear nerve [IV]** contains motor fibers (GSE) for the superior oblique from the nucleus of trochlear nerve in the brainstem.
The **abducent nerve [VI]** contains motor fibers (GSE) from the nucleus of abducent nerve for the lateral rectus.

* EDINGER-WESTPHAL nucleus

## Clinical Remarks

**Lesions of individual cranial nerves that innervate extra-ocular muscles** lead to the paralysis of the corresponding extra-ocular muscles with resulting deviations of the eyeballs. The direction and extent of this deviation of the eye depends on the stronger action of the still intact extra-orbital muscles (and corresponding intact cranial nerve[s]) as opposed to the paralysed muscle(s). For more details → p. 113.
A complete **oculomotor nerve paresis** results in ptosis, mydriasis, the inability to accommodate, and a bulbus pointing down and outwards (down and out).
An **abducent nerve paresis** is particularly frequent due to the long extradural course of the abducent nerve [VI] and its passage through the cavernous sinus. When the patient is asked to move the affected eye to the temporal side, the eyeball remains pointing straight ahead since the lateral rectus is paralyzed.

## Trigeminal nerve [V]

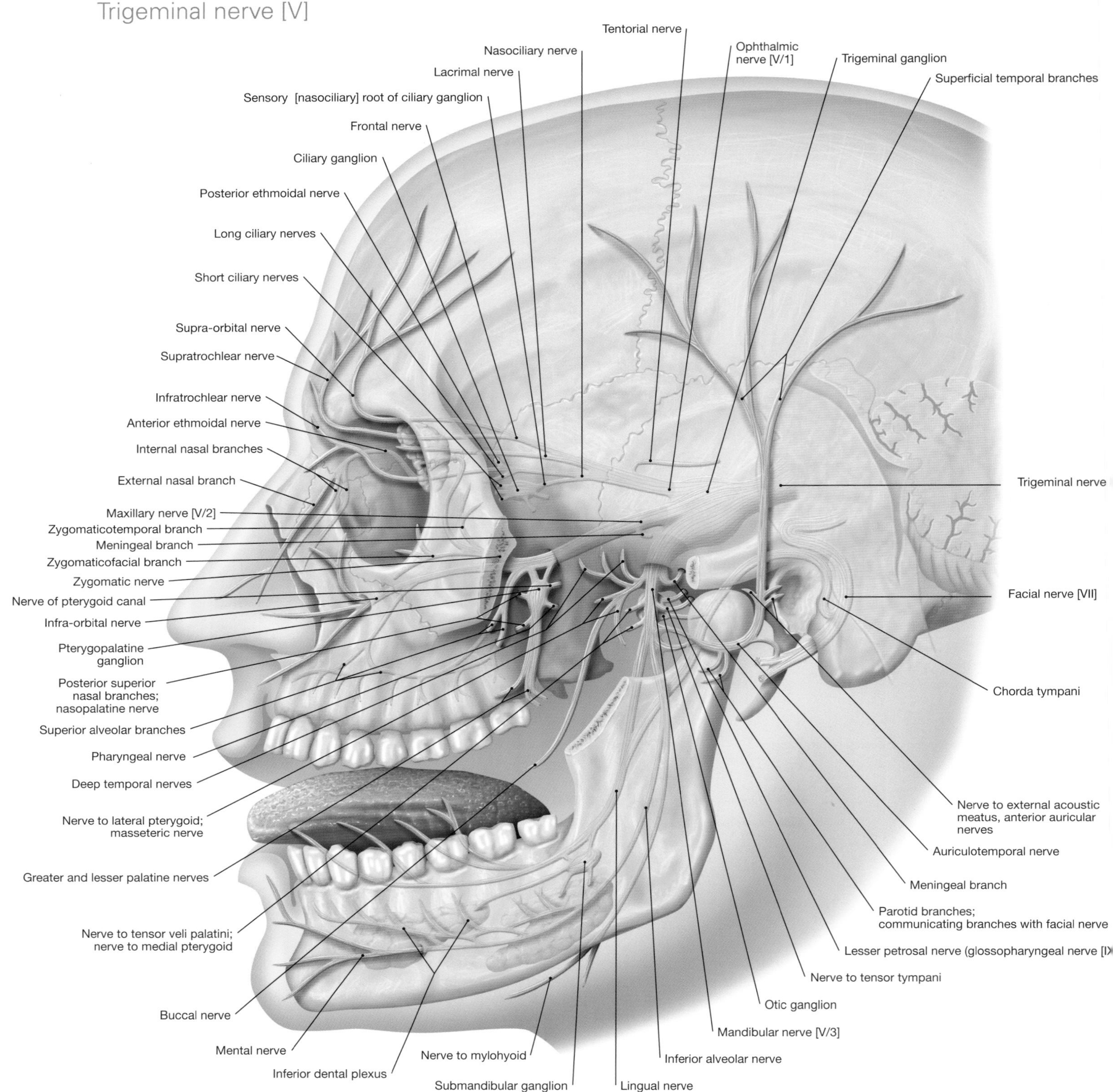
Tentorial nerve
Nasociliary nerve
Ophthalmic nerve [V/1]
Trigeminal ganglion
Lacrimal nerve
Superficial temporal branches
Sensory [nasociliary] root of ciliary ganglion
Frontal nerve
Ciliary ganglion
Posterior ethmoidal nerve
Long ciliary nerves
Short ciliary nerves
Supra-orbital nerve
Supratrochlear nerve
Infratrochlear nerve
Anterior ethmoidal nerve
Internal nasal branches
External nasal branch
Trigeminal nerve
Maxillary nerve [V/2]
Zygomaticotemporal branch
Meningeal branch
Zygomaticofacial branch
Zygomatic nerve
Facial nerve [VII]
Nerve of pterygoid canal
Infra-orbital nerve
Pterygopalatine ganglion
Posterior superior nasal branches; nasopalatine nerve
Chorda tympani
Superior alveolar branches
Pharyngeal nerve
Deep temporal nerves
Nerve to lateral pterygoid; masseteric nerve
Nerve to external acoustic meatus, anterior auricular nerves
Auriculotemporal nerve
Greater and lesser palatine nerves
Meningeal branch
Parotid branches; communicating branches with facial nerve
Nerve to tensor veli palatini; nerve to medial pterygoid
Lesser petrosal nerve (glossopharyngeal nerve [IX
Nerve to tensor tympani
Otic ganglion
Buccal nerve
Mandibular nerve [V/3]
Mental nerve
Nerve to mylohyoid
Inferior alveolar nerve
Inferior dental plexus
Submandibular ganglion
Lingual nerve

**Fig. 12.144 Trigeminal nerve [V], left side;** lateral view.
The trigeminal nerve [V] is the nerve of the first pharyngeal arch and divides into the three main branches: ophthalmic nerve [V/1] (bright green), maxillary nerve [V/2] (orange), and mandibular nerve [V/3] (turquoise). It mainly carries general somato-afferent (GSA) fibers, some special viscero-efferent (SVE) fibers, and motor fibers (V/3).
The **ophthalmic nerve [V/1]** innervates the eye (including cornea and conjunctiva), the skin of the upper eyelid, forehead, back of the nose, the nasal and paranasal mucosa. Parasympathetic fibers innervate the lacrimal gland and associate with the peripheral course of the ophthalmic nerve [V/1].
The **maxillary nerve [V/2]** innervates the skin of the anterior temporal region and the upper cheek as well as the skin below the eye. In addition, this nerve provides sensory fibers to the palate, the teeth of the upper jaw, the gingiva, and the mucosa of the maxillary sinus.
The **mandibular nerve [V/3]** innervates the masticatory muscles, two muscles at the floor of the mouth (mylohyoid and anterior belly of the digastric), as well as the tensor veli palatini and tensor tympani. It also contributes sensory branches to the skin of the posterior temporal region, the cheek, and the chin, and innervates the teeth and gingiva of the lower jaw. Parasympathetic fibers for the large salivary glands as well as taste fibers for the tongue associate with branches of the mandibular nerve [V/3]. The latter also provides sensory fibers for the anterior two-thirds of the tongue.

→ T 58e

## Trigeminal nerve [V]

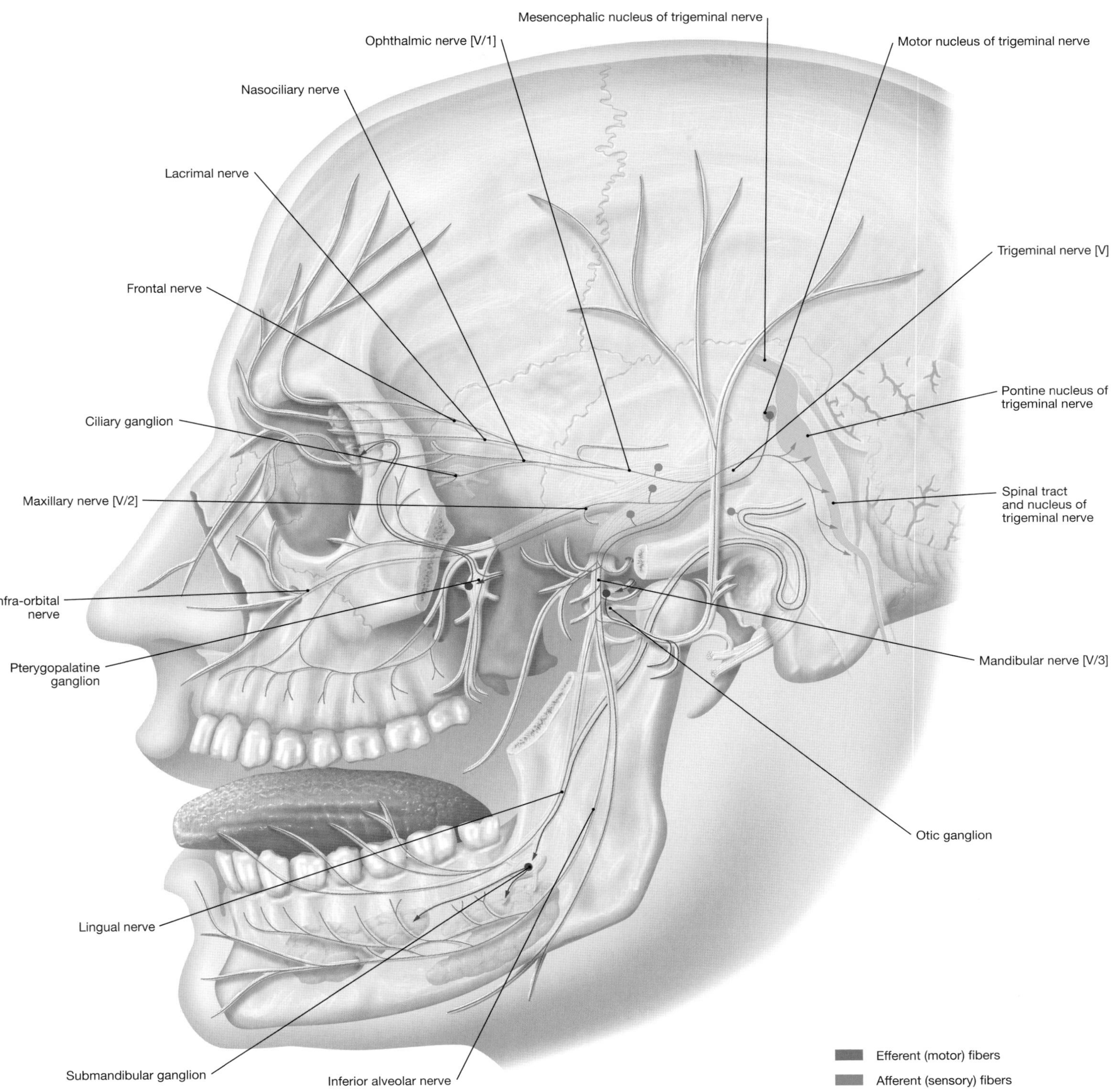

Mesencephalic nucleus of trigeminal nerve
Ophthalmic nerve [V/1]
Motor nucleus of trigeminal nerve
Nasociliary nerve
Lacrimal nerve
Trigeminal nerve [V]
Frontal nerve
Pontine nucleus of trigeminal nerve
Ciliary ganglion
Spinal tract and nucleus of trigeminal nerve
Maxillary nerve [V/2]
Infra-orbital nerve
Pterygopalatine ganglion
Mandibular nerve [V/3]
Otic ganglion
Lingual nerve
Submandibular ganglion
Inferior alveolar nerve
Efferent (motor) fibers
Afferent (sensory) fibers
Parasympathetic fibers


**Fig. 12.145 Fiber qualities of the trigeminal nerve [V], left side;** lateral view.

**Nuclei of origin** and **terminal nuclei** of the trigeminal nerve [V] are the mesencephalic nucleus of trigeminal nerve (somato-sensory), the pontine (principal sensory) nucleus of trigeminal nerve (somato-sensory), the spinal nucleus of trigeminal nerve (general somato-afferent, GSA), and the motor nucleus of trigeminal nerve (specific viscero-efferent, SVE).

The trigeminal nerve [V] consists of a **sensory root** (major portion) and a **motor root** (minor portion). After exiting the pons, the trigeminal nerve passes over the clivus and reaches the trigeminal ganglion (semilunar ganglion, clinical term: GASSERIAN ganglion, contains pseudounipolar neurons which provide the pontine and spinal nuclei of trigeminal nerve with protopathic and epicritic sensory stimuli) and divides into its three main branches ophthalmic [V/1], maxillary [V/2], and mandibular [V/3] nerves.

## Trigeminal nerve [V]

| Branches of the Ophthalmic Nerve [V/1] (exclusively somato-efferent) | | |
|---|---|---|
| **Main Branch** | **Minor Branches** | **Innervation Area** |
| Recurrent meningeal branch [tentorial branch] | | Parts of the meninges |
| Frontal nerve | Supra-orbital nerve | Skin of forehead and mucosa of the frontal sinus |
| | Supratrochlear nerve | Skin and conjunctiva at the nasal corner of the eye |
| Lacrimal nerve | | Lacrimal gland (postganglionic parasympathetic fibers from the zygomatic nerve for secretory innervation associate with the lacrimal nerve), skin and connective tissue of the nasal corner of the eye |
| Nasociliary nerve | (→Table below) | Nasal sinuses, anterior part of the nasal cavity and iris, ciliary body, cornea of the eye (→Table below) |

| Branches of the Nasociliary Nerve (from V/1) [14] | | |
|---|---|---|
| **Branch** | **Course** | **Innervation Area** |
| Sensory root of ciliary ganglion [communicating branch with ciliary ganglion] | Contributes the sensory component for the ciliary ganglion which generates the short ciliary nerves | Eyeball and its conjunctiva (jointly with the long ciliary nerves) |
| Long ciliary nerves | Associate with the optic nerve and course with the short ciliary nerves from the ciliary ganglion to the eyeball; they also contain sympathetic fibers from the carotid plexus | Eyeball and its conjunctiva; the sympathetic fibers innervate the dilatator pupillae |
| Posterior ethmoidal nerve | Passes through the identically named foramen to reach the posterior ethmoidal cells and the sphenoidal sinus | Mucosa of the posterior ethmoidal cells and the sphenoidal sinus |
| Anterior ethmoidal nerve | Passes through the identically named foramen back into the anterior cranial fossa, courses through the cribriform plate into the nasal cavity; ends with external nasal branches in the skin of the dorsum of the nose | Mucosa of the anterior nasal cavity and the anterior ethmoidal cells, skin of the dorsum of the nose |
| Infratrochlear nerve | Courses to the nasal corner of the eye inferior to the trochlea | Skin of the nasal corner of the eye |

| Branches of the Maxillary Nerve [V/2] (exclusively somato-afferent) | | |
|---|---|---|
| **Main Branch** | **Minor Branches** | **Innervation Area** |
| Meningeal branch | | Parts of the meninges |
| Zygomatic nerve | Zygomaticotemporal branch | Skin of the temporal region |
| | Zygomaticofacial branch | Skin of the upper cheek region; for the secretory innervation of the lacrimal gland, postganglionic parasympathetic fibers associate with the zygomatic nerve which contributes to the lacrimal nerve |
| Ganglionic branches for the pterygopalatine ganglion | (→ Table, at top of p. 305) | Contribute sensory fibers for the pterygopalatine ganglion, innervation of palate and nose (→ Table at top of p. 305), sympathetic and parasympathetic fibers for the nasal and palatine glands (special viscero-efferent) and taste fibers |
| Infra-orbital nerve | Superior alveolar nerves with posterior, medial and anterior alveolar branches | Mucosa of the maxillary sinus, teeth of the upper jaw and corresponding gingiva |
| | | Skin and conjunctiva of the lower eyelid, lateral skin area of the nasal wings, skin of upper lip and lateral cheek region between lower eyelid and upper lip |

## Trigeminal nerve [V]

| Branches of the Ganglionary Branches to the Pterygopalatine Ganglion (from V/2) [14] | | |
|---|---|---|
| **Branch** | **Course** | **Innervation Area** |
| Greater palatine nerve | Passes across the greater palatine canal and through the greater palatine foramen | Mucosa of the hard palate, palatine glands, palatine taste buds |
| Lesser palatine nerves | Exit the greater palatine canal through the lesser palatine foramina | Mucosa of the soft palate, palatine tonsil, palatine glands, palatine taste buds |
| Superior, lateral, and medial posterior nasal branches | Pass through the sphenopalatine foramen into the nasal cavity and branch off the nasopalatine nerve which reaches the hard palate through the incisive canal | Mucosa of the nasal conchae, nasal septum, mucosa of the anterior part of the hard palate, upper incisors and gingiva, nasal glands |

| Branches of the Mandibular Nerve [V/3] (somato-afferent and viscero-efferent) | | |
|---|---|---|
| **Main Branch** | **Minor Branches** | **Innervation Area** |
| Meningeal branch | | Parts of the meninges |
| Masseteric nerve | | Masseter |
| Deep temporal nerves | | Temporalis |
| Nerve to lateral pterygoid | | Lateral pterygoid |
| Nerve to medial pterygoid | | Medial pterygoid |
| Nerve to tensor veli palatini | | Tensor veli palatini |
| Nerve to tensor tympani | | Tensor tympani |
| Buccal nerve | | Skin and mucosa of the cheek and gingiva of the lower jaw |
| Auriculotemporal nerve | Parotid branches | Associated postganglionic parasympathetic fibers from the otic ganglion innervate the parotid gland |
| | Communicating branches with facial nerve | Associated postganglionic parasympathetic fibers from the otic ganglion innervate the parotid gland |
| | Nerve to external acoustic meatus | External acoustic meatus, tympanic membrane |
| | Anterior auricular nerves | Skin anterior to the auricle |
| | Superficial temporal nerves | Skin of the posterior temporal region |
| Lingual nerve | Branches to isthmus fauces | Mucosa of the soft palate |
| | Sublingual nerve | Mucosa of the floor of the mouth |
| | | Sensory innervation of the anterior two-thirds of the tongue, taste fibers of the anterior two-thirds of the tongue, association of preganglionic parasympathetic fibers derived from the chorda tympani for the submandibular ganglion |
| Inferior alveolar nerve | | Teeth and gingiva of the lower jaw |
| | Nerve to mylohyoid | Mylohyoid and anterior belly of the digastric |
| | Mental nerve | Skin of the chin |

## Trigeminal nerve [V]

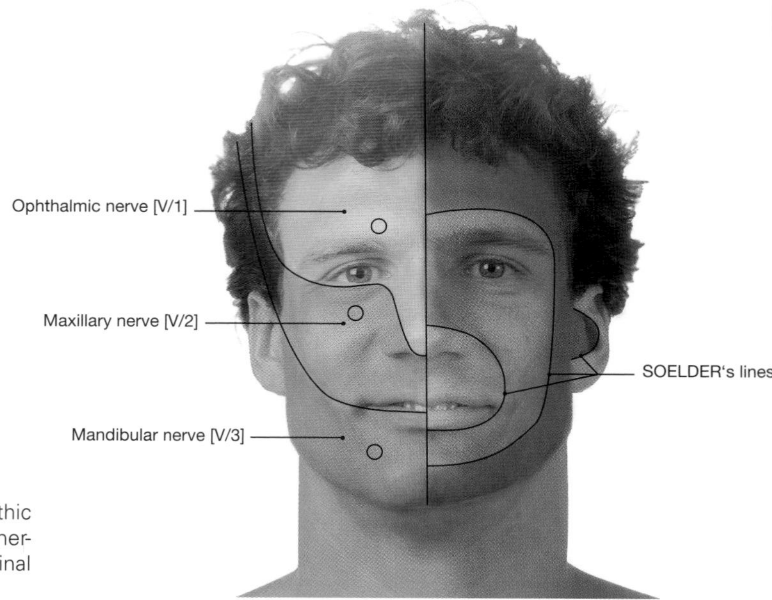
Ophthalmic nerve [V/1]
Maxillary nerve [V/2]
Mandibular nerve [V/3]
SOELDER's lines

**Fig. 12.146 Innervation areas of the facial skin, exit points for nerves, and protopathic sensibility.**
On the left side of the face, the somatotopic order of the protopathic sensibility is demonstrated. The right side of the face shows the innervation areas and exit points for the three branches of the trigeminal nerve.

### Clinical Remarks

Often **lesions of the trigeminal nerve [V]** are associated with deficiencies in blood supply, with selective or partial nuclear areas rather than the complete trigeminal nerve [V] being affected. These lesions can for example manifest as an ipsilateral palsy of the masticatory muscles or a selective loss of the epicritic sensory quality. The afferent fibers with protopathic sensibility reach the spinal nucleus of trigeminal nerve in a somatotopic order (→ Fig. 12.146). A defined segment of the spinal nucleus of trigeminal nerve innervates a concentric area of the facial skin. To assess the extent of a nuclear lesion, one can test the protopathic sensibility along the concentric **SOELDER's lines.**

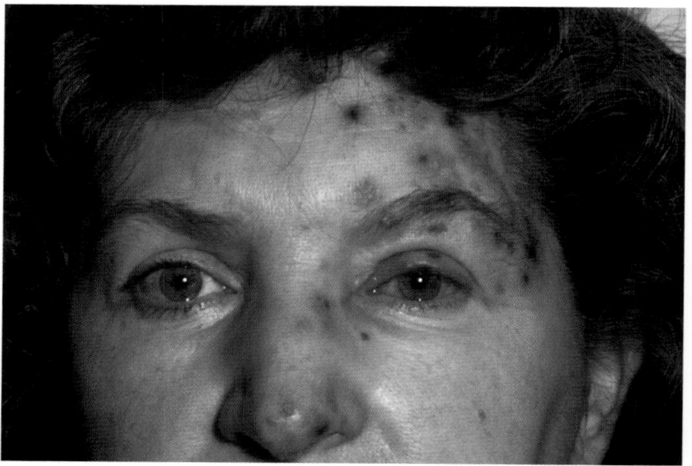

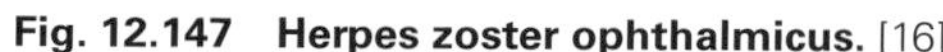

**Fig. 12.147 Herpes zoster ophthalmicus.** [16]
Patient with (herpes) zoster ophthalmicus (skin in the innervation area of the first trigeminal branch is affected by the infection with varicella zoster virus, facial herpes zoster). The involvement of the surface epithelium of the eye (cornea and conjunctiva) is particularly dangerous (risk of blindness) and painful. The redness of the conjunctiva and the narrowing of the eyelids are clearly visible.

### Clinical Remarks

Loss of sensibility in the innervation area of a trigeminal branch suggests a **peripheral lesion** of the nerve. For the ophthalmic nerve [V/1] and the maxillary nerve [V/2] potential causes are a cavernous sinus thrombosis (→ p. 223), tumors of the cranial base, and skull fractures. Sensory deficiencies in the region of the mandible or paralysis of masticatory muscles often have an iatrogenic cause (dental work).
The frequent and still not fully understood **trigeminal neuralgia** presents with hypersensitivity of the trigeminal nerve [V] and paroxysmal episodes of intense, stabbing pain in the sensory innervation area of the affected trigeminal branch. Even light touch of the area of the corresponding exit point of the branch (→ Fig. 12.146) can trigger pain.
Infections of the first trigeminal branch by varicella zoster virus (→ Fig. 12.147) can cause a post-zoster neuralgia of the ophthalmic nerve [V/1], known as **herpes zoster ophthalmicus.**

## Facial nerve [VII]

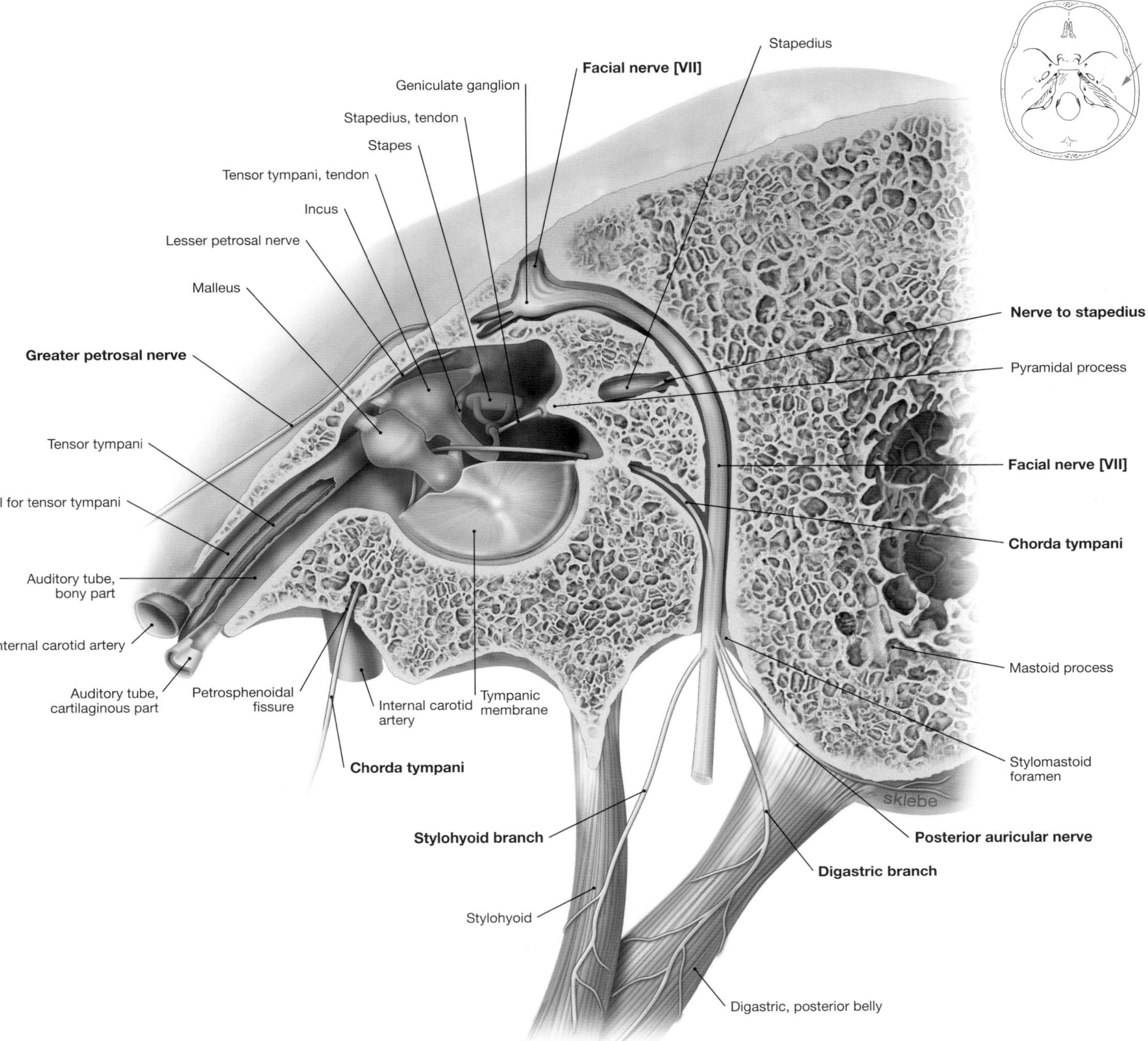
Stapedius
Facial nerve [VII]
Geniculate ganglion
Stapedius, tendon
Stapes
Tensor tympani, tendon
Incus
Lesser petrosal nerve
Malleus
Greater petrosal nerve
Tensor tympani
anal for tensor tympani
Auditory tube, bony part
Internal carotid artery
Auditory tube, cartilaginous part
Petrosphenoidal fissure
Internal carotid artery
Tympanic membrane
Chorda tympani
Nerve to stapedius
Pyramidal process
Facial nerve [VII]
Chorda tympani
Mastoid process
Stylomastoid foramen
Posterior auricular nerve
Digastric branch
Stylohyoid branch
Stylohyoid
Digastric, posterior belly
sklebe

**Fig. 12.148 Course of the facial nerve [VII];** vertical section through the facial canal; view from the left side.
Approximately 1 cm after the facial nerve [VII] enters the petrosal part of the temporal bone through the internal acoustic pore (not shown), the nerve makes a sharp bend, known as the external genu of the facial nerve. Here, the geniculate ganglion is located. The main stem of the facial nerve runs within a bony canal towards the stylomastoid foramen. Along its way through the petrous bone, the facial nerve [VII] releases the greater petrosal nerve, nerve to stapedius, and the chorda tympani (→ Table, p. 310).

→ T 58g

## Clinical Remarks

The close topographic relationship between the facial canal and the tympanic cavity puts the facial nerve [VII] at risk during petrous bone fractures, middle ear and mastoid infections, and surgical interventions involving the middle and inner ear. The symptoms depend on the location of the lesion. **Lesions located close to or anterior to the geniculate ganglion** result in paralysis of all mimic muscles. Furthermore, the stapedius muscle is paralysed (hyperacusis) and gustatory impairment, diminished tear production as well as reduced nasal and salivary secretion occur.
If the **lesion locates below the branching point of the nerve to stapedius,** paralysis of the mimic muscles occurs and the chorda tympani fibers for taste and glandular secretion are affected. Isolated injury to the chorda tympani is possible during middle ear infections (→ p. 147) or surgical procedures conducted in the middle and inner ear because of its unprotected course between the malleus and incus in the tympanic cavity of the middle ear.
The biggest problem in patients with peripheral facial palsy is **lagophthalmos** (due to the paralysis of the orbicularis oculi, the eye cannot be closed properly; → Fig. 12.151c) causing the cornea to dry out (blindness due to lack of blinking and reduced production of lacrimal fluid).

## Facial nerve [VII]

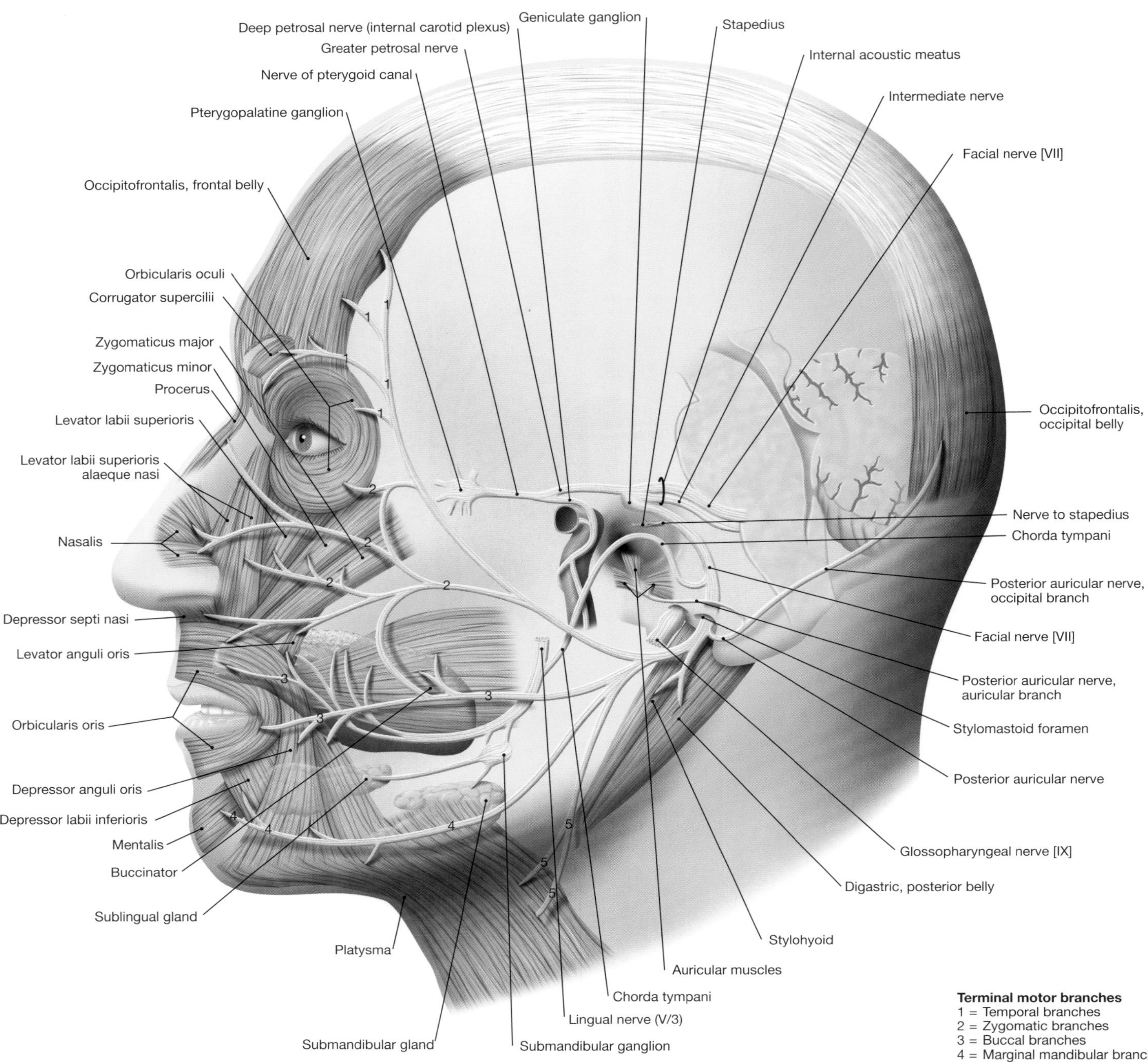
Deep petrosal nerve (internal carotid plexus)
Geniculate ganglion
Stapedius
Greater petrosal nerve
Internal acoustic meatus
Nerve of pterygoid canal
Intermediate nerve
Pterygopalatine ganglion
Facial nerve [VII]
Occipitofrontalis, frontal belly
Orbicularis oculi
Corrugator supercilii
Zygomaticus major
Zygomaticus minor
Procerus
Levator labii superioris
Occipitofrontalis, occipital belly
Levator labii superioris alaeque nasi
Nerve to stapedius
Chorda tympani
Nasalis
Posterior auricular nerve, occipital branch
Depressor septi nasi
Facial nerve [VII]
Levator anguli oris
Posterior auricular nerve, auricular branch
Orbicularis oris
Stylomastoid foramen
Depressor anguli oris
Posterior auricular nerve
Depressor labii inferioris
Mentalis
Glossopharyngeal nerve [IX]
Buccinator
Digastric, posterior belly
Sublingual gland
Stylohyoid
Platysma
Auricular muscles
Chorda tympani
Lingual nerve (V/3)
Submandibular gland
Submandibular ganglion
Terminal motor branches
1 = Temporal branches
2 = Zygomatic branches
3 = Buccal branches
4 = Marginal mandibular branches
5 = Cervical branches

**Fig. 12.149 Facial nerve [VII], left side;** lateral view.
The facial nerve [VII], the intermediate nerve (a part of the facial nerve [VII] but often viewed as a separate nerve), and the vestibulocochlear nerve [VIII] jointly exit the cerebellopontine angle. Shortly thereafter, the intermediate nerve and facial nerve [VII] unite. The facial nerve [VII] and vestibulocochlear nerve [VIII] project towards the petrous part of the temporal bone and enter the bone through the internal acoustic pore and meatus. Upon release of the cochlear and vestibular nerve, the facial nerve [VII] enters the facial canal (→ also Fig. 12.153). Here the facial nerve makes a posterior inferior turn in an almost right angle (external genu of the facial nerve; → Fig. 12.148). The geniculate ganglion is located just prior to the location of the turn of the facial nerve. Along its course within the facial canal, this cranial nerve provides a number of branches (→ Table, p. 310). Upon exiting the cranial base through the stylomastoid foramen, the facial nerve turns rostral, provides additional branches, and then enters the parotid gland. Here, the nerve divides into its terminal motor branches (intraparotid plexus; → Table, p. 310).

→ T 58g

## Facial nerve [VII]

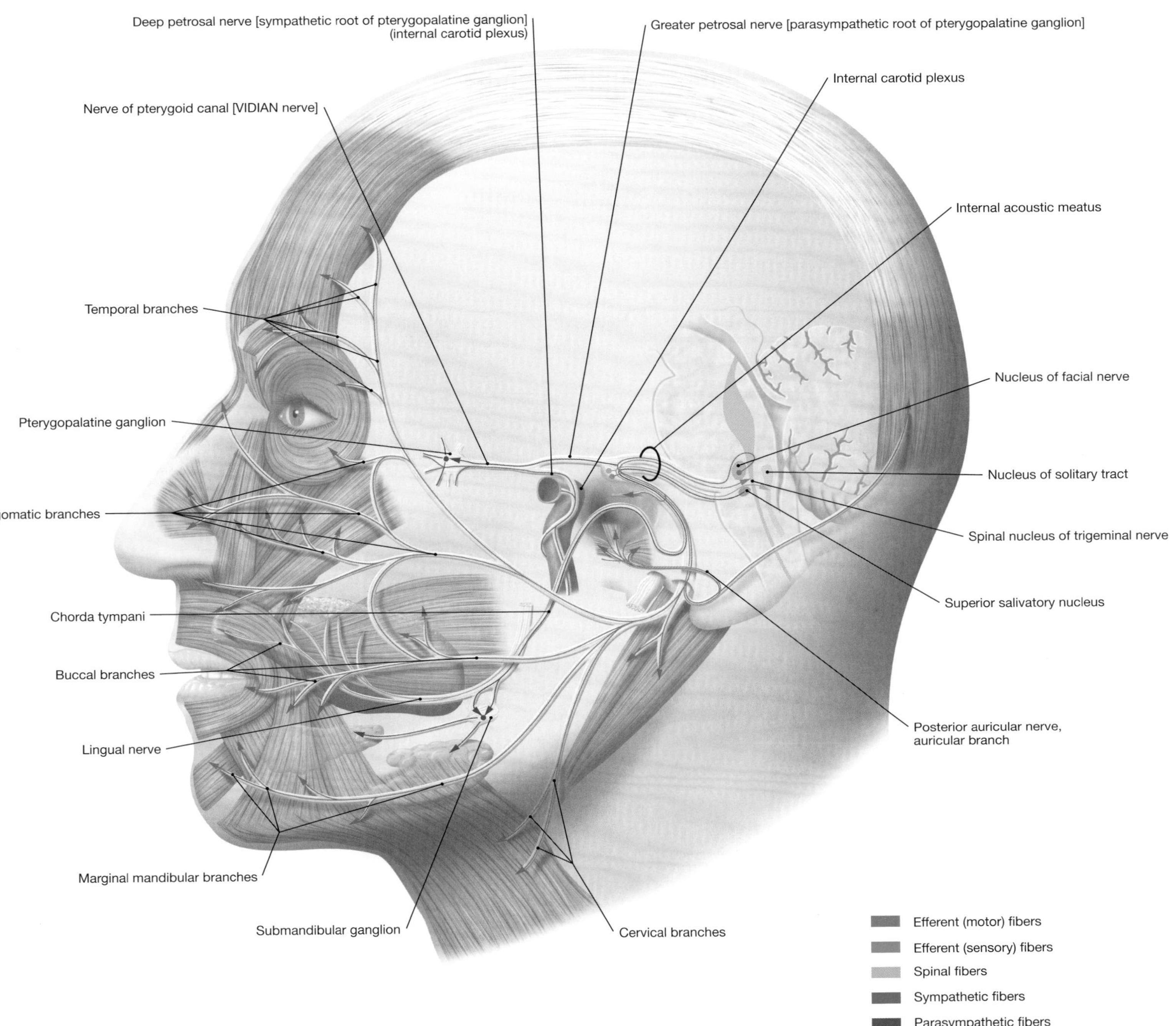
Deep petrosal nerve [sympathetic root of pterygopalatine ganglion] (internal carotid plexus)
Greater petrosal nerve [parasympathetic root of pterygopalatine ganglion]
Internal carotid plexus
Nerve of pterygoid canal [VIDIAN nerve]
Internal acoustic meatus
Temporal branches
Nucleus of facial nerve
Pterygopalatine ganglion
Nucleus of solitary tract
Zygomatic branches
Spinal nucleus of trigeminal nerve
Superior salivatory nucleus
Chorda tympani
Buccal branches
Posterior auricular nerve, auricular branch
Lingual nerve
Marginal mandibular branches
Submandibular ganglion
Cervical branches
Efferent (motor) fibers
Efferent (sensory) fibers
Spinal fibers
Sympathetic fibers
Parasympathetic fibers

**Fig. 12.150 Fiber qualities of the facial nerve [VII], left side;** lateral view.

The facial nerve [VII] is the nerve of the second pharyngeal arch and has several different fiber qualities.

Its **motor fibers** (special viscero-efferent, SVE) derive from the motor **nucleus of facial nerve.** These fibers course around the nucleus of abducent nerve in a posterior arch (internal genu of the facial nerve). The upper part of the nucleus contains the neurons for the innervation of the mimic muscles for the forehead and external orbit, whereas the lower part of the nucleus harbors the neurons innervating all mimic muscles located below the eye. The upper nuclear portion receives double innervation from both cortical hemispheres (→ Fig. 12.152). Thus, it receives corticonuclear fibers from the ipsilateral and contralateral sides. By contrast, the lower portion of the motor nucleus of facial nerve exclusively receives corticonuclear fibers from the contralateral sides.

**Preganglionic parasympathetic fibers** derive from the **superior salivatory nucleus** (general viscero-efferent, GVE). They run with the intermedius part across the facial nerve [VII], course via the greater petrosal nerve to the pterygopalatine ganglion or associate with the chorda tympani and reach the submandibular ganglion via the lingual nerve (from V/3). Synapsing onto the **postganglionic fibers** occurs in these ganglia. These postganglionic fibers project into the lacrimal, nasal and palatine glands, and into the sublingual and submandibular gland (→ trigeminal nerve [V], p. 302).

Special viscero-afferent (SVA) fibers of the anterior two-thirds of the tongue for the perception of taste project into the upper part of the **nucleus of solitary tract.** These fibers reach the facial nerve [VII] via the lingual nerve and chorda tympani and then enter the brainstem.

General somato-afferent fibers (GSA) from the posterior wall of the external acoustic meatus and partially from behind the ear, the auricle, and the tympanic membrane join the vagus nerve [X] (communicating branches with vagus nerve) for a short distance. However, these GSA fibers separate from the vagus nerve while still in the petrous part and associate with the facial nerve [VII]. The perikarya of both the GSA fibers and the gustatory fibers locate in the geniculate ganglion. They reach the spinal nucleus of trigeminal nerve via the intermediate part of the facial nerve [VII].

## Facial nerve [VII]

| Branches of the Facial Nerve [VII] [28] | | |
|---|---|---|
| **Branch** | **Course** | **Innervation Area** |
| Greater petrosal nerve [parasympathic pterygopalatine root] | Exits the facial nerve at the external genu of the facial nerve [VII] and courses through the canal of greater petrosal nerve into the middle cranial fossa; passes through the foramen lacerum to enter the pterygoid canal. Here, it forms the nerve of pterygoid canal together with the sympathetic deep petrosal nerve, which then projects to the pterygopalatine ganglion (synapses of parasympathetic fibers) | **GVE** (via branches of the maxillary nerve [V/2]): lacrimal, nasal, palatine, pharyngeal glands<br>**SVA** (via branches of the mandibular nerve [V/3]): taste buds of the palate |
| Nerve to stapedius | Exits in the lower part of the facial canal | **SVE:** stapedius |
| Chorda tympani | Shortly before the distal end of the facial canal it engages in a retrograde course through its own bony canal to enter the tympanic cavity, which it traverses freely between the handle of malleus and the long limb of the incus behind the tympanic membrane; after passing through the petrotympanic fissure, it associates with the lingual nerve (from V/3) | **GVE** (via the lingual nerve, synapsing in the submandibular ganglion): submandibular and sublingual gland<br>**SVA** (via lingual nerve): anterior two-thirds of the tongue |
| Posterior auricular nerve | Branches off shortly after exiting the facial canal | **SVE:** occipitofrontalis, muscles of the outer ear |
| Digastric branch and stylohyoid branch | Small branches to the muscles | **SVE:** posterior belly of digastric, stylohyoid |
| Intraparotid plexus | Branches with motor fibers to the mimic muscles divide the parotid gland into a temporofacial part and a cervicofacial part; these motor branches subdivide into five terminal branches: temporal branches, zygomatic branches, buccal branches, marginal mandibular branches, cervical/colli branches (→ Fig. 8.81) | **SVE:** mimic muscles, including buccinator and platysma |

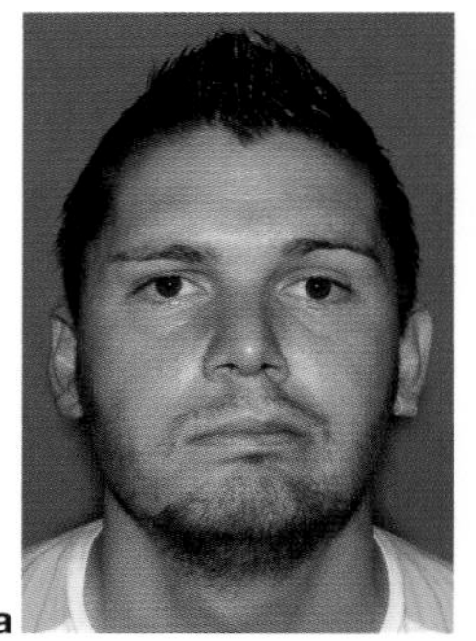
a

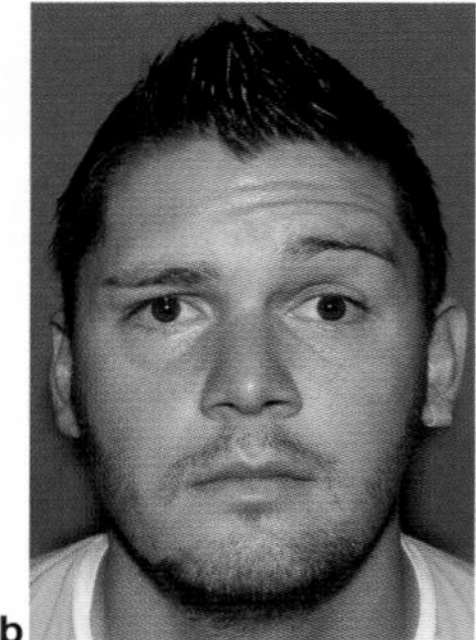
b

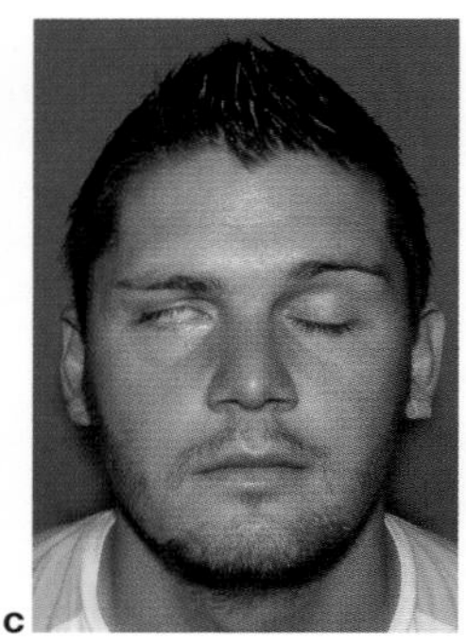
c

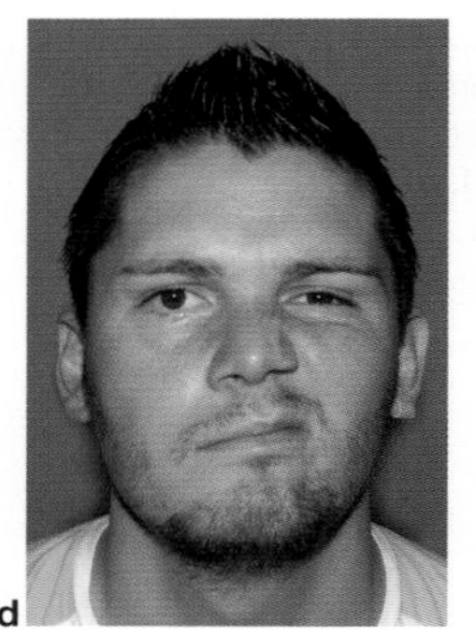
d

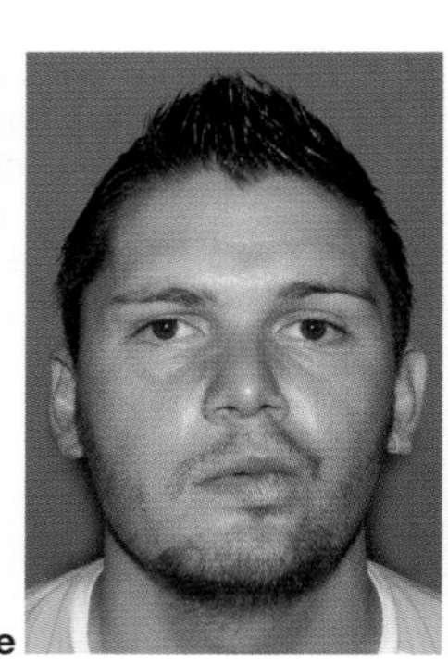
e

**Figs. 12.151a to e Peripheral paralysis of the facial nerve [VII], right side**

- **a** Admission status of the patient. Skin folds on the right side of the face have disappeared.
- **b** When the patient is asked to raise the eyebrows, only the left side of the forehead displays wrinkles (paralysis of the occipitofrontalis, evidence for a peripheral facial palsy).
- **c** When the patient is asked to shut both eyes, this is not accomplished at the side of the damaged facial nerve (lagophthalmos). When eyelids are closed, the eyeball automatically turns upwards. Due to the inability to close the eye properly, the white sclera of the eye becomes visible at the side of facial palsy (BELL's phenomenon).
- **d** When the patient is asked to wrinkle his nose this is impossible on the right side of the face.
- **e** When the patient is asked to whistle, no tone is produced but the air escapes through the lips at the paralysed side.

## Clinical Remarks

**Central facial palsy** (also named lower facial palsy) is caused by a **supranuclear lesion** (lesion of the corticonuclear fibers, e.g. through infarction in the internal capsule). In contrast to an infranuclear lesion and due to the bilateral innervation of the mimic muscles of the eye and forehead, only the lower contralateral part of the face displays motor defects (→ Fig. 12.152).
An **infranuclear lesion** (inferior to the motor nucleus of facial nerve), e.g. caused by a malignant parotid tumor, results in the paralysis of all motor branches of the facial nerve [VII] on the affected side **(peripheral facial palsy).**
An **acousticus neurinoma** (→ p. 313) derives from SCHWANN's cells of the vestibulocochlear nerve [VIII] or the facial nerve [VII]. Sooner or later, this slowly growing benign tumor will displace and damage both nerves. A peripheral facial palsy results and all topodiagnostic tests (→ p. 311) are negative. The diagnosis is concluded by MRI or CT imaging.

## Facial nerve [VII]

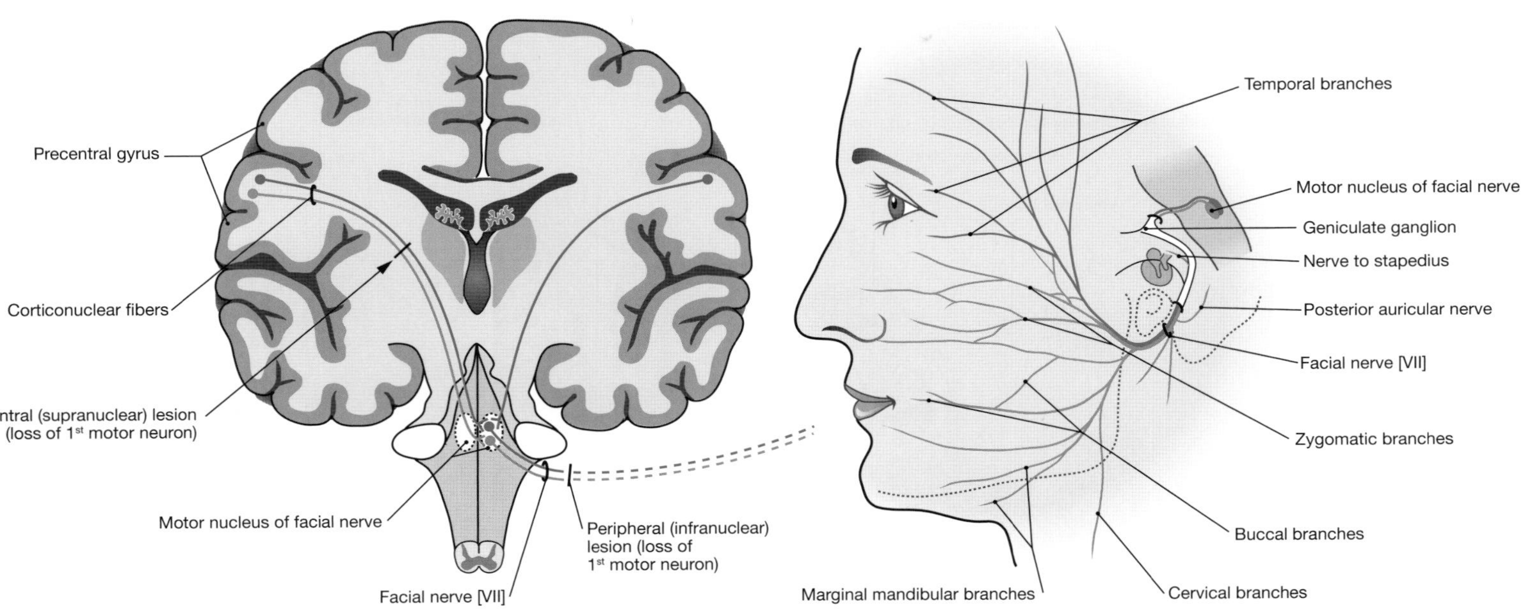
Precentral gyrus
Corticonuclear fibers
entral (supranuclear) lesion (loss of 1st motor neuron)
Motor nucleus of facial nerve
Facial nerve [VII]
Peripheral (infranuclear) lesion (loss of 1st motor neuron)
Temporal branches
Motor nucleus of facial nerve
Geniculate ganglion
Nerve to stapedius
Posterior auricular nerve
Facial nerve [VII]
Zygomatic branches
Buccal branches
Marginal mandibular branches
Cervical branches

**Fig. 12.152 Corticonuclear connections and peripheral course of the facial nerve [VII].** (according to [2])
On the left side, the central connections to the motor nucleus of facial nerve are shown in a simplified schematic representation. The corticonuclear tracts to the upper part of the nucleus (for temporal branches; green) derive from both hemispheres. The lower part of the nucleus (for zygomatic, buccal, marginal mandibular, and cervical/colli branches) connects exclusively with the contralateral hemisphere (red).
On the right side, the peripheral efferent fibers (SVE) derived from the upper and lower part of the motor nucleus of facial nerve are shown.

## Clinical Remarks

**Localization of the Lesion in Peripheral Facial Palsy**
With the advent of modern high resolution imaging procedures, the importance of classical topodiagnostic procedures has diminished because of their unspecific and low prognostic value when compared to electrodiagnostic procedures. However, the individual tests have clinical relevance.

- The SCHIRMER's test provides information about the normal production of lacrimal fluid (→ Fig. 9.27).
- The stapedius reflex test determines the function of the nerve to stapedius.
- Gustometry (testing taste perception) assesses the functionality and intactness of the chorda tympani.
- Nerve excitability tests allow the electrical stimulation of mimic muscles.
- The difference of the conduction velocity of electrical potentials on the healthy and damaged side is determined by electroneurography.

| Site of the Lesion | Topodiagnostic Procedure | Cause of Lesion |
|---|---|---|
| Inferior to the nuclear area within the brainstem | MRI, CT, SCHIRMER's test (functional test for the lacrimal gland) | e.g. acousticus neurinoma |
| After greater petrosal nerve has branched off | Stapedius reflex test | e.g. otitis media (middle ear infection) |
| After chorda tympani has branched off | Gustometry (testing taste perception) | e.g. otitis media (middle ear infection) |
| After passing through the stylomastoid foramen | Testing facial motor functions | e.g. malignant parotid tumor |

## Vestibulocochlear nerve [VIII]

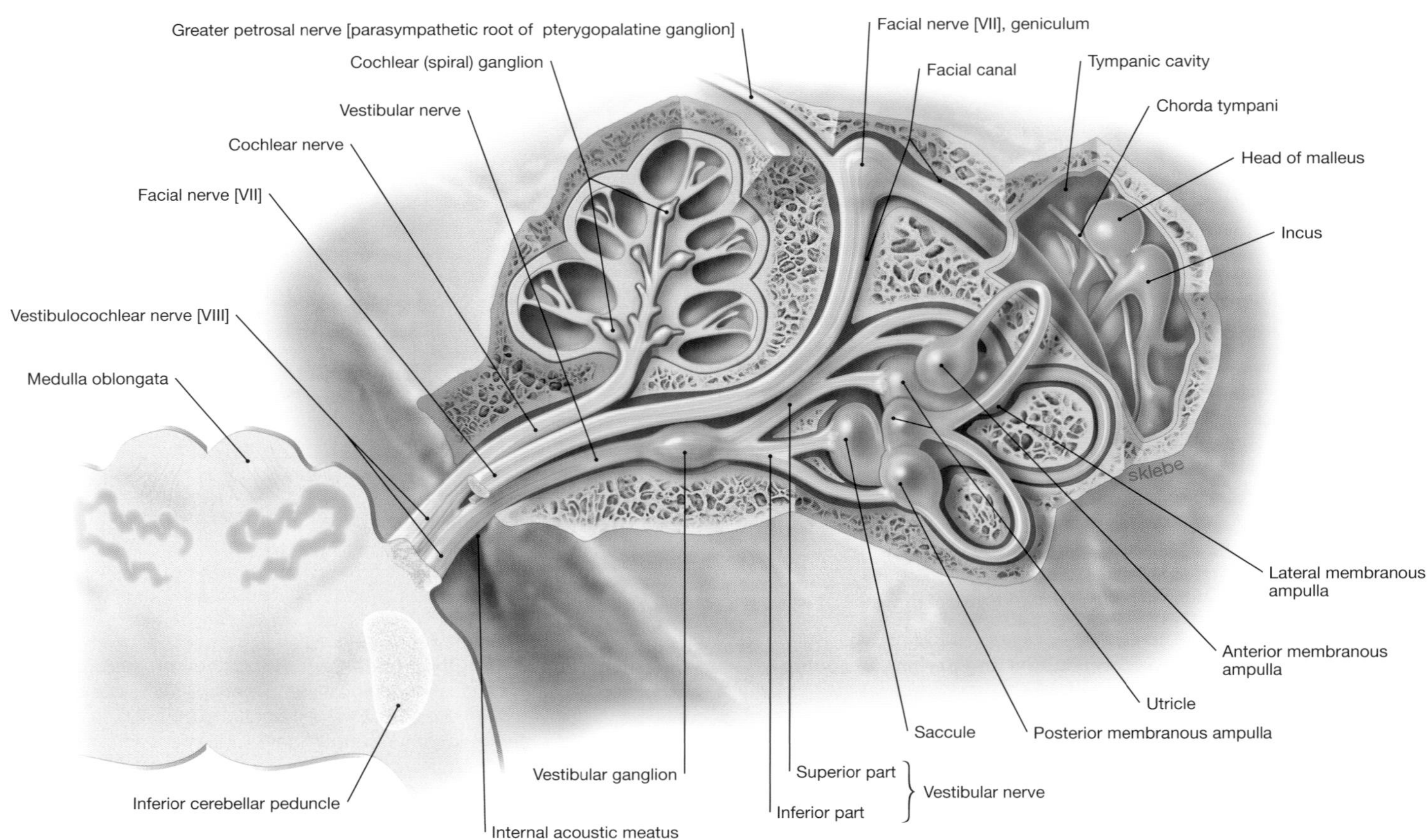
Greater petrosal nerve [parasympathetic root of pterygopalatine ganglion]
Cochlear (spiral) ganglion
Vestibular nerve
Cochlear nerve
Facial nerve [VII]
Vestibulocochlear nerve [VIII]
Medulla oblongata
Facial nerve [VII], geniculum
Facial canal
Tympanic cavity
Chorda tympani
Head of malleus
Incus
Lateral membranous ampulla
Anterior membranous ampulla
Utricle
Saccule
Posterior membranous ampulla
Vestibular ganglion
Superior part
Inferior part
Vestibular nerve
Inferior cerebellar peduncle
Internal acoustic meatus
sklebe

**Fig. 12.153 Vestibulocochlear nerve [VIII], course in the petrous part of the temporal bone;** superior view; the petrous part has been opened.

The **cochlear nerve** is composed of nerve fibers generated in the organ of CORTI of the cochlea. The perikarya of these fibers are located in the cochlear (spiral) ganglion within the modiolus (bipolar neurons) and the central axons form the cochlear nerve. The vestibular organ also possesses bipolar neurons. Like the cochlear neurons, they receive sensory input from hair cells. Their perikarya reside in the vestibular ganglion which is located at the floor of the internal acoustic meatus. The central neuronal projections form the **vestibular nerve.** The nerve merges with the cochlear nerve to form the vestibulocochlear nerve [VIII] (clinically frequently referred to as stato-acoustic nerve) at the internal acoustic meatus and enters the brainstem at the cerebellopontine angle.

Also demonstrated is the course of the facial nerve [VII] in the internal acoustic meatus and the facial canal. In addition, the geniculate ganglion, the separation of the greater petrosal nerve and the course of the facial nerve [VII] in the tympanic cavity are shown. The chorda tympani runs between the malleus and the incus.

→ T 58h

## Vestibulocochlear nerve [VIII]

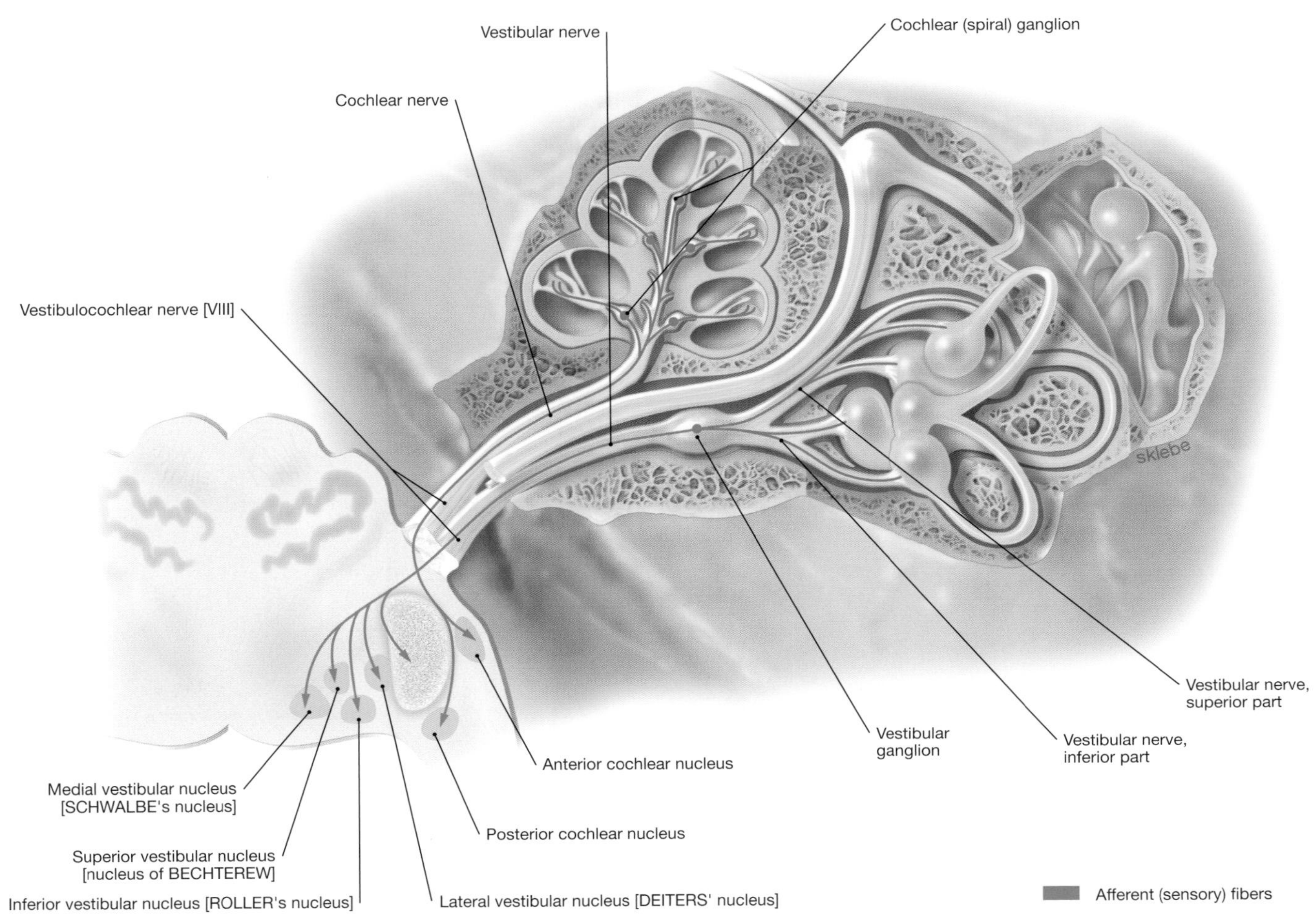
Vestibular nerve
Cochlear (spiral) ganglion
Cochlear nerve
Vestibulocochlear nerve [VIII]
Vestibular nerve, superior part
Vestibular ganglion
Vestibular nerve, inferior part
Anterior cochlear nucleus
Medial vestibular nucleus [SCHWALBE's nucleus]
Posterior cochlear nucleus
Superior vestibular nucleus [nucleus of BECHTEREW]
Inferior vestibular nucleus [ROLLER's nucleus]
Lateral vestibular nucleus [DEITERS' nucleus]
Afferent (sensory) fibers

**Fig. 12.154 Fiber qualities of the vestibulocochlear nerve [VIII];** superior view; petrous part of the temporal bone has been opened.
The inner hair cells of the organ of CORTI and hair cells of the semicircular canals as well as utricle and saccule of the vestibular apparatus transmit sensory information to the specific somato-afferent neuronal fibers (SSA). These fibers constitute the peripheral projections of bipolar neurons (1st neuron of the central auditory and vestibular tracts). The perikarya of these bipolar neurons reside in the cochlear (spiral) ganglion and the vestibular ganglion, respectively. The **central projections** of the **cochlear ganglion** merge to form the **cochlear nerve,** course through the internal acoustic meatus, and reach the brainstem via the cerebellopontine angle. Here they connect with the anterior and posterior cochlear nuclei. The **central projections of the 1st neuron of the vestibular tract** (SSA) form the **vestibular nerve** and also pass through the cerebellopontine angle into the medulla oblongata. Here they project to the medial vestibular nucleus (SCHWALBE's nucleus), superior vestibular nucleus (nucleus of BECHTEREW), inferior vestibular nucleus (ROLLER's nucleus), and lateral vestibular nucleus (DEITERS' nucleus).

## Clinical Remarks

A sudden decrease in hearing, tinnitus, disturbances in balance, and vertigo can all be the first signs of an **acousticus neurinoma.** This is a benign tumor composed of connective and neuronal tissues. In most cases, the tumor derives from SCHWANN's cells of the vestibular part of the vestibulocochlear nerve [VIII] **(vestibular schwannoma)** and locates in the cerebellopontine angle or the internal acoustic meatus. In 5% of cases, the acousticus neurinoma occurs bilaterally. Due to the joint course with the facial nerve [VII], a peripheral facial palsy can result.

## Glossopharyngeal nerve [IX]

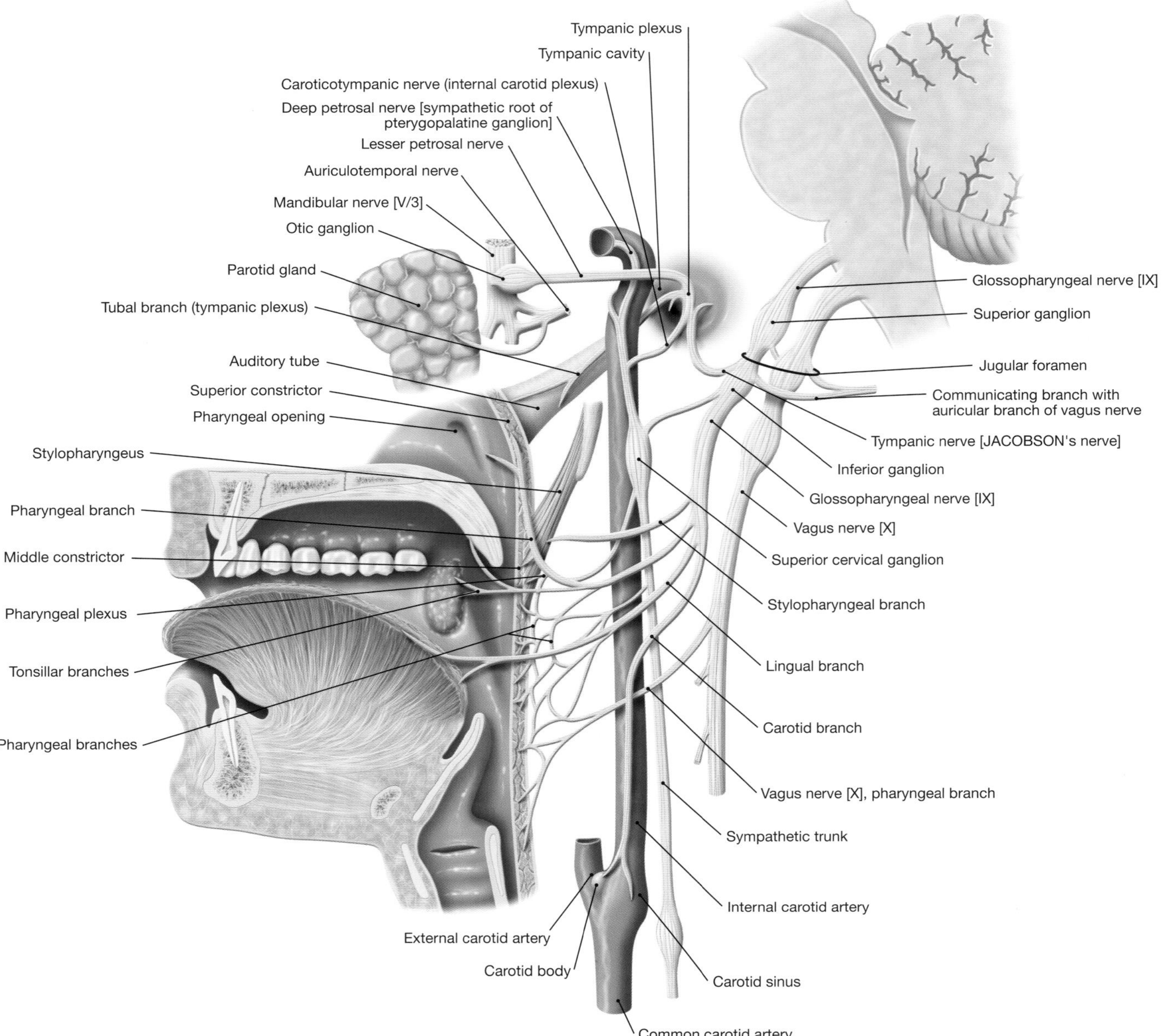
Tympanic plexus
Tympanic cavity
Caroticotympanic nerve (internal carotid plexus)
Deep petrosal nerve [sympathetic root of pterygopalatine ganglion]
Lesser petrosal nerve
Auriculotemporal nerve
Mandibular nerve [V/3]
Otic ganglion
Parotid gland
Tubal branch (tympanic plexus)
Auditory tube
Superior constrictor
Pharyngeal opening
Stylopharyngeus
Pharyngeal branch
Middle constrictor
Pharyngeal plexus
Tonsillar branches
Pharyngeal branches
Glossopharyngeal nerve [IX]
Superior ganglion
Jugular foramen
Communicating branch with auricular branch of vagus nerve
Tympanic nerve [JACOBSON's nerve]
Inferior ganglion
Glossopharyngeal nerve [IX]
Vagus nerve [X]
Superior cervical ganglion
Stylopharyngeal branch
Lingual branch
Carotid branch
Vagus nerve [X], pharyngeal branch
Sympathetic trunk
Internal carotid artery
External carotid artery
Carotid body
Carotid sinus
Common carotid artery

**Fig. 12.155 Glossopharyngeal nerve [IX];** schematic median section; view from the left side.

The glossopharyngeal nerve [IX], the vagus nerve [X], and the accessory nerve [XI] exit the brainstem in the retro-olivary sulcus and pass through the jugular foramen at the cranial base. Within the foramen lies the smaller of two ganglia, the superior ganglion, followed immediately by the caudal inferior ganglion. Once the glossopharyngeal nerve has passed through the cranial base, it courses caudally in between the internal jugular vein and the internal carotid artery and by arching forward and running between the stylopharyngeus and styloglossus enters the root of the tongue. In its course, the **tympanic nerve** branches off and projects to the tympanic cavity. Here the tympanic nerve divides into the intramucosal tympanic plexus and exits the tympanic cavity as **lesser petrosal nerve.** The lesser petrosal nerve runs parallel to the greater petrosal nerve at the anterior aspect of the petrous bone and passes through the foramen lacerum to reach the otic ganglion. Fibers of the glossopharyngeal nerve [IX] passing through this ganglion innervate the parotid gland.

Additional **branches** are the muscular branches to stylopharyngeus and the pharyngeal branches to the superior constrictor, palatoglossus, and palatopharyngeus, as well as sensory fibers to the pharyngeal mucosa and to the pharyngeal glands.

Together with the sympathetic trunk and the vagus nerve [X], additional fibers generate the **pharyngeal plexus** which innervates the inferior constrictor, levator veli palatini, and uvula.

The tonsillar branches supply sensory fibers to the palatine tonsil and the mucosa of the isthmus faucium, the lingual branches contain gustatory (taste) fibers for the posterior third of the tongue. The carotid branch transmits sensory input from mechano- and chemoreceptors at the carotid sinus and carotid body to the brainstem.

→ T 58i

## Glossopharyngeal nerve [IX]

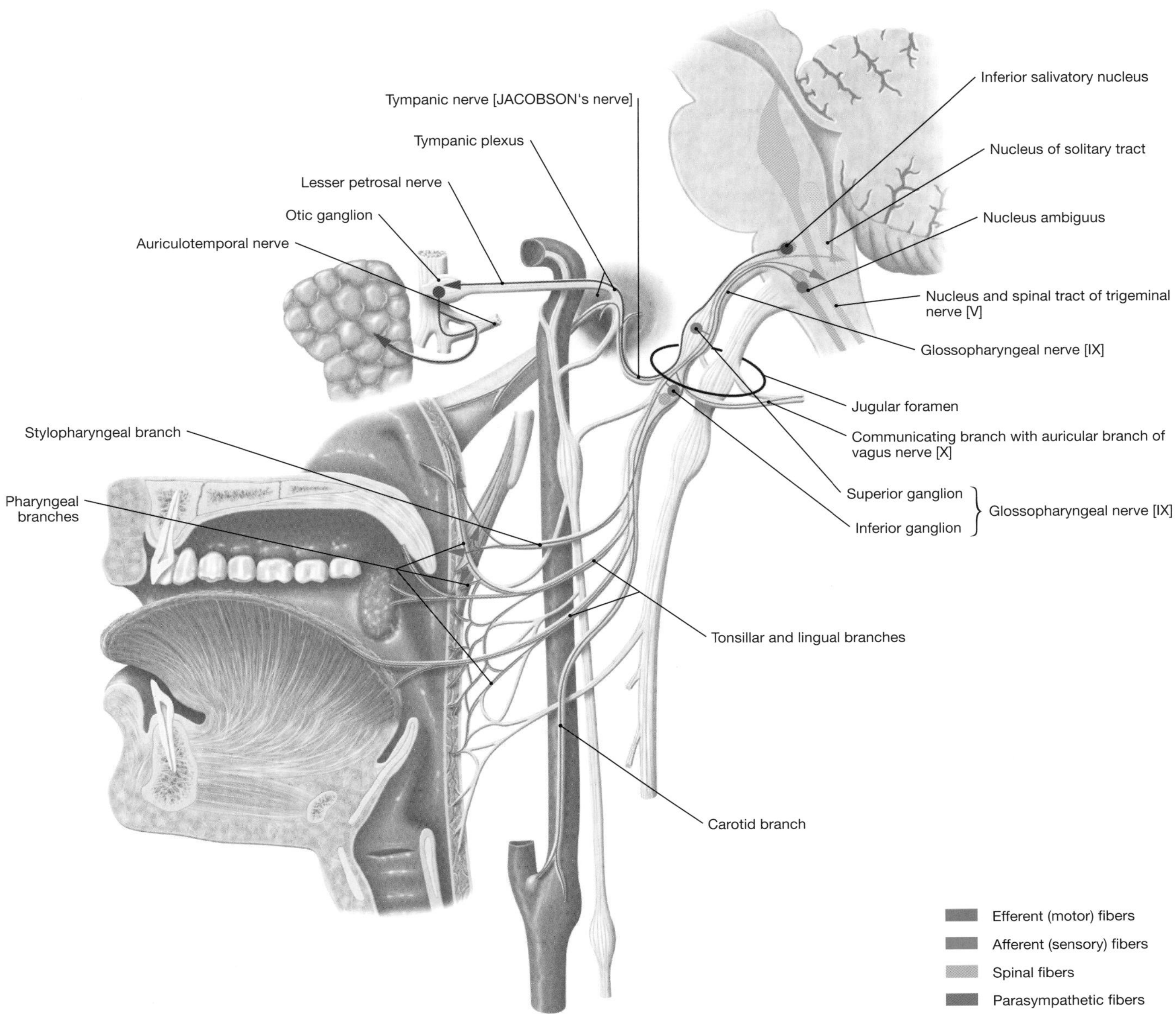
Tympanic nerve [JACOBSON's nerve]
Tympanic plexus
Lesser petrosal nerve
Otic ganglion
Auriculotemporal nerve
Inferior salivatory nucleus
Nucleus of solitary tract
Nucleus ambiguus
Nucleus and spinal tract of trigeminal nerve [V]
Glossopharyngeal nerve [IX]
Jugular foramen
Communicating branch with auricular branch of vagus nerve [X]
Superior ganglion
Inferior ganglion
Glossopharyngeal nerve [IX]
Stylopharyngeal branch
Pharyngeal branches
Tonsillar and lingual branches
Carotid branch
Efferent (motor) fibers
Afferent (sensory) fibers
Spinal fibers
Parasympathetic fibers

**Fig. 12.156 Fiber qualities of the glossopharyngeal nerve [IX];** schematic median section, view from the left side.
**Motor** fibers (SVE) of the glossopharyngeal nerve [IX] derived from the nucleus ambiguus and from the vagus nerve [X] (also from the nucleus ambiguus, SVE) jointly innervate the muscles of the soft palate.
**Parasympathetic** fibers (GVE) from the inferior salivatory nucleus project to the otic ganglion via the tympanic nerve, tympanic plexus, and lesser petrosal nerve. In the otic ganglion, the preganglionic fibers synapse to postganglionic neurons. The postganglionic fibers associate with the auriculotemporal nerve (from V/3) and the facial nerve [VII] to reach the parotid gland. Additional parasympathetic fibers (GVE) reach the pharyngeal glands. Numerous **general somato-afferent** fibers (GSA) that project to the spinal nucleus of trigeminal nerve derive from the tympanic cavity, the pharyngeal mucosa, and the posterior third of the tongue.
**General viscero-afferent** fibers (GVA) transmit the sensory input of mechanoreceptors in the carotid sinus (determine blood pressure) and of chemoreceptors in the carotid body (measure partial pressure of $O_2$ and $CO_2$ and pH of the blood). The brainstem integrates this sensory input and issues reflexive changes in the frequency of breathing and of the central blood pressure.
Specific viscero-afferent fibers (SVA) conduct taste sensations to the nuclei of solitary tract of the posterior third of the tongue.

## Clinical Remarks

**Lesions of the glossopharyngeal nerve [IX]** result in swallowing difficulties (paralysis of the superior constrictor, failure to form the PASSAVANT's ridge), a deviation of the uvula to the healthy side (paralysis of the levator veli palatini, palatoglossus, palatopharyngeus, uvulae), an impaired sensibility of the pharyngeal region (lack of gag reflex), a lack of taste sensation at the posterior third of the tongue, as well as disturbances in the secretion by the parotid gland. In most cases, damage to the glossopharyngeal nerve [IX] is not an isolated event. Frequently, fractures, aneurysms, tumors, and thrombosis of cerebral blood vessels supplying the brain in the region of the jugular foramen also affect the vagus nerve [X] and accessory nerve [XI].

## Vagus nerve [X]

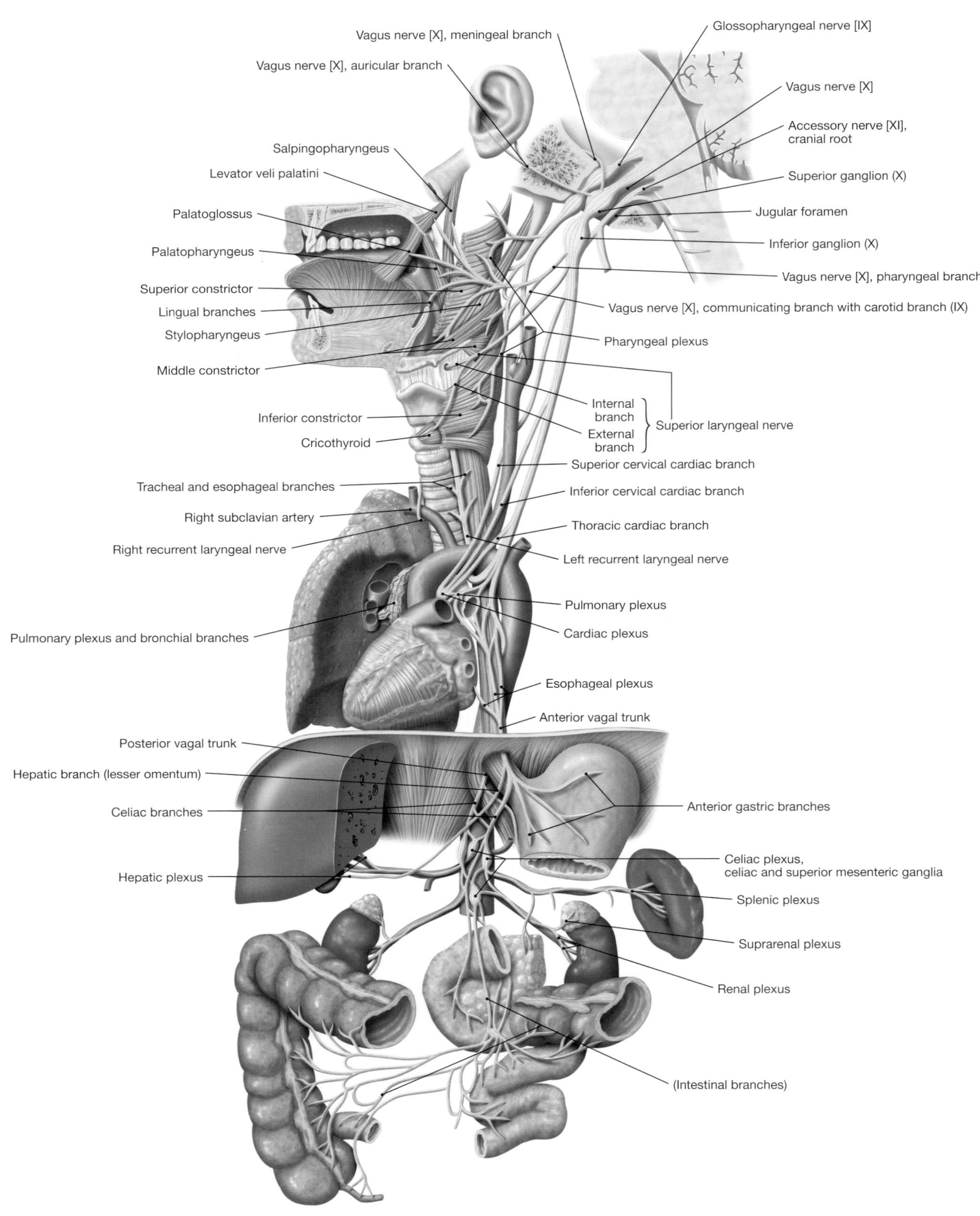
Vagus nerve [X], meningeal branch
Glossopharyngeal nerve [IX]
Vagus nerve [X], auricular branch
Vagus nerve [X]
Accessory nerve [XI], cranial root
Salpingopharyngeus
Levator veli palatini
Superior ganglion (X)
Palatoglossus
Jugular foramen
Inferior ganglion (X)
Palatopharyngeus
Vagus nerve [X], pharyngeal branch
Superior constrictor
Vagus nerve [X], communicating branch with carotid branch (IX)
Lingual branches
Stylopharyngeus
Pharyngeal plexus
Middle constrictor
Internal branch
External branch
Superior laryngeal nerve
Inferior constrictor
Cricothyroid
Superior cervical cardiac branch
Tracheal and esophageal branches
Inferior cervical cardiac branch
Right subclavian artery
Thoracic cardiac branch
Right recurrent laryngeal nerve
Left recurrent laryngeal nerve
Pulmonary plexus
Pulmonary plexus and bronchial branches
Cardiac plexus
Esophageal plexus
Anterior vagal trunk
Posterior vagal trunk
Hepatic branch (lesser omentum)
Anterior gastric branches
Celiac branches
Celiac plexus,
celiac and superior mesenteric ganglia
Hepatic plexus
Splenic plexus
Suprarenal plexus
Renal plexus
(Intestinal branches)

**Fig. 12.157 Vagus nerve [X];** schematic median section in the region of the head.
For a detailed description of the course of the vagus nerve [X] → p. 318.

→ T 58j

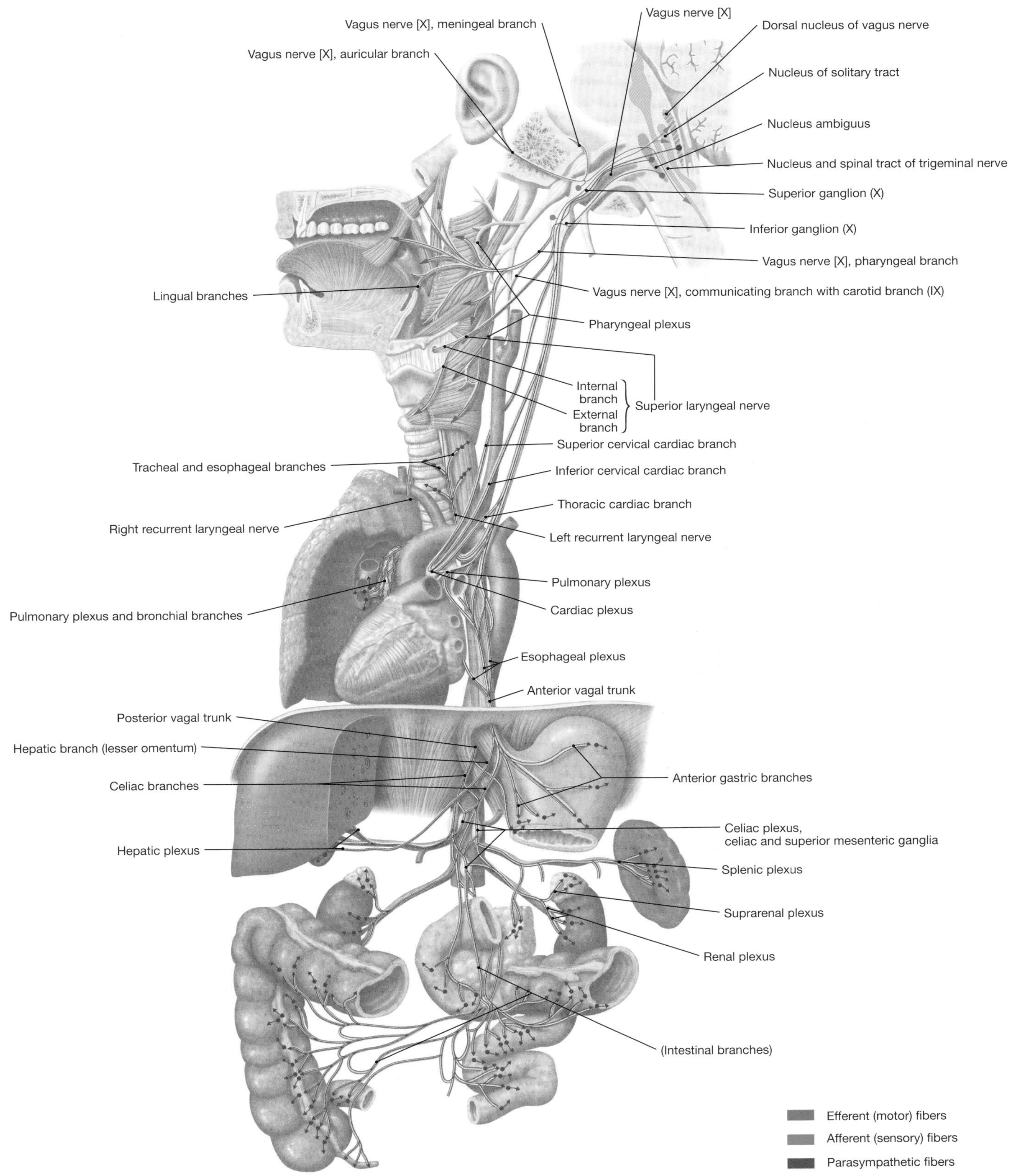
Vagus nerve [X], meningeal branch
Vagus nerve [X], auricular branch
Vagus nerve [X]
Dorsal nucleus of vagus nerve
Nucleus of solitary tract
Nucleus ambiguus
Nucleus and spinal tract of trigeminal nerve
Superior ganglion (X)
Inferior ganglion (X)
Vagus nerve [X], pharyngeal branch
Vagus nerve [X], communicating branch with carotid branch (IX)
Lingual branches
Pharyngeal plexus
Internal branch
External branch
Superior laryngeal nerve
Superior cervical cardiac branch
Tracheal and esophageal branches
Inferior cervical cardiac branch
Thoracic cardiac branch
Right recurrent laryngeal nerve
Left recurrent laryngeal nerve
Pulmonary plexus
Pulmonary plexus and bronchial branches
Cardiac plexus
Esophageal plexus
Anterior vagal trunk
Posterior vagal trunk
Hepatic branch (lesser omentum)
Celiac branches
Anterior gastric branches
Celiac plexus,
celiac and superior mesenteric ganglia
Hepatic plexus
Splenic plexus
Suprarenal plexus
Renal plexus
(Intestinal branches)
Efferent (motor) fibers
Afferent (sensory) fibers
Parasympathetic fibers

**Fig. 12.158 Fiber qualities of the vagus nerve [X];** schematic median section in the region of the head.
For a detailed description of the fiber qualities of the vagus nerve [X] → p. 318.

## Vagus nerve [X]

**Vagus nerve [X] → Fig. 12.157**
Together with the glossopharyngeal nerve [IX] and the accessory nerve [XI], the vagus nerve [X] exits the brainstem in the retro-olivary sulcus and traverses the cranial base through the jugular foramen. The **superior ganglion** locates in the jugular foramen and releases the meningeal branch which re-enters the cranial cavity to provide sensory innervation to the meninges of the posterior cranial fossa. Also branching off is the auricular branch for the innervation of the outer wall of the external acoustic meatus. The **inferior ganglion** locates slightly below the jugular foramen.
The vagus nerve [X] crosses the neck and the thoracic cavity and enters the abdominal cavity. In its course, the vagus nerve [X] progressively loses its appearance as a coherent nerve. At the level of the esophagus, two distinct trunks can still be discerned (anterior and posterior vagal trunk), but from the stomach onward the fibers distribute more widely and form multiple **plexus** to reach the liver, pancreas, spleen, kidney, adrenal gland, small intestine, and colon. The fibers of the vagus nerve [X] terminate at the level of the CANNON-BÖHM point (left colic flexure).
In its **cervical passage,** the vagus nerve [X] provides pharyngeal branches to the **pharyngeal plexus.** This plexus also receives contributions from the glossopharyngeal nerve [IX] and from sympathetic fibers (innervation of the middle and inferior constrictor, levator veli palatini, uvula – motor function [SVE], pharyngeal glands – parasympathetic function [GVE], and pharyngeal mucosa – sensory function [GVA]). Additional vagal branches are the lingual branch (taste fibers from the root of the tongue and epiglottis, SVA), the superior laryngeal nerve (with the external branch for the cricothyroid and inferior constrictor as well as the internal branch for the sensory innervation of the laryngeal mucosa above the vocal cords) and the superior and inferior cervical cardiac branches to the cardiac plexus at the heart (which affects the regulation of the blood pressure).
In its **thoracic part,** the vagus nerve [X] releases the recurrent laryngeal nerve. The latter loops around the aortic arch on the left side and the subclavian artery on the right side and projects back cranially to the larynx. Here the recurrent laryngeal nerve innervates all laryngeal muscles (with the exception of the cricothyroid) and the mucosa below the vocal cords. Additional thoracic vagal branches include the thoracic cardiac branches for the cardiac plexus at the heart. The bronchial branches reach the pulmonary plexus and innervate muscles and glands of the bronchial tree. The pulmonary vagal innervation registers the tension within the lung tissue and adjusts breathing by a reflectory neuronal feedback loop.
Right and left vagus nerve [X] form a web-like plexus (esophageal plexus) at the middle part of the esophagus. The plexus eventually contributes to the formation of the anterior vagal trunk (mainly fibers of the left vagus nerve [X]) and the posterior vagal trunk (mainly fibers of the right vagus nerve [X]). Both trunks accompany the esophagus during its passage through the diaphragm into the **abdominal cavity.** From the stomach onwards, the trunks diversify further to create numerous plexuses for the above-mentioned abdominal organs.

**Fiber qualities in the vagus nerve [X] → Fig. 12.158**
**Parasympathetic** fibers (GVE) of the vagus nerve [X] originate from the dorsal (posterior) nucleus of vagus nerve in the medulla oblongata and innervate glands and smooth muscles of the viscera.
**General viscero-afferent** fibers (GVA) of the same organs project into the dorsal (posterior) nucleus of vagus nerve and the nucleus of solitary tract.
**Specific viscero-efferent** fibers (SVE) originate in the nucleus ambiguus and innervate the skeletal muscles of the palate, pharynx, larynx, and esophagus.
**General viscero-afferent** fibers (GVA) from the mucosa of the same structures project into the dorsal (posterior) nucleus of vagus nerve and the nucleus of solitary tract.
**General somato-afferent** fibers (GSA) of the external acoustic meatus and the meninges of the posterior cranial fossa project into the spinal nucleus of trigeminal nerve.
**Gustatory fibers** (SVA) at the root of the tongue and the epiglottis connect with the nucleus of solitary tract.

| **N. vagus [X]** | |
|---|---|
| Nuclei (quality) | • Nucleus ambiguus (SVE)<br>• Solitary nucleus (SVA, GVA)<br>• Spinal nucleus of trigeminal nerve (GSA)<br>• Dorsal (posterior) nucleus of vagus nerve (GVE, GVA) |
| Exit points in the brain | • Medulla oblongata: retro-olivary sulcus |
| Position within the subarachnoid space | • Basal cistern |
| Passage through the cranial base | • Jugular foramen |
| Innervation area | **Motor:**<br>• Pharyngeal muscles (caudal part), levator veli palatini, uvula<br>• Laryngeal muscles<br>**Specific sensory:**<br>• Root of the tongue<br>**Sensory:**<br>• Dura mater of the posterior cranial fossa<br>• External acoustic meatus (sickle-shaped deep part)<br>• Tympanic membrane (outer surface)<br>**Parasympathetic:**<br>• Organs of the neck, thorax, and abdomen up to the CANNON-BÖHM point |

## Vagus nerve [X]

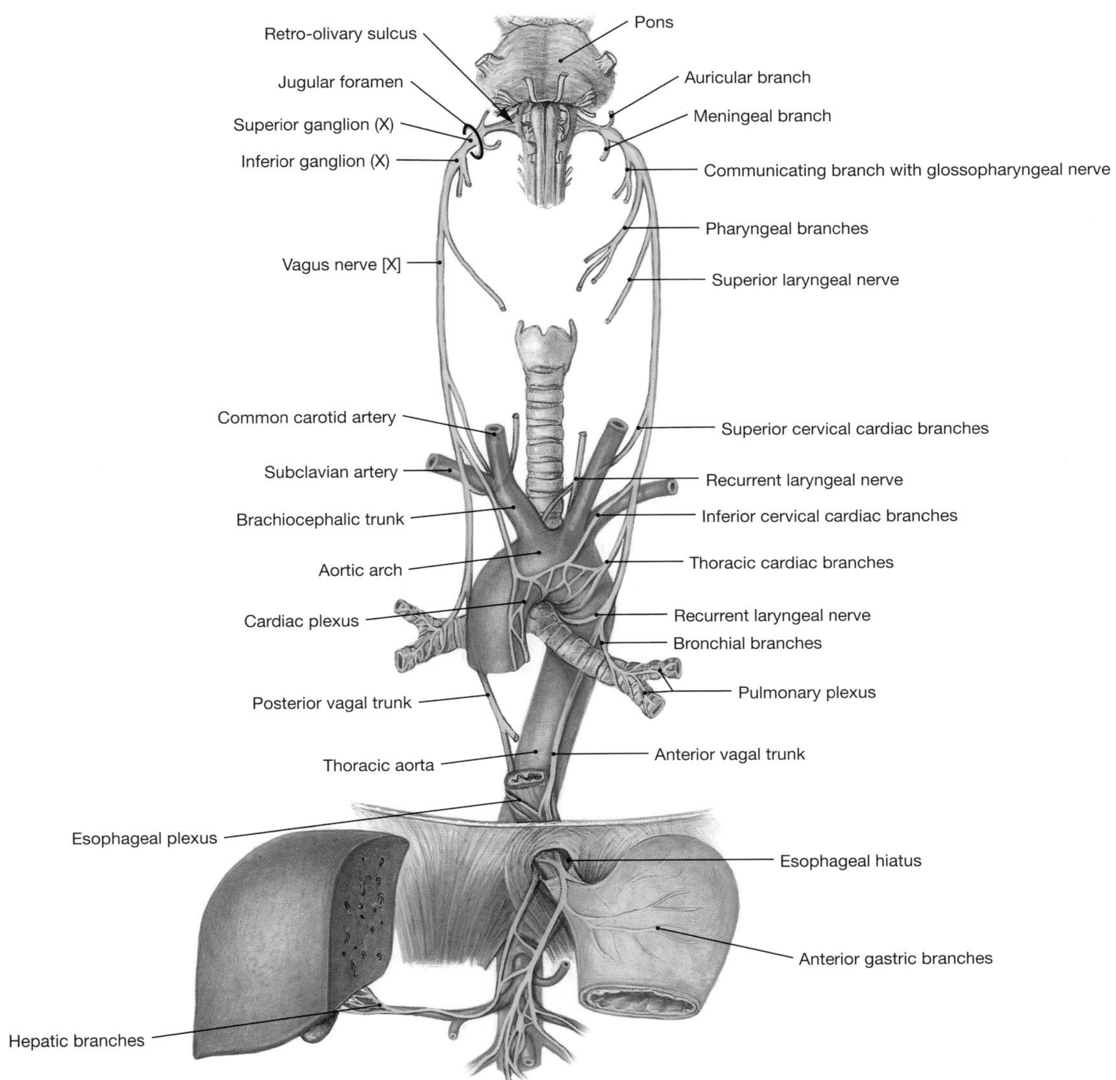
Retro-olivary sulcus
Pons
Jugular foramen
Auricular branch
Meningeal branch
Superior ganglion (X)
Inferior ganglion (X)
Communicating branch with glossopharyngeal nerve
Pharyngeal branches
Vagus nerve [X]
Superior laryngeal nerve
Common carotid artery
Superior cervical cardiac branches
Subclavian artery
Recurrent laryngeal nerve
Brachiocephalic trunk
Inferior cervical cardiac branches
Aortic arch
Thoracic cardiac branches
Cardiac plexus
Recurrent laryngeal nerve
Bronchial branches
Pulmonary plexus
Posterior vagal trunk
Thoracic aorta
Anterior vagal trunk
Esophageal plexus
Esophageal hiatus
Anterior gastric branches
Hepatic branches

**Fig. 12.159 Vagus nerve [X];** both nerve branches; anterior view. The image emphasizes the slightly different course of the right and left vagus nerve and the course of their branches until the anterior and posterior vagal trunks enter the abdominal cavity.

→T 58j

## Clinical Remarks

Complete **lesions of the vagus nerve [X]** mainly occur at the jugular foramen. Frequently, the glossopharyngeal nerve [IX] and the accessory nerve [XI] are also affected. Depending on the location of the lesion, the symptoms include a difficulty in swallowing and deviation of the uvula to the healthy side (damage of the pharyngeal plexus), sensory deficits in the pharynx and the epiglottis (lack of gag reflex, gustatory impairment), hoarseness (paralysis of laryngeal muscles), tachycardia and arrhythmia (innervation of the heart). The unilateral damage has little effect on the autonomic vagal functions. However, bilateral damage of the vagus nerve can result in severe respiratory and circulatory problems that can cause the death of a patient.

## Accessory nerve [XI]

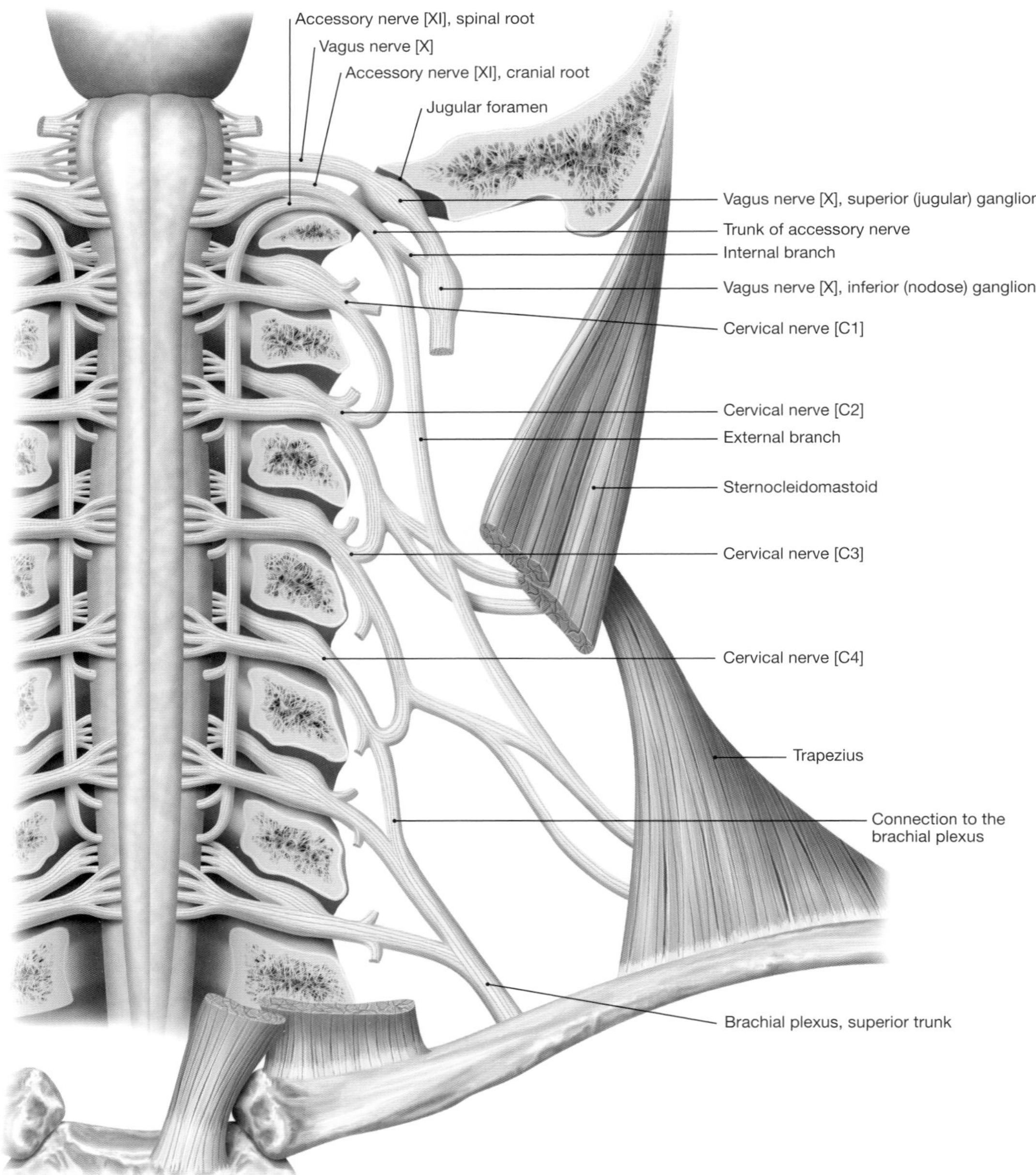
Accessory nerve [XI], spinal root
Vagus nerve [X]
Accessory nerve [XI], cranial root
Jugular foramen
Vagus nerve [X], superior (jugular) ganglion
Trunk of accessory nerve
Internal branch
Vagus nerve [X], inferior (nodose) ganglion
Cervical nerve [C1]
Cervical nerve [C2]
External branch
Sternocleidomastoid
Cervical nerve [C3]
Cervical nerve [C4]
Trapezius
Connection to the brachial plexus
Brachial plexus, superior trunk

**Fig. 12.160 Accessory nerve [XI];** anterior view; vertebral canal and skull have been opened.

The accessory nerve [XI] exits the brainstem in the retro-olivary sulcus together with the glossopharyngeal nerve [IX] and the vagus nerve [X] and all three cranial nerves traverse the cranial base through the jugular foramen. The accessory nerve [XI] has two different roots. The **cranial root** of the accessory nerve [XI] originates from the nucleus ambiguus in the medulla oblongata. At the level of the jugular foramen, it joins the **spinal root** of the accessory nerve [XI] which consists of fibers derived from the anterior and posterior segmental roots in the cervical spinal cord. According to current textbook knowledge, the fibers of the cranial root form the internal branch and converge on the vagus nerve [X] inferior to the jugular foramen (according to newer preliminary findings which require further analysis, the accessory nerve [XI] has no cranial root and no connection to the vagus nerve [X]). The cranial root participates in the innervation of the pharyngeal and laryngeal muscles and, strictly speaking, is not part of the accessory nerve [XI]. The fibers of the spinal root project caudally to the sternocleidomastoid, course through the lateral cervical triangle to the anterior margin of the trapezius, and innervate both muscles.

→ T 58k

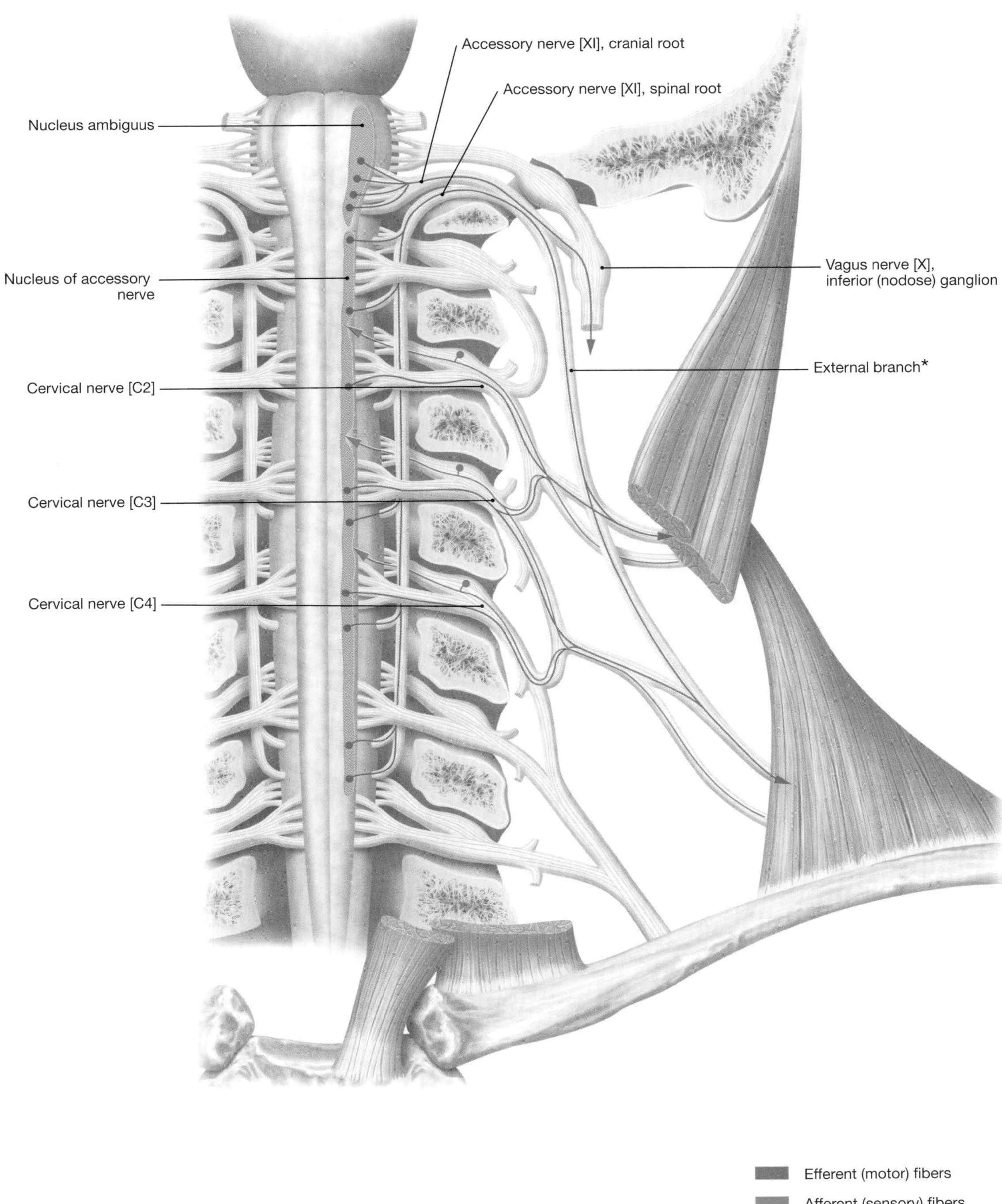
Accessory nerve [XI], cranial root
Accessory nerve [XI], spinal root
Nucleus ambiguus
Nucleus of accessory nerve
Vagus nerve [X], inferior (nodose) ganglion
External branch*
Cervical nerve [C2]
Cervical nerve [C3]
Cervical nerve [C4]
Efferent (motor) fibers
Afferent (sensory) fibers

**Fig. 12.161 Fiber qualities of the accessory nerve [XI];** anterior view, vertebral canal and skull have been opened.
The accessory nerve [XI] innervates the sternocleidomastoid and trapezius with **specific viscero-efferent** fibers (SVE) from the nucleus of accessory nerve.

* for sternocleidomastoid and trapezius

## Clinical Remarks

**Lesions of the accessory nerve [XI]** are frequent due to its superficial course in the lateral triangle of the neck. Iatrogenic lesions (as consequence of medical actions, e.g. extirpation of lymph nodes) are particularly common. Injuries to the neck are another cause for nerve lesions. If the accessory nerve [XI] is injured superior to the sternocleidomastoid, the patient is incapable of turning the head to the healthy side (paralysis of the sternocleidomastoid). In addition, an elevation of the arm above the horizontal plane is impossible (paralysis of the trapezius). In most cases, however, the lesion locates inferior to the branches supplying the sternocleidomastoid in the lateral triangle of the neck. The shoulder on this side drops deeper compared to the healthy side and elevation of the arm above the horizontal plane becomes challenging.

## Hypoglossal nerve [XII]

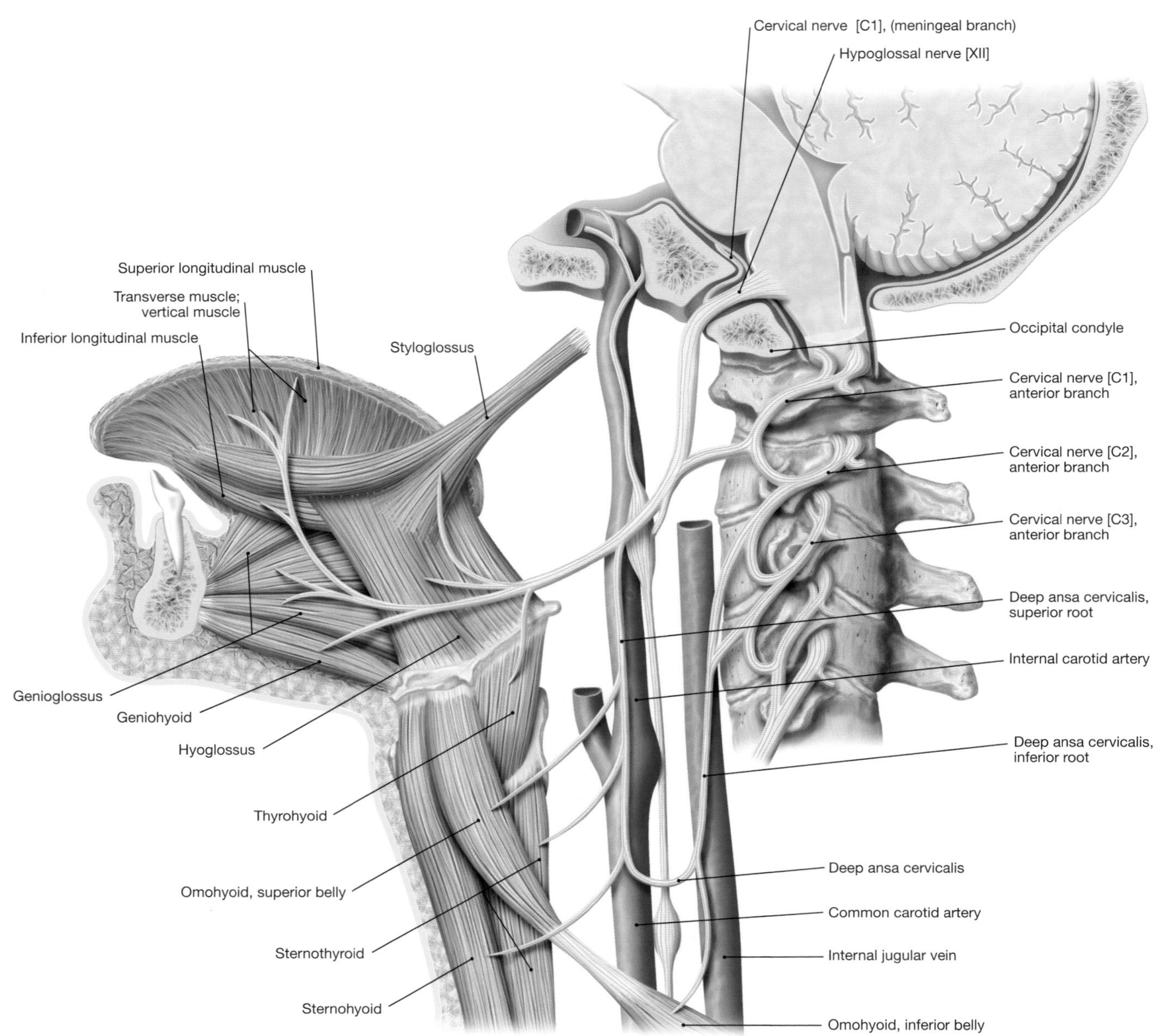
Cervical nerve [C1], (meningeal branch)
Hypoglossal nerve [XII]
Superior longitudinal muscle
Transverse muscle; vertical muscle
Inferior longitudinal muscle
Styloglossus
Occipital condyle
Cervical nerve [C1], anterior branch
Cervical nerve [C2], anterior branch
Cervical nerve [C3], anterior branch
Deep ansa cervicalis, superior root
Internal carotid artery
Genioglossus
Geniohyoid
Hyoglossus
Deep ansa cervicalis, inferior root
Thyrohyoid
Omohyoid, superior belly
Deep ansa cervicalis
Common carotid artery
Sternothyroid
Internal jugular vein
Sternohyoid
Omohyoid, inferior belly

**Fig. 12.162 Hypoglossal nerve [XII]; schematic median section;** view from the left side.

The nucleus of hypoglossal nerve in the medulla oblongata provides the fibers for the hypoglossal nerve [XII]. The fibers exit the brainstem as multiple small bundles between the pyramid and olive in the anterolateral sulcus. They join to form the hypoglossal nerve [XII] which passes through the **hypoglossal canal.** Inferior to the cranial base, fibers of the spinal nerves C1 and C2 accompany the hypoglossal nerve for a short distance and part again, first as superior root (limb) of the **deep ansa cervicalis** and then as a branch to the geniohyoid. Together with fibers from C2 and C3, these fibers form the deep ansa cervicalis and, in addition, innervate the geniohyoid. Posterior to the vagus nerve [X] in the neurovascular bundle behind the pharynx, the hypoglossal nerve [XII] passes caudally and, in an arch-shaped bend of 90°, turns rostrally and medially. It runs at the upper margin of the carotid triangle, crosses the external carotid artery at the branching point of the lingual artery and reaches the tongue between the hyoglossus and mylohyoid. The hypoglossal nerve [XII] innervates all internal muscles of the tongue and the styloglossus, hyoglossus, and genioglossus.

→ T 58l

## Hypoglossal nerve [XII]

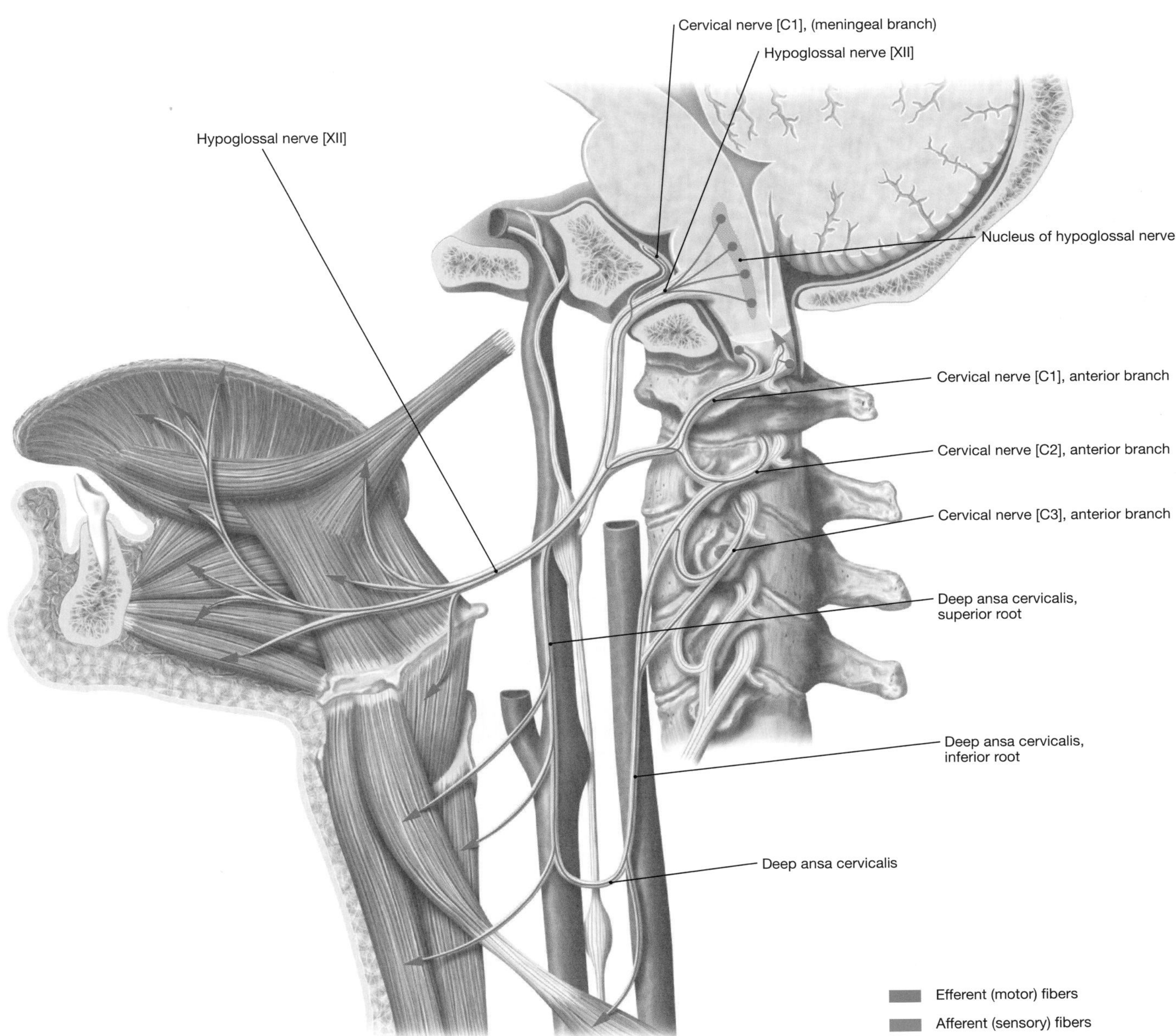
Cervical nerve [C1], (meningeal branch)
Hypoglossal nerve [XII]
Hypoglossal nerve [XII]
Nucleus of hypoglossal nerve
Cervical nerve [C1], anterior branch
Cervical nerve [C2], anterior branch
Cervical nerve [C3], anterior branch
Deep ansa cervicalis, superior root
Deep ansa cervicalis, inferior root
Deep ansa cervicalis
Efferent (motor) fibers
Afferent (sensory) fibers

**Fig. 12.163 Fiber qualities of the hypoglossal nerve [XII];** schematic median section; view from the left side.
The hypoglossal nerve [XII] consists of general somato-efferent fibers (GSE) from the nucleus of hypoglossal nerve and innervates the internal muscles of the tongue and the styloglossus, hyoglossus, and genioglossus.

## Clinical Remarks

A unilateral **lesion of the hypoglossal nerve [XII],** e.g. caused by a fracture of the cranial base, causes the tongue to deviate towards the affected side because the intact lingual muscles of the opposite side push the tongue to the paretic side. In the case of a persistent paralysis of lingual muscles, signs of muscle atrophy are visible on the paretic side. In addition, dysphagia (difficulty in swallowing) and dysarthria (poor articulation) are the result of a paralysis of lingual muscles.

## Spinal cord segments

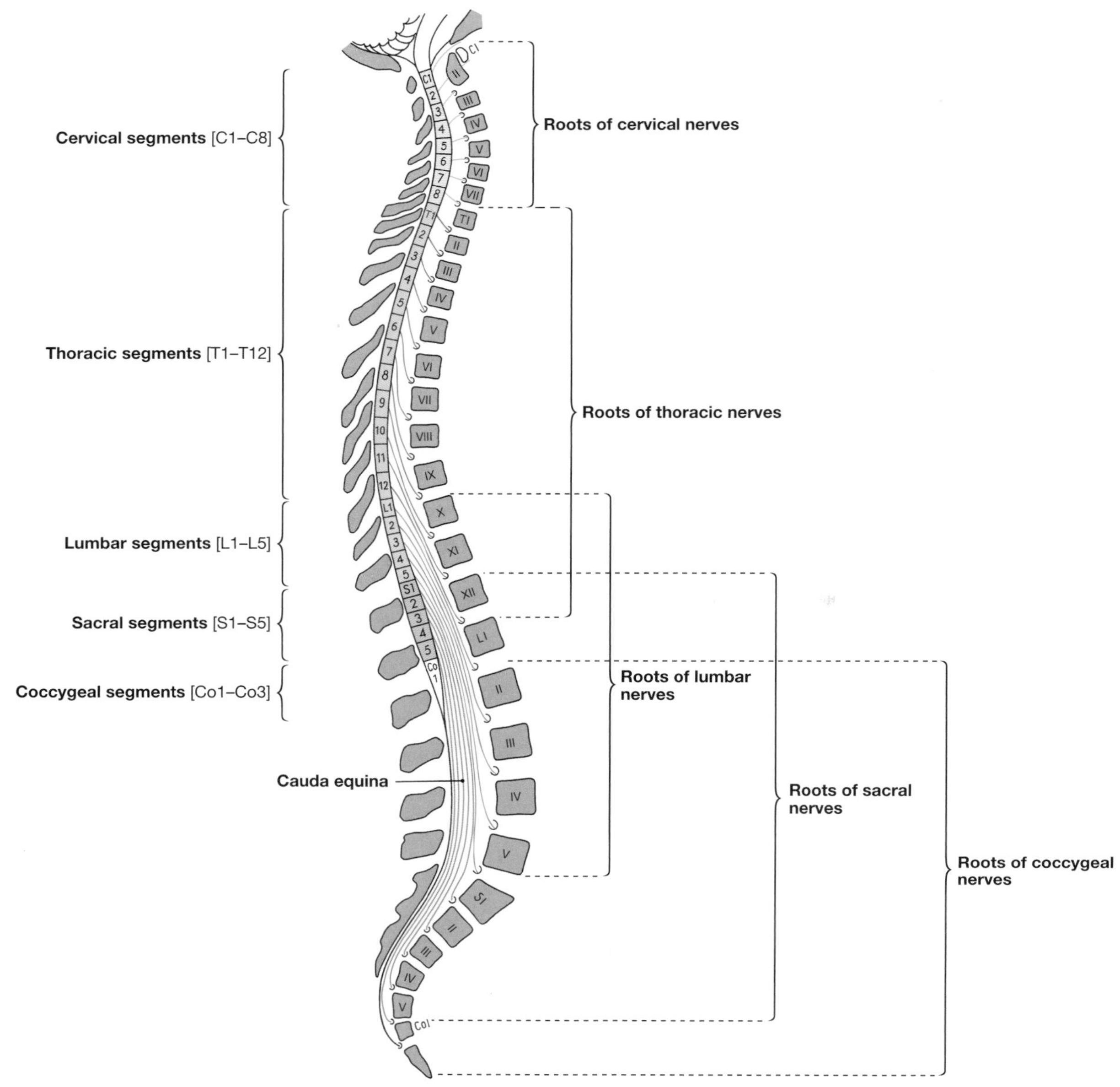
Cervical segments [C1–C8]
Thoracic segments [T1–T12]
Lumbar segments [L1–L5]
Sacral segments [S1–S5]
Coccygeal segments [Co1–Co3]
Cauda equina
Roots of cervical nerves
Roots of thoracic nerves
Roots of lumbar nerves
Roots of sacral nerves
Roots of coccygeal nerves

**Fig. 12.164 Spinal cord segments;** schematic median section; view from the left side; regional segments highlighted in different colors. The spinal cord is composed of eight cervical segments (C1–C8), twelve thoracic segments (T1–T12), five lumbar segments (L1–L5), five sacral segments (S1–S5), and one to three coccygeal segments (Co1–Co3). In the adult, the spinal cord extends only to the level of the lumbar vertebra LI–LII.

As the spinal cord does not follow the faster growth of the vertebral column, the course of the spinal roots towards their corresponding segmental intervertebral foramina becomes steeper and longer from cranial to caudal within the vertebral canal. Below LI–LII the arrangement of spinal nerves in the vertebral canal resembles a horse tail, thus, the name cauda equina.

### Clinical Remarks

Any narrowing of the vertebral canal causes an irritation of the corresponding segmental neurons. Tumors or median disc prolapses inferior to the spinal cord segment S3 can result in a **conus medullaris syndrome** (lesion of spinal cord segments S3–Co3) or **cauda equina syndrome** (CES; lesion of the spinal nerve roots in the area of the cauda equina). The symptoms are sensory deficiencies (saddle anesthesia), flaccid paralysis, incontinence, and impotence.

## Spinal cord segments

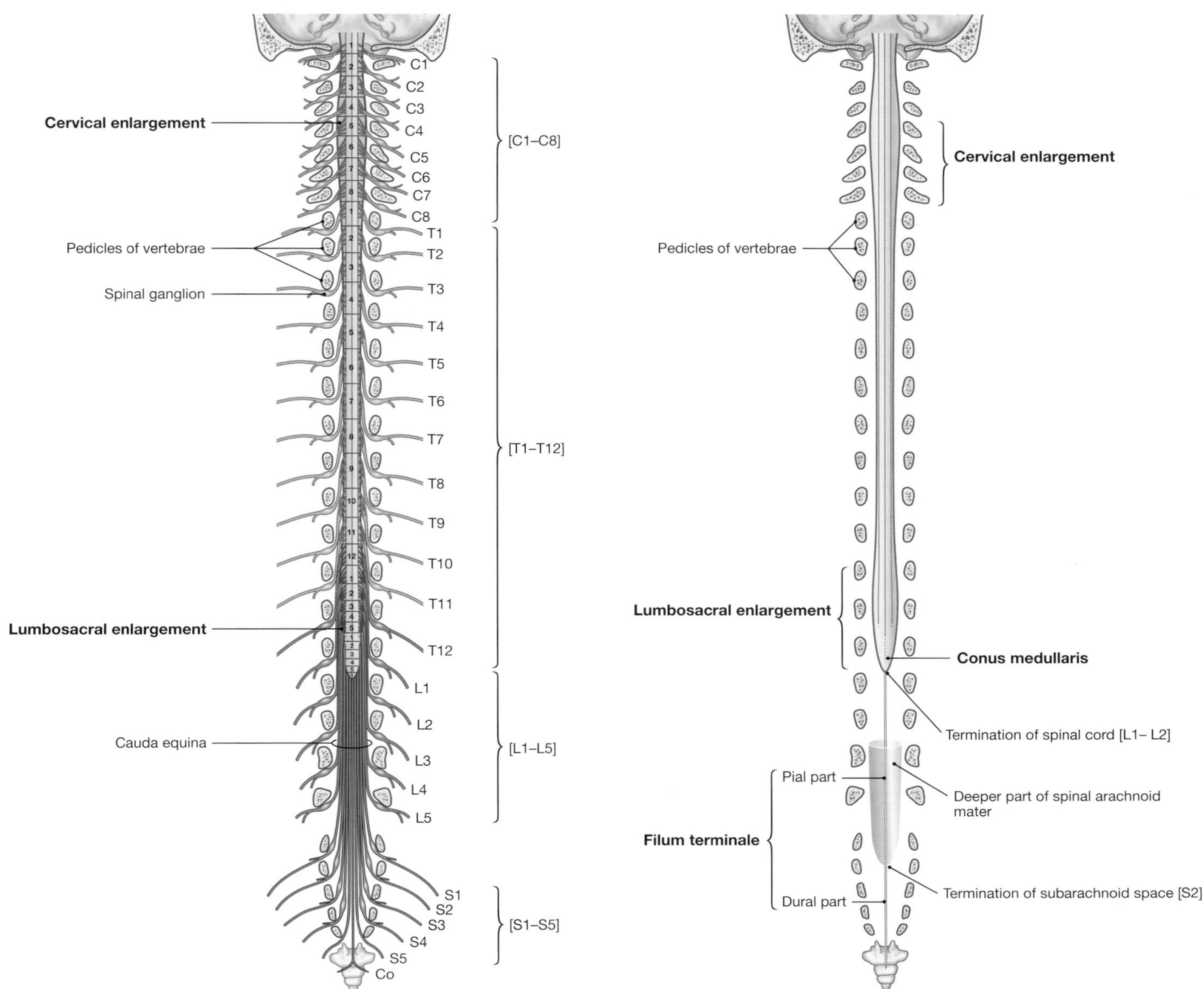
Cervical enlargement
Pedicles of vertebrae
Spinal ganglion
Lumbosacral enlargement
Cauda equina
C1
C2
C3
C4
C5
C6
C7
C8
T1
T2
T3
T4
T5
T6
T7
T8
T9
T10
T11
T12
L1
L2
L3
L4
L5
S1
S2
S3
S4
S5
Co
[C1–C8]
[T1–T12]
[L1–L5]
[S1–S5]
Cervical enlargement
Pedicles of vertebrae
Lumbosacral enlargement
Conus medullaris
Termination of spinal cord [L1– L2]
Pial part
Deeper part of spinal arachnoid mater
Filum terminale
Dural part
Termination of subarachnoid space [S2]

**Fig. 12.165 Spinal cord segments;** schematic frontal section; ventral view. [8]
As the spinal cord does not follow the faster growth of the vertebral column and is much shorter than the vertebral column, the course of the spinal roots towards their corresponding segmental intervertebral foramina becomes steeper and longer from cranial to caudal and more oblique for those fibers located more lateral within the vertebral canal. In adults, the spinal cord ends at the level of LI–LII (ranging from TXII to LII/LIII). Therefore, the anterior and posterior roots locate at higher segments of the vertebral column than the corresponding spinal nerve exiting the vertebral canal. Inferior to the conus medullaris (medullary cone), the anterior and posterior roots of the bundled lumbar, sacral, and coccygeal nerves extend caudally to reach their intervertebral foramina to exit the vertebral canal. This collection of nerve roots is named the cauda equina.

**Fig. 12.166 Spinal cord;** ventral view. [8]
The spinal cord is the part of the CNS located in the upper two-thirds of the vertebral canal. In the adult, it extends from the foramen magnum to approximately the level of LI/LII. In the newborn, the spinal cord reaches to the level of LIII or even LIV. The distal end has the shape of a conus medullaris. This **medullary cone** contains a fine network of connective tissue (filum terminale or terminal filum), derived from parts of the pia mater, which extends caudally into the vertebral canal. The diameter of the spinal cord increases in the areas with spinal nerve roots dedicated for the extremities. The upper **(cervical) enlargement** (C5–T1) contains neurons for the innervation of the upper extremities, the lower **(lumbosacral) enlargement** lies at the level of the spinal nerve roots L1–S3 and serves for the innervation of the lower extremities.

## Somatic and visceral nerve plexuses

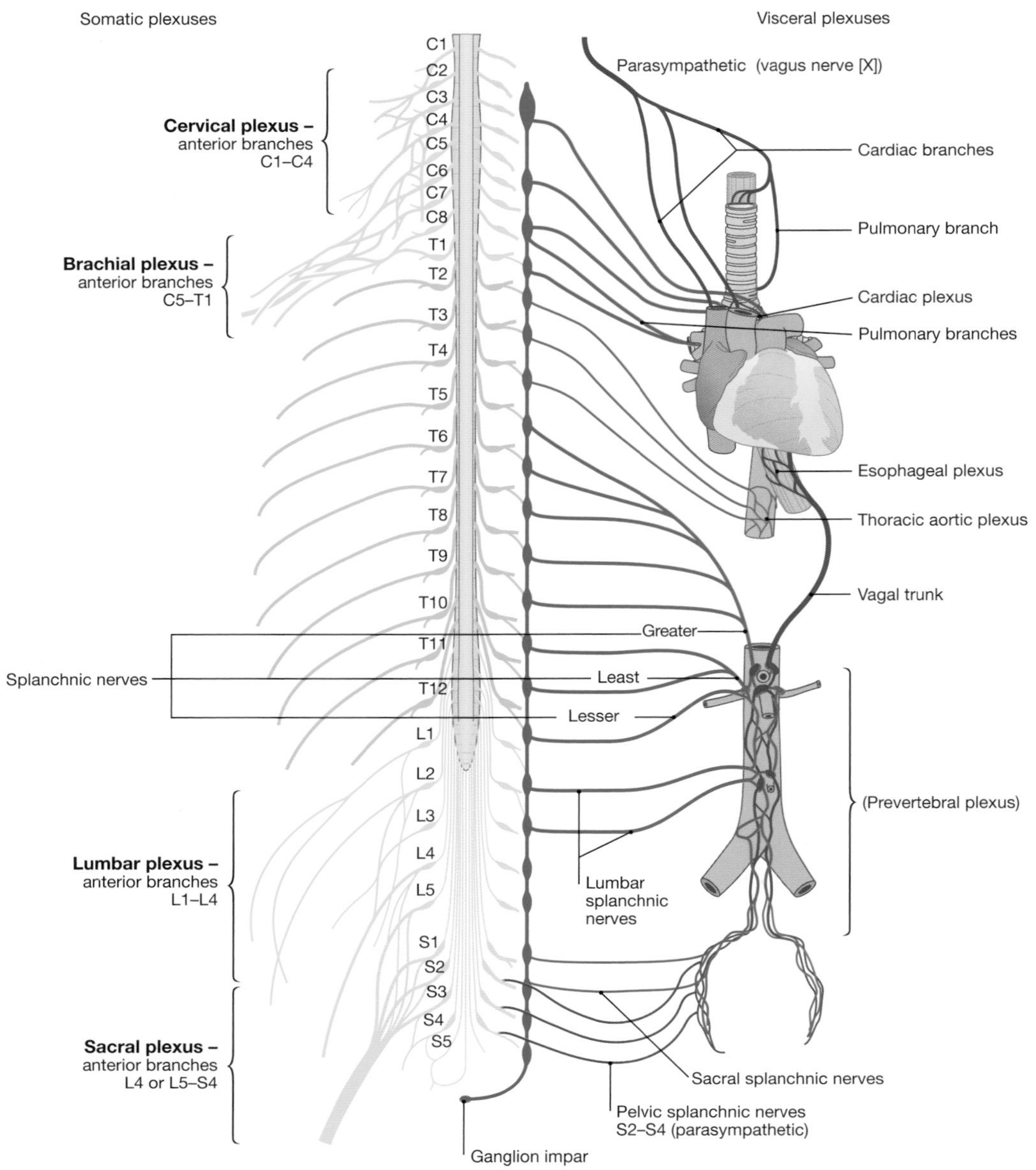
Somatic plexuses
Visceral plexuses
C1
C2
C3
C4
C5
C6
C7
C8
T1
T2
T3
T4
T5
T6
T7
T8
T9
T10
T11
T12
L1
L2
L3
L4
L5
S1
S2
S3
S4
S5
Cervical plexus – anterior branches C1–C4
Brachial plexus – anterior branches C5–T1
Lumbar plexus – anterior branches L1–L4
Sacral plexus – anterior branches L4 or L5–S4
Splanchnic nerves
Parasympathetic (vagus nerve [X])
Cardiac branches
Pulmonary branch
Cardiac plexus
Pulmonary branches
Esophageal plexus
Thoracic aortic plexus
Vagal trunk
Greater
Least
Lesser
(Prevertebral plexus)
Lumbar splanchnic nerves
Sacral splanchnic nerves
Pelvic splanchnic nerves S2–S4 (parasympathetic)
Ganglion impar

**Fig. 12.167 Somatic and visceral nerve plexuses.** [8]
The nature of nerve plexuses can be somatic (left side of the image) or visceral (right side of the image) and include fibers of different qualities and levels. Nerves that originate from a plexus project towards different target tissues and organs. The plexuses of the enteric nervous system can generate reflex activities independent of the CNS.
The extensive **somatic plexuses** ooriginate from the anterior branches of the spinal nerves: cervical plexus (C1–C4), brachial plexus (C5–T1), lumbar plexus (L1–L4), sacral plexus (L4–S4), and coccygeal plexus (S5–Co). With the exception of the spinal nerve T1, all anterior branches of the thoracic spinal nerves are independent and do not participate in the formation of the plexuses.
The **visceral plexuses** form in conjunction with the viscera and normally contain efferent (sympathetic and parasympathetic) and afferent parts. Visceral plexuses are the cardiac and pulmonal plexus in the thorax and the anterior prevertebral plexus to the aorta in the abdominal cavity, which extends caudally to the lateral walls of the pelvis. The prevertebral plexus projects efferent fibers to all abdominal and pelvic organs and receives afferences from the same organs.

### Clinical Remarks

**Referred pain,** sometimes also named reflective pain, is viewed as a misinterpretation by the brain of pain derived from inner organs. In the case of referred pain, visceral pain is not felt at the site of origin but is projected to a distant area of the skin **(HEAD's zone).** Normally, referred pain involves a region with a low number of sensory afferences, such as the intestine. These visceral afferences converge at the same level in the spinal cord with those of a specific cutaneous area that comprises a high number of sensory afferences. The brain erroneously localizes the visceral pain to the corresponding skin area. A typical example is the pain referred into the left shoulder and/or arm during angina pectoris or myocardial infarction.

## Spinal nerves

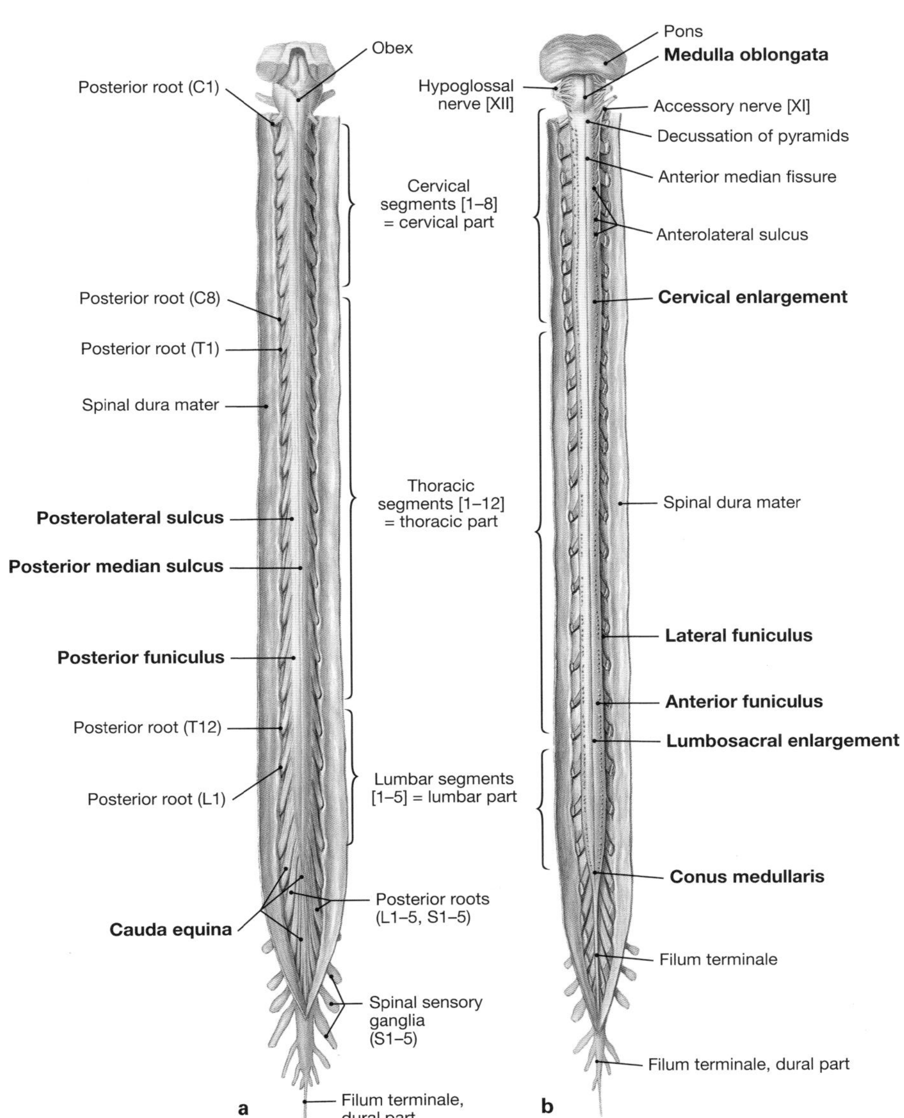
Obex
Posterior root (C1)
Hypoglossal nerve [XII]
Cervical segments [1–8] = cervical part
Posterior root (C8)
Posterior root (T1)
Spinal dura mater
Thoracic segments [1–12] = thoracic part
Posterolateral sulcus
Posterior median sulcus
Posterior funiculus
Posterior root (T12)
Posterior root (L1)
Lumbar segments [1–5] = lumbar part
Posterior roots (L1–5, S1–5)
Cauda equina
Spinal sensory ganglia (S1–5)
Filum terminale, dural part
a
Pons
Medulla oblongata
Accessory nerve [XI]
Decussation of pyramids
Anterior median fissure
Anterolateral sulcus
Cervical enlargement
Spinal dura mater
Lateral funiculus
Anterior funiculus
Lumbosacral enlargement
Conus medullaris
Filum terminale
Filum terminale, dural part
b

**Figs. 12.168a and b Spinal cord and spinal nerves;** the vertebral canal and the dural sac have been opened.
**a** Dorsal view
**b** Ventral view

The spinal cord has the shape of a sword and a diameter of 1–1.5 cm. It extends from the medulla oblongata of the brainstem. Its cervical and lumbar segments increase in diameter to form the cervical enlargement (C5–T1) and the lumbosacral enlargement (L2–S3). These are the location of multiple neurons and nerve fibers concerned mainly with the innervation of the extremities. The conus medullaris is the caudal tip of the spinal cord.

The surface of the spinal cord displays characteristic **longitudinal grooves.** In the midline on the ventral side this is the anterior median fissure and on the posterior side the posterior median sulcus. The anterior funiculus located to both sides of the anterior median fissure, is followed by the ventrolateral sulcus which separates the anterior funiculus from the lateralis funiculus. On the dorsal side and bilaterally to the posterior median sulcus are the posterior funiculi. The latter are separated from the lateral funiculi by the posterolateral sulci.

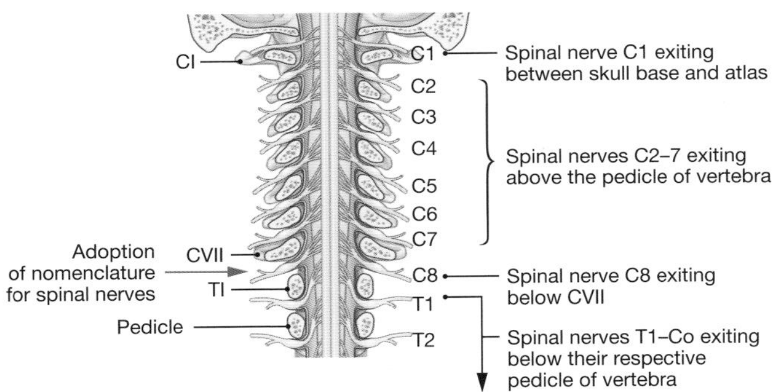
CI
C1
Spinal nerve C1 exiting between skull base and atlas
C2
C3
C4
C5
C6
C7
Spinal nerves C2–7 exiting above the pedicle of vertebra
Adoption of nomenclature for spinal nerves
CVII
TI
C8
Spinal nerve C8 exiting below CVII
T1
T2
Pedicle
Spinal nerves T1–Co exiting below their respective pedicle of vertebra

**Fig. 12.169 Nomenclature of the spinal nerves.** [8]
In contrast to the other spinal cord segments, the number of spinal cord segments in the **cervical spinal cord** is not identical with the number of vertebrae. The cervical region has eight cervical segments but only seven cervical vertebrae. The first pair of cervical nerves exits between the cranial base and the atlas (CI vertebra). The spinal nerve pairs C2–C7 each exit **superior** to the corresponding pedicle of vertebral arch. At the transition from the 7th cervical vertebra to the 1st thoracic vertebra, the nomenclature changes since the 8th spinal nerve exits inferior to the 7th cervical vertebra. All pairs of spinal nerves T1–Co that follow will always exit **inferior** to the corresponding vertebral arch.

## Arteries of the spinal cord

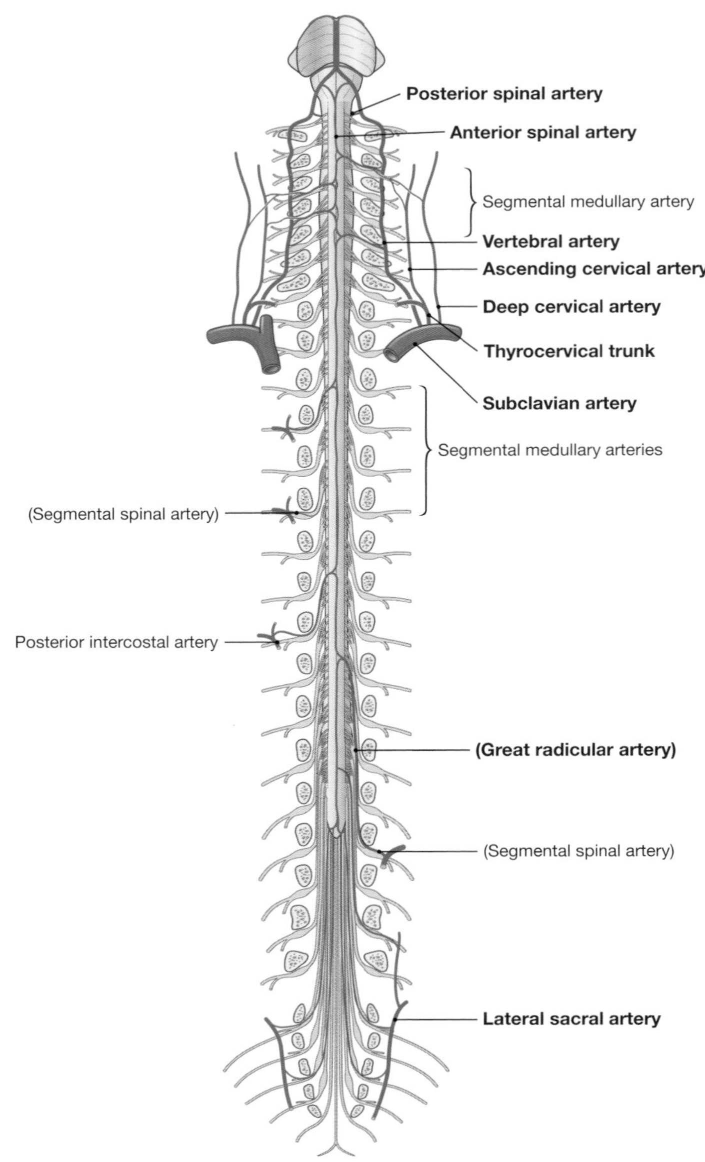
Posterior spinal artery
Anterior spinal artery
Segmental medullary artery
Vertebral artery
Ascending cervical artery
Deep cervical artery
Thyrocervical trunk
Subclavian artery
Segmental medullary arteries
(Segmental spinal artery)
Posterior intercostal artery
(Great radicular artery)
(Segmental spinal artery)
Lateral sacral artery

**Fig. 12.170 Arteries of the spinal cord;** ventral view; not all segmental spinal arteries are shown. [8]
There are three sources of arterial supply for the spinal cord:
- through the **subclavian artery** (cervical) via the anterior spinal artery and anterior and posterior radicular branches from the vertebral arteries, the ascending cervical artery, and the deep cervical artery
- through the **thoracic aorta** (thoracic part) via the supreme intercostal artery and the posterior intercostal arteries
- through the **abdominal aorta** (lumbosacral part) via lumbar arteries

The internal iliac artery supplies the cauda equina through the iliolumbar artery and the lateralis sacral artery. All these arteries provide spinal branches.
The largest spinal branch is the great radicular artery (artery of ADAMKIEWICZ; vertebra TXII–LII) which is usually found on the left side of the body.

## Clinical Remarks

The anterior spinal artery (supply area → Fig. 12.171) can be occluded by thrombosis, tumors, etc. This results in an **anterior spinal artery syndrome.** Damage of the anterior horns occurs at the level of the occlusion, resulting in a flaccid paresis of the muscles and muscles parts innervated by the corresponding spinal cord segment. Simultaneously, the tracts in the anterolateral funiculus become nonfunctional. Those body regions innervated by the spinal cord segments below the site of injury will display spastic parapareses, loss of pain and temperature perception but preservation of touch, vibration, and postural sensation, as well as deficits in micturition, defecation, and sexual functions.
Blockage of the blood supply from the largest of the anterior radicular vessels, the great radicular artery (artery of ADAMKIEWICZ), results in a **greater radicular artery syndrome.** Depending on the level of the blockage, paraplegia in the lower thoracic or upper lumbar regions with complete loss of the entire caudally located spinal cord functions is observed.

## Arteries and meninges of the spinal cord

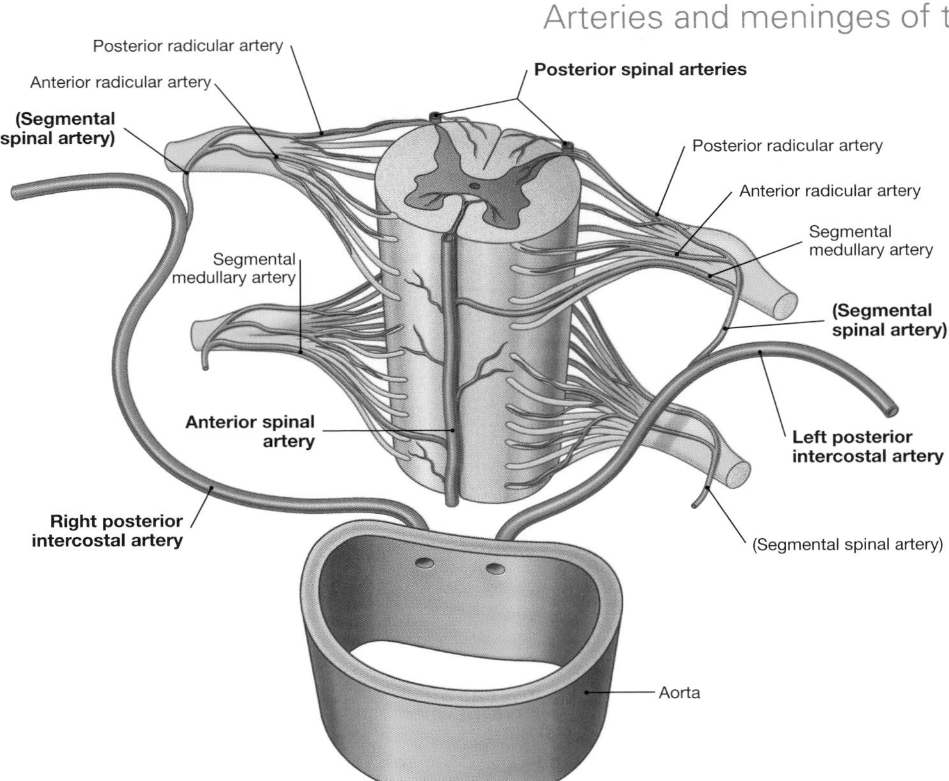
Posterior radicular artery
Anterior radicular artery
(Segmental spinal artery)
Posterior spinal arteries
Posterior radicular artery
Anterior radicular artery
Segmental medullary artery
Segmental medullary artery
(Segmental spinal artery)
Anterior spinal artery
Left posterior intercostal artery
Right posterior intercostal artery
(Segmental spinal artery)
Aorta

**Fig. 12.171 Segmental arterial supply of the spinal cord.** [8]
Blood supply to the spinal cord is achieved through the **anterior spinal artery** and the **posterior spinal arteries,** longitudinal blood vessels running alongside the spinal cord which originate in the cervical region. Additional contributors are feeder arteries (spinal segmental arteries from the vertebral arteries, the deep cervical arteries, the intercostal arteries and the lumbar arteries) which enter the vertebral canal through the intervertebral foramina and divide into **anterior** and **posterior radicular branches** at the level of each spinal cord plane. The anterior and posterior radicular branches follow the spinal nerves and supply them with blood. At different planes, the spinal segmental arteries release segmental **medullary arteries** which project to and anastomose with the longitudinal arteries.

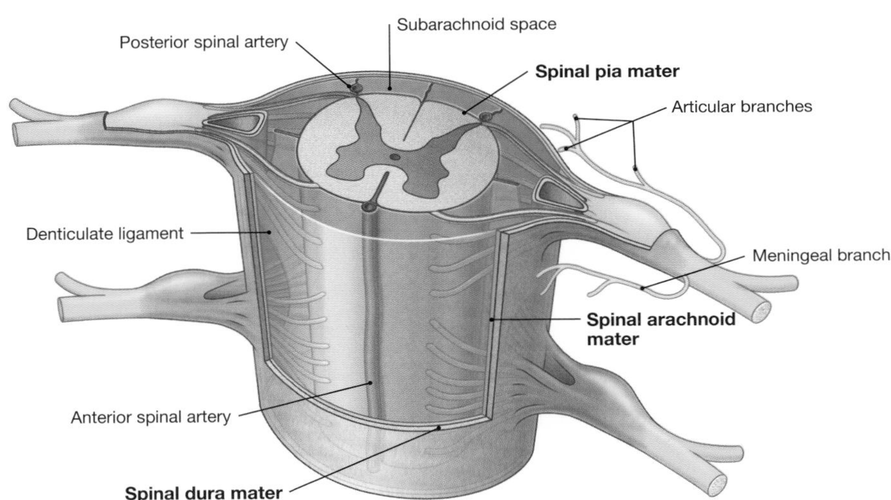
Posterior spinal artery
Subarachnoid space
Spinal pia mater
Articular branches
Denticulate ligament
Meningeal branch
Spinal arachnoid mater
Anterior spinal artery
Spinal dura mater

**Fig. 12.172 Meninges of the spinal cord;** oblique ventral view. [8]
Like the brain, the spinal cord is surrounded by the three meninges, which provide protection and suspension of this CNS structure within the vertebral canal.
The **spinal dura mater** is the strongest of the three meninges and is located farthest to the outside. The laterally exiting spinal nerves and their roots are surrounded by a tubular dural sheath which radiates into and fuses with the nerve sheath (epineurium) of the spinal nerves. Inside the dura follows the spinal arachnoid mater which is separated from the spinal pia mater by the subarachnoid space filled with cerebrospinal fluid (CSF). Delicate trabeculations (arachnoid trabeculae, not shown) connect the spinal arachnoid mater of one side with the spinal pia mater on the other side. This connective tissue also surrounds the blood vessels located within the subarachnoid space.
The **spinal pia mater** is a membrane rich in blood vessels and tightly attached to the surface of the spinal cord. It extends deeply into the anterior median fissure, creates a sheath-like lining around the anterior and posterior roots of the spinal nerves and accompanies them on their way through the subarachnoid space.
In the exit and entry areas of the radices, the spinal pia mater transitions into the **spinal arachnoid mater.** The denticulate ligaments are lateral extensions of the spinal pia mater to the spinal arachnoid and dura mater along both sides of the spinal cord. They serve to attach the spinal cord in the center of the subarachnoid space.

## Venous plexus of the spinal cord

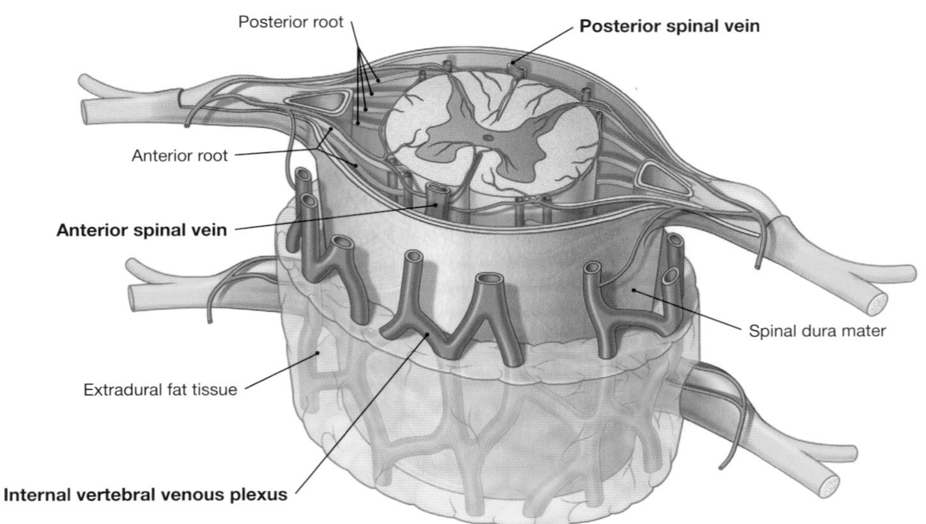
Posterior root
Posterior spinal vein
Anterior root
Anterior spinal vein
Spinal dura mater
Extradural fat tissue
Internal vertebral venous plexus

**Fig. 12.173 Veins of the vertebral canal;** oblique ventral view. [8]
The veins draining the spinal cord mainly form longitudinal collecting vessels running alongside the spinal cord. Two pairs of longitudinal veins group around the exit and entry points of the anterior root and posterior root out of and into the spinal cord, respectively. In addition, the **anterior spinal vein** and **posterior spinal vein** course alongside the anterior median fissure and the posterior median sulcus, respectively. These veins drain into the **internal vertebral venous plexus** in the epidural space of the vertebral canal. The venous plexus connects with segmental veins which, like the azygos system, drain into the large collecting veins of the body. The internal vertebral venos plexus also communicates with intracranial veins.

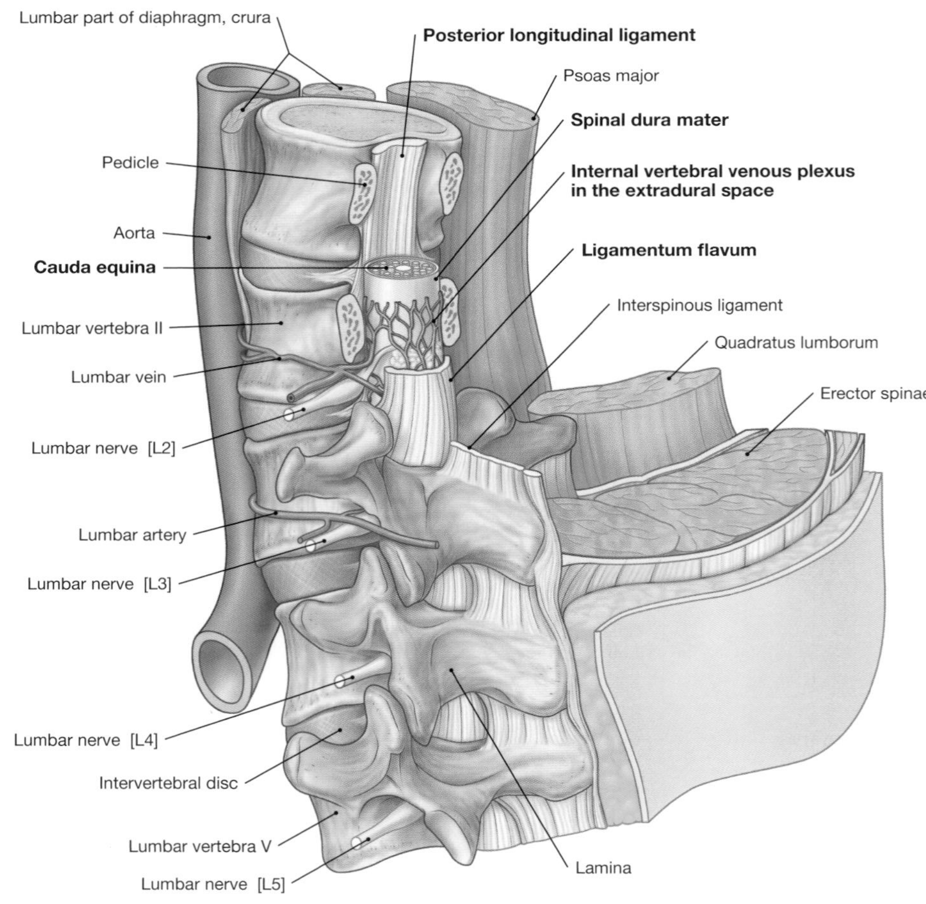
Lumbar part of diaphragm, crura
Posterior longitudinal ligament
Psoas major
Spinal dura mater
Pedicle
Internal vertebral venous plexus in the extradural space
Aorta
Ligamentum flavum
Cauda equina
Interspinous ligament
Quadratus lumborum
Lumbar vertebra II
Erector spinae
Lumbar vein
Lumbar nerve [L2]
Lumbar artery
Lumbar nerve [L3]
Lumbar nerve [L4]
Intervertebral disc
Lumbar vertebra V
Lamina
Lumbar nerve [L5]

**Fig. 12.174 Position of the spinal cord within the vertebral canal;** dorsolateral view. [8]
The dural tube positions ventral to the posterior longitudinal ligament and is surrounded by the internal vertebral venos plexus. The vertebral arches of the first two lumbar vertebrae have been removed. The topographic relationship of the nerve root to the intervertebral disc below the spinal nerve L2 is shown. The ligamentum flavum provides the dorsal cover for the dural tube.

Clinics

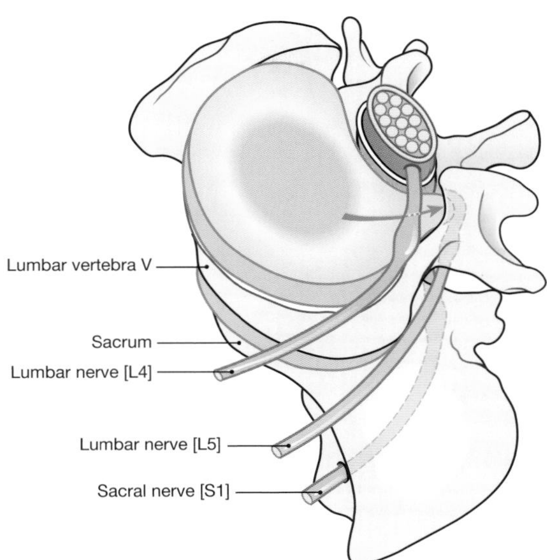
Lumbar vertebra V
Sacrum
Lumbar nerve [L4]
Lumbar nerve [L5]
Sacral nerve [S1]

**Fig. 12.175 Schematic representation of a mediolateral herniation of the intervertebral disc between the 4th and 5th lumbar vertebrae;** lateroventral superior view. [23]

This disc prolapse results in the compression of the spinal nerve root L5 located one segment below; the more medially positioned L4 root exiting in the same segment remains unaffected.

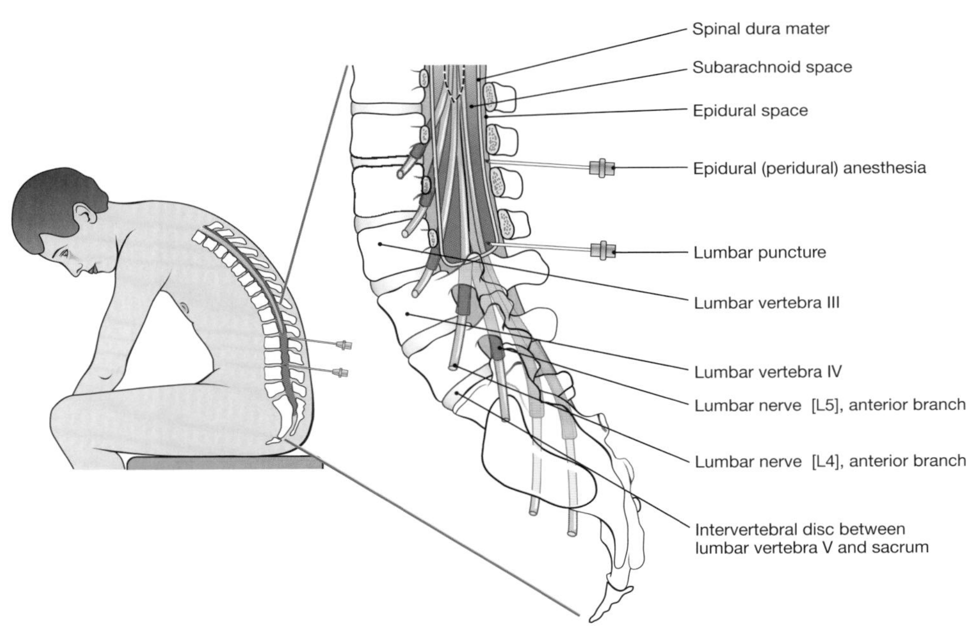
Spinal dura mater
Subarachnoid space
Epidural space
Epidural (peridural) anesthesia
Lumbar puncture
Lumbar vertebra III
Lumbar vertebra IV
Lumbar nerve [L5], anterior branch
Lumbar nerve [L4], anterior branch
Intervertebral disc between
lumbar vertebra V and sacrum

**Fig. 12.176 Epidural (peridural) anesthesia and spinal anesthesia.** [23]

Anesthetics are injected into the epidural space (epidural or peridural anesthesia) to anesthetize individual spinal nerves. The local adipose tissue prevents the anesthetic from affecting other spinal cord segments.

In contrast to the epidural anesthesia, in **spinal anesthesia** the anesthetics are applied directly into the subarachnoid space. The medication mixes with the cerebrospinal fluid but, as a result of g-force, remains below the injection site (in an upright sitting patient) and, thus, exclusively anesthetizes nerve fibers located below the injection site.

For **lumbar puncture,** the back must be maximally bent forward and the needle is inserted between the spinous processes of the lumbar vertebrae III and IV or IV and V. Then, the needle is pushed forward carefully until the spinal dura mater is punctured and the tip of the needle rests in the subarachnoid space. Now, cerebrospinal fluid (CSF) can be drawn for diagnostic purposes or an anesthetic can be applied.

## Spinal cord and vertebral canal, imaging

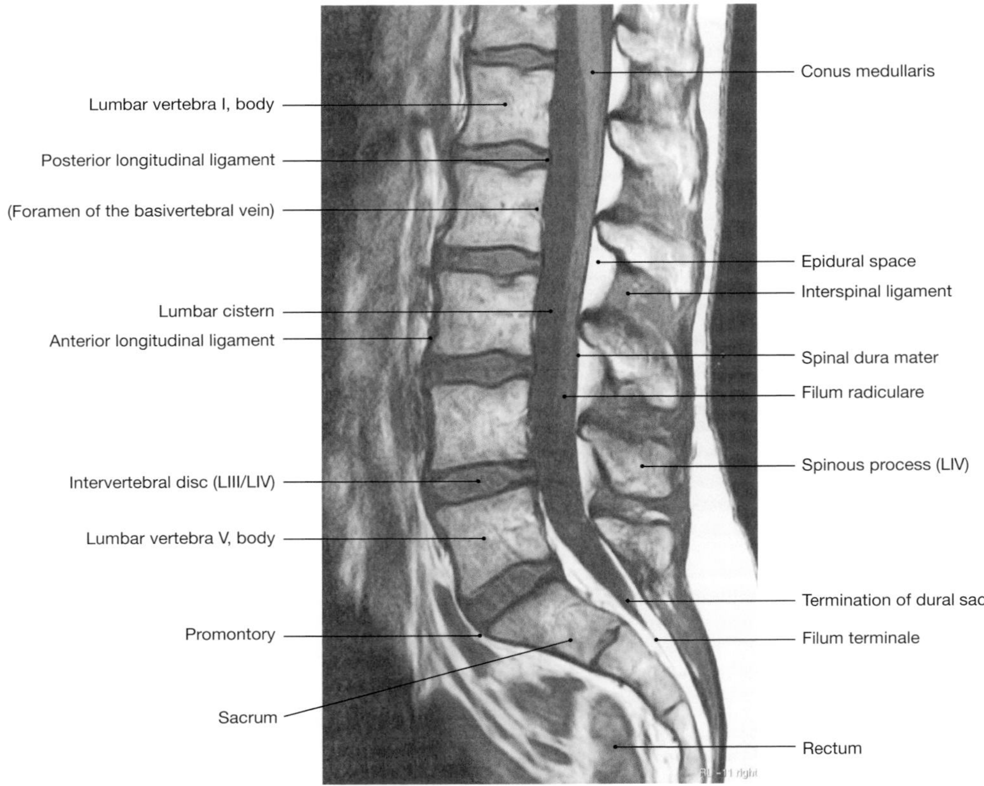
Lumbar vertebra I, body
Posterior longitudinal ligament
(Foramen of the basivertebral vein)
Lumbar cistern
Anterior longitudinal ligament
Intervertebral disc (LIII/LIV)
Lumbar vertebra V, body
Promontory
Sacrum
Conus medullaris
Epidural space
Interspinal ligament
Spinal dura mater
Filum radiculare
Spinous process (LIV)
Termination of dural sac
Filum terminale
Rectum

**Fig. 12.177 Lumbar part of the vertebral column;** magnetic resonance tomographic image (MRI), T1-weighted; median section of the lumbar and lower thoracic parts of the vertebral column. [27]

The border between the end of the spinal cord at the level of LI/LII and the beginning of the cauda equina, which only partially occupies the vertebral canal, is clearly visible.

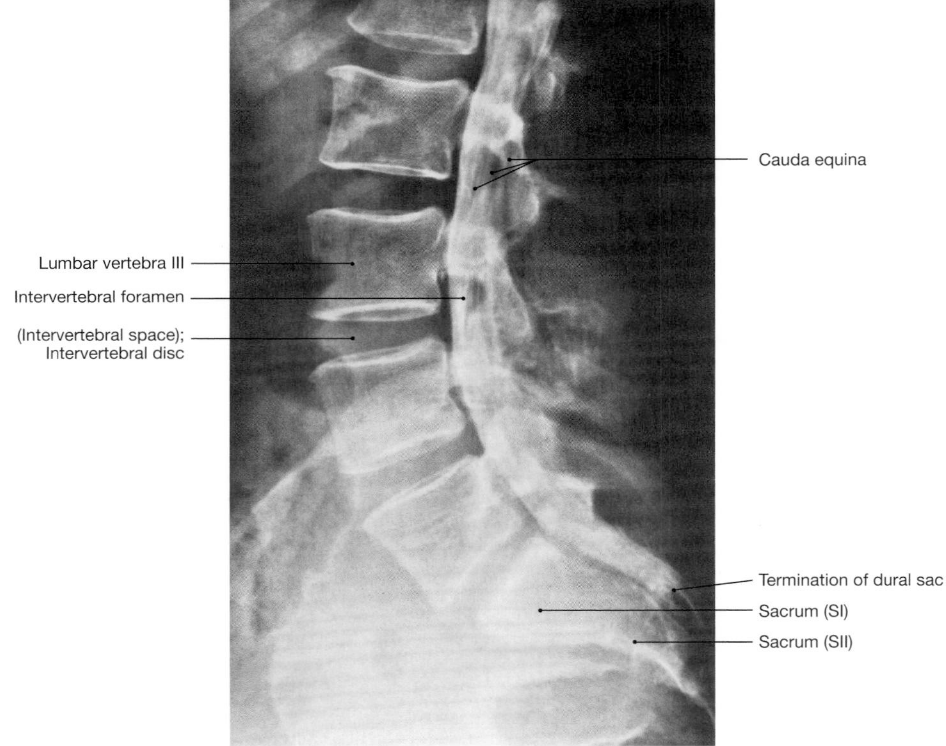
Cauda equina
Lumbar vertebra III
Intervertebral foramen
(Intervertebral space); Intervertebral disc
Termination of dural sac
Sacrum (SI)
Sacrum (SII)

**Fig. 12.178 Myelography of the lumbosacral transition;** radiograph in lateral beam projection. [27]
The contrast medium has distributed within the subarachnoid space.

The dural sac (subarachnoid space) terminates at the level of the 2nd sacral vertebra (SII).

Clinics

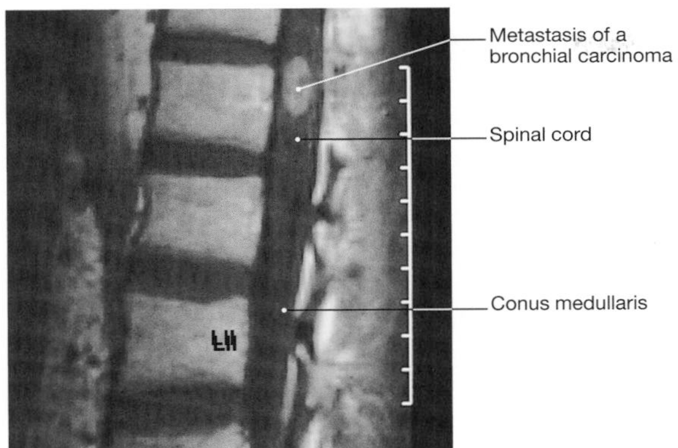
Metastasis of a bronchial carcinoma
Spinal cord
Conus medullaris

**Fig. 12.179 Vertebral canal with spinal cord;** magnetic resonance tomographic image (MRI); median section of the lower thoracic and lumbar parts of the vertebral column, paraplegia due to a spinal tumor. [23]
In the MRI images, the tumor presents as a white mass against the surrounding spinal cord. This is a metastasis of a known bronchial carcinoma. The patient was admitted with complete paraplegia of the lower extremities and loss of all sensory functions below dermatome L2.

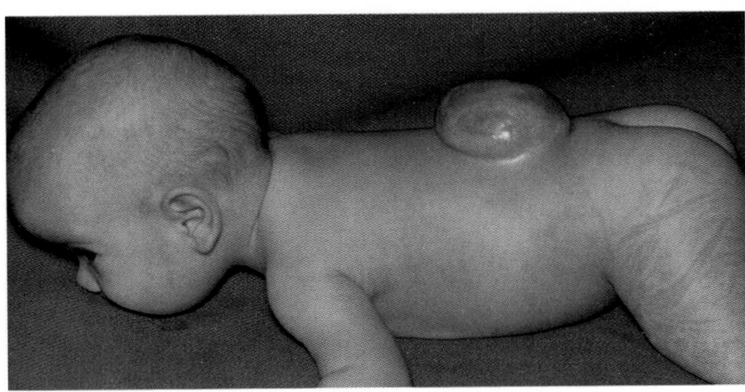

**Fig. 12.180 Spina bifida cystica.** [20]
Infant with spina bifida cystica (meningomyelocele) in the lumbar region.

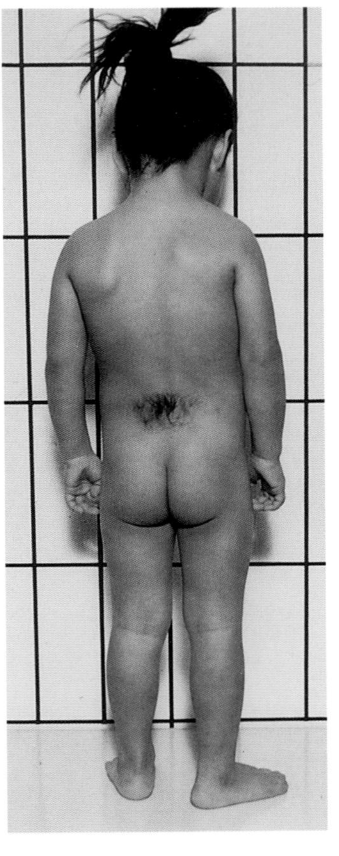

**Fig. 12.181 Spina bifida occulta.** [20]
The hairy skin area in the lumbosacral region is the visible sign of the underlying spina bifida occulta.

## Clinical Remarks

**Damage or compression of the spinal cord** can be caused by intramedullary (→ Fig. 12.179) or extramedullary tumors, medial disc prolapses, dorsal spondylophytes, or traumatic injury. A complete paraplegia results in the loss of all qualities of sensation, motor function, and autonomic functions below the site of the lesion. In the early stages, a flaccid paralysis develops below the lesion (spinal shock), which then converts into a spastic paralysis.
The **BROWN-SÉQUARD's syndrome** describes a spinal hemiplegia with spastic paresis below the site of the lesion plus a dissociated impairment of sensor functions with loss of proprioception, vibration and epicritic sensibility (dorsal tracts) on the site of the injury and loss in pain and temperature sensation on the contralateral side (lateral tracts; → Fig. 12.192).
**Spina bifida** is a congenital defective closure of the vertebral column and spinal cord caused by teratogenic factors (e.g. alcohol, medication) or missing induction of the chorda dorsalis.

The **spina bifida occulta** is the mildest form (→ Fig. 12.181) and exclusively involves the vertebral arches. In most cases, unfused arches are found in one or two vertebrae and the corresponding overlying skin is often covered with hair and is more intensely pigmented. Usually, these patients show no symptoms.
In the case of a **spina bifida cystica** (→ Fig. 12.180), the vertebral arches of a number of neighboring vertebrae are not closed; a cyst-like protrusion of the spinal meninges extends into the defect (meningocele). A meningomyelocele exists if the meningeal cyst contains spinal cord and nerves (coincides with functional deficits).
**Spina bifida aperta** (rachischisis, myeloschisis) is the most severe form of spina bifida with underlying defect in the proper closure of the neural folds. With no skin cover to protect it, the undifferentiated neural plate is exposed on the back. Newborns with such defects usually die shortly after birth.

## Spinal cord, sections

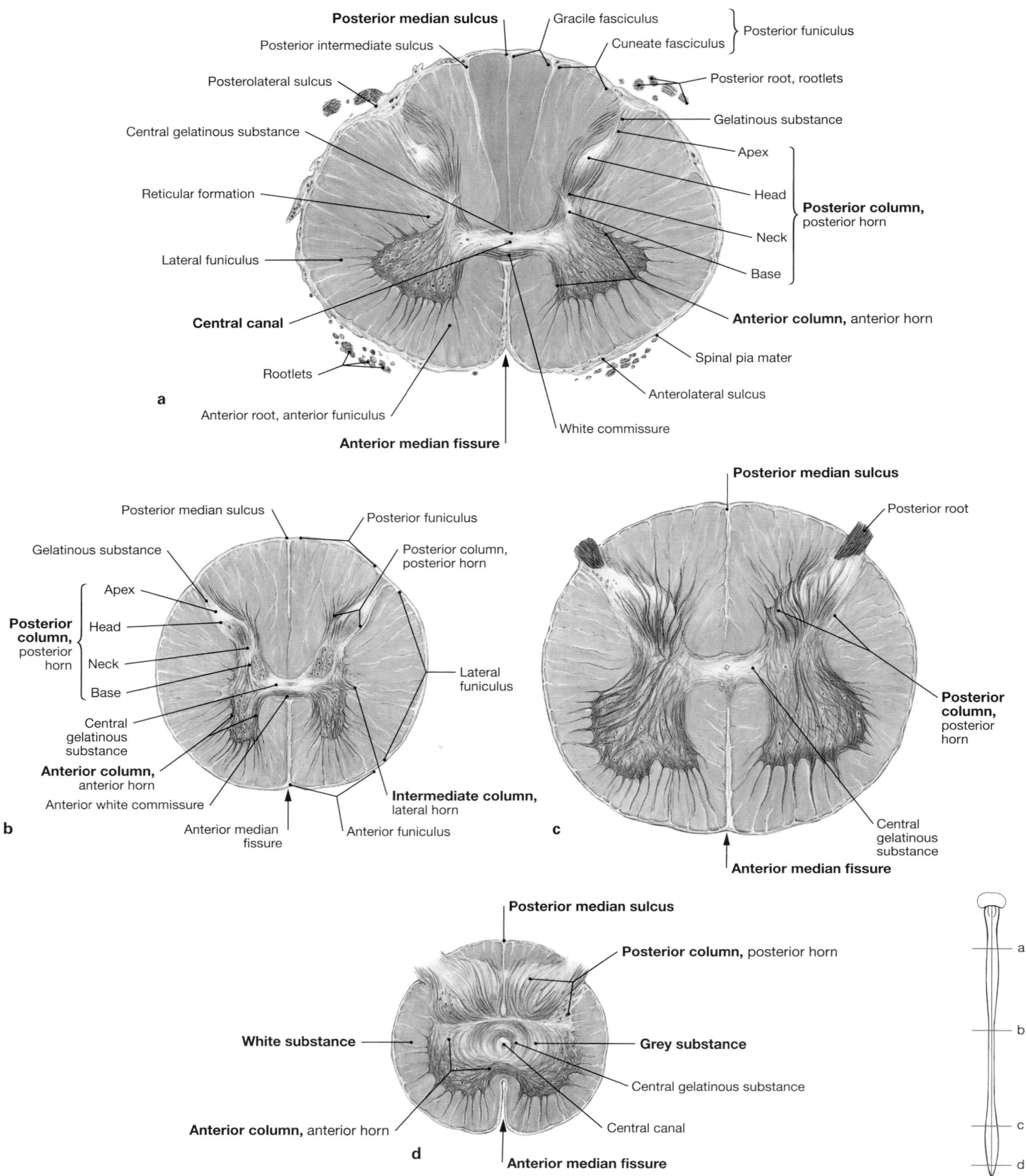

Posterior median sulcus
Gracile fasciculus
Cuneate fasciculus
Posterior funiculus
Posterior intermediate sulcus
Posterolateral sulcus
Posterior root, rootlets
Gelatinous substance
Central gelatinous substance
Apex
Head
Posterior column, posterior horn
Reticular formation
Neck
Base
Lateral funiculus
Anterior column, anterior horn
Central canal
Spinal pia mater
Rootlets
Anterolateral sulcus
a
Anterior root, anterior funiculus
White commissure
Anterior median fissure
Posterior median sulcus
Posterior funiculus
Gelatinous substance
Posterior column, posterior horn
Apex
Posterior column, posterior horn
Head
Neck
Base
Lateral funiculus
Central gelatinous substance
Anterior column, anterior horn
Intermediate column, lateral horn
Anterior white commissure
b
Anterior median fissure
Anterior funiculus
Posterior median sulcus
Posterior root
Posterior column, posterior horn
c
Central gelatinous substance
Anterior median fissure
Posterior median sulcus
Posterior column, posterior horn
White substance
Grey substance
Central gelatinous substance
Anterior column, anterior horn
Central canal
d
Anterior median fissure
a
b
c
d


**Figs. 12.182a to d Spinal cord;** cross-sections; myelin stain; approximately 500%.
**a** Cervical part
**b** Thoracic part
**c** Lumbar part
**d** Sacral part

The spinal cord has a symmetrical mirror-image structure and all spinal cord segments (**a–d**) consist of gray and white matter. The **gray matter** consists mainly of the perikarya of neurons, it has the shape of a butterfly in cross-sectional images, and is surrounded by **white matter.** The latter is mainly composed of neuronal fibers and glia cells and divides into tracts (funiculi). The center of the butterfly structure contains the **central canal.** Although part of the inner CSF space, this canal has a caudal blind end, preventing the circulation of the cerebrospinal fluid. The wings of the butterfly represent **columns:** an anterior (ventral) column, an intermediate column (zone), and a posterior (dorsal) column. These columns form the anterior (ventral) horn, lateral horn, and posterior (dorsal) horn. The gray commissures (not shown) connect the intermediate columns from both sides.

## Functional organization of the spinal cord

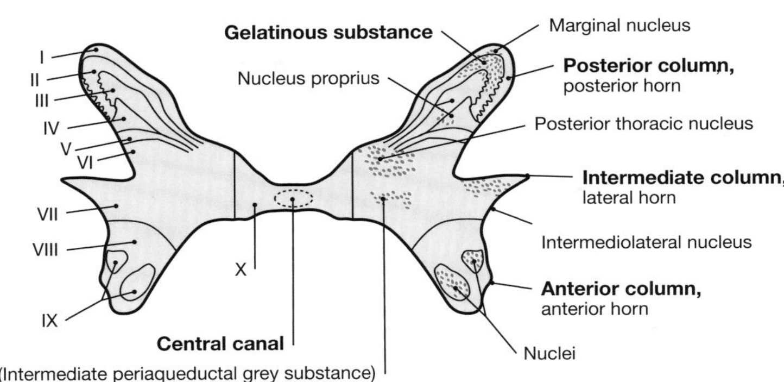
Gelatinous substance
Marginal nucleus
Nucleus proprius
Posterior column,
posterior horn
Posterior thoracic nucleus
Intermediate column,
lateral horn
Intermediolateral nucleus
Anterior column,
anterior horn
Nuclei
Central canal
(Intermediate periaqueductal grey substance)
I
II
III
IV
V
VI
VII
VIII
IX
X

**Fig. 12.183 Spinal cord;** laminar organization of the gray matter according to its cytoarchitecture [according to REXED, 1952], exemplified by the tenth thoracic segment (T10).
Histologically (cytoarchitecturally), the gray matter divides into a number of **layers** (spinal laminae) which are numbered I to X from dorsal to ventral (extent and number of the layers vary in different segments of the spinal cord). In addition, various **nuclei** are distinguished and can stretch over more than one cytoarchitectural neuronal layer. The structure of the spinal laminae reflects functional aspects.

The paired **posterior (dorsal) horns** (spinal laminae I–VI: posterior (dorsal) thoracic nucleus [CLARKE's column], nucleus proprius, gelatinous substance) contain relais neurons for the transmission of afferent sensory input (sensory information from the skin, proprioceptive information, perception of pain from the periphery). The **two lateral horns** (spinal lamina VII) harbor neurons (intermediolateral nucleus) for autonomic efferences. The paired **anterior (ventral) horns** form the anterior (ventral) columns (spinal laminae VIII, IX) and contain the efferent neurons (somato-efferent root cells) for the muscles.

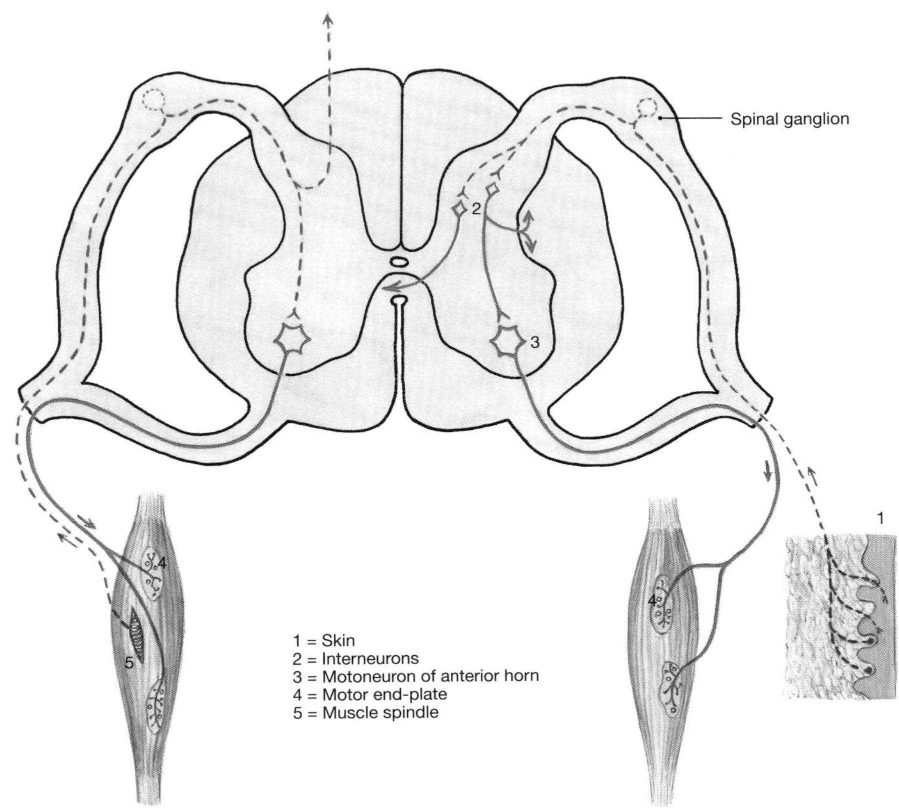
Spinal ganglion
1
2
3
4
5
1 = Skin
2 = Interneurons
3 = Motoneuron of anterior horn
4 = Motor end-plate
5 = Muscle spindle

**Fig. 12.184 Reflexes of the spinal cord.**
The spinal cord contains a **system that connects it with supraspinal centers** and a **local autonomic system** capable of eliciting spinal reflexes without the input from supraspinal neuronal structures. Spinal reflexes for example are important in keeping an adequate muscle tonus during different activities or to protect against harmful stimuli (e.g. withdrawal reflex from a painful stimulus).
The type of connectivity and complexity distinguishes two forms of **reflex circuitry:** monosynaptic and polysynaptic reflexes. Supraspinal centers can modify polysynaptic reflexes.

Left side of the image: reflex circuitry of a monosynaptic, bineuronal, proprioceptive reflex (a typical stretch reflex like the knee-jerk [(patellar)] reflex, etc., collectively named myotactic or deep tendon reflexes [DTRs]).
Right side of the image: complex reflex circuitry of a polysynaptic, polyneuronal reflex (typical flexor or withdrawal reflexes are initiated by cutaneous receptors and include the abdominal, cremaster reflex, foot sole reflex etc.).

## Functional organization of the spinal cord

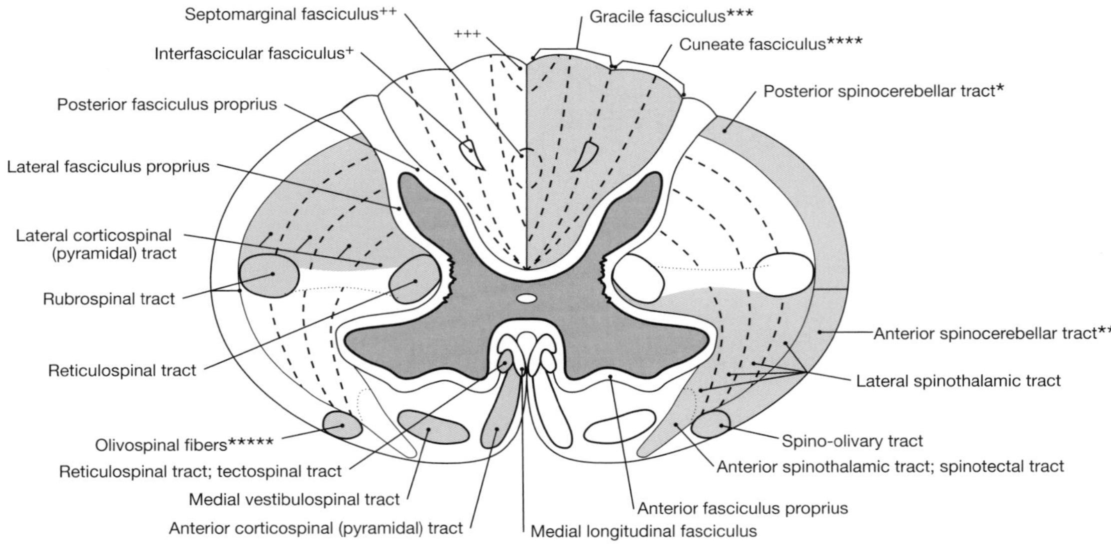
Septomarginal fasciculus++
+++
Gracile fasciculus***
Cuneate fasciculus****
Interfascicular fasciculus+
Posterior spinocerebellar tract*
Posterior fasciculus proprius
Lateral fasciculus proprius
Lateral corticospinal (pyramidal) tract
Rubrospinal tract
Anterior spinocerebellar tract**
Reticulospinal tract
Lateral spinothalamic tract
Olivospinal fibers*****
Spino-olivary tract
Reticulospinal tract; tectospinal tract
Anterior spinothalamic tract; spinotectal tract
Medial vestibulospinal tract
Anterior fasciculus proprius
Anterior corticospinal (pyramidal) tract
Medial longitudinal fasciculus

**Fig. 12.185 Spinal cord;** schematic organization of the white matter exemplified by a lower cervical segment.
Afferent (= ascending) pathways in blue; efferent (= descending) pathways in red.
The regions indicated with +, ++, and +++ designate descending collateral tracts of the posterior fasciculi.

* clinical term: FLECHSIG's tract
** clinical term: GOWERS' tract
*** clinical term: GOLLS' tract
**** clinical term: BURDACH's tract
***** The actual existence of these fibers has not definitely been documented.
\+ SCHULTZE's comma tract (cervical part)
\++ oval bundle of FLECHSIG (thoracic part)
\+++ triangle of PHILIPPE-GOMBAULT (lumbar and sacral parts)

**Important Stretch Reflexes of the Spinal Cord** [14]

| Reflex | Segment | Reflex Trigger | Target Organ | Nerve (afferent and efferent limb) |
|---|---|---|---|---|
| Biceps | C5, C6 | Tapping the biceps tendon | Biceps brachii | Musculocutaneus nerve |
| Brachioradialis | C5, C6 | Tapping the brachioradialis insertion tendon or the periosteum | Brachioradialis, brachialis, biceps brachii | Radial nerve, musculocutaneus nerve |
| Triceps | C6–C8 | Tapping the triceps tendon | Triceps brachii | Radial nerve |
| Knee-jerk (patellar) | L2–L4 | Tapping the patellar ligament | Quadriceps femoris | Femoral nerve |
| Ankle-jerk (ACHILLES) | L5–S2 | Tapping the ACHILLES tendon | Triceps surae | Tibial nerve |

**Important Flexor Reflexes of the Spinal Cord** [14]

| Reflex | Segment | Reflex Trigger | Target Organ | Afferent Limb | Efferent Limb |
|---|---|---|---|---|---|
| Abdominal | T8–T12 | Stroking of the abdominal skin | Abdominal muscles | Intercostal nerves (T8–T11), iliohypogastric nerve, ilioinguinal nerve | |
| Cremaster | L1, L2 | Stroking of the skin at the inside of the thigh | Cremaster | Femoral branch and genital branch of the genitofemoral nerve | |
| Foot sole | S1, S2 | Stroking of the lateral side of the foot sole | Flexor muscles of the toes (2–5) | Plantar nerves of the tibial nerve | Tibial nerve |
| Anal | S3–S5 | Stroking of the anal region | External sphincter ani | Anococcygeal nerves | Pudendal nerve |

## Tracts of the spinal cord

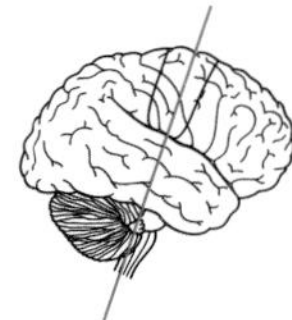

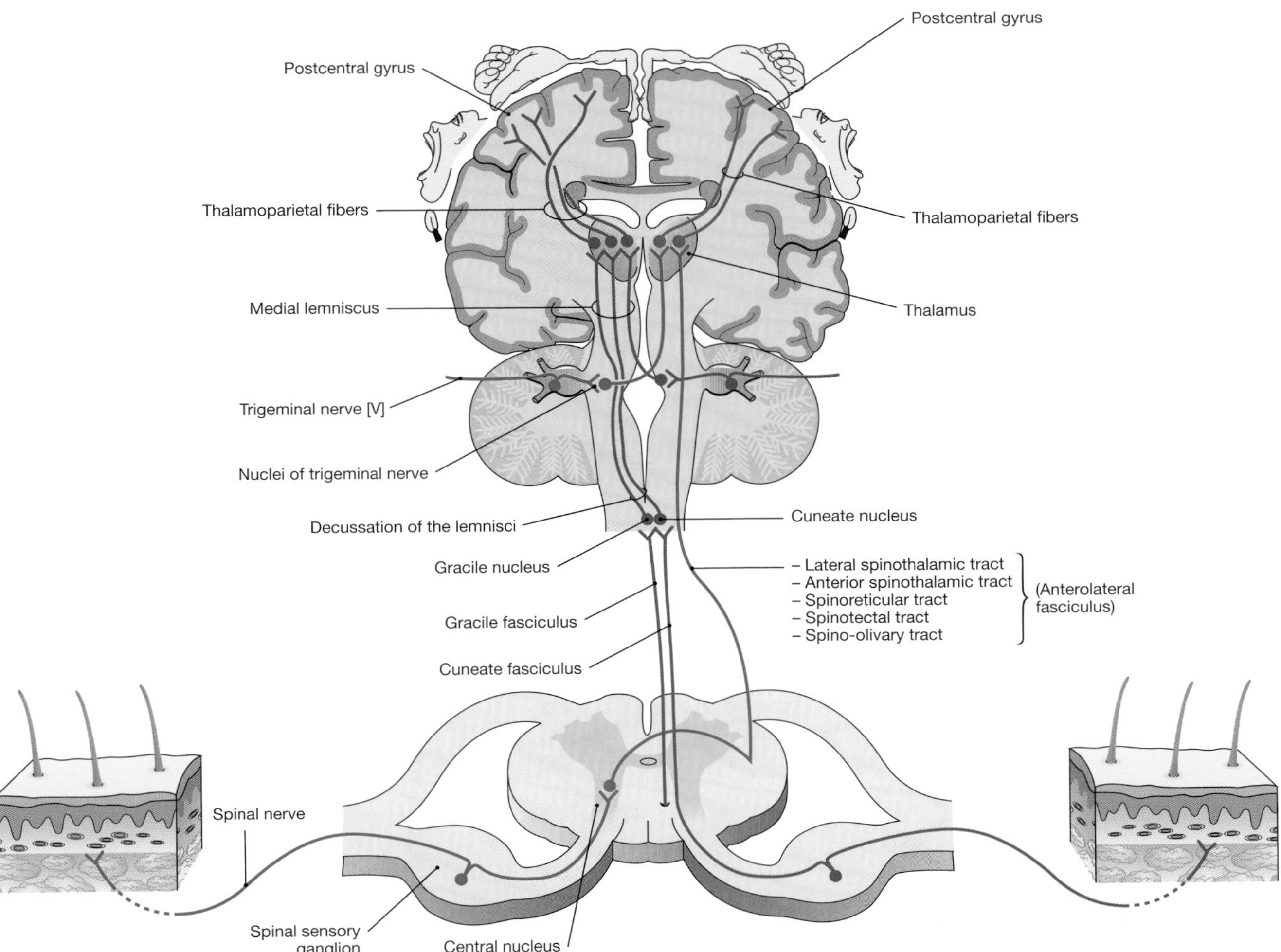
Postcentral gyrus
Postcentral gyrus
Thalamoparietal fibers
Thalamoparietal fibers
Thalamus
Medial lemniscus
Trigeminal nerve [V]
Nuclei of trigeminal nerve
Decussation of the lemnisci
Cuneate nucleus
Gracile nucleus
– Lateral spinothalamic tract
– Anterior spinothalamic tract
– Spinoreticular tract
– Spinotectal tract
– Spino-olivary tract
(Anterolateral fasciculus)
Gracile fasciculus
Cuneate fasciculus
Spinal nerve
Spinal sensory ganglion
Central nucleus

**Fig. 12.186 Pathways for epicritic (blue) and protopathic (green) sensibility (afferent tracts).**

Pathway of **epicritic sensibility** (touch pathway, serves the perception of precise differentiation of pressure and touch as well as proprioception):

- **1st neuron** (uncrossed): from receptors (exteroceptors) in the skin and the mucosa, the periosteum, the joints and the muscle spindles etc., to the gracile and cuneate nuclei in the medulla oblongata via the gracile fasciculus and cuneate fasciculus in the posterior (dorsal) funiculus (perikarya in the spinal ganglia); additional descending collaterals
- **2nd neuron** (crossed): from the medulla oblongata (cuneate nucleus, gracile nucleus) to the thalamus (medial lemniscus, perikarya in cuneate and gracile nucleus)
- **3rd neuron** (uncrossed): from the thalamus (posterolateral ventral nucleus) to the cerebral cortex, particularly to the postcentral gyrus (thalamocortical fibers, perikarya in the thalamus)

Pathway for **protopathic sensibility** (pain pathway, serves the pain, temperature and general pressure sensation):

- **1st neuron** (uncrossed): from receptors (exteroceptors) of the skin and the mucosa etc., to the posterior (dorsal) horn, spina laminae I to V (perikarya in the dorsal root ganglia)
- **2nd neuron** (crossed, some fibers possibly uncrossed): from the posterior (dorsal) horn to the thalamus, in the reticular formation and to the tectum of midbrain (anterior and lateral spinothalamic tract, spinoreticular tract, spinotectal tract; perikarya in the posterior (dorsal) column)
- **3rd neuron** (uncrossed): from the thalamus among others to the cerebral cortex, particularly to the postcentral gyrus (thalamocortical fibers, perikarya in the thalamus)

## Tracts of the spinal cord

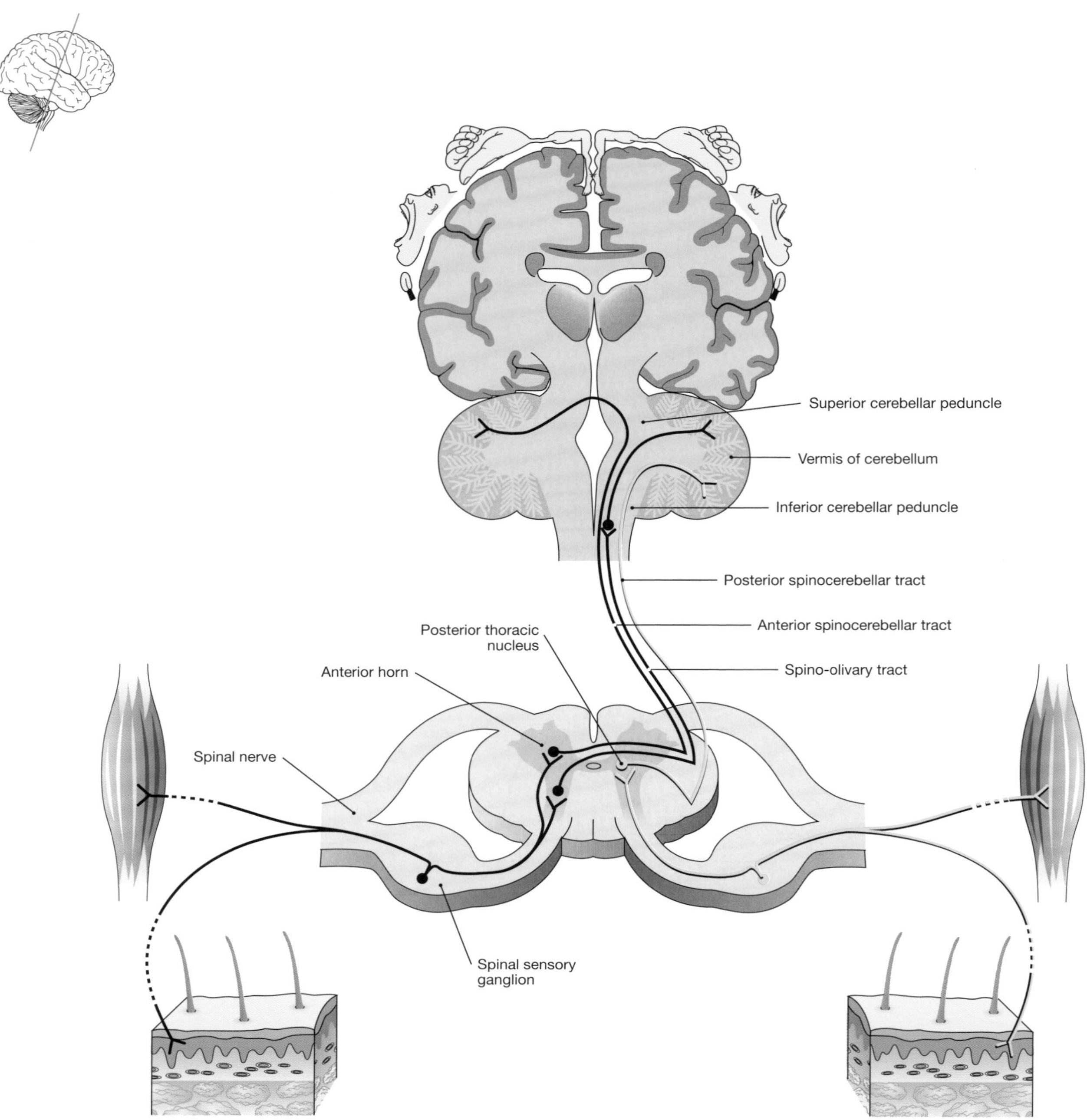
Superior cerebellar peduncle
Vermis of cerebellum
Inferior cerebellar peduncle
Posterior spinocerebellar tract
Anterior spinocerebellar tract
Posterior thoracic nucleus
Anterior horn
Spino-olivary tract
Spinal nerve
Spinal sensory ganglion

**Fig. 12.187 Pathway of unconscious proprioception (afferent tract).**
Pathway of unconscious proprioception (unconscious, but precise spatial differentiation as a prerequisite for movement coordination by the cerebellum) via the **anterior spinocerebellar tract** (black):

- **1st neuron** (uncrossed): from receptors (proprioceptors) in muscles, tendons, and in the connective tissue to the nuclei in the intermediate zone and the anterior (ventral) column (perikarya in the spinal ganglia).
- **2nd neuron** (two times crossed): from the anterior (ventral) horn within the anterior spinocerebellar tract of the anterolateral tract via the superior cerebellar peduncle to the cerebellum (perikarya in the intermediate zone and the anterior (ventral) horn).

Pathway of unconscious proprioception via the **posterior spinocerebellar tract** (yellow):

- **1st neuron** (uncrossed): from end organs (proprioceptors) in muscles, tendons, and in the connective tissue to the nuclei of the posterior column and to the thoracic nucleus (perikarya in the dorsal root ganglia).
- **2nd neuron** (uncrossed): from the posterior horn and the thoracic nucleus within the posterior spinocerebellar tract of the lateral tract via the inferior cerebellar peduncle to the cerebellum (perikarya in the thoracic nucleus and at the base of the posterior (dorsal) column).

## Tracts of the spinal cord

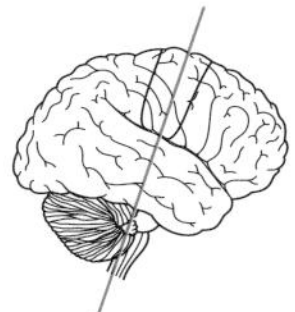

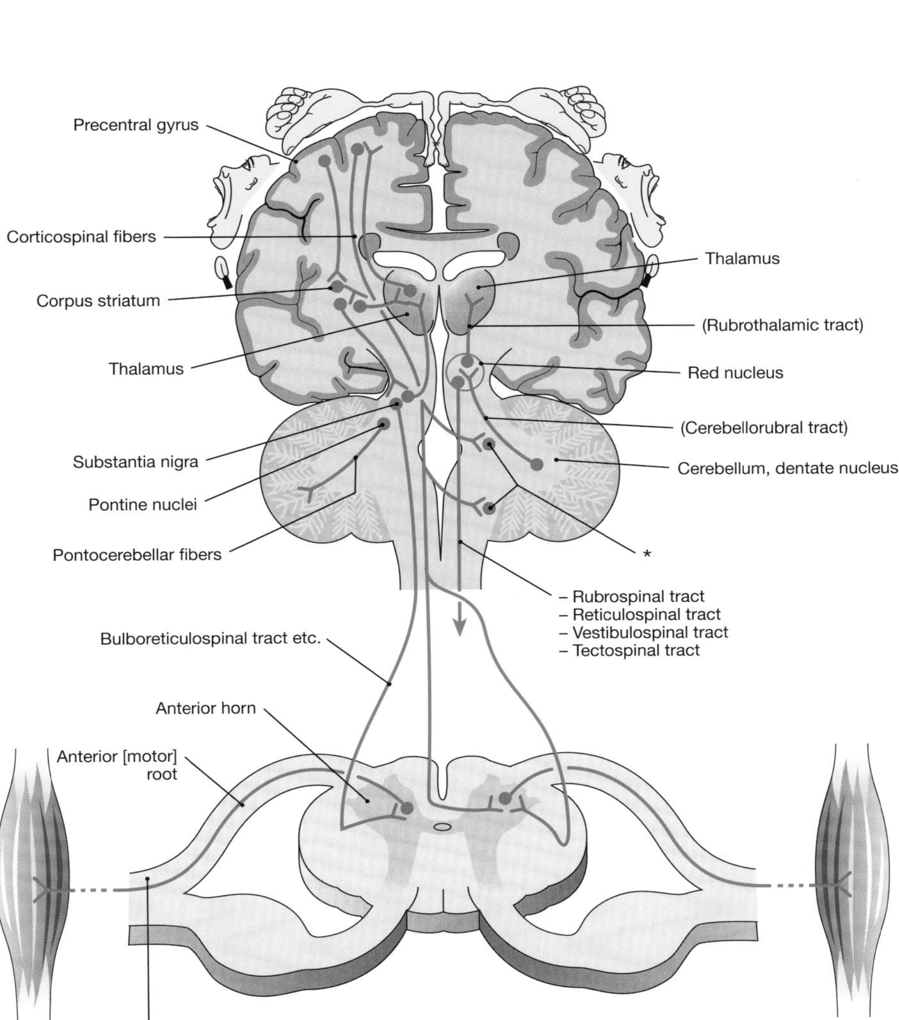
Precentral gyrus
Corticospinal fibers
Corpus striatum
Thalamus
Substantia nigra
Pontine nuclei
Pontocerebellar fibers
Bulboreticulospinal tract etc.
Anterior horn
Anterior [motor] root
Spinal nerve
Thalamus
(Rubrothalamic tract)
Red nucleus
(Cerebellorubral tract)
Cerebellum, dentate nucleus
*
– Rubrospinal tract
– Reticulospinal tract
– Vestibulospinal tract
– Tectospinal tract

**Fig. 12.188 Pathways of the motor system (efferent tracts).**
The motor system comprises a large number of nuclear regions and tracts. The "final motor pathway" are the motoneurons. Despite the extraordinary complexity of these circuits, the traditional organization will be maintained for didactic reasons.

**Pyramidal tract:**

- (Central) Neuron (crossed): from the cerebral cortex through the internal capsule and the cerebral peduncles to interneurons within the anterior and posterior columns (lateral corticospinal tract, anterior corticospinal tract, perikarya in the precentral gyrus).
- (Peripheral) Neuron (final motor pathway, $\alpha$-motoneurons): from the anterior (ventral) horn to the motor end plates of the skeletal muscles (motoneurons, perikarya in the anterior (ventral) horn).

**Cranial nerves:**

- From the anterior corticospinal tract of the pyramidal tract fibers branch off for the nuclei of the cranial nerves (corticonuclear fibers and bulbar corticonuclear fibers).

**Extrapyramidal motor system:**

- Central neurons: (crossed and uncrossed): from the cerebral cortex, particularly the precentral gyrus and the adjacent anterior cortical areas including synapses to the basal ganglia, thalamus, subthalamic nucleus, red nucleus, substantia nigra, cerebellum, etc. and feedback loops to interneurons of the anterior column (rubrospinal tract, reticulospinal tract, medial and lateral vestibulospinal tracts, tectospinal tract).
- Peripheral neuron (motor end pathway, $\alpha$-motoneurons): from the anterior (ventral) horn to the motor end plates of the skeletal muscles (motoneurons, perikarya in the anterior (ventral) horn).

* motor nuclei of cranial nerves

## Tracts of the spinal cord, clinics

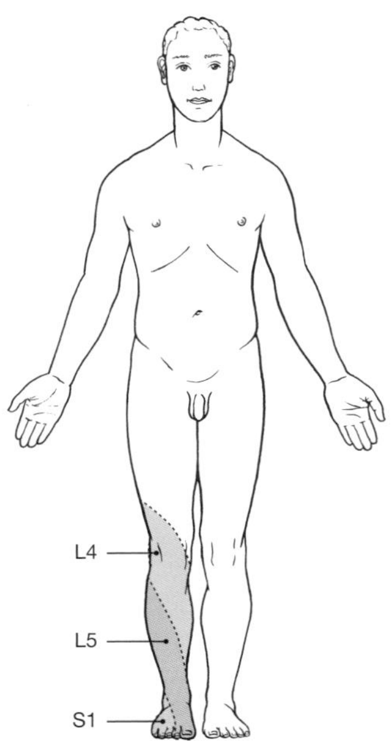
L4
L5
S1

**Fig. 12.189 Dysfunctional cutaneous innervation due to palsy of certain, frequently affected spinal nerves.**
A disc prolapse frequently affects the spinal nerves L4, L5, and S1.

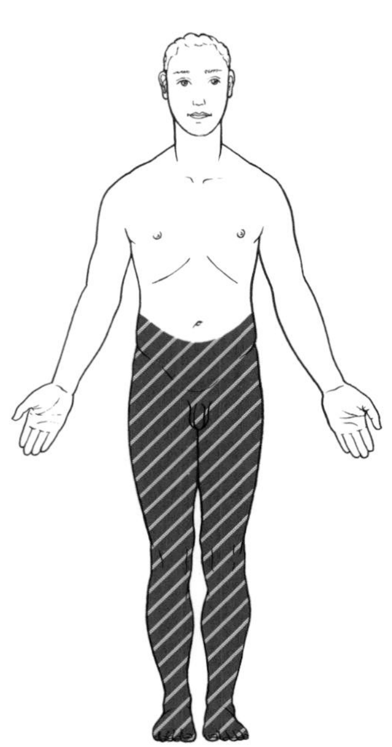

**Fig. 12.190 Complete paraplegia at the level of the 11th thoracic segment (T11).**
Paralysis of the whole motor and sensory system in the hatched area.

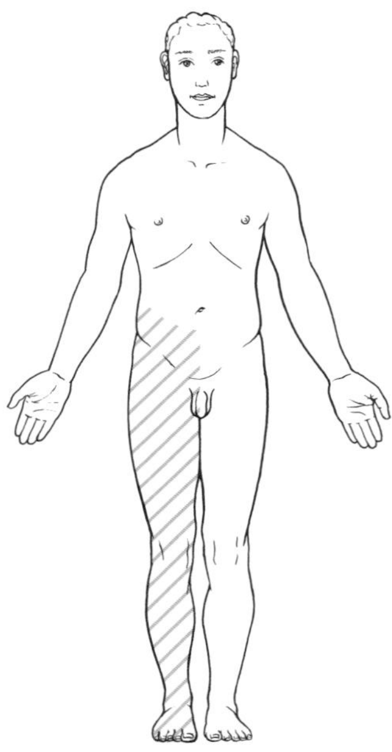

**Fig. 12.191 Paralysis of the tracts of the right posterior funiculus at the level of the 11th thoracic segment (T11).**
Loss of fine tactile sensation as well as loss of postural sense and vibration (gross touch sensation remains functionally normal).

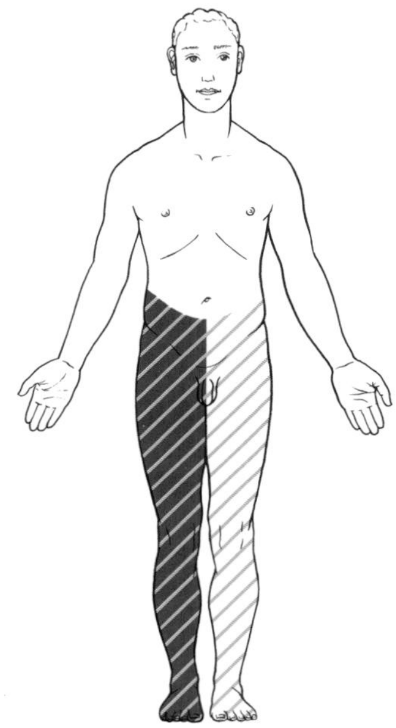

**Fig. 12.192 Hemiplegia (BROWN-SÉQUARD) due to a hemilateral right-sided disruption of the spinal cord at the level of the 11th thoracic segment (T11).**
On the right side (ipsilateral): loss of motor function (initially flaccid, later spastic); loss of fine discriminative tactile sensation as well as loss of postural sense and vibration (gross touch sensation remains functionally normal). On the left side (contralateral): loss of pain and temperature sensation (→ Fig. 12.186).

## Autonomic nervous system, functional overview

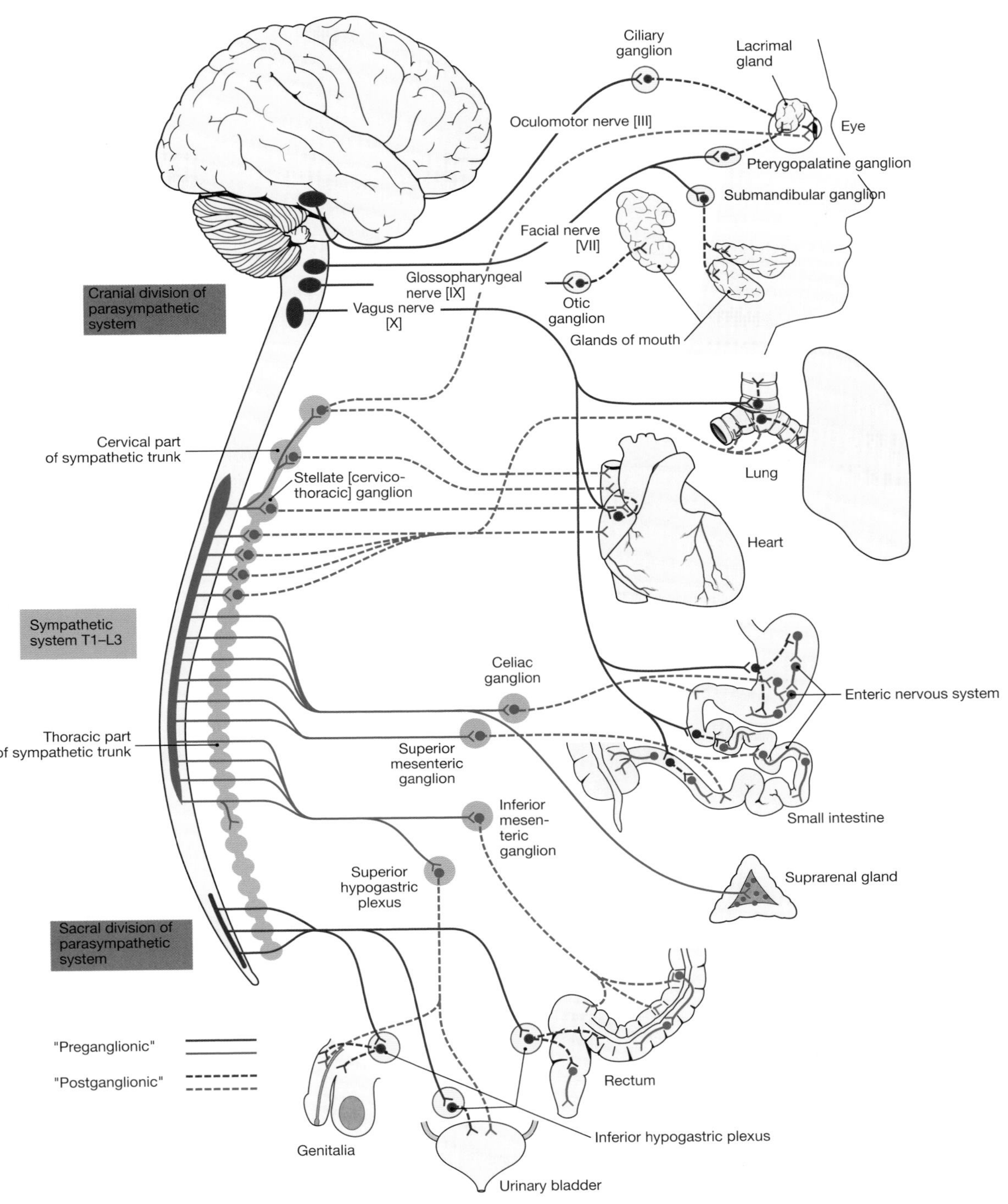
Ciliary ganglion
Lacrimal gland
Oculomotor nerve [III]
Eye
Pterygopalatine ganglion
Submandibular ganglion
Facial nerve [VII]
Glossopharyngeal nerve [IX]
Vagus nerve [X]
Otic ganglion
Glands of mouth
Cranial division of parasympathetic system
Cervical part of sympathetic trunk
Stellate [cervico-thoracic] ganglion
Lung
Heart
Sympathetic system T1–L3
Celiac ganglion
Enteric nervous system
Thoracic part of sympathetic trunk
Superior mesenteric ganglion
Inferior mesen-teric ganglion
Small intestine
Superior hypogastric plexus
Suprarenal gland
Sacral division of parasympathetic system
"Preganglionic"
"Postganglionic"
Rectum
Genitalia
Inferior hypogastric plexus
Urinary bladder

**Fig. 12.193 Autonomic nervous system (sympathetic and parasympathetic part).** [22]
The autonomic nervous system comprises the sympathetic (green), parasympathetic (purple), and the enteric nervous system (blue).
The neurons of the **sympathetic** part locate in the intermediolateral horn of the thoracolumbar section of the spinal cord. Their axons project to the sympathetic chain of ganglia and to the ganglia of the enteric system. Here they synapse to postganglionic neurons which project to the target organs. The sympathetic activation serves to mobilize the body in case of an emergency. The adrenal medulla is part of the sympathetic system and secretes adrenaline and noradrenaline.

Nuclear areas of the **parasympathetic** part locate in the brainstem and the sacral part of the spinal cord. Their axons project to ganglia adjacent to the target organs which locate in the head, thorax, and the abdominal cavity. Here synapsing onto postganglionic neurons occurs, which reach the target organs via short axons. The parasympathetic system has important roles in food intake and digestion, sexual arousal, and opposes the sympathetic system.
The **enteric nervous system** regulates the intestinal activity and is modulated by sympathetic and parasympathetic influences.

## Central motor system

| Components of the Motor System and their Functions [14] | |
|---|---|
| **Components** | **Functions** |
| Spinal cord | • Autonomous execution of elementary functions (stretch and flexor reflexes) → spinal basic system<br>• Target organ for supraspinal motor commands |
| Centers in the brainstem (i.e. red nucleus, reticular formation, lower olivary nuclear complex, pontine nuclei) | • Particulary involuntary motor regulation of posture and gait as well as coordination of movements (→ ordered sequence of voluntary movements) through numerous nuclear regions and the extrapyramidal tracts arising from them<br>• Contributing to the fine-tuning of voluntary movements<br>• Centers for the motor regulation of ocular movements |
| Cerebellum | • Control of equilibrium<br>• Control of stance and precision movements<br>• Coordination and timing of precision movements (fine-tuning and modulation) |
| Basal ganglia (striatum, pallidum, subthalamic nucleus and substantia nigra) | • Programming of precision movements (fine-tuning and modulation) |
| Motor cortex regions and pyramidal tract | • Initiation of movement strategies and programs through association areas and secondary motor cortex areas<br>• Execution of voluntary movements via the precentral motor cortex → pyramidal tract → spinal cord |

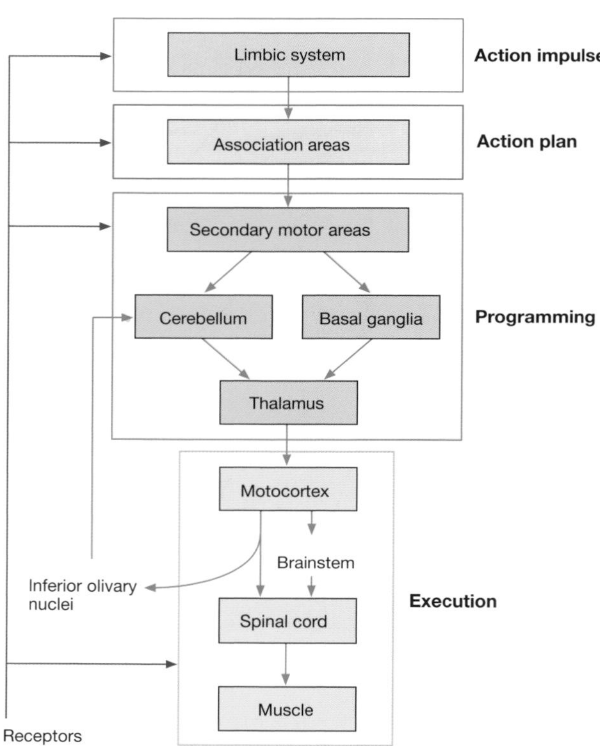
Limbic system
Action impulse
Association areas
Action plan
Secondary motor areas
Cerebellum
Basal ganglia
Programming
Thalamus
Motocortex
Brainstem
Inferior olivary nuclei
Spinal cord
Execution
Muscle
Receptors

**Fig. 12.194 Simplified schematic representation of the organization of the somatomotor system.** [14]

The current assumption is that the inner **motivation** for motor activity (the initial motor action impulse) initiates in the limbic system. From here, these impulses reach association areas (e.g. in the prefrontal cortex) and a **strategic action plan** for this movement is created. The realization requires the inclusion of secondary motor areas which plan the details of the intended movement and fine-tune the motion program through feedback from the cerebellum and the basal ganglia. Once the **planning phase** of the intended movement is completed, the so modulated motion program is transmitted to the thalamus and from here to the motor areas, particularly to the motor cortex that signals the beginning of the **execution phase.** The pyramidal tract originates at the motor cortex and projects into the spinal cord, where the information reaches the muscles. The inferior olivary nucleus and the cerebellum receive copies of the motion program to initiate modulations and/or corrections of the motor action in a timely fashion. In addition, extensive sensory feedback loops exist between peripheral receptor systems and all structures involved in the motion program to ensure a smooth execution of the motor action.

# Appendix

# Picture Credits

The editors sincerely thank all clinical colleagues that made ultrasound, computed tomographic and magnetic resonance images as well as endoscopic and intraoperative pictures available:

Prof. Altaras, Center for Radiology, University of Giessen (Figs. 2.18; 2.39; 2.40)
Prof. Brueckmann and Dr. Linn, Neuroradiology, Institute for Diagnostic Radiology, University of Munich (Fig. 4.148)
Prof. Daniel, Department of Cardiology, University of Erlangen (Fig. 10.39)
Prof. Galanski and Dr. Schäfer, Department of Diagnostic Radiology, Hannover Medical School (Figs. 2.97; 5.3; 5.103; 6.31; 6.129)
Prof. Gebel, Department of Gastroenterology and Hepatology, Hannover Medical School (Figs. 6.73; 6.75; 6.76; 6.94; 6.95; 7.25)
Dr. Greeven, St. Elisabeth Hospital, Neuwied (Figs. 4.96; 8.96)
Prof. Hoffmann and Dr. Bektas, Clinic for Abdominal and Tranplantation Surgery, Hannover Medical School (Fig. 4.41)
Prof. Hohlfeld, Clinic for Pneumology, Hannover Medical School (Fig. 5.71)
Prof. Jonas, Urology, Hannover Medical School (Fig. 7.33)
Prof. Kampik and Prof. Müller, Ophthalmology, University of Munich (Fig. 9.66)
Dr. Kirchhoff and Dr. Weidemann, Department of Diagnostic Radiology, Hannover Medical School (Figs. 6.131; 6.133; 7.26)
Prof. Kleinsasser, Clinic and Polyclinic of Oto-Rhino-Laryngology, Plastic and Aesthetic Surgery, University Hospital Wuerzburg (Figs. 11.41; 11.42; 11.43)
PD Dr. Kutta, Clinic and Polyclinic for Oto-Rhino-Laryngology, University Hospital Hamburg-Eppendorf (Figs. 8.101; 10.16; 11.16)
Dr. Meyer, Department of Gastroenterology and Hepatology, Hannover Medical School (Figs. 6.22; 6.32; 7.104)
Prof. Pfeifer, Radiology Innenstadt, Institute for Diagnostic Radiology, University of Munich (Figs. 2.63–2.65; 2.67–2.70; 3.52; 3.54; 3.55; 4.97; 4.99; 4.100; 4.105; 4.106)
Prof. Possinger and Prof. Bick, Medical Clinic and Polyclinic II, Division of Hematology and Oncology, Charité Campus Mitte, Berlin (Fig. 2.141)
Prof. Ravelli †, formerly Institute of Anatomy, University of Innsbruck (Fig. 2.62)
Prof. Reich, Orofacial Surgery, University of Bonn (Figs. 8.60; 8.61)
Prof. Reiser and Dr. Wagner, Institute for Diagnostic Radiology, University of Munich (Figs. 2.71; 12.105; 12.106; 12.110; 12.111)
Dr. Scheibe, Department of Surgery, Rosman Hospital, Breisach (Fig. 4.79)
Prof. Scheumann, Clinic for Abdominal and Tranplantation Surgery, Hannover Medical School (Fig. 11.58)
Prof. Schillinger, Department of Gynaecology, University of Freiburg (Fig. 1.49)
Prof. Schliephake, Orofacial Surgery, University of Goettingen (Figs. 8.156; 8.157)
Prof. Schloesser, Center for Gynaecology, Hannover Medical School (Fig. 7.79)
cand. med. Carsten Schroeder, Kronshagen (Fig. 9.27)
Prof. Schumacher, Neuroradiology, Department of Radiology, University of Freiburg (Fig. 12.5)
Dr. Sel, University Hospital and Polyclinic for Ophthalmology, University Hospital Halle (Saale) (Fig. 9.64)
Dr. Sommer and PD Dr. Bauer, Radiologists, Munich (Figs. 4.101; 4.102)
PD Dr. Vogl, Radiology, University of Munich (Figs. 9.69; 9.70)
Prof. Witt, Department of Neurosurgery, University of Munich (Fig. 3.116)
Prof. Zierz and Dr. Jordan, University Hospital and Polyclinic for Neurology, University Hospital Halle (Saale) (Figs. 8.82, 12.151)

**Additional illustrations were obtained from the following textbooks:**


1 Benninghoff-Drenckhahn: Anatomie, Band 1 (Drenckhahn D., editor), 17. Aufl., Urban & Fischer 2008
2 Benninghoff-Drenckhahn: Anatomie, Band 2 (Drenckhahn D., editor), 16. Aufl., Urban & Fischer 2004
3 Benninghoff-Drenckhahn: Taschenbuch Anatomie (Drenckhahn D., Waschke, J., editors), Urban & Fischer 2007
4 Berchtold, R., Bruch, H.-P., Trentz, O. (editors): Chirurgie, 6. Aufl., Urban & Fischer 2008
5 Böcker, W., Denk, H., Heitz, P. U., Moch, H. (editors): Pathologie, 4. Aufl., Urban & Fischer 2008
6 Classen, M., Diehl, V., Kochsiek, K., Berdel, W. E., Böhm, M., Schmiegel, W. (editors): Innere Medizin, 5. Aufl., Urban & Fischer 2003
7 Classen, M., Diehl, V., Kochsiek, K., Hallek, M., Böhm, M. (editors): Innere Medizin, 6. Aufl., Urban & Fischer 2009
8 Drake, R. L., Vogl, A. W., Mitchell, A., Paulsen, F. (editors): Gray's Anatomie für Studenten, 1. Aufl., Urban & Fischer 2007
9 Drake, R. L., Vogl, A. W., Mitchell, A.: Gray's Anatomy for Students, 2nd ed., Churchill Livingstone 2010
10 Drake, R. L., Vogl, A. W., Mitchell, A.: Gray's Atlas der Anatomie, Urban & Fischer 2009
11 Fleckenstein, P., Tranum-Jensen, J.: Röntgenanatomie, Urban & Fischer 2004
12 Forbes, A., Misiewicz, J., Compton, C., Quraishy, M., Rubesin, S., Thuluvath, P.: Atlas of Clinical Gastroenterology, 3rd ed., Mosby 2004
13 Franzen, A.: Kurzlehrbuch Hals-Nasen-Ohren-Heilkunde, 3. Aufl., Urban & Fischer 2007
14 Garzorz, N.: BASICS Neuroanatomie, Urban & Fischer 2008
15 Kanski, J. J.: Klinische Ophthalmologie, 5. Aufl., Urban & Fischer 2003
16 Kanski, J. J.: Klinische Ophthalmologie, 6. Aufl., Urban & Fischer 2008
17 Kauffmann, G. W., Moser, E., Sauer, R. (editors): Radiologie, 3. Aufl., Urban & Fischer 2006
18 Lippert, H.: Lehrbuch Anatomie, 7. Aufl., Urban & Fischer 2006
19 Mettler, F. A. (editor): Klinische Radiologie, Urban & Fischer 2005
20 Moore, K., Persaud, T. V. N., Viebahn, C. (editors): Embryologie, 5. Aufl., Urban & Fischer 2007
21 Schulze, S.: Kurzlehrbuch Embryologie, Urban & Fischer 2006
22 Speckmann, E.-J., Hescheler, J., Köhling, R. (editors): Physiologie, 5. Aufl., Urban & Fischer 2008
23 Trepel, M.: Neuroanatomie, 4. Aufl., Urban & Fischer 2008
24 Welsch, U.: Sobotta Lehrbuch Histologie, 2. Aufl., Urban & Fischer 2005
25 Welsch, U., Deller, T.: Sobotta Lehrbuch Histologie, 3. Aufl., Urban & Fischer 2010
26 Welsch, U.: Atlas Histologie, 7. Aufl., Urban & Fischer 2005
27 Wicke, L.: Atlas der Röntgenanatomie, 7. Aufl., Urban & Fischer 2005
28 Rengier, F.: BASICS Leitungsbahnen, Urban & Fischer 2009


**The following illustrators have developed the new illustrations:**

Dr. Katja Dalkowski: Figs. 8.42, 9.52, 10.12, 10.15, 10.26, 10.50, 11.63, 11.76, 12.10, 12.51, 12.87, 12.89, 12.91, 12.98, 12.152, 12.175, 12.176

Sonja Klebe: Figs. 8.153, 8.163, 9.22, 10.9, 11.9, 11.14, 11.31, 11.35, 11.37, 11.39, 11.81, 12.11, 12.12, 12.99, 12.100, 12.138, 12.139, 12.141, 12.142, 12.148, 12.153, 12.154

Jörg Mair: Figs. 9.19, 11.69, 12.1, 12.131, 12.142, 12.143, 12.144, 12.145, 12.149, 12.150, 12.155, 12.156, 12.157, 12.158, 12.160, 12.161, 12.162, 12.163

Stephan Winkler: Figs. 8.57, 8.144

## 1. List of abbreviations

Singular:

| | | |
|---|---|---|
| A. | = | Arteria |
| Lig. | = | Ligamentum |
| M. | = | Musculus |
| N. | = | Nervus |
| Proc. | = | Processus |
| R. | = | Ramus |
| V. | = | Vena |
| Var. | = | Variation |

Plural:

| | | |
|---|---|---|
| Aa. | = | Arteriae |
| Ligg. | = | Ligamenta |
| Mm. | = | Musculi |
| Nn. | = | Nervi |
| Procc. | = | Processus |
| Rr. | = | Rami |
| Vv. | = | Venae |

♀ = female
♂ = male

Percentages:
In the light of the large variation in individual body measurements, the percentages indicating size should only be taken as approximate values.

## 2. General terms of direction and position

The following terms indicate the position of organs and parts of the body in relation to each other, irrespective of the position of the body (e.g. supine or upright) or direction and position of the limbs. These terms are relevant not only for human anatomy but also for clinical medicine and comparative anatomy.

**General terms**

*anterior – posterior* = in front – behind (e.g. anterior and posterior tibial artery)
*ventral – dorsal* = towards the belly – towards the back
*superior – inferior* = above – below (e.g. superior and inferior nasal concha)
*cranial – caudal* = towards the head – towards the tail
*medius, intermedius* = located between two other structures (e.g. the middle nasal concha is located between the superior and inferior nasal concha)
*median* = located in the midline (anterior median fissure of the spinal cord). The median plane is a sagittal plane which divides the body into right and left halves.
*medial – lateral* = located near to the midline – located away from the midline of the body (e.g. medial and lateral inguinal fossa)
*frontal* = located in a frontal plane, but also towards the front (e.g. frontal process of the maxilla)
*longitudinal* = parallel to the longitudinal axis (e.g. superior longitudinal muscle of the tongue)
*sagittal* = located in a sagittal plane
*transverse* = transverse direction (e.g. transverse process of a thoracic vertebra)

**Terms of direction and position for the limbs**

*proximal – distal* = located towards or away from the attached end of a limb or the origin of a structure (e.g. proximal and distal radio-ulnar joint)

for the upper limb:
*radial – ulnar* = on the radial side – on the ulnar side (e.g. radial and ulnar artery)

for the hand:
*palmar – dorsal* = towards the palm of the hand – towards the back of the hand (e.g. palmar aponeurosis, dorsal interosseous muscle)

for the lower limb:
*tibial – fibular* = on the tibial side – on the fibular side (e.g. anterior tibial artery)

for the foot:
*plantar – dorsal* = towards the sole of the foot – towards the back of the foot (e.g. lateral and medial plantar arteries, dorsalis pedis artery)

## 3. Use of brackets

[ ]: Latin terms in square brackets refer to alternative terms as given.

( ): Round brackets are used in different ways:
- for terms also listed in round brackets in the Terminologia Anatomica
- for terms not included in the official nomenclature but which the editors consider important and clinically relevant, e.g. (zygomatico-alveolar crest)
- to indicate the origin of a given structure, e.g. spinal branch (vertebral artery).

## A

# Index

# Index

## F

## J



## K



## L

## M

## N



## O

## P

# Index

# Index

## T

## U



## V

## W



## Z